Veterinary Microbiology

Veterinary Microbiology

Editor:

Patricia Marques, Ph.D.

Delve Publishing
www.delvepublishing.com

Veterinary Microbiology

Editor: Patricia Marques, Ph.D.

708 3rd Avenue, 6th Floor
New York, NY 10017
United States of America

www.delvepublishing.com

ISBN: 978-1-68095-871-3

Library of Congress Control Number: 2016951622

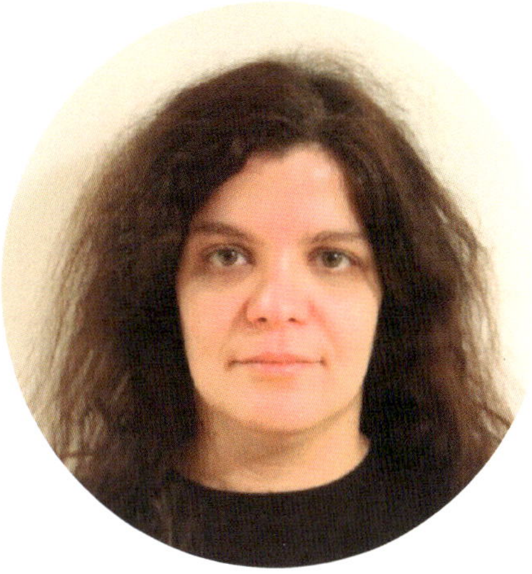

About the Editor

Patricia Marques, Ph.D.

Patricia obtained her PhD form University College Dublin in 2010. Her interests are on Microbiology and Parasitology. She is currently working as a Postdoc at University of Maryland Baltimore, USA on Chlamydia infections

Contents

Section X: Brucella Abortus - Abortion

List of Contributors

Aneta Nowakiewicz
Sub-Department of Veterinary Microbiology, Institute of Biological Bases of Animal Diseases, Faculty of Veterinary Medicine University of Life Sciences, Lublin, Poland

Przemysław Zięba
State Veterinary Laboratory, Lublin, Poland

Grażyna Ziółkowska
Sub-Department of Veterinary Microbiology, Institute of Biological Bases of Animal Diseases, Faculty of Veterinary Medicine University of Life Sciences, Lublin, Poland

Sebastian Gnat
Sub-Department of Veterinary Microbiology, Institute of Biological Bases of Animal Diseases, Faculty of Veterinary Medicine University of Life Sciences, Lublin, Poland

Marta Muszyńska
State Veterinary Laboratory, Lublin, Poland

Krzysztof Tomczuk
Sub-Department of Parasitology and Invasive Diseases, Institute of Biological Bases of Animal Diseases, Faculty of Veterinary Medicine, University of Life Sciences, Lublin, Poland

Barbara Majer Dziedzic
Sub-Department of Veterinary Microbiology, Institute of Biological Bases of Animal Diseases, Faculty of Veterinary Medicine University of Life Sciences, Lublin, Poland

Łukasz Ulbrych
Warta Mouth National Park, Górzyca, Poland

Aleksandra Trościańczyk
Sub-Department of Veterinary Microbiology, Institute of Biological Bases of Animal Diseases, Faculty of Veterinary Medicine University of Life Sciences, Lublin, Poland

Brian Austin
Institute of Aquaculture, Pathfoot Building, University of Stirling, Stirling FK9 4LA, Scotland, UK

Massimo Palmarini
The Scripps Research Institute, United States of America

Evelien De Clercq
Department of Molecular Biotechnology, Faculty of Bioscience Engineering, Ghent University, Coupure Links 653, B-9000 Ghent, Belgium

Bert Devriendt
Laboratory of Immunology, Faculty of Veterinary Medicine, Ghent University, Salisburylaan 133, B-9820 Merelbeke, Belgium

Lizi Yin
Department of Molecular Biotechnology, Faculty of Bioscience Engineering, Ghent University, Coupure Links 653, B-9000 Ghent, Belgium
College of Veterinary Medicine, Sichuan Agricultural University, Ya'an 625014, China

Koen Chiers
Department of Pathology, Bacteriology and Poultry Diseases, Faculty of Veterinary Medicine, Ghent University, Salisburylaan 133, B-9820 Merelbeke, Belgium

Eric Cox
Laboratory of Immunology, Faculty of Veterinary Medicine, Ghent University, Salisburylaan 133, B-9820 Merelbeke, Belgium

Daisy Vanrompay
Department of Molecular Biotechnology, Faculty of Bioscience Engineering, Ghent University, Coupure Links 653, B-9000 Ghent, Belgium

Martina Jelocnik
Institute for Health and Biomedical Innovation, Queensland University of Technology, Kelvin Grove, Queensland 4059, Australia

David Forshaw
Department of Agriculture and Food Western Australia, Albany, Western Australia 6330, Australia

Jennifer Cotter
Department of Agriculture and Food Western Australia, Albany, Western Australia 6330, Australia

Danny Roberts
Department of Agriculture and Food Western Australia, Albany, Western Australia 6330, Australia

Peter Timms
Institute for Health and Biomedical Innovation, Queensland University of Technology, Kelvin Grove, Queensland 4059, Australia
Faculty of Science, Health, Education and Engineering, University of the Sunshine Coast, Sippy Downs 4556, Australia

Adam Polkinghorne
Institute for Health and Biomedical Innovation, Queensland University of Technology, Kelvin Grove, Queensland 4059, Australia
Faculty of Science, Health, Education and Engineering, University of the Sunshine Coast, Sippy Downs 4556, Australia

Stina Englund
National Veterinary Institute, 751 89 Uppsala, Sweden

Carl Hård af Segerstad
National Veterinary Institute, 751 89 Uppsala, Sweden

Frida Arnlund
Stavby-Väsby 86, 747 94 Alunda, Sweden

Eva Westergren
National Veterinary Institute, 751 89 Uppsala, Sweden

Magdalena Jacobson
Department of Clinical Sciences, Faculty of Veterinary Medicine and Animal Science, Swedish University of Agricultural Sciences, 750 07 Uppsala, Sweden.

Hannah Lenzko
Institute of Molecular Pathogenesis, Friedrich Loeffler Institute, Naumburger Straße 96a, 07743 Jena, Germany

Udo Moog
Animal Health Service, Thüringer Tierseuchenkasse, Victor-Goerttler-Straße 4, 07745 Jena, Germany

Klaus Henning
Institute of Epidemiology, Friedrich Loeffler Institute, Seestraße 55, 16868 Wusterhausen, Germany

Robert Lederbach
State Office of Food Safety and Consumer Protection, Department of Veterinary examination, Tennstedter Street 8/9, 99947 Bad Langensalza, Germany

Roland Diller
Institute of Bacterial Infections and Zoonoses, Friedrich Loeffler Institute, Naumburger Straße 96a, 07743 Jena, Germany

Christian Menge
Institute of Molecular Pathogenesis, Friedrich Loeffler Institute, Naumburger Straße 96a, 07743 Jena, Germany

Konrad Sachse
Institute of Molecular Pathogenesis, Friedrich Loeffler Institute, Naumburger Straße 96a, 07743 Jena, Germany

Lisa D Sprague
Institute of Bacterial Infections and Zoonoses, Friedrich Loeffler Institute, Naumburger Straße 96a, 07743 Jena, Germany

Ann-Charlotte Godin
Division of Ruminant Medicine and Veterinary Epidemiology, Department of Clinical Sciences, Faculty of Veterinary Medicine and Animal Science, Swedish University of Agricultural Sciences (SLU), SE-750 07, Uppsala, Sweden

Camilla Björkman
Division of Ruminant Medicine and Veterinary Epidemiology, Department of Clinical Sciences, Faculty of Veterinary Medicine and Animal Science, Swedish University of Agricultural Sciences (SLU), SE-750 07, Uppsala, Sweden

Stina Englund
Department of Animal Health and Antimicrobial strategies, Section of Antibiotics, National Veterinary Institute (SVA), SE-751 89, Uppsala, Sweden

KarlErik Johansson
Division of Bacteriology and Food Safety, Department of Biomedical Sciences and Veterinary Public Health, Faculty of Veterinary Medicine and Animal Science, Swedish University of Agricultural Sciences (SLU), SE-750 07, Uppsala, Sweden
Department of Bacteriology; National Veterinary Institute (SVA), SE-751 89, Uppsala, Sweden

Rauni Niskanen
Division of Ruminant Medicine and Veterinary Epidemiology, Department of Clinical Sciences, Faculty of Veterinary Medicine and Animal Science, Swedish University of Agricultural Sciences (SLU), SE-750 07, Uppsala, Sweden

Stefan Alenius
Division of Ruminant Medicine and Veterinary Epidemiology, Department of Clinical Sciences, Faculty of Veterinary Medicine and Animal Science, Swedish University of Agricultural Sciences (SLU), SE-750 07, Uppsala, Sweden

Dirk Theegarten
Institute of Pathology and Neuropathology, University Duisburg-Essen Medical School, Hufelandstr. 55, D-45122 Essen, Germany

Konrad Sachse
Institute of Bacterial Infections and Zoonoses, Friedrich-Loeffler-Institute, Naumburger Str. 96a, D-07743 Jena, Germany

Britta Mentrup
Institute of Pathology and Neuropathology, University Duisburg-Essen Medical School, Hufelandstr. 55, D-45122 Essen, Germany

Kerstin Fey
Clinic for Horses, Internal Medicine, Justus-Liebig-University, Frankfurter Str. 126, D-35392 Gießen, Germany

Helmut Hotzel
Institute of Molecular Pathogenesis, FriedrichLoeffler-Institute, Naumburger Str. 96a, D-07743 Jena, Germany

Olaf Anhenn
Institute of Pathology and Neuropathology, University Duisburg-Essen Medical School, Hufelandstr. 55, D-45122 Essen, Germany
Clinic for Internal Medicine, General Hospital Hagen, Grünstr. 35, D-58095 Hagen, Germany
Department of Pneumology, Ruhrlandklinik, University Duisburg-Essen Medical School, Tüschener Weg 40, D-45239 Essen, Germany

Naíla C do Nascimento
Department of Veterinary Pathobiology, Purdue University, 725 Harrison Street, 47907 West Lafayette, IN, USA

Andrea P dos Santos
Department of Veterinary Pathobiology, Purdue University, 725 Harrison Street, 47907 West Lafayette, IN, USA

Yuefeng Chu
Department of Veterinary Pathobiology, Purdue University, 725 Harrison Street, 47907 West Lafayette, IN, USA
State Key Laboratory of Veterinary Etiological Biology, Lanzhou Veterinary Research Institute of CAAS, Lanzhou, China

Ana MS Guimaraes
Department of Veterinary Pathobiology, Purdue University, 725 Harrison Street, 47907 West Lafayette, IN, USA
Present address: Department of Animal Health and Preventive Veterinary Medicine, College of Veterinary Medicine and Animal Science of University of São Paulo, São Paulo, Brazil

Aubrey N Baird
Department of Veterinary Clinical Sciences, Purdue University, 625 Harrison Street, 47907 West Lafayette, IN, USA

Ann B Weil
Department of Veterinary Clinical Sciences, Purdue University, 625 Harrison Street, 47907 West Lafayette, IN, USA

Joanne B Messick
Department of Veterinary Pathobiology, Purdue University, 725 Harrison Street, 47907 West Lafayette, IN, USA

Kinga M Sulyok
Institute for Veterinary Medical Research, Centre for Agricultural Research, Hungarian Academy of Sciences, Hungária körút

21, Budapest 1143, Hungary

Zsuzsa Kreizinger
Institute for Veterinary Medical Research, Centre for Agricultural Research, Hungarian Academy of Sciences, Hungária körút 21, Budapest 1143, Hungary

Lilla Fekete
Institute for Veterinary Medical Research, Centre for Agricultural Research, Hungarian Academy of Sciences, Hungária körút 21, Budapest 1143, Hungary

Veronika Hrivnák
Institute for Veterinary Medical Research, Centre for Agricultural Research, Hungarian Academy of Sciences, Hungária körút 21, Budapest 1143, Hungary

Tibor Magyar
Institute for Veterinary Medical Research, Centre for Agricultural Research, Hungarian Academy of Sciences, Hungária körút 21, Budapest 1143, Hungary

Szilárd Jánosi
Veterinary Diagnostic Directorate, National Food Chain Safety Office, Tábornok utca 2, Budapest 1143, Hungary

Nóra Schweitzer
Veterinary Diagnostic Directorate, National Food Chain Safety Office, Tábornok utca 2, Budapest 1143, Hungary

Ibolya Turcsányi
Veterinary Diagnostic Directorate, National Food Chain Safety Office, Tábornok utca 2, Budapest 1143, Hungary

László Makrai
Faculty of Veterinary Science, Szent István University, Hungária körút 23-25, Budapest 1143, Hungary.

Károly Erdélyi
Veterinary Diagnostic Directorate, National Food Chain Safety Office, Tábornok utca 2, Budapest 1143, Hungary

Miklós Gyuranecz
Institute for Veterinary Medical Research, Centre for Agricultural Research, Hungarian Academy of Sciences, Hungária körút 21, Budapest 1143, Hungary

Kinga M Sulyok
Institute for Veterinary Medical Research, Centre for Agricultural Research, Hungarian Academy of Sciences, Hungária körút 21, Budapest 1143, Hungary

Zsuzsa Kreizinger
Institute for Veterinary Medical Research, Centre for Agricultural Research, Hungarian Academy of Sciences, Hungária körút 21, Budapest 1143, Hungary

Lilla Fekete
Institute for Veterinary Medical Research, Centre for Agricultural Research, Hungarian Academy of Sciences, Hungária körút 21, Budapest 1143, Hungary

Szilárd Jánosi
Veterinary Diagnostic Directorate, National Food Chain Safety Office, Tábornok utca 2, Budapest 1143, Hungary

Nóra Schweitzer
Veterinary Diagnostic Directorate, National Food Chain Safety Office, Tábornok utca 2, Budapest 1143, Hungary

Ibolya Turcsányi
Veterinary Diagnostic Directorate, National Food Chain Safety Office, Tábornok utca 2, Budapest 1143, Hungary

László Makrai
Faculty of Veterinary Science, Szent István University, Hungária körút 23-25, Budapest 1143, Hungary.

Károly Erdélyi
Veterinary Diagnostic Directorate, National Food Chain Safety Office, Tábornok utca 2, Budapest 1143, Hungary

Miklós Gyuranecz
Institute for Veterinary Medical Research, Centre for Agricultural Research, Hungarian Academy of Sciences, Hungária körút 21, Budapest 1143, Hungary

Jaime Ariza-Miguel
Agricultural Technological Institute of Castilla and Leon (ITACyL), Ministry of Agriculture and Livestock. Castilla y Leon, Carretera de Burgos km. 119, C.P. 47071, Valladolid, Spain

David Rodríguez-Lázaro
Agricultural Technological Institute of Castilla and Leon (ITACyL), Ministry of Agriculture and Livestock. Castilla y Leon, Carretera de Burgos km. 119, C.P. 47071, Valladolid, Spain

Marta Hernández
Agricultural Technological Institute of Castilla and Leon (ITACyL), Ministry of Agriculture and Livestock. Castilla y Leon, Carretera de Burgos km. 119, C.P. 47071, Valladolid, Spain

Frantisek Vitula
Department of Veterinary Ecology and Environmental Protection, Faculty of Veterinary Hygiene and Ecology, University of Veterinary and Pharmaceutical Sciences, Brno, Czech Republic

Lucie Peckova
Department of Veterinary Ecology and Environmental Protection, Faculty of Veterinary Hygiene and Ecology, University of Veterinary and Pharmaceutical Sciences, Brno, Czech Republic

Hana Bandouchova
Department of Veterinary Ecology and Environmental Protection, Faculty of Veterinary Hygiene and Ecology, University of Veterinary and Pharmaceutical Sciences, Brno, Czech Republic

Miroslav Pohanka
Centre of Advanced Studies, Faculty of Military Health Sciences, University of Defence, Hradec Kralove, Czech Republic

Ladislav Novotny
Department of Pathological Morphology and Parasitology, Faculty of Veterinary Medicine, University of Veterinary and Pharmaceutical Sciences, Brno, Czech Republic

David Jira
Department of Veterinary Ecology and Environmental Protection, Faculty of Veterinary Hygiene and Ecology, University of Veterinary and Pharmaceutical Sciences, Brno, Czech Republic

Jiri Kral
Department of Veterinary Ecology and Environmental Protection, Faculty of Veterinary Hygiene and Ecology, University of Veterinary and Pharmaceutical Sciences, Brno, Czech Republic

Karel Ondracek
Department of Veterinary Ecology and Environmental Protection, Faculty of Veterinary Hygiene and Ecology, University of Veterinary and Pharmaceutical Sciences, Brno, Czech Republic

Jitka Osickova
Department of Veterinary Ecology and Environmental Protection, Faculty of Veterinary Hygiene and Ecology, University of Veterinary and Pharmaceutical Sciences, Brno, Czech Republic

Dagmar Zendulkova
Department of Infectious Diseases and Microbiology, Faculty of Veterinary Medicine, University of Veterinary and Pharmaceutical Sciences, Brno, Czech Republic

Katerina Rosenbergova
Department of Infectious Diseases and Microbiology, Faculty of Veterinary Medicine, University of Veterinary and Pharmaceutical Sciences, Brno, Czech Republic

Frantisek Treml
Department of Infectious Diseases and Microbiology, Faculty of Veterinary Medicine, University of Veterinary and Pharmaceutical Sciences, Brno, Czech Republic

Jiri Pikula
Department of Veterinary Ecology and Environmental Protection, Faculty of Veterinary Hygiene and Ecology, University of Veterinary and Pharmaceutical Sciences, Brno, Czech Republic

Branko Kokotovic
National Veterinary Institute, New Technical University of Denmark, Bülowsvej 27, DK-1790 Copenhagen V, Denmark

Niels F Friis
National Veterinary Institute, New Technical University of Denmark, Bülowsvej 27, DK-1790 Copenhagen V, Denmark

Peter Ahrens
National Veterinary Institute, New Technical University of Denmark, Bülowsvej 27, DK-1790 Copenhagen V, Denmark

Szilvia Vincze
Institute of Microbiology and Epizootics, Veterinary Faculty, Free University Berlin, Germany

Ivonne Stamm
Vet Med Labor GmbH, Division of IDEXX Laboratories, Ludwigsburg, Germany

Peter A. Kopp
Vet Med Labor GmbH, Division of IDEXX Laboratories, Ludwigsburg, Germany

Julia Hermes
Department of Infectious Diseases Epidemiology, Robert Koch Institute, Berlin, Germany

Cornelia Adlhoch
Department of Infectious Diseases Epidemiology, Robert Koch Institute, Berlin, Germany

Torsten Semmler
Institute of Microbiology and Epizootics, Veterinary Faculty, Free University Berlin, Germany

Lothar H. Wieler
Institute of Microbiology and Epizootics, Veterinary Faculty, Free University Berlin, Germany

Antina Lu¨bke-Becker
Institute of Microbiology and Epizootics, Veterinary Faculty, Free University Berlin, Germany

Birgit Walther
Institute of Microbiology and Epizootics, Veterinary Faculty, Free University Berlin, Germany

Tara C. Smith
Center for Emerging Infectious Diseases, Department of Epidemiology, University of Iowa College of Public Health, University of Iowa, Iowa City, Iowa, United States of America

Wondwossen A. Gebreyes
Department of Veterinary Preventive Medicine, Ohio State University, Columbus, Ohio, United States of America

Melanie J. Abley
Department of Veterinary Preventive Medicine, Ohio State University, Columbus, Ohio, United States of America

Abby L. Harper
Center for Emerging Infectious Diseases, Department of Epidemiology, University of Iowa College of Public Health, University of Iowa, Iowa City, Iowa, United States of America

Brett M. Forshey
Center for Emerging Infectious Diseases, Department of Epidemiology, University of Iowa College of Public Health, University of Iowa, Iowa City, Iowa, United States of America

Michael J. Male
Center for Emerging Infectious Diseases, Department of Epidemiology, University of Iowa College of Public Health, University of Iowa, Iowa City, Iowa, United States of America

H. Wayne Martin
Department of Veterinary Population Medicine, College of Veterinary Medicine, University of Minnesota, St. Paul, Minnesota, United States of America

Bayleyegn Z. Molla
Department of Veterinary Preventive Medicine, Ohio State University, Columbus, Ohio, United States of America

Srinand Sreevatsan
Department of Veterinary Population Medicine, College of Veterinary Medicine, University of Minnesota, St. Paul, Minnesota, United States of America

Siddhartha Thakur

Department of Population Health and Pathobiology, College of Veterinary Medicine, North Carolina State University, Raleigh, North Carolina, United States of America

Madhumathi Thiruvengadam
Department of Veterinary Population Medicine, College of Veterinary Medicine, University of Minnesota, St. Paul, Minnesota, United States of America

Peter R. Davies
Department of Veterinary Population Medicine, College of Veterinary Medicine, University of Minnesota, St. Paul, Minnesota, United States of America

Carmen S. Arriola
School of Veterinary Medicine, San Marcos Major National University, Lima, Peru
Department of International Health, Johns Hopkins Bloomberg School of Public Health, Johns Hopkins University, Baltimore, Maryland, United States of America

Mariella E. Gu¨ ere
School of Veterinary Medicine, San Marcos Major National University, Lima, Peru

Jesper Larsen
Department of Microbiological Surveillance and Research, Statens Serum Institut, Copenhagen, Denmark

Robert L. Skov
Department of Microbiological Surveillance and Research, Statens Serum Institut, Copenhagen, Denmark

Robert H. Gilman
Department of International Health, Johns Hopkins Bloomberg School of Public Health, Johns Hopkins University, Baltimore, Maryland, United States of America

Armando E. Gonzalez
School of Veterinary Medicine, San Marcos Major National University, Lima, Peru

Ellen K. Silbergeld
Department of Environmental Health Sciences, Johns Hopkins Bloomberg School of Public Health, Johns Hopkins University, Baltimore, Maryland, United States of America

Haitske Graveland
Division of Environmental Epidemiology, Institute for Risk Assessment Sciences, Utrecht University, Utrecht, The Netherlands

Jaap A. Wagenaar
Department of Infectious Diseases and Immunology, Faculty of Veterinary Medicine, Utrecht University, Utrecht, The Netherlands

Hans Heesterbeek
Department of Farm Animal Health, Faculty of Veterinary Medicine, Utrecht University, Utrecht, The Netherlands

Dik Mevius
Department of Infectious Diseases and Immunology, Faculty of Veterinary Medicine, Utrecht University, Utrecht, The Netherlands
Central Veterinary Institute of Wageningen UR, Lelystad, The Netherlands

Engeline van Duijkeren
Department of Infectious Diseases and Immunology, Faculty of Veterinary Medicine, Utrecht University, Utrecht, The Netherlands

Dick Heederik
Division of Environmental Epidemiology, Institute for Risk Assessment Sciences, Utrecht University, Utrecht, The Netherlands
Julius Center for Health Sciences and Primary Care, University Medical Center, Utrecht, The Netherlands

Salvatore Virdis
Department of Animal Biology, University of Sassari, via Vienna 2, 07100 Sassari, Italy

Christian Scarano
Department of Animal Biology, University of Sassari, via Vienna 2, 07100 Sassari, Italy

Francesca Cossu
Department of Animal Biology, University of Sassari, via Vienna 2, 07100 Sassari, Italy

Vincenzo Spanu
Department of Animal Biology, University of Sassari, via Vienna 2, 07100 Sassari, Italy

Carlo Spanu
Department of Animal Biology, University of Sassari, via Vienna 2, 07100 Sassari, Italy

Enrico Pietro Luigi De Santis
Department of Animal Biology, University of Sassari, via Vienna 2, 07100 Sassari, Italy

R. Köck
Institute of Hygiene, University Hospital Münster, Robert-Koch-Str. 41, 48149 Münster, Germany
Institute of Medical Microbiology, University Hospital Münster, Domagkstr. 10, 48149 Münster, Germany

J. Harlizius
Chamber for Agriculture North Rhine-Westphalia, Animal Health Services, Siebengebirgsstr. 200, 53229 Bonn, Germany

N. Bressan
Institute of Hygiene, University Hospital Münster, Robert-Koch-Str. 41, 48149 Münster, Germany

R. Laerberg
Institute of Hygiene, University Hospital Münster, Robert-Koch-Str. 41, 48149 Münster, Germany

L. H. Wieler
Institute of Microbiology and Epizootics, Free University Berlin, Philippistr. 13, 10115 Berlin, Germany

W. Witte
Robert-Koch Institute, Burgstr. 27, 38855 Wernigerode, Germany

R. H. Deurenberg
Department of Medical Microbiology, University Hospital Maastricht, 6202 AZ Maastricht, The Netherlands

A. Voss
Department of Medical Microbiology, Canisius-Wilhelmina Hospital and Radboud University Nijmegen Medical Centre, Geert-Groote-Plein 10, 6500 HB Nijmegen, The Netherlands

K. Becker
Institute of Medical Microbiology, University Hospital Münster, Domagkstr. 10, 48149 Münster, Germany

A. W. Friedrich
Institute of Hygiene, University Hospital Münster, Robert-Koch-Str. 41, 48149 Münster, Germany

Tara C. Smith
Department of Epidemiology, University of Iowa College of Public Health, Iowa City, Iowa, United States of America
Center for Emerging Infectious Diseases, University of Iowa College of Public Health, Iowa City, Iowa, United States of America

Michael J. Male
Department of Epidemiology, University of Iowa College of Public Health, Iowa City, Iowa, United States of America
Center for Emerging Infectious Diseases, University of Iowa College of Public Health, Iowa City, Iowa, United States of America

Abby L. Harper
Department of Epidemiology, University of Iowa College of Public Health, Iowa City, Iowa, United States of America
Center for Emerging Infectious Diseases, University of Iowa College of Public Health, Iowa City, Iowa, United States of America

Jennifer S. Kroeger
Department of Medicine, University of Iowa Carver College of Medicine, Iowa City, Iowa, United States of America

Gregory P. Tinkler
Center for Emerging Infectious Diseases, University of Iowa College of Public Health, Iowa City, Iowa, United States of America

Erin D. Moritz
Department of Epidemiology, University of Iowa College of Public Health, Iowa City, Iowa, United States of America
Center for Emerging Infectious Diseases, University of Iowa College of Public Health, Iowa City, Iowa, United States of America

Ana W. Capuano
Department of Epidemiology, University of Iowa College of Public Health, Iowa City, Iowa, United States of America
Center for Emerging Infectious Diseases, University of Iowa College of Public Health, Iowa City, Iowa, United States of America

Loreen A. Herwaldt

Department of Epidemiology, University of Iowa College of Public Health, Iowa City, Iowa, United States of America
Department of Medicine, University of Iowa Carver College of Medicine, Iowa City, Iowa, United States of America
Program of Hospital Epidemiology, University of Iowa Hospitals and Clinics, Iowa City, Iowa, United States of America

Daniel J. Diekema
Department of Medicine, University of Iowa Carver College of Medicine, Iowa City, Iowa, United States of America
Program of Hospital Epidemiology, University of Iowa Hospitals and Clinics, Iowa City, Iowa, United States of America
Department of Pathology, University of Iowa Carver College of Medicine, Iowa City, Iowa, United States of America

Tobias Revold
Department of Companion Animal Clinical Sciences, Norwegian Univer sity of Life Sciences (previously Norwegian School of Veterinary Science), Ullevålsveien 72, 0033 Oslo, Norway

Takele Abayneh
Department of Companion Animal Clinical Sciences, Norwegian Univer sity of Life Sciences (previously Norwegian School of Veterinary Science), Ullevålsveien 72, 0033 Oslo, Norway
School of Veterinary Medicine, Addis Ababa University, DebreZeit, Ethiopia

Hege BrunHansen
Department of Companion Animal Clinical Sciences, Norwegian Univer sity of Life Sciences (previously Norwegian School of Veterinary Science), Ullevålsveien 72, 0033 Oslo, Norway

Signe L. Kleppe
Department of Companion Animal Clinical Sciences, Norwegian Univer sity of Life Sciences (previously Norwegian School of Veterinary Science), Ullevålsveien 72, 0033 Oslo, Norway
Aktiv Dyreklinikk, 1484 Hakadal, Norway

ErnstOtto Ropstad
Department of Companion Animal Clinical Sciences, Norwegian Univer sity of Life Sciences (previously Norwegian School of Veterinary Science), Ullevålsveien 72, 0033 Oslo, Norway

Robert A. Hellings
Rikstoto clinic Bjerke, Økern, 0510 Oslo, Norway

Henning Sørum
Department of Companion Animal Clinical Sciences, Norwegian Univer sity of Life Sciences (previously Norwegian School of Veterinary Science), Ullevålsveien 72, 0033 Oslo, Norway

Rocio Crespo
Avian Health and Food Safety Laboratory, Washington Animal Disease Diagnostic Laboratory, Washington State University, 2607 West Pioneer, Puyallup, WA 98371, USA

Michael M Garner
Northwest ZooPath, 654 W. Main St., Monroe, WA 98272, USA

Sharon G Hopkins
Public Health–Seattle & King County, 401 5th Avenue, Ste 1100, Seattle, WA 98104, USA

Devendra H Shah
Department of Veterinary Microbiology, Washington State University, Pullman, WA 99164-7040, USA
Pathology and Paul Allen School for Global Animal Health, Washington State University, Pullman, WA 99164-7040, USA

Karen Hunt
Teagasc Food Research Centre, Moorepark, Fermoy, Co. Cork, Ireland
Veterinary Sciences Centre, School of Agriculture, Food Science and Veterinary Medicine, University College Dublin, Belfield, Dublin

Niall Drummond
Cork County Council Veterinary Food Safety Laboratories, Iniscarra, Co. Cork, Ireland

Mary Murphy
Cork County Council Veterinary Food Safety Laboratories, Iniscarra, Co. Cork, Ireland

Francis Butler
Veterinary Sciences Centre, School of Agriculture, Food Science and Veterinary Medicine, University College Dublin, Belfield, Dublin

Jim Buckley

Cork County Council Veterinary Food Safety Laboratories, Iniscarra, Co. Cork, Ireland

Kieran Jordan
Teagasc Food Research Centre, Moorepark, Fermoy, Co. Cork, Ireland

Vincent P Richards
Department of Population Medicine and Diagnostic Sciences, College of Veterinary Medicine, Cornell University, Ithaca, NY 14853, USA

Ruth N Zadoks
Quality Milk Production Services, College of Veterinary Medicine, Cornell University, Ithaca, NY 14853, USA
Current address: Moredun Research Institute, Pentlands Science Park, Bush Loan, Penicuik and Royal (Dick) School of Veterinary Studies, University of Edinburgh, Scotland, UK

Paulina D Pavinski Bitar
Department of Population Medicine and Diagnostic Sciences, College of Veterinary Medicine, Cornell University, Ithaca, NY 14853, USA

Tristan Lefébure
Department of Population Medicine and Diagnostic Sciences, College of Veterinary Medicine, Cornell University, Ithaca, NY 14853, USA
Current address: Université de Lyon, Université Lyon 1, National Centre for Scientific Research, Ecology and Natural Hydrosystèmes anthropized, Villeurbanne, France

Ping Lang
Current address: Department of Plant Pathology & Plant-Microbe Biology, Cornell University, Ithaca, NY 14853, USA

Brenda Werner
Quality Milk Production Services, College of Veterinary Medicine, Cornell University, Ithaca, NY 14853, USA

Linda Tikofsky
Quality Milk Production Services, College of Veterinary Medicine, Cornell University, Ithaca, NY 14853, USA
Current address: 4055 McIntyre Road, Trumansburg, NY 14886, USA

Paolo Moroni
Quality Milk Production Services, College of Veterinary Medicine, Cornell University, Ithaca, NY 14853, USA
Università degli Studi di Milano, Department of Health, Animal Science and Food Safety, Via Celoria 10, 20133 Milan, Italy

Michael J Stanhope
Department of Population Medicine and Diagnostic Sciences, College of Veterinary Medicine, Cornell University, Ithaca, NY 14853, USA

Philip N Ward
Nuffield Department of Clinical Laboratory Sciences, Oxford University, John Radcliffe Hospital, Headington, Oxford, OX3 9DU, UK

Matthew TG Holden
The Wellcome Trust Sanger Institute, Wellcome Trust Genome Campus, Hinxton, Cambridge, CB10 1SA, UK

James A Leigh
The School of Veterinary Medicine and Science, The University of Nottingham, Sutton Bonington Campus, Sutton Bonington, Leicestershire, LE12 5RD, UK

Nicola Lennard
The Wellcome Trust Sanger Institute, Wellcome Trust Genome Campus, Hinxton, Cambridge, CB10 1SA, UK

Alexandra Bignell
The Wellcome Trust Sanger Institute, Wellcome Trust Genome Campus, Hinxton, Cambridge, CB10 1SA, UK

Andy Barron
The Wellcome Trust Sanger Institute, Wellcome Trust Genome Campus, Hinxton, Cambridge, CB10 1SA, UK

Louise Clark
The Wellcome Trust Sanger Institute, Wellcome Trust Genome Campus, Hinxton, Cambridge, CB10 1SA, UK

Michael A Quail
The Wellcome Trust Sanger Institute, Wellcome Trust Genome Campus, Hinxton, Cambridge, CB10 1SA, UK

John Woodward
The Wellcome Trust Sanger Institute, Wellcome Trust Genome Campus, Hinxton, Cambridge, CB10 1SA, UK

Bart G Barrell
The Wellcome Trust Sanger Institute, Wellcome Trust Genome Campus, Hinxton, Cambridge, CB10 1SA, UK

Sharon A Egan
The School of Veterinary Medicine and Science, The University of Nottingham, Sutton Bonington Campus, Sutton Bonington, Leicestershire, LE12 5RD, UK

Terence R Field
Institute for Animal Health, Compton Laboratory, Compton, Newbury, Berks, RG20 7NN, UK

Duncan Maskell
Dept. of Veterinary Medicine, The University of Cambridge, Cambridge, CB3 0ES, UK

Michael Kehoe
Institute for Cell and Molecular Biosciences, The Medical School, University of Newcastle upon Tyne, Framlington Place, Newcastle upon Tyne, NE2 4HH, UK

Christopher G Dowson
Department of Biological Sciences, University of Warwick, Coventry, CV4 7AL, UK

Neil Chanter
Centre for Preventative Medicine, Animal Health Trust, Newmarket, Suffolk, CB8 7UU, UK

Adrian M Whatmore
Department of Biological Sciences, University of Warwick, Coventry, CV4 7AL, UK
Veterinary Laboratories Agency, Weybridge, UK

Stephen D Bentley
The Wellcome Trust Sanger Institute, Wellcome Trust Genome Campus, Hinxton, Cambridge, CB10 1SA, UK

Julian Parkhill
The Wellcome Trust Sanger Institute, Wellcome Trust Genome Campus, Hinxton, Cambridge, CB10 1SA, UK

Andreas Sjödin
Division of CBRN Security and Defence, FOI - Swedish Defence Research Agency, Umeå, Sweden

Kerstin Svensson
Division of CBRN Security and Defence, FOI - Swedish Defence Research Agency, Umeå, Sweden

Caroline Öhrman
Division of CBRN Security and Defence, FOI - Swedish Defence Research Agency, Umeå, Sweden

Jon Ahlinder
Division of CBRN Security and Defence, FOI - Swedish Defence Research Agency, Umeå, Sweden

Petter Lindgren
Division of CBRN Security and Defence, FOI - Swedish Defence Research Agency, Umeå, Sweden

Samuel Duodu
Section for Bacteriology, Norwegian Veterinary Institute, Oslo, Norway

Anders Johansson
Department of Clinical Microbiology, Umeå University, SE-901 85, Umeå, Sweden

Duncan J Colquhoun
Section for Bacteriology, Norwegian Veterinary Institute, Oslo, Norway

Pär Larsson
Division of CBRN Security and Defence, FOI - Swedish Defence Research Agency, Umeå, Sweden

Mats Forsman
Division of CBRN Security and Defence, FOI - Swedish Defence Research Agency, Umeå, Sweden

Rakel Arrazuria
Animal Health Department, NEIKER- Basque Institute for Agricultural Research and Development, Berreaga, 1, 48160 Derio,

Bizkaia, Spain

Iker A Sevilla
Animal Health Department, NEIKER- Basque Institute for Agricultural Research and Development, Berreaga, 1, 48160 Derio, Bizkaia, Spain

Elena Molina
Animal Health Department, NEIKER- Basque Institute for Agricultural Research and Development, Berreaga, 1, 48160 Derio, Bizkaia, Spain

Valentín Pérez
Department of Animal Health, Faculty of Veterinary Medicine, University of León, León, Spain

Joseba M Garrido
Animal Health Department, NEIKER- Basque Institute for Agricultural Research and Development, Berreaga, 1, 48160 Derio, Bizkaia, Spain

Ramón A Juste
Animal Health Department, NEIKER- Basque Institute for Agricultural Research and Development, Berreaga, 1, 48160 Derio, Bizkaia, Spain

Natalia Elguezabal
Animal Health Department, NEIKER- Basque Institute for Agricultural Research and Development, Berreaga, 1, 48160 Derio, Bizkaia, Spain

Mohamed E. Hamid
Department of Clinical Microbiology and Parasitology, College of Medicine, King Khalid University, Abha 61321, Saudi Arabia

Casey L Cazer
College of Veterinary Medicine, Cornell University, Ithaca, NY 14853, USA

Rebecca M Mitchell
Department of Population Medicine and Diagnostic Sciences, Cornell University College of Veterinary Medicine, Animal Health Diagnostic Center, Ithaca, NY 14853, USA

Kellie M Cicconi-Hogan
Department of Population Medicine and Diagnostic Sciences, Cornell University College of Veterinary Medicine, Animal Health Diagnostic Center, Ithaca, NY 14853, USA

Michael Gamroth
Department of Animal and Range Sciences, Oregon State University, Corvallis, OR 97331, USA

Roxann M Richert
Department of Dairy Science, University of WI, Madison, WI 53706, USA

Pamela L Ruegg
Department of Dairy Science, University of WI, Madison, WI 53706, USA

Ynte H Schukken
Department of Population Medicine and Diagnostic Sciences, Cornell University College of Veterinary Medicine, Animal Health Diagnostic Center, Ithaca, NY 14853, USA

Ocean R. Cohen
Department of Infectious Disease and Global Health, Tufts Cummings School of Veterinary Medicine, North Grafton, Massachusetts, United States of America

Jennifer A. Steele
Department of Infectious Disease and Global Health, Tufts Cummings School of Veterinary Medicine, North Grafton, Massachusetts, United States of America

Quanshun Zhang
Department of Infectious Disease and Global Health, Tufts Cummings School of Veterinary Medicine, North Grafton, Massachusetts, United States of America

Diane J. Schmidt
Department of Infectious Disease and Global Health, Tufts Cummings School of Veterinary Medicine, North Grafton, Massachusetts, United States of America

Yuankai Wang
Department of Infectious Disease and Global Health, Tufts Cummings School of Veterinary Medicine, North Grafton, Massachusetts, United States of America

Philip E. S. Hamel
Department of Infectious Disease and Global Health, Tufts Cummings School of Veterinary Medicine, North Grafton, Massachusetts, United States of America

Gillian Beamer
Department of Infectious Disease and Global Health, Tufts Cummings School of Veterinary Medicine, North Grafton, Massachusetts, United States of America

Bingling Xu
Department of Infectious Disease and Global Health, Tufts Cummings School of Veterinary Medicine, North Grafton, Massachusetts, United States of America

Saul Tzipori
Department of Infectious Disease and Global Health, Tufts Cummings School of Veterinary Medicine, North Grafton, Massachusetts, United States of America

Sandra Janezic
National Laboratory for Health, Environment and Food, Maribor, Slovenia

Valerija Zidaric
National Laboratory for Health, Environment and Food, Maribor, Slovenia

Bart Pardon
Department of Large Animal Internal Medicine, Faculty of Veterinary Medicine, Ghent University, Merelbeke, Belgium

Alexander Indra
Austrian Agency for Health and Food Safety (AGES), Vienna, Austria

Branko Kokotovic
Technical University of Denmark, National Veterinary Institute, Copenhagen, Denmark

Jose Luis Blanco
Complutense University, Madrid, Spain

Christian Seyboldt
Friedrich-Loeffler-Institut, Federal Research Institute for Animal Health, Institute of Bacterial Infections and Zoonoses, Jena, Germany

Cristina Rodriguez Diaz
University of Liege, Faculty of Veterinary Medicine, Liege, Belgium

Ian R Poxton
University of Edinburgh, Edinburgh, UK

Vincent Perreten
University of Bern, Institute of Veterinary Bacteriology, Bern, Switzerland

Ilenia Drigo
IZSVe, Treviso, Italy

Alena Jiraskova
Charles University in Prague, 1st Faculty of Medicine, Prague, Czech Republic

Matjaz Ocepek
University of Ljubljana, Veterinary Faculty, Ljubljana, Slovenia

J Scott Weese
University of Guelph, Ontario Veterinary College, Ontario, Canada

J Glenn Songer
Department of Veterinary Science and Microbiology, University of Arizona, Tucson, USA

Mark H Wilcox

Department of Medical Microbiology, Leeds Teaching Hospitals, Leeds, UK

Maja Rupnik
National Laboratory for Health, Environment and Food, Maribor, Slovenia
University of Maribor, Medical Faculty, Maribor, Slovenia
Centre of Excellence for Integrated Approaches in Chemistry and Biology of Proteins, Ljubljana, Slovenia

Stefanie Verherstraeten
Department of Pathology, Bacteriology and Avian Diseases, Faculty of Veterinary Medicine, Ghent University, Salisburylaan 133, Merelbeke B-9820, Belgium

Evy Goossens
Department of Pathology, Bacteriology and Avian Diseases, Faculty of Veterinary Medicine, Ghent University, Salisburylaan 133, Merelbeke B-9820, Belgium

Bonnie Valgaeren
Department of Internal Medicine and Clinical Biology of Large Animals, Faculty of Veterinary Medicine, Ghent University, Salisburylaan 133, Merelbeke B-9820, Belgium

Bart Pardon
Department of Internal Medicine and Clinical Biology of Large Animals, Faculty of Veterinary Medicine, Ghent University, Salisburylaan 133, Merelbeke B-9820, Belgium

Leen Timbermont
Department of Pathology, Bacteriology and Avian Diseases, Faculty of Veterinary Medicine, Ghent University, Salisburylaan 133, Merelbeke B-9820, Belgium

Karen Vermeulen
Department of Pathology, Bacteriology and Avian Diseases, Faculty of Veterinary Medicine, Ghent University, Salisburylaan 133, Merelbeke B-9820, Belgium

Stijn Schauvliege[3],
Department of Surgery and Anesthesia of Domestic Animals, Faculty of Veterinary Medicine, Ghent University, Salisburylaan 133, Merelbeke B9820, Belgium

Freddy Haesebrouck
Department of Pathology, Bacteriology and Avian Diseases, Faculty of Veterinary Medicine, Ghent University, Salisburylaan 133, Merelbeke B-9820, Belgium

Richard Ducatelle
Department of Pathology, Bacteriology and Avian Diseases, Faculty of Veterinary Medicine, Ghent University, Salisburylaan 133, Merelbeke B-9820, Belgium

Piet Deprez
Department of Internal Medicine and Clinical Biology of Large Animals, Faculty of Veterinary Medicine, Ghent University, Salisburylaan 133, Merelbeke B-9820, Belgium

Filip Van Immerseel
Department of Pathology, Bacteriology and Avian Diseases, Faculty of Veterinary Medicine, Ghent University, Salisburylaan 133, Merelbeke B-9820, Belgium

Gloria Chan
Department of Population Medicine, University of Guelph, Guelph, ON N1G 2W1, Canada

Abdolvahab Farzan
Department of Population Medicine, University of Guelph, Guelph, ON N1G 2W1, Canada

Glenn Soltes
Department of Pathobiology, University of Guelph, Guelph, ON N1G 2W1, Canada

Vivian M Nicholson
Department of Pathobiology, University of Guelph, Guelph, ON N1G 2W1, Canada

Yanlong Pei
Department of Pathobiology, University of Guelph, Guelph, ON N1G 2W1, Canada

Robert Friendship
Department of Population Medicine, University of Guelph, Guelph, ON N1G 2W1, Canada

John F Prescott
Department of Pathobiology, University of Guelph, Guelph, ON N1G 2W1, Canada

Marcio C Costa
Department of Pathobiology, Ontario Veterinary College, University of Guelph, Guelph, Canada

Richard Reid-Smith
Public Health Agency of Canada, Guelph and Saskatoon, Guelph, Canada

Sheryl Gow
Feedlot Health Management Services Ltd., Okotoks, Canada

Sherry J Hannon
Feedlot Health Management Services Ltd., Okotoks, Canada

Calvin Booker
Feedlot Health Management Services Ltd., Okotoks, Canada

Joyce Rousseau
Department of Pathobiology, Ontario Veterinary College, University of Guelph, Guelph, Canada

Katharine M Benedict
Department of Clinical Sciences, Colorado State University, Fort Collins, CO, USA

Paul S Morley
Department of Clinical Sciences, Colorado State University, Fort Collins, CO, USA

J Scott Weese
Department of Pathobiology, Ontario Veterinary College, University of Guelph, Guelph, Canada

T. Getachew
National Animal Health Diagnostic and Investigation Center (NAHDIC), Ethiopian Ministry of Livestock and Fisheries Development, Sebeta, Ethiopia

G. Getachew
National Animal Health Diagnostic and Investigation Center (NAHDIC), Ethiopian Ministry of Livestock and Fisheries Development, Sebeta, Ethiopia

G. Sintayehu
National Animal Health Diagnostic and Investigation Center (NAHDIC), Ethiopian Ministry of Livestock and Fisheries Development, Sebeta, Ethiopia

M. Getenet
National Animal Health Diagnostic and Investigation Center (NAHDIC), Ethiopian Ministry of Livestock and Fisheries Development, Sebeta, Ethiopia

A. Fasil
National Animal Health Diagnostic and Investigation Center (NAHDIC), Ethiopian Ministry of Livestock and Fisheries Development, Sebeta, Ethiopia

Elaine MS Dorneles
Department of Preventive Veterinary Medicine, Veterinary School, Applied Bacteriology Laboratory, Federal University of Minas Gerais, Belo Horizonte, MG, Brazil

Nammalwar Sriranganathan
Department of Biomedical Sciences and Pathobiology, Center for Molecular Medicine and Infectious Diseases, Regional College of Veterinary Medicine, Virginia Polytechnic Institute and State University, Blacksburg, VA, USA

Andrey P. Lage
Department of Preventive Veterinary Medicine, Veterinary School, Applied Bacteriology Laboratory, Federal University of Minas Gerais, Belo Horizonte, MG, Brazil

Miklós Gyuranecz
Institute for Veterinary Medical Research, Centre for Agricultural Research, Hungarian Academy of Sciences, Budapest 1143, Hungária körút 21, Hungary

Brandy D Rannals

Center for Microbial Genetics & Genomics, Northern Arizona University, 1298 S. Knoles Drive, Flagstaff, AZ 86011-4073, USA

Christina A Allen
Center for Microbial Genetics & Genomics, Northern Arizona University, 1298 S. Knoles Drive, Flagstaff, AZ 86011-4073, USA

Szilárd Jánosi
Veterinary Diagnostic Directorate, National Food Chain Safety Office, Budapest 1143, Tábornok utca 2, Hungary

Paul S Keim
Center for Microbial Genetics & Genomics, Northern Arizona University, 1298 S. Knoles Drive, Flagstaff, AZ 86011-4073, USA

Jeffrey T Foster
Center for Microbial Genetics & Genomics, Northern Arizona University, 1298 S. Knoles Drive, Flagstaff, AZ 86011-4073, USA

Natacha Wu
Centre for Fish and Wildlife Health (FIWI), Institute of Animal Pathology, Vetsuisse Faculty, University of Bern, Bern, Switzerland

Carlos Abril
Institute of Veterinary Bacteriology, Centre for Zoonoses, Bacterial Animal Diseases and Antimicrobial Resistance (ZOBA), Vetsuisse Faculty, University of Bern, Bern, Switzerland
Suisselab AG, Schützenmattstrasse 10, 3052 Zollikofen, Switzerland

Andreas Thomann
Institute of Veterinary Bacteriology, Centre for Zoonoses, Bacterial Animal Diseases and Antimicrobial Resistance (ZOBA), Vetsuisse Faculty, University of Bern, Bern, Switzerland

Eleonore Grosclaude
Service de la Consommation et des Affaires Vétérinaires, Geneva, Switzerland

Marcus G Doherr
Veterinary Public Health Institute, Vetsuisse Faculty, University of Bern, Bern, Switzerland

Patrick Boujon
Present address: Galli-Valerio Institute, Laboratory of veterinary analyzes, Lausanne, Switzerland

Marie-Pierre Ryser-Degiorgis
Centre for Fish and Wildlife Health (FIWI), Institute of Animal Pathology, Vetsuisse Faculty, University of Bern, Bern, Switzerland

Betsy J Bricker
Bacterial Diseases of Livestock Research Unit, National Animal Disease Center, Agricultural Research Service, United States Department of Agriculture, 2300 Dayton Rd, Ames, IA, 50010, USA

Darla R Ewalt
Diagnostic Bacteriology Laboratory, National Veterinary Services Laboratories, Animal and Plant Health Inspection Service, United States Department of Agriculture, 1800 Dayton Rd, Ames, IA, 50010, USA

Md. Arifur Rahman
Department of Medicine, Faculty of Veterinary Science, Bangladesh Agricultural University (BAU), Mymensingh 2202, Bangladesh

Md. Mahbub Alam
Department of Medicine, Faculty of Veterinary Science, Bangladesh Agricultural University (BAU), Mymensingh 2202, Bangladesh

Md. Aminul Islam
Department of Medicine, Faculty of Veterinary Science, Bangladesh Agricultural University (BAU), Mymensingh 2202, Bangladesh

A. K. Fazlul Haque Bhuiyan
Department of Animal Breeding and Genetics, Faculty of Animal Husbandry, BAU, Mymensingh 2202, Bangladesh

A. K. M. Anisur Rahman
Department of Medicine, Faculty of Veterinary Science, Bangladesh Agricultural University (BAU), Mymensingh 2202, Bangladesh

Angela Hilbert
Institut für Epidemiologie, Friedrich-Loeffler-Institut, National Reference Laboratory for Q-fever, Wusterhausen, Germany

Gernot Schmoock
Institute of Bacterial Infections and Zoonoses, Friedrich Loeffler Institute, Jena, Germany

Hannah Lenzko
Institute of Molecular Pathogenesis, Friedrich Loeffler Institute, Jena, Germany

Udo Moog
Animal Health Service, Thüringer Tierseuchenkasse, Jena, Germany

Roland Diller
Institute of Bacterial Infections and Zoonoses, Friedrich Loeffler Institute, Jena, Germany

Andreas Fröhlich
Institute of Epidemiology, Friedrich Loeffler Institute, National Reference Laboratory for Q-fever, Wusterhausen, Germany

Lothar Hoffmann
Thuringian State Office of Food Safety and Consumer Protection, Bad Langensalza, Germany

Steffen Horner
Thuringian State Office of Food Safety and Consumer Protection, Bad Langensalza, Germany

Michael Elschner
Thuringian Ministry for Health, Family and Health, Erfurt, Germany

Herbert Tomaso
Institute of Bacterial Infections and Zoonoses, Friedrich Loeffler Institute, Jena, Germany

Klaus Henning
Institute of Epidemiology, Friedrich Loeffler Institute, National Reference Laboratory for Q-fever, Wusterhausen, Germany

Heinrich Neubauer
Institut für Bakterielle Infektionen und Zoonosen, Friedrich-Loeffler-Institut, Jena, Germany

Lisa D Sprague
Institute of Bacterial Infections and Zoonoses, Friedrich Loeffler Institute, Jena, Germany

Francisco Ruiz-Fons
Neiker Basque Institute for Agricultural Research and Development, Department of Animal Health, Berreaga 1, 48160 Derio, Bizkaia, Spain

Ianire Astobiza
Neiker Basque Institute for Agricultural Research and Development, Department of Animal Health, Berreaga 1, 48160 Derio, Bizkaia, Spain

Jesús F Barandika
Neiker Basque Institute for Agricultural Research and Development, Department of Animal Health, Berreaga 1, 48160 Derio, Bizkaia, Spain

Ana Hurtado
Neiker Basque Institute for Agricultural Research and Development, Department of Animal Health, Berreaga 1, 48160 Derio, Bizkaia, Spain

Raquel Atxaerandio
Neiker Basque Institute for Agricultural Research and Development, Department of Animal Health, Berreaga 1, 48160 Derio, Bizkaia, Spain

Ramón A Juste
Neiker Basque Institute for Agricultural Research and Development, Department of Animal Health, Berreaga 1, 48160 Derio, Bizkaia, Spain

Ana L García-Pérez
Neiker Basque Institute for Agricultural Research and Development, Department of Animal Health, Berreaga 1, 48160 Derio, Bizkaia, Spain

Rebecca T Trout Fryxell
Department of Entomology and Plant Pathology, University of Tennessee, Knoxville, TN, USA

C Dayton Steelman
Department of Entomology, University of Arkansas, Fayetteville, AR, USA

Allen L Szalanski
Department of Entomology, University of Arkansas, Fayetteville, AR, USA

Ken L Kvamme
Department of Anthropology, University of Arkansas, Fayetteville, AR, USA

Peggy M Billingsley
Department of Forensic and Investigative Genetics, University of North Texas Health Science Center, Ft. Worth, TX, USA

Philip C Williamson
Department of Forensic and Investigative Genetics, University of North Texas Health Science Center, Ft. Worth, TX, USA

Laia Solano-Gallego
Department of Animal Medicine and Surgery, Faculty of Veterinary Medicine, Autonomous University of Barcelona (UAB), Cerdanyola 08193, Barcelona, Spain
Royal Veterinary College, University of London, Hatfield, United Kingdom

Alessandra Caprì
Veterinary Clinic Camagna, Reggio Calabria, Italy
Dip.to of Veterinary Sciences, University Centre Annunziata, Messina, Italy

Maria Grazia Pennisi
Dip.to of Veterinary Sciences, University Centre Annunziata, Messina, Italy

Marco Caldin
Veterinary Laboratory San Marco, Padova, Italy

Tommaso Furlanello
Veterinary Laboratory San Marco, Padova, Italy

Michele Trotta
Veterinary Laboratory San Marco, Padova, Italy

Miriam Wächter
Comparative Tropical Medicine and Parasitology, Ludwig-Maximilians-University Munich, Leopoldstrasse 5, 80802 Munich, Germany

Silke Wölfel
Department of Virology and Rickettsiology, Bundeswehr Institute of Microbiology, Neuherbergstrasse 11, 80937 Munich, Germany
DZIF German Centre for Infection Research–Ludwig-Maximilians-University Munich, Geschwister-Scholl-Platz 1, 80539 Munich, Germany

Martin Pfeffer
Institute of Animal Hygiene and Veterinary Public Health, University of Leipzig, An den Tierkliniken 1, 04103 Leipzig, Germany

Gerhard Dobler
Department of Virology and Rickettsiology, Bundeswehr Institute of Microbiology, Neuherbergstrasse 11, 80937 Munich, Germany
DZIF German Centre for Infection Research–Ludwig-Maximilians-University Munich, Geschwister-Scholl-Platz 1, 80539 Munich, Germany

Barbara Kohn
Small Animal Clinic, Faculty of Veterinary Medicine, Freie Universität Berlin, Oertzenweg 19b, 14163 Berlin, Germany

Andreas Moritz
Department of Veterinary Clinical Sciences, Clinical Pathology and Clinical Pathophysiology, Justus-Liebig-University, Frankfurterstrasse 126, 35392 Gießen, Germany

Stefan Pachnicke
Bayer Vital GmbH, 51368 Leverkusen, Germany

Cornelia Silaghi
Current affiliation: National Centre for Vector Entomology, Institute of Parasitology, University of Zurich, Winterthurerstrasse 266a, 8057 Zurich, Switzerland
Comparative Tropical Medicine and Parasitology, Ludwig-Maximilians-University Munich, Leopoldstrasse 5, 80802 Munich, Germany

Ferran Segura
Department of Infectious Diseases, Corporació Sanitària Parc Taulí - Institut Universitari Parc Taulí – Universitat Autonoma de Barcelona, Sabadell, Spain
Department of Medicine, Universitat Autonoma de Barcelona, Bellaterra, Spain

Immaculada Pons
Department of Infectious Diseases, Corporació Sanitària Parc Taulí - Institut Universitari Parc Taulí – Universitat Autonoma de Barcelona, Sabadell, Spain

Jaime Miret
Animal Shelter Company (Vallès Oriental), Granollers, Spain

Júlia Pla
Veterinary Clinic "Centre", Sabadell, Spain

Anna Ortuño
Department of Animal Health, Universitat Autonoma de Barcelona, Bellaterra, Spain

María-Mercedes Nogueras
Department of Infectious Diseases, Corporació Sanitària Parc Taulí - Institut Universitari Parc Taulí – Universitat Autonoma de Barcelona, Sabadell, Spain

Oleg Mediannikov
URMITE, UMR IRD 198/CNRS 6236, Medical Faculty, Mediterranean University, Marseille, France and Dakar, Senegal

Georges Diatta
URMITE, UMR IRD 198/CNRS 6236, Medical Faculty, Mediterranean University, Marseille, France and Dakar, Senegal

Florence Fenollar
URMITE, UMR IRD 198/CNRS 6236, Medical Faculty, Mediterranean University, Marseille, France and Dakar, Senegal

Cheikh Sokhna
URMITE, UMR IRD 198/CNRS 6236, Medical Faculty, Mediterranean University, Marseille, France and Dakar, Senegal

Jean-Franc¸ois Trape
URMITE, UMR IRD 198/CNRS 6236, Medical Faculty, Mediterranean University, Marseille, France and Dakar, Senegal

Didier Raoult
URMITE, UMR IRD 198/CNRS 6236, Medical Faculty, Mediterranean University, Marseille, France and Dakar, Senegal

Ángel Sainz
Department of Animal Medicine and Surgery, Veterinary Clinic Hospital, Faculty of Veterinary Medicine, Universidad Complutense de Madrid, Madrid Spain

Xavier Roura
Hospital Clinic Veterinari, Universitat Autònoma de Barcelona, Barcelona, Spain

Guadalupe Miró
Department of Animal Health, Veterinary Clinic Hospital, Faculty of Veterinary Medicine, Universidad Complutense de Madrid, Madrid, Spain

Agustín Estrada-Peña
Department of Animal Pathology, Faculty of Veterinary Medicine, University of Zaragoza, Zaragoza, Spain

Barbara Kohn
Small Animal Clinic, Faculty of Veterinary Medicine, Freie Universität Berlin, Berlin, Germany

Shimon Harrus
Koret School of Veterinary Medicine, The Hebrew University of Jerusalem, Rehovot, Israel

Laia Solano-Gallego
Department of Animal Medicine and Surgery, Faculty of Veterinary Medicine, Autonomous University of Barcelona, Bellaterra,

Spain

Viktor Dyachenko
Institute for Infectious Diseases and Zoonoses, Department for Veterinary Sciences, Faculty for Veterinary Medicine, LMU Munich, Veterinärstraße 13, 80539 Munich, Germany

Nikola Pantchev
IDEXX Vet Med Lab, Moerikestraße. 28/3, 71636 Ludwigsburg, Germany

Hans-Joerg Balzer
IDEXX Vet Med Lab, Moerikestraße. 28/3, 71636 Ludwigsburg, Germany

Ariane Meyersen
Small Animal Clinic, Hörder Bahnhofstraße 5, 44263 Dortmund-Hörde, Germany

Reinhard K Straubinger
Institute for Infectious Diseases and Zoonoses, Department for Veterinary Sciences, Faculty for Veterinary Medicine, LMU Munich, Veterinärstraße 13, 80539 Munich, Germany

Manuela Oliveira
CIESA / Faculty of Veterinary Medicine, University of Lisbon, Technical University Avenue, 1300-477 Lisbon, Portugal

Cynthia Barroco
CIESA / Faculty of Veterinary Medicine, University of Lisbon, Technical University Avenue, 1300-477 Lisbon, Portugal

Carla Mottola
CIESA / Faculty of Veterinary Medicine, University of Lisbon, Technical University Avenue, 1300-477 Lisbon, Portugal

Raquel Santos
CIESA / Faculty of Veterinary Medicine, University of Lisbon, Technical University Avenue, 1300-477 Lisbon, Portugal

Abdelhak Lemsaddek
BioFIG, Centre for Biodiversity Genomics Integrative and Functional, Faculty of Science, University of Lisbon, 1749-016 Lisbon, Portugal

Luis Tavares
CIESA / Faculty of Veterinary Medicine, University of Lisbon, Technical University Avenue, 1300-477 Lisbon, Portugal

Teresa Semedo-Lemsaddek
CIESA / Faculty of Veterinary Medicine, University of Lisbon, Technical University Avenue, 1300-477 Lisbon, Portugal

Anja Berger
National Consiliary Laboratory for Diphtheria, Oberschleißheim, Germany
Bavarian Health and Food Safety Authority, Oberschleißheim

Ingrid Huber
Bavarian Health and Food Safety Authority, Oberschleißheim

Sophie-Susann Merbecks
Public Health Laboratory of Saxony, Germany

Ingrid Ehrhard
Public Health Laboratory of Saxony, Germany

Regina Konrad
National Consiliary Laboratory for Diphtheria, Oberschleißheim, Germany
Bavarian Health and Food Safety Authority, Oberschleißheim

Stefan Hörmansdorfer
Bavarian Health and Food Safety Authority, Oberschleißheim

Michael Hogardt
National Consiliary Laboratory for Diphtheria, Oberschleißheim, Germany
Bavarian Health and Food Safety Authority, Oberschleißheim

Andreas Sing
National Consiliary Laboratory for Diphtheria, Oberschleißheim, Germany
Bavarian Health and Food Safety Authority, Oberschleißheim

Geraldine Boseret
Epidemiology and Risk Analysis Applied to Veterinary Sciences (UREAR-ULg), Department of Infectious and Parasitic Diseases, Faculty of Veterinary Medicine, University of Liège, 4000 Liège, Belgium

Bertrand Losson
Parasitology, Department of Infectious and Parasitic Diseases, Faculty of Veterinary Medicine, University of Liège, 4000 Liège, Belgium

Jacques G Mainil
Bacteriology and Pathology of Bacterial Diseases, Department of Infectious and Parasitic Diseases, Faculty of Veterinary Medicine, University of Liège, 4000 Liège, Belgium

Etienne Thiry
Veterinary Virology and Animal Viral Diseases, Department of Infectious and Parasitic Diseases, Faculty of Veterinary Medicine, University of Liège, 4000 Liège, Belgium

Claude Saegerman
Epidemiology and Risk Analysis Applied to Veterinary Sciences (UREAR-ULg), Department of Infectious and Parasitic Diseases, Faculty of Veterinary Medicine, University of Liège, 4000 Liège, Belgium

Michael J Day
School of Veterinary Sciences, University of Bristol, Langford BS40 5DU, UK

Preface

Micro-organisms and their activities are vitally important to virtually all processes on Earth. Micro-organisms matter because they affect every aspect of our lives – they are in us, on us and around us. Microbiology is the study of all living organisms that are too small to be visible with the naked eye. This includes bacteria, archaea, viruses, fungi, prions, protozoa and algae, collectively known as 'microbes'. These microbes play key roles in nutrient cycling, biodegradation/biodeterioration, climate change, food spoilage, the cause and control of disease, and biotechnology. Microbes influence all living things and contribute to all manner of chemical and physical processes. Because these activities are so diverse, the science of microbiology is multidisciplinary, calling on the skills and knowledge of individuals specializing in many different fields of life science, environmental science, and engineering. Microbiology arose, and continues to profit from, several previously independent scientific and medical disciplines, including bacteriology, virology, public health science, clinical microbiology, immunology, parasitology, vaccinology, and a host of other areas of inquiry. The field of Veterinary Microbiology comprises the study of four big areas, bacteria, virus, fungi and parasites. Veterinary Microbiology is concerned with microbial (bacterial, fungal, viral) diseases of domesticated vertebrate animals (livestock, companion animals, fur-bearing animals, game, poultry, fish) that supply food, other useful products or companionship. This book will only concentrate on bacteria. An Introduction about reservoirs, and bacterial pathogenesis is given in Section 1. Intracellular bacteria (Chlamydia and Mycoplasma) that can cause different diseases depending on species and host are discussed in Sections 2 and 3. The next Section (Section 4) is dedicated to Staphylococcus aureus that cause Respiratory disease. Listeria monocytogenes, a Foodborne bacteria, is discussed in Section 5. Sections 6 to 11 are about different agents of disease (Tularemia, Tuberculosis, Botulism, Abortion and Q fever, respectively). The next 3 Sections (Sections 12 to 14) concentrate on tick-borne bacteria (Borrelia, Rickttesia, Anaplasma and Ehrlichia). Section 15 discusses Corynebacterium an emerging bacteria. Most of this bacteria are zoonotic, they can infect both humans and animals, Section 16 focuses on the study of zoonoses.

Editor

Patricia Marques, Ph.D.

INTRODUCTION

Microbiology is the study of living organisms of microscopic size. The term 'Microbiology' was introduced by French chemist Louis Pasteur (1822-95). Sedilot first used the term Microbe in 1878. Microorganisms include bacteria, viruses, fungi and protozoa. Microbes were probably the first living things to appear on the earth and the study of fossil remains indicates that microbial infections and epidemic diseases existed thousands of years ago.

Egyptian writing between 2000 B.C. and 1500 B.C. dates the earliest records and refer to descriptions of diseases such as anthrax, tuberculosis, sheep pox and rabies and the attempts to control the deadly and serious infectious diseases at that time. Greek and Roman empires recognized the economic impact of animal health in relation to food and human welfare, introduced regulations to control the diseases and initiated the study of diseases.

However, the evident of real study of microbes and their host pathogen interaction has to await the development of microscopes, staining methods, cultivation of microbes in pure culture, cell culture, identification of microbes, development of modern era molecular diagnostics and effective vaccines.

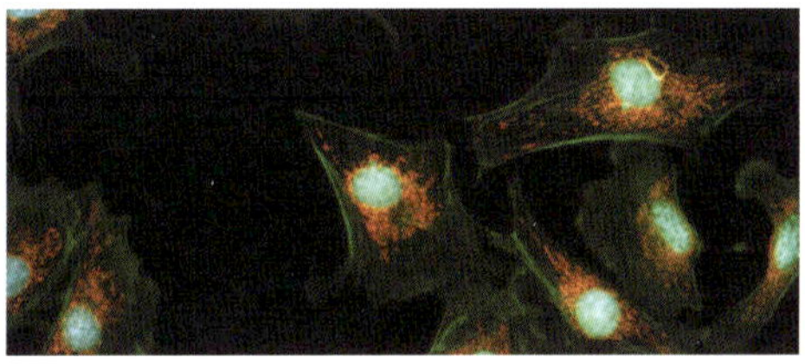

Brief about Microbiology

Microbiology is the study of microscopic organisms, those being unicellular (single cell), multicellular (cell colony), or acellular (lacking cells). Microbiology encompasses numerous sub-disciplines including virology, mycology, parasitology, and bacteriology.

Eukaryotic micro-organisms possess membrane-bound cell organelles and include fungi and protists, whereas prokaryotic organisms—all of which are microorganisms—are conventionally classified as lacking membrane-bound organelles and include eubacteria and archaebacteria. Microbiologists traditionally relied on culture, staining, and microscopy. However, less than 1% of the microorganisms present in common environments can be cultured in isolation using current means. Microbiologists often rely on extraction or detection of nucleic acid, either DNA or RNA sequences.

Viruses have been variably classified as organisms, as they have been considered either as very simple microorganisms or very complex molecules. Prions, never considered microorganisms, have been investigated by virologists, however, as the clinical effects traced to them were originally presumed due to chronic viral infections, and virologists took search—discovering "infectious proteins".

As an application of microbiology, medical microbiology is often introduced with medical principles of immunology as microbiology and immunology. Otherwise, microbiology, virology, and immunology as basic sciences have greatly exceeded the medical variants, applied sciences

Branches

The branches of microbiology can be classified into pure and applied sciences. Microbiology can be also classified based on taxonomy, in the cases of bacteriology, mycology, protozoology, and phycology. There is considerable overlap between the specific branches of microbiology with each other and with other disciplines, and certain aspects of these branches can extend beyond the traditional scope of microbiology.

Types

The field of microbiology can be generally divided into several subdisciplines:

Microbial physiology: The study of how the microbial cell functions biochemically. Includes the study of microbial growth, microbial metabolism and microbial cell structure.

Microbial genetics: The study of how genes are organized and regulated in microbes in relation to their cellular functions. Closely related to the field of molecular biology.

Medical microbiology: The study of the pathogenic microbes and the role of microbes in human illness. Includes the study of microbial pathogenesis and epidemiology and is related to the study of disease pathology and immunology.

Veterinary microbiology: The study of the role in microbes in veterinary medicine or animal taxonomy.

Environmental microbiology: The study of the function and diversity of microbes in their natural environments. Includes the study of microbial ecology, microbially-mediated nutrient cycling, geomicrobiology, microbial diversity and bioremediation. Characterisation of key bacterial habitats such as the rhizosphere and phyllosphere, soil and groundwater ecosystems, open oceans or extreme environments (extremophiles).

Evolutionary microbiology: The study of the evolution of microbes. Includes the study of bacterial systematics and taxonomy.

Industrial microbiology: The exploitation of microbes for use in industrial processes. Examples include industrial fermentation and wastewater treatment. Closely linked to the biotechnology industry. This field also includes brewing, an important application of microbiology.

Aeromicrobiology: The study of airborne microorganisms.

Food microbiology: The study of microorganisms causing food spoilage and foodborne illness. Using microorganisms to produce foods, for example by fermentation.

Pharmaceutical microbiology: the study of microorganisms causing pharmaceutical contamination and spoilage.

Oral microbiology: the study of microorganisms of the mouth in particular those causing caries and periodontal disease.

Benefits

While some fear microbes due to the association of some microbes with various human illnesses, many microbes are also responsible for numerous beneficial processes such as industrial fermentation (e.g. the production of alcohol, vinegar and dairy products), antibiotic production and as vehicles for cloning in more complex organisms such as plants. Scientists have also exploited their knowledge of microbes to produce biotechnologically important enzymes such as Taq polymerase, reporter genes for use in other genetic systems and novel molecular biology techniques such as the yeast two-hybrid system.

Bacteria can be used for the industrial production of amino acids. Corynebacterium glutamicum is one of the most important bacterial species with an annual production of more than two million tons of amino acids, mainly L-glutamate and L-lysine. Since some bacteria have the ability to synthesize antibiotics, they are used for medicinal purposes, such as Streptomyces to make aminoglycoside antibiotics.

A variety of biopolymers, such as polysaccharides, polyesters, and polyamides, are produced by microorganisms. Microorganisms are used for the biotechnological production of biopolymers with tailored properties suitable for high-value medical application such as tissue engineering and drug delivery. Microorganisms are used for the biosynthesis of xanthan, alginate, cellulose, cyanophycin, poly (gamma-glutamic acid), levan, hyaluronic acid, organic acids, oligosaccharides and polysaccharide, and polyhydroxyalkanoates.

Microorganisms are beneficial for microbial biodegradation or bioremediation of domestic, agricultural and industrial wastes and subsurface pollution in soils, sediments and marine environments. The ability of each microorganism to degrade toxic waste depends on the nature of each contaminant. Since sites typically have multiple pollutant types, the most effective approach to microbial biodegradation is to use a mixture of bacterial and fungal species and strains, each specific to the biodegradation of one or more types of contaminants.

Symbiotic microbial communities are known to confer various benefits to their human and animal hosts health including aiding digestion, production of beneficial vitamins and amino acids, and suppression of pathogenic microbes. Some benefit may be conferred by consuming fermented foods, probiotics (bacteria potentially beneficial to the digestive system) and/or prebiotics (substances consumed to promote the growth of probiotic microorganisms). The ways the microbiome influences human and animal health, as well as methods to influence the microbiome are active areas of research.

Research has suggested that microorganisms could be useful in the treatment of cancer. Various strains of non-pathogenic clostridia can infiltrate and replicate within solid tumors. Clostridial vectors can be safely administered and their potential to deliver therapeutic proteins has been demonstrated in a variety of preclinical models.

Veterinary physician

A veterinary physician, colloquially called a vet, shortened from veterinarian (American English, Australian English) or veterinary surgeon (British English), is a professional who practices veterinary medicine by treating disease, disorder, and injury in animals.

In many countries, the local nomenclature for a veterinarian is a regulated and protected term, meaning that members of the public without the prerequisite qualifications and/or licensure are not able to use the title. In many cases, the activities that may be undertaken by a veterinarian (such as treatment of illness or surgery in animals) are restricted only to those professionals who are registered as a veterinarian. For instance, in the United Kingdom, as in other jurisdictions, animal treatment may only be performed by registered veterinary physicians (with a few designated exceptions, such as paraveterinary workers), and it is illegal for any person who is not registered to call themselves a veterinarian or prescribe any treatment.

Most veterinary physicians work in clinical settings, treating animals directly. These veterinarians may be involved in a general practice, treating animals of all types; they may be specialized in a specific group of animals such as companion animals, livestock, zoo animals or equines; or may specialize in a narrow medical discipline such as surgery, dermatology or internal medicine. As with other healthcare professionals, veterinarians face ethical decisions about the care of their patients. Current debates within the profession include the ethics of certain procedures believed to be purely cosmetic or unnecessary for behavioral issues, such as declawing of cats, docking of tails, cropping of ears and debarking on dogs.

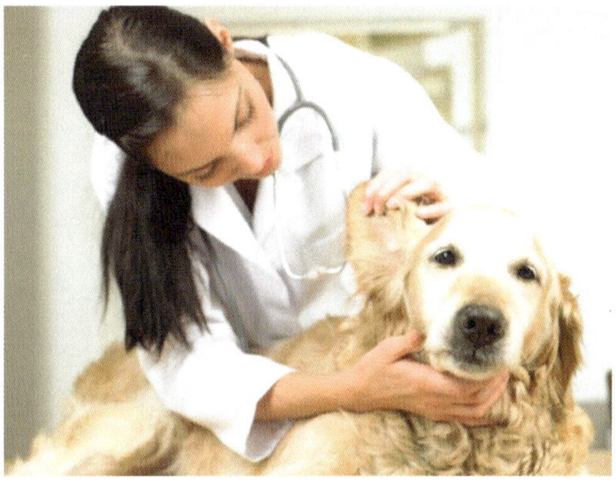

Veterinary medicine

Veterinary medicine is the branch of medicine that deals with the prevention, diagnosis and treatment of disease, disorder and injury in non-human animals. The scope of veterinary medicine is wide, covering all animal species, both domesticated and wild, with a wide range of conditions which can affect different species.

Veterinary medicine is widely practiced, both with and without professional supervision. Professional care is most often led by a veterinary physician (also known as a vet, veterinary surgeon or veterinarian), but also by paraveterinary workers such as veterinary nurses or technicians. This can be augmented by other paraprofessionals with specific specialisms such as animal physiotherapy or dentistry, and species relevant roles such as farriers.

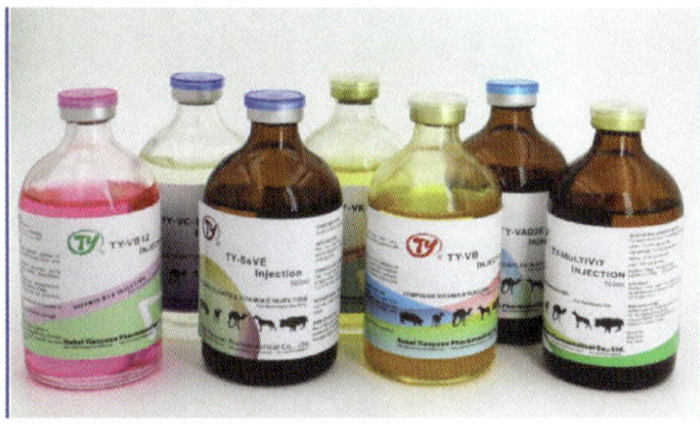

Veterinary science helps human health through the monitoring and control of zoonotic disease (infectious disease transmitted from non-human animals to humans), food safety, and indirectly through human applications from basic medical research. They also help to maintain food supply through livestock health monitoring and treatment, and mental health by keeping pet's healthy and long living. Veterinary scientists often collaborate with epidemiologists, and other health or natural scientists depending on type of work. Ethically, veterinarians are usually obliged to look after animal welfare.

Animal Microbiology

Microbiology is often incorrectly classed as the study of germs or of bacteria. While some microbiologists may specifically study viruses, also called virology, or bacteria, also called bacteriology, microbiology encompasses the whole of studying microscopic organisms. This includes the study of bacteria, protozoa, fungi, some types of algae, and often viruses.

The origins of this field can be traced to scientists positing that small unseeable things might affect other organisms. Anton van Leeuwenhoek was able to observe tiny bacteria in a primitive microscope in the 17th century. Many cite microbiology of medical origin as having been founded by Louis Pasteur and Robert Koch in the mid to late 19th century.

Later discoveries in the 20th century, like the discovery of viruses, proved of immense importance to medicine. Most medical professionals today credit this field with some of the most important work related to human illness that has ever been conducted.

Medical microbiology is only one facet of the field. Other subsections of study include applications of the science to physiology, genetics, environmental studies, evolutionary biology, and pharmaceutical studies.

In each case, microbes are studied and knowledge about them contributes to these other disciplines. For example, understanding the basic make-up of microbes and how they develop and die is part of physiological microbiology. As well, evaluation of how microbes interact with each other in a complex environment enhances our understanding of our environment.

Microbiology in simple applications can also help people understand some of the basic functions of baking ingredients. For example, studies into the behavior of yeast allows people to understand how to effectively use yeast to bake bread. It also helps to explain why a loaf may fall flat.

Scientists in microbiology see the world as composed of almost uncountable numbers of tiny unseen parts that influence us in many ways. The field is constantly uncovering more that may be of benefit to all humans interacting with their environment.

Microbiology is only getting started as a science. Scientists estimate that about 99% of the microbes existing on earth have not yet been studied. This suggests that greater application of this science may further help us understand some of the mysteries of life that still daunt us.

Diagnostic Microbiology

Diagnostic microbiology is a specialty in the sciences which focuses on applying microbiology to medical diagnosis. Like other microbiologists, diagnostic microbiologists tend to work in a lab environment which allows them access to a variety of equipment which they can use to identify and study the organisms they encounter. People in this field can work in labs which handle diagnostic testing for hospitals and clinics, and they can also work in research and development, helping to develop new diagnostic techniques and treatments for microbial infection.

Microbes such as bacteria, protozoans, and fungi play a role in many disease processes. When a patient presents with a condition which is caused by an infection, the doctor usually wants to determine which organism is responsible so that the best treatment can be selected. A diagnostic microbiologist takes a sample collected from the patient and cultures it to see what grows, returning results to the doctor.

In addition to being involved in the identification of a disease-causing organism, diagnostic microbiology can also be a part of developing a treatment plan. Many microbes have developed resistance to medications, for example, so a microbiologist might be asked to test various medications with the cultured organism to find the most effective treatment. A clinical microbiologist can also be asked to look for signs of multiple infectious organisms, or to provide insight into the pathology of the infection.

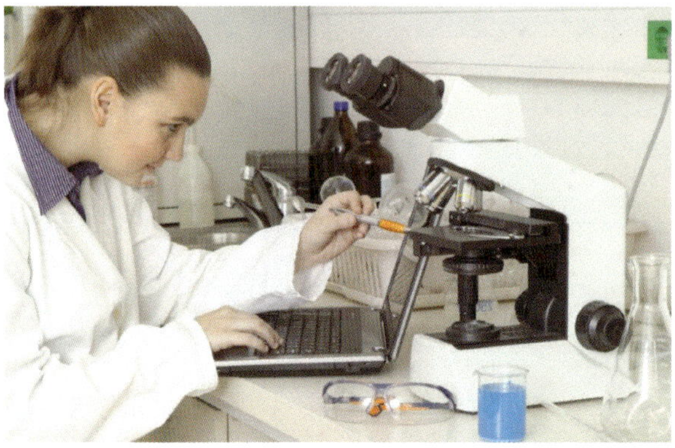

Diagnostic microbiology can also be applied to epidemiology. Clinical microbiologists are usually involved in the early stages of tracking and studying epidemics, to identify the organisms involved, find connections between them, and help to develop an approach to stop the epidemic and treat people who have been infected. Their skills are also put to use to determine who belongs in the epidemic and who does not, using their diagnostic skills to trace infections as they spread and to distinguish between people with ordinary infections and people caught up in an infectious epidemic.

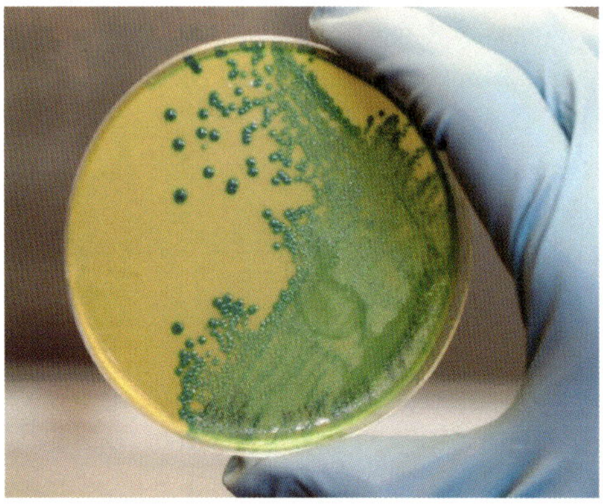

Scope of Veterinary Microbiology

Veterinary microbiology is concerned with the etiology (causation), pathogenesis (Mechanism of attack on tissues), laboratory diagnosis and treatment of infection in the individual and with the epizootology (study of mass disease among the animals) and prevention and control of infection in the community. Hence, it has close links with other veterinary disciplines such as pathology, medicine, surgery, pharmacology and preventive medicine.

Microbiology has a close link with curative medicine in regard to the precise diagnosis and the rational treatment of infectious diseases. If a clinician is unable to identify/anticipate the organism in the absence of typical clinical symptoms then it becomes all the more necessary to go in for microbiological investigations. Due to the common symptoms irrespective of pathogens, the veterinarian needs the casting vote of microbiologist.

Role of microbiology is unparallel in the suggestion of exact/suitable drug by performing drug sensitivity test. In other words, vets have to identify and treat specific infections rather than clinical syndromes.

Knowledge of veterinary microbiology is essential for the development of rapid, sensitive diagnostics and suitable, effective vaccines for diseases of livestock.

Theories of Disease causation

Ancient man had thought the infectious diseases to be cause of divine wrath and supernatural powers. From merely times, there have been many suggestions/ theories put forth for the cause of disease.

1. Theurgical theory of disease

Disease was due to wrath of divine spirits for punishment of individual sins.

2. Miasmatic theory

Disease was due to emanations from the earth, influence of stars, the moon and the wind, the water and seasons (4 elements).

3. Bible

Jews required leprous people to be segregated indicates that they were aware of the fact ' that disease spread by contact', but the cause always was considered to be supernatural. Infected were required to shield their faces with their hand.

4. Hippocrates

Related the disease to different water, direction of wind, and slope of land. Didn't think that disease caused by transmissible agents.

5. Pore theory

- Asclepiades (124 B.C.), Themison and Thessalus.
- According to this, symmetry or proportion of pores resulted in health and disease.
- Pores should be changed in afflicted parts to assure recovery from diseases.

6. Galen (120-200 A.D.)

Excess or defraction of 4 elements resulted in disease.

7. Boccaccio (1313-75)

Infectious nature of disease.Transmission of plague-Two hogs dragged off a poor man died of plague . Rooted and tossed of their jaws and fell down taking as poison

8. Fracastorius (1478-1553)

Advanced concept of contagium vivum as the possible cause of disease (infectious). Earliest doctrine of infection (Closest to truth). Was based on observations on epidemics of plague, syphilis, typhus of man and FMD in Italy.

- Contagion (The direct cause, such as a bacterium or virus, of a communicable disease) was attributed to:
- Contagion by contact
- Contagion by fomite
- Contagion by distance

- Contagion by seminaria (seeds of disease)

9. Athanasius Kircher (1602-80)

Reported minute 'WORMS' in the blood of plague patient, but the equipment available to him it is more likely to that what he observed were only blood cells. Credit of using microscope of magnification 32 power.

10. Von Plenciz (1762)

Each disease caused by separate agent.

11. Spontaneous Generation Theory

Aristotle (384-322 B.C.) proposed that some of the simple invertebrates could arise by spontaneous generation. In 1748, the English Priest, John Needham conducted the experiment by boiling mutton broth and then tightly stoppered the flasks. On incubation, could found growth of microorganism in the flasks. Proposed that organic matter contained a vital force that confers the properties of life on non-living matter. Few years later, Lazzaro Spallanzani (1729-1799)improved the experiment of John Needham and used sealed flasks containing the seed of microorganisms and water and placed the flask in a boiling water for quarter to one hour, no growth was seen as long as long as the flask remained sealed. Spallanzani proposed that external air carries the germs and required for growth of organisms already in the culture medium-modified proposal of spontaneous generation.

SECTION I: INTRODUCTION

CHAPTER 1 FREE-LIVING SPECIES OF CARNIVOROUS MAMMALS IN POLAND: RED FOX, BEECH MARTEN, AND RACCOON AS A POTENTIAL RESERVOIR OF SALMONELLA, YERSINIA, LISTERIA SPP. AND COAGULASE-POSITIVE STAPHYLOCOCCUS

Aneta Nowakiewicz, Przemysław Zięba, Grażyna Ziółkowska, Sebastian Gnat, Marta Muszyńska, Krzysztof Tomczuk, Barbara Majer Dziedzic, Łukasz Ulbrych, Aleksandra Trościańczyk

INTRODUCTION

Free-living animals have always been a significant source of infectious diseases transmitted to humans. Zoonoses whose reservoir is this group of animals are currently a serious problem [1], particularly as an increasing number of pathogens appear to be of animal origin. Free-living carnivorous animals are a permanent biocoenotic element that is highly diverse in terms of adaptation to the environment; in general, they have outstanding migratory potential associated with an active search for food. These predators not only live in environments without people, but also appear in areas populated by humans, particularly in the winter or spring when there is considerably less available food [2]. Species such as the red fox, beech marten, or raccoon constitute a relatively large percentage of the population of free-living carnivorous animals in Poland. The red fox *Vulpes vulpes* (Linnaeus, 1758) is a common species all over Europe and its population in Poland is estimated at 200,000–250,000 individuals [3]. Its high level of synanthropization, manifested as gradual colonization of suburban and urban areas, may significantly increase the possibility of contact with humans and thus the probability of transfer of pathogenic agents onto both humans and other domesticated animals [4,5]. The beech marten *Martes foina* (Erxleben, 1777) inhabits most regions of Europe and is found all over Poland, where its population is difficult to estimate, but it is probably approx. 100,000. The species is closely associated with environments populated by humans [6]. Both the red fox and the beech marten are common in Europe. In Poland, they have a status of game species with a closed period [6]. The raccoon *Procyon lotor* (Linnaeus, 1758) is the most recently recorded alien species in Poland. It originally lived in North America. In 1934, raccoons were introduced in Germany and the first record of the presence of the raccoon in Poland dates back to 1970. Since then, the raccoon population has grown fairly rapidly, particularly in northern and western Poland. Raccoons are now a permanent component of both the natural environment [7] and urban areas (large and smaller cities) in this part of the country [8], but research conducted in 2005–2009 also showed isolated cases of the presence of individuals of this species in other regions of Poland. The most serious problem is their invasion into protected natural areas, which is one of the reasons why raccoons are game animals that can be hunted year round with no closed season.

A characteristic trait of these species of free-living animals is a broad-spectrum diet, including all vertebrates, numerous invertebrates, and carrion. Carnivorous animals at

Citation: Nowakiewicz A, Zięba P, Ziółkowska G, Gnat S, Muszyńska M, Tomczuk K, et al. (2016) Free-Living Species of Carnivorous Mammals in Poland: Red Fox, Beech Marten, and Raccoon as a Potential Reservoir of Salmonella, Yersinia, Listeria spp. and Coagulase-Positive Staphylococcus. PLoS ONE 11(5): e0155533. doi:10.1371/journal.pone.0155533.

the top of the food chain can therefore become carriers of a broad spectrum of microbes that are potentially pathogenic for humans. The clear tendency towards synanthropization in these species suggests the possibility of direct contact with the living environment of humans, which may increase the likelihood of transmission and spread of microbes, including those posing a threat to public health [5,9]

Analysis of these species in terms of carriage of zoonotic diseases in Poland primarily focuses on detection of the rabies virus. Monitoring for this virus, particularly in foxes, which are its main reservoir in Europe [10], is legally sanctioned. The importance of these animals as a potential source of parasitoses of animal origin, such as *Echinococcus multilocularis* in foxes [1, 11] and *Baylisascaris procyonis* in raccoons [12] has also been confirmed.

Data on the occurrence and isolation of other microorganisms in wildlife animals are fragmentary and either concern single cases of isolation or occurrence in other free-living animals species, e.g. isolation of *Mycobacterium bovis* from wild boar [13], prevalence of *Salmonella* in free-living birds [14], or detection of the HEV virus in wild boar [15].

The objective of the study was to examine red fox, beech marten, and raccoon populations for the occurrence of bacteria that may be potentially pathogenic agents for humans and for other animal species and to determine their virulence potential.

MATERIAL AND METHODS

Animals used in the study and sample collection

Samples in the form of rectal swabs were collected from May 2011 to April 2015 in western Poland (52.593333, 14.748333) and in southern and south-eastern Poland (51.216667, 22.9) from the following free-living species: the red fox *Vulpes vulpes* (n = 286), beech marten *Martes foina* (n = 65), and raccoon *Procyon lotor* (n = 70). The samples were taken from foxes that were killed under a program monitoring the effectiveness of rabies vaccination [16] and from martens supplied to the laboratory due to suspected infection of rabies, according to regulations on combating infectious diseases in animals. The animals were not sacrificed solely for the sake of the sampling for the research conducted in this study. Since cases of rabies in animals are still detected in Poland, in the case of suspected symptoms of rabies, free-living animals, including foxes and martens, shall be subject to diagnostics observation by qualified veterinary staff and, in the case of death during the observation, these animals are transferred for rabies testing to an official laboratory. In addition, in the case of foxes, there is mandatory assessment of the effectiveness of the vaccination against rabies and, therefore, every year a certain number of animals must be shot by hunters and delivered to an official laboratory for appropriate tests [16]. Because the material was obtained from dead animals analyzed at the State Veterinary Laboratory on the basis of the Act on protection of animal health and combating infectious diseases in animals (Dz.U. [Journal of Laws] 2004 no. 69 item 625), no approval of the ethics commission was required.

Bacteriological examination of the samples was performed only after virological tests had been completed with negative results. Until that time, they were stored at -80°C for maximum 30 days.

Samples from the raccoons were taken from individuals captured in the environment (Warta Mouth National Park) in restraining traps and then the animals were subjected to euthanasia by qualified veterinary staff (prior pharmacological premedication) under the project LIFE+ No: LIFE09 NAT/PL/000263 entitled 'Protection of water and marsh birds in five National Parks–reconstructing habitats and curbing the influence of invasive species' [17]. As an invasive species in Poland, the raccoon may pose a threat to native species in some specific areas (e.g. national parks or nature reserves) and a specified part of the invasive animal population need to be caught and euthanized for biodiversity conservation. The material was collected in sterile conditions at the State Veterinary Laboratory immediately after the dead animals were delivered, and bacteriological analysis was performed within 24 h.

The direction of the research was chosen on the basis of the available literature on potential bacterial threats to human health in the environment [18, 19, 20].

The samples were initially incubated in 2 mL of buffered peptone water (24 h at 37°C). *Salmonella* were isolated according to the Polish standard [21]. Five typical colonies were selected from each culture for further identification. Bacterial species were confirmed using a commercial test (ENTEROtest 24N, Erba Lachema, Brno, Czech Republic) and serotyping was performed using commercial sera for O and H antigens (SIFIN, Berlin, Germany), according to the Kauffman-White classification [22].

Listeria spp. were isolated according to the Polish standard [23]. One typical colony was selected from each culture for further identification. Species identification was based on PCR-restriction fragment length polymorphism according to Paillard et al. [24]. All isolates of *L. monocytogenes* were tested by PCR for the presence of the following virulence genes: *inl*A, *inl*C, *inl*J (internalins), *iap* (protein p60), *hly*A (listeriolysin O—LLO), *plc*A (phosphatidylinositol-phospholipase C–PI-PLC), *act*A (surface protein ActA), and *prf*A (virulence regulator PrfA). PCR primers and conditions followed those described in previously established protocols [25].

The *Yersinia* spp. isolation procedure consisted in cold incubation at 5°C for 7 d in Tripticase Soy Broth (Biocorp, Warsaw, Poland) followed by inoculation on Yersinia CIN Lab Agar (Biocorp, Warsaw, Poland) at 25°C for 24 h. Colonies that were morphologically similar to *Yersinia* spp. were subcultured for biochemical examination with the commercial test ENTEROtest 24N (Erba Lachema, Brno, Czech Republic). Genotypic species identification (based on analysis of the 16S rRNA gene) and the pathogenicity of *Y. enterocolitica* strains (the presence of the *ail* gene) were determined by duplex PCR according to Wannet et al. [26].

Staphylococcus spp. were isolated according to the Polish standard [27]. One typical colony was selected from each culture for further identification. Species identification of isolates was carried out with the commercial kit STAPHYtest 24 (Erba Lachema, Brno, Czech Republic). Species identification of coagulase-positive isolates was confirmed according to Sasaki et al. [28]. In addition, tests were performed for the presence of coagulase (using rabbit coagulase plasma, Biocorp, Warsaw, Poland) and for the presence of DNAse (DNA-se test Lab Agar Biocorp, Warsaw Poland). All *S. aureus* isolates were tested by PCR for the presence of genes coding for staphylococcal enterotoxins (*sea*, *seb*, *sec*, *sed*, *see*, *seg*, *seh*, *sei*, *sej*, *sen*, *seo*, and *sem*) [29], leukocidin genes (*luk*S/F-PV and *luk*M), leukotoxin genes *luk*E/D [29], hemolysin genes (*hla*, *hlb* and *hld*) [29], and the *tst* gene encoding toxic shock syndrome toxin (TSST-1) [30].

Statistical analysis was performed in R (ver. 3.1.1; Vienna, Austria). Confidence intervals (95%) for individual groups of microorganisms and animal species and analysis of statistical significance were performed using Student's T-test. The degree of variation in the frequency of appearance of potentially pathogenic bacteria with respect to the total number of isolates in each group of animals was tested by ANOVA. Statistical comparison of the potential epidemiological threat presented by individuals of different species was tested by Tukey's HSD test. In both cases, the null and alternative hypotheses were based on average numbers of pathogenic bacteria in the analyzed groups of animal species.

RESULTS

The tests conducted on 421 animals made it possible to distinguish 328 isolates belonging to the genera *Salmonella*, *Staphylococcus*, *Listeria*, and *Yersinia* (Table 1).

Table 1: Species of bacteria isolated from free-living animals

Species/serotype of bacteria	Number of positive isolates (%)			
	Vulpes vulpes (n = 286)	*Martes foina* (n = 65)	*Procyon lotor* (n = 70)	Total (n = 421)
Salmonella enterica subsp *enterica*	**7 (2.45)**	**6 (9.2)**	**2 (2.85)**	**15 (3.56)**
serotype Typhimurium,	3 (1.04)	3 (4.6)	1 (1.42)	7 (1.66)
Saintpaul	1 (0.35)	1 (1.5)		2 (0.47)
Infantis	1 (0.35)			1 (0.24)
Mbandaka,	1 (0.35)			1 (0.24)
Newport	1 (0.35)	1 (1.5)	1 (1.42)	3 (0.71)
Enteritidis		1 (1.5)		1 (0.24)
Salmonella enterica subsp *diarizonae*	**2 (0.69)**		**1 (1.42)**	**3 (0.71)**
Salmonella enterica subsp *houtenae*			**1 (1.42)**	**1 (0.24)**
***Salmonella* spp total**	**9 (3.15)**	**6 (9.23)**	**4 (5.7)**	**19 (4.51)**
Staphylococcus aureus	28 (9.8)	8 (12.3)	4 (5.71)	40 (9.5)
Staphylococcus pseudintermedius	172 (60.1)	10 (15.38)		182 (43.23)
Staphylococcus delphini B	2 (0.69)	7 (10.76)		9 (2.13)
Staphylococcus delphini A		2 (3.07)	21 (30)	23 (5.46)
***Staphylococcus* coagulase-positive strains total**	**202 (70.62)**	**27 (41.53)**	**25 (35.71)**	**254 (60.33)**
Listeria monocytogenes	13 (4.5)	4 (6.15)	3 (4.28)	20 (4.75)
Listeria inocua	5 (1.74)			5 (1.18)
Listeria ivanovii	1 (0.35)			1 (0.24)
Listeria velshimerii	3 (1.04)		2 (2.85)	5 (1.18)
***Listeria* spp total**	**22 (7.69)**	**4 (6.15)**	**5 (7.14)**	**31 (7.36)**
Yersinia enterocolitica	6 (2.09)	2 (3.07)	2 (2.85)	10 (2.37)
Yersinia kristensenii			1 (1.42)	1 (0.24)
Yersinia frederiksenii	10 (3.49)	3 (4.61)		13 (3.08)
***Yersinia* spp total**	**16 (5.59)**	**5 (7.69)**	**3 (4.28)**	**24 (5.7)**

doi:10.1371/journal.pone.0155533.t001

http://dx.doi.org/10.1371/journal.pone.0155533.t001

The percentages of individual genera and groups of bacteria in the biota of the animals were varied and the samples isolated from each animal were positive for no more than three different bacterial species. The coagulase-positive *Staphylococcus* spp. were isolated most frequently (60.33%; CI: 27.8–35.53), while the presence of the other bacteria was detected in a smaller number of animals: *Listeria* spp. 7, 36%; (CI: 4.71–5.65), *Yersinia* spp. 5.7% (CI: 3.12–5.58), and *Salmonella* spp. 4.51% (CI: 1.31–6.2) (Table 1).

Of the total pool of 328 isolates, 90 isolates (21.34%) belonging to taxa posing the greatest potential threat to human health (considered mainly as foodborne pathogens) were selected for further analysis, including statistical analysis. This group included the following isolates: *Salmonella* spp. (n = 19), *Listeria monocytogenes* and *L. ivanovii* (n = 21), *Yersinia enterocolitica* (n = 10), and *Staphylococcus aureus* (n = 40). Irrespective of the animal species, *S. aureus* was isolated most frequently, accounting for 44.4% (CI: 42.23–46.57); *Listeria monocytogenes* and *L. ivanovii* (23.3%; CI: 22.83–23.77) and *Salmonella* spp. (21.11%; CI: 17.86–24.36) were isolated less frequently. *Y. enterocolitica* was the least frequent from the selected species of bacteria, accounting for 11.1% (CI: 10.71–11.5) of potentially pathogenic isolates. In general, one potentially pathogenic species was isolated from a single individual, except for 10 animals (6 foxes, 3 martens, and 1 raccoon), which were carriers of two different potentially pathogenic bacterial species at the same time. In most cases, the presence of *S. aureus* (80%; 8/10) was accompanied by *Salmonella* spp. (40%; 4/10), *L. monocytogenes* (10%; 1/10), or *Y. enterocolitica* (10%; 1/10). In one case, *L. monocytogenes* and *Y. enterococlitica* were isolated from a single individual (a fox) and, in another case, two different subspecies of *Salmonella* (*S.* subsp. *enterica* and *S.* subsp. *houtenae*) were isolated from a raccoon (Table 2).

Table 2: Distribution of potentially pathogenic bacteria in the free-living animal species studied

Potentially pathogenic species/serotype	Host species		
	Vulpes vulpes (n = 286)	*Martes foina* (n = 65)	*Procyon lotor* (n = 70)
S. enterica subsp *enterica* serotype Typhimurium + *S. aureus*	1	1	
Salmonella enterica subsp. *enterica* serotype Saintpaul + *S. aureus*		1	
S. enterica subsp. *diarizonae* + *S. aureus*	1		
L. monocytogenes + *S. aureus*	2		
L. monocytogenes + *Y. enterocolitica*	1		
Y. enterocolitica + *S. aureus*	1	1	
S. enterica subsp. *enterica* serotype Typhimurium + *S. enterica* subsp *houtenae*			1
Total mixed	6	3	1
Salmonella enterica subsp *enterica*			
serotype Typhimurium,	2	2	
Saintpaul	1		
Infantis	1		
Mbandaka,	1		
Newport	1	1	1
Enteritidis	1		
Salmonella enterica spp *diarizonae*	1	1	
Staphylococcus aureus	23	5	4
Listeria monocytogenes	10	4	3
Listeria ivanovii	1		
Yersinia enterocolitica	4	1	2
Total	51 (12,11)	18 (4,27)	12 (2,85)

doi:10.1371/journal.pone.0155533.t002

http://dx.doi.org/10.1371/journal.pone.0155533.t002

Taking into account the differences in the sizes of the samples from the different animal species (Student's T-test; $p < 0.05$), we showed that on average for the entire group of animals (n = 421) the percentage of carriage of potentially pathogenic bacteria was 6.33%. The percentage of animals in which the presence of potentially pathogenic isolates was noted varied in the different groups; the highest percentage of individuals was noted in the group of foxes (n = 51; 12.11%; CI: 10.17–14.06), but it was much lower, i.e. 4.27% (CI: 2.93–5.15) and 2.85% (CI: 2.08–3.62), in the martens (n = 18) and raccoons (n = 12) (Table 2).

In the next stage of the study, the potential virulence of the isolates tested (*L. monocytogenes*, *S. aureus* and *Y. enterocolitica*) was analyzed on the basis of selected genes characteristic for a given bacterial species. The profiles of the virulence genes tested within the individual bacterial species were highly heterogeneous; 8 different profiles were found in the case of *L. monocytogenes* and 20 for *S. aureus* (Tables 3 and 4).

Table 3: Virulence profiles of *L. monocytogenes* **is**olated from free-living animals

Number of *L. monocytogenes* isolates (n)%	Species host (n = 20)	Internalin genes	other genes detected
(7) 35	Fox(5),Marten (2)	*inlA, inlC, inlJ*	*hlyA, iap, plcA, prfA, actA*
(1)5	Fox(1)	*inlA, inlC, inlJ*	*hlyA, iap, plcA, prfA*
(2)10	Fox(2)	*inlA, inlC, inlJ*	*hlyA, iap, plcA, prfA*
(3) 15	Fox(1), Marten (1),Raccoon (1)	*inlA, inlC, inlJ*	*hlyA, iap, actA*
(2)10	Fox (1), Raccoon (1)	*inlA, inlC, inlJ*	*hlyA, iap, prfA*
(1)5	Fox (1)	*inlA, inlC, inlJ*	*hlyA, iap*
(1)5	Fox (1)	*inlA, inlC*	*hlyA, iap, plcA, prfA, actA*
(3) 15	Fox (1),Marten (1)Raccoon (1)	*inlA, inlC*	*hlyA, iap, prfA, actA*

doi:10.1371/journal.pone.0155533.t003

http://dx.doi.org/10.1371/journal.pone.0155533.t003

Table 4: Virulence profiles of *S. aureus* **is**olated from free-living animals

Number of *S. aureus* isolates (n) %	Species host (n = 40)	Enterotoxins genes detected	other toxins genes detected
(7)17.5	Fox(6),Marten (1)	*see, sei*	*hla, hld,hlb,luk*ED
(2) 5	Marten (1), Raccoon (1)	*see, sei*	*hla, hld, luk*ED
(1) 2.5	Marten (1)	[*seg, sei, sem, sen, seo*]	*tst, hla, hld, luk*ED
(2) 5	Fox(2)	[*seg, sei, sem, sen, seo*]	*hla, hld, luk*ED
(4) 10	Marten (2), Fox (2)	*sea, seb, seg, sed*	*hla, hld, luk*ED
(1) 2.5	Fox (1)	[*seg, sei, sem, sen, seo*]*sec*	*hla, hld,hlb, luk*ED
(1) 2.5	Fox (1)	[*sem, sen, sei*]	*tst,hla, hld, luk*ED
(1) 2.5	Fox (1)	*sea, see, sed*	*hla, hld, luk*ED
(1) 2.5	Fox (1)	*sea, see*	*hla, hld, hlb, luk*ED
(1) 2.5	Fox (1)	*sed, sej*	*hla, hld, luk*ED
(2) 5	Fox (2)	*seh*	*hla, hld,hlb, luk*ED
(2) 5	Fox (1), Marten (1)	*seh*	*hla, hld*
(1) 2.5	Fox (1)	*sei*	*hla, hld, luk*ED
(1) 2.5	Fox (1)	*sej*	*hla, hld, luk*ED
(1) 2.5	Raccoon (1)	*see*	*hla, hld, luk*ED
(1) 2.5	Raccoon (1)	*see*	*hla, hld*
(2) 5	Fox (2)	*sec*	*hla, hld, luk*ED
(2) 5	Fox (2)		*hla, hld, luk*ED
(5) 12.5	Fox (3), Marten (2)		*hla, hld*
(2) 5	Fox (1), Raccoon (1)		

doi:10.1371/journal.pone.0155533.t004

http://dx.doi.org/10.1371/journal.pone.0155533.t004

The distribution of the particular virulence genes in the pool of 20 isolates of *L. monocytogenes*was varied, both quantitatively and qualitatively; the presence of all genes tested (*inl*A, *inl*C, *inl*J, *hly*A, *iap*, *plc*A, *prf*A and *act*A) was noted in 35% of the isolates, while the number of genes in the other isolates ranged from 5 to 7. The *inl*A, *inl*C, *hly*A and *iap* genes were present in all the tested isolates of *L. monocytogenes*, while genes *inl*J, *plc*A, *prf*A and *act*A occurred with varying frequency: 80% (CI: 78.23–81.77), 55% (CI: 53.31–59.69), 70% (CI: 68.65–71.35), and 80% (CI: 78.51–81.49), respectively. The virulence profiles of the 40 *S. aureus* isolates were determined on the basis of the presence of toxin-encoding genes (Table 4).

Most of the isolates (95%; CI: 93.41–96.59) contained hemolysin-encoding genes *hla* and *hld*, whereas gene *hlb* was noted in only 32.5% (CI: 30.27–34.73) of the isolates. The *luk*ED gene encoding bicomponent leucotoxins was detected in 70% (CI: 68.29–71.71) of *S. aureus*isolates. Two strains, from a fox and a marten, showed the presence of the gene encoding TSST-1. Genes encoding enterotoxins were detected in 77.5% (CI: 79.88–79.12) of the isolates, including five (12.5%) with *egc*-like variants (Table 4). No genes encoding leukocidins (*luk*S/F-PV and *luk*M) were observed in any of the *S. aureus* isolates.

In the case of *Y. enterocolitica*, the presence of the *ail* gene was found in 60% of isolates (Table 5); only isolates from martens were all positive for this gene.

Table 5: Number and prevalence of pathogenic *Yersinia enterocolitica* in free-living animals

Animal species (positive isolation of *Y. enterocolitica*)	positive PCR amplification results (%)	
	16S rRNA gene (330bp)	*ail* gene (425bp)
Vulpes vulpes (n = 6)	6 (100)	3 (50)
Martes foina (n = 2)	2 (100)	2 (100)
Procyon lotor (n = 2)	2 (100)	1 (50)
Total (n = 10)	10 (100)	6 (60)

doi:10.1371/journal.pone.0155533.t005

http://dx.doi.org/10.1371/journal.pone.0155533.t005

DISCUSSION

Free-living animals, particularly predatory species, are a significant link in the epidemiological chain of most zoonoses, mainly as a reservoir for transmission of zoonotic agents to humans and domestic animals [1]. In Poland, there has been little comprehensive research of this issue; more extensive research has been conducted only in a deer population [31]. Our analysis focused on evaluating the degree of carriage of potentially pathogenic bacteria of the genera *Salmonella*, *Yersinia*, and *Listeria* as well as coagulase–positive *Staphylococcus* in three most common carnivorous animal species in Poland.

Foxes, which constituted the largest group of animals in the present study, belong to species with a strong focus on synanthropization. Due to the fact that intensive vaccination against rabies used in the recent years led to a significant increase in their population, the animals began to change their habitat and move to regions populated by humans more densely (high availability of food resources). A significant percentage of the samples (40%) were taken from foxes suspected of having rabies, and the animals came mainly from urban and suburban areas, where the human population density ranged from 200 to 2000 persons/km^2. The other samples came from foxes culled as part of monitoring tests, and these animals were obtained from rural areas (with a density of 20–100 persons/km^2) and uninhabited or sparsely populated areas with a density of less than 20 persons/km^2.

In the case of the marten, all animals were from both rural and urban areas inhabited by humans (including urban green areas such as parks and gardens). This is not a surprising phenomenon, because the beech marten is closely related to the human environment, nesting in places such as farm buildings and houses. Although raccoons have been caught in the National Park, it should be emphasized that this area is directly adjacent to the urban area (e.g. Kostrzyn city). Analysis of the direct impact of this species of animals on humans should take into account the fact that raccoons, as synanthropic animals, strongly penetrate the direct human environment [32,33] and have a very high potential of migration and a very dynamic growth of the population size [34].

The presence of these animals in the human environments is not only connected with the possibility of transferring microorganisms by direct contact, both in urban and rural human populations as well as in groups of increased risk (forest guards, veterinary staff, hunters, wildlife officers), but also by indirect contamination of the environment by feces. Pathogens found in feces can contaminate water and soil, and in this way they can contaminate the food of plant origin (e.g. raw fruit and vegetables) [35]. According to the report of the European Commission of Health and Consumer Protection [36], all bacterial species examined in this study as potential foodborne pathogens can contaminate agricultural produce and have a capacity to cause outbreaks.

The considerable percentage of the positive isolations of *Salmonella* spp. (4.51%) was generally consistent with the results of studies carried out in similar animal populations in Italy, Spain, Norway, the USA, and Japan, which suggests the need for international monitoring of free-living animals in this regard. In the case of detection of *Salmonella* carriage, continual monitoring is currently only required for farm animals [37], while research on other groups of animals is fragmentary; in Poland, it has concerned mainly living birds and cold-blooded vertebrates [14, 38].

The degree of *Salmonella* spp. carriage is varied and depends in part on the host species (host-restricted, host-adapted, and ubiquitous). In the pool of the animals analyzed, the highest percentage of positive isolations was obtained in the martens (9.2%). Similar results were noted in Italy [39], whereas in Spain [40] no positive isolations of *Salmonella* were found in this species. In the case of foxes, the frequency of *Salmonella* isolation was lower than that reported by other authors (5.2% to 12.5%) [39, 40, 41], which may be linked to a certain seasonality of *Salmonella* occurrence in foxes [42] and to climatic determinants influencing the survival and distribution of these bacteria in the environment [43].

As a reservoir of *Salmonella* spp., the raccoon ranked between the two species discussed above; the percentage of positive isolates was 5.7%, which was consistent with other research [32, 44]. It is interesting that two subspecies of *Salmonella*, *S. enterica* subsp. *enterica* and *S. enterica* subsp. *houtenae*, were both present in the biota of the digestive tract of a single individual. A similar phenomenon was observed in a previous study [38], which clearly suggests the need to include more than one colony isolated from a given sample in the isolation and identification of *Salmonella*. Among the six *S. enterica* subsp. *enterica* serotypes isolated in our study, four (*S.* Typhimurium, *S.* Infantis, *S.* Newport, and *S.* Enteritidis) are included among the 10 serotypes of non-typhoidal *Salmonella*, which are most often responsible for infections in humans in Europe, including Poland [45]. In Poland, *Salmonella*Typhimurium is the second most frequently isolated serotype in cases of salmonellosis in humans [46] and carriage in farm animals [47] and free-living birds [14]; as shown in the present study, it is also the most frequently isolated serotype among *S. enterica* subsp. *enterica* in free-living carnivorous animals.

Due to the fact that *Salmonella* is a multi-host pathogen and can persist in the environment for long periods, there are only a few cases documenting a direct relationship between the wildlife source and the occurrence of salmonellosis in humans [48, 49] or livestock [5], similar to the documented cases of direct contamination of fresh produce by free-living animals [49].

However, the possibility of *Salmonella* circulation between humans and free-living animals (or livestock as an indirect link) is very complex, and in many stages both direct and indirect contact can lead to transmission of *Salmonella* [35]. Likewise, the source of contamination of the free-living animals analyzed in the present study is not exactly known. Probably, the carriage may be linked to the type of animal diet covering e.g. small rodents or free-living birds. Many authors have shown a significant role of mice, rats, hedgehogs, amphibians, reptiles, and free-living birds as a reservoir of *Salmonella* [14, 50, 51].

Another group of bacteria with considerable zoonotic potential that was isolated from carnivorous species of free-living animals was *Yersinia* spp. (5.7%). According to the European Centre for Disease Prevention and Control [37], *Y. enterocolitica* is the cause of 96.5% of cases of yersiniosis in humans, while the second pathogenic species belonging to this genus, *Y. pseudotuberculosis*, is responsible for only 1.9% of infections. The main route of infection is foodborne transmission. Infection may also occasionally result from indirect contact with infected animals, including free-living animals (e.g. via water, soil, and vegetables contaminated by such animals) [52]. Most studies on the occurrence of *Yersinia* spp. among free-living animals have concerned wild boars as a potential (analogously to the pig) reservoir of *Y. enterocolitica* [53, 54]. Other species of free-living animals have rarely been studied and these have usually been small groups of animals [55, 56]. An exception is a study by Lee et al. [32] carried out in a raccoon population, in which *Y. pseudotuberculosis* was found to be the dominant isolated species. In our study, the degree of carriage of *Yersinia* spp., irrespective of the host species (fox, marten, or raccoon), was similar, i.e. 5.7%, and 41.6% of all *Yersinia*isolates were *Y. enterocolitica*. The other species, *Y. kristensenii* and *Y. frederiksenii*, accounted for 4.2% and 54.1% of all *Yersinia* isolates. As their role in the pathogenesis of infections has not been established [52], they were not included in further analyses. Detection of the presence of the *ail* gene, responsible for attachment and invasion, in 60% of the *Y. enterocolitica* isolates confirms the potential health risk for humans and animals posed by the presence of these bacteria in the digestive tract of these carnivorous animal species. Direct contact with infected (carrier) individuals or the environment contaminated these bacteria may be an important element of the epidemiological chain, not only in the case of yersiniosis but also listeriosis [57, 58].

Among all species of *Listeria* spp., mainly *Listeria monocytogenes* and *L. ivanovii* are regarded as potentially pathogenic, with the latter species primarily associated with infections in animals [25, 59, 60]. Among all the strains of *Listeria* isolated in the present study, *L. monocytogenes*comprised the largest group (20/31), and the overall percentage of isolation was similar to results obtained by other authors in wildlife animals [61, 62]. *L. monocytogenes* is pathogenic for human population groups, but poses the greatest threat to infants, pregnant women, and elderly immunosuppressed individuals [63]. Pathogenic strains must be differentiated from non-pathogenic ones, particularly in the case of isolation from the environment. Virulence and pathogenicity factors of *L. monocytogenes* strains, such as internalin, listeriolysin O, actin, phosphatidylinositol phospholipase C, IAP proteins associated with invasiveness, and virulence regulators have been found both among strains isolated from disease cases, such as miscarriage in women [64], and in environmental strains [25]. Markers identifying strains as virulent include the presence of the gene encoding internalin lmo2821 (*inl*J), which is a marker differentiating virulent strains causing mouse mortality from non-virulent strains [65]. This gene was found in 80% of *L. monocytogenes* isolates from the animals in our study. The gene encoding phosphatidylinositol phospholipase C (PI-PLC), which has been detected only in pathogenic strains of *L. monocytogenes* and *L. ivanovii* [64], seems to be equally significant. In the present study, the gene encoding PI-PLC was present in 55% of *L. monocytogenes*isolates—only those from foxes and martens. The other virulence genes identified (inl*A*, inl*C*, prf*A*, act*A*, hly*A*, and *iap*) occurred in varying numbers and configurations in all strains from which *L. monocytogenes* was isolated (8 separate profiles), with the full panel of virulence genes noted in 7 of the 20 isolates. These results indicate that these isolates possess all the properties of a virulent strain and are very likely to pose a direct threat to the health of humans and animals (including livestock).

The most frequently isolated group of bacteria in the pool of the animals studied was coagulase-positive *Staphylococcus*

(60.33%). These are commonly occurring bacteria colonizing the bodies of humans and animals, and their interaction with the host can be either commensal or opportunistic [66]. *S. aureus* is responsible for most infections induced by this group of bacteria in humans [67] and constitutes one of the important causes of foodborne diseases [68, 69, 70]. Among all coagulase-positive *Staphylococcus* species, *S. aureus* is the main described cause of staphylococcal foodborne outbreaks [70]. Other species, especially belonging to the *Staphylococcus intermedius* group, have low enterotoxigenic potential and only occasionally induce cases of disease [71]. *S. aureus* compared with other genera, i.e. *Salmonella*, *Campylobacter*, or *Shigella*, seems to account for a small percentage among documented bacterial causes of foodborne diseases reported to public health agencies, but the true number of cases of *S. aureus* foodborne disease may be much higher for various reasons, most often associated with a lack of laboratory confirmation of the presence of SEs in clinical stool samples [68]. Therefore, *S. aureus* should also be included in analysis of the presence of potential pathogens in free-living animals. A broad and diverse panel of factors allowing *S. aureus* to adapt particularly well to the human body [72] by colonizing and/or infecting it may also be active in the case of other mammalian hosts [73]. In our study, *S. aureus* was isolated at a similar level from all the animal species and, as in studies by other authors [74, 75, 76], it was not a dominant species among coagulase-positive *Staphylococcus* spp. The vast majority of isolates (38/40) had genes encoding virulence factors occurring in varying configurations (number/type of gene). Among the 40 *S. aureus* isolated in this study, 31 were characterized by the presence of genes encoding at least one type of enterotoxin (SEs). Enterotoxins belonging to the family of pyrogenic toxin superantigens (PTSAg) have been linked to food poisoning and, as superantigens (SAg), can lead to potentially lethal toxic shock syndrome [70]. In five strains, there were also enterotoxin gene cluster (*egc*) or *egc*-like variants, which were detected in over half of all *S. aureus* strains, both commensal and invasive [77]. Novrousian et al. [77] demonstrated that the presence of an *egc* locus can facilitate colonization by *S. aureus* of mucosal surfaces and increase weight loss in an experimental model of *S. aureus* infection. The *hla* and *hld* genes encoding hemolysins α and δ, leukotoxin LukE-LukD (30/40), and hemolysin β (11/40) were noted most frequently. The virulence factors such as leucotoxins have been demonstrated to kill human neutrophils, but only LukE-LukD leucotoxin exhibited lytic activity against red blood cells [78]. Genes encoding leukotoxin LukE-LukD were present in most *S. aureus* strains isolated from cases of mastitis in cows [79] and in blood isolated from humans with *S. aureus* bacteremia [80]. Hemolysins, especially α-hemolysin, are important virulence factors in several animal models of infection, including pneumonia and mastitis [81] The presence of the *hla*, *hld*, and *hlb* genes and the enterotoxin gene cluster has also been shown in *S. aureus* strains from cases of mastitis in cows in Poland [82, 83].

The presence of the *tst* gene encoding toxic shock syndrome toxin-1 (TSST-1) in two (5%) strains isolated from a fox and a marten in the present study is noteworthy. TSST-1 has also properties of a superantigen and its presence is connected with toxic shock syndrome (TSS), a rare but important cause of morbidity and mortality [84]. The presence of this toxin is also related to the etiology of many other diseases or syndromes in humans [73]. The *tst* gene has not been detected so far in isolates from companion animals and livestock (dogs, cats, pigs, or chickens) in Poland [82], but it has been present in isolates from neonatal intensive care units in Polish hospitals, usually in combination with the enterotoxin gene cluster (*egc*) and *egc*-like variants [85]. This phenomenon may indicate that the presence of *S. aureus tst* gene positive strains in free-living animals may be associated rather with their exposure to direct human sources (e.g. sewage, waste from hospitals), as in the case of our previous studies on isolation of a community-acquired methicillin-resistant *S. aureus* (CA-MRSA) strain from a marten [86].

In the case of free-living animals, the level of carriage of specific microbes is most often analyzed [41, 53, 86, 87, 88]. Confirmed cases of illness are noted less frequently (salmonellosis, listeriosis, yersiniosis, or local and generalized *S. aureus* infection) [33, 48, 89, 90] and the primary source of infection/carriage of these animals is analyzed extremely rarely [91]. Due to their varied diet, carnivorous animals may constitute an accumulation vector by eating small mammals, birds, and even insects that may be carriers of pathogens and transmit them in contact with humans or domestic animals. Most animals (foxes and martens), in the present study came from areas that include provinces with the largest number of farms producing organic food, including farm animal. One of the requirements for organic farming is to keep farm animals with outdoor access, which greatly increases the possibility of contact of free-living animals with farm animals and, thus, the potential transmission of pathogens [35].

Apart from the transfer from free-living animals to humans, a reverse phenomenon can occur. As a result of increasing anthropogenic changes in the environment leading to greater interpenetration of communities of humans and free-living animals, exposure of animals to pathogens that are present in the human environment or livestock (waste, manure from farm animals) can occur. Messenger et al. [92] showed that 50% of all recorded infections in animals related to reverse zoonosis apply to free living animals, where direct contact was suggested as the most frequent transmission route.

The present study showed that predatory species of free-living animals can be a significant reservoir of potentially pathogenic bacteria. Among the species analyzed (the red fox, beech marten, and raccoon), the fox may pose the greatest threat, due to its continually growing population size and occurrence all over Poland, as well as the statistically significantly higher frequency of isolation of bacteria that are potentially pathogenic for humans and other animals. To analyze the importance and participation of free-living carnivorous animals in the chain of transmission and spread of the microorganisms analyzed in the present study, additional research should be carried out covering the lower floors of the food chain (small mammals and birds, amphibians, reptiles, insects) and the natural habitat of carnivorous animals (water, soil, plants). Moreover, given the virulence potential of the isolated strains (the presence of virulence genes), it is clear that expanding epidemiological monitoring to include free-living animals must be considered.

AUTHOR CONTRIBUTIONS

Conceived and designed the experiments: AN PZ GZ SG KT ŁU MM BMD AT. Performed the experiments: AN PZ GZ SG

KT ŁU MM BMD AT. Analyzed the data: AN PZ GZ SG KT. Contributed reagents/materials/analysis tools: AN PZ GZ SG KT ŁU MM BMD AT. Wrote the paper: AN PZ GZ SG KT ŁU MM BMD AT.

REFERENCES

1. Kruse H, Kirkemo AM, Handeland K. Wildlife as source of zoonotic infections. Emerg Infect Dis. 2004; 10: 2067–2072. pmid:15663840 doi: 10.3201/eid1012.040707
2. Wereszczuk A. Occurrence of wild mammals and birds in villages–the use of camera traps in the evaluation of species composition. Chrońmy Przyr Ojcz. 2015; 71: 9–16.
3. Kamieniarz R, Panek M. Game animals in Poland at the turn of the 20th and 21st century. The research Station in Czempiń– OHZ PZŁ. Raport Game Animals in Poland. 2008. (In Polish with English summary) Available: http://www.czempin.pzlow.pl/palio/html.wmedia?_Instance=pzl_www&_Connector=palio&_ID=3991&_CheckSum=-1363983456
4. Duscher GG, Leschnik M, Fuehrer H-P, Joachim A. Wildlife reservoirs for vector-borne canine, feline and zoonotic infections in Austria. Int J Parasitol. 2015; 4: 88–96. doi: 10.1016/j.ijppaw.2014.12.001
5. Navarro-Gonzalez N, Casas-Díaz E, Porrero CM, Mateos A, Domínguez L, Lavín S, et al. Food-borne zoonotic pathogens and antimicrobial resistance of indicator bacteria in urban wild boars in Barcelona, Spain. Vet Microbiol. 2013; 167: 686–689 doi: 10.1016/j.vetmic.2013.07.037. pmid:23992794
6. Sumiński P, Goszczyński J, Romanowski J. Ssaki drapieżne Europy. Warsaw: Państwowe Wydawnictwo Rolnicze i Leśne; 1993.
7. Gabryś G, Nowaczyk J, Ważna A, Kościelska A, Nowakowska K, Cichocki J. Expansion of the raccoon Procyon lotor in Poland. Acta Biol. 2014; 21: 169–181.
8. Bartoszewicz M, Okarma H, Szczęsna J, Zalewski A. Ecology of raccoon (Procyon lotor L. 1758) from western Poland. Ann Zool Fenn. 2008; 45: 291–298. doi: 10.5735/086.045.0409
9. Daszak P, Cunningham AA, Hyatt AD. Wildlife ecology—emerging infectious diseases of wildlife—threats to biodiversity and human health. Science. 2000; 287: 443–449 pmid:10642539 doi: 10.1126/science.287.5452.443
10. European Commission Health & Consumer Protection Directorate-General: Report of the Scientific Committee on Animal Health and Animal Welfare: The oral vaccination of foxes against rabies. 2002.
11. Karamon J, Kochanowski M, Sroka J, Cencek T, Różycki M, Chmurzyńska E, et al. The prevalence of Echinococcus multilocularis in red foxes in Poland—current results (2009–2013). Parasitol Res. 2014; 113: 317–322 doi: 10.1007/s00436-013-3657-z. pmid:24221887
12. Karamon J, Kochanowski M, Cencek T, Bartoszewicz M, Kusyk P. Gastrointestinal helminths of raccoons (Procyon lotor) in western Poland (Lubuskie province)—with particular regard to Baylisascaris procyonis. B Vet I Pulawy. 2014; 58: 547–552. doi: 10.2478/bvip-2014-0084
13. Krajewska M, Lipiec M, Zabost A, Augustynowicz-Kopeć E, Szulowski K. Bovine tuberculosis in a wild boar (Sus scrofa) in Poland. J Wild Dis. 2014; 50: 1001–1002. doi: 10.7589/2013-07-187
14. Krawiec M, Kuczkowski M, Kruszewicz AG, Wieliczko A. Prevalence and genetic characteristics of Salmonella in free-living birds in Poland. BMC Vet Res. 2015; 11: 15. doi: 10.1186/s12917-015-0332-x. pmid:25636375
15. Larska M, Krzysiak MK, Jabłoński A, Kęsik J, Bednarski M, Rola J. Hepatitis E virus antibody prevalence in wildlife in Poland. Zoonoses and Public Health. 2015; 62: 105–110. doi: 10.1111/zph.12113. pmid:24655475
16. Polish Veterinary Inspection. Animal Health–Regulatory Committee-presentations: Rabies–Poland, 09–10 Sept. 2015. Available: http://ec.europa.eu/food/animals/health/regulatory_committee/presentations_en.htm
17. Zalewski A. Protection of water and marsh birds in five national parks—reconstructing habitats and curbing the influence of invasive species. Project LIFE09 NAT/PL/000263. Available: http://ec.europa.eu/environment/life/project/Projects/index.cfm?fuseaction=search.dspPage&n_proj_id=3868
18. EFSA and ECDC (European Food Safety Authority and European Centre for Disease Prevention and Control): The European Union summary report on trends and sources of zoonoses, zoonotic agents and food-borne outbreaks in 2013. EFSA J. 2015; 13: 162
19. European Centre for Disease Prevention and Control Annual epidemiological report 2014 Food- and waterborne diseases and zoonoses. Available: http://ecdc.europa.eu/en/publications/surveillance_reports/annual_epidemiological_report/Pages/epi_index.aspx
20. Scallan E, Hoekstra RM, Angulo RJ, Tauxe RV, Widdowson M-A, Roy SL, et al. Foodborne Illness Acquired in the United States—Major Pathogens. Emerg Infect Dis. 2011; 17 doi: 10.3201/eid1701.P11101.
21. Polish Committee for Standardization: Microbiology of food and animal feeding stuffs—Horizontal method for the detection of Salmonella spp. PN-EN ISO 6579:2003. Polish Committee for Standardization, Warsaw, Poland, 2003.
22. Popoff M, Le Minor L. Antigenic formulae of the Salmonella serovars. WHO Collaborating Centre for Reference and Research on Salmonella. Institut Pasteur, Paris, France, 2001.
23. Polish Committee for Standardization: Microbiology of food and animal feeding stuffs—Horizontal method for detecting the presence and enumeration of Listeria monocytogenes. PNEN ISO 11290–1:1999. Polish Committee for Standardization, Warsaw, Poland, 1999.
24. Paillard D, Dubois V, Duran R, Nathier F, Guittet C, Caumette P, et al. Rapid identification of Listeria species by using restriction fragment length polymorphism of PCR-amplified 23S rRNA gene fragments. Appl Environ Microbiol. 2003; 69: 6386–6392. pmid:14602590 doi: 10.1128/aem.69.11.6386-6392.2003

25. Soni DK, Singh RK, Singh DV, Dubey SK. Characterization of Listeria monocytogenes isolated from Ganges water, human clinical and milk samples at Varanasi, India. Infect Genet Evol. 2013: 14: 83–91. doi: 10.1016/j.meegid.2012.09.019. pmid:23201044

26. Wannet WJB, Reessink M, Brunings HA, Maas HME. Detection of pathogenic Yersinia enterocolitica by a rapid and sensitive duplex PCR assay. J Clin Microbiol. 2001; 39: 4483–4486. pmid:11724866 doi: 10.1128/jcm.39.12.4483-4486.2001

27. Polish Committee for Standardization: Microbiology of food and animal feeding stuffs—Horizontal method for the enumeration of coagulase-positive staphylococci (Staphylococcus aureus and other species)—Part 1: Method Rusing Baird-Parker agar. PN-EN ISO 6888–1:2001. Polish Committee for Standardization, Warsaw, Poland, 2001.

28. Sasaki T, Tsubakishita S, Tanaka Y, Sakusabe A, Ohtsuka M, Hirotaki S, et al. Multiplex-PCR method for species identification of coagulase-positive staphylococci. J Clin Microbiol. 2010; 48: 765–769. doi: 10.1128/JCM.01232-09. pmid:20053855

29. Jarraud S, Mougel C, Thioulouse J, Lina G, Meugnier H, Forey F, et al. Relationships between Staphylococcus aureus genetic background, virulence factors, agr groups (alleles), and human disease. Infect Immun. 2002; 70: 631–641. pmid:11796592 doi: 10.1128/iai.70.2.631-641.2002

30. Hwang SY, Kim SH, Jang EJ, Kwon NH, Park YK, Koo HC, et al. Novel multiplex PCR for the detection of the Staphylococcus aureus superantigen and its application to raw meat isolates in Korea. Int J Food Microbiol. 2007; 117: 99–105. pmid:17439826 doi: 10.1016/j.ijfoodmicro.2007.02.013

31. Gnat S, Trościańczyk A, Nowakiewicz A, Majer-Dziedzic B, Ziółkowska G, Dziedzic R, et al. Experimental studies of microbial populations and incidence of zoonotic pathogens in the faeces of red deer (Cervus elaphus). Lett Appl Microbiol. 2015; 61: 446–452. doi: 10.1111/lam.12471. pmid:26222832

32. Lee K, Iwata T, Nakadai A, Kato T, Hayama S, Taniguchi T, et al. Prevalence of Salmonella, Yersinia and Campylobacter spp. in feral raccoons (Procyon lotor) and masked palm civets (Paguma larvata) in Japan. Zoonoses Public Health. 2011; 58: 424–431. doi: 10.1111/j.1863-2378.2010.01384.x. pmid:21824337

33. Hamir AN. Systemic Staphylococcus aureus infection in a free-ranging raccoon (Procyon lotor). J Wildlife Dis. 2010; 46: 665–668 doi: 10.7589/0090-3558-46.2.665

34. Bartoszewicz, M. 2011 [cited 11 April 2016]. In: NOBANIS–Invasive Alien Species Fact Sheet–Procyon lotor–Online Database of the European Network on Invasive Alien Species. Available: https://www.nobanis.org/fact-sheets/ NOBANIS)

35. Hilbert F, Smulders FJM, Chopra-Dewasthaly R, Paulsen P. Salmonella in the wildlife-human interface. Food Res Int. 2012; 45: 603–608 doi: 10.1016/j.foodres.2011.08.015

36. European Commision of Health and Consumer Protection. Report of the Scientific Committee on Food: Risk profile on the microbiological contamination of fruits and vegetables eaten raw 2002. Available: http://ec.europa.eu/food/fs/sc/scf/out125_en.pdf

37. European Centre for Disease Prevention and Control: Annual epidemiological report 2014 –food- and waterborne diseases and zoonoses. Stockholm, ECDC, 2014.

38. Nowakiewicz A, Ziółkowska G, Zięba P, Stępniewska K, Tokarzewski S. Russian tortoises (Agrionemys horsfieldi) as a potential reservoir for Salmonella spp. Res Vet Sci. 2012; 92: 187–190. doi: 10.1016/j.rvsc.2011.03.019. pmid:21486674

39. Botti V, Navillod FV, Domenis L, Orusa R, Pepe E, Robetto S, et al. Salmonella spp. and antibiotic-resistant strains in wild mammals and birds in north-western Italy from 2002 to 2010. Veter Ital. 2013; 49: 195–202.

40. Millán J, Aduriz G, Moreno B, Juste RA, Barral M. Salmonella isolates from wild birds and mammals in the Basque country (Spain). Rev Sci Tech Off Int Epiz. 2004; 23: 905–911. doi: 10.20506/rst.23.3.1529

41. Chiari M, Ferrari N, Giardiello D, Lanfranchi P, Zanoni M, Lavazza A, et al. Isolation and identification of Salmonella spp. from red foxes (Vulpes vulpes) and badgers (Meles meles) in northern Italy. Acta Vet Scand. 2014; 56: 86. doi: 10.1186/s13028-014-0086-7. pmid:25492524

42. Handeland K, Nesse LL, Lillehaug A, Vikøren T, Djønne B, Bergsjø B. Natural and experimental Salmonella Typhimurium infections in foxes (Vulpes vulpes). Vet Microbiol. 2008; 132: 129–134. doi: 10.1016/j.vetmic.2008.05.002. pmid:18547749

43. Maurer JJ, Martin G, Hernandez S, Cheng Y, Gerner-Smidt P, Hise KB, et al. Diversity and persistence of Salmonella enterica strains in rural landscapes in the Southeastern United States. Plos Med. 2015. doi: 10.1371/journal.pone.0128937.

44. Compton JA, Baney JA, Donaldson SC, Houser BA, Julian GJ, Yahner RH, et al. Salmonella infections in the common raccoon (Procyon lotor) in Western Pennsylvania. J Clin Microbiol. 2008; 46: 3084–3086. doi: 10.1128/JCM.00685-08. pmid:18596136

45. Hendriksen R S, Vieira AR, Karlsmose S, Lo Fo Wong DMA, Jensen AB, Wegener HC, et al. Global monitoring of Salmonella serovar distribution from the World Health Organization Global Foodborne Infections Network Country Data Bank: results of quality assured laboratories from 2001 to 2007. Foodborne Pathog Dis. 2011; 8, doi: 10.1089/fpd.2010.0787.

46. Hoszowski A, Samcik I, Lalak A, Skarżyńska M, Wnuk D, Zając M, et al. Charakterystyka jednofazowych izolatów Salmonella enterica serowar Typhimurium (1,4,[5],12:i:-). Med Weter. 2014; 70: 117–121.

47. Hoszowski A, Wasyl D. Salmonella serovars found in animals and feeding stuffs in 2001 and their antimicrobial resistance. B Vet I Pulawy 2002; 46: 165–178.

48. Simpson VR. Wild animals as reservoirs of infectious diseases in the UK. Vet J. 2002; 163: 128–146. pmid:12093188 doi: 10.1053/tvjl.2001.0662

49. Jay-Russell MT. What is the risk from wild animals in food-borne pathogen contamination of plants? CAB Rev. 2013; 8; 040. Available: http://www.wifss.ucdavis.edu/wp-content/uploads/documents/foodSafety/CABReviewWildlife.pdf

50. Keymer IF, Gibson EA, Reynolds DJ. Zoonoses and other findings in hedgehogs (Erinaceus europaeus): a survey of mortality and review of the literature. Vet Rec. 1991; 128: 245–249 pmid:2035215 doi: 10.1136/vr.128.11.245

51. Wales AD, Carrique-Mas JJ, Rankin M, Bell B, Thind BB, Davies RH. Review of the carriage of zoonotic bacteria by arthropods with special reference to Salmonella in mites, flies and litter beetles. Zoonoses Public Health. 2010; 57: 299–314. doi: 10.1111/j.1863-2378.2008.01222.x. pmid:19486496

52. Sabina Y, Rahman A, Ray RC, Montet D Yersinia enterocolitica: mode of transmission, molecular insights of virulence, and pathogenesis of infection. J Pathog. 2011, doi: 10.4061/2011/429069.

53. Bancerz-Kisiel A, Szczerba-Turek A, Platt-Samoraj A, Socha P, Szweda W. Application of multiplex PCR for the evaluation of the occurrence of ail, ystA, and ystB genes in Yersinia enterocolitica strains isolated from wild boars (Sus scrofa). B Vet I Pulawy. 2009; 53: 351–355. doi: 10.1111/j.1439-0450.2006.00969.x

54. Sannö A, Aspán A, Hestvik G, Jacobson M. Presence of Salmonella spp., Yersinia enterocolitica, Yersinia pseudotuberculosis and Escherichia coli O157:H7 in wild boars. Epidemiol Infect. 2014; 142: 2542–2547. doi: 10.1017/S0950268814000119. pmid:24512817

55. Kaneko KI, Hashimoto N. Occurrence of Yersinia enterocolitica in wild animals. Appl Environ Microb. 1981; 41: 635–638.

56. Nikolova S, Tzvetkov Y, Najdenski H, Vesselinova A. Isolation of pathogenic yersiniae from wild animals in Bulgaria. J Vet Med B. 2001; 48: 203–209. doi: 10.1046/j.1439-0450.2001.00448.x

57. Zadernowska A, Chajęcka-Wierzchowska W, Łaniewska-Trokenheim Ł. Yersinia enterocolitica: a dangerous, but often ignored, foodborne pathogen. Food Rev Int. 2014; 30: 53–70. doi: 10.1080/87559129.2013.853775

58. Vackachan MB, Latha C, Sunil B, Menon VK. Prevalence of Listeria spp. in soils of central Kerala, India. Int J Curr Microbiol App Sci. 2015; 4: 938–943.

59. Orsi RH, den Bakker HC, Wiedmann M. Listeria monocytogenes lineages: Genomics, evolution, ecology, and phenotypic characteristics. Int J Med Microbiol. 2011; 301: 79–96 doi: 10.1016/j.ijmm.2010.05.002. pmid:20708964

60. Jadhav S, Bhave M, Palombo EA. Methods used for the detection and subtyping of Listeria monocytogenes. See comment in PubMed Commons belowJ Microbiol Methods. 2012; 88: 327–341 doi: 10.1016/j.mimet.2012.01.002. pmid:22261140

61. Yoshida T, Sugimoto T, Sato M, Hirai K. Incidence of Listeria monocytogenes in wild animals in Japan. J Vet Med Sci. 2000; 62: 673–675. pmid:10907701 doi: 10.1292/jvms.62.673

62. Lyautey E, Hartmann A, Pagotto F, Tyler K, Lapen DR, Wilkes G et al. Characteristics and frequency of detection of fecal Listeria monocytogenes shed by livestock, wildlife, and humans. See comment in PubMed Commons belowCan J Microbiol. 2007; 53: 1158–67. doi: 10.1139/w07-084

63. Liu D, Lawrence ML, Ainsworth AJ, Austin FW. Toward an improved laboratory definition of Listeria monocytogenes virulence. Int J Food Microbiol. 2007; 118: 101–115. pmid:17727992 doi: 10.1016/j.ijfoodmicro.2007.07.045

64. Kaur S, Malik SVS, Vaidya VM, Barbuddhe SB. Listeria monocytogenes in spontaneous abortions in humans and its detection by multiplex PCR. J Appl Microbiol. 2007; 103: 1889–1896. pmid:17953598 doi: 10.1111/j.1365-2672.2007.03414.x

65. Liu D, Lawrence M, Austin FW, Ainsworth AJ. A multiplex PCR for species- and virulence-specific determination of Listeria monocytogenes. J Microbiol Meth. 2007; 71: 133–140. doi: 10.1016/j.mimet.2007.08.007

66. Hanselman BA, Kruth SA, Rousseau J, Weese JS. Coagulase positive staphylococcal colonization of humans and their household pets. Can Vet J. 2009; 50: 954–958. pmid:19949556

67. Liu GY. Molecular pathogenesis of Staphylococcus aureus infection. Pediatr Res. 2009; 65: 71–77. doi: 10.1203/pdr.0b013e31819dc44d

68. Kadariya J, Smith TC, Thapaliya D. Staphylococcus aureus and staphylococcal food-borne disease: an ongoing challenge in public health. BioMed Res Int. 2014; Available online: doi: 10.1155/2014/827965.

69. Sofos JN. Bacterial Foodborne Diseases. Proceedings, The 15th Congress of FAVA. FAVA -OIE Joint Symposium on Emerging Diseases 2008

70. Hennekinne JA, De Buyser ML, Dragacci S. Staphylococcus aureus and its food poisoning toxins: characterization and outbreak investigation. FEMS Microbiol Rev. 2012; 36: 815–36 doi: 10.1111/j.1574-6976.2011.00311.x. pmid:22091892

71. Bennett RW. Atypical toxigenic Staphylococcus and non-Staphylococcus aureus species on the horizon? An update. J Food Protect. 1996; 59: 1123–1126.

72. Murugaiyan J, Walther B, Stamm I Abou-Elnaga Y, Brueggemann-Schwarze S, Vincze S, et al. Species differentiation within the Staphylococcus intermedius group using a refined MALDI-TOF MS database. Clin Microbiol Infect. 2014; 20: 1007–1014. doi: 10.1111/1469-0691.12662. pmid:24807701

73. Dinges MM, Orwin PM, Schlievert PM. Exotoxins of Staphylococcus aureus. Clin Microbiol Rev. 2000; 13: 16–34. pmid:10627489 doi: 10.1128/cmr.13.1.16-34.2000

74. Gomez-Sanz E, Torres C, Lozano C, Zarazaga M. High diversity of Staphylococcus aureus and Staphylococcus pseudintermedius lineages and toxigenic traits in healthy pet-owning household members. Underestimating normal household contact? Comp Immunol Microb. 2013; 36: 83–94. doi: 10.1016/j.cimid.2012.10.001

75. Porrero CM, Mentaberre G, Sanchez S, Fernandez Llario P, Gomez-Barrero S, Navarro-Gonzalez N, et al. Methicillin-resistant Staphylococcus aureus (MRSA) carriage in different free-living animals species in Spain. Vet J. 2013; 198: 127–130. doi: 10.1016/j.tvjl.2013.06.004. pmid:23846031

76. Gomez P, Gonzalez-Barrio D, Benito D, Garcia JT, Vinuela J, Zarazaga M, et al. Detection of methicillin-resistant Staphylococcus aureus (MRSA) carrying the mecC gene in wild small mammals in Spain. J Antimicrob Chemoth. 2014; 69: 2061–2064. doi: 10.1093/jac/dku100

77. Nowrouzian FL, Ali A, Badiou C, Dauwalder O, Lina G, Josefsson E. Impacts of enterotoxin gene cluster-encoded superantigens on local and systemic experimental Staphylococcus aureus infections. Eur J Clin Microbiol Infect Dis. 2015; 34:1443–1449 doi: 10.1007/s10096-015-2371-4. pmid:25864191

78. Yoong P, Torres VJ. The effects of Staphylococcus aureus leukotoxins on the host: cell lysis and beyond. Curr Opin Microbiol. 2013; 16: 63–69. doi: 10.1016/j.mib.2013.01.012. pmid:23466211

79. Fueyo JM, Mendoza MC, Rodicio MR, Muniz J, Alvarez MA, Martın MC. Cytotoxin and pyrogenic toxin superantigen gene profiles of Staphylococcus aureus associated with subclinical mastitis in dairy cows and relationships with macrorestriction genomic profiles. J Clin Microbiol 2005; 43: 1278–1284. pmid:15750096 doi: 10.1128/jcm.43.3.1278-1284.2005

80. Eiff C, Friedrichb AW, Petersa G, Beckera K. Prevalence of genes encoding for members of the staphylococcal leukotoxin family among clinical isolates of Staphylococcus aureus. Diag Micr Infec Dis. 2004; 49: 157–162. doi: 10.1016/j.diagmicrobio.2004.03.009

81. Schwan WR, Langhorne MH, Ritchie HD, Stover CK. Loss of hemolysin expression in Staphylococcus aureus agr mutants correlates with selective survival during mixed infections in murine abscesses and wounds. FEMS Immunol Med. Mic. 2003; 38: 23–28 doi: 10.1016/s0928-8244(03)00098-1

82. Garbacz K, Piechowicz L, Mroczkowska A. Distribution of toxin genes among different spa types and phage types of animal Staphylococcus aureus. Arch Microbiol. 2015; 197: 935–940. doi: 10.1007/s00203-015-1127-y. pmid:26108193

83. Puacz E, Ilczyszyn WM, Kosecka M, Buda A, Dudziak W, Polakowska K, et al. Clustering of Staphylococcus aureus bovine mastitis strains from regions of Central-Eastern Poland based on their biochemical and genetic characteristics. Pol J Ve. Sci. 2015; 18: 333–342. doi: 10.1515/pjvs-2015-0043

84. Murray RJ. Recognition and management of Staphylococcus aureus toxin-mediated disease. See comment in PubMed Commons belowIntern Med J. 2005; 35 Suppl 2: 106–119.

85. Romaniszyn D, Różańska A, Wójkowska-Mach J, Chmielarczyk A, Pobiega M, Adamski P, et al. Epidemiology, antibiotic consumption and molecular characterization of Staphylococcus aureus infections–data from the Polish Neonatology Surveillance Network, 2009–2012. BMC Infect Dis. 2015; 15: 169. doi: 10.1186/s12879-015-0890-3. pmid:25888217

86. Nowakiewicz A, Ziółkowska G, Zięba P, Gnat S, Wojtanowicz-Markiewicz K, Trościańczyk A. Coagulase-positive Staphylococcus isolated from wildlife: Identification, molecular characterization and evaluation of resistance profiles with focus on a methicillin-resistant strain. Comp Immunol Microb. 2016; 44: 21–28 doi: 10.1016/j.cimid.2015.11.003

87. Zaytseva E, Ermolaeva S, Somov GP. Low genetic diversity and epidemiological significance of Listeria monocytogenes isolated from wild animals in the far east of Russia. Infect Genet Evol. 2007;7: 736–742 pmid:17716956 doi: 10.1016/j.meegid.2007.07.006

88. Hoelzer K, Moreno Switt AI, Wiedmann M. Animal contact as a source of human non-typhoidal salmonellosis Vet Res. 2011; 42: 34 doi: 10.1186/1297-9716-42-34. pmid:21324103

89. Hamir AN, Mattson DE, Sonn RJ, Stasko J, Habecker PL. Concurrent candidiasis, listeriosis and adenovirus infections in a raccoon (Procyon lotor). Vet Rec. 2000; 146: 320–322 pmid:10766117 doi: 10.1136/vr.146.11.320

90. Rothenburger JL, Bennett KR, Bryan L, Bollinger TK. Septicemic listeriosis in wild hares from Saskatchewan, Canada. J Wildlife Dis. 2015; 51: 503–508. doi: 10.7589/2014-06-159

91. Tizard I. Salmonellosis in wild birds. Seminars in Avian and Exotic Pet Medicine. 2004; 13: 50–66 doi: 10.1053/j.saep.2004.01.008

92. Messenger AM, Barnes AN, Gray GC. Reverse zoonotic disease transmission (zooanthroponosis): A systematic review of seldom- documented human biological threats to animals. PLoS One 2014; 9: e89055 doi: 10.1371/journal.pone.0089055. pmid:24586500

CHAPTER 2

TAXONOMY OF BACTERIAL FISH PATHOGENS

Brian Austin

INTRODUCTION

"What's in a name?" (William Shakespeare; Romeo and Juliet)

The Swedish botanist Carl Linnaeus (1707-1778), who was also known as Carolus Linnaeus and Carl von Linné, is undoubtedly the Father of Taxonomy, and was responsible for developing a system for naming and ranking living organisms. His lasting contribution was the development of a simplified naming system in Latin with consistency across all living organisms, i.e. the binomial system, in which each organism has a unique two-word name - incorporating genus and species. A simplistic view is that Linnaeus made order out of chaos. Yet, for Linnaeus and his contemporaries, the process was comparatively easy, and involved only large organisms, which were clearly visible to the naked eye (= macro-organisms) and easily seen morphological characteristics (= a category of phenotypic characters). Thus, these early classifications (= the process of arranging organisms into groups) were based on limited but easily visible data, and the outcomes were largely obvious, for example a dog is notably different from a horse and would therefore belong in separate species.

The founding father of microbiology, the Dutch textile merchant and lens maker, Antonie van Leeuwenhoek (1632-1723), observed small organisms initially from the proximity of his teeth (= bacteria and protozoa?), and these entities were termed "animalcules", which he wrote about in a letter to the Royal Society of London in 1676. His careful illustrations suggested morphological variation between the cells. Yet, another two centuries were to pass before serious attempts at naming and ordering bacteria started. Thus, bacterial taxonomy has progressed from the simplistic approach involving a small number of readily observable characteristics, such as morphology as deduced from observation using light microscopes, to the modern applications of molecular biology.

With improvements in knowledge, there have been refinements in taxonomic processes and an increase in reliability. It should be remembered that taxonomy (= the theory of classification, nomenclature and identification) is a man-made process, i.e. the organisms included in any classification have not chosen to be placed in the groups that have been created by human beings. Nevertheless if done properly, taxonomy has value in:

- Understanding biodiversity, namely the range of organisms in a given habitat
- Communication between scientists, thus enabling exchange of information about similar organisms
- Cataloguing information - the name is the key to a catalogue of information about the organism
- Enabling identification, such that new isolates may be readily and reliably identified
- Providing an insight into evolutionary pathways (= phylogenetics).

To be effective, taxonomy should be

- based on a high information content
- reproducible, and
- stable,
- otherwise confusion will surely result.

Since the start of bacterial taxonomic processes in the nineteenth century, there has been a progression in the type of information used in the procedure. It may be argued that early bacteriologists had considerable taxonomic insight judging from the conclusions reached from the comparatively simple data that were available. However, taxonomy is a dynamic science, with new developments/methods being incorporated into processes including the descriptions of bacterial species. Since the 1950 s, bacterial taxonomy has evolved rationally, encompassing numerical methods [1, 2], chemotaxonomy (e.g. [3, 4]), and molecular techniques [5]. Taxonomy has progressed from a highly artificial process involving limited amounts of phenotypic data to the recognition of more natural relationships between organisms, based on comparatively large amounts of varied and reliable data covering multiple aspects of the biology of an organism, and including phenotypic,

Citation: Brian Austin, Taxonomy of bacterial fish pathogens, DOI: 10.1186/1297-9716-42-20.

chemotaxonomic, genotypic and phylogenetic date, i.e. a polyphasic approach. However, the current dominance of 16S rRNA gene sequencing although revolutionising some aspects of bacterial classification needs to be treated cautiously as overreliance on the approach may lead to erroneous conclusions [5]. Nevertheless, it is apparent that sequencing methods are instrumental with the explosion of new species names, which have greeted the arrival of the twenty-first century. Whereas, the information content of many of the new species descriptions is generally high, an unwelcome trend is that many new taxa (= taxonomic groups) are described solely after the study of only single strains. Therefore, the diversity/variability within the new taxon cannot be adequately assessed. Also, it is impossible to determine whether a single strain is effectively an outlier or a median representative of the group (in future years, will it be regarded as typical or atypical of the group?). However, taxonomy is often ignored by many microbiologists in other specialisms, and there may well be concern that basic principles could be forgotten, e.g. is the purity and authenticity of cultures always verified before use? Where culturing is not possible, there is the possibility of analyzing the nucleic acids, determining species composition, and even proposing new taxa, i.e. by the use of culture-independent approaches.

BACTERIAL FISH PATHOGENS

There has been a steady increase in the numbers of bacterial species associated with fish diseases, with new pathogens regularly recognised in the scientific literature [6]. However, the names of many bacterial fish pathogens have been subjected to taxonomic change over time, with some species split, for example *Vibrio anguillarum* biotype 2 becoming re-classified as a separate species *V. ordalii*[7, 8]. In other cases, different nomenspecies have been combined, for example *V. carchariae, V. harveyi* and *V. trachuri* into *V. harveyi*, which had precedence because it was the first name to be proposed, albeit as the luminous *Achromobacter harveyi*[9, 10, 11]. The oldest known fish pathogen, *V. anguillarum*, has undergone name changes to *Beneckea*[12] and *Listonella*[13]; neither of which was widely accepted. However, *Listonella* remains a valid name and is mentioned in the current edition of Bergey's Manual of Systematic Bacteriology, and *Beneckea*has been consigned to the history books. A positive aspect of sequencing methods is that there has been a progression towards the Orwellian notion of "Order out of Chaos" even if scientists do not always appreciate the significance of the data.

ISOLATION OF FISH PATHOGENS: THE CULTURE-DEPENDENT APPROACH

With the rapid development in molecular biology, it is not always necessary to culture an organism in order to enable its study, including the allocation of a species name. Thus, the concept of culture-independent techniques was developed and refined. Sensitivity and specificity increased, but without culturing there was an inability to carry out associated studies, such as the determination of pathogenicity factors. The attraction of culture-dependent approaches is that a pure culture may be obtained and deposited in culture collections as reference material for use by others. This raises a concern about the usefulness of cultures. An assumption is made that pathological material may be used for the recovery of a pure culture of the aetiological agent. This will depend on using appropriate media and incubation conditions, and assumes that the organism is in a form that may be cultured and that the microbiologist picks the "correct" colony. If mixed growth occurs or if the pathogen is largely overgrown by opportunists/secondary invaders/ saprophytes, then there is concern that the actual pathogen will be missed. In addition, infections resulting from two or more organisms working synergistically will undoubtedly be mis-diagnosed if the diagnostician chooses only one culture for study. However, there are only a comparatively few indications of disease resulting from multiple species, such as *Aeromonas hydrophila* with *A. salmonicida*[6]. It is speculative how many diagnoses (if any) are made of contaminants rather than the actual pathogen. Moreover, it is surprising that only two species of anaerobic bacteria, namely *Clostridium botulinum* and *Eubacterium tarantellae*, have been implicated as fish pathogens [6]. Of course, this could reflect the general lack of use of appropriate anaerobic procedures by microbiologists rather than the absence of anaerobic pathogens.

APPROACHES TO CHARACTERIZATION

Phenotype

Traditionally, bacteria were characterized phenotypically, and undoubtedly for some groups, e.g. the Enterobacteriaceae, a wealth of knowledge emerged particularly from the 1950's onwards. Currently, emphasis on phenotype has declined with a concomitant move towards molecular-based approaches. Nevertheless, phenotypic data have a role in polyphasic studies whereby many facets of the biology of an organism are studied [14]. Phenotyping leads the way with diagnoses worldwide; emphasis often being placed on commercial kits and the use of manufacturer's probabilistic databases to achieve an acceptable identification. Although the approach has standardized diagnoses, the weakness is that most identification systems have been developed for medically important bacteria that grow within 24-48 h at 35-37°C. Consequently, the reliability of these kits for use with fish pathogens which need lower incubation temperatures for longer periods needs to be questioned [6, 15]. In particular, the API 20E system includes the use of sugar fermentation reactions, which may be influenced by the presence of plasmids [6]. Moreover, there may be confusion over the interpretation of the profiles. For example, some of the profiles of *A. hydrophila* are similar to those of *A. allosaccharophila* and *A. sobria; Yersinia ruckeri* may be confused with *Hafnia alvei;* moreover *Tenacibaculum maritimum* and *Pseudomonas anguilliseptica* are indistinguishable by API 20E [6]. Problems may result when data from rapid commercial kits are used in conjunction with conventional diagnostic schemes, which have been developed for traditional and often laborious phenotypic characters. Also, some of the traditional tests, e.g. the Voges Proskauer reaction, are not noted for their reproducibility and may introduce errors into the taxonomic process and lead to mis-identification [16].

Undoubtedly, selective media have proved useful for the recovery of some fish pathogens, with an example including selective kidney disease medium (SKDM) for *Renibacterium salmoninarum*[17]. However, selective media are only available for a minority of all fish pathogens, therefore recovery is dependent on more general culturing methods. Specially developed diagnostic procedures have aided identification of some group, e.g. the glucose motility deep cultures have benefitted the recovery and identification of *V. anguillarum*[18].

Immunological methods

The development and availability of standardized immunological (antibodies and kits) reagents have improved diagnoses considerably [6, 19, 20], and enhanced the reliability of methods for the detection of pathogens, including *Mycobacterium* spp., *Photobacterium damselae* subsp. *piscicida*[21], *Piscirickettsia salmonis*[22], *R. salmoninarum*[23] and *Streptococcus iniae*[24]. Tentative diagnoses, including of asymptomatic infections, may result from use of monospecific polyclonal or monoclonal antibodies in a range of antibody-based procedures, including the indirect fluorescent antibody test (iFAT), whole-cell (slide) agglutination, precipitin reactions, complement fixation, immunodiffusion, antibody-coated latex particles, co-agglutination using antibody-coated staphylococcal cells, passive haemagglutination, immuno-India ink technique (Geck) or enzyme linked immunosorbent assay (ELISA; reviewed by [25]), the latter of which may also be used for serology, i.e. detecting antibodies in the host to specific pathogens [26]. Antibody-based methods are used effectively for detecting exposure to fish viruses, such as Koi herpes virus [27], but bacterial pathogens pose a more complicated picture with cross reactivities likely unless specific known molecules/antigens are used to coat the ELISA plates rather than whole pathogens [19]. Techniques are often sensitive, specific, rapid and reliable, and in some cases may be used in the field [6]. This is in marked contrast to molecular biology, which may be much slower and relies on specialist, well equipped laboratories.

Chemotaxonomy

Chemotaxonomy involves the investigation of chemical constituents of bacteria, and is particularly useful for the study of Gram-positive bacteria. The molecules studied include fatty acids, polar lipids, lipopolysaccharide (nature of the chain length of the fatty acid and the sugar in the Lipid A moiety; [28]), menaquinones, naphthoquinones, ubiquinones, mycolic acids, peptidoglycan, polyamines, teichoic and teichuronic acids and isoprenoid quinones [29]. Mycolic acids, which are useful taxonomic markers, are present in Gram-positive bacteria with high G+C ratios of their DNA [4], and have been reported for a range of fish pathogens, including *Mycobacterium chelonei* subsp. *piscarium*[3] and *M. shottsii*[30]. The length of the mycolate side chain has been correlated to 16S rRNA gene sequence homology [31]. Specific examples for which reliable chemotaxonomic data exist for Gram-positive bacterial fish pathogens are detailed below:

Lactococccus piscium

The long chain cellular fatty acids of *Lactococcus piscium* were reported to be straight chain saturated, mono-unsaturated and cyclopropane-ring types. The major acids corresponded to hexadecanoic acid, Δ 11-octadecanoic acid and Δ 11-methylenoctadecanoic acid [32].

Mycobacterium neoarum

The cell wall chemotype has been given as IVA, with glycolated muramic acids, mycolic acids and MK-9, as the predominant isoprenoid quinone, being present [33].

Nocardia

Nocardia salmonicida contains LL-diaminopimelic acid (DAP) and glycine but not meso-DAP, arabinose or galactose in the cell wall (i.e. Type I). The major cellular fatty acids are hexdecanoic, octadecanoic, octadecanoic and 10-methyloctadecanoic acid [34].

N. seriolae contains *meso-* diaminopimelic acid, arabinose and galactose, indicative of chemotype IVA. Mycolic acids containing 44-58 carbon atoms are present. The cellular fatty acids are dominated by *n*- $C_{16:0}$, *n*-$C_{16:1}$ and *n*- $C_{18:1}$; 10-methyl-$C_{19:0}$ is also present as a major component in some isolates. The predominant isoprenoid quinone is tetrahydrogenated menaquinone with eight isoprene units [34].

Renibacterium salmoninarum

Chemotaxonomic traits of *R. salmoninarum* have been highlighted in part because of the comparative difficulty with obtaining conventional phenotypic test results. Thus, the cell wall peptidoglycan was deduced to contain D-alanine, D-glutamic acid, glycine and lysine as the diamino acids [35]. The principal cell wall sugar was glucose, although arabinose, mannose and rhamnose were also present; mycolic acids were absent [36]. Methyl-branched fatty acids form > 92% of the total fatty acid component of the cells, with 12-methyltetradecanoic (anteiso-C_{15}), 13-methyldecanoic (iso-C_{15}) and 14-methylhexadecanoic (anteiso-C_{17}) as the major components. Straight chain fatty acids generally account for 1% of the total fatty acids, and unsaturated fatty acids are not detected at all. Over 81% of the total fatty acids are composed of the lower melting point anteiso acids, which may contribute to membrane fluidity at low temperatures. Unsaturated menaquinones with nine isoprene units are present. All strains contain diphosphatydylglycerol, 2 major and 6 or 7 minor glycolipids and two unidentified minor phospholipids [37].

Molecular/genetic methods

Molecular/genetic methods involving 16S rRNA gene sequencing [38], reverse transcriptase-sequencing [39, 40] and polymerase chain reaction (PCR)-based gene sequencing [41] have been useful additions to the armoury of techniques applicable to bacterial taxonomy [29, 31]. DNA hybridization, which is regarded as the "gold standard" for demonstrating the presence or absence of new species, was introduced into bacterial taxonomy during the 1960s (e.g. [42]). Genotypic classification involving sequencing of the 16S and 23S RNA genes (the latter is less popular) is regarded as the definitive standard for determining phylogenetic relationships of bacteria [29, 38]. In particular, the genes are regarded as having all the attributes of useful, relevant and stable biological markers being present and homologous in all bacteria. Also, they are not prone to the effects of gene transfer [29]. Yet, the exact homology values have a profound effect on interpretation of the outputs. Thus, homology values of ≤ 98.7% (97% according to [31]) indicates membership of different species, and this correlates well with DNA hybridization results. Yet, occasionally higher homology values may be attributed to distinct species groupings [43]. By themselves, 16S rRNA gene sequences are insufficient to describe a new species, but may be used indicatively and in conjunction with DNA:DNA hybridization [31]. However, sequencing has permitted the recognition of new variants. For example, sequencing revealed a new variant among Israeli isolates of *Streptococcus iniae*[44]. Moreover, 16S rRNA cataloguing has been useful in providing information about the position of species in existing classifications. Thus, small-subunit rRNA sequencing and DNA:DNA hybridization revealed that *Pasteurella piscicida* was related to *Photobacterium damsela* leading to the proposal that the pathogen be re-classified as *Ph. damsela(e)* subsp. *piscicida*[45]. Furthermore, *R. salmoninarum* was deduced to be a member of the actinomycete subdivision, being related to *Arthrobacter, Brevibacterium, Cellulomonas, Jonesia, Micrococcus, Promicromonospora, Stomatococcus*and *Terrabacter*[46, 47]. The evolutionary relationship of *R. salmoninarum* to *Arthrobacter* was reinforced as the result of genome sequencing, which suggested that the genome of the former had been reduced significantly since its divergence from a common ancestor [48].

Nucleic acid fingerprinting methods, including amplified fragment-length polymorphism PCR (AFLP), pulsed field gel electrophoresis (PFGE), random amplified polymorphic DNA (RAPD), rep-PCR (repetitive element primed PCR), REP-PCR (repetitive extragenic palindromic-PCR), ERIC-PCR (enterobacterial repetitive intergenic consensus sequences-PCR), BOX-PCR (derived from the boxA element) and ribotyping, provide information at or below the subspecies level [31]. Of these, AFLP and ribotyping are extremely useful and standardized.

It is unfortunate that with the increasing use of molecular methods, the description of bacterial groups has been often met with the use of minimal phenotypic data, which causes problems for diagnostics especially in laboratories, which are not equipped for molecular biology [6]. In these situations where distinguishing phenotypic feature have not been or could not be provided then the species should be referred to as a geno[mo] species. Nevertheless, molecular methods have revolutionized taxonomy, and led to the description of an increasing number of new taxa. The methodologies may be culture-independent, allowing for the study of uncultured organisms but there are issues with genomic fluidity [29]. «*Candidatus*" describes uncultured prokaryotes for which phylogenetic relationships have been determined, and authenticity confirmed by methods such as in situ probing [29].

Sequencing of the 16S rDNA is becoming an accepted procedure for the identification of fish pathogens, for example *V. harveyi*[49] and confirming its synonymy with *V. carchariae*[9, 10], and has been instrumental in the recognition of new pathogens, including *Streptococcus dysgalactiae*[50], *S. parauberis* (previously recognised as *S. uberis* genotype II; [51]) and *Vagococcus salmoninarum*[8, 52], and confirmed the presence of *Lactococcus garvieae* in Taiwan [53].

DNA:DNA and RNA:DNA hybridization, 16S RNA cataloguing, and 5S and 16S rRNA sequencing techniques have been used with increasing regularity and success. A review of PCR with emphasis on validation of the techniques and problems with diagnosis has been published [54]. PCR has been used successfully to identify hard-to-isolate fish pathogens, such as *Mycobacterium* spp. in sea bass (*Dicentrarchus labrax)*[55] and *M. chelonei* in a cichlid oscar *(Astronotus ocellatus)*[56]. Moreover, PCR has been useful with distinguishing different species from within the same genus, such as *Lactococcus garvieae* from *L. lactis*[57], from related genera, i.e. *L. garvieae, S. difficilis, S. iniae* and *S. parauberis*[58], and with an admirable level of specificity [59].

The sensitivity of PCR is clearly a positive attribute particularly with slow growing and/or nutritionally fastidious pathogens that are otherwise difficult to study in the laboratory. Of relevance, a PCR was developed [60, 61], which detected only 22 cells of *R. salmoninarum;* a sensitivity of 10 cells was reported by others [62]. Similarly, PCR detected only 10^2 colony forming units (CFU) of *N. seriolae* in yellowtail [63].

A recent development is multi locus sequence analysis (MLSA), which permits the genotypic examination of micro-organisms by comparison of the sequences of multiple, i.e. 12 or more, house-keeping genes. The benefit of using multiple genes is that the outputs are more informative and less likely to generate results that are distorted by recombination of single loci [29]. The resulting phylogenetic trees are capable of recognizing deeply branching clusters and permit the delineation of groups within a species or genus [64].

NEW SPECIES OF FISH PATHOGENS RECOGNIZED BY 16S RRNA SEQUENCING

16S rRNA sequencing has helped the description of fish pathogens where phenotypic characterization alone does not permit their incorporation in classifications. For example, a new disease of Atlantic salmon (*Salmo salar*) was linked to the *Streptobacillus moniliformis* and the fusobacteria group on the basis of sequence homology; biochemical traits did not permit identification [65]. The newly described cause of a mycobacteriosis in Chesapeake Bay (USA) striped bass *(Morone saxatilis)* was equated to a new species, *M. shottsii*, with confirmation by 16S rRNA sequence homology in which the pathogen was linked most closely to *M. marinum* and *M. ulcerans* (similarity = 99.2%) [30]. In one study, *M. gordonae* was identified by 16S rRNA sequencing [66]. Furthermore, phylogenetic analysis based on 16S rRNA gene sequencing together with partial sequences from the 65 kDa heat-shock protein (hsp65) and the beta-subunit of the bacterial RNA polymerase (*rpoB*) genes and the 16S-23S internal transcribed spacer 1 (ITS 1) region named other novel mycobacteria as *M. stomatepiae* and *M. barombii*[67].

During an examination of 16S rRNA sequences, two isolates of motile aeromonads from diseased elvers in Spain were described as a new species, *Aeromonas allosaccharophila*[68], albeit phenotypically heterogeneous [69]. This heterogenicity has caused problems for reliable phenotypic-based diagnoses.

Francisella became recognized as the cause of a new disease of Atlantic cod (*Gadus morhua*) in Norway in which the affected fish displayed white granuloma in the viscera and skin. Isolates were recovered, and determined to possess the key phenotypic characters of *Francisella*, viz. non-motile, strictly aerobic Gram-negative intracellular coccobacilli which produced H_2S from cysteine-containing media [70]. 16S rRNA sequencing revealed a 99.17% homology to *Francisella philomiragia*[71], although a slightly higher value of 99.3% was published [70] with the proposal for a new subspecies, i.e. *Francisella philomiragia* subsp. *noatunensis*, to accommodate the organisms. There was 92.2-99.0% homology with *Francisella philomiragia*housekeeping genes, *groEL, shdA, rpoB, rpoA, pgm* and *atpA*. A DNA:DNA hybridization of 68% was recorded between the fish pathogen and *Francisella philomiragia*[70].

Pasteurella skyensis was recovered from diseased Atlantic salmon in Scotland, linked to the family Pasteurellaceae by phenotypic analysis, and elevated to a new species largely as a result of 16S rRNA sequencing that identified the closest neighbour as *Pasteurella phocoenarum* (homology = 97.1%; [72]).

Piscirickettsia salmonis was named to accommodate isolates from diseased salmon in Chile, of which LF-89 was studied in detail [73] with 16S rRNA conforming to the gamma subdivision of the Proteobacteria with similarities to the family Rickettsiales, and in particular *Wolbachia persica* (similarity = 86.3%) and *Coxiella burnetii* (similarity = 87.5%) more than to representatives of *Ehrlichia, Rickettsia* or *Rochalimaea* leading to the description of a new genus and species [73]. Other rickettsias not conforming exactly with *Piscirickettia salmonis* have been described. For example, an organism recovered from white sea bass (*Atractascion nobilis*) was reported to have a 96.3-98.7% 16S rDNA homology with *Piscirickettsia salmonis*[74], which was considered by the authors to be too low for a confirmed identity. A Tasmanian isolate from Atlantic salmon was distinct from *Piscirickettsia* in terms of sequence alignment of the 16S rRNA, and for the present regarded as a rickettsial-like organism (RLO; [75]).

Pseudomonas plecoglossicida, the causal agent of bacterial ascites of ayu *(Plecoglossus altivelis)*, was described as a new species as a result of 16S rRNA gene sequence analysis confirming distinctiveness from *P. putida* biovar A. DNA:DNA hybridization confirmed the isolates to be a new centre of variation insofar as < 50% homology was recorded with other pseudomonads, including *P. putida*[76].

Streptococcus phocae was recognized as a cause of systemic disease in Atlantic salmon farmed in Chile. Phenotypic testing linked the pathogen with the streptococci, notably *Gemella*, but analysis of 16S rRNA genes provided a link to *S. phocae*[77].

Tenacibaculum soleae was recovered from diseased sole *(Solea senegalensis)* in Spain, and confirmed as a new species largely on account of 16S rRNA homology values of 94.8-96.7% with other members of the genus [78].

Two groups of bacteria were recovered from Atlantic salmon with winter ulcer disease/syndrome [79], of which one cluster was found to be closest to *Moritella marina* (43% re-association by DNA:DNA hybridization), and was named as *V. viscosus*. By 16S rDNA sequencing, the closest match was with *Moritella*[79] and *M. marina* (99.1% sequence homology) so that the organism was re-classified to *Moritella*, but as a new species, as *M. viscosa*[80], despite the high sequence homology [29]. Separately, 19 Icelandic and one Norwegian isolate from shallow skin lesions on Atlantic salmon, and the type strain of *V. marinus* NCIMB 1144 were identified as *V. marinus* after an examination of phenotypic data and analyses by numerical taxonomy [81]. On the basis of 16S rRNA sequencing, the species was transferred to *Moritella* as *M. marina*[82].

New and uncultured fish pathogens: " *Candidatus"*

Molecular techniques have permitted the recognition of uncultured pathogens belonging to new groupings for which the name of "*Candidatus*" has been used. "*Candidatus* arthromitus" has been recovered from rainbow trout (*Oncorhynchus mykiss*) with summer enteritic syndrome, which is a gastro-enteritis [83, 84]. The organism was observed in histological preparations to which nested polymerase chain reaction was used, with confirmation by sequencing [85]. "*Candidatus* piscichlamydia salmonis" was detected by RT-DGGE in intracellular inclusions, i.e. epitheliocysts, in Atlantic salmon with proliferative gill inflammation [86]. «*Candidatus* clavochlamydia salmonicola" is an intracellular organism, causing epitheliocystis in Atlantic salmon, which was recognized as novel as a result of 16S rRNA sequencing [87].

TAXONOMIC DEVELOPMENTS ASSOCIATED WITH SPECIFIC BACTERIAL FISH PATHOGENS

From the early literature, a question-mark has hung over the reliability of some bacterial names insofar as there was often negligible evidence to support the use of those names. Concern may also be expressed about the value of studies based on only single isolates where concern about the reasons for choice of the culture may be aired. Some of the controversy surrounding specific diseases/pathogens follows:

Motile aeromonas septicaemia

Aeromonas hydrophila (= *A. formicans* and *A. liquefaciens)* would appear to have worldwide distribution and to be a pathogen, causing motile aeromonas septicaemia, of many species of freshwater fish. Indeed, there are reports of a spread into marine fish, notably ulcer disease of cod [88]. Since its initial recognition in the literature, a wealth of knowledge has been accumulated about many facets of its biology (see [6]). A new variant *A. hydrophila* subsp. *dhakenis*, which was originally recovered from children with diarrhoeae in Bangladesh, was determined to be pathogenic to rainbow trout [89]. However overall, there has been some doubt about the role of *A. hydrophila* as a pathogen, and in some cases it may well be present in fish tissue only as a secondary invader [6]. Moreover with developments in the taxonomy of motile aeromonads [90], the accuracy of some of the early published identifications may be justifiably questioned. Could other motile aeromonads be associated with fish disease and may have been confused previously with *A. hydrophila*[89]?

It is clear that there is phenotypic, serological and genotypic heterogeneity within the descriptions of fish pathogenic *A. hydrophila* [e.g. 91, 92], and other motile aeromonads have been implicated as the aetiological agents of (fish) diseases. Thus, 8 isolates reported as pathogenic to eel in Spain were identified by numerical taxonomy as *A. jandaei*[93, 94]. Certainly, the current approach of allocating species names as a result of the examination of 16S rRNA gene sequences has encompassed fish pathogenic motile aeromonads. For example, isolates from diseased fish which were recovered in *Aeromonas* DNA Hybridization Group 2 (= *A. hydrophila)* were equated with a new group, *A. bestiarum*[95]. Subsequently, *A. sobria* (*A. sobria* biovar sobria and *A. veronii* biovar sobria were reported as pathogenic to rainbow trout [89]. Indeed, *A. sobria* has been previously found to have a role as a fish pathogen, with isolates recovered from wild spawning gizzard shad (*Dorosoma cepedianum)* in Maryland, USA during 1987 [15, 96]. Also, *A. veronii* has been recovered from Siberian sturgeon (*Acipenser baerii*) with identification of the pathogen resulting from phenotyping and 16S rRNA gene sequencing [97].

Aeromonas salmonicida

Aeromonas salmonicida is one of the oldest described fish pathogens, being isolated initially from diseased hatchery-maintained brown trout (*Salmo trutta*) in Germany, and named as "Bacillus der Forellenseuche" or bacillus of trout contagious disease. The history of the organism reveals a plethora of synonyms including *Bacillus devorans*, *Bacterium salmonica*, *Bacterium salmonicida*, *Bacillus truttae* and *Bacillus salmonicida*[6]. The 7th edition of *Bergey's Manual of Determinative Bacteriology* (1957) placed the pathogen in the genus *Aeromonas* within the family Pseudomonadaceae [98]. Later, there was a transfer to the family Vibrionaceae and subsequently to its own family, i.e. the Aeromonadaceae [99]. Re-classification was based primarily on phenotyping [100]. Thus in 1953, the first detailed description of the pathogen was published, and from an examination of 10 isolates, it was concluded that *Bacterium salmonicida* was homogeneous in cultural and biochemical characteristics [100]. Numerous studies have addressed the homogeneity of the species (e.g. [101]). The basic description is of an organism, which comprises non-motile (motility and *flaA* and *flaB* flagellar genes have been reported [52, 82]), fermentative, Gram-negative rods, which produce a brown water-soluble pigment on tryptone-containing agar, do not grow at 37°C, and produce catalase and oxidase [6]. Cultures have the ability to dissociate into rough, smooth and G-phase (= intermediate) colonies [102]. The pathogen has spread from its dominance in salmonids to cyprinids and marine flatfish [6]. An ongoing issue surrounds the intraspecies structure, i.e. the validity of subspecies *achromogenes, masoucida, pectinolytica, salmonicida*and *smithia*, and the status of so-called atypical isolates.

A. salmonicida subsp. *salmonicida*, isolates of which have been obtained almost exclusively from outbreaks of furunculosis in salmonids, is regarded as homogeneous, and is referred to as "typical" [103]; all other isolates are considered as heterogeneous and "atypical" [6]. So called atypical strains may demonstrate weak, slow or non-pigment production [104, 105], catalase [106] or oxidase-negativity [e.g. 106, 107], nutritional fastidiousness for blood products [108], slow growth, i.e. ≥ 5 days compared with 1-2 days for typical isolates [106, 108], and be pathogenic for fish other than salmonids, e.g. cyprinids (e.g. [106, 108, 109]) and marine flatfish, namely dab (*Limanda limanda*), plaice (*Pleuronectes platessa*), flounder (*Platichthys flesus*) and turbot (*Scophthalmus maximus*) [110, 111, 112], and cause ulceration rather than furunculosis [6, 113]. The deviation in characteristics from the typical to atypical isolates has made typing difficult [114, 115, 116]. Even 16S rDNA sequencing has not helped with the clustering of atypical forms (e.g. [117]).

Smith [118] recognized heterogeneity in the species description of *A. salmonicida*. She examined six isolates of non-pigmented *A. salmonicida*, which were clustered as Group I in her numerical taxonomy study, for which a separate new species name was proposed, i.e. *A. achromogenes*, but the proposal was not adopted widely. A second non-pigmented group was described by Kimura [119], and named as *A. salmonicida* subsp. *masoucida*. Schubert [120] considered these non-pigmented isolates as subspecies, and coined the names of *A. salmonicida* subsp. *achromogenes* and *A. salmonicida* subsp. *masoucida*, respectively. Pigmented strains (= typical) were classified as *A. salmonicida* subsp. *salmonicida*[120]. The precise relationship of the subspecies has been the subject of detailed discussion. In particular, it was contended that subsp. *achromogenes* and *masoucida* were more closely related to *A. hydrophila* than to *A. salmonicida*[121]. Later, it was mooted that subsp. *masoucida* bridged typical *A. salmonicida* and *A. hydrophila*[122]. Yet, *A. salmonicida* subsp. *masoucida* is non-motile, sensitive to *A. salmonicida* bacteriophages, possesses an antigenic profile specific to *A. salmonicida*, and shares a DNA homology of 103% with *A. salmonicida*[92]. By PCR, a combination of *achromogenes* with *masoucida* could be justified, but this was not substantiated by ribotyping and RAPD analyses [114]. Phenotypic data suggest a case for combining subsp. *masoucida* with *salmonicida*, and subsp. *achromogenes* with *Haemophilus piscium*, which is the causal agent of ulcer disease of trout [123]. Examination of the small subunit rRNA gene sequences revealed 99.9% homology of an authentic strain of *H. piscium* with *A. salmonicida* subsp. *salmonicida*[124]. So far, the comparative uniqueness of subsp. *smithia*has been indicated from several studies (e.g. [114]). The complication is with aberrant strains of *A. salmonicida* from fish species other than salmonids.

DNA homology was used to reveal that all isolates of *A. salmonicida* (including *A. salmonicida* subsp. *masoucida)* were highly related, i.e. 96-106% homology, when hybridized against *A. salmonicida* subsp. *salmonicida*[92]. It was opined that *A. salmonicida* subsp. *masoucida* and some atypical isolates did not warrant separate subspecies status, because they were regarded as variants of other well-recognized groups. Also as a result of genotypic analyses, it was reported that typical and atypical isolates of *A. salmonicida* were very closely related, with minimal divergence [125]. Using DNA:DNA re-association, it was concluded that typical *A. salmonicida* were recovered in a homogeneous group, whereas the atypical representatives were more diverse [126]. From numerical taxonomy and DNA:DNA hybridization, similar conclusions resulted regarding the homogeneity of typical isolates of *A. salmonicida*[101]. However using 16S rRNA sequencing techniques, it was reported that subspecies *achromogenes* and *masoucida* were indistinguishable, and only differed from subspecies *salmonicida* by two bases [68].

The relation of *A. salmonicida* to other aeromonads has been discussed. Eddy [127] focused on the inability of *A. salmonicida* to produce 2,3-butanediol from glucose, and the absence of motility, which were in contrast to the genus description [128]. A new genus, i.e. *Necromonas*, was proposed with two species, namely *N. salmonicida* for the typical isolates and *N. achromogenes* for the non-pigmented strains [118]. This proposal was not formally widely accepted, although Cowan [129] used the suggestion in his landmark identification scheme for medically important bacteria. Subsequent serological and bacteriophage sensitivity data supported the relationship between *A. salmonicida* and the motile aeromonads. Common antigens between *A. hydrophila* and *A. salmonicida* subsp. *masoucida* and other isolates of *A. salmonicida* were reported [122, 130]. Furthermore, serological cross-reactions between *A. salmonicida* and motile aeromonads were discussed [131]. Moreover, *A. hydrophila* cultures were found to be sensitive to *A. salmonicida* bacteriophages [132, 133]. The outcome of all the studies is that DNA homology supports the classification of *A. salmonicida*in the genus *Aeromonas* (e.g. [92, 122, 126]).

There are certainly outstanding questions about the validity and taxonomic placing of *Haemophilus piscium*[123], but an authentic reference strain was not deposited any in any recognized culture collection at the time of its first isolation. Later, it was concluded that the organism was not a *bona fide Haemophilus*because of the lack of requirement for haemin or NAD [134]. In particular *H. piscium* differed from the type species of the genus, *H. influenzae*, in the inability to reduce nitrate or alkaline phosphatase and to grow at 37°C, in conjunction with a higher G+C ratio of the DNA. It was commented that there was only a low similarity between *H. piscium* and other *Haemophilus* spp. in a numerical taxonomic study [135]. A link with atypical, achromogenic *A. salmonicida* was made [122]. This link was reinforced by bacteriophage sensitivity, when it was concluded that *H. piscium* is an atypical *A. salmonicida*[136]. Other workers have supported this view (e.g. [114]). However with the absence of an authentic, original type strain, the definitive taxonomic position of *H. piscium* is only speculative.

A lack of congruence has been reported between the results of molecular (PCR, RAPD and ribotyping) and phenotypic methods in taxonomy of aeromonads [114]. Moreover, there are problems of inter-laboratory differences and lack of standardisation in test methods [137]. The outcome is that the definitive classification of *A. salmonicida* has not been achieved, to date.

Enteric redmouth (ERM)

There has been discussion about the taxonomic position of the aetiological agent of ERM. Strong agglutination with *Salmonella enterica* subsp *arizonae* O group 26, and a weak reaction with O group 29 was reported [138]. In addition, biochemical similarities with enterics, notably *Enterobacter liquefaciens, Serratia marcescens*subsp. *kiliensis* as well as *Salmonella enterica* subsp. *arizonae* were mentioned [138]. Serological cross-reactions were also recorded with *Hafnia alvei*[139]. Nevertheless, a new species, i.e. *Yersinia ruckeri* was described although there was only a 30-31% DNA homology with *Y. enterocolitica* and *Y. pseudotuberculosis*[140]. This compares to DNA homologies of 24-28% and 31% with *Serratia marcescens*and *Serratia liquefaciens*, respectively [141]. Indeed, it has been suggested that the causal agent of ERM should belong in a new genus of the Enterobacteriaceae [142]. A complication developed when a new non-motile form of the pathogen was recovered from rainbow trout. By 16S rRNA sequencing and a homology of 100%, the organisms were linked to *Y. ruckeri* but regarded as a new biogroup [143]. Similar non-motile variants were also recovered from previously vaccinated rainbow trout in Spain [144].

Vibriosis

The causal agent of "red-pest" in eels was first designated as *Bacterium anguillarum*[6]. Subsequently, an outbreak among eels in Sweden led to the use of the name *Vibrio anguillarum*. Numerous studies have pointed to heterogeneity in *V. anguillarum* initially with the delineation of two sub-groupings/ biotypes (e.g. [12]). This increased to 3 [145] and then 4 sub-groups/phena within the species definition [146, 147]. Ribotyping has confirmed the heterogeneity [148], although a single taxon, homogeneous by ribotyping but heterogeneous by LPS profiles, plasmid composition, serogrouping, and BIOLOG-GN fingerprints and API 20E profiles was described [149, 150]. Biotype II became recognized as a separate species, i.e. *V. ordalii*[151], which is homogeneous by plasmid profiling, ribotyping and serogrouping, accommodates two LPS groups, but is heterogeneous by BIOLOG-GN fingerprints and API 20E profiles [150].

Serology has been widely used for diagnosis, but has complicated the understanding of *V. anguillarum*[151], and the establishment of serotypes has to some extent traversed species boundaries. With *V. anguillarum*, serogroup 02 and 05, there are common antigens with *V. ordalii*[152] and *V. harveyi*[149], respectively. Initially, three serotypes were recognised for isolates from salmonids from the northwest USA, Europe, and the Pacific-northwest (USA) [103]. This number increased to 6 [128], and then 10 [153] and upwards [148, 154]. Serogroup O1 dominates the number of isolates available for study and the relative importance to fish pathology [149, 155, 156, 157]. Serogroup O2 has been further subdivided into serogroup O2a and O2b [158].

V. anguillarum was re-classified initially to *Beneckea*[12] and then to a newly proposed genus *Listonella*[13], but the changes were not widely accepted.

THE ROLE OF PHYLOGENETICS IN BACTERIAL FISH PATHOLOGY

The techniques described above are relevant for the taxonomy of bacterial fish pathogens. Yet, molecular methods, namely sequencing of the 16S rRNA gene, permit the study of evolutionary relationships, i.e. phylogenetics, which may be viewed as phylogenetic trees, which are interpreted by cladistics and used in defining taxa. The approach is essential in the study of the evolutionary tree of life, but is it strictly necessary for fish pathology and the recognition of species? One concern is the comparative fluidity by which genes may be exchanged, such as by horizontal gene transfer, and the impact of this movement on the outcome of the taxonomic/ phylogenetic process.

CONCLUSIONS

There has been a resurgence of interest in bacterial taxonomy partially because of the current focus on biodiversity and the development of reliable molecular methods [159], notably 16S rRNA sequencing. Undoubtedly, these molecular approaches have led to greater confidence and accuracy in the reporting of bacterial names. Nevertheless, it is conceded that bacterial taxonomy is a specialist subject, which is not of interest to all fish pathologists. However, it cannot be overstated that there is a real value for good taxonomy as a means of communication. In terms of fish pathology, taxonomy enables the recognition of new pathogens, improvements in the understanding of relationships between taxa, an appreciation of variation within existing nomenspecies including the recognition of new subspecies and biogroups, and facilitates accurate commentary about all aspects of biology from epizootiology to pathogenicity (e.g. [160]), although the position of so-called atypical isolates in taxonomic hierarchies is often difficult to determine [161].

For the future, a range of new techniques, including in situ hybridization, probe hybridization, microarray techniques and restriction enzyme digestion, are entering taxonomic use, and are likely to be used in fish pathology. The impact of these new approaches is difficult to predict, but will undoubtedly be incorporated in some fish bacteriology laboratories.

REFERENCES

1. Sneath PHA: The application of computers to taxonomy. J Gen Microbiol. 1957, 17: 201-226.
2. Sokal RR, Michener CD: Numerical Taxonomy. 1958, WH Freeman, London
3. Arakawa CK, Fryer JL: Isolation and characterization of a new subspecies of *Mycobacterium chelonei* infections for salmonid fish. Helgoländer Meeresuntersuch. 1984, 37: 329-342.
4. Brennan PJ: *Mycobacterium* and other actinomycetes. Microbial Lipids. Edited by: Ratledge C, Wilkinson SG. 1988, Academic Press, London, 1: 203-298.
5. Kämpfer P: The characterization of prokaryote strains for taxonomic purposes. Int J Syst Evol Microbiol. 2010, 60: 7-10.1099/ijs.0.020768-0.
6. Austin B, Austin DA: Bacterial Fish Pathogens: Disease in Farmed and Wild Fish. 2007, Springer-Praxis, Goldalming, 4
7. Schiewe MH, Trust TJ, Crosa JH: *Vibrio ordalii* sp. nov.: a causative agent of vibriosis in fish. Curr Microbiol. 1981, 6: 343-348. 10.1007/BF01567009.
8. Schmidtke LM, Carson J: Characteristics of *Vagococcus salmoninarum* isolated from diseased salmonid fish. J Appl Bacteriol. 1994, 77: 229-236.
9. Gauger E, Gómez-Chiarri M: 16S ribosomal DNA sequencing confirms the synonymy of *Vibrio harveyi* and *V. carchariae*. Dis Aquat Org. 2002, 52: 39-46. 10.3354/dao052039.
10. Pedersen K, Verdonck L, Austin B, Austin DA, Blanch AR, Grimont PAD, Jofre J, Koblavi S, Larsen JL, Tiainen T, Vigneulle M, Swings J: Taxonomic evidence that *Vibrio carchariae* Grimes et al. 1985 is a junior synonym of *Vibrio harveyi* (Johnson and Shunk 1936) Baumann et al. 1981. Int J Syst Bacteriol. 1998, 48: 749-758. 10.1099/00207713-48-3-749.
11. Thompson FL, Hoste B, Vandemeulebroecke K, Engelbeen K, Denys R, Swings J: *Vibrio trachuri* Iwamoto et al., 1995 is a junior synonym of *Vibrio harveyi* (Johnson and Shunk 1936) Baumann et al. 1981. Int J Syst Evol Microbiol. 2002, 52: 973-976. 10.1099/ijs.0.02046-0.
12. Baumann P, Bang SS, Baumann L: Phenotypic characterization of *Beneckea anguillara* biotypes I and II. Curr Microbiol. 1978, 1: 85-88. 10.1007/BF02605421.
13. MacDonell MT, Colwell RR: Phylogeny of the Vibrionaceae and recommendations for two new genera, *Listonella* and *Shewanella*. Syst Appl Microbiol. 1985, 6: 171-182.
14. Vandamme P, Pot B, Gillis M, de Vos P, Kersters K, Swings J: Polyphasic taxonomy, a consensus approach to bacterial systematics. Microbiol Rev. 1996, 60: 407-438.
15. Toranzo AE, Santos Y, Nieto TP, Barja JL: Evaluation of different assay systems for identification of environmental *Aeromonas* strains. Appl Environ Microbiol. 1986, 51: 652-656.
16. Sneath PHA, Johnson R: The influence of numerical taxonomic similarities of errors in microbiological tests. J Gen Microbiol. 1972, 72: 377-392.
17. Austin B, Embley TM, Goodfellow M: Selective isolation of *Renibacterium salmoninarum*. FEMS Microbiol Lett. 1983, 17: 111-114. 10.1111/j.1574-6968.1983.tb00383.x.
18. Walters GR, Plumb JA: Modified oxidation/fermentation medium for use in the identification of bacterial fish pathogens. J Fish Res Bd Can. 1978, 35: 1629-1630. 10.1139/f78-253.
19. Adams A, Thompson KD: Recent applications of biotechnology to novel diagnostics for aquatic animals. Rev Sci Tech. 2008, 27: 197-209.
20. Goerlich R, Schlüsener HJ, Lehmann J, Greuel E: The application of monoclonal antibodies to diagnosis of *Aeromonas salmonicida* infections in fishes. Bull Europ Assoc Fish Pathol. 1984, 4: 66-
21. Jung TS, Thompson KD, Adams A, Morris DJ, Snedden K: The production of monoclonal antibodies against *Photobacterium damselae* subsp. *piscicida* and their application in immunohistochemistry. J Fish Dis. 2001, 24: 64-67. 10.1046/j.1365-2761.2001.00260.x.
22. Steiropoulos NA, Yuksel SA, Thompson KD, Adams A, Ferguson HW: Detection of *Rickettsia*-like organisms (RLOs) in European sea bass *(Dicentrarchus labrax*, L) by immunohistochemistry, using rabbit anti-*Rickettsia salmonis* serum. Bull Eur Assoc Fish Pathol. 2002, 22: 428-432.
23. Adams A, Thompson KD, Morris D, Farias C, Chen SC: Development and use of monoclonal antibody probes for immunohistochemistry, ELISA and IFAT to detect bacterial and parasitic fish pathogens. Fish Shellfish Immunol. 1995, 5: 537-547. 10.1016/S1050-4648(95)80040-9.
24. Klesius P, Evans J, Shoemaker C, Yeh H, Goodwin AE, Adams A, Thompson KD: Rapid detection and identification of *Streptococcus iniae* using a monoclonal antibody-based indirect fluorescent antibody technique. Aquaculture. 2005, 258: 180-186. 10.1016/j.aquaculture.2005.06.040.

25. Adams A: Advances in disease diagnosis, vaccine development and other emerging methods to control pathogens. Edited by: Burnell G, Allan G. 2009, New Technologies in Aquaculture, Improving Production, Efficiency, Quality and Environmental Management, Woodhead, England, Chapter 7: 197-211.

26. Saeed MO, Plumb JA: Serological detection of *Edwardsiella ictaluri* Hawke lipopolysaccharide antibody in serum of channel catfish *Ictalurus punctatus* Rafinesque. J Fish Dis. 1987, 10: 205-209. 10.1111/j.1365-2761.1987.tb01062.x.

27. Adkinson MA, Gilad O, Hedricks RP: An enzyme linked immunosorbent assay (ELISA) for detection of antibodies to the Koi herpes virus (KHV) in the serum of Koi *Cyprinus carpio*. Fish Pathol. 2005, 40: 53-62. 10.3147/jsfp.40.53.

28. Mayer H, Masoud H, Urbanik-Sypniewska T, Weckesser J: Lipid A composition and phylogeny of Gram-negative bacteria. Bull Jap Fed Cult Collect. 1989, 5: 19-25.

29. Scheifer KH: Classification of bacteria and Archaea: past, present and future. Syst Appl Microbiol. 2009, 32: 533-542. 10.1016/j.syapm.2009.09.002.

30. Rhodes MW, Kator H, Kotob S, van Berkum P, Kaattari I, Vogelbein W, Quinn F, Floyd MM, Butler WR, Ottinger CA: *Mycobacterium shottsii* sp nov., a slowly growing species isolated from Chesapeake Bay striped bass (*Morone saxatilis)*. Int J Syst Evol Microbiol. 2003, 53: 421-424. 10.1099/ijs.0.02299-0.

31. Tindall BJ, Rosselló-Móra R, Busse HJ, Ludwig W, Kämpfer P: Notes on the characterization of prokaryote strains for taxonomic purposes. Int J Syst Evol Microbiol. 2010, 60: 249-266. 10.1099/ijs.0.016949-0.

32. Williams AM, Fryer JL, Collins MD: *Lactococcus piscium* sp. nov. a new *Lactococcus* species from salmonid fish. FEMS Microbiol Lett. 1990, 68: 109-114. 10.1111/j.1574-6968.1990.tb04132.x.

33. Backman S, Ferguson HW, Prescott JF, Wilcock BP: Progressive panophthalmitis in chinook salmon, *Oncorhynchus tshawytscha* (Walbaum): a case report. J Fish Dis. 1990, 13: 345-353. 10.1111/j.1365-2761.1990.tb00793.x.

34. Isik K, Chun J, Hah YC, Goodfellow M: *Nocardia salmonicida* nom. rev., a fish pathogen. Int J Syst Bacteriol. 1999, 49: 833-837. 10.1099/00207713-49-2-833.

35. Fiedler F, Draxl R: Biochemical and immunochemical properties of the cell surface of *Renibacterium salmoninarum*. J Bacteriol. 1986, 168: 799-804.

36. Sanders JE, Fryer JL: *Renibacterium salmoninarum* gen. nov., sp. nov., the causative agent of bacterial kidney disease in salmonid fishes. Int J Syst Bacteriol. 1980, 30: 496-502. 10.1099/00207713-30-2-496.

37. Embley TM, Goodfellow M, Minnikin DE, Austin B: Fatty acid, isoprenoid quinone and polar lipid composition in the classification of *Renibacterium salmoninarum*. J Appl Bacteriol. 1983, 55: 31-37.

38. Fox GE, Pechman KR, Woese CR: Comparative cataloging of 16S ribosomal ribonucleic acid: molecular approach to procaryotic systematics. Int J Syst Bacteriol. 1977, 27: 44-57. 10.1099/00207713-27-1-44.

39. Lane DJ, Field KG, Olsen GJ, Pace NR: Reverse transcriptase sequencing of ribosomal RNA for phylogenetic analysis. Meth Enzymol. 1988, 167: 138-144. full_text.

40. Sanger F, Nicklen S, Coulson AR: DNA sequencing with chain-terminating inhibitors. Proc Natl Acad Sci USA. 1977, 74: 5463-5467. 10.1073/pnas.74.12.5463.

41. Saiki RK, Gelfand DH, Stoffel S, Scharf SJ, Higuchi R, Horn GT, Mullis KB, Erlich HA: Primer-directed enzymatic amplification of DNA with a thermostable DNA polymerase. Science. 1988, 239: 487-491. 10.1126/science.2448875.

42. De Ley J, Park IW, Tijtgat R, van Ermengem J: DNA homology and taxonomy of *Pseudomonas* and *Xanthomonas*. J Gen Microbiol. 1966, 42: 43-56.

43. Fox GE, Wisotzkey JD, Jurtshuk P: How close is close: 16S rRNA sequence identity may not be sufficient to guarantee species identity. Int J Syst Bacteriol. 1992, 42: 166-170. 10.1099/00207713-42-1-166.

44. Kvitt H, Colorni A: Strain variation and geographic endemism in *Streptococcus iniae*. Dis Aquat Org. 2004, 61: 67-73. 10.3354/dao061067.

45. Gauthier G, Lafay B, Ruimy R, Breittmayer V, Nicolas JL, Gauthier M, Christen R: Small-subunit rRNA sequences and whole DNA relatedness concur for the re-assignment of *Pasteurella piscicida* (Snieszko et al.) Janssen and Surgalla to the genus *Photobacterium* as *Photobacterium damsela* subsp. *piscicida* comb. nov. Int J Syst Bacteriol. 1995, 45: 139-144. 10.1099/00207713-45-1-139.

46. Gutenberger SK, Giovannoni SJ, Field KG, Fryer JL, Rohovec JS: A phylogenetic comparison of the 16S rRNA sequence of the fish pathogen, *Renibacterium salmoninarum*, to Gram-positive bacteria. FEMS Microbiol Lett. 1991, 77: 151-156. 10.1111/j.1574-6968.1991.tb04339.x.

47. Stackebrandt E, Wehmeyer U, Nader H, Fiedler F: Phylogenetic relationship of the fish pathogenic *Renibacterium salmoninarum* to *Arthrobacter, Micrococcus* and related taxa. FEMS Microbiol Lett. 1988, 50: 117-120. 10.1111/j.1574-6968.1988.tb02922.x.

48. Wiens GD, Rockey DD, Wu ZN, Chang J, Levy R, Crane S, Chen DS, Capri GR, Burnett JR, Sudheesh PS, Schipma MJ, Burd H, Bhattacharyya A, Rhodes LD, Kaul R, Strom MS: Genome sequence of the fish pathogen *Renibacterium salmoninarum* suggests reductive evolution away from an environmental *Arthrobacter* ancestor. J Bacteriol. 2008, 190: 6970-6982. 10.1128/JB.00721-08.

49. Ransangan J, Mustafa S: Identification of *Vibrio harveyi* isolated from diseased Asian sea bass *Lates calcarifer* by use of 16S ribosomal DNA sequencing. J Aquat Anim Health. 2009, 21: 150-155. 10.1577/H09-002.1.

50. Nomoto R, Munasinghe LI, Shimahara Y, Yasuda H, Nakamura A, Misawa N, Itami T, Yoshida T: Lancefield group C *Streptococcus dysgalactiae* infection responsible

for fish mortalities in Japan. J Fish Dis. 2004, 27: 679-686. 10.1111/j.1365-2761.2004.00591.x.

51. Doménech A, Fernández-Garayzábal JF, Pascual C, Garcia JA, Cutuli MT, Moreno MA, Collins MD, Dominguez L: Streptococcosis in cultured turbot, *Scophthalmus maximus* (L.), associated with *Streptococcus parauberis*. J Fish Dis. 1996, 19: 33-38. 10.1111/j.1365-2761.1996.tb00117.x.

52. Wallbanks S, Martinez-Murcia AJ, Fryer JL, Phillips BA, Collins MD: 16S rRNA sequence determination for members of the genus *Carnobacterium* and related lactic acid bacteria and description of *Vagococcus salmoninarum* sp. nov. Int J Syst Bacteriol. 1990, 40: 224-230. 10.1099/00207713-40-3-224.

53. Chen SC, Liaw LL, Su HY, Ko SC, Wu CY, Chaung HC, Tsai YH, Yang KL, Chen YC, Chen TH, Lin GR, Cheng SY, Lin YD, Lee JL, Lai CC, Weng YJ, Chu SY: *Lactococcus garvieae*, a cause of disease in grey mullet, *Mugil cephalus* L., in Taiwan. J Fish Dis. 2002, 25: 727-732. 10.1046/j.1365-2761.2002.00415.x.

54. Hiney MP, Smith PR: Validation of polymerase chain reaction-based techniques for proxy detection of bacterial fish pathogens: framework, problems and possible solutions for environmental applications. Aquaculture. 1998, 162: 41-68. 10.1016/S0044-8486(98)00207-5.

55. Knibb W, Colorni A, Ankaoua M, Lindell D, Diamant A, Gordin H: Detection and identification of a pathogenic marine mycobacterium from the European seabass *Dicentrarchus labrax* using polymerase chain reaction and direct sequencing of 16S rRNA sequences. Mol Mar Biol Biotechnol. 1993, 2: 225-232.

56. McCormick JI, Hughes MS, McLoughlin MF: Identification of *Mycobacterium chelonae* in a cichlid oscar *Astronotus ocellatus* Cuvier, by direct cycle sequencing of polymerase chain reaction amplified 16S rRNA gene sequences. J Fish Dis. 1995, 18: 459-461. 10.1111/j.1365-2761.1995.tb00337.x.

57. Zlotkin A, Eldar A, Ghittino C, Bercovier H: Identification of *Lactococcus garvieae* by PCR. J Clin Microbiol. 1998, 36: 983-985.

58. Mata AI, Gibello A, Casamayor A, Blanco MM, Domínquez L, Fernández-Garayzábal JF: Multiplex PCR assay for the detection of bacterial pathogens associated with warm-water streptococcosis in fish. Appl Environ Microbiol. 2004, 70: 3183-3187. 10.1128/AEM.70.5.3183-3187.2004.

59. Aoki T, Park CI, Yamashita H, Hirono I: Species-specific polymerase chain reaction primers for *Lactococcus garvieae*. J Fish Dis. 2000, 23: 1-6. 10.1046/j.1365-2761.2000.00207.x.

60. León G, Maulén N, Figueroa J, Villanueva J, Rodríguez C, Vera MI, Krauskopf M: A PCR based assay for the identification of the fish pathogen *Renibacterium salmoninarum*. FEMS Microbiol Lett. 1994, 115: 131-136.

61. León G, Martinez MA, Etchegaray JP, Vera MI, Figueroa J, Krauskopf M: Specific DNA probes for the identification of the fish pathogen, *Renibacterium salmoninarum*. Wld J Microbiol Biotechnol. 1994, 10: 149-153. 10.1007/BF00360876.

62. Magnüssen HB, Fridjónsson ÓH, Andrésson ÓS, Benediktsdóttir E, Gudmundsdóttir S, Andrésdottír V: *Renibacterium salmoninarum*, the causal agent of bacterial kidney disease in salmonid fish, detected by nested reverse transcription-PCR of 16S rRNA sequences. Appl Environ Microbiol. 1994, 60: 4580-4583.

63. Miyoshi Y, Suzuki S: PCR method to detect *Nocardia seriolae* in fish samples. Fish Pathol. 2003, 38: 93-97. 10.3147/jsfp.38.93.

64. Soria-Carrasco V, Talavera G, Igea J, Castresana J: The K tree score: quantification of differences in the relative branch length and topology of phylogenetic trees. Bioinformatics. 2007, 23: 2954-2956. 10.1093/bioinformatics/btm466.

65. Maher M, Palmer R, Gannon F, Smith T: Relationship of a novel bacterial fish pathogen to *Streptobacillus moniliformis*and the fusobacteria group, based on 16S ribosomal RNA analysis. Syst Appl Microbiol. 1995, 18: 79-84.

66. Sakai M, Konno T, Tassakka ACMAR, Ponpornpisit A, Areechon N, Katagiri T, Yoshida T, Endo M: Characterization of a *Mycobacterium* sp. isolated from guppy *Poecilia reticulata*, using 16S ribosomal RNA and its internal transcribed spacer sequences. Bull Eur Assoc Fish Pathol. 2005, 25: 64-69.

67. Pourahmad F, Cervellione F, Thompson KD, Taggart JB, Adams A, Richards RH: *Mycobacterium stomatepiae* sp. nov., a slowly growing non-chromogenic species isolated from fish. Int J Syst Evol Microbiol. 2008, 58: 2821-2827. 10.1099/ijs.0.2008/001164-0.

68. Martinez-Murcia AJ, Esteve C, Garay E, Collins MD: *Aeromonas allosaccharophila* sp. nov., a new mesophilic member of the genus *Aeromonas*. FEMS Microbiol Lett. 1992, 91: 199-206. 10.1111/j.1574-6968.1992.tb05209.x.

69. Huys G, Kämpfer P, Swings J: New DNA-DNA hybridization and phenotypic data on the species *Aeromonas ichthiosmia*and *Aeromonas allosaccharophila*: A. *ichthiosmia is a later synonym of A. veronii* Hickman-Brenner et al. 1987. Syst Appl Microbiol. 2001, 24: 177-182. 10.1078/0723-2020-00038.

70. Mikalsen J, Olsen AB, Tengs T, Colquohoun DJ: *Francisella philomiragia* subsp *noatunensis* subsp nov., isolated from farmed Atlantic cod (*Gadus morhua* L.). Int J Syst Evol Microbiol. 2007, 57: 1960-1965. 10.1099/ijs.0.64765-0.

71. Nylund A, Ottem KF, Watanabe K, Karlsbakk E, Krossoy B: *Francisella* sp (Family Francisellaceae) causing mortality in Norwegian cod *(Gadus morhua)* farming. Arch Microbiol. 2006, 185: 383-392. 10.1007/s00203-006-0109-5.

72. Birkbeck TH, Laidler LA, Grant AN, Cox DI: *Pasteurella skyensis* sp nov., isolated from Atlantic salmon *(Salmo salar* L.). Int J Syst Evol Microbiol. 2002, 52: 699-704. 10.1099/ijs.0.01884-0.

73. Fryer JL, Lannan CN, Giovannoni SJ, Wood ND: *Piscirickettsia salmonis* gen. nov., the causative agent of an epizootic disease in salmonid fishes. Int J Syst Bacteriol. 1992, 42: 120-126. 10.1099/00207713-42-1-120.

74. Arkush KD, Mcbride AM, Mendonca HL, Okihiro MS, Andree KB, Marshall S, Henriquez V, Hedrick RP: Genetic characterization and experimental pathogenesis of *Piscirickettsia salmonis* isolated from white seabass *Atractascion nobilis*. Dis Aquat Org. 2005, 63: 139-149. 10.3354/dao063139.

75. Corbeil S, Hyatt AD, Crane MStJ: Characterisation of an emerging rickettsia-like organism in Tasmanian farmed Atlantic salmon *Salmo salar*. Dis Aquat Org. 2005, 64: 37-44. 10.3354/dao064037.

76. Nishimori E, Kita-Tsukamoto K, Wakabayashi H: *Pseudomonas plecoglossicida* sp nov., the causative agent of bacterial haemorrhagic ascites of ayu, *Plecoglossus altivelis*. Int J Syst Evol Microbiol. 2000, 50: 83-89. 10.1099/00207713-50-1-83.

77. Romalde JL, Ravelo C, Valdes I, Magariños B, de la Fuente E, Martin CS, Avendano-Herrera R, Toranzo AE: *Streptococcus phocae*, an emerging pathogen for salmonid culture. Vet Microbiol. 2008, 130: 198-207. 10.1016/j.vetmic.2007.12.021.

78. Pineiro-Vidal M, Carballas C, Gomez-Barreiro O, Riaza A, Santos Y: *Tenacibaculum soleae* sp nov., isolated from diseased sole *(Soleae senegalensis* Kaup). Int J Syst Evol Microbiol. 2008, 58: 881-885. 10.1099/ijs.0.65539-0.

79. Lunder T, Sorum H, Holstad G, Steigerwalt AG, Mowinckel P, Brenner DJ: Phenotypic and genotypic characterization of *Vibrio viscosus* sp nov and *Vibrio wodanis* sp nov isolated from Atlantic salmon *(Salmo salar)* with "winter ulcer". Int J Syst Evol Microbiol. 2000, 50: 427-450. 10.1099/00207713-50-2-427.

80. Benediktsdóttir E, Verdonck L, Spröer C, Helgason S, Swings J: Characterization of *Vibrio viscosus* and *Vibrio wodanis*isolated from different geographical locations: a proposal for re-classification of *Vibrio viscosus* as *Moritella viscose*comb. nov. Int J Syst Evol Microbiol. 2000, 50: 479-488. 10.1099/00207713-50-2-479.

81. Benediktsdóttir E, Helgason S, Sigurjónsdóttir H: *Vibrio* spp. isolated from salmonids with shallow skin lesions and reared at low temperature. J Fish Dis. 1988, 21: 19-28.

82. Urakawa H, Kita-Tsukamoto K, Stevens SE, Ohwada K, Colwell RR: A proposal to transfer *Vibrio marinus* (Russell 1891) to a new genus *Moritella* gen. nov. as *Moritella marina* comb. nov. FEMS Microbiol Lett. 1998, 165: 373-378. 10.1111/j.1574-6968.1998.tb13173.x.

83. Del-Pozo J, Crumlish M, Ferguson HW, Turnbull JF: Retrospective cross-sectional study on «*Candidatus arthromitus*" associated rainbow trout gastroenteritis (RTGE) in the UK. Aquaculture. 2009, 290: 22-27. 10.1016/j.aquaculture.2009.02.009.

84. Michel C, Bernardet JF, Daniel P, Chilmonczyk S, Urdaci M, de Kinkelin P: Clinical and aetiological aspects of a summer enteritic syndrome associated with the sporulating segmented filamentous bacterium "*Candidatus Arthromitus*" in farmed rainbow trout, *Oncorhynchus mykiss* (Walbaum). J Fish Dis. 2002, 25: 533-543. 10.1046/j.1365-2761.2002.00400.x.

85. Del-Pozo J, Turnbull J, Ferguson H, Crumlish M: A comparative molecular study of the presence of «*Candidatus arthromitus*" in the digestive system of rainbow trout, *Oncorhynchus mykiss* (Walbaum), healthy and affected with rainbow trout gastroenteritis. J Fish Dis. 2010, 33: 241-250. 10.1111/j.1365-2761.2009.01117.x.

86. Stevenson RMW, Daly JG: Biochemical and serological characteristics of Ontario isolates of *Yersinia ruckeri*. Can J Fish Aquat Sci. 1982, 39: 870-876. 10.1139/f82-118.

87. Karlsen M, Nylund A, Watanabe K, Helvik JV, Nylund S, Plarre H: Characterization of "*Candidatus Clavochlamydia salmonicola*": an intracellular bacterium infecting salmonid fish. Environ Microbiol. 2008, 10: 208-218.

88. Larsen JL, Jensen NJ: An *Aeromonas* species implicated in ulcer-disease of the cod (*Gadus morhua*). Nord Veterinaermed. 1977, 29: 199-211.

89. Orozova P, Barker M, Austin DA, Austin B: Identification and pathogenicity to rainbow trout, *Oncorhynchus mykiss*(Walbaum), of some aeromonads. J Fish Dis. 2009, 32: 865-871. 10.1111/j.1365-2761.2009.01065.x.

90. Carnahan AM, Altwegg M: Taxonomy. The Genus Aeromonas. Edited by: Austin B, Altwegg M, Gosling PJ, Joseph S, Wiley, Chichester. 1996, 1-38.

91. Allen DA, Austin B, Colwell RR: *Aeromonas media*, a new species isolated from river water. Int J Syst Bacteriol. 1983, 33: 599-604. 10.1099/00207713-33-3-599.

92. MacInnes JI, Trust TJ, Crosa JH: Deoxyribonucleic acid relationships among members of the genus *Aeromonas*. Can J Microbiol. 1979, 25: 579-586. 10.1139/m79-083.

93. Esteve C: Numerical taxonomy of *Aeromonadaceae* and *Vibrionaceae* associated with reared fish and surrounding fresh and brackish water. System Appl Microbiol. 1995, 18: 391-402.

94. Esteve C, Biosca EG, Amaro C: Virulence of *Aeromonas hydrophila* and some other bacteria isolated from European eels *Anguilla anguilla* reared in fresh water. Dis Aquat Org. 1993, 16: 15-20. 10.3354/dao016015.

95. Ali A, Carnahan AM, Altwegg M, Lüthy-Hotenstein J, Joseph SW: *Aeromonas bestiarum* sp. nov. (formerly genomospecies DNA group 2 *A. hydrophila)* a new species isolated from non-human sources. Med Microbiol Lett. 1996, 5: 156-165.

96. Toranzo AE, Baya AM, Romalde JJ, Hetrick FM: Association of *Aeromonas sobria* with mortalities of adult gizzard shad, *Dorosoma cepedianum* Lesueur. J Fish Dis. 1989, 12: 439-448. 10.1111/j.1365-2761.1989.tb00555.x.

97. Ma Z, Yang H, Li T, Luo L, Gao JL: Isolation and identification of pathogenic *Aeromonas veronii* isolated from infected Siberian sturgeon (*Acipenser baerii*). Wei Sheng Wu Xue Bao. 2009, 49: 1289-1294. (article in Chinese)

98. Snieszko SF: Genus IV. *Aeromonas* Kluyver and van Niel 1936, Bergey's Manual of Determinative Bacteriology. Edited by: Breed RS, Murray EGD, Smith NR. 1957, Williams and Wilkins, Baltimore, 189-193. 7

99. Colwell RR, MacDonell MT, De Ley J: Proposal to recognize the family Aeromonadaceae fam. nov. Int J Syst Bacteriol. 1986, 36: 473-477. 10.1099/00207713-36-3-473.

100. Griffin PJ, Snieszko SF, Friddle SB: A more comprehensive description of *Bacterium salmonicida*. Trans Am Fish Soc. 1953, 82: 129-138. 10.1577/1548-8659(1952)82[129:AMCDOB]2.0.CO;2.

101. Austin DA, McIntosh D, Austin B: Taxonomy of fish associated *Aeromonas* spp., with the description of *Aeromonas salmonicida* subsp. *smithia* subsp. nov. Syst Appl Microbiol. 1989, 11: 277-290.

102. Duff DCB: Dissociation in *Bacillus salmonicida*, with special reference to the appearance of the G form of culture. J Bacteriol. 1937, 34: 49-67.

103. Pacha RE, Kiehn ED: Characterization and relatedness of marine vibrios pathogenic to fish: physiology, serology and epidemiology. J Bacteriol. 1969, 100: 1242-1247.

104. Koppang EO, Fjølstad M, Melgård B, Vigerust M, Sørum H: non-pigment-producing isolates of *Aeromonas salmonicida*subspecies *salmonicida:* isolation, identification, transmission and pathogenicity in Atlantic salmon, *Salmo salar* L. J Fish Dis. 2000, 23: 39-48. 10.1046/j.1365-2761.2000.00205.x.

105. Nakatsugawa T: Atypical *Aeromonas salmonicida* isolted from cultured shotted halibut. Fish Pathol. 1994, 29: 193-198. 10.3147/jsfp.29.193.

106. Kaku Y, Yamada Y, Wakabayashi H: Characterization of atypical *Aeromonas salmonicida* isolated from an epizootic ulcerative disease in carp (*Cyprinus carpio*). Fish Pathol. 1999, 34: 155-162. 10.3147/jsfp.34.155.

107. Wiklund T, Bylund G: Skin ulcer disease of flounder *Platichthys flesus* in the northern Baltic Sea. Dis Aquat Org. 1993, 17: 165-174. 10.3354/dao017165.

108. Austin B: Recovery of «atypical» isolates of *Aeromonas salmonicida*, which grow at 37°C, from ulcerated non-salmonids in England. J Fish Dis. 1993, 16: 165-168. 10.1111/j.1365-2761.1993.tb00862.x.

109. Goodwin AE, Merry GE: Are all Koi ulcer cases associated with infection by atypical *Aeromonas salmonicida*? Polymerase chain reaction assays of Koi carp skin swabs submitted by hobbyists. J Aquat Anim Health. 2009, 21: 98-103. 10.1577/H08-042.1.

110. Pedersen K, Kofod H, Dalsgaard I, Larsen JL: Isolation of oxidase-negative *Aeromonas salmonicida* from disease turbot *Scophthalmus maximus*. Dis Aquat Org. 1994, 18: 149-154. 10.3354/dao018149.

111. Wiklund T, Dalsgaard I, Eerola E, Olivier G: Characteristics of "atypical" cytochrome-oxidase negative *Aeromonas salmonicida* isolated from ulcerated flounder *(Platichthys flesus* (L.). J Appl Bacteriol. 1994, 76: 511-520.

112. Wiklund T, Dalsgaard I: Atypical *Aeromonas salmonicida* associated with ulcerated flatfish species in the Baltic Sea and the North Sea. J Aquat Anim Health. 1995, 7: 218-224. 10.1577/1548-8667(1995)007<0218:AASAWU>2.3.CO;2.

113. Goldschmidt-Clermont E, Hochwartner O, Demarta A, Caminada AP, Frey J: Outbreaks of an ulcerative and haemorrhagic disease in Arctic char *Salvelinus alpinus* caused by *Aeromonas salmonicida* subsp *smithia*. Dis Aquat Org. 2009, 86: 81-86. 10.3354/dao02110.

114. Austin B, Austin DA, Dalsgaard I, Gudmundsdóttir BK, Høie S, Thornton JM, Larsen JL, O'Hici B, Powell R: Characterization of atypical *Aeromonas salmonicida* by different methods. Syst Appl Microbiol. 1998, 21: 50-64.

115. Høie S, Dalsgaard I, Aase IL, Heum M, Thornton JM, Powell R: Polymerase chain reaction (PCR) based typing analysis of atypical isolates of the fish pathogen *Aeromonas salmonicida*. Syst Appl Microbiol. 1999, 22: 403-411.

116. Lund V, Jenssen LM, Wesmajervi MS: Assessment of genetic variability and relatedness among atypical *Aeromonas salmonicida* from marine fishes, using AFLP fingerprinting. Dis Aquat Org. 2002, 50: 119-126. 10.3354/dao050119.

117. Yamada Y, Kaku Y, Wakabayashi H: Phylogenetic intrarelationships of atypical *Aeromonas salmonicida* isolated in Japan as determined by 16S rDNA sequencing. Fish Pathol. 2000, 35: 35-40. 10.3147/jsfp.35.35.

118. Smith IW: The classification of *Bacterium salmonicida*. J Gen Microbiol. 1963, 33: 263-274.

119. Kimura T: A new subspecies of *Aeromonas salmonicida* as an etiological agent of furunculosis on "Sakuramasu" *(Oncorhynchus masou)* and pink salmon *(O. gorbuscha)* rearing for maturity. Fish Pathol. 1969, 3: 34-44. 10.3147/jsfp.3.2_34. Part 1. On the serological properties

120. Schubert RHW: Genus II. *Aeromonas* Kluyver and van Niel 1936, 398, Bergey's Manual of Determinative Bacteriology. Edited by: Buchanan RE, Gibbons NE. 1974, Williams and Wilkins, Baltimore, 345-348. 8th

121. Popoff M: Bacterioses, generalities - *Aeromonas* et Aeromonose. Mimeograph. 1970, Institut National de la Recherche Agronomique, 1-38.

122. Paterson WD, Douey D, Desautels D: Relationships between selected strains of typical and atypical *Aeromonas salmonicida, Aeromonas hydrophila*, and *Haemophilus piscium*. Can J Microbiol. 1980, 26: 588-598. 10.1139/m80-104.

123. Snieszko SF, Griffin P, Friddle SB: A new bacterium *(Haemophilus piscium* n. sp.) from ulcer disease of trout. J Bacteriol. 1950, 59: 699-710.

124. Thornton JM, Austin DA, Austin B, Powell R: Small subunit rRNA gene sequences of *Aeromonas salmonicida* subsp. *smithia* and *Haemophilus piscium* reveal pronounced similarities with *A. salmonicida* subsp. *salmonicida*. Dis Aquat Org. 1999, 35: 155-158. 10.3354/dao035155.

125. McCarthy DH: Some ecological aspects of the bacterial fish pathogen - *Aeromonas salmonicida*. Aquatic Microbiology Symp Soc Appl Bacteriol. 1980, 6: 299-324.

126. Belland RJ, Trust TJ: DNA:DNA reassociation analysis of *Aeromonas salmonicida*. J Gen Microbiol. 1988, 134: 307-315.

127. Eddy BP: Cephalotrichous, fermentative Gram-negative bacteria: the genus *Aeromonas*. J Appl Bacteriol. 1960, 23: 216-248.

128. Kluyver AJ, Van Niel CB: Prospects for a natural system of classification of bacteria. Z Bakteriol Parasiten, Infekt Hyg, Orig. 1936, 94: 369-403. 2 Abt

129. Cowan ST: Cowan and Steel's Manual for the Identification of Medical Bacteria. 1974, Cambridge University Press, Cambridge, 2

130. Kimura T: A new subspecies of *Aeromonas salmonicida* as an etiological agent of furunculosis on "Sakuramasu" *(Oncorhynchus masou)* and pink salmon *(O. gorbuscha)* rearing for maturity. Part 2. On the morphological and physiological properties. Fish Pathol. 1969, 3: 45-52. 10.3147/jsfp.3.2_45.

131. Liu PV: Observations on the specificities of extra-cellular antigens of the genera *Aeromonas* and *Serratia*. J Gen Microbiol. 1961, 24: 145-153.

132. Popoff M: Étude sur les *Aeromonas salmonicida*. II. Caracterisation des bactériophages actifs sur les "*Aeromonas salmonicida*" et lysotypie. Ann Recherch Vét. 1971, 2: 33-45.

133. Popoff M: Intérêt diagnostique d'un bactériophage spécifique des *Aeromonas salmonicida*. Ann Rech Vét. 1971, 2: 137-139.

134. Kilian M: A taxonomic study of the genus *Haemophilus*, with the proposal of a new species. J Gen Microbiol. 1976, 93: 9-62.

135. Broom AK, Sneath PHA: Numerical taxonomy of *Haemophilus*. J Gen Microbiol. 1981, 126: 123-149.

136. Trust TJ, Ishiguro EE, Atkinson HM: Relationship between *Haemophilus piscium* and *Aeromonas salmonicida* revealed by *Aeromonas hydrophila* bacteriophage. FEMS Microbiol Lett. 1980, 9: 199-201. 10.1111/j.1574-6968.1980.tb05636.x.

137. Dalsgaard I, Gudmundsdóttir BK, Helgason S, Høie S, Thoresen OF, Wichardt UP, Wiklund T: Identification of atypical *Aeromonas salmonicida*: inter-laboratory evaluation and harmonization of methods. J Appl Microbiol. 1998, 84: 999-1006. 10.1046/j.1365-2672.1998.00435.x.

138. Ross AJ, Rucker RR, Ewing WH: Description of a bacterium associated with redmouth disease of rainbow trout (*Salmo gairdneri*). Can J Microbiol. 1966, 12: 763-70. 10.1139/m66-103.

139. Steinum T, Sjastad K, Falk K, Kvellestad A, Colquhuin DJ: An RT PCR-DGGE survey of gill-associated bacteria in Norwegian seawater-reared Atlantic salmon suffering proliferative gill inflammation. Aquaculture. 2009, 293: 172-179. 10.1016/j.aquaculture.2009.05.006.

140. Ewing WH, Ross AJ, Brenner DJ, Fanning GR: *Yersinia ruckeri* sp. nov., the redmouth (RM) bacterium. Int J Syst Bacteriol. 1978, 28: 37-44. 10.1099/00207713-28-1-37.

141. Steigerwalt AG, Fanning GR, Fife-Asbury MA, Brenner DJ: DNA relatedness among species of *Enterobacter* and *Serratia*. Can J Microbiol. 1976, 22: 121-137. 10.1139/m76-018.

142. Bercovier H, Mollaret HH: Genus XIV. *Yersinia* van Loghem 1944, 15AL. Bergey's Manual of Systematic Bacteriology. Edited by: Krieg NR, Holt JG. 1984, Williams and Wilkins, Baltimore, I: 489-506.

143. Austin DA, Robertson PAW, Austin B: Recovery of a new biogroup of *Yersinia ruckeri* from diseased rainbow trout *(Oncorhynchus mykiss*, Walbaum). Syst Appl Microbiol. 2005, 26: 127-131. 10.1078/072320203322337416.

144. Fouz B, Zarza C, Amaro C: First description of non-motile *Yersinia ruckeri* serovar I strains causing disease in rainbow trout, *Oncorhynchus mykiss* (Walbaum), cultured in Spain. J Fish Dis. 2006, 29: 339-346. 10.1111/j.1365-2761.2006.00723.x.

145. Smith IW: A disease of finnock due to *Vibrio anguillarum*. J Gen Microbiol. 1961, 74: 247-252.

146. Kaper JB, Lockman H, Remmers EF, Kristensen K, Colwell RR: Numerical taxonomy of vibrios isolated from estuarine environments. Int J Syst Bacteriol. 1983, 33: 229-255. 10.1099/00207713-33-2-229.

147. Pazos F, Santos Y, Magariños B, Bandín I, Núñez S, Toranzo AE: Phenotypic characteristics and virulence of *Vibrio anguillarum* - related organisms. Appl Environ Microbiol. 1993, 59: 2969-2976.

148. Olsen JE, Larsen JL: Ribotypes and plasmid content of *Vibrio anguillarum* strains in relation to serovar. Appl Environ Microbiol. 1993, 59: 3863-3870.

149. Austin B, Alsina M, Austin DA, Blanch AR, Grimont F, Grimont PAD, Jofre J, Koblavi S, Larsen JL, Pedersen K, Tiainen T, Verdonck L, Swings J: Identification and typing of *Vibrio anguillarum* a comparison of different methods. Syst Appl Microbiol. 1995, 18: 285-302.

150. Austin B, Austin DA, Blanch AR, Cerdà M, Grimont F, Grimont PAD, Jofre J, Koblavi S, Larsen JL, Pedersen K, Tiainen T, Verdonck L, Swings J: A comparison of methods for the typing of fish-pathogenic *Vibrio* spp. Syst Appl Microbiol. 1997, 20: 89-101.

151. Schiewe MH: Taxonomic status of marine vibrios pathogenic for salmonid fish. Dev Biol Stand. 1981, 49: 149-158.

152. Muthiara LW, Raymond BT, Dekievit TR, Stevenson RHW: Antibody specificities of polyclonal rabbit and rainbow trout antisera against *Vibrio ordalii* and serotype O:2 strains of *Vibrio anguillarum*. Can J Microbiol. 1993, 39: 492-499. 10.1139/m93-070.

153. Sørensen UBS, Larsen JL: Serotyping of *Vibrio anguillarum*. Appl Environ Microbiol. 1986, 51: 593-597.

154. Grisez L, Ollevier F: Comparative serology of the marine fish pathogen *Vibrio anguillarum*. Appl Environ Microbiol. 1995, 61: 4367-4373.

155. Pedersen K, Dalsgaard I, Larsen JL: Characterization of atypical *Aeromonas salmonicida* isolates by ribotyping and plasmid profiling. J Appl Bacteriol. 1996, 80: 37-44.

156. Pedersen K, Tiainen T, Larsen JL: Plasmid profiles, restriction length polymorphisms and O-serotypes among *Vibrio anguillarum* isolates. Epidemiol Infect.

1996, 117: 471-478. 10.1017/S0950268800059136.

157. Kitao T, Aoki T, Fukodome M, Kawano K, Wada Y, Mizuno Y: Serotyping of *Vibrio anguillarum* isolated from diseased freshwater fish in Japan. J Fish Dis. 1983, 6: 175-181. 10.1111/j.1365-2761.1983.tb00064.x.

158. Tiainen T, Pedersen K, Larsen JL: Immunological reactivity of *Vibrio anguillarum* sero-subgroups O2a and O2b, and comparison of their lipopolysaccharide profiles. Curr Microbiol. 1997, 34: 38-42. 10.1007/s002849900141.

159. O›Hici B, Olivier G, Powell R: Genetic diversity of the fish pathogen *Aeromonas salmonicida* demonstrated by random amplified polymorphic DNA and pulsed-field gel electrophoresis analyses. Dis Aquat Org. 2000, 39: 109-119.

160. Umelo E, Trust TJ: Identification and molecular characterization of two tandomly located flagellin genes from *Aeromonas salmonicida* A449. J Bacteriol. 1997, 179: 5292-5299.

161. McIntosh D, Austin B: Atypical characteristics of the salmonid pathogen *Aeromonas salmonicida*. J Gen Microbiol. 1991, 137: 1341-1343.

CHAPTER 3 A VETERINARY TWIST ON PATHOGEN BIOLOGY

Massimo Palmarini

The recent epidemics of bovine spongiform encephalopathy, foot and mouth disease, and avian influenza have focused the attention of the general public and scientific community on veterinary pathogens. Studies on naturally occurring infectious diseases of domestic animals, although perceived to be mostly relevant for animal health, have often unveiled new paradigms on the biology of infectious agents, inspired the identification of novel human pathogens, and occasionally launched entire new disciplines. This article aims to provide some examples that illustrate how veterinary diseases (focusing on viral diseases in particular) have provided novel comparative and biological platforms (Figure 1).

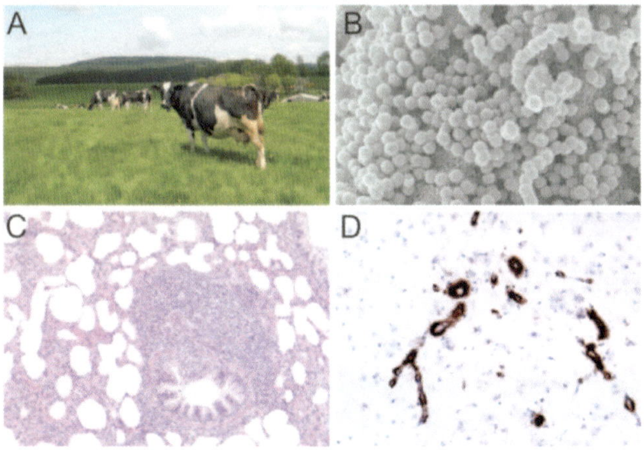

Figure 1: Novel Biological Platforms Unveiled in the Barnyard

Studies on viruses of veterinary interest have revealed many fundamental aspects of pathogen biology. (A) Dairy cows grazing the Scottish hills. (B) Rous sarcoma virus particles budding from the surface of chicken fibroblasts as imaged by scanning electron microscopy. (C) Histology from a lung section of a sheep affected by maedi-visna virus showing chronic interstitial pneumonia. (D) Immunohistochemistry showing disease-associated prion protein (PrP) vascular amyloid in the cerebellar cortex of a sheep affected by scrapie.

The discipline of animal virology itself began with the discovery of the causative agents of major infectious diseases of domestic animals: foot and mouth disease initially [1], followed by the recognition of "filterable agents" in rabbit myxomatosis, African horse sickness, avian influenza (fowl plague), and avian leukosis [2,3]. Soon after, Peyton Rous [4,5] demonstrated the viral etiology of avian sarcoma, a discovery met with great skepticism at the time, as it was not believed that cancer could be infectious. Curiously, modern cancer genetics was essentially initiated with studies on the very same virus (Rous sarcoma virus) discovered by Rous (Figure 1B). The genome of Rous sarcoma virus, in addition to the canonical retroviral structural and enzymatic genes, was found to contain a cell-derived gene, *v-src*, which is both the first discovered oncogene and the first tyrosine kinase [6–9]! Over the years, avian retroviruses have been instrumental to the discovery of many other oncogenes such as *myc, jun, myb, rel, erbA,* and others that are now considered "usual suspects" in cancer initiation and progression [10].

The above examples are described in most biology textbooks along with the pioneer studies of Jenner, Koch, and Pasteur on cowpox, anthrax, and rabies. However, there are instances where studies on viral diseases of domestic animals had a profound impact on biology and medicine that is not often appreciated outside veterinary science. Rinderpest (also known as "cattle plague"), for example, has a rich and long history of scientific landmarks [11]. The consequences of rinderpest for agriculture were so serious that in the 18th century, Pope Clement XI instructed his physician, Giovanni Maria Lancisi, to devise measures to control the disease. Lancisi declared that the disease "was caused by exceedingly fine and pernicious particles that pass from one body to another". He made the suggestion to "destroy all ill and suspect animals . . . rather than allowing the contagion to increase . . ." and to bury the whole animals in lime [11]. These principles constituted a milestone in controlling the spread of contagious diseases by restrictions on animal movements, quarantine, and removal of affected animals.

Citation: Palmarini M (2007) A Veterinary Twist on Pathogen Biology. PLoS Pathog 3(2): e12. doi:10.1371/journal.ppat.0030012.

In 1762, the first veterinary school in the world opened in Lyon (France) in order to teach the principles put forward by Lancisi, who is appropriately considered the first modern hygienist. Three hundred years later, we have faced and controlled the epidemic of foot and mouth disease in the United Kingdom by using essentially the same measures devised by Lancisi to control rinderpest.

Rinderpest is associated with other scientific milestones. A self-taught Dutch farmer, Geert Reinders, during a rinderpest epidemic in 1768, was the first to grasp the concept of "maternal immunity" and to notice that cattle which had experienced the natural illness (or mild symptoms) were protected from subsequent infection and disease [3,12]. This observation was published well before Jenner›s landmark studies on cowpox [3,12]. Curiously, the clinical thermometer was developed in order to diagnose fever in cattle suspected to be affected by rinderpest as an additional tool to control the disease [12].

Studies during the 1940s and 1950s by Björn Sigurdsson on a small group of diseases of sheep bred in Iceland [13] constitute a true biological "treasure". Maedi-visna, ovine pulmonary adenocarcinoma (OPA), and paratuberculosis were introduced into Iceland after the import of a small number of rams from Germany in 1933. These diseases spread in the Icelandic flocks despite the fact that imported rams were regularly kept in quarantine on the island before putting them in contact with the local sheep population. Maedi-visna, OPA, and paratuberculosis had been described before [14,15], but the unique epidemiological and geographical circumstances surrounding the Icelandic epidemics stimulated Sigurdsson to develop the concept of "slow diseases" of sheep, in which an infectious agent could induce disease in its host months or even years after initial infection. Sigurdsson also recognized scrapie, present since 1878 in Iceland, as one of the slow diseases of sheep [13].

Over the intervening years, these relatively obscure diseases of small ruminants had several claims to fame in the biomedical arena. Maedi-visna, for example, a disease characterized mainly by pneumonia and encephalitis, was subsequently discovered to be caused by a retrovirus [16]. This retrovirus, maedi-visna virus (Figure 1C), was considered the prototype of the *Lentivirus* genus within the Retroviridae family. The name "lentivirus" derives from the Latin for "slow" and refers to the term coined by Sigurdsson. Another lentivirus, HIV, would emerge afterwards as the cause of AIDS and soon became the most studied virus in human history. Early studies on HIV-1, now the new lentivirus prototype, in the 1980s took some advantage on data accumulated on maedi-visna virus and on another animal lentivirus, equine infectious anemia virus [17–20].

Scrapie, another of the slow diseases of sheep, was the first disease described [15] within the group of the transmissible spongiform encephalopathies (TSEs) (Figure 1D). The apparent lack of nucleic acids in the infectious material associated with scrapie and other TSEs has represented a wonderful biological puzzle, culminating in the award of the Nobel prize to Stanley Prusiner for the prion theory [21]. TSEs have also been diagnosed in humans and include kuru, Gerstmann-Sträussler-Scheinker syndrome, fatal familial insomnia, Creutzfeldt-Jakob disease, and the new variant Creutzfeldt-Jakob disease. Kuru, the first recognized human TSE, was originally described by Carleton Gajdusek and Vincent Zigas in members of the Fore tribe in the Papua New Guinea at the end of the 1950s. Interestingly, the first hint that kuru and scrapie might be similar diseases was made serendipitously by a veterinary pathologist, William Hadlow, who was attending an exhibit on kuru at the Wellcome Medical Museum in London [22]. The vacuolated neuronal cell bodies were unusual in human pathology but well characterized in sheep with scrapie. Seven years after this connection was made, Gajdusek and colleagues described the experimental transmission of kuru in chimpanzees inoculated with brain tissues from persons who had died of the disease [23].

Of course, when the bovine spongiform encephalopathy epidemic spread across the UK in the 1990s [24] and public health concerns started to rise, the early studies on scrapie provided a critical intellectual framework (although possibly misleading with respect to potential human transmission) to understand the biology of bovine spongiform encephalopathy and the zoonotic variant Creutzfeldt-Jakob disease [25,26].

The other slow disease of sheep, OPA, is probably best known to the general public for being the cause of the demise of Dolly, the first mammal cloned by nuclear transfer. However, the causative agent of OPA, a retrovirus known as Jaagsiekte sheep retrovirus (JSRV), has been found to be the only oncogenic retrovirus (and the only oncogenic virus in general) to possess a structural protein (the viral envelope) functioning as a dominant oncogene in vitro and in vivo [27–29]. In addition, the JSRV/OPA model sparked fundamental studies on the biological roles of endogenous retroviruses in mammalian evolution. Endogenous retroviruses are ancient remains of retrovirus infections stably integrated in the genome of every animal species. Studies on sheep endogenous retroviruses related to JSRV demonstrated in experiments in vivo that endogenous retroviruses can play a fundamental role in host placentation and conceptus development [30].

Many viruses of domestic animals have also inspired, directly or indirectly, discoveries of related human viruses. Feline leukemia virus [31,32] was taken as an example that retroviruses horizontally transmitted could cause tumours in outbred animal species; this fuelled the chase for human retroviruses, eventually leading to the discovery of human T lymphotropic virus [33,34].

An interesting example of viruses identified in animals before being found in humans is provided by rotaviruses, the main cause of diarrhea in infants and children throughout the world and in the developing countries in particular [35–37]. The causal association between rotaviruses and diarrhea was made in calves well before it was realized for humans [37,38]. Mebus and colleagues demonstrated that diarrhea in calves was caused by rotaviruses [39,40] and established a cell culture system to propagate them [41]. In addition, studies in both calves and lambs were key to realizing the importance of local immunity and colostrum-derived antibodies in the resistance to rotavirus infection [42,43]. All of these studies have had a profound impact in understanding and preventing human rotavirus infection.

Studies on animal papillomaviruses of rabbits, cattle, and dogs have provided the intellectual background for the identification of human papillomaviruses as etiological agents of the overwhelming majority of cervical cancers and some cutaneous cancers [44–48]. The success of the recently highly publicized vaccine against human papillomavirus is based on the proof of principle gained in vaccine development against animal papillomaviruses [49].

Animal viruses are also important causes of zoonosis. The recent zoonotic episodes of Nipah virus, Hendra virus [50], and, more importantly, avian influenza [51–53], are a growing list of examples on infectious agents that can pass from animals to humans without previous "warning", a particularly worrisome scenario given that 75% of human infections are estimated to be zoonotic in origin [54].

This article has no pretensions to be exhaustive but aims to show how research on pathogens of veterinary interest needs to be fostered, not only for its direct relevance to animal health, but for its significance to comparative medicine and public health. Veterinary scientists play important roles in the study of infectious diseases and can operate at the interface between basic, applied, and clinical research since they are equipped with a unique combination of expertise in biology, ecology, and husbandry [55]. The understanding of complex emerging diseases needs collaborative efforts between experts in public health, the environment, and animal health, where veterinary scientists can provide a critical contribution [56].

Unfortunately, in the last two decades there has been a steady decline worldwide in the number of veterinary graduates undertaking a career in research, which is a cause of great concern. Veterinary schools and veterinary research institutes should create an environment where hypothesis-driven research is encouraged and maintained, and its importance continuously highlighted to funding agencies, policy makers, veterinary students, and the scientific community as a whole.

ACKNOWLEDGMENTS

This article was inspired by the Research Committee of the Royal College of Veterinary Surgeons (RCVS). I would like to thank J. Parkins, M. Johnson, M. De las Heras, and L. González for kindly providing the images represented in Figure 1. I would also like to thank my colleagues S. Wotton and S. Campo at the Institute of Comparative Medicine of the University of Glasgow Veterinary School, and U. Agrimi, B. Blacklaws, C. Brown, I. Capua, L. González, M. Sharp, and D. Snodgrass for useful comments and suggestions.

REFERENCES

1. Loeffler F, Frosch P (1897) Summarischer bericht über die ergebnisse der untersuchungen der Kommission zur Erforschung der maul und klauenseuche bei dem Institut für Infektionskrankheiten. Dt Med Wschr 98: 80–84.
2. Ellerman V, Bang O (1908) Experimentelle leukamie bei huhnern. Fizentralblatt bakteriologie. Zentralblatt der Bakteriologie 46: 595–609.
3. Horzinek MC (1997) The birth of virology. Antonie Van Leeuwenhoek 71: 15–20.
4. Rous P (1911) Transmission of a malignant new growth by means of a cell-free filtrate. JAMA 56: 198.
5. Rous P (1911) A sarcoma of the fowl transmissible by an agent separable from the tumour cells. J Exp Med 13: 397–411.
6. Duesberg PH, Vogt PK (1970) Differences between the ribonucleic acids of transforming and nontransforming avian tumor viruses. Proc Natl Acad Sci U S A 67: 1673–1680.
7. Stehelin D, Guntaka RV, Varmus HE, Bishop JM (1976) Purification of DNA complementary to nucleotide sequences required for neoplastic transformation of fibroblasts by avian sarcoma viruses. J Mol Biol 101: 349–365.
8. Stehelin D, Varmus HE, Bishop JM, Vogt PK (1976) DNA related to the transforming gene(s) of avian sarcoma viruses is present in normal avian DNA. Nature 260: 170–173.
9. Czernilofsky AP, Levinson AD, Varmus HE, Bishop JM, Tischer E, et al. (1980) Nucleotide sequence of an avian sarcoma virus oncogene (src) and proposed amino acid sequence for gene product. Nature 287: 198–203.
10. Rosenberg N, Jolicoeur P (1997) Retroviral pathogenesis. In: Coffin JM, Hughes S, Varmus HE, editors. Retroviruses. New York: Cold Spring Harbor Laboratory Press. pp. 475–585.
11. Barrett T, Pastoret PP, Taylor W (2005) Rinderpest and peste des petits ruminants: Virus plagues of large and small ruminants. London: Academic Press.
12. Spinage C (2003) Cattle plague: A history. New York: Kluwer/Plenum Publishers. 770 p.
13. Sigurdsson B (1954) Rida, a chronic encephalitis of sheep: With general remarks on infections which develop slowly and some of their special characteristics. Br Vet J 110: 341–354.
14. McFadyean J (1894) Verminous pneumonia in the sheep. J Comp Pathol Ther 7: 31–42.
15. Stockman S (1913) Scrapie: An obscure disease of sheep. J Comp Pathol 26: 317–327.
16. Lin FH, Thormar H (1970) Ribonucleic acid-dependent deoxyribonucleic acid polymerase in visna virus. J Virol 6: 702–704.
17. Clements JE, Gdovin SL, Montelaro RC, Narayan O (1988) Antigenic variation in lentiviral diseases. Annu Rev Immunol 6: 139–159.
18. Narayan O, Zink MC, Huso D, Sheffer D, Crane S, et al. (1988) Lentiviruses of animals are biological models of the human immunodeficiency viruses. Microb Pathog 5: 149–157.
19. Haase AT (1986) Pathogenesis of lentivirus infections. Nature 322: 130–136.
20. Thormar H (2005) Maedi-visna virus and its relationship to human immunodeficiency virus. AIDS Rev 7: 233–245.
21. Prusiner SB (1991) Molecular biology of prion diseases. Science 252: 1515–1522.
22. Hadlow WJ (1999) Reflections on the transmissible spongiform encephalopathies. Vet Pathol 36: 523–529.
23. Liberski PP, Gajdusek DC (1997) Kuru: Forty years later, a historical note. Brain Pathol 7: 555–560.

24. Hope J, Reekie LJ, Hunter N, Multhaup G, Beyreuther K, et al. (1988) Fibrils from brains of cows with new cattle disease contain scrapie-associated protein. Nature 336: 390–392.

25. Wilesmith JW (1988) Bovine spongiform encephalopathy. Vet Rec 122: 614.

26. Wilesmith JW, Wells GA, Cranwell MP, Ryan JB (1988) Bovine spongiform encephalopathy: Epidemiological studies. Vet Rec 123: 638–644.

27. Maeda N, Palmarini M, Murgia C, Fan H (2001) Direct transformation of rodent fibroblasts by Jaagsiekte sheep retrovirus DNA. Proc Natl Acad Sci U S A 98: 4449–4454.

28. Wootton SK, Halbert CL, Miller AD (2005) Sheep retrovirus structural protein induces lung tumours. Nature 434: 904–907.

29. Caporale M, Cousens C, Centorame P, Pinoni C, De las Heras M, et al. (2006) Expression of the Jaagsiekte sheep retrovirus envelope glycoproteins is sufficient to induce lung tumor in sheep. J Virol 80: 8030–8037.

30. Dunlap KA, Palmarini M, Varela M, Burghardt RC, Hayashy K, et al. (2006) Endogenous retroviruses regulate peri-implantation conceptus growth and differentiation. Proc Natl Acad Sci U S A 103: 14390–14395.

31. Jarrett WF, Crawford EM, Martin WB, Davie F (1964) A virus-like particle associated with leukemia (lymphosarcoma). Nature 202: 567–569.

32. Jarrett WF, Martin WB, Crighton GW, Dalton RG, Stewart MF (1964) Transmission experiments with leukemia (lymphosarcoma). Nature 202: 566–567.

33. Gallo RC, Kalyanaraman VS, Sarngadharan MG, Sliski A, Vonderheid EC, et al. (1983) Association of the human type C retrovirus with a subset of adult T-cell cancers. Cancer Res 43: 3892–3899.

34. Gallo RC (2005) History of the discoveries of the first human retroviruses: HTLV-1 and HTLV-2. Oncogene 24: 5926–5930.

35. Parashar UD, Bresee JS, Gentsch JR, Glass RI (1998) Rotavirus. Emerg Infect Dis 4: 561–570.

36. Parashar UD, Kilgore PE, Holman RC, Clarke MJ, Bresee JS, et al. (1998) Diarrheal mortality in US infants. Influence of birth weight on risk factors for death. Arch Pediatr Adolesc Med 152: 47–51.

37. Kapikian AZ, Hoshino Y, Chanok RM (2001) Rotaviruses. In: Knipe DM, Howley PM, editors. Fields virology. 4th edition. Philadelphia: Lippincott Williams & Wilkins. pp. 1787–1833.

38. Bishop RF, Davidson GP, Holmes IH, Ruck BJ (1973) Virus particles in epithelial cells of duodenal mucosa from children with acute non-bacterial gastroenteritis. Lancet 2: 1281–1283.

39. Mebus CA, Underdahl NR, Rhodes MB, Twiehaus MJ (1969) Further studies on neonatal calf diarrhea virus. Proc Annu Meet U S Anim Health Assoc 73: 97–99.

40. Mebus CA, Underdahl NR, Rhodes M, Twiehaus M (1969) Calf diarrhea (scours): Reproduced with a virus from field outbreak. Univ Nebraska Res Bull 233: 1–16.

41. Mebus CA, Kono M, Underdahl NR, Twiehaus MJ (1971) Cell culture propagation of neonatal calf diarrhea (scours) virus. Can Vet J 12: 69–72.

42. Snodgrass DR, Wells PW (1976) Rotavirus infection in lambs: Studies on passive protection. Arch Virol 52: 201–205.

43. Woode GN, Jones J, Bridger J (1975) Levels of colostral antibodies against neonatal calf diaahoea virus. Vet Rec 97: 148–149.

44. Nicholls PK, Stanley MA (1999) Canine papillomavirus—A centenary review. J Comp Pathol 120: 219–233.

45. Rous P, Kidd JG (1938) The carcinogenic effect of a papillomavirus on the tarred skin of rabbits. J Exp Med 67: 399–439.

46. Jarrett WF, Murphy J, O›Neil BW, Laird HM (1978) Virus-induced papillomas of the alimentary tract of cattle. Int J Cancer 22: 323–328.

47. Campo MS (2002) Animal models of papillomavirus pathogenesis. Virus Res 89: 249–261.

48. Gissmann L, Boshart M, Durst M, Ikenberg H, Wagner D, et al. (1984) Presence of human papillomavirus in genital tumors. J Invest Dermatol 83: 26s–28s.

49. Giles M, Garland SM (2006) HPV vaccines. In: Campo MS, editor. Papillomavirus biology: From natural history to vaccine and beyond. Norfolk: Caister Academic Press. pp. 341–356.

50. Eaton BT, Broder CC, Middleton D, Wang LF (2006) Hendra and Nipah viruses: Different and dangerous. Nat Rev Microbiol 4: 23–35.

51. Fauci AS (2006) Emerging and re-emerging infectious diseases: Influenza as a prototype of the host-pathogen balancing act. Cell 124: 665–670.

52. Webster RG, Peiris M, Chen H, Guan Y (2006) H5N1 outbreaks and enzootic influenza. Emerg Infect Dis 12: 3–8.

53. Capua I, Alexander DJ (2004) Human health implications of avian influenza viruses and paramyxoviruses. Eur J Clin Microbiol Infect Dis 23: 1–6.

54. Taylor LH, Latham SM, Woolhouse ME (2001) Risk factors for human disease emergence. Philos Trans R Soc Lond B Biol Sci 356: 983–989.

55. Brown C (2006) Avian influenza: Virchow›s reminder. Am J Pathol 168: 6–8.

56. Capua I, Brown I, Johnson M, Senne D, Swayne D (2006) Veterinary virologists share avian flu data. Science 312: 1597.

SECTION II: CHLAMYDIA SPP. – INTRACELLULAR BACTERIA

CHAPTER 4

THE IMMUNE RESPONSE AGAINST CHLAMYDIA SUIS GENITAL TRACT INFECTION PARTIALLY PROTECTS AGAINST RE-INFECTION

Evelien De Clercq, Bert Devriendt, Lizi Yin, Koen Chiers, Eric Cox and Daisy Vanrompay

INTRODUCTION

Chlamydia suis is widespread in commercial pig production and causes important economic losses [1]. *C. suis*infections are associated with a variety of diseases including conjunctivitis [2], rhinitis [3], pneumonia [3],[4], enteritis [5],[6], periparturient dysgalactiae syndrome (PDS) [7] and numerous reproductive disorders [1],[7]-[10] such as abortion, mummification, perinatal and neonatal mortality, repeat breeding, vaginal discharge and endometritis in addition to orchitis, epididymitis and urethritis in boars [11]. *C. suis* has also been detected in the semen of boars, suggesting the possibility of venereal transmission during mating or artificial insemination [1],[12],[13]. Furthermore, *C. suis* has frequently been identified in asymptomatic carriers [14]-[16].

Experimental infection of gnotobiotic and conventionally raised pigs with *C. suis* proved its pathogenic potential for the porcine respiratory system [3],[4],[17], gastrointestinal tract [5],[6],[18] and eyes [2]. In contrast, the exact role of *C. suis* in reproductive problems still has to be defined. To our knowledge, experimental genital tract infection of pigs with *C. suis* has never been performed before. Nevertheless, considering the possibility of venereal transmission, genital *C. suis* infections and re-infections are probably common in breeder sows, since they are mated or inseminated a minimum of twice a year and generally two to three inseminations per oestrus are carried out. In the present study, conventionally raised *Chlamydia*-negative pigs were intravaginally infected and/or re-infected with *C. suis* strain S45, the type strain of this species. The aim of this study was to reveal the characteristic features of a genital *C. suis* infection and re-infection in female pigs by studying the immune response, pathological changes, replication of chlamydiae in the genital tract and excretion of viable bacteria.

MATERIALS AND METHODS

Chlamydia suis

C. suis strain S45 (kindly donated by A. Andersen, National Animal Disease Center, USDA Agriculture Research Service, Ames, Iowa) was used to infect the pigs. This strain was isolated in the late 1960s from feces of an asymptomatic Austrian pig [19]. The bacteria were grown in McCoy cells using standard techniques [20]. The 50% Tissue Culture Infective Dose ($TCID_{50}$) was determined by the method of Spearman and Kaerber [21]. $TCID_{50}$/mL is routinely used for titrating intracellular organisms like viruses in cell cultures and it correlates with IFU/mL as examined by Beeckman et al. [22].

Citation: Evelien De Clercq, Bert Devriendt, Lizi Yin, Koen Chiers, Eric Cox and Daisy Vanrompay, The immune response against Chlamydia suis genital tract infection partially protects against re-infection, DOI: 10.1186/s13567-014-0095-6.

Infection experiment

Fifteen 9-week-old conventionally bred female pigs (Belgian Landrace) were randomly divided into three groups of five pigs. Antibodies against *Chlamydiaceae* were absent as determined by a *C. suis* ELISA using purified elementary bodies (EBs) of strain S45. Nasal, rectal and vaginal swabs did not contain chlamydial bacteria as determined by culture on McCoy cells. The animals were housed in isolation units and fed *ad libitum* with a commercial starting diet. At day 0, all pigs were anesthetized by intramuscular injection of Zoletil® 100 (Virbac Animal Health, Louvain La Neuve, Belgium) in 2% Xylazine-M® (VMD, Arendonk, Belgium). The control group and the infection group were inoculated with phosphate-buffered saline (PBS). The re-infection group was infected by intravaginal injection of 1×10^7 $TCID_{50}$ of *C. suis* strain S45. Intravaginal inoculation was performed by inserting an artificial insemination pipette connected to a syringe into the vagina and injecting the bacterial suspension in 1 mL PBS or injecting simply 1 mL PBS (controls). At day 56, pigs were anesthetized again, whereafter the control group was inoculated with PBS and the infection group and the re-infection group were infected intravaginally with *C. suis* strain S45 (1×10^7 $TCID_{50}$). All groups were euthanized at day 77 by intravenous injection of an overdose of pentobarbital (70 mg/kg; Nembutal®, Ceva Santé Animale, Maassluis, the Netherlands) followed by exsanguination.

Vaginal swabs in 2 mL *Chlamydia* transport medium for chlamydial isolation and in 2 mL PBS with protease inhibitor for mucosal antibody detection were collected weekly. Swabs were stored at −80 °C until analysis. Blood for antibody detection was sampled from the jugular vein (*v. jugularis*) weekly. Blood samples were stored overnight at room temperature and centrifuged (9300 × *g*, 20 °C, 10 min) for serum collection. Sera were stored at −20 °C until tested. At euthanasia, pigs were examined for gross lesions that were scored as none (0), slight (1), moderate (2) or severe (3). Samples of the spleen, liver, caecum, urethra, vagina, cervix, corpus uteri, uterine tubes, oviducts and ovaries were imbedded in methylcellulose medium, frozen in liquid nitrogen and stored at −80 °C until preparation of cryostat tissue sections for localization and quantification of the infection. Samples from the same tissues were taken for histopathology. The experimental procedure was approved by the animal care and ethical committee of Ghent University (EC2012/078).

Chlamydial antigen detection

Vaginal swabs in *Chlamydia* transport medium were shaken for 1 h at 4 °C, centrifuged and cultured in McCoy cells grown on 13 mm cover slips in *Chlamydia* Trac Bottles (International Medical, Brussels, Belgium) as described by Vanrompay et al. [20]. Additionally, cells were washed twice with 1 mL phosphate buffer supplemented with 0.003% DEAE-dextran before the inoculum was added to the cells. Chlamydial growth was monitored using the IMAGEN™ direct immunofluorescence staining (Oxoid, Drongen, Belgium) at 6 days post inoculation. Cryostat tissue sections (5 μm) were also stained by use of the IMAGEN™ immunofluorescence test. All slides were examined by immunofluorescence microscopy (BX41 Olympus, 600×). Positive cells were counted in five microscopic fields. The calculated mean was presented as a score ranging from 0 to 6. Score 0 indicated a negative result. Score 1 and 2 indicated 1 to 5 and 6 to 10 elementary bodies (EBs) per microscopic field in the absence of inclusions, respectively. Score 3 represented more than 10 elementary bodies and 1 inclusion-positive cell per microscopic field. Score 4, 5 and 6 indicated 1 to 5, 6 to 10 and more than 10 inclusion-positive cells per microscopic field, respectively.

Antibody responses

Sera were heat inactivated at 56 °C during 30 min and subsequently pretreated with kaolin to reduce background activity [23]. Vaginal swabs in PBS with protease inhibitor were shaken for 1 h at room temperature and centrifuged. Isotype-specific serum and mucosal antibody titers were determined in an ELISA using purified S45 EBs as antigen. Maxisorp 96-well microtiter plates were coated with purified *C. suis*strain S45 EBs (1×10^7 $TCID_{50}$ per well) diluted in PBS. Plates were blocked overnight (4 °C) with PBS supplemented with 5% bovine serum albumin (BSA). Serum and mucosal antibody titers were determined using twofold dilution series in dilution buffer (PBS + 3% BSA + 0.05% Tween®20), starting at a dilution of 1:15. Antibody isotype titers were determined using monoclonal antibodies against swine IgA (mAb 27.8.1), IgG (mAb 23.3.1b) and IgM (mAb 28.4.1) [24] at a dilution of 1:15, 1:20 and 1:50, respectively, followed by an 1:5000 dilution of biotinylated anti-mouse IgG (H + L) (Dako, Glostrup, Denmark). Subsequently, the plates were incubated with 1:2500 diluted peroxidase-labeled streptavidin (Zymed Laboratories, San Francisco, USA). Finally, the substrate and chromogene ABTS (2, 2′-Azino-di(3-ethylbenzthiazoline-6-sulfonate); KPL, Maryland, USA) was added. Antibody titers were defined as the reciprocal of the highest dilution that gave an absorbance reading at 405 nm above the cut-off value (mean absorbance of seronegative pig serum + twice the standard deviation). Positive and negative control sera and mucosal secretions originated from a former experimental infection in pigs [25].

Proliferative responses of PBMC and MC

At 7 and 10 days post infection (dpi) or re-infection, peripheral blood mononuclear cells (PBMC) were isolated from heparinized blood samples collected from the jugular vein. Isolation of PBMC was performed by density gradient centrifugation (500 × *g*, 18 °C, 25 min) on Lymphoprep™ (Axis-Shield, Oslo, Norway). After lysis of erythrocytes in ammonium chloride, the cells were washed and resuspended in leukocyte medium (RPMI-1640 (Life Technologies, Merelbeke, Belgium) supplemented with 5% heat-inactivated fetal calf serum (Life Technologies), 5×10^{-5} M β-mercaptoethanol (Life Technologies), 1% non-essential amino acids (Life Technologies), 1% sodium pyruvate (Life Technologies), 1% L-glutamine (Life Technologies), 1% penicillin-streptomycin and 1% kanamycin). At euthanasia, monomorphonuclear cells (MC) were isolated from the spleen, the cervical lymph node (*cervicalis superficialis)* and the pelvic lymph nodes (*iliaci mediales*, *iliaci laterales, sacrales* and *anorectales*). Isolation of MC was performed by tearing the tissues apart, after the surrounding fat was removed. Subsequently, the erythrocytes were lysed with ammonium chloride. After centrifugation (270

× *g*, 4 °C, 10 min), the cells were washed and resuspended in leukocyte medium without β-mercaptoethanol. PBMC or MC were grown in 96-well tissue culture plates at a concentration of 5 × 10^5cells/well. Proliferation was tested by adding 10^5 viable *C. suis* purified S45 EBs, 10 μg concanavalin A (ConA) (positive control) or medium (negative control) to the wells. Each condition was tested in duplicate. The cells were incubated at 37 °C in a humidified atmosphere with 5% CO_2. ConA- or antigen-induced proliferation was measured by incorporation of 1 μCi/well of ^{3}H-thymidine (Amersham ICN, Bucks, UK) during the last 16 h of culture, on day 3 and day 4, respectively. Cells were harvested onto glass fiber filter strips (Perkin Elmer, Life Science, Oosterhout, The Netherlands) with a cell harvester (Skatron, Liers, Norway). Radioactivity incorporated into the DNA was measured with a β-scintillation counter (Perkin Elmer). The stimulation index (SI) was defined as the ratio of the mean counts per minute of stimulated PBMC or MC versus the mean counts per minute of the negative control.

Flow cytometric analysis

PBMC and MC from the spleen, cervical and pelvic lymph nodes were isolated as described above. Flow cytometry was used to analyze the immune cell (sub)populations in the blood at different time points post infection and of the spleen, cervical and pelvic lymph nodes at euthanasia. T cell populations ($CD3^+CD4^+CD8^-$, $CD3^+CD4^-CD8^+$, $CD3^+CD4^+CD8^+$, $CD3^+CD4^-CD8^-$, T cells with a γδ T cell receptor), B cells ($MHCII^+CD21^+$, $MHCII^+IgM^+$), monocytes ($MHCII^+SWC3^+$), NK cells ($CD3^-CD4^-CD8^+$) and plasmacytoid dendritic cells (pDC) ($CD3^-CD4^+CD8^-$) were quantified. However, for the lymphoid tissues the $CD3^-CD4^+CD8^-$ population does not exist entirely of pDC, but also contains an unknown lineage, presumably of myeloid origin [26]. Based on the used markers, it was impossible to distinguish between both populations. PBMC and MC (10^6 cells) were incubated for 20 min in staining buffer (RPMI-1640 + 1% heat-inactivated FCS) with optimal concentrations of mAbs (Table 1). Cells stained with isotype-matched irrelevant mAbs were used to analyze aspecific binding. Subsequently, the cells were washed with staining buffer and incubated (20 min) with the appropriate isotype-specific Alexa-647-, FITC- or PE- conjugated antibodies (Life Technologies). Cells were washed with staining buffer and with PBS and were resuspended in PBS. Data were acquired on a FACSCanto flow cytometer (Beckton Dickinson, Erembodegem, Belgium) with a minimum event count of 50 000 and analyzed with FACSDiva® software. Doublets were excluded based on FSC-H/FSC-A and SSC-H/SSC-A plots.

Table 1: Monoclonal antibodies used in flow cytometry

Specificity	Clone	Isotype	Reference
CD3	PTT3	IgG1	[27]
CD4	74-12-4	IgG2b	[28]
CD8α	11/295/33	IgG2a	[29]
CD8β	PG164A	IgG2a	[30]
CD21	BB6-11C9	IgG1	[30]
IgM	28.4.1	IgG1	[24]
MHCII	MSA3	IgG2a	[31]
SWC3a	74-22-15	IgG1	[28]
TCR1-N4 (δ chain)	PGBL22A	IgG1	[32]

Cytokine secretion by PBMC and MC

PBMC and MC isolated from the spleen, pelvic lymph nodes and the *cervicales superficiales dorsales* lymph nodes were planted in 24-well microtiter plates at a concentration of 10^7 cells/well. Subsequently, the cells were stimulated by adding 10^5 viable purified S45 EBs to each well. Supernatant was collected 16, 24, 48 and 72 h later. The concentration of IL-1β, IL-4, IL-6, IL-8, IL-10, IL-12p40, IFN-γ and TNF-α in the supernatant was determined using commercially available ELISA kits (DuoSet® ELISA Development System, R&D Systems, Abingdon, UK). Assays were performed according to the manufacturer's guidelines.

Histopathology

Samples were fixed in 10% phosphate-buffered formalin, dehydrated and embedded in paraffin, sectioned at 5 μm and stained with haematoxylin and eosin. The samples were studied blindly. Slides were examined microscopically (Leitz). The microscopic findings were either graded (none (0), minimal (1), slight (2), moderate (3), marked (4) or severe (5) histological change) or indicated as present or absent without a grade.

Statistical analysis

Statistical analyses were performed using SPSS 22 and results for all groups were compared by use of the non-parametric Mann–Whitney U test. Results were considered significantly different if $P < 0.05$.

RESULTS

Macroscopic lesions

The mean scores for macroscopic lesions, determined at necropsy, are presented in Table 2. Macroscopic lesions were absent in all but one pig of the control group. One control animal had a severely inflamed vagina, cervix and uterus caused by an abnormal vaginal anatomy. Therefore, that animal was excluded from the experiment. All infected and re-infected animals showed gross pathology. The macroscopic lesions were generally more severe for the infection group than for the re-infection group. Four pigs (80%) of the infection group showed moderate to severe congestion of the genital tract. The genital tract of the remaining pig (20%) of the infection group was slightly congested. In the re-infection group, all but one animal (80%) showed only slight congestion of the genital tract. In the other re-infected pig, a severely congested genital tract was noticed. In 60% of the pigs of the infection group, a large amount of clear watery exudate was present in almost the entire genital tract, whereas only one animal (20%) of the re-infection group showed a moderate amount of watery exudate in the cervix. The pelvic lymph nodes were enlarged in 80% of the animals of both infected groups. Congestion of the pelvic lymph nodes could only be detected in four pigs (80%) of the infection group. Macroscopic lesions in the mesovarium and pelvic lymph nodes were significantly different between the groups.

Table 2: Mean scores ± standard deviation (% of positive animals) for macroscopic lesions in the infection and the re-infection group at euthanasia [*]

Tissue	Macroscopic lesion	Infection group	Re-infection group
Vagina	Congestion	0.0 ± 0.00	0.2 ± 0.45 (20)
	Serous exudate	0.6 ± 1.34 (20)	0.0 ± 0.00
Cervix	Congestion	0.6 ± 1.34 (20)	0.2 ± 0.45 (20)
	Serous exudate	1.0 ± 1.41 (40)	0.4 ± 0.89 (20)
Uterus	Congestion	0.8 ± 1.10 (40)	1.0 ± 1.22 (60)
	Hypertrophy	0.6 ± 1.34 (20)	0.0 ± 0.00
	Serous exudate	1.6 ± 1.52 (60)	0.0 ± 0.00
Uterine tubes	Congestion	1.2 ± 1.10 (60)	0.4 ± 0.55 (40)
	Hypertrophy	0.6 ± 1.34 (20)	0.0 ± 0.00
	Serous exudate	1.2 ± 1.64 (40)	0.0 ± 0.00
Oviducts	Serous exudate	0.6 ± 1.34 (20)	0.0 ± 0.00
Ovaries	Congestion	0.4 ± 0.89 (20)	0.0 ± 0.00
Lig. Latum uteri	Congestion	0.8 ± 0.84 (60)	0.4 ± 0.55 (40)
Mesovarium	Congestion	1.6 ± 1.34 (80)[a]	0.2 ± 0.45 (20)
Mesosalpinx	Congestion	1.4 ± 1.52 (60)	0.2 ± 0.45 (20)
Spleen	Congestion	0.4 ± 0.89 (20)	0.0 ± 0.00
	Enlargement	0.0 ± 0.00	1.0 ± 1.41 (40)
Liver	Congestion	0.2 ± 0.45 (20)	0.0 ± 0.00
Pelvic lymph nodes	Congestion	1.6 ± 1.14 (80)[a,c]	0.0 ± 0.00[c]
	Enlargement	2.2 ± 1.3 (80)[a]	2.0 ± 1.22 (80)[b]
Cervical lymph node	Enlargement	1.8 ± 1.64 (60)	0.4 ± 0.89 (20)

[*]The mean score ± SD in the control group was 0.0 ± 0.00 for all tissues.

[a]$P < 0.05$ for a comparison of the control group and the infection group.

[b]$P < 0.05$ for a comparison of the control group and the re-infection group.

[c]$P < 0.05$ for a comparison of the infection group and the re-infection group.

Chlamydia suis vaginal excretion

The presence of viable *C. suis* in vaginal swabs was examined using culture in McCoy cells. Figure 1 shows the culture scores for vaginal swabs collected at different time points post infection. All swabs taken at day 0 of the experiment were *Chlamydiaceae* negative. Vaginal swab samples of the control group remained negative throughout the experiment. Vaginal *C. suis* shedding was detected in the infection group from day 59, three days after infection of those animals, onwards. In the re-infection group, *C. suis* excretion was consistently high from day 3 to day 28 post primo-infection. After 28 dpi, mean culture scores decreased gradually until re-infection. Thereafter shedding was again consistently high. Before primo-infection of the infection group, the mean excretion scores of the re-infection group were statistically higher than those of the other groups. From day 59 onwards, vaginal shedding was significantly higher in the infection group and the re-infection group than in the control group. After primo-infection of the infection group, the mean culture scores of both infected groups did only differ statistically at day 66, when the infection group had the highest score, and at day 70, when the re-infection group had the highest score.

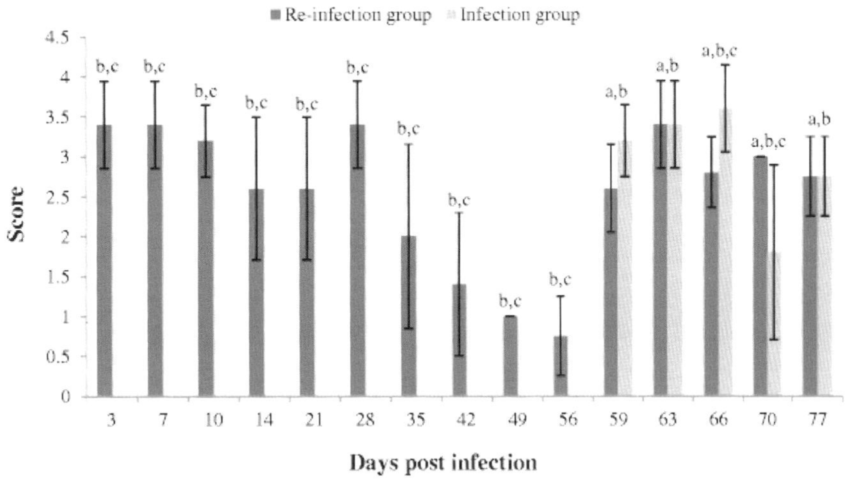

Figure 1: Mean scores ± standard deviation for vaginal *C. suis* shedding from 3 to 77 dpi in the infection and the re-infection group. The mean score ± SD in the control group was 0.0 ± 0.00 for all time points. [a]$P < 0.05$ for a comparison of the control group and the infection group. [b]$P < 0.05$ for a comparison of the control group and the re-infection group. [c]$P < 0.05$ for a comparison of the infection group and the re-infection group.

Chlamydial antigen detection in the urogenital tract

Table 3 presents the mean scores for the presence of *Chlamydiaceae* in urogenital tissues collected at euthanasia, 21 days after infection or re-infection of the infection group and the re-infection group, respectively. All tissue samples from the non-infected pigs were negative, as were the spleen, the liver and the caecum of both infected groups. An ascending chlamydial infection occurred in all pigs of the infection group and in 4 of 5 pigs of the re-infection group, as chlamydial EBs and/or intracellular inclusions were detected in the upper genital tract of those animals. Intracellular chlamydial inclusions, indicating the presence of replicating chlamydiae, were detected in the urethra (20%), vagina (40%), cervix (60%), right uterine horn (20%), oviducts (20%) and ovaries (40%) of the infection group. In the re-infection group, chlamydial replication could only be observed in the urethra of one pig (20%), the vagina of two pigs (40%) and the right oviduct of one pig (20%). Overall, more chlamydial EBs and inclusions, demonstrated by higher mean scores, occurred in the urogenital tract of the infection group than of the re-infection group. Statistical analysis revealed significant differences between the mean scores of the right uterine horn and the left oviduct of both infected groups. Furthermore, mean scores for the presence of *Chlamydiaceae* in the vagina, right uterine horn, left oviduct and right ovary of the infection group were statistically higher than for the control group. In the re-infection group, the level of *Chlamydia* replication in the vagina and the urethra was significantly higher than in the non-infected pigs.

Table 3: Mean scores ± standard deviation for the presence of *C. suis* in urogenital tissues of the infection and the re-infection group at euthanasia *

Tissue	Infection group	Re-infection group
Vagina	1.80 ± 1.10[a]	2.00 ± 1.41[b]
Cervix	2.00 ± 1.87	0.40 ± 0.55
Corpus uteri	0.80 ± 0.45	0.20 ± 0.45
Uterine horn R	1.40 ± 0.89[a,c]	0.40 ± 0.55[c]
Uterine horn L	0.20 ± 0.45	0.40 ± 0.55
Oviduct R	0.80 ± 1.30	0.80 ± 1.30
Oviduct L	1.40 ± 0.89[a,c]	0.50 ± 0.58[c]
Ovary R	1.60 ± 1.34[a]	0.20 ± 0.45
Ovary L	0.80 ± 1.30	0.00 ± 0.00
Urethra	1.20 ± 1.30	1.20 ± 1.10[b]

*The mean score ± SD in the control group was 0.00 ± 0.00 for all tissues.

[a]$P < 0.05$ for a comparison of the control group and the infection group.

[b]$P < 0.05$ for a comparison of the control group and the re-infection group.

[c]$P < 0.05$ for a comparison of the infection group and the re-infection group.

Antibody responses

The *C. suis* S45-specific IgM, IgG and IgA antibody titers in serum (Table 4) and vaginal swab samples (Table 5) were determined following primo- and re-infection. The control pigs had no chlamydial antibodies in both serum and vaginal secretion throughout the experiment. Before infection, no serum or vaginal antibodies were detected in the animals of the infection and the re-infection group. Primo-infection induced IgM and IgG, but no IgA antibodies in serum and vaginal secretion. *C. suis* S45-specific serum IgM and IgG were observed from 7 days post primo-infection onwards and mean titers peaked at 14 or 21 dpi. Vaginal antichlamydial IgM and IgG antibodies appeared at 14 and at 14 and 21 days post primo-infection, respectively. Seven days after re-infection, mean *C. suis*-specific serum IgM and IgG titers had increased again and they kept on rising towards euthanasia. Antichlamydial mucosal IgM and IgG antibodies were detected from 7 to 14 and from 7 to 21 days post re-infection, respectively. Moreover, *C. suis*-specific serum and vaginal IgA antibodies appeared from 14 days following re-infection onwards. Compared to the antibody responses after primo-infection, re-infection with *C. suis* S45 induced lower IgM antibody titers and higher antichlamydial IgG and IgA titers, which is illustrative for a secondary antibody response.

Table 4: Mean *C. suis* S45-specific IgM, IgG and IgA serum titers of the infection (I) and the re-infection (R) group ± standard deviation *

Dpi	Procedure	Serum IgM		Serum IgG		Serum IgA
		Infection group	Re-infection group	Infection group	Re-infection group	Re-infection group
0	Infection R	0 ± 0.00	0 ± 0.00	0 ± 0.00	0 ± 0.00	0 ± 0.00
7		0 ± 0.00[c]	30 ± 0.00[b,c]	0 ± 0.00[c]	48 ± 16.43[b,c]	0 ± 0.00
14		0 ± 0.00[c]	168 ± 98.59[b,c]	0 ± 0.00[c]	240 ± 0.00[b,c]	0 ± 0.00
21		0 ± 0.00[c]	60 ± 0.00[b,c]	0 ± 0.00[c]	144 ± 90.99[b,c]	0 ± 0.00
28		0 ± 0.00	0 ± 0.00	0 ± 0.00[c]	36 ± 13.42[b,c]	0 ± 0.00
35		0 ± 0.00	0 ± 0.00	0 ± 0.00[c]	48 ± 16.43[b,c]	0 ± 0.00
42		0 ± 0.00	0 ± 0.00	0 ± 0.00[c]	36 ± 13.42[b,c]	0 ± 0.00
49		0 ± 0.00	0 ± 0.00	0 ± 0.00[c]	54 ± 39.12[b,c]	0 ± 0.00
56	Infection I & R	0 ± 0.00	0 ± 0.00	0 ± 0.00[c]	48 ± 16.43[b,c]	0 ± 0.00
63		30 ± 0.00[a]	30 ± 0.00[b]	45 ± 21.21[a,c]	264 ± 131.45[b,c]	0 ± 0.00
70		216 ± 53.67[a,c]	42 ± 16.43[b,c]	120 ± 0.00[a,c]	336 ± 131.45[b,c]	30 ± 0.00[b,c]
77	Euthanasia	72 ± 26.83[a]	60 ± 0.00[b]	195 ± 178.12[a,c]	816 ± 321.99[b,c]	60 ± 0.00[b,c]

*The mean IgM, IgG and IgA serum antibody titers ± SD in the control group and the mean IgA serum titers ± SD in the infection group were 0 ± 0.00 for all time points. Antibody titers were defined as the reciprocal of the highest dilution that gave an absorbance reading at 405 nm above the cut-off value (mean absorbance of seronegative pig serum + twice the standard deviation).

[a]$P < 0.05$ for a comparison of the control group and the infection group.

[b]$P < 0.05$ for a comparison of the control group and the re-infection group.

[c]$P < 0.05$ for a comparison of the infection group and the re-infection group.

Table 5: Mean *C. suis* S45-specific IgM, IgG and IgA mucosal (vaginal) titers of the infection (I) and the re-infection (R) group ± standard deviation *

Dpi	Procedure	Mucosal IgM		Mucosal IgG		Mucosal IgA
		Infection group	Re-infection group	Infection group	Re-infection group	Re-infection group
0	Infection R	0 ± 0.00	0 ± 0.00	0 ± 0.00	0 ± 0.00	0 ± 0.00
7		0 ± 0.00	0 ± 0.00	0 ± 0.00	0 ± 0.00	0 ± 0.00
14		0 ± 0.00[c]	60 ± 0.00[b,c]	0 ± 0.00[c]	54 ± 13.42[b,c]	0 ± 0.00
21		0 ± 0.00	0 ± 0.00	0 ± 0.00[c]	30 ± 0.00[b,c]	0 ± 0.00
28-49		0 ± 0.00	0 ± 0.00	0 ± 0.00	0 ± 0.00	0 ± 0.00

56	Infection I & R	0 ± 0.00	0 ± 0.00	0 ± 0.00	0 ± 0.00	0 ± 0.00
63		0 ± 0.00^{c}	30 ± 0.00^{b,c}	0 ± 0.00^{c}	48 ± 16.43^{b,c}	0 ± 0.00
70		48 ± 16.43^{a,c}	24 ± 13.42^{b,c}	60 ± 0.00^{a,c}	96 ± 32.86^{b,c}	24 ± 13.42^{b,c}
77	Euthanasia	0 ± 0.00	0 ± 0.00	96 ± 32.86^{a,c}	48 ± 16.43^{b,c}	30 ± 0.00^{b,c}

*The mean IgM, IgG and IgA mucosal antibody titers ± SD in the control group and the mean IgA mucosal titers ± SD in the infection group were 0 ± 0.00 for all time points. Antibody titers were defined as the reciprocal of the highest dilution that gave an absorbance reading at 405 nm above the cut-off value (mean absorbance of seronegative pig serum + twice the standard deviation).

$^{a}P < 0.05$ for a comparison of the control group and the infection group.

$^{b}P < 0.05$ for a comparison of the control group and the re-infection group.

$^{c}P < 0.05$ for a comparison of the infection group and the re-infection group.

Proliferative responses of PBMC and MC

Proliferative responses of PBMC to *C. suis* strain S45 were determined 7 and 10 days post primo-infection of the re-infection group, and again at day 63 and day 66, 7 and 10 days post infection or re-infection of the infection group and the re-infection group, respectively. At day 7 and 10, the proliferative activities of PBMC of all groups were statistically the same (data not shown). At day 63, the mean stimulation index (SI ± SD) of the PBMC for the control group, the infection group and the re-infection group were 2.03 ± 1.42, 2.15 ± 1.23 and 8.80 ± 5.46, respectively. The PBMC of the re-infection group showed significantly higher proliferative responses than the PBMC of the other groups. At day 66, the mean SI ± SD of the PBMC for the control, the infection and the re-infection group were 7.42 ± 2.87, 2.24 ± 1.35 and 7.29 ± 3.39. The proliferative activity of PBMC of the infection group was statistically lower than for the control group and the re-infection group. However, at day 66, the PBMC of the control group showed significantly higher proliferative responses to the positive control ConA, a T cell mitogen, than the PBMC of the other groups (data not shown). This indicates that the PBMC of the control group had a higher proliferative capacity than the other groups at that time and explains the high SI following stimulation with *C. suis* for the control group. At euthanasia, proliferative responses of MC from the spleen, cervical and pelvic lymph nodes were statistically the same for all groups (data not shown).

Immune cell populations

Blood immune cell populations were analyzed by flow cytometry at 7 and 10 days post primo-infection of the re-infection group and again at day 63 and day 66, 7 and 10 days post infection or re-infection of the infection group and the re-infection group, respectively. Seven days post primo-infection of the re-infection group, the infected animals had a significantly lower mean percentage of $CD4^{+}$ T cells than the non-infected animals. At day 10, a significantly lower percentage of T cells was noticed in the re-infection group than in the infection group. At day 63, the re-infected animals had significantly higher mean percentages of T cells, B cells and monocytes, but a significantly lower mean percentage of pDC as compared to the control group or the infection group. Within total T cells, significantly less $CD4^{+}CD8^{-}$ T cells were present in the re-infection group than in the infection group. At day 66, the re-infection group had significantly higher percentages of B cells and $CD4^{-}CD8^{+}$ T cells. At that time, a significantly lower percentage of monocytes was detected in the infection group than in the other groups. Furthermore, immune cell populations in the spleen, cervical and pelvic lymph nodes were analyzed at euthanasia. For the spleen, the mean percentage of T cells was significantly lower in the re-infection group than in the other groups and within total T cells significantly less $CD4^{+}CD8^{+}$ and $CD4^{-}CD8^{+}$ T cells and significantly more $CD4^{+}CD8^{-}$ T cells were present in the re-infection group. Moreover, the re-infection group had significantly lower mean percentages of B cells and monocytes in the spleen as compared to the control group, but a significantly higher percentage of $CD3^{-}CD4^{+}CD8^{-}$ spleen MC, which contain pDC, than the other groups. The mean percentage of NK cells in the spleen was significantly higher for the infection group. For the cervical lymph nodes, significantly higher mean percentages of $CD4^{+}CD8^{-}$ T cells, B cells and monocytes, besides a significantly lower mean percentage of $CD3^{-}CD4^{+}CD8^{-}$ MC, containing pDC, were noticed in the non-infected animals. For the pelvic lymph nodes, the control pigs had significantly higher mean percentages of γδ T cells, IgM^{+} B cells and monocytes. The mean percentage of NK cells was significantly higher for the infection group than for the re-infected animals. Within total T cells, significantly more $CD4^{-}CD8^{+}$ T cells were detected in the re-infection group than in the other groups.

Cytokine secretion by PBMC and MC

Results for cytokine detection at 16 h and 72 h post stimulation are presented. Data of cytokine production at 24 h and 48 h post stimulation are not shown, since the results were either without statistical differences between the groups or with statistical differences similar to these observed at 72 h post stimulation. Compared to the amount of cytokines produced at 16 h following stimulation, PBMC and MC had produced generally more IFN-γ, TNF-α, IL-6 and IL-10 and less IL-1β at 72 h after stimulation. Only the data of cytokine secretion at 72 h post stimulation are discussed in detail.

At 7 dpi, the PBMC of the re-infection group produced significantly more TNF-α, IL-1β, IL-6 and IL-12p40 than the PBMC of the other groups. At day 10, cytokine production by PBMC was statistically the same for all groups. At day 63, seven days post infection or re-infection of the infection group and the re-infection group, respectively, the mean concentrations of IFN-γ, TNF-α, IL-1β, IL-6, IL-10 and IL-12p40 for the re-infection group were significantly higher than the concentrations produced by the PBMC of the other groups. At day 66, the PBMC of the re-infected animals had produced significantly more TNF-α, IL-1β, IL-6 and IL-10 than the PBMC of the other animals. Furthermore, significantly more IL-8 and IL-12p40 was produced by the blood mononuclear cells from the re-infection group when compared to the infection group. For the infection group, mean IL-1β and IL-10 concentrations in PBMC culture media were significantly lower than for the control group.

At euthanasia, spleen MC of the infection group had produced significantly less IFN-γ, TNF-α, IL-1β, IL-6, IL-8 and IL-12p40 than MC of the other groups. The production of TNF-α, IL-6 and IL-8 by cervical lymph node MC was significantly higher for the control animals than for the infection or the re-infection group. Mean IL-6 amounts produced by MC isolated from the pelvic lymph nodes were significantly higher for the control group than for both infected groups. The MC from pelvic lymph nodes of the infection group produced significantly less IL-4 than the MC of the control group.

Histopathology

An overview of the mean scores of the histopathological lesions found in the urogenital tract of the pigs at euthanasia is presented in Table 6. Histopathological findings consisted of: (a) intraluminal proteinaceous fluid; (b) the presence of a superficial layer of exfoliated (epithelial) cells and/or inflammatory cells: cells and debris laying on the surface of the epithelium; (c) interepithelial inflammatory cells, thus indicating the presence of migrating lymphocytes or polymorphonuclear cells in the epithelium; (d) degeneration (vacuolation) and/or apoptosis (cell death) of epithelial cells; (e) infiltration of inflammatory cells in the lamina propria with infiltration of the connective tissue layer beneath the epithelium with polymorphonuclear cells (pmc), a feature of more acute inflammation, or with mononuclear cells (mnc) (lymphocytes and/or plasma cells), a feature of more subacute to chronic inflammation; (f) oedema in the lamina propria: presence of loosely arranged fibers in the connective tissue and/or eosinophilic fluid between the fibers; (g) infiltration of inflammatory cells (pmc or mnc) in the muscular layer, (h) or in the serosa. In the corpus uteri, both uterine horns and the right oviduct mononuclear inflammatory cells increased slightly in the mucosa with infection with *C. suis* S45 (infection group) and even more when animals were re-infected (re-infection group). The inflammatory cells in the infection group were more periglandularly clustered in the deep mucosa, whereas in the re-infection group the inflammation was more diffusely present throughout the mucosa. No lesions were noted in both ovaries and the lesions observed in the left oviduct, the cervix, the vagina and the urethra did not differ statistically between the different groups. In the liver of two pigs of the re-infection group slight to moderate, focal to multifocal granulomatous inflammations within the portal areas were noticed. The same animals presented also minimal to slight diffuse follicular hyperplasia in the spleen, a feature of immunological stimulation. The spleen and liver samples from the remaining pigs and all caecum samples showed no histopathological changes.

Table 6: Mean scores ± standard deviations for histopathological findings [#]

Tissue	Histopathological findings	Control group	Infection group	Re-infection group
Vagina	Exfoliation*	0.5 ± 1.00	0.2 ± 0.45	0.0 ± 0.00
	Interepithelial inflammatory cells	0.0 ± 0.00	0.4 ± 0.55	0.2 ± 0.45
	Degeneration and/or apoptosis of epithelial cells	0.0 ± 0.00	0.4 ± 0.55	0.4 ± 0.55
	Infiltration of mnc in the lamina propria	1.5 ± 0.58	1.4 ± 0.55	1.2 ± 0.45
Cervix	Interepithelial inflammatory cells	1.0 ± 0.82	0.8 ± 0.84	1.2 ± 0.84
	Degeneration and/or apoptosis of epithelial cells	0.0 ± 0.00	0.2 ± 0.45	0.0 ± 0.00
	Infiltration of mnc in the lamina propria	2.0 ± 0.82	1.4 ± 0.55	1.8 ± 0.84
Corpus	Interepithelial inflammatory cells	1.0 ± 0.00	1.2 ± 0.45	1.2 ± 0.45
uteri	Degeneration and/or apoptosis of epithelial cells	0.3 ± 0.50	0.2 ± 0.45	0.0 ± 0.00
	Infiltration of mnc in the lamina propria	1.0 ± 0.00[b]	1.2 ± 1.30	2.0 ± 0.71[b]
	Oedema lamina propria	2.3 ± 0.96	1.8 ± 1.30	1.4 ± 1.34
Uterine	Exfoliation*	0.0 ± 0.00	0.0 ± 0.00	0.4 ± 0.89
Horn R	Interepithelial inflammatory cells	1.3 ± 0.50	1.2 ± 0.45	1.2 ± 0.45
	Degeneration and/or apoptosis of epithelial cells	0.3 ± 0.50	0.4 ± 0.55	0.0 ± 0.00
	Infiltration of mnc in the lamina propria	1.3 ± 0.50[b]	2.2 ± 1.10	2.6 ± 0.55[b]
	Oedema lamina propria	1.5 ± 0.58	1.6 ± 1.34	1.2 ± 1.30

Uterine	Exfoliation*	0.0 ± 0.00	0.4 ± 0.89	0.0 ± 0.00
Horn L	Interepithelial inflammatory cells	1.8 ± 0.50	1.8 ± 0.45	1.2 ± 0.45
	Degeneration and/or apoptosis of epithelial cells	0.3 ± 0.50	0.8 ± 0.45	0.8 ± 0.45
	Infiltration of mnc in the lamina propria	1.3 ± 0.50[b]	2.2 ± 1.10	2.4 ± 0.55[b]
	Oedema lamina propria	1.0 ± 0.82	1.4 ± 0.55	1.0 ± 0.00
Oviduct R	Intraluminal proteinaceous fluid	4 of 4	4 of 5	4 of 5
	Exfoliation*	0.5 ± 0.58	0.0 ± 0.00	0.0 ± 0.00
	Infiltration of mnc in the lamina propria	1.0 ± 0.00[b]	1.4 ± 0.55[c]	2.2 ± 0.45[b,c]
Oviduct L	Intraluminal proteinaceous fluid	1 of 4	1 of 5	2 of 5
	Exfoliation*	0.3 ± 0.50	0.2 ± 0.45	0.4 ± 0.55
	Interepithelial inflammatory cells	0.0 ± 0.00	0.4 ± 0.55	0.6 ± 0.55
	Infiltration of pmc in the lamina propria	0.3 ± 0.50	0.0 ± 0.00	0.0 ± 0.00
	Infiltration of mnc in the lamina propria	1.3 ± 0.50	1.4 ± 0.89	1.4 ± 0.55
Urethra	Interepithelial inflammatory cells	0.3 ± 0.50	0.2 ± 0.45	0.0 ± 0.00
	Infiltration of mnc in the lamina propria	1.0 ± 0.00	0.8 ± 1.30	1.4 ± 1.52

[#]The mean scores ± SD for the histopathological parameters which are not shown in the table, were 0.0 ± 0.00 for the three groups.

*Superficial layer of exfoliated (epithelial) cells and/or inflammatory cells.

pmc: polymorphonuclear inflammatory cells; mnc: mononuclear inflammatory cells.

[b]$P < 0.05$ for a comparison of the control group and the re-infection group.

[c]$P < 0.05$ for a comparison of the infection group and the re-infection group.

DISCUSSION

Genital *C. suis* infections are likely to be transmitted venereally, since these bacteria have been detected in the semen of boars [1],[12],[13]. However, non-sexual transmission cannot be ruled out, for instance by fecal contamination of the vagina. In fact, *C. suis* has been commonly detected in the gastrointestinal tract of pigs [33], and in most of the cases it is associated with subclinical infections. Therefore, the gastrointestinal tract could serve as a reservoir for chlamydial genital tract infection [34]. In this study, female pigs were successfully infected in the genital tract with *C. suis* strain S45, which was isolated from feces of an asymptomatic pig. This indeed suggests that persistent intestinal *C. suis* infections are able to cause pathology in the genital tract of pigs.

In the present study, all infected animals showed gross pathology at necropsy. However, the pigs that were infected once had significantly more severe lesions than the re-infected animals. Moreover, more chlamydial EBs and inclusions were found in the urogenital tract of the infection group than in the re-infected pigs. For the infection group, chlamydial replication occurred throughout the urogenital tract and even in the ovaries, whereas for the re-infection group, inclusions were scarce. This indicates that a certain level of protection against re-infection was developed following primo-infection. This presumption is in accordance with human epidemiologic studies suggesting that prior genital infection with *Chlamydia trachomatis*, which is phylogenetically highly related to *C. suis*, confers some short term protection against re-infection [35],[36]. Moreover, in all evaluated animal models of genital chlamydial infection, including the mouse [37], guinea pig [38] and macaque [39], it has been demonstrated that at least partial immunity to re-infection develops. Nevertheless, vaginal inoculation with *C. suis* resulted in an ascending infection in both groups. Likewise, *C. trachomatis* was able to ascend in the genital tract of pigs after intravaginal inoculation [40]. No chlamydial bacteria were detected outside the urogenital tract. With the exception of the lymphogranuloma venereum strains, *C. trachomatis* also does not disseminate beyond the urogenital tract [41].

Infection of the female porcine genital tract with *C. suis* resulted microscopically in a slight increase of mononuclear inflammatory cells in the mucosa of the corpus uteri, both uterine horns and the right oviduct. Surprisingly, this histopathological finding was even more prominent when animals were re-infected, which is not in accordance with the less severe macroscopic lesions and the lower mean scores for the presence of chlamydial bacteria observed in this group. However, these mononuclear cells, including lymphocytes and plasma cells, may indicate the mobilization of memory cells in response to re-infection and can contribute to protective immunity against infection. In the future, we will include immunohistochemistry to obtain in situ information on the cells contributing to this partial protection. Schautteet et al. [42] also observed that protection against gross lesions was correlated with a higher infiltration of mononuclear inflammatory cells in the genital tract mucosa of pigs intravaginally infected with *C. trachomatis*.

Vaginal chlamydial excretion was observed in all infected animals from three dpi onwards. There were no differences noticed between shedding after primo-infection and re-infection. Interestingly, vaginal excretion started to decrease gradually at four weeks post primo-infection and one out of five animals stopped shedding chlamydial bacteria at 56 dpi. Since the animals were infected again at that moment, we could not determine whether the pigs were able to resolve a genital *C. suis* infection spontaneously after a certain period of time. Also, it would have been interesting to follow up the animals for a longer period than three weeks post re-infection in order to assess whether chlamydial excretion stops earlier post re-infection than post primo-infection.

Primo-infection with *C. suis* induced antichlamydial IgM and IgG, but no IgA antibodies in sera and vaginal secretions. Compared to the antibody responses after primo-infection, re-infection with *C. suis* resulted in lower IgM antibody titers and higher IgG and IgA titers in sera and genital secretions, which is illustrative for a secondary antibody response. Furthermore, re-infection was, in contrast to primo-infection, able to induce *C. suis*-specific proliferation of PBMC after 7 and 10 days, which indicates the mobilization of memory cells in response to re-infection. Re-infection was associated with a shift to more B cells, monocytes and $CD4^{-}CD8^{+}$ T cells, but less pDC and $CD4^{+}CD8^{-}$ T cells within PBMC. However, the immune responses detected in the blood do not necessarily reflect the immune responses induced at the local site of infection. Again, immunohistochemistry might assist in determining the local responses. The shifts in immune cell populations from the spleen, cervical and pelvic lymph nodes are presumably not resulting from *C. suis*-specific MC since their proliferative responses were not statistically different between groups.

Primary genital *C. suis* infection of the re-infection group (nine-week-old pigs) resulted in increased secretion of TNF-α, IL-1β, IL-6 and IL-12p40 by PBMC, whereas primo-infection of the infection group (seventeen-week-old animals) decreased the IL-1β, IL-8 and IL-10 secretion by PBMC. This discrepancy could be due to age differences between both groups at the moment of the primo-infection. In pigs, various aspects of the immune system change with age such as the level of NK cells, which was shown to be higher in younger pigs [43],[44]. Since NK cells produce cytokines like TNF-α, this can explain the higher cytokine production following primo-infection at nine weeks of age. Furthermore, it was demonstrated that neonatal porcine blood DCs were more responsive to stimulation with toll-like receptor ligands than adult porcine blood DCs, since they showed higher expression levels of cytokines and chemokines following stimulation [45]. After re-infection, higher concentrations of IFN-γ and IL-10 were produced by PBMC, next to higher amounts of the cytokines upregulated after primo-infection.

Our data suggest that antibody producing B cells, mononuclear phagocytes, $CD8^{+}$ T cells, and IFN-γ may contribute to protection against a genital *C. suis* infection. The role of IL-10 is less clear. Antibodies, and especially mucosal antibodies, albeit not considered as crucial, may contribute to protection by neutralization and opsonization of extracellular *Chlamydia*. Indeed, antibodies clearly play an important role in resistance to genital *Chlamydia muridarum* re-infection in mice [46]. Moreover, mucosal antichlamydial IgA antibodies have been associated with the resolution of *C. muridarum* and *C. trachomatis* infection in mice and women, respectively [47],[48]. The Th1-type cytokine IFN-γ was also shown to be essential for the resolution of *C. muridarum* infection [49],[50]. IFN-γ produced by NK cells, $CD4^{+}$ Th1 cells and $CD8^{+}$ cytotoxic T cells is known to up-regulate and/or induce expression of major histocompatibility complex (MHC) class I and II molecules on a number of cells, including antigen presenting cells. In addition, IFN-γ favours immunoglobulin class switching to the IgG2a isotype and activation of cytotoxic T lymphocytes, which induce apoptosis in infected cells. IL-10, as the main anti-inflammatory cytokine, plays important roles in immune-homeostasis after microbe elimination [51]. IL-10 expression results in an inhibition of antigen presentation and MHCII expression on the surface of infected cells. However, as an anti-inflammatory cytokine, it also deactivates macrophages and interferes with the Th1 response through inhibition of the NF-κB pathway [52]. Interestingly, Moore-Connors et al. [53] showed that *C. muridarum* induces a novel $CD43^{-}CD1d^{hi}CD5^{+}$ IL-10-producing regulatory B cell population (Bregs) during a genital infection in mice. These IL-10 producing B cells displayed *bona fide*regulatory Breg activity by potently suppressing IFN-γ production in vitro in an IL-10-dependent manner. We do not know if these IL-10 producing $CD43^{-}CD1d^{hi}CD5^{+}$ Bregs do exist in the pig and if they can be induced by *C. suis*, but it could be a possible explanation for our observation that $CD4^{+}$ Th1 cells, which are generally considered as crucial immune effectors in antichlamydial immunity, were less dominantly present.

In conclusion, we demonstrated that *C. suis* strain S45 is pathogenic for the female porcine urogenital tract. Chlamydial replication occurred throughout the urogenital tract, causing inflammation and pathology. Furthermore, genital infection elicited both cellular and humoral immune responses. Compared to the primo-infection of pigs with *C. suis*, re-infection was characterized by less severe macroscopic lesions and significantly less chlamydial EBs and inclusions in the urogenital tract. This indicates the development of a certain degree of protection following the initial infection. Protective immunity against re-infection coincided with higher antichlamydial IgG and IgA antibody titers in sera and vaginal secretions, higher proliferative responses of peripheral blood mononuclear cells (PBMC), higher percentages of blood B lymphocytes, monocytes and $CD8^{+}$ T cells and upregulated production of IFN-γ and IL-10 by PBMC.

DECLARATIONS

Acknowledgements

The research was financed by the Special Research Fund of Ghent University. Arthur Andersen (National Animal Disease Center, USDA Agriculture Research Service, Ames, Iowa) is acknowledged for providing *C. suis*strain S45. We gratefully thank A. Dumont, S. Tshitenge-Mulume, S. Brabant and G. De Smet for technical assistance in the laboratory. I. Kalmar, J. Geldhof and R. Cooman are acknowledged for their veterinary assistance during the animal experiment.

Authors' contributions

EDC carried out the majority of the experiments, was responsible for data collection and analysis and drafted the manuscript. BD supervised the flow cytometric analysis and participated in interpretation of these data. LY prepared and stained all cryosections and performed the interpretation of the stainings. He also participated during the autopsies. KC participated in histopathological analysis. EC participated in the coordination of the study and in helpful discussions. DV conceived of the study, participated during autopsies, assisted during interpretation of all data and critically revised the manuscript. All authors read and approved the final manuscript.

REFERENCES

1. Schautteet K, De Clercq E, Miry C, Van Groenweghe F, Delava P, Kalmar I, Vanrompay D: Tetracycline-resistant *Chlamydia suis* in cases of reproductive failure on Belgian, Cypriote and Israeli pig production farms. J Med Microbiol. 2013, 62: 331-334. 10.1099/jmm.0.042861-0.
2. Rogers DG, Andersen AA: Conjunctivitis caused by a swine *Chlamydia trachomatis*-like organism in gnotobiotic pigs. J Vet Diagn Invest. 1999, 11: 341-344. 10.1177/104063879901100408.
3. Rogers DG, Andersen AA, Hunsaker BD: Lung and nasal lesions caused by a swine chlamydial isolate in gnotobiotic pigs. J Vet Diagn Invest. 1996, 8: 45-55. 10.1177/104063879600800108.
4. Reinhold P, Kirschvink N, Theegarten D, Berndt A: An experimentally induced *Chlamydia suis* infection in pigs results in severe lung function disorders and pulmonary inflammation. Vet Res. 2008, 39: 35-10.1051/vetres:2008012.
5. Rogers DG, Andersen AA: Intestinal lesions caused by two swine chlamydial isolates in gnotobiotic pigs. J Vet Diagn Invest. 1996, 8: 433-440. 10.1177/104063879600800405.
6. Guscetti F, Schiller I, Sydler T, Heinen E, Pospischil A: Experimental enteric infection of gnotobiotic piglets with *Chlamydia suis* strain S45. Vet Microbiol. 2009, 135: 157-168. 10.1016/j.vetmic.2008.09.038.
7. Eggemann G, Wendt M, Hoelzle LE, Jäger C, Weiss R, Failing K: Prevalence of *Chlamydia* infections in breeding sows and their importance in reproductive failure. Dtsch Tierarztl Wochenschr. 2000, 107: 3-10. (in German)
8. Woollen N, Daniels EK, Yeary T, Leipold HW, Phillips RM: Chlamydial infection and perinatal mortality in a swine herd. J Am Vet Med Assoc. 1990, 197: 600-601.
9. Schiller I, Koesters R, Weilenmann R, Thoma R, Kaltenboeck B, Heitz P, Pospischil A: Mixed infections with porcine *Chlamydia trachomatis/pecorum* and infections with ruminant *Chlamydia psittaci* serovar 1 associated with abortions in swine. Vet Microbiol. 1997, 58: 251-260. 10.1016/S0378-1135(97)00154-5.
10. Kauffold J, Melzer F, Berndt A, Hoffmann G, Hotzel H, Sachse K: Chlamydiae in oviducts and uteri of repeat breeder pigs. Theriogenology. 2006, 66: 1816-1823. 10.1016/j.theriogenology.2006.04.042.
11. Sarma DK, Tamuli MK, Rahman T, Boro BR, Deka BC, Rajkonwar CK: Isolation of *chlamydia* from a pig with lesions in the urethra and prostate gland. Vet Rec. 1983, 112: 525-10.1136/vr.112.22.525-a.
12. Kauffold J, Melzer F, Henning K, Schulze K, Leiding C, Sachse K: Prevalence of chlamydiae in boars and semen used for artificial insemination. Theriogenology. 2006, 65: 1750-1758. 10.1016/j.theriogenology.2005.10.010.
13. Teankum K, Pospischil A, Janett F, Bürgi E, Brugnera E, Hoelzle K, Polkinghorne A, Weilenmann R, Zimmermann DR, Borel N, Polkinghorne A, Weilenmann R, Zimmermann DR, Borel N: Detection of chlamydiae in boar semen and genital tracts. Vet Microbiol. 2006, 116: 149-157. 10.1016/j.vetmic.2006.03.021.
14. Hoelzle LE, Steinhausen G, Wittenbrink MM: PCR-based detection of chlamydial infection in swine and subsequent PCR-coupled genotyping of chlamydial omp1-gene amplicons by DNA-hybridization, RFLP-analysis, and nucleotide sequence analysis. Epidemiol Infect. 2000, 125: 427-439. 10.1017/S0950268899004446.
15. Camenisch U, Lu ZH, Vaughan L, Corboz L, Zimmermann DR, Wittenbrink MM, Pospischil A, Sydler T: Diagnostic investigation into the role of *Chlamydiae* in cases of increased rates of return to oestrus in pigs. Vet Rec. 2004, 155: 593-596. 10.1136/vr.155.19.593.
16. Englund S, Af Segerstad CH, Arnlund F, Westergren E, Jacobson M: The occurrence of Chlamydia spp. in pigs with and without clinical disease. BMC Vet Res. 2012, 8: 9-10.1186/1746-6148-8-9.
17. Sachse K, Grossmann E, Berndt A, Schütt C, Henning K, Theegarten D, Anhenn O, Reinhold P: Respiratory chlamydial infection based on experimental aerosol challenge of pigs with *Chlamydia suis*. Comp Immunol Microbiol Infect Dis. 2004, 27: 7-23. 10.1016/S0147-9571(02)00079-6.
18. Rogers DG, Andersen AA: Intestinal lesions caused by a strain of *Chlamydia suis* in weanling pigs infected at 21 days of age. J Vet Diagn Invest. 2000, 12: 233-239. 10.1177/104063870001200306.
19. Kolbl O: Untersuchungen uber das Vorkommen von Miyagawanellen beim Schwein. Wien Tierarztl Monatsschr. 1969, 56: 355-361. (in German)
20. Vanrompay D, Ducatelle R, Haesebrouck F: Diagnosis of avian chlamydiosis: specificity of the modified Giménez staining on smears and comparison of the sensitivity of isolation in eggs and three different cell cultures. Zentralbl Veterinarmed B. 1992, 39: 105-112. 10.1111/j.1439-0442.1992.tb00162.x.
21. Mayr A, Bachmann P, Bibrack B, Wittman G: Zellkulturen — Bebrütete Hühnereier — Versuchstiere. Virol Arbeitsmethoden. 1974, VEB Gustav Fischer Verlag, Jena, 35-
22. Beeckman DS, Meesen G, Van Oostveldt P, Vanrompay D: Digital titration: automated image acquisition and analysis of load and growth of Chlamydophila psittaci. Microsc Res Tech. 2009, 72: 398-402. 10.1002/jemt.20694.

23. Novak M, Moldoveanu Z, Schafer DP, Mestecky J, Compans RW: Murine model for evaluation of protective immunity to influenza virus. Vaccine. 1993, 11: 55-60. 10.1016/0264-410X(93)90339-Y.

24. Van Zaane D, Hulst MM: Monoclonal antibodies against porcine immunoglobulin isotypes. Vet Immunol Immunopathol. 1987, 16: 23-36. 10.1016/0165-2427(87)90171-1.

25. Schautteet K, De Clercq E, Jönsson Y, Lagae S, Chiers K, Cox E, Vanrompay D: Protection of pigs against genital *Chlamydia trachomatis* challenge by parenteral or mucosal DNA immunization. Vaccine. 2012, 30: 2869-2881. 10.1016/j.vaccine.2012.02.044.

26. Mair KH, Sedlak C, Käser T, Pasternak A, Levast B, Gerner W, Saalmüller A, Summerfield A, Gerdts V, Wilson HL, Meurens F: The porcine innate immune system: an update. Dev Comp Immunol. 2014, 45: 321-343. 10.1016/j.dci.2014.03.022.

27. Yang H, Oura CA, Kirkham PA, Parkhouse RM: Preparation of monoclonal anti-porcine CD3 antibodies and preliminary characterization of porcine T lymphocytes. Immunology. 1996, 88: 577-585. 10.1046/j.1365-2567.1996.d01-682.x.

28. Pescovitz MD, Lunney JK, Sachs DH: Preparation and characterization of monoclonal antibodies reactive with porcine PBL. J Immunol. 1984, 133: 368-375.

29. Saalmüller A, Aasted B, Canals A, Dominguez J, Goldman T, Lunney JK, Maurer S, Pescovitz MD, Pospisil R, Salmon H: Analyses of mAb reactive with porcine CD8. Vet Immunol Immunopathol. 1994, 43: 249-254. 10.1016/0165-2427(94)90144-9.

30. Saalmüller A: Characterization of swine leukocyte differentiation antigens. Immunol Today. 1996, 17: 352-354. 10.1016/S0167-5699(96)90273-X.

31. Lunney JK, Walker K, Goldman T, Aasted B, Bianchi A, Binns R, Licence S, Bischof R, Brandon M, Blecha F: Overview of the First International Workshop to Define Swine Leukocyte Cluster of Differentiation (CD) Antigens. Vet Immunol Immunopathol. 1994, 43: 193-206. 10.1016/0165-2427(94)90136-8.

32. Davis WC, Zuckermann FA, Hamilton MJ, Barbosa JI, Saalmüller A, Binns RM, Licence ST: Analysis of monoclonal antibodies that recognize gamma delta T/null cells. Vet Immunol Immunopathol. 1998, 60: 305-316. 10.1016/S0165-2427(97)00107-4.

33. Schiller I, Koesters R, Weilenmann R, Kaltenboeck B, Pospischil A: Polymerase chain reaction (PCR) detection of porcine *Chlamydia trachomatis* and ruminant *Chlamydia psittaci* serovar 1 DNA in formalin-fixed intestinal specimens from swine. Zentralbl Veterinarmed B. 1997, 44: 185-191.

34. Yeruva L, Spencer N, Bowlin AK, Wang Y, Rank RG: Chlamydial infection of the gastrointestinal tract: a reservoir for persistent infection. Pathog Dis. 2013, 68: 88-95. 10.1111/2049-632X.12052.

35. Barnes R, Roddy R, Stamm W: Serovars of *Chlamydia trachomatis* causing repeated genital infections. Chlamydial Infect Proc Sixth Int Symp Hum Chlamydial Infect. Edited by: Oriel D, Ridgeway G, Schachter J, Taylor-Robinson D, Ward M. 1986, 503-507.

36. Rietmeijer CA, Van Bemmelen R, Judson FN, Douglas JM: Incidence and repeat infection rates of *Chlamydia trachomatis*among male and female patients in an STD clinic: implications for screening and rescreening. Sex Transm Dis. 2002, 29: 65-72. 10.1097/00007435-200202000-00001.

37. Barron AL, Rank RG, Moses EB: Immune response in mice infected in the genital tract with mouse pneumonitis agent (*Chlamydia trachomatis* biovar). Infect Immun. 1984, 44: 82-85.

38. Rank RG, Batteiger BE, Soderberg LS: Susceptibility to reinfection after a primary chlamydial genital infection. Infect Immun. 1988, 56: 2243-2249.

39. Wolner-Hanssen P, Patton DL, Holmes KK: Protective immunity in pig-tailed macaques after cervical infection with *Chlamydia trachomatis*. Sex Transm Dis. 1991, 18: 21-25. 10.1097/00007435-199101000-00005.

40. Vanrompay D, Hoang TQ, De Vos L, Verminnen K, Harkinezhad T, Chiers K, Morre SA, Cox E: Specific-pathogen-free pigs as an animal model for studying *Chlamydia trachomatis* genital infection. Infect Immun. 2005, 73: 8317-8321. 10.1128/IAI.73.12.8317-8321.2005.

41. Morrison RP, Caldwell HD: Immunity to murine chlamydial genital infection. Infect Immun. 2002, 70: 2741-2751. 10.1128/IAI.70.6.2741-2751.2002.

42. Schautteet K, Stuyven E, Cox E, Vanrompay D: Validation of the Chlamydia trachomatis genital challenge pig model for testing recombinant protein vaccines. J Med Microbiol. 2011, 60: 117-127. 10.1099/jmm.0.024448-0.

43. Sutherland MA, Rodriguez-Zas SL, Ellis M, Salak-Johnson JL: Breed and age affect baseline immune traits, cortisol, and performance in growing pigs. J Anim Sci. 2005, 83: 2087-2095.

44. Talker SC, Käser T, Reutner K, Sedlak C, Mair KH, Koinig H, Graage R, Viehmann M, Klingler E, Ladinig A, Ritzmann M, Saalmüller A, Gerner W: Phenotypic maturation of porcine NK- and T-cell subsets. Dev Comp Immunol. 2013, 40: 51-68. 10.1016/j.dci.2013.01.003.

45. Auray G, Facci MR, Van Kessel J, Buchanan R, Babiuk LA, Gerdts V: Porcine neonatal blood dendritic cells, but not monocytes, are more responsive to TLRs stimulation than their adult counterparts. PLoS One. 2013, 8: e59629-10.1371/journal.pone.0059629.

46. Morrison SG, Morrison RP: A predominant role for antibody in acquired immunity to chlamydial genital tract reinfection. J Immunol. 2005, 175: 7536-7542. 10.4049/jimmunol.175.11.7536.

47. Morrison RP, Feilzer K, Tumas DB: Gene knockout mice establish a primary protective role for major histocompatibility complex class II-restricted responses in *Chlamydia trachomatis* genital tract infection. Infect Immun. 1995, 63: 4661-4668.

48. Brunham RC, Kuo CC, Cles L, Holmes KK: Correlation of host immune response with quantitative recovery

of *Chlamydia trachomatis* from the human endocervix. Infect Immun. 1983, 39: 1491-1494.

49. Cotter TW, Ramsey KH, Miranpuri GS, Poulsen CE, Byrne GI: Dissemination of *Chlamydia trachomatis* chronic genital tract infection in gamma interferon gene knockout mice. Infect Immun. 1997, 65: 2145-2152.

50. Perry LL, Feilzer K, Caldwell HD: Immunity to *Chlamydia trachomatis* is mediated by T helper 1 cells through IFN-gamma-dependent and -independent pathways. J Immunol. 1997, 158: 3344-3352.

51. Hakimi H, Zare-Bidaki M, Zainodini N, Assar S, Arababadi MK: Significant roles played by IL-10 in *Chlamydia* infections. Inflammation. 2014, 37: 818-823. 10.1007/s10753-013-9801-1.

52. Moore KW, De Waal MR, Coffman RL, O'Garra A: Interleukin-10 and the interleukin-10 receptor. Annu Rev Immunol. 2001, 19: 683-765. 10.1146/annurev.immunol.19.1.683.

53. Moore-Connors JM, Kim HS, Marshall JS, Stadnyk AW, Halperin SA, Wang J: CD43-, but not CD43+, IL-10-producing CD1dhiCD5+ B cells suppress type 1 immune responses during*Chlamydia muridarum*genital tract infection. in press.,

CHAPTER 5

MOLECULAR AND PATHOLOGICAL INSIGHTS INTO CHLAMYDIA PECORUM-ASSOCIATED SPORADIC BOVINE ENCEPHALOMYELITIS (SBE) IN WESTERN AUSTRALIA

Martina Jelocnik, David Forshaw, Jennifer Cotter, Danny Roberts, Peter Timms and Adam Polkinghorne

Keywords: Sporadic bovine encephalomyelitis, *Chlamydia pecorum,* Cattle, MLSA, Histopathology, Immunohistochemistry

BACKGROUND

Cases of *Chlamydia pecorum* infection in Australian livestock are not well documented with only sporadic reports of chlamydiosis described by district veterinarians in agriculturally productive areas in Australia [1, 2, 3]. In cattle, *C. pecorum* is known to cause sporadic bovine encephalomyelitis (SBE), characterised by systemic infection involving the central nervous system. Cattle with SBE present with fever, followed by depression, limb stiffness, diarrhoea and staggering [2, 4]. The disease is often fatal without rapid antimicrobial treatment in high doses [5]. *C. pecorum* can also cause other diseases in ruminants including infertility, vaginitis [6], enteritis [7], mastitis [8], pneumonia [9], conjunctivitis and arthritis [10]. The majority of *C. pecorum* infections in cattle appear to be subclinical and asymptomatic while exerting chronic pathological effects on the health of infected animals [10, 11]. A common feature of these infections has been the consistent presence of *C. pecorum* in the gastrointestinal tract [5, 10, 12]. It has been suggested that the major route of transmission is the faecal-oral route, although infected animals also shed chlamydiae from genital [13], ocular and nasal sites [14].

Citation: Martina Jelocnik, David Forshaw, Jennifer Cotter, Danny Roberts, Peter Timms and Adam Polkinghorne, Molecular and pathological insights into Chlamydia pecorum-associated sporadic bovine encephalomyelitis (SBE) in Western Australia, DOI: 10.1186/1746-6148-10-121.

The detection of *C. pecorum* from different anatomical sites in infected animals associated with a range of diseases other than SBE, has raised questions over the pathogenic potential of *C. pecorum* and the exact relationship between different strains and disease. Molecular markers have been used to discriminate between livestock *C. pecorum* strains with different disease presentations [15, 16]. Yousef Mohamad et al. (2008), using Multi Virulence Locus Sequence Typing (MVLST) of *C. pecorum* strains isolated from a range of hosts and disease states, showed significant genetic diversity within these strains and some evidence of separation of livestock *C. pecorum* strains associated with morbidity from those isolated from the faeces of healthy cows. More recently, we evaluated the use of Multi Locus Sequence Analysis (MLSA) of *C. pecorum*house-keeping genes to understand the molecular epidemiology of *C. pecorum* infections in Australian livestock [15]. This analysis revealed (i) identical *C. pecorum* sequence types (STs) at ocular and/or urogenital anatomical sites and/or in association with diseases such as conjunctivitis, polyarthritis as well as no disease; and (ii) mixed different *C. pecorum* STs at different anatomical sites within the same animal. The latter observation highlighted the importance of sampling and molecular typing of *C. pecorum* from all potential infection sites within the same host to discriminate between strains with different pathogenic potential.

In the current report, we apply our MLSA scheme alongside pathological and immunohistochemical descriptions to characterise the relationship between *C. pecorum* types and disease in an outbreak of SBE in Western Australian (WA)

cattle. We describe histopathological changes in internal organs of affected calves and demonstrate systemic dissemination and tissue invasion of a *C. pecorum* by immunohistochemistry and PCR. Using molecular typing we detected one *C. pecorum* genotype (denoted with ST 23), associated with these SBE cases from WA, as well as other SBE cases from Australia, England and the USA. Interestingly, MLSA also identified the presence of a second genetically distinct *C. pecorum* type in the gastrointestinal tract of calves affected by SBE.

CASE PRESENTATION

Clinical history

Affected animals were two Murray Grey calves, 12 and 16 weeks old, at pasture on a property at Gairdner on the south coast of Western Australia. Six calves, aged 12 – 16 weeks, from a herd of 80 had died over the preceding two month period. The attending veterinarian was told that calves died in similar circumstances every year with animals becoming progressively duller over 3–4 days before dying. Calf WA/B31, a 12 week old Murray Grey heifer calf, was markedly depressed, unresponsive to external stimuli, blind and markedly dehydrated. Calf WA/B65, a 16 week old Murray Grey heifer calf, was markedly depressed with a stiff legged gait. Blood samples for serological and molecular analyses were taken from both calves and they were then euthanized with intravenous pentobarbitone. Both were necropsied and a range of tissues (brain, heart, liver, lung, skeletal muscle, small intestine, abomasum, mesenteric lymph node, kidney and forestomach) preserved in 10% buffered formalin for histopathology. From WA/B31, aerobic bacterial cultures were performed on a brain swab, joint swab, lung and liver. From WA/B65, aerobic bacterial cultures were performed on swabs of brain, joint, heart and abdomen. Impression smears were made of submitted fresh brain and lung of WA/B65 and fixed in acetone for immunofluorescence testing.

Twenty four swabs from the conjunctiva, vulva and rectum of 10 unaffected cohorts from the same herd were also collected for *C. pecorum* specific qPCR.

Significant necropsy findings of euthanized calves

Calf WA/B31 - The liver of was slightly swollen and the lungs reddened and firm with approximately 5% of ventral lobes affected. Joints were not grossly swollen but examination of a carpus and stifle revealed excess clear fluid. No abnormalities were noted in the brain.

Calf WA/B65 - Massive opaque white fluid exudation into pleural, pericardial and peritoneal cavities was observed. Fibrin coated serosal surfaces and fibrin clumps were seen free in the fluid. The lungs appeared collapsed but no obvious consolidation was noted. There was excess clear joint fluid in the carpal joints examined. No abnormalities were noted in the brain.

Significant histopathological changes

In both calves, most medium and small vessels throughout the brain had perivascular, mostly mononuclear cell cuffs up to four cells thick. Occasional vessels contained fibrinocellular thrombi and multifocal aggregates of polymorphonuclear neutrophils (PMNs) infiltrated the parenchyma, some well-preserved but others with advanced karryorhexis and karyolysis and multiple well circumscribed random foci of malacia were present. Rare basophilic intracytoplasmic inclusions were present in endothelium or mononuclear cells in inflammatory foci. There were extensive areas of glial cell proliferation surrounding these lesions and patchy gliosis throughout, most pronounced in the brain stem. There was a diffuse, mostly mononuclear, meningeal cell infiltrate most pronounced in the cerebellum where meningeal vessels had prominent lymphocytic perivascular cuffs with lesser numbers of macrophages and PMNs. The morphologic diagnosis was multifocal, severe, subacute, meningoencephalitis with vasculitis, fibrinocellular thrombosis and malacia.

Calf WA/B31

Heart, liver, lung, skeletal muscle, small intestine, abomasum, lymph node, kidney and forestomach were examined.

In the epicardium, there was diffuse, focally intense, infiltration of PMNs with lesser numbers of macrophages and lymphocytes accompanied by mild to moderate oedema. Activated mesothelial cells over inflamed areas were cuboidal with expanded cytoplasm and enlarged nuclei. The morphologic diagnosis was diffuse, focally severe, subacute epicarditis.

Areas of lung seen to be red and firm were atelectatic and there was diffuse congestion with increased mononuclear cells and smaller numbers of PMNs in alveolar septa. The morphologic diagnosis was mild acute interstitial pneumonia.

No significant lesions were detected in other organs.

Calf WA/B65

Liver, kidney, heart, spleen, lung, forestomach and brain were examined.

Pleural, epicardial and pericardial surfaces were heavily infiltrated by mixed inflammatory cells, predominantly PMNs and lymphoplasmacytic cells. On the serosal surfaces of abdominal organs, activated mesothelial cells proliferated with numerous cells sloughing into the overlying fibrinous exudate within which there was much streaming basophilic material (presumed DNA from degenerating cells) and infiltrating leukocytes. In places there was an intense mononuclear cell infiltrate below the fibrinous exudate. The morphologic diagnosis was severe diffuse subacute fibrinonecrotic pleuritis, epicarditis and pericarditis. No significant lesions were detected in other organs.

Immunohistochemistry (IHC)

Selected sections of brain ileum, spleen and lung were labelled using a commercial mouse monoclonal protein A purified genus-specific epitope of the *Chlamydia* lipopolysaccharide antigen (Progen Biotechnik catalogue number ACI-C). Briefly, after deparaffinization of 5 micrometer thick sections in xylene and rehydration through graded ethanol to water, antigen retrieval was performed by a 5 minute enzyme digestion (Proteinase K, Dako S3004). After endogenous peroxidase activity was inhibited by incubation for 5–10 minutes with 3% hydrogen peroxide (Dako S 2023), slides were incubated at 4°C overnight with the primary antibody diluted 1:50 in the supplied antibody diluent. After rinsing in Tris Buffered Saline, specific labelling was developed using a proprietary system (Envision™+Dual Link, single reagent HRP Rabbit/Mouse, Dako K 4063 or K4061). Following rinsing in purified water, sections were counterstained with haematoxylin. As well as the sections from cases WA/B65 and WA/B31, brain sections from two further cases were retrieved from the archives of the Department of Agriculture and Food, Western Australia (DAFWA) where a diagnosis of SBE had previously been made on the basis of histopathology and serological positivity by complement fixation.

Control sections of normal bovine brain and single sections from single archived cases of the common bovine neurological conditions; polioencephalomalacia, lead poisoning, listeriosis, salt poisoning, histophilosis and bacterial meningitis were also tested.

Similar results were obtained upon examination of brain sections from calves WA/B31, WA/B65 and the two cases from the DAFWA archives.Calf WA/B31: There was intense but sporadic labelling of the cytoplasm of endothelial cells and intravascular mononuclear cells (Figures 1B) within inflammatory lesions and less intense speckled cytoplasmic staining of mononuclear cells in areas of malacia. There was rare intense labelling of single endothelial cells in blood vessels away from the foci of inflammation and in the meninges. In a single section of ileum from calf WA/B31, rare individual cells within the intestinal epithelium and endothelium of vessels in the lamina propria were labelled (Figure 1A).Calf WA/B65: Within the severe exudative pleuritis, there was labelling of mononuclear cell (macrophage or mesothelia) cytoplasm in a zone below the surface fibrin exudation in patchy but extensive zones (Figure 2B) and of the cytoplasm of individual mesothelial cells of the spleen (Figure 2A). No labelling was seen in the parenchyma of lung or spleen.

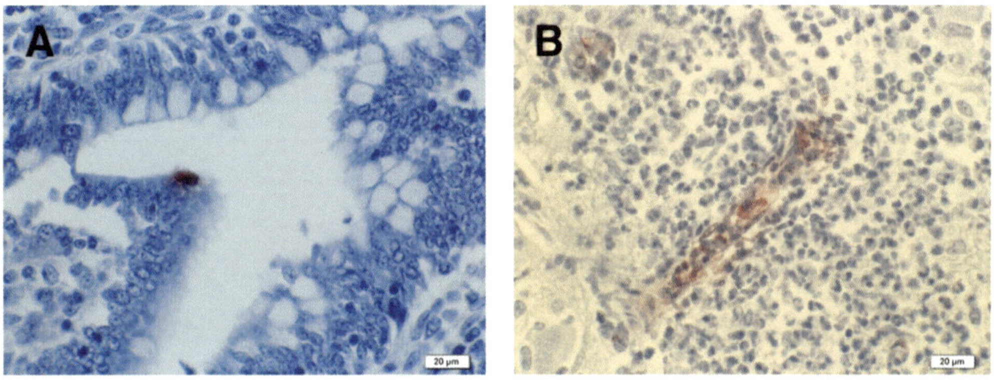

Figure 1: Calf WA/B31 immunohistochemical staining using commercial monoclonal antibody to chlamydial LPS. **A)** Ileum – Brown intracytoplasmic labelling of individual intestinal epithelial cells. **B)** Brain – Brown intracytoplasmic labelling of endothelium and intravascular mononuclear cells, in a focus of inflammation.

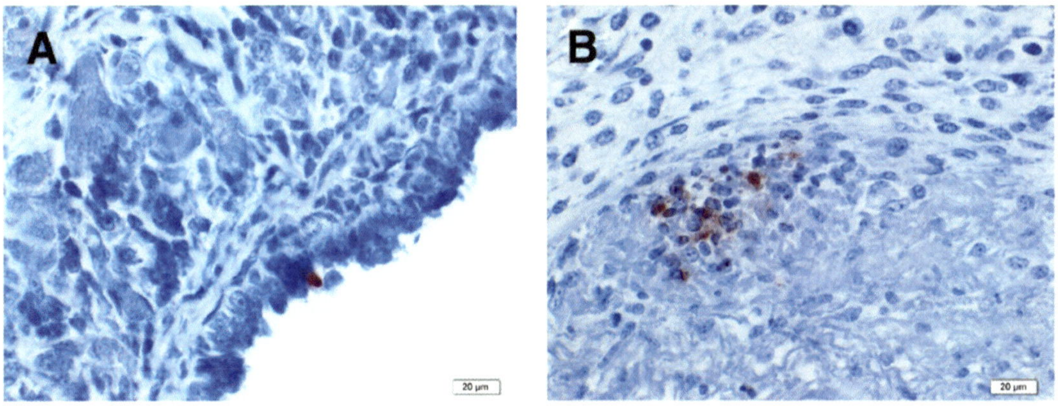

Figure 2: Calf WA/B65 immunohistochemical staining using commercial monoclonal antibody to chlamydial LPS. **A)**Spleen – Brown intra-cytoplasmic labelling of activated mesothelial cells. **B)** Lung – Brown intracytoplasmic labelling of mononuclear cells beneath layer of fibrin in overlying pleura.

There was no labelling of control sections of normal bovine brain (data not shown) nor of single sections from archived cases of the common bovine neurological conditions as previously described.

Other relevant test results

Immunocytochemistry – Acetone fixed impression smears of pleura and brain were stained with a fluorescein conjugated commercial monoclonal antibody to *Chlamydia* group specific lipopolysaccharide (Imagen, Oxoid catalogue no K610111-2) and examined with a fluorescent microscope. Punctate fluorescence was noted in the brain smear but not the lung smear.

Serology - Using the *Chlamydia* complement fixation test (CFT) which detects and measures antibodies (Ab) to the chlamydial genus specific lipopolysaccharide (LPS) antigen [17], antibodies were detected in serum from calf WA/B65 at a 1/64 dilution. Serum from calf WA/B31 was not tested.

Bacteriology - There were no significant bacterial isolates from brain swab, joint swab, lung and liver neither from calf WA/B31 nor from swabs of abdomen, pericardium, brain and a joint of calf WA/B65.

*C. pecorum*species-specific quantitative PCR (qPCR) screening

In order to confirm the presence of *C. pecorum* in association with these cases of SBE, DNA was extracted using a QIAmp DNA kit (Qiagen, Doncaster, Australia) from lungs, livers, heart, brain, cerebrospinal fluid (CSF), kidney, mesenteric lymph node, ileal tissue and clotted blood of the two affected calves (B31 and B65) and from swabs collected from asymptomatic animals, as per manufacturer's instructions. The testing of these swabs has been considered by the Queensland University of Technology (QUT) Animal Ethics Committee and approved under Tissue Use Notification #1100000362. This was used as a template for a previously described *C. pecorum*-specific qPCR, targeting a 202 bp region of the *C. pecorum* 16S ribosomal RNA (rRNA) [18]. The presence of *C. pecorum* DNA and the relative infectious loads in each tissue sample analysed are described in Table 1. With the exception of one sample (CSF in WA/Bovine 31), *C. pecorum* was detected in all tissues from both animals, with infectious loads ranging from very low as observed in kidneys and lymph node, to high as observed in brain, heart and lungs (Table 1). Nine of the 10 cohort animals with no apparent disease had < 15 *C. pecorum* 16S rDNA copies/µl of template, with *C. pecorum* DNA detected in six animals at ocular and vulval sites and three animals at one site only (ocular or vulval) (data not shown). The highest *C. pecorum* DNA positivity (70%), albeit at low infectious loads, was detected in vulval swabs, while no *C. pecorum* DNA was detected in the four available rectal swabs.

Table 1: *C. pecorum* screening results for samples taken from the two SBE diseased calves

Host	Anatomical site	*C. pecorum*qPCR screen	*C. pecorum*infectious load*
WA/B31	Lung A	POS	1.7×10^4
	Lung B	POS	1.5×10^4
	Liver**	POS	1.1×10^5
	CSF	NEG	Nil
	Ileal tissue**	POS	1.8×10^3
	Mesenteric lymph node**	POS	6.3×10^1
WA/B65	Lung	POS	2.6×10^4
	Liver**	POS	3.2×10^3
	Brain	POS	4.0×10^5
	Heart**	POS	9.7×10^3
	Blood Clot	POS	7.2×10^2
	Kidney**	POS	1.8×10^1

*Mean No. of copies of 202 bp *C. pecorum* 16S ribosomal DNA PCR product per microliter of the tissue extracted DNA; ** Tissues in which no significant lesions were identified.

*C. pecorum*MLSA from SBE field cases

To assess the phylogenetic relationships among *C. pecorum* strains detected in the two calves analysed in this study, we analysed concatenated sequence sets against the available HK gene sequences from seven other bovine *C. pecorum* isolates described worldwide and in association with several different aetiologies, utilising Bayesian methods. PCR amplification was successful for all samples except the WA/B31 lymph node and the WA/B65 clot and kidney samples.

The complete list of bovine *C. pecorum* isolates whose sequences were analysed in this study is described in (Table 2). In addition to the Australian samples from calves screened and typed in this study, HK gene fragment sequences from cases of SBE from the USA and England and from cases of pneumonia, arthritis, conjunctivitis and healthy faecal *C. pecorum* isolates were obtained from the *Chlamydiales* MLST website http://pubmlst.org/chlamydiales/[19], while the HK gene fragments sequences for the Italian bovine metritis PV3056/3 isolate were obtained from Genbank (accession number CP004033.1). Fragments of seven HK genes (*eno*A, *opp*A_3, gid*A*, *hem*N, *hfl*X, *fum*C and *gat*A) and *C. pecorum* specific primers to amplify them were previously used for typing Australian koala and livestock *C. pecorum* isolates. The PCRs and DNA sequencing of each *C. pecorum* HK gene was performed as previously described [15]. HK gene sequences of the bovine *C. pecorum* isolates described here are available in Genbank (KF714242 – KF714290). Additionally, we have identified allele numbers and STs for the Australian *C. pecorum* from the two calves, analysed in this study at http://pubmlst.org/chlamydiales/ [19] (Additional file 1: Table S2).

Table 2: *C. pecorum* bovine isolates used in the study

Isolate ID.	Country	Pathology	Isolate reference
66P130	USA	Healthy (faeces)	[20]
BE53	England	Healthy (faeces)	[16]
E58	USA	Encephalomyelitis	[4]
FC-Stra	USA	Conjunctivitis	[21]
L14	USA	Pneumonia	[21]
LW623	USA	Arthritis	[21]
PV3056/3	Italy	Metritis	[22]
NSW/Bov/SBE	AUS	Encephalomyelitis	[15]
SBE	England	Encephalomyelitis	[16]
WA/B31/Ileal	AUS	SBE	This work
WA/B31/Liver	AUS	SBE	This work
WA/B31/Lung	AUS	SBE	This work
WA/B65/Brain	AUS	SBE	This work
WA/B65/Heart	AUS	SBE	This work
WA/B65/Liver	AUS	SBE	This work
WA/B65/Lung	AUS	SBE	This work

Chromatograms and sequences of the seven HK gene fragments were analysed using the Geneious Pro 6.0.4 software package [23], as previously described [15]. Sequences of individual genes and concatenated gene sets were aligned using ClustalW [24]. The level of individual HK fragments as well as the concatenated sequences polymorphisms were determined by analysing the number of synonymous (d_s) and non-synonymous (d_n) substitutions per site, Jukes-Cantor corrected, and the number of segregating sites (Δnt), haplotypes and haplotype diversity (H) using DnaSP 5.0 (Additional file 2: Table S1) [25]. As observed in Additional file 2: Table S1, HK gene fragments and/or concatenated sequences are both under negative evolutionary selection with low d_n/d_s ratios ranging from 0.0 – 0.15, with the number of synonymous substitutions per synonymous site (d_s) occurring 3.7 times more than non-synonymous substitutions per non-synonymous site (d_n). As such, sequences of the HK genes, being representative of overall bacterial chromosomal change, can provide effective phylogenetic resolution of bacterial strains [26].

Best-fit models of nucleotide substitution for constructing phylogenies of our data sets were estimated by considering eleven substitution models using jModelTest v.2.1.1 [27]. A mid-point phylogenetic tree containing all 16 bovine *C. pecorum* strains was constructed based on concatenated MLSA sequences, using the program MrBayes [28] with the HKY85+I+G model, as implemented in Geneious Pro 6.0.4. Run parameters included four Markov Chain Monte Carlo (MCMC) chains with a million generations, sampled every 100 generations and with the first 1000 trees were discarded as burn-in.

Phylogenetic analysis revealed the presence of two genetically distinct *C. pecorum* STs in the samples analysed from the two animals (Figure 3). The predominant *C. pecorum* ST, detected in the brain, heart, lungs and liver from calves WA/B65 and WA/B31 was identical to the previously reported HK gene fragment sequences of the *C. pecorum* E58 SBE type strain, another SBE strain described in England and an Australian SBE strain (NSW/Bov/SBE), grouping them together in a well-supported Clade 3 (Figure 3). The second *C. pecorum* ST detected (WA/B31/Ileal) was found only in the ileal sample from calf WA/B31. This ST was clearly distinct from the other ST detected in these animals, differing by a total of 16 nucleotides, and clearly grouping in a well-supported clade together with other previously typed faecal (BE53 and 66P130) and cervical (PV3056/3) *C. pecorum* bovine genotypes (Figure 3). Phylogenetic analysis also revealed that both STs detected in these cases were also clearly distinct from a Clade 1 consisting of bovine isolates (Fc-Stra, L14 and LW623) previously associated with pathologies such as conjunctivitis, pneumonia and arthritis, respectively (Figure 3). MLSA of *C. pecorum* positive swab samples of healthy cohorts was not performed due to the low *C. pecorum* load. The phylogenetic distinction of the two *C. pecorum* genotypes observed in calf WA/B31, was supported by allele and ST identification with the ST from liver and lung determined as ST23, a ST previously described from Australian and the USA SBE isolates (NSW/Bov/SBE and E58), while the second *C. pecorum* ST from the ileal sample was assigned a novel ST since these sequences had not been previously reported (Additional file 1: Table S2).

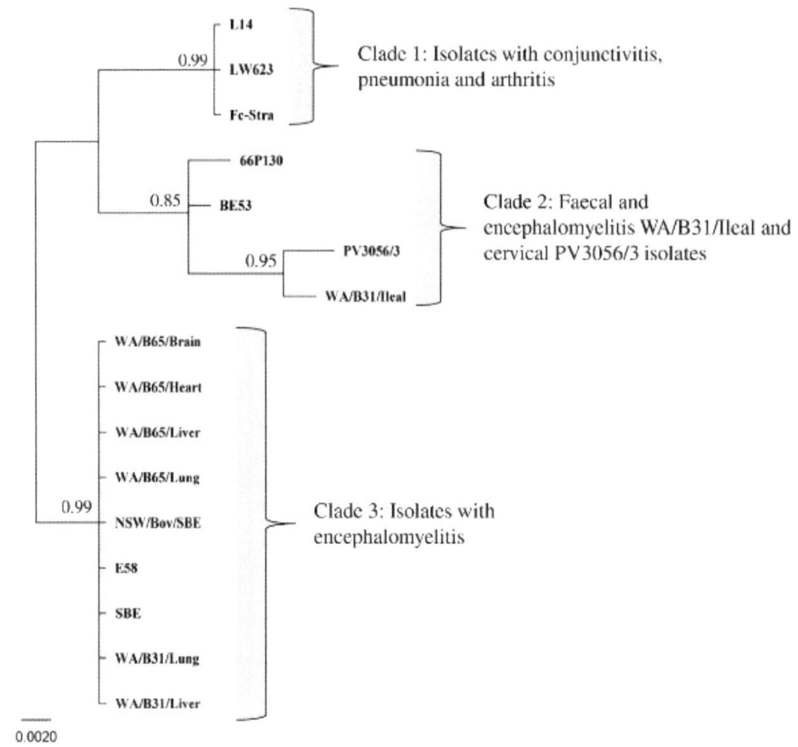

Figure 3: Mid-point rooted Bayesian phylogenetic analysis of concatenated sequences of the seven HK gene fragments of the 16 bovine *C. pecorum* isolates used in this study. Posterior probabilities of> 0.85 are displayed on the tree nodes.

We utilised pathological techniques to identify cases of SBE as well as a species-specific qPCR and a recently described *C. pecorum* MLSA scheme to molecularly characterise the strains of *C. pecorum* detected. This analysis revealed systemic dissemination of *C. pecorum* with associated pathologic changes. Molecular typing revealed the presence of two genetically distinct *C. pecorum* STs providing evidence for the presence of *C. pecorum* strains with different pathogenic potentials infecting cattle.

Histopathological findings were consistent with previous descriptions [2]. *Chlamydia*-specific IHC, targeting the genus-specific *Chlamydia*l polysaccharide (LPS), of affected tissues resulted in sporadic intense specific intracellular labelling of endothelium, intravascular mononuclear cells and mononuclear cells within inflammatory foci. Patchy intense labelling was seen in mononuclear cells (presumed macrophages or mesothelial cells) in superficial chronic exudative serosal lesions and individual mesothelial cells stained in less exudative lesions. These observations suggest that the initial site of infection in the brain is endothelium and in serosa, mesothelium. Detected antigen was not widespread in the tissues but appeared in clusters of cells. In one section of ileum (Figure 1A), rare individual cells within the intestinal epithelium and endothelial cells stained, suggesting a low level of infection in these sites. In the absence of *C. pecorum* specific antibody assays, we utilised highly sensitive *C. pecorum*-specific qPCR screening [18] to confirm these *Chlamydia*-specific IHC results in examined tissues. In contrast to these results, comparative screening by qPCR revealed a high average load of 10^4*C. pecorum* 16S rDNA copies/µl of template in all tissues except the CSF sample. In several recent surveillance studies, PCR screening for *C. pecorum* has been shown to be an effective tool for assessing the overall herd prevalence from screening a limited selection of animals [29, 30]. In Australian veterinary diagnostic laboratories, PCR testing for *Chlamydia* is not routinely performed but the results of this current study suggest that this should be reconsidered.

We also performed *C. pecorum* species-specific qPCR screening of asymptomatic in-contact animals. Nine out of 10 animals from the same mob were PCR positive for *C. pecorum* at ocular and vulval sites; however, the infectious load was very low (<15 *C. pecorum* 16S rDNA copies/µl of template). This observation is consistent with previous reports describing low levels of *C. pecorum* in vaginal swabs from cattle with no apparent disease [6, 12, 29]. The rectal swabs from in-contact animals in the current study were notably negative, raising questions about shedding, transmission and genetic relationships of strains particularly given the assumption that the gastrointestinal tract is the preferred site of infection for *Chlamydiae*[31]. Although unlikely, we cannot discount the presence of PCR inhibitors in these samples despite the fact that *C. pecorum*shedding in faecal samples of Australian cattle and sheep was previously observed and detected [15, 32]. Unfortunately, molecular typing could not be performed on these swabs as the amount of *C. pecorum*positive DNA was insufficient for PCR amplification of the MLSA house-keeping genes. It has been hypothesised that subclinical infections may develop into diseases such as SBE by dissemination into other susceptible tissues via haematogenous spread [2], although the factors that determine this dissemination and disease development are unclear.

Previous observations that one animal can harbour two distinct *C. pecorum* genotypes from different anatomical sites [15], raised questions over the identity and genetic relationships between *C. pecorum*detected from multiple sites in both diseased and healthy animals in this study. To investigate this, we applied our *C. pecorum* MLSA scheme to reconstruct phylogenetic relationships [15] between the strains detected in the diseased calves and others previously described. This analysis revealed that Calf WA/31 harboured two distinct *C. pecorum* strain types, one in the gastrointestinal site (WA/B31/Ileal), apparently not associated with pathology and the other disseminated in multiple organs (WA/B31/Lung and Liver) and associated with severe pathology (Figure 3). These latter isolates had 100% sequence identity to other *C. pecorum* SBE isolates (E58, NSW/Bov/SBE and SBE), with a clear separation from isolates detected in bovine faeces. This observation of a phylogenetic distinction between SBE and faecal isolates has been previously described using an alternative multi-locus virulence typing scheme [16]. This is the first study to describe this observation in a single animal, however, further reinforcing that bacterial genetic differences may indeed be associated with differences in tissue tropism/ pathogenicity [22]. As already mentioned, *C. pecorum* positive vaginal and ocular samples of healthy companion animals could not be typed due to very low levels of *C. pecorum*; however we hypothesise that if the MLSA was applied on these samples they would most likely cluster with the previously typed faecal isolates from healthy animals.

While the molecular evidence continues to mount for the existence of *C. pecorum* with different pathogenic potentials [22], this data needs to be supported by experimental infection studies. Rodolakis and colleagues in 1989, isolated intestinal *C. psittaci* strains (now reclassified as *C. abortus* and *C. pecorum*) from the faeces of healthy ruminants and showed in a mouse model that they were less "pathogenic" than strains isolated from animals with disease. Eight of 10 intestinal strains were non- invasive including the *C. pecorum* strains, while the majority of strains from diseased hosts, including *C. abortus*, successfully colonised the placenta and foetuses of pregnant mice [33]. To the best of our knowledge, more recent studies are currently lacking but will be required to experimentally verify the molecular evidence presented in this study. Molecular typing and experimental infection studies of the "true" pathogenic potential of *C. pecorum* will be particularly important in light of the growing number of studies which have linked *C. pecorum* infection to adverse but sub-clinical health consequences in dairy cattle [11, 34].

CONCLUSION

A combination of histopathological methods and molecular typing provided a new insight into the pathogenesis and epidemiology of SBE. Little is known about the prevalence and impact of *C. pecorum*infections on Australian livestock however this study provides a starting point for further investigations into cases of SBE in other regions of Australia and the relationship between *C. pecorum* infections and other health problems in Australian cattle. The detection of multiple genetically distinct *C. pecorum* strains that cluster with other disease associated or faecal strains reported in the rest of the world hint at a complex epidemiology in Australian animals that will require a combination of (i) large-scale 'on-farm' epidemiological studies; and (ii) further experimental infection studies with suspected "pathogenic" and "non-pathogenic" *C. pecorum* strains if we are to improve the diagnosis, treatment and control of these infections in livestock.

DECLARATIONS

Acknowledgments

This work was funded by an ARC Discovery Project grant (DP130102066) awarded to PT and AP. This study made use of several bovine *C. pecorum* MLST sequences available from the *Chlamydiales* MLST website (http://pubmlst.org/ chlamydiales/). We thank Dr. Yvonne Pannekoek, University of Amsterdam, The Netherlands for permission to include these sequences in our study. We thank Eileen Roulis for technical assistance with preparation of figures.

Authors' contributions

MJ performed the molecular testing, data analyses and drafted the manuscript. DF performed the necropsy, histology and immunochemistry and assisted with preparation of the manuscript. JC and DR performed all field work. PT and AP conceived the study, assisted with data analysis and drafting of the manuscript. All authors read and approved the final manuscript.

REFERENCES

1. Watt B: Chlamydial infection in sheep. Proceedings of the 92nd District Veterinarian's Conference: 2011; Dubbo. New South Wales, Australia: District Veterinarian's Association; 2011:109-113.
2. Kessell AE, Finnie JW, Windsor PA: Neurological diseases of ruminant livestock in Australia. III: bacterial and protozoal infections. Aust Vet J. 2011, 89 (8): 289-296. 10.1111/j.1751-0813.2011.00807.x.
3. Durham PJK, Paine GD: Serological survey for antibodies to infectious agents in beef cattle in northern South Australia. Aust Vet J. 1997, 75 (2): 139-140. 10.1111/j.1751-0813.1997.tb14176.x.
4. McNutt SH, Waller EF: Sporadic Bovine Encephalomyelitis (Buss Disease). Cornell Vet. 1940, 30: 437-448.
5. Kaltenboeck B, Hehnen HR, Vaglenov A: Bovine *Chlamydophila* spp. infection: Do we underestimate the impact on fertility?. Vet Res Commun. 2005, 29 (1): 1-15.
6. DeGraves FJ, Gao D, Hehnen H-R, Schlapp T, Kaltenboeck B: Quantitative detection of Chlamydia psittaci and C. pecorum by high-sensitivity Real-Time PCR reveals high prevalence of vaginal infection in cattle. J Clin Microbiol. 2003, 41 (4): 1726-1729. 10.1128/JCM.41.4.1726-1729.2003.
7. Reggiardo C, Fuhrmann TJ, Meerdink GL, Bicknell EJ: Diagnostic features of *Chlamydia* infection in dairy calves. J Vet Diagn Invest. 1989, 1 (4): 305-308. 10.1177/104063878900100405.
8. Biesenkamp-Uhe C, Li Y, Hehnen H-R, Sachse K, Kaltenboeck B: Therapeutic Chlamydophila abortus and C. pecorum vaccination transiently reduces bovine mastitis associated with Chlamydophila infection. Infect Immun. 2007, 75 (2): 870-877. 10.1128/IAI.00691-06.
9. Wheelhouse N, Longbottom D, Willoughby K: *Chlamydia* in cases of cattle pneumonia in Scotland. Vet

Rec. 2013, 172 (4): 110-10.1136/vr.f469.

10. Reinhold P, Sachse K, Kaltenboeck B: *Chlamydiaceae* in cattle: commensals, trigger organisms, or pathogens?. Vet J. 2011, 189 (3): 257-267. 10.1016/j.tvjl.2010.09.003.

11. Poudel A, Elsasser TH, Rahman KS, Chowdhury EU, Kaltenboeck B: Asymptomatic endemic *Chlamydia pecorum*infections reduce growth rates in calves by up to 48 percent. PLoS One. 2012, 7 (9): e44961-10.1371/journal.pone.0044961.

12. Jee J, Degraves FJ, Kim T, Kaltenboeck B: High prevalence of natural *Chlamydophila* species infection in calves. J Clin Microbiol. 2004, 42 (12): 5664-5672. 10.1128/JCM.42.12.5664-5672.2004.

13. Kauffold J, Henning K, Bachmann R, Hotzel H, Melzer F: The prevalence of chlamydiae of bulls from six bull studs in Germany. Anim Reprod Sci. 2007, 102 (1–2): 111-121.

14. Lenzko H, Moog U, Henning K, Lederbach R, Diller R, Menge C, Sachse K, Sprague L: High frequency of chlamydial co-infections in clinically healthy sheep flocks. BMC Vet Res. 2011, 7 (1): 29-10.1186/1746-6148-7-29.

15. Jelocnik M, Frentiu FD, Timms P, Polkinghorne A: Multi-locus sequence analysis provides insights into the molecular epidemiology of *Chlamydia pecorum* infections in Australian sheep, cattle and koalas. J Clin Microbiol. 2013, 51 (8): 2625-2632. 10.1128/JCM.00992-13.

16. Yousef Mohamad K, Roche SM, Myers G, Bavoil PM, Laroucau K, Magnino S, Laurent S, Rasschaert D, Rodolakis A: Preliminary phylogenetic identification of virulent *Chlamydophila pecorum* strains. Infect Genet Evol. 2008, 8 (6): 764-771. 10.1016/j.meegid.2008.06.009.

17. Timms P: Chlamydial infections in birds and animals. Australia and New Zealand Standard Diagnostic Procedures. The Subcommittee on Animal Health Laboratory Standards; Department of Agriculture, Australian Government; 2010:1-14.

18. Wan C, Loader J, Hanger J, Beagley KW, Timms P, Polkinghorne A: Using quantitative polymerase chain reaction to correlate *Chlamydia pecorum* infectious load with ocular, urinary and reproductive tract disease in the koala (*Phascolarctos cinereus*). Aust Vet J. 2011, 89 (10): 409-412. 10.1111/j.1751-0813.2011.00827.x.

19. Jolley K, Maiden M: BIGSdb: scalable analysis of bacterial genome variation at the population level. BMC Bioinformatic. 2010, 11 (1): 595-10.1186/1471-2105-11-595.

20. Kaltenboeck B, Kousoulas KG, Storz J: Structures of and allelic diversity and relationships among the major outer membrane protein (*omp*A) genes of the four chlamydial species. J Bacteriol. 1993, 175 (2): 487-502.

21. Perez-Martinez JA, Storz J: Antigenic diversity of *Chlamydia psittaci* of mammalian origin determined by microimmunofluorescence. Infect Immun. 1985, 50 (3): 905-910.

22. Sait M, Livingstone M, Clark EM, Wheelhouse N, Spalding L, Markey B, Magnino S, Lainson FA, Myers GS, Longbottom D: Genome sequencing and comparative analysis of three *Chlamydia pecorum* strains associated with different pathogenic outcomes. BMC Genomics. 2014, 15 (1): 23-10.1186/1471-2164-15-23.

23. Biomatters: Geneious v7.0. 2013, http://www.geneious.com/.

24. Larkin MA, Blackshields G, Brown NP, Chenna R, McGettigan PA, McWilliam H, Valentin F, Wallace IM, Wilm A, Lopez R, Thompson JD, Gibson TJ, Higgins DG: Clustal W and Clustal X version 2.0. Bioinformatics. 2007, 23 (21): 2947-2948. 10.1093/bioinformatics/btm404.

25. Librado P, Rozas J: DnaSP v5: a software for comprehensive analysis of DNA polymorphism data. Bioinformatics. 2009, 25 (11): 1451-1452. 10.1093/bioinformatics/btp187.

26. Maiden MCJ, van Rensburg MJJ, Bray JE, Earle SG, Ford SA, Jolley KA, McCarthy ND: MLST revisited: the gene-by-gene approach to bacterial genomics. Nat Rev Micro. 2013, 11 (10): 728-736. 10.1038/nrmicro3093.

27. Darriba D, Taboada GL, Doallo R, Posada D: jModelTest 2: more models, new heuristics and parallel computing. Nat Meth. 2012, 9 (8): 772.

28. Huelsenbeck JP, Ronquist F: MRBAYES: Bayesian inference of phylogenetic trees. Bioinformatics. 2001, 17 (8): 754-755. 10.1093/bioinformatics/17.8.754.

29. Petit T, Spergser J, Aurich J, Rosengarten R: Prevalence of *Chlamydiaceae* and *Mollicutes* on the genital mucosa and serological findings in dairy cattle. Vet Microbiol. 2008, 127 (3–4): 325-333.

30. Godin A-C, Bjorkman C, Englund S, Johansson K-E, Niskanen R, Alenius S: Investigation of *Chlamydophila* spp. in dairy cows with reproductive disorders. Acta Vet Scand. 2008, 50 (1): 39-10.1186/1751-0147-50-39.

31. Yeruva L, Spencer N, Bowlin AK, Wang Y, Rank RG: Chlamydial infection of the gastrointestinal tract: a reservoir for persistent infection. Path dis. 2013, 68 (3): 88-95. 10.1111/2049-632X.12052.

32. St George TD: The isolation of *chlamydiae* from faeces of sheep in Australia. Aust Vet J. 1971, 47: 74.

33. Rodolakis A, Bernard F, Lantier F: Mouse models for evaluation of virulence of *Chlamydia psittaci* isolated from ruminants. Res Vet Sci. 1989, 46 (1): 34-39.

34. Reinhold P, Jaeger J, Liebler-Tenorio E, Berndt A, Bachmann R, Schubert E, Melzer F, Elschner M, Sachse K: Impact of latent infections with *Chlamydophila* species in young cattle. Vet J. 2008, 175 (2): 202-211. 10.1016/j.tvjl.2007.01.004.

CHAPTER 6

THE OCCURRENCE OF CHLAMYDIA SPP. IN PIGS WITH AND WITHOUT CLINICAL DISEASE

Stina Englund, Carl Hård af Segerstad, Frida Arnlund, Eva Westergren and Magdalena Jacobson

BACKGROUND

The *Chlamydiaceae* family including the genera *Chlamydia* is a well-recognised cause of disease in many animal species including cats, ruminants, birds and humans [1, 2]. Within the genera, nine distinct species have been identified. Four of these have been described in pigs (*Chlamydia (C.) abortus, C. psittaci, C. pecorum*, and *C. suis*) and related to reproductive disorders, conjunctivitis, enteritis, pneumonia, polyarthritis, pleuritis and polyserositis [1, 3, 4, 5]. The epidemiology, clinical, and zoonotic importance of these species are however largely unknown [6, 7, 8]. However, *C. suis* seems to be both common and widespread, often occurring in mixed infections with *C. abortus* and *C. pecorum* [2].

In gnotobiotic pig challenge studies from USA, *C. suis* caused dose-dependent diarrhoea in young piglets. Histologically, villi atrophy, tip erosions, necrosis, inflammatory changes and lymphangitis were noted in the distal small intestine. Chlamydial antigens were demonstrated in enterocytes and chlamydiae were re-isolated from tissue specimens and faecal swabs [9, 10]. However, weaned pigs developed microscopical lesions but remained clinically healthy [11]. Similar lesions have also been demonstrated in clinical cases of diarrhoea in weaned pigs [12]. However, other studies have not been able to confirm a causal relationship [3, 8].

A few studies have addressed conjunctivitis [13]. Chlamydiae were seen in eight pigs by ultrastructural examination and were isolated in two pigs [4], and subclinical conjunctivitis was experimentally induced in 3-day-old gnotobiotic piglets [14].

Isolation is the gold standard for diagnosis but many strains are difficult to cultivate [2, 5]. Other methods includes serology, immunohistochemistry, histology, and PCR on faeces, mucosal swabs or tissue specimens [2]. Because of cross-reactivity, some tests may lack sensitivity and specificity [5, 12, 15]. In a study comparing four diagnostic methods, *C. suis* were demonstrated in 42% of the samples by PCR and in 33% by culture. The sensitivity was 94.4% and specificity 81.0%, whereas the two ELISAs performed considerably weaker. PCR was concluded to be a reliable, highly sensitive and specific tool for detection of *C. suis* [16].

The present study aimed to investigate the presence of *Chlamydia* spp in the intestines of growing pigs and in conjunctival swabs from finisher pigs, and relate those findings to the occurrence of clinical signs.

METHODS

The study was approved by the Ethical Committee for Animal Experiments, Uppsala, Sweden. All herd owners had given an informed consent prior to the study.

Citation: Stina Englund, Carl Hård af Segerstad, Frida Arnlund, Eva Westergren and Magdalena Jacobson, The occurrence of Chlamydia spp. in pigs with and without clinical disease, DOI: 10.1186/1746-6148-8-9.

Herds and animals

DNA from enteric specimens originated from a previous study on growing pigs with diarrhoea [17]. The samples originated from the major pig producing areas of Sweden, *i.e.* in the south-western and eastern parts of the country, and included 36 pigs from six herds with poor performance and diarrhoea in growing pigs, and 12 pigs from four herds with good performance and no diarrhoea. From each of the poor performance herds, three case and three control pigs were chosen, and from each of the four good performance herds, three control pigs were chosen. The case pigs had diarrhoea that had commenced within 2 days and no other diseases were evident. The control pigs were matched to the case pigs for age and sex, but showed no signs of clinical disease. The control pigs had a mean age of 72 days and a mean weight of 18.7 kg, and the case pigs had a mean weight of 12.1 kg. The pigs submitted from the good performance herds had a mean age of 67 days and a mean weight of 23.1 kg. All animals were weaned at approximately 5 weeks of age and none of the pigs had been treated with antibiotics. The pigs were transported to the laboratory and euthanized within 15 min prior to necropsy.

Further, animals from three finisher herds were sampled based on the present occurrence of conjunctivitis. The pigs originated from several piglet-producing herds and were introduced to the finisher herds at 25-30 kg. b.w., *i.e.* 4-14 weeks prior to sampling. They were kept 10 pigs per pen in units of 300 pigs each. In two herds, 7 case and 7 control pigs were selected from each of 3 units, and in one herd, 20 case and 20 control pigs from one unit were selected. The case pigs were selected based on clinical signs of moderate to severe conjunctivitis, defined as hyperaemia and chemosis with epiphora and/or muco-purulent secretion. The control pigs were selected from the same pens as the case pigs but showed no or only mild conjunctivitis, *i.e.* none to slight hyperaemia in the conjunctiva and no chemosis or epiphora.

Necropsy and sampling

The necropsies were carried out at the Department of Pathology at the National Veterinary Institute, Uppsala, or at AnalyCen, Skara. The animals were stunned with electricity, weighed and exsanguinated, and necropsy was immediately performed. All gross lesions were noted, and specimens for histological examination were taken from ileum and from all macroscopically visible lesions. The samples were fixed in 10% buffered formalin, embedded in paraffin blocks, sectioned and stained with haematoxylin and eosin according to standard protocols.

The finisher pigs were snared and sterile cotton swabs were rubbed against the conjunctiva in the conjunctival sac in the left and right eye, respectively. The swabs were placed in sterile tubes and transported to the laboratory.

Polymerase chain reaction

Intestinal samples were prepared from a 0.5 cm^3 piece of frozen mucosa from the distal ileum. DNA was extracted by phenol/chloroform and precipitated by ethanol [18, 19]. DNA from the conjunctival swabs was extracted according to K. Sachse [20] and all samples were analysed by real-time PCR according to Everett and others [21]. The primers TQF and TQR targeted the 23 S ribosomal DNA and detected all members of the family *Chlamydiaceae*. Multiple negative controls were included and DNA from *Cp. abortus* and *C. suis* (kindly provided by K. Sachse, Friedrich-Loeffler-Institute, Jena, Germany) were used as positive controls.

To detect false negative PCR results due to inhibiting agents, an internal amplification control (mimic) was constructed and used as previously described [22]. The primers used in the mimic producing PCR were TQFActin (5›GAAAAGAACCCT TGTTAAGGGAGCCATGTACCCTGGCATTG-3›) and TQRActin (5›-CTTAACTCCCTG GCTCATCAT GGATCCACACGGAGTACTTGC-3›). The sequence of the ROX-labelled mimic probe used in real-time PCR was 5›-CCGACAGGATGCAGAAGGAGATCA-3›.

The conjunctival swabs were analysed both undiluted and diluted 1:100 in accordance with the standard protocol applied at the NVI, and a positive reaction in at least one of these dilutions was regarded as positive. In the statistical analyses, threshold values below Ct 36 were regarded as positive whereas values between Ct 36 and Ct 38 were regarded as doubtful. The results were calculated separately for the respective thresholds. Values above Ct 38 were regarded as negative or were excluded in the calculations. The difference in detection rate of *Chlamydia* spp. between pigs with moderate to severe conjunctivitis and the control pigs were analysed by chi-square test.

DNA sequence analysis

Sequence analysis was performed on 19 samples from the intestinal specimens giving a strong positive reaction in the PCR. PCR was performed with primers 16SF2 and 23R according to Everett and Andersen [23] on DNA samples from seven case pigs and six control pigs from poor performance herds and six pigs from good performance herds. The predicted PCR product of 600 bp as well as one PCR product of larger and one of smaller size was purified prior to sequencing by using the GFX PCR DNA and Gel Band Purification Kit (Amersham Bioscience Europe, GmbH Germany). The purified products were sequenced with the same primers used in the PCR and by using the BigDye Terminator v3.1 Cycle Sequencing Kit (Applied Biosystems, Foster City, CA, USA) in combination with ethanol/EDTA/sodium acetate precipitation, according to the protocol supplied. Thermocycling was performed in a GeneAmp 2700 Thermocycler (Applied Biosystems). The sequencing products were subjected to electrophoretic separation and on-line detection on an ABI PRISM 3100 Genetic Analyzer (Applied Biosystems), followed by BLAST search.

Immunohistochemistry

Paraffin-embedded intestinal specimens were available from 44 of the 48 growing pigs. 4-μm thick sections of the formalin-fixed, paraffin-embedded blocks where cut and placed onto positively charged slides (Polysine™, Menzel-Gläser, Braunschweig, Germany). Prior to immunostaining, deparaffinisation and hydration where done in xylene and graded ethanol to distilled water. After hydration, a blocking for endogenous peroxidase where done in 0.03% H_2O_2 in Tris-buffered saline (TBS) and nonspecific binding sites where blocked with 2% bovine serum albumin (BSA). Antigen retrieval was performed by heat induced epitope retrieval (HIER) in retrieval buffer pH = 9 (TBS-EDTA), using microwave as heat source. HIER was performed by heating the Polysine™-slides immersed in retrieval buffer for 7 min at 750 W followed by 14 min at 340 W. After completed heating procedure, the slides remained in the retrieval buffer at room temperature for 20 min. The slides where incubated with a mouse monoclonal antibody against Chlamydia, clone ACI (Progen Biotechnik Gmbh, Germany) diluted 1:100. Visualisation of the bound primary antibody was achieved by using Dako EnVision™ + System utilising an HCP-labelled anti-mouse monoclonal antibody (Glostrup, Denmark), and the presence of the relevant antigen was detected with 3,3›-diaminobenzidine (DAB, NVI, Sweden). Slides were weakly counterstained with haematoxylin. The staining included at least one positive and one negative control section. The positive control originated from previously confirmed routine cases. The results were graded as negative (-), sparse (+), moderate (++) or abundant (+++) occurrence.

RESULTS

Necropsy

No gross lesions were observed in the pigs from the good performance herds. In the pigs from the poor performance herds, five control pigs and 20 pigs with diarrhoea had macroscopic lesions consistent with *Lawsonia (L.) intracellularis* infection and one had a parasitic colitis. By histology, lesions that may be consistent with chlamydial infection [9] were noted in 20 pigs: Villus atrophy was noted in six pigs with diarrhoea and in ten control pigs from the poor performance herds. Epithelial exocytosis or necroses were noted in five pigs with diarrhoea, in one control pig from the poor performance herds, and in one pig from the good performance herds (Table 1).

Table 1: The findings in intestinal specimens from growing pigs with diarrhoea (case), clinically healthy control pigs from the same poor performance herds (casecontrol), and from healthy pigs originating from good performance herds (control), examined by immunohistochemistry (IHC), necropsy, and PCR

		Case	**Casecontrol**	**Control**
		(n = 18)	**(n = 18)**	**(n = 12)**
IHC	-	1 (7%)	9 (53%)	2 (17%)
	+	5 (33%)	3 (18%)	7 (58%)
	++	7 (47%)	4 (24%)	3 (25%)
	+++	2 (13%)	1 (6%)	0
	missing	3	1	-
Necropsy	Villi atrophy	6 (33%)	10 (56%)	0
	Villi necrosis	5 (28%)	1 (6%)	1 (8%)
PCR	positive	18 (100%)	18 (100%)	10 (83%)
	inhibited	0	0	2 (17%)

The percentage given within brackets is calculated on the actual number of analyses performed in each group, *i.e.* the "missing samples" are excluded

Microbiological analyses

In the previous study [17], *Brachyspira pilosicoli* were demonstrated in eight case pigs and five control pigs, *Campylobacter jejuni*; in one case pig and four control pigs, *Yersinia enterocolitica* in three case and five control pigs, haemolytic *Escherichia (E.) coli* in two case and two control pigs, *Clostridium perfringens* in two case pigs, and *L. intracellularis* were previously demonstrated in 11 case and eight control pigs from the poor performance herds. In addition, haemolytic *E. coli* had been demonstrated in two pigs from the good performance herds. Rotavirus had been demonstrated in one case pig. Coronavirus was not included in the study, since Sweden has previously been shown to be free from transmissible gastroenteritis and porcine epidemic diarrhoea. *Balantidium coli* were demonstrated in one case and three control pigs from the poor performance herds, and in one pig from the good performance herds.

Real-time PCR and DNA sequence analysis

Of the 48 enteric samples analysed, 46 were positive for *Chlamydiaceae* (Table 1). Two samples could not be evaluated due to amplification inhibition. The major band of 600 b.p. found in all samples was confirmed as *C. suis* in the 19 samples subjected to sequence analysis. The larger PCR product described in the Methods' section was 98-100% identical to *Escherichia coli* whereas the smaller PCR product did not match any sequence in the BLAST search.

In the PCR analyses on the conjunctival swabs, one pig with conjunctivitis and three control animals together with their matched counterparts were excluded from the statistical calculations, since the PCR was partially or totally inhibited. Thus, in total, 116 conjunctival swabs were included in the statistical analyses. Of these, three samples from pigs with conjunctivitis gave weakly positive reactions (Ct > 38 in undiluted samples) and were judged as negative.

Employing a cut-off value of Ct 36, 45 samples from pigs with conjunctivitis and 35 control pigs were determined as positive by PCR. Using a cut-off value of Ct 38, 48 samples from pigs with conjunctivitis and 42 control pigs were determined as positive. A statistically significant difference ($P = 0.03$) was detected between pigs with and without conjunctivitis when a Ct value of 36 was employed. The difference was mainly related to one of the herds (18 positive pigs with conjunctivitis and 12 positive control pigs). When a Ct of 38 was employed, no significant differences were noted.

Immunohistochemistry

The results are shown in Table 1. Among the case pigs, 6 (40%) were negative or were carrying a low-grade infection. Among the control pigs from good performance herds, 9 (75%) were negative or sparsely (+) infected. The two control specimens in which the PCR analyses had been inhibited were graded as + and ++, respectively, by immunohistochemistry. A significant ($P < 0.05$) relationship was detected between the presence of clinical signs and a high degree (++ or +++) of infection. No relationship was detected between the occurrence of histological lesions and the demonstration of chlamydial antigen by immunohistochemistry.

DISCUSSION

The pig intestine is considered as the natural reservoir for *C. suis*, and the microbe seems generally to be well adapted to its host [1]. In the present study, *Chlamydia* spp. were demonstrated in high prevalence in all herds investigated. This is consistent with the few studies that have previously addressed the occurrence of *Chlamydia* spp. in pig herds. Overall, it was not possible to relate the demonstration of the microbe to the presence of diarrhoea. However, based on the immunohistochemistry, pigs with diarrhoea might have been more heavily infected than the healthy pigs. This is in consistency with the results from another study on 447 pigs submitted for necropsy, where it was not possible to relate the presence of *Chlamydia* spp. to the occurrence of diarrhoea, but in 12 cases, it was the only pathogen found [6]. Similar experiences have also been noted in calves and sheep [24, 25, 26].

In the study by Becker *et al.* [13], *C. suis* was significantly ($P < 0.0001$) related to conjunctivitis in extensive pig production systems, whereas in intensive farming systems, high prevalences (88-90%) were found in both pigs with conjunctivitis and in clinically asymptomatic pigs. This is in accordance with the findings in the present study. Becker *et al.* discussed, that environmental factors might predispose to infection. However, in one of the herds in the present study, factors such as emission of ammonium and carbon dioxide gases, air movements and overcrowding were investigated, but it was not possible to relate any environmental factor to the occurrence of conjunctivitis (data not shown). However, in one stable a high relative humidity (83%) was noted that might facilitate microbial survival. In the present study, the pigs originated from several piglet producing herds and it should be emphasized that intensive farming systems with the mixing of pigs from several sources also imply increased opportunities for microbial spread among animals of different immunological status. In fact, in one herd a significant relationship was noted between conjunctivitis and the presence of *Chlamydia* spp. when the lower threshold value was applied in the real-time PCR. This might further indicate that the infectious load is important in the development of disease.

Although *Chlamydia* spp. was demonstrated in the ileal sections by immunohistochemistry in the present study, lesions compatible to those described in gnotobiotic pigs [9] were only noted in 50% of the pigs. Several authors speculate that the development of lesions may depend on different factors such as the virulence of the strain, the infectious dose, the route of infection, or the age and the immunological status of the host [1, 6, 8, 10, 11, 27]. Since young, naive pigs seem to develop lesions in response to an experimental infection [9], host immunity might be induced at an early age in the field [11, 28]. It is also possible that co-infections with other presumptive pathogens might act synergistically to exacerbate the lesions or that lesions induced by one microbe might increase the susceptibility to other infections. Several pathogens have been discussed in this respect [3, 6, 11, 13, 29, 30]. Most of the intestinal lesions described in the present study were shown to be related to infections with *L. intracellularis* or *B. pilosicoli* [17].

Some studies also report the occurrence of mixed infection with several chlamydial species [3, 31, 32, 33]. In wild boars, *C. psittaci* was the dominating species but *C. suis* and *C. abortus* was also demonstrated by sequencing [31]. In the present study, preliminary data obtained by PCR-RFLP indicated the co-infection by other species [34]. However, sequencing of the amplicons revealed the involvement of *C. suis* only, whereas other bands detected by PCR originated from *E. coli* and un-identified bacterial species. The results underline the difficulties involved in the diagnosis and a large variation in reported prevalences between various detection methods exist [3, 15, 16, 35]. In the present study, the problem was circumvented by the use of an internal probe and a high melting temperature in the real-time PCR, combined with sequencing of the amplicons that assured a high specificity.

CONCLUSIONS

Chlamydia suis was found in high prevalences in growing pigs with or without diarrhoea, and in finisher pigs with or without conjunctivitis. Overall, no correlation to clinical signs was detected. However, a correlation was noted between samples with a high degree of infection and the presence of clinical signs. It is possible, that the intensive pig producing systems investigated in the present study might predispose for the transmission and survival of the microbe, thus increasing the infectious load and the risk for disease in the pig. Interestingly, no other species of the *Chlamydiaceae* family were detected, as also supported by the findings in other animal species in Swedish surveys [36].

DECLARATIONS

Acknowledgements

We wish to thank Marianne Persson for skilful technical assistance. We also wish to thank the herd owners who kindly supplied the pigs and allowed us to enter the herds.

Authors' contributions

SE was responsible for the PCR investigation and sequencing of DNA from the intestinal specimens, analysis and interpretation of these data, and revised the manuscript. CHS made an intellectual contribution by drafting the manuscript and revising it critically. FA was responsible for collecting of the conjunctival swabs, PCR analysis and interpretation of these data, and revised the manuscript. EW was responsible for the immunohistochemical analyses, interpretations of these data, and revised the manuscript. MJ was planning the studies, collected and prepared the intestinal specimens, and was responsible for drafting and writing the manuscript. All authors read and approved the final manuscript.

REFERENCES

1. Shewen PE: Chlamydial infection in animals: a review. Can Vet J. 1980, 21: 2-11.
2. Schautteet K, Vanrompay D: Chlamydiaceae infections in pig. Vet Res. 2011, 42: 1-10.
3. Hoelzle LE, Steinhausen G, Wittenbrink MM: PCR-based detection of chlamydial infection in swine and subsequent PCR-coupled genotyping of chlamydial *omp*--gene amplicons by DNA-hybridization, RFLP-analysis, and nucleotide sequence analysis. Epidemiol Inf. 2000, 125: 427-439. 10.1017/S0950268899004446.
4. Rogers DG, Andersen AA, Hogg A, Nielsen DL, Huebert MA: Conjunctivitis and keratoconjunctivitis associated with chlamydiae in swine. J Am Vet Med A. 1993, 203 (9): 1321-1323.
5. Longbottom D: Chlamydial infections of domestic ruminants and swine: new nomenclature and new knowledge. Vet J. 2004, 168: 9-11. 10.1016/S1090-0233(03)00106-0.
6. Nietfeld JC, Leslie-Steen P, Zeman DH, Nelson D: Prevalence of intestinal chlamydial infection in pigs in the midwest, as determined by immunoperoxidase staining. Am J Vet Res. 1997, 58 (3): 260-264.
7. Szeredi L, Schiller I, Sydler T, Guscetti F, Heinen E, Corboz L, Eggenberger E, Jones GE, Pospischil A: Intestinal *Chlamydia*in finishing pigs. Vet Pathol. 1996, 33 (4): 369-374. 10.1177/030098589603300401.
8. Zahn I, Szeredi L, Schiller I, Straumann Kunz U, Bürgi E, Guscetti F, Heinen E, Corboz L, Sydler T, Pospischil A: Immunohistologischer Nachweis von *Chlamydia psittaci/pecorum* und *C. trachomatis* im Ferkel-Darm. J Vet Med B. 1995, 42: 266-276. 10.1111/j.1439-0450.1995.tb00710.x.
9. Rogers DG, Andersen AA: Intestinal lesions caused by two swine chlamydial isolates in gnotobiotic pigs. J Vet Diagn Invest. 1996, 8: 433-440. 10.1177/104063879600800405.
10. Guscetti F, Schiller I, Sydler T, Heinen E, Pospischil A: Experimental enteric infection of gnotobiotic piglets with *Chlamydia suis* strain S45. Vet Microbiol. 2009, 135: 157-168. 10.1016/j.vetmic.2008.09.038.
11. Rogers DG, Andersen AA: Intestinal lesions caused by a strain of *Chlamydia suis* in weanling pigs infected at 21 days of age. J Vet Diagn Invest. 2000, 12: 233-239. 10.1177/104063870001200306.
12. Nietfeld JC, Janke BH, Leslie-Steen P, Robison DJ, Zeman DH: Small intestinal *Chlamydia* infection in piglets. J Vet Diagn Invest. 1993, 5: 114-117. 10.1177/104063879300500129.
13. Becker A, Lutz-Wohlgroth L, Brugnera E, Lu ZH, Zimmermann DR, Grimm F, Grosse Beilage E, Kaps S, Spiess B, Pospischil A, Vaughan L: Intensively kept pigs pre-disposed to chlamydial associated conjunctivitis. J Vet Med A. 2007, 54: 307-313. 10.1111/j.1439-0442.2007.00963.x.
14. Rogers DG, Andersen AA: Conjunctivitis caused by a swine *Chlamydia trachomatis*-like organism in gnotobiotic pigs. J Vet Diagn Invest. 1999, 11: 341-344. 10.1177/104063879901100408.
15. Rohde G, Straube E, Essig A, Reinhold P, Sachse K: Chlamydial zoonoses. Dtsch Ärtzebl Int. 2010, 107 (10): 174-180.
16. Sachse K, Grossmann E, Jäger C, Diller R, Hotzel H: Detection of *Chlamydia suis* from clinical specimens: comparison of PCR, antigen ELISA, and culture. J Microbiol Meth. 2003, 54: 233-238. 10.1016/S0167-7012(03)00040-X.
17. Jacobson M, Hård af Segerstad C, Gunnarsson A, Fellström C, de Verdier Klingenberg K, Wallgren P, Jensen-Waern M: Diarrhoea in the growing pig--a comparison of clinical, morphological and microbial findings between animals from good and poor performance herds. Res Vet Sci. 2003, 74: 163-169. 10.1016/S0034-5288(02)00187-X.
18. Jacobson M, Aspan A, Heldtander Königsson M, Hård af Segerstad C, Wallgren P, Fellström C, Jensen-Waern M, Gunnarsson A: Routine diagnostics of *Lawsonia intracellularis* performed by PCR, serological and post mortem examination, with special emphasis on sample preparation methods for PCR. Vet Microbiol. 2004, 102 (3-4): 189-201. 10.1016/j.vetmic.2004.04.014.
19. Johansson K-E, Persson A, Persson M: Diagnosis of contagious caprine and contagious bovine pleuropneumonia by PCR and restriction enzyme analysis. Int Symp Diagn Contr Livestock Dis Nucl Tech Int Atomic Energy Agency: 1998. 1998, Vienna, Italy, 137-158.
20. Sachse K, Hotzel H: Detection and differentiation of *Chlamydiae* by nested PCR. Meth Mol Biol. 2003, 216: 123-136.
21. Everett KD, Hornung LJ, Andersen AA: Rapid detection of the *Chlamydiaceae* and other families in the order *Chlamydiales*: three PCR tests. J Clin Microbiol. 1999, 37 (3): 575-580.
22. Englund S, Bölske G, Ballagi-Pordány A, Johansson K-E: Detection of *Mycobacterium avium* subsp. *paratuberculosis* in tissue samples by single, fluorescent and nested PCR based on the IS*90* gene. Vet Microbiol. 2001, 81: 257-271. 10.1016/S0378-1135(01)00348-0.
23. Everett KD, Andersen AA: Identification of nine species of the *Chlamydiaceae* using PCR-RFLP. Int J Syst Bacteriol. 1999, 49: 803-813. 10.1099/00207713-49-2-803.
24. Storz J, Eugster AK, Altera KP, Olander HJ: Behavior of different bovine chlamydial agents in newborn calves. J Comp Pathol. 1971, 81: 299-307. 10.1016/0021-9975(71)90104-6.
25. Doughri AM, Young S, Storz J: Pathologic changes in intestinal chlamydial infection of newborn calves. Am J Vet Res. 1974, 35 (7): 939-944.

26. Lenzko H, Moog U, Henning K, Lederbach R, Diller R, Menge C, Sachse K, Sprague LD: High frequency of chlamydial co-infections in clinically healthy sheep flocks. BMC Vet Res. 2011, 7: 29-10.1186/1746-6148-7-29. [http://www.biomedcentral.com/1746-6148/7/29]

27. Reinhold P, Kirschvink N, Theegarten D, Berndt A: An experimentally induced *Chlamydia suis* infection in pigs results in severe lung function disorders and pulmonary inflammation. Vet Res. 2008, 39: 1-19. 10.1051/vetres:2007039.

28. Guscetti F, Schiller I, Sydler T, Corboz L, Pospischil A: Experimental *Chlamydia psittaci* serotype 1 enteric infection in gnotobiotic piglets: Histopathological, immunohistochemical and microbiological findings. Vet Microbiol. 1998, 62: 251-263. 10.1016/S0378-1135(98)00221-1.

29. Pospischil A, Wood RL: Intestinal *Chlamydia* in pigs. Vet Pathol. 1987, 24: 568-570.

30. Koudela B, Vitovec J, Sterba J: Concurrent infection of enterocytes with *Eimeria scabra* and other enteropathogens in swine. Vet Parasitol. 1990, 35: 71-77. 10.1016/0304-4017(90)90117-T.

31. Hotzel H, Berndt A, Melzer F, Sachse K: Occurrence of *Chlamydiaceae* spp. in a wild boar (*Sus scrofa* L.) population in Thuringia (Germany). Vet Microbiol. 2004, 103: 121-126. 10.1016/j.vetmic.2004.06.009.

32. Schiller I, Koesters R, Weilenmann R, Thoma R, Kaltenboeck B, Heitz P, Pospischil A: Mixed infections with porcine *Chlamydia trachomatis/pecorum* and infections with ruminant *Chlamydia psittaci* serovar 1 associated with abortions in swine. Vet Microbiol. 1997, 58: 251-260. 10.1016/S0378-1135(97)00154-5.

33. Pantchev A, Sting R, Bauerfeind R, Tyczka J, Sachse K: Detection of all *Chlamydophila* and *Chlamydia* spp. of veterinary interest using species-specific real-time PCR assays. Comp Immunol, Microbiol Inf Dis. 2010, 33 (6): 473-484. 10.1016/j.cimid.2009.08.002.

34. Jacobson M, Englund S: The occurrence of *Chlamydia* species in intestinal specimens from Swedish grower pigs. The 20th International Pig Veterinary Society Congress: 2008. 2008, Durban, South Africa, 186.

35. Wendt M, Eggermann G, Wittenbrink MM, Jäger C, Weiss R, Failing K: Prevalence of Chlamydial infection in breeding sows. Proceedings of the 15th International Pig Veterinary Society Congress: 1998. 1998, Birmingham, England, 379.

36. Godin A-C, Björkman C, Englund S, Johansson K-E, Niskanen R, Alenius S: Investigation of *Chlamydophila* spp. in dairy cows with reproductive disorders. Acta Vet Scand. 2008, 50: 39-10.1186/1751-0147-50-39. [http://www.actavetscand.com/content/50/1/39]

CHAPTER 7

HIGH FREQUENCY OF CHLAMYDIAL CO-INFECTIONS IN CLINICALLY HEALTHY SHEEP FLOCKS

Hannah Lenzko, Udo Moog, Klaus Henning, Robert Lederbach, Roland Diller, Christian Menge, Konrad Sachse and Lisa D Sprague

BACKGROUND

Two species of the genus *Chlamydophila (C.)* have been reported to cause infections in sheep, *C.abortus*, and *C. pecorum*. Enzootic abortion of ewes (EAE) or ovine enzootic abortion, induced by *C. abortus* is particularly feared, not only because of the major financial losses it can produce in the affected flocks [1] but also due to its zoonotic potential. Exposure of pregnant women to infected sheep can lead to severe septicaemia in the mother resulting in spontaneous abortion or stillbirth of the child [2, 3]. Ewes are usually infected via the oro-pharyngeal or respiratory route. Infected animals generally show no signs of disease until the following pregnancy, when chlamydiae invade and colonise the placental tissues [4, 5]. EAE is a notifiable disease in Germany and also notifiable to the OIE.

Occasional cases of aborted lambs caused by *C. pecorum* have also been reported [6]. In susceptible animals, especially lambs, infection can induce, according to the subtype, pneumonia, polyarthritis, conjunctivitis, and enteritis [6]. Infection occurs through inhalation, ingestion, and direct contact. Rodolakis et al. [7] mention the occurrence of clinically inapparent *C. pecorum* infections in both abortion affected and non-affected flocks of small ruminants. The agent is not known to cause disease in humans [8].

There are very few detailed epidemiological data regarding the distribution of ovine chlamydial infections in countries outside the UK. Most of the few existing German studies are outdated and based on materials submitted for routine laboratory examination. Moreover, virtually all data have been obtained from serological studies, which are unable to discriminate among *Chlamydiaceae* spp. and interpretation of the results is cumbersome due to the variety of applied techniques [9, 10, 11, 12]. Accordingly, the aim of this study was to estimate the chlamydial sero- and antigen prevalence in sheep flocks using the state of Thuringia as a model example.

METHODS

Sheep flocks and sampling procedures

Flocks with an average abortion rate lower than 1% and distributed throughout the state of Thuringia were chosen at random (Table 1). The flocks had to contain more than 100 ewes, and not been vaccinated against chlamydia in the past ten years. Flocks were kept on pasture, lambing took place indoors. The sample size was calculated as such that an estimated seroprevalence of 10% and an estimated antigen prevalence of 25% at flock-level would be detected with 95% confidence [13].

Citation: Hannah Lenzko, Udo Moog, Klaus Henning, Robert Lederbach, Roland Diller, Christian Menge, Konrad Sachse and Lisa D Sprague, High frequency of chlamydial co-infections in clinically healthy sheep flocks, DOI: 10.1186/1746-6148-7-29.

Table 1: Summary of the sampled flocks and collected samples

				# of samples taken						
flock #	**flock size (ewes)**	**vaccine Status**	**abortion rate (%)§**	**1^{st}serum d1/2 p.p.**	**2nd serum d21 p.p.**	**vaginal swab/ PCR**	**vaginal swab/ culture**	**rectal swab**	**afterbirth**	**foetus/foetal swab**
1	500	-	0	-	29	11	11	11	-	-
2	1000	-	0	29	25	11	11	11	9	-
3	1800	-	< 1	29	27	11	11	11	12	4
4	1300	-	0	29	29	11	11	11	-	-
5	1200	-	3	29	6	11	11	11	3	4
6	500	-	0	29	27	11	11	11	-	-
7	450	-	0	29	25	11	11	11	9	-
8	1100	-	< 1	30	30	11	11	11	-	-
9	1800	-	0	29	29	11	11	11	-	-
10	550	-	0	29	29	11	11	11	3	-
11	700	-	< 1	29	29	11	11	11	-	-
12	330	-	0	30	29	11	11	11	2	-
13*	2500	+	2	30	30	11	11	11	11	-
14	400	-	< 1	29	28	11	11	11	-	-
15	700	-	< 1	29	28	11	11	11	-	-
16	750	-	< 1	29	29	11	11	11	-	-
17	900	-	< 1	29	29	11	11	11	3	-
18	250	-	< 1	29	29	11	11	11	-	-
19*	450	+	< 1	29	27	11	11	11	1	-
20	1000	-	< 1	29	25	11	11	11	-	-
21	500	-	< 1	29	29	11	11	11	-	-
22	406	-	< 1	29	29	11	11	11	-	-
23	700	-	< 1	29	29	11	11	11	-	-
24	700	-	0	29	19	11	11	11	-	-
25	550	-	< 1	29	25	11	11	11	-	-
26	1000	-	1	29	29	11	11	11	-	-
27	317	-	< 1	29	29	11	11	11	-	-
28*	350	+	6	29	29	11	11	11	1	2
29	420	-	0	29	27	11	11	11	-	-
30*	1178	+	< 1	29	25	11	11	11	-	-
31*	500	+	< 1	29	29	11	11	11	-	-
32	120	-	0	29	29	11	11	11	4	-
33	115	-	< 1	29	28	11	11	11	11	-
34	400	-	< 1	29	29	11	11	11	1	-
35	650	-	< 1	29	29	11	11	11	-	-
36*	133	+	0	29	28	11	11	11	-	-
37	377	-	< 1	29	26	11	11	11	2	-
38*	409	+	< 1	29	28	11	11	11	-	-
39**	25	-	0	25	24	11	11	11		
40	460	-	< 1	29	-	11	11	11	-	-
total				**1130**	**1059**	**440**	**440**	**440**	**72**	**10**

§according to the sheep farmers and the Thuringian sheep health authority

*due to a vaccination history not included in the prevalence study but analysed separately

**excluded from the prevalence study due to flock size

Sera and swabs were collected during the lambing seasons by and under the supervision of a veterinarian (UM) from the Thuringian sheep health service during his flock management visits between February 2009 to June 2009 (flocks 1-13) and December 2009 to April 2010 (flocks 14-40). In practice, the sampling was carried out as follows: Paired serum samples were collected from 29 ewes per flock on day 1 or day 2 post partum and three weeks later. Additionally, two vaginal and one rectal swab were obtained from 11/29 ewes. Afterbirths and foetuses occurring in the flocks were collected when available. A total of 2189 serum samples, 880 vaginal swabs, 440 rectal swabs, 72 afterbirths and 10 foetuses/foetal/pharyngeal swabs were collected (Table 1). Due to the later discovery of a vaccination history, seven flocks (13, 19, 28, 30, 31, 36, and 38) were excluded from the prevalence study and analysed separately. An eighth flock (39) was excluded due to the small flock size. For the prevalence study a total of 1740 serum samples, 704 vaginal swabs, 352 rectal swabs, 59 afterbirths, and 8 foetuses/ foetal/pharyngeal swabs from 32 flocks were evaluated.

Sample preparation and conservation

Blood was drawn from the jugular vein with a 14 gauge needle into 7.5 mL serum Monovettes (Kabe GmbH, Nümbrecht-Elsenroth, Germany) and stored upright at RT for 12 h. The Monovettes were then centrifuged at 1500 × *g* for 10 min, the supernatant serum removed and stored at -20°C until further use. Vaginal swabs (Nerbe plus GmbH, Winsen/Luhe, Germany) collected for subsequent cell culture cultivation were transferred to 1 mL of sucrose phosphate glutamate buffer (SPG, 218 mM sucrose, 38 mM KH_2PO_4, 7 mM K_2HPO_4, 5 mM L-glutamic acid) supplemented with 0.1% (w/v) bovine serum albumin V, and stored at -80°C. Vaginal swabs collected for nucleic acid extraction were transferred to 200 µl lysis buffer [(6 M guanidiumisothiocyanate, 10 mM urea, 20% (v/v) Triton X-100 and 10 mM Tris HCl (pH 4.4); Roche Diagnostics, Mannheim, Germany)] and stored at 4°C. Afterbirths and organ samples from aborted foetuses were stored at -80°C until further use.

ELISA

Serum samples were tested for the presence of chlamydial antibodies using the CHECKIT™ Chlamydia Test Kit (Idexx GmbH, Ludwigsburg, Germany) according to the manufacturer's instructions. All measurements were performed in duplicate and matching serum pairs were analysed on the same microtitre plate. Results were normalised using the positive and negative control sera provided in the kit and expressed as percentage of the positive control according to the following formula: [(OD sample - OD negative control)/ (OD positive control - OD negative control)] × 100. Sera with values below 30% were considered negative, sera with values between 30 and 40% were considered inconclusive, and sera with values greater 40% were considered as positive. Animals were considered to have seroconverted when a change from negative to positive between the first and second serum sampling was observed.

Cell culture and isolation of chlamydiae

Buffalo Green Monkey (BGM) cells in Minimal Essential Medium (MEM) supplemented with 5% foetal calf serum were seeded into trac bottles containing glass cover slips (Dunn Labortechnik GmbH, Asbach, Germany) and maintained in a humidified atmosphere with 5% CO_2 at 37°C. The cell monolayers were assessed for confluent growth on the day of inoculation.

Vaginal swabs were ultrasonicated (ten 6 s impulses at an amplitude of 80%; Branson 450D digital sonifier), and between 30 and 300 µL of the solution used for inoculation of five trac bottles per sample. Organ samples were thawed, mechanically disrupted, resuspended in 3 mL PBS, and ultrasonicated (two 30 s impulses at an amplitude of 80%). The resulting suspension was centrifuged for 15 min at 500 × *g* and the supernatant used for inoculation of five trac bottles containing Nephros LP medium (BioWhittacker, Walkersville, USA) with nystatin (25 E/mL), 0.4% (v/v) gentamicin (40 µg/mL), and 0.1% (v/v) vancomycin-HCl (25 µg/mL). Upon inoculation, the trac bottles were centrifuged for 60 min at 3,400 × *g* and 37°C and subsequently incubated for 2 h. After replacement of medium, the cells were incubated for a further 18 h after which medium was again renewed. Between two to ten days after inoculation, one cover slip was fixed in methanol, and the monolayer was stained for 15 min at 37°C with 25 µL of the test reagent provided in the IMAGEN™ Chlamydia kit (Oxoid Ltd., Cambridge, UK). This kit uses a *Chlamydiaceae*-specific monoclonal fluorescent antibody recognising surface LPS from all known chlamydial species. Specimens were considered positive if they showed inclusions of typical chlamydial morphology in the form of bright apple-green, smooth-edged spots. If no specific fluorescent reaction was observed after two passages, specimens were considered negative.

DNA extraction from samples

DNA from vaginal, rectal, foetal, and foetal organs swabs as well as from pharyngeal swabs of premature born live lambs was isolated using the High Pure PCR Template Preparation Kit™ (Roche Diagnostics) according to the manufacturer's instructions. Organ samples were cut into 50 mg sections, mechanically disrupted and digested over night in 200 µL lysis buffer with 40 µL proteinase K (20 mg/mL) (Roche Diagnostics) at 37°C.

Polymerase chain reaction (PCR)

Real-time PCR

Real-time PCR assays for *Chlamydiaceae, C. abortus, C. pecorum*, and *C. psittaci* were conducted as duplex amplifications in Thermo-Fast 96-well microplates (Biodeal, Markkleeberg, Germany) using a Stratagene Mx3000P Thermocycler (Agilent Technologies, Santa Clara, CF, USA) according to the method of [14]. Each reaction included an internal amplification control as described by [15], using primers EGFP1-F (GAC CAC TAC CAG CAG AAC AC), and EGFP10-R (CTT GTA CAG CTC GTC CAT GC) at a final concentration of 300 nM each, as well as TaqMan probe EGFP-HEX (HEX-AGC ACC CAG TCC GCC CTG AGC A-BHQ1) at 200 nM. Plasmid IC2 (0.5 µl, 10,000 copies) served as the internal control template (Intype IC-DNA, Labordiagnostik Leipzig, Germany). The final 25 µl reaction mixture included 12.5 µl of TaqMan GenEx Master Mix supplemented with

ROX (Applied Biosystems, Darmstadt, Germany), 0.8 μM primers, and 0.2 μM probes and 1 μl of sample DNA. Cycling parameters were as follows: initial denaturation step at 95°C for 10 min, 45 cycles of 95°C for 15 s and 60°C for 60 s (annealing and extension). The cycle threshold value (Ct) was calculated by the instrument›s software MxPro3000P v 4.01.

Nested PCR

Samples with Ct values between 38 and 40 in the *Chlamydiaceae*-specific real-time PCR were additionally analysed with a modified version of a nested PCR procedure. This PCR targets the variable domains (VD) III and IV of the *ompA* specific for all *Chlamydiaceae* [16]. Conventional PCR was carried out in a T3 Thermocycler (Biometra GmbH, Göttingen, Germany). The amplification product obtained by the outer primer pair 191CHOMP/CHOMP371 and the inner primer pair 201CHOMP/CHOMP336s was subsequently used for sequencing when species-specific assays were negative. For the outer PCR, 35 cycles were completed, each consisting of 15 s denaturation at 95°C, 30 s annealing at 50°C, and 30 s elongation at 72°C. A final elongation step of 30 s at 72°C completed the run. The same conditions also applied to the inner PCR, except that the annealing conditions were 30 s at 60°C and only 20 cycles were run. From each PCR reaction, 15 μL were analysed by agarose gel electrophoresis (2% w/v in Tris Borate EDTA buffer).

Biotinylation PCR

For subsequent species-specific microarray hybridization, DNA of randomly selected samples was amplified and biotin-labelled according to the method described by [17] using the primers U23F-19 and 23R-22. The temperature-time profile was 60°C/60 s for the initial denaturation, 40 cycles of 94°C/30 s, 55°C/60 s, 72°C/45 s and a final extension step at 72°C/240 s. From each PCR reaction, 10 μL were analysed by agarose gel electrophoresis (1.5% w/v in Tris Borate EDTA buffer).

DNA samples for successive *C. psittaci* genotyping were amplified and biotinylated by means of a duplex PCR procedure described by [18]. This PCR uses two primer pairs, VD1-f/VD2-r, and 201CHOMP/ompA-rev, which encompass all the variable domains of the *ompA* of *C. psittaci*. The following PCR cycling conditions were used: initial denaturation at 96°C/60 s, 40 cycles of 94°C/30 s, 50°C/60 s, 72°C/30 s and a final extension step at 72°C/240 s. From each PCR reaction, 10 μL were analysed by agarose gel electrophoresis (1.5% w/v in Tris Borate EDTA buffer).

PCR-RFLP

In order to differentiate *C. abortus* field strains from the vaccine strain a PCR-Restriction Fragment Length Polymorphism (RFLP) assay was conducted as described by [19] using the primer pairs CAB153-F/CAB153-R, CAB636-F/CAB636-R and CAB648-F/CAB648-R. Due to three point mutations in the coding sequences of the vaccine strain 1B, specific restriction sites are lost thus enabling the differential identification of field strains. PCR cycling conditions were: an initial 15 min denaturation step at 95°C followed by 30 cycles 95°C/30 s, 60°C/30 s (CAB636-F/R and CAB648-F/R), 58°C/30 s (CAB153-F/R), 72°C/3 s and a final extension step at 72°C/10 min. Next, 10 μL of each PCR product was digested with 2 U of the respective enzyme, i.e. *Sfc*I for CAB153, *Hae*III for CAB636 and *Sau*3A for CAB648, at 37°C over night. Ten μL of the amplification products and restriction fragments (Table 2) were analysed by agarose gel electrophoresis (2% w/v in Tris Borate EDTA buffer).

Table 2: PCR-RFLP pattern of *C.abortus* vaccine strain and *C. abortus* field strains

coding sequence	restriction enzyme	fragment size vaccine (bp)	fragment size field strain (bp)
CAB153	*Sfc*I	319	177 + 142
CAB636	*Hae*III	118	74 + 44
CAB648	*Sau*3A	87 + 90	87 + 69 + 21

Identification of chlamydiae and genotyping of *C. psittaci*using DNA microarray assays

Selected samples were examined by means of the ArrayTube™ (AT) DNA microarray assay (Alere, formerly Clondiag, Jena, Germany) as described by Borel et al. (2008) to corroborate the results obtained in the species-specific real-time PCRs. Hybridization signals were measured at room temperature with the ATR-01 array tube reader and analysed using the Iconoclust software version 2.2 (both Alere).

In addition to *ompA* sequence alignments and BLAST search, a DNA microarray genotyping assay based on the ArrayTube™ technology was used to determine the genotype of the *C. psittaci* strains according to the procedures described by [18].

ompA Sequencing

In cases of inconclusive PCR results, i.e. positive in the *Chlamydiaceae* or nested PCR but with CT values > 38 in the species-specific PCR, samples were analysed by means of partial sequencing of the *ompA*. Amplicons were purified and concentrated using the DNA Clean & Concentrator™-5 kit (ZymoResearch, Freiburg, Germany) according to the manufacturer's instructions. Sequencing of the amplicons using the primer pair 201CHOMP/CHOMP336s was performed at Eurofins MWG Operon (Ebersberg, Germany). Species identity based on the *ompA* FASTA sequences was established following a BLAST search.

Statistical analyses

In order to assess how the sampling point influenced the isolated species and the frequency of detection the Wilcoxon rank-sum test was used. For the analysis of how flock size correlated with finding ELISA (2nd serum sample) and/or PCR positive animals the Spearman-Rho coefficient was calculated. In both tests, a p-value < 0.05 was considered to be statistically significant. All tests were conducted using the statistical package SPSS, release 12.0.1 for Windows (SPSS Inc., Chicago, IL., USA).

RESULTS

Serology

A flock was considered sero-positive if at least one animal was tested positive in the ELISA. With the exception of two flocks (12, 40) all unvaccinated flocks were serologically positive (94%; CI 95). Moreover, seroconversion in the tested ewes was seen in 15/32 (47%) flocks (Table 3). All vaccinated flocks were serologically positive (7/7) and seroconversion of single animals was observed in three (43%) flocks (Table 4).

Table 3: Summation of positive sera from the unvaccinated flocks

		# positive sera vs. # sera tested		# of animals	
flock #	abortion rate (%)	1st serum d1/2 p.p.	2nd serum d21 p.p.	positive/ # total	sero-conversion/ # total
1	0	0	4/29	4/29	-
2	0	5/29	2/25	5/29	0/25
3	< 1	6/29	5/27	6/29	0/29
4	0	11/29	10/29	11/29	0/29
5	3	11/29	4/6	13/29	**2/6**
6	0	1/29	2/27	2/29	**1/27**
7	0	6/29	6/25	9/29	**3/25**
8	< 1	6/30	5/30	6/30	0/30
9	0	7/29	12/29	14/29	**6/29**
10	0	1/29	1/29	1/29	0/29
11	< 1	3/29	5/29	5/29	**2/29**
12	0	0/30	0/29	0/30	0/29
14	< 1	1/29	2/28	2/29	**1/28**
15	< 1	9/29	9/28	9/29	0/28
16	< 1	8/29	8/29	9/29	**1/29**
17	< 1	15/29	16/29	16/29	**1/29**
18	< 1	1/29	1/29	1/29	0/29
20	< 1	8/29	6/25	8/29	0/29
21	< 1	3/29	2/29	3/29	0/29
22	< 1	8/29	9/29	10/29	**1/29**
23	< 1	7/29	7/29	8/29	**1/29**
24	0	2/29	1/19	2/29	0/19
25	< 1	5/29	4/25	5/29	0/25
26	1	6/29	6/29	6/29	0/29
27	< 1	4/29	5/29	6/29	**2/29**
29	0	3/29	2/27	3/29	0/27
32	0	1/29	2/29	2/29	**1/29**
33	< 1	2/29	2/28	2/29	0/28
34	< 1	3/29	6/29	7/29	**4/29**
35	< 1	5/29	10/29	10/29	**5/29**
37	< 1	1/29	2/26	2/29	**1/26**
40	< 1	0/29	-	0/29	-

Table 4: Summary of positive sera from the vaccinated flocks

	abortion rate[§]			# positive sera vs. # sera tested		# of animals	
flock #	prior to vaccination	upon vaccination	vaccination*	1st serum d1/2 p.p.	2nd serum d21 p.p.	total	sero-conversion
13	1-10%	0.8-2%	since 1995 all teggs	3/30	4/30	4/30	**1/30**
19	7%	< 1%	in 2004 complete flock; since 2005 all teggs	6/29	4/27	6/29	0/27
28	2009: 17%	6%	since 1998 all teggs; in 2009 complete flock	9/29	9/29	9/29	0/29
30	< 1%	< 1%	since 1980 all teggs	2/29	0/25	2/29	0/25
31	< 1%	< 1%	since 2002 all teggs	2/29	2/29	2/29	0/29
36	< 1%	0	since 1995 all teggs	2/29	3/28	4/29	**2/28**
38	2003: 49%	< 1%	in 2003 complete flock; since 2004 all teggs	3/29	4/28	4/29	**1/28**

*Ovilis Enzovax (Intervet Deutschland GmbH, Unterschleißheim, Germany)

[§] according to the sheep farmers and the Thuringian sheep health authority

Isolation of chlamydiae

A total of 23 PCR positive vaginal swabs (flocks 1-8, 11, 14, 17, 18, 23, 26, 27, 28, 34-36, 38, 40) and three afterbirths (flocks 17, 28, 23) were analysed. *C. abortus* was isolated and propagated from three vaginal swabs taken from flocks 5 (abortion), 17 and 35 (both normal births) and from a placenta in flock 28 (abortion). The latter was a field strain as determined by PCR-RFLP. *C. pecorum* was isolated and propagated from a vaginal swab in flock 14 (normal birth). Vaginal swabs taken in flocks 3, 7, 11, 34, and 38 (normal births), initially showed signs of chlamydial growth and were positive for *C. abortus* in the species-specific real-time PCR, however, no isolates could be obtained.

Detection of chlamydiae by means of PCR

Unvaccinated flocks were considered antigen positive if at least one animal was tested positive for chlamydial DNA (Tables 5, 6). *Chlamydiaceae*-specific real-time or conventional PCR revealed the presence of chlamydia in 25/32 flocks (78%; CI 95%). Species-specific real-time PCR detected *C. abortus* in 15/32 flocks (47%), *C. pecorum* in 13/32 flocks (41%), and *C. psittaci* in 8/32 flocks (25%). In 10/32 flocks (31%) more than one chlamydial species was found, i.e. the combination *C. abortus* and *C. psittaci* (flocks 1, 3, 4, 5, 8, 11), *C. psittaci* and *C. pecorum* (flocks 1, 2, 6) or *C. abortus* and *C. pecorum* (flocks 11, 17, 19). In three (9%) of these flocks (1, 5, 8) all three species were detected (Tables 5, 6). Simultaneous detection of more than one chlamydial species per swab occurred in 9/32 flocks (28%) (flocks 1, 2, 3, 4, 5, 8, 11, 17, and 19).

Table 5: Compilation of the PCR, sequencing, and microarray results from the vaginal swabs of the unvaccinated flocks

	Chlamydiaceae detection method [# positive vs. # tested sample]			*Chlamydiaceae* species identification detection method [# positive vs. # tested sample]			species detected[$]				
flock #	23 S RT PCR[§]	nested PCR	positive vaginal swabs	species-specific RT PCR	sequencing CHOMP	microarray	ps	pc	ab	m	
1	2/11	2/11	3/11	3/11	1/11	1/11	2	-	-	1	ab,ps
2	0/11	1/11	1/11	1/11	-	-	1	-	-	-	ps
3	1/11	1/11	2/11	2/11	-	-	1	-	-	1	ab,ps
4	0/11	1/11	1/11	0/11	1/11	-	1	-	-	-	ps
5	6/11	3/11	9/11	9/11	-	1/11	-	-	3	6	ab,ps
6	5/11	0/11	5/11	3/11	2/11	-	5	-	-	-	ps

7	1/11	3/11	4/11	2/11	4#/11	-	3	-	-	-	ps, su#
8	1/11	0/11	1/11	1/11	-	-	-	-	-	1	ab,ps
9	neg.	-	0/11	-	-	-	-	-	-	-	-
10	neg.	-	0/11	-	-	-	-	-	-	-	-
11	1/11	0/11	1/11	1/11	-	1/11	-	-	1	-	ab
12	neg.	-	0/11	-	-	-	-	-	-	-	-
14	1/11	0/11	1/11	1/11	-	1/11	-	1	-	-	pc
15	neg.	-	0/11	-	-	-	-	-	-	-	-
16	neg.	-	0/11	-	-	-	-	-	-	-	-
17	11/11	-	11/11	11/11	-	-	-	-	11	-	ab
18	0/11	1/11	1/11	0/11	1/11	-	-	-	1	-	ab
20	neg.	-	0/11	-	-	-	-	-	-	-	-
21	neg.	-	0/11	-	-	-	-	-	-	-	-
22	neg.	-	0/11	-	-	-	-	-	-	-	-
23	1/11	-	1/11	1/11	-	1/11	-	-	1	-	ab
24	neg.	-	0/11	-	-	-	-	-	-	-	-
25	neg.	-	0/11	-	-	-	-	-	-	-	-
26	0/11	2/11	2/11	1/11	1/11	-	-	-	2	-	ab
27	1/11	-	1/11	1/11	-	-	-	-	1	-	ab
29	neg.	-	0/11	-	-	-	-	-	-	-	-
32	neg.	-	0/11	-	-	-	-	-	-	-	-
33	neg.	-	0/11	-	-	-	-	-	-	-	-
34	6/11	0/11	6/11	6/11	-	-	-	-	6	-	ab
35	1/11	1/11	2/11	2/11	-	1/11	-	-	2	-	ab
37	neg.	-	0/11	-	-	-	-	-	-	-	-
40	1/11	-	1/11	1/11	-	-	-	1	-	-	pc

§0 = ct > 38; ab: $C. abortus; ps: *C. psittaci*; pc: *C. pecorum*; su:#*C. suis*; m: mixed infection;

- : not determined; neg.: negative;

Table 6: Compilation of the PCR, sequencing, and microarray results from the rectal swabs of the unvaccinated flocks

	Chlamydiaceae			***Chlamydiaceae*species identification**							
	detection method [# positive vs. # tested sample]			**detection method [# positive vs. # tested sample]**			**species detected$**				
flock #	**23 S RT PCR§**	**nested PCR**	**positive rectal swabs**	**species-specific RT PCR**	**sequencing CHOMP**	**DNA microarray**	**ps**	**pc**	**ab**	**m**	
1	1/11	7/11	8/11	8/11	-	1/11	1	-	-	7	ab,ps,pc
2	0/11	2/11	2/11	1/11	2/11	-	1	-	-	1	ps,pc
3	1/11	2/11	3/11	3/11	1/11	-	1	-	-	2	ab,ps
4	3/11	0/11	3/11	3/11	-	1/11	-	-	1	2	ab,ps
5	7/11	0/11	7/11	7/11	-	1/11	-	-	2	5	ab,ps,pc
6	3/11	0/11	3/11	3/11	-	-	-	3	-	-	pc
7	0/11	1/11	1/11	1/11	-	-	1	-	-	-	ps
8	1/11	1/11	1/11	1/11	-	-	-	1	-	-	pc
9	neg.	-	0/11	-	-	-	-	-	-	-	-
10	0/11	1/11	1/11	1/11	-	-	-	-	1	-	ab

11	0/11	2/11	2/11	2/11	-	-	-	-	1	1	ab,pc
12	neg.	-	0/11	-	-	-	-	-	-	-	-
14	1/11	0/11	1/11	1/11	-	-	-	1	-	-	pc
15	neg.	-	0/11	-	-	-	-	-	-	-	-
16	1/11	3/11	4/11	3/11	1/11	-	-	1	3	-	ab,pc
17	9/11	1/11	11/11	11/11	-	-	-	-	4	7	ab,pc
18	neg.	-	0/11	-	-	-	-	-	-	-	-
20	neg.	-	0/11	-	-	-	-	-	-	-	-
21	0/11	1/11	1/11	1/11	-	-	-	1	-	-	pc
22	neg.	-	0/11	-	-	-	-	-	-	-	-
23	0/11	2/11	3/11	1/11	-	-	-	-	3	-	ab
24	neg.	-	0/11	-	-	-	-	-	-	-	-
25	1/11	1/11	2/11	2/11	-	-	-	2	-	-	pc
26	neg.	-	0/11	-	-	-	-	-	-	-	-
27	neg.	-	0/11	-	-	-	-	-	-	-	-
29	1/11	0/11	1/11	1/11	-	-	-	1	-	-	pc
32	neg.	-	0/11	-	-	-	-	-	-	-	-
33	2/11	3/11	4/11	3/11	1/11	-	-	-	4	-	ab
34	0/11	1/11	1/11	1/11	-	-	-	-	1	-	ab
35	0/11	2/11	2/11	1/11	1/11	-	-	-	2	-	ab
37	1/11	0/11	1/11	1/11	-	-	-	1	-	-	pc
40	neg.	-	0/11	-	-	-	-	-	-	-	-

§ 0 = ct > 38; ab: $ *C. abortus*; ps: *C. psittaci*; pc: *C. pecorum*; m: mixed infection;

- : not determined; neg.: negative;

Of the 53 positive vaginal swabs, 28 were positive for *C. abortus*, two for *C. pecorum*, and 13 for *C. psittaci*. Nine swabs were positive for more than one chlamydial species. One swab was positive for *Chlamydia suis* as determined by *omp*A sequencing. The species distribution obtained from the 62 positive rectal swabs was 22 for *C. abortus*, 11 for *C. pecorum*, four for *C. psittaci*, and 25 for more than one chlamydial species. The frequency of detected positive *C. psittaci* samples, *C. pecorum* samples (both $p \leq 0.05$) and samples with multiple chlamydial species ($p \leq 0.01$) differed significantly between vaginal and rectal swabs (Tables 5, 6). In the vaccinated flocks chlamydial DNA was detected by means of species-specific real-time PCR in 4/7 (57%) flocks (19, 28, 36, 38) which on further analysis proved to be specific for *C. abortus*. Subsequent PCR-RFLP revealed all *C. abortus* isolates to be field strains (data not shown). *C. pecorum* was additionally found in flock 28 and a *C. abortus/C. pecorum* mixed infection was detected in flock 19 (Tables 7, 8).

Table 7: Compilation of the PCR, sequencing and microarray results from the vaginal swabs of the vaccinated flocks

	Chlamydiaceae detection method [# positive vs. # tested sample]			***Chlamydiaceae*species identification** detection method [# positive vs. # tested sample]			**species detected$**				
flock #	**23 S RT PCR§**	**nested PCR**	**positive rectal swabs**	**species-specific RT PCR**	**sequencing CHOMP**	**DNA microarray**	**ps**	**pc**	**ab**	**m**	
13	neg.	-	0/11	-	-	-	-	-	-	-	-
19	1/11	0/11	1/11	1/11	-	-	-	-	-	1	ab,pc
28	3/11	1/11	4/11	4/11	-	-	-	1	3	-	ab,pc
30	neg.	-	0/11	-	-	-	-	-	-	-	-
31	neg.	-	0/11	-	-	-	-	-	-	-	-
36	neg.	-	0/11	-	-	-	-	-	-	-	-
38	neg.	-	0/11	-	-	-	-	-	-	-	-

§ 0 = ct > 38; ab: $ *C. abortus*; ps: *C. psittaci*; pc: *C. pecorum*; m: mixed infection;

- : not determined; neg.: negative;

Table 8: Compilation of the PCR, sequencing, and microarray results from the rectal swabs of the vaccinated flocks

	Chlamydiaceae detection method [# positive vs. # tested sample]			***Chlamydiaceae*species identification** detection method [# positive vs. # tested sample]			**species detected$**				
flock #	**23 S RT PCR§**	**nested PCR**	**positive vaginal swabs**	**species-specific RT PCR**	**sequencing CHOMP**	**DNA microarray**	**ps**	**pc**	**ab**	**m**	
13	neg.	-	0/11	-	-	-	-	-	-	-	-
19	neg.	-	0/11	-	-	-	-	-	-	-	-
28	2/11	0/11	2/11	2/11	-	-	-	-	2	-	ab
30	neg.	-	0/11	-	-	-	-	-	-	-	-
31	neg.	-	0/11	-	-	-	-	-	-	-	-
36	1/11	0/11	1/11	1/11	-	1/11	-	-	1	-	ab
38	2/11	-	2/11	2/11	-	-	-	-	2	-	ab

§ 0 = ct > 38; ab: $ *C. abortus*; ps: *C. psittaci*; pc: *C. pecorum*; m: mixed infection;

- : not determined; neg.: negative;

Detection of chlamydiae in afterbirths and foetuses/foetal samples

C. psittaci was detected in seven afterbirths from ewes in flocks 2, 3 and 7. *C. abortus* was found in nine afterbirths from animals in flocks 5, 17, 28 and 33 and in all ten foetal samples. One positive swab obtained from an aborted foetus in flock 3 could not be allocated to any specific chlamydial species. Two pharyngeal swabs from premature born lambs in flock 5 contained *C. psittaci* and *C. abortus* (Table 9).

Table 9: Chlamydial species detected in ovine afterbirths and foetus/foetal/pharyngeal swabs

Chlamydiaceae							***Chlamydiaceae*species identification**				
	detection method [# positive vs. # tested sample]						**detection method [# positive vs. # tested sample]**				**detected species$**
	23 S RT PCR§		**nested PCR**		**afterbirths**	**foetus/ foetal swab&**	**species-specific RT-PCR**		**sequencing CHOMP**	**DNA microarray**	
flock #	**a**	**fs**	**a**	**fs**			**a**	**fs**			
2	0/9	-	1/9	-	1/9	-	1/9	-	1/9	-	ps
3	1/12	3/4	6/12	4/4	6/12	4/4	2/12	4/4	4/12	1/4	5x ps; 1x-; 2x ab; 2x ab/ps
5	3/3	4/4	-	4/4	3/3	4/4	3/3	4/4	-	-	ab
7	0/9	-	1/9	-	1/9	-	1/9	-	-	-	ps
10	0/3	-	-	-	0/3	-	-	-	-	-	-
12	0/2	-	-	-	0/2	-	-	-	-	-	-
13*	0/11	-	-	-	0/11	-	-	-	-	-	-
17	2/3	-	1/3	-	3/3	-	2/3	-	1/3	-	ab
19*	0/1	-	-	-	0/1	-	-	-	-	-	-
28*	1/1	-	-	-	1/1	2/2	1/1	2/2	-	1/4	ab
32	0/4	-	-	-	0/4	-		-	-	-	-
33	2/11	-	-	-	2/11	-	2/11	-	-	-	ab

34	0/1	-	-	-	0/1	-		-	-	-	-
37	0/2	-	-	-	0/2	-	-	-	-	-	-

§ 0 = ct > 38; a: afterbirth; fs: foetal swab;

*vaccinated flock; $ ab: *C. abortus*; ps: *C. psittaci*; pc: *C. pecorum*;

& pharyngeal swabs from premature born lambs; - : not determined;

Identification of chlamydiae by means of a DNA microarray assay

DNA obtained from seven vaginal swabs from ewes in flocks 1, 5, 11, 14, 23, 35 and 37, as well as three rectal swabs from ewes in flocks 1, 4, and 5, was additionally analysed by means of the microarray assay. *C. abortus*was detected in nine samples (flocks 1, 11, 23, 35 and 37), *C. pecorum* was found in one sample (flock 14) (Table 5), thus corroborating the results from the species-specific PCRs. The presence of *C. abortus* in a foetal tissue from an aborted lamb in flock 3 and in a foetal sample from flock 28 was additionally confirmed via microarray testing (Table 9).

Genotyping of C. psittaci

The *C. psittaci* DNA was extracted from four vaginal swabs, one rectal swab (abortion) and from one afterbirth obtained from ewes in flocks 1, 2, 3, 6, and 7 was analysed with the DNA microarray genotyping assay which assigned all samples to the genotype A-VS1.

Sequencing

Partial sequencing of the *omp*A confirmed the presence of *C. psittaci* in four vaginal swabs deriving from ewes in flocks 1, 4, 6, and 7 and in 5 afterbirths from flocks 2 and 3. The presence of *C. abortus* was confirmed in two vaginal swabs and three rectal swabs taken from ewes in flocks 16, 18, 26, 33, and 35 (Table 5, 6) as well as in one afterbirth in flock 17 (Table 9).

Correlation between flock size and finding chlamydia-positive animals

Spearman's Rho revealed a correlation between flock size and ELISA positive animals (correlation coefficient: 0.179; $p \leq 0.01$) and between flock size and PCR positive animals (correlation coefficient: 0.119; $p \leq 0.05$).

DISCUSSION

Epidemiological data regarding the distribution of ovine chlamydiosis in Germany are scarce and are based solely on materials submitted for routine laboratory examination [9, 10, 11, 12]. Results obtained from such studies are frequently biased, since the materials are not randomly sampled. The present study, therefore, aimed at estimating the chlamydial sero- and antigen prevalence in randomly chosen unvaccinated sheep flocks in the state of Thuringia with an average abortion status lower than 1%.

Assuming a seroprevalence of 10% at flock level, we found that 94% of the tested flocks were serologically positive with ongoing infection, i.e. animals that had undergone seroconversion during the study period, in nearly half (47%) of the flocks. A study conducted by [12] in the state of Baden-Württemberg on an arbitrary panel of sera, vaginal, foetal, and placental swabs from flocks with increased abortion rates, revealed the presence of chlamydial infection in up to 91% of the flocks. Other studies estimating the seroprevalence of *C. abortus* in small ruminants found rates ranging from 4.8% in Sardinia [20], to 29% in Switzerland [21], 36% in Slovakia [22] and 47% in north eastern Turkey [23]. However, due to numerous parameters such as differences in study design and inclusion criteria (e.g. high abortion rates), flock size and management, prevalence of other abortifacient agents (e.g. *Brucellae, Salmonellae, Toxoplasma, Coxiella (C.) burnetii*) and the detection methods applied (CFT, competitive ELISA), it is virtually impossible to compare the present study's seroprevalence findings with the afore mentioned studies. Although no clinical signs were detected in our examined herds, seroconversion occurred around time of lambing. We observed seropositive animals at both sampling times, indicating chlamydial circulation within the herds resulting in the infection of naïve or seronegative animals.

On the basis of an estimated 25% antigen prevalence, PCR analyses revealed the presence of chlamydia in 78% of the flocks in the present study. A German study found chlamydial antigen prevalence in sheep to range between 50 and 71% [12] while a British study found prevalences of chlamydial infection to vary between 5-50% [24]. Other studies found prevalence rates in small ruminants to be around 11% in southern Italy [25], 7% in Anatolia [26] and 24% in Tunisia [27]. Prevalence was either determined by antigen ELISA, cultivation, conventional or multiplex PCR. All studies were carried out on samples from flocks with higher abortion rates than in our study.

The species most frequently found in our study was *C. abortus* (50%), directly followed by *C. pecorum* (47%). Remarkably, *C. psittaci* was detected in 25% of the tested flocks. Mixed infections occurred in 25% of the tested flocks. The likelihood of detecting chlamydia by using swabs appears to be independent of the sampling site, i.e. vagina or rectum. However, the frequency of individual species detected differed significantly between vaginal and rectal swab samples. Vaginal swabs were more reliable at finding *C. psittaci*whereas *C. pecorum* and samples with mixed infections were detected significantly more often in rectal swabs. We therefore recommend taking samples from both sites so that infections with neither chlamydial species are missed. The finding that no significant differences with regard to the sampling site were observed for the detection of *C. abortus* is noteworthy and supports the possibility of intestinal infection and/or faecal-oral transmission, as already postulated by others [28, 7, 8]. The higher detection rate of *C. pecorum* in rectal swabs appears to reflect its assumed habitat, since sheep frequently harbour this agent in their intestine [8]. The discovery of eighteen *C. psittaci* positive swabs and seven positive afterbirths was unexpected. Only two recent reports mention the sporadic isolation of *C. psittaci* strains from sheep [29, 30]. We were not able to obtain any *C. psittaci* isolates, most likely due to the low concentration of the agent in the samples as determined by real-time PCR. Other factors explaining this failure could be due to sampling technique or sample transport, low viability or amount of inocula [31, 32, 33]. Therefore, in order to confirm the real-time PCR results and to determine the genotype, we additionally analysed these samples by means of sequencing and DNA microarray. We exclude cross-contamination during sampling, as flocks were sampled on different days and in different parts of Thuringia. Moreover, in order to minimise carry over between the samples from different flocks during preparation in the laboratory, collected samples were processed and analysed flock-wise. Finally, real-time PCR revealed not only different species but also varying Ct values for the respective species within an analysed flock, which indicates differences in chlamydial loads among individual animals.

The seven *C. psittaci* positive afterbirths could all be allocated to the respective ewes. One ewe in flock 2 was positive in both serum samples but PCR negative pointing towards a recent chlamydial infection. In flock 3, one ewe had a *C. psittaci* positive vaginal swab but was serologically negative, indicating an acute, possibly intrauterine infection. A second ewe in flock 3 was PCR positive for a mixed infection with *C. psittaci* and *C. abortus* but serologically negative, also indicating a possible acute infection. Of the three ewes in flock 3, one was neither serologically nor PCR positive; the remaining two were serologically negative. This also applied to the ewe in flock 7. Since no swabs had been taken from the last three animals, we cannot exclude the possibility of an acute chlamydial infection. A further possibility explaining the presence of *C. psittaci* in the afterbirths might be contamination of the lambing quarters with avian faeces, since birds, i.e. sparrows and pigeons, had free access to them. However, the detection of *C. psittaci* in vaginal and rectal swabs indicates that these infections indeed occurred in the flocks examined. It is conceivable that the agent was transmitted to the ewes through contact with the birds. Others have reported cross-infections between cattle, sheep, and kestrels [34]. In any case, the significance of *C. psittaci* in sheep in terms of their virulence and possible zoonotic impact is still unclear and more studies are needed for clarification.

We were intrigued to find one flock (12) to be presumably free of chlamydial infection, as none of the tested animals was positive in the ELISA or in the PCR analyses. This comparatively small flock had a good hygiene regime, as assessed by the Thuringian sheep health authority according to the criteria defined in [35, 36] and only introduced vaccinated rams into the flock. When looking at the flock size we noticed that increasing flock size indeed influenced the probability of finding chlamydia positive animals. It is obvious that competent flock management and high standards of hygiene are easier to maintain in smaller flocks than in larger ones. However, when looking at the vaccinated flocks, flock size was not the main criterion for healthy flocks. High rates of abortion in the smaller flocks prior to vaccination not only indicate poor flock management but also inadequate standards of hygiene. Moreover, vaccination might even mask shortcomings in hygiene.

We were somewhat surprised at the low number of seropositve animals in the vaccinated flocks and the ongoing infection in three of the flocks. A Swiss study reports the unexpectedly low rate of seroconversion after vaccination and attribute it to individual immunoreactions of the sheep [37]. The identification of wild type *C. abortus* isolates in vaccinated flocks has also been described by others [38]. Although vaccination could not eliminate *C. abortus* from the flocks, it did reduce the rate of abortion considerably, especially in flocks 28 and 38. Vaccination in combination with good flock management and hygiene appear to be a feasible approach to contain chlamydial infection within a flock [39].

Our study has shown that serological testing is an adequate technique for monitoring sheep flocks for the presence of chlamydia. However, in order to obtain a realistic picture on the distribution of the various species present in a flock, serology is not sufficient. The ELISA technique which was used in our study, for example, can not discriminate between *C. abortus, C. pecorum*, and *C. psittaci* [40, 41]. Standardised or harmonised and commercially available testing systems for serology capable of differentiating *C. abortus, C. pecorum*, and *C. psittaci* would considerably improve the informative value of prevalence studies. Though sampling for DNA analysis is tedious, it does provide additional information with regard to species distribution.

CONCLUSIONS

Our data show that unexpectedly high chlamydia prevalence rates exist in flocks with low abortion status and corroborate the findings by others [42, 43]. This could imply that other factors, such as the virulence of the chlamydial strains, individual animal or breed related immunity, and presence of other microorganisms and parasites (e.g. salmonella, coxiella, toxoplasmas) might additionally be responsible for eliciting abortions. In order to determine these, future studies should compare clinically healthy chlamydia-positive flocks with flocks with clinically manifest chlamydial infection and flocks with reproductive disorders without chlamydial infections. Isolation and characterisation of ovine *C. psittaci* strains are required to assess their clinical impact and possible zoonotic potential.

DECLARATIONS

Acknowledgements

We are greatly indebted to all the sheep farmers who joined the study. We thank Dr. R. Teuscher for his active support. Prof. Dr. H. Neubauer is thanked for providing the ELISA kits and critical reading of the manuscript. We appreciate the help of Dr. M. J. Sprague for his critical reading of the manuscript. C. Grajetzki and S. Bettermann are thanked for their technical assistance.

This study was supported by the German Ministry for Education and Research (BMBF), Zoonotic chlamydiae - Models of chronic and persistent infections in humans and animals Grant # 01 KI 0720

Authors' contributions

HL: collected and processed the samples and evaluated the data. UM: collected the samples and helped with the contacting of the sheep farmers. KH: helped with the ELISA and cultivation of the chlamydial isolates. RL: examined the foetuses and afterbirths. RD: designed the study and carried out the statistical analyses. CM: contributed to the interpretation of the data and helped with editing and revision of the manuscript; KS: contributed to the study design, obtained the funding, and evaluated the microarray, DNA sequencing, and PCR results and helped with the revision of the manuscript. LDS: contributed to the study design, evaluated the data, drafted, and wrote the manuscript. All authors read and approved the final manuscript.

REFERENCES

1. Longbottom D, Coulter LJ: Animal chlamydioses and zoonotic implications. J Comp Pathol. 2003, 128: 217-244. 10.1053/jcpa.2002.0629.
2. Pospischil A, Thoma R, Hilbe M, Grest P, Zimmermann D, Gebbers JO: Abortion in humans caused by *Chlamydophila abortus (Chlamydia psittaci* serovar 1). Schweiz Arch Tierheilkd. 2002, 144: 463-466. 10.1024/0036-7281.144.9.463.
3. Baud D, Regan L, Greub G: Emerging role of Chlamydia and Chlamydia-like organisms in adverse pregnancy outcomes. Curr Opin Infect Dis. 2008, 21: 70-76. 10.1097/QCO.0b013e3282f3e6a5.
4. Buxton D, Barlow RM, Finlayson J, Anderson IE, Mackellar A: Observations on the pathogenesis of *Chlamydia psittaci*infection of pregnant sheep. J Comp Pathol. 1990, 102: 221-237.
5. Buxton D, Anderson IE, Longbottom D, Livingstone M, Wattegedera S, Entrican G: Ovine chlamydial abortion: characterization of the inflammatory immune response in placental tissues. J Comp Pathol. 2002, 127: 133-141. 10.1053/jcpa.2002.0573.
6. Berri M, Rekiki A, Boumedine KS, Rodolakis A: Simultaneous differential detection of *Chlamydophila abortus, Chlamydophila pecorum*, and *Coxiella burnetii* from aborted ruminant's clinical samples using multiplex PCR. BMC Microbiol. 2009, 9: 130-10.1186/1471-2180-9-130.
7. Rodolakis A, Salinas J, Papp J: Recent advances on ovine chlamydial abortion. Vet Res. 1998, 29: 275-288.
8. Nietfeld JC: Chlamydial infections in small ruminants. Vet Clin North Am Food Anim Pract. 2001, 17: 301-314.
9. Matschullat G: Causes of miscarriage in sheep. Tierärztliche Umschau. 1984, 39: 45.
10. Plagemann O: The most frequent infectious causes of abortion in sheep in north Bavaria with special reference to Chlamydia and Salmonella infections. Tierärztl Praxis. 1989, 17: 145-148.
11. Lehmann C, Elze K: Results of microbiological investigations of abortions in horses, cattle, pigs and sheep in Germany. Tierärztliche Umschau. 1997, 52: 495-505.
12. Sting R, Nagel C, Steng G: Significance of causes of infectious abortion in sheep flocks in northern Baden-Württemberg with special reference to *Chlamydia psittaci*. Berl Munch Tierarztl Wochenschr. 1997, 110: 5-11.
13. Lorenz R: Krankheitsüberwachung in Tierbeständen - Ein Leitfaden zur Bestimmung von Stichprobenumfängen. 1990, Auswertungs- und Informationsdienst für Ernährung, Landwirtschaft und Forsten (AID e.V.), Bonn
14. Pantchev A, Sting R, Bauerfeind R, Tyczka J, Sachse K: Detection of all *Chlamydophila* and *Chlamydia spp.* of veterinary interest using species-specific real-time PCR assays. Comp Immunol Microbiol Infect Dis. 2010, 33: 473-484. 10.1016/j.cimid.2009.08.002.
15. Hoffmann B, Depner K, Schirrmeier H, Beer M: A universal heterologous internal control system for duplex real-time RT-PCR assays used in a detection system for pestiviruses. Journal of Virological Methods. 2006, 136: 200-209. 10.1016/j.jviromet.2006.05.020.
16. Sachse K, Hotzel H: Detection and differentiation of Chlamydiae by nested PCR. Methods Mol Biol. 2003, 216: 123-136.
17. Borel N, Kempf E, Hotzel H, Schubert E, Torgerson P, Slickers P, Ehricht R, Tasara T, Pospischil A, Sachse K: Direct identification of chlamydiae from clinical samples using a DNA microarray assay: a validation study. Mol Cell Probes. 2008, 22: 55-64. 10.1016/j.mcp.2007.06.003.
18. Sachse K, Laroucau K, Vorimore F, Magnino S, Feige J, Müller W, Kube S, Hotzel H, Schubert E, Slickers P, Ehricht R: DNA microarray-based genotyping of *Chlamydophila psittaci* strains from culture and clinical samples. Vet Microbiol. 2009, 135: 22-30. 10.1016/j.vetmic.2008.09.041.
19. Laroucau K, Vorimore F, Sachse K, Vretou E, Siarkou VI, Willems H, Magnino S, Rodolakis A, Bavoil PM: Differential identification of *Chlamydophila abortus* live vaccine strain 1B and *C. abortus* field isolates by PCR-RFLP. Vaccine. 2010, 28: 5653-5656. 10.1016/j.vaccine.2010.06.064.
20. Masala G, Porcu R, Sanna G, Tanda A, Tola S: Role of *Chlamydophila abortus* in ovine and caprine abortion in Sardinia, Italy. Vet Res Commun. 2005, 29: 117-123.
21. Borel N, Doherr MG, Vretou E, Psarrou E, Thoma R, Pospischil A: Seroprevalences for ovine enzootic abortion in Switzerland. Prev Vet Med. 2004, 65: 205-216. 10.1016/j.prevetmed.2004.08.005.
22. Trávníč M, Kováčová D, Bhide MR, Zubrický P, Čisláková L: Detection of IgG Antibodies against *Chlamydophila abortus* in Sheep with Reproductive Disorders. Acta Vet Brno. 2003, 72: 95-99. 10.2754/avb200372010095.
23. Gokce HI, Kacar C, Genc O, Sozmen M: Seroprevalance of *Chlamydophila abortus* in aborting ewes and dairy cattle in the north-east part of Turkey. Bulletin of the Veterinary Institute in Pulawy. 2007, 51: 9-13.
24. Clarkson MJ, Philips HL: Isolation of faecal chlamydia from sheep in Britain and their characterization by cultural properties. The Veterinary Journal. 1997, 153: 307-310. 10.1016/S1090-0233(97)80064-0.
25. Greco G, Totaro M, Madio A, Tarsitano E, Fasanella A, Lucifora G, Buonavoglia D: Detection of *Chlamydophila abortus* in sheep and goat flocks in southern Italy by PCR using four different primer sets. Vet Res Commun. 2005, 29: 107-115.

26. Güler L, Hadimli HH, Erganiş O, Ateş M, Ok U, Gündüz K: Field evaluation of a PCR for the diagnosis of chlamydial abortion in sheep. Vet Rec. 2006, 159: 742-745. 10.1136/vr.159.22.742.

27. Rekiki A, Sidi-Boumedine K, Souriau A, Jemli J, Hammami S, Rodolakis A: Isolation and characterisation of local strains of *Chlamydophila abortus (Chlamydia psittaci* serotype 1) from Tunisia. Vet Res. 2002, 33: 215-222. 10.1051/vetres:2002009.

28. Amin JD, Wilsmore AJ: In vitro survival of the BS isolate of *Chlamydia psittaci* (ovis) in ruminal and abomasal contents. Res Vet Sci. 1995, 59: 136-138. 10.1016/0034-5288(95)90047-0.

29. Sachse K, Laroucau K, Hotzel H, Schubert E, Ehricht R, Slickers P: Genotyping of *Chlamydophila psittaci* using a new DNA microarray assay based on sequence analysis of *omp*A genes. BMC Microbiol. 2008, 8: 63-10.1186/1471-2180-8-63.

30. Song L, Li Y, Liu G, He J, Zhu H, Duan Q: Genotyping of *Chlamydophila psittaci*strains derived from avian and mammalian species. Vet Res Commun. 2009.

31. Rota TR: Techniques for culturing and determining antimicrobial susceptibility of *Chlamydia trachomatis*. Arch Androl. 1980, 4: 63-69. 10.3109/01485018008988281.

32. Suchland RJ, Geisler WM, Stamm WE: Methodologies and cell lines used for antimicrobial susceptibility testing of *Chlamydia* spp. Antimicrobial Agents Chem. 2003, 47: 636-642. 10.1128/AAC.47.2.636-642.2003.**View**

33. Malathi J, Shyamala G, Madhavan HN: Relative susceptibility of six continuous cell lines for cultivation of *Chlamydia trachomatis* strains. Indian J Med Microbiol. 2004, 22: 169-171.

34. Lemus JA, Fargallo JA, Vergara P, Parejo D, Banda E: Natural cross chlamydial infection between livestock and free-living bird species. PLoS One. 2010, 5 (10): e13512-10.1371/journal.pone.0013512.

35. Worbes H: Hygiene der Schafhaltung. Lehrbuch der Schafkrankheiten. Edited by: Ganter M. 2001, Berlin, Wien: Blackwell Wissenschafts Verlag, 441-452. 4

36. Programm zur Förderung der Tiergesundheit in den Schaf- und Ziegenbeständen in Thüringen. Thüringer Staatsanzeiger. 2008, 16: 564-565.

37. Gerber A, Thoma R, Vretou E, Psarrou E, Kaiser C, Doherr MG, Zimmermann DR, Polkinghorne A, Pospischil A, Borel N: Ovine Enzootic Abortion (OEA): a comparison of antibody responses in vaccinated and naturally-infected Swiss sheep over a two year period. BMC Vet Res. 2007, 3: 24-10.1186/1746-6148-3-24.

38. Wheelhouse N, Aitchison K, Laroucau K, Thomson J, Longbottom D: Evidence of *Chlamydophila abortus* vaccine strain 1B as a possible cause of ovine enzootic abortion. Vaccine. 2010, 28: 5657-5663. 10.1016/j.vaccine.2010.04.114.

39. Longbottom D, Livingstone M: Vaccination against chlamydial infections of man and animals. The Veterinary Journal. 2006, 171: 263-275. 10.1016/j.tvjl.2004.09.006.

40. Wilson K, Livingstone M, Longbottom D: Comparative evaluation of eight serological assays for diagnosing *Chlamydophila abortus* infection in sheep. Vet Microbiol. 2009, 135: 38-45. 10.1016/j.vetmic.2008.09.043.

41. Vretou E, Radouani F, Psarrou E, Kritikos I, Xylouri E, Mangana O: Evaluation of two commercial assays for the detection of *Chlamydophila abortus* antibodies. Vet Microbiol. 2007, 20: 153-161.

42. Gut-Zangger P, Vretou E, Psarrou E, Pospischil A, Thoma R: Chlamydia abortion in sheep: possibilities for serological diagnosis using a competitive ELISA and insight into the epidemiologic situation in Switzerland. Schweiz Arch Tierheilkd. 1999, 141: 361-366.

43. Polkinghorne A, Borel N, Becker A, Lu ZH, Zimmermann DR, Brugnera E, Pospischil A, Vaughan L: Molecular evidence for chlamydial infections in the eyes of sheep. Vet Microbiol. 2009, 135: 142-146. 10.1016/j.vetmic.2008.09.034

CHAPTER 8

INVESTIGATION OF CHLAMYDOPHILA SPP. IN DAIRY COWS WITH REPRODUCTIVE DISORDERS

Ann-Charlotte Godin, Camilla Björkman, Stina Englund, KarlErik Johansson, Rauni Niskanen and Stefan Alenius

BACKGROUND

Chlamydia are obligate, intracellular, gram-negative bacteria that cause a wide range of diseases in humans, other mammals and birds. The two species *Chlamydophila (Cp.) abortus* (formerly *Chlamydia (C.) psittaci*serotype 1) and *Cp. pecorum* (formerly *C. pecorum*) are known to infect ruminants [1]. It has also been reported that *Cp. psittaci* may infect cattle [2, 3, 4]. In many sheep-producing countries *Cp. abortus* is known to cause Ovine Enzootic Abortion (OEA) [5]. The zoonotic potential of *Cp. abortu* s is well known and poses a threat to mainly pregnant women, handling sheep and goats [6]. Chlamydial infection in cattle has been associated with reproductive disorders including abortion, endometritis, repeat breeding, vaginitis, seminal vesiculitis, weak calves and perinatal mortality [7, 8, 9, 10, 11]. Moreover, symptoms such as pneumonia, conjunctivitis, enteritis, polyarthritis and encephalitis have been reported [12, 13, 14]. It has been suggested that both *Cp. abortus and Cp. pecorum* are ubiquitous in cattle [10, 15, 16].

Reproductive disorders and infertility are major causes of culling in dairy herds. The diagnostic rate of abortions is usually below 35% [17, 18]. In Sweden, 97% of all dairy herds are free of Bovine viral diarrhoea virus (BVDV) [19] and the prevalence of *Neospora (N.) caninum* infection is 2% [20]. Furthermore, Sweden is free from *Brucella abortus*, *Leptospira* spp. and Bovine herpes virus 1 (IBR/IPV) [21]. The prevalence of chlamydial infections and their effect on reproduction in Swedish cattle is unclear and has not previously been investigated. The aim of this study was therefore to investigate the prevalence of antibodies against *Chlamydophila* spp., preferably *Cp. abortus* and the occurrence of chlamydial agents in Swedish dairy herds with a history of reproductive disorders.

METHODS

Animals and samples

Seventy dairy herds from different parts of Sweden that experienced reproductive disorders, mainly abortions, during January 2000 to December 2006 were included in this study. Herd sizes ranged from 19 to 215 cows and all herds were free of BVDV and *N. caninum*. As part of the diagnosis investigations, blood samples were collected by local veterinarians and sent by mail to the laboratory. Samples were collected from 4 to 15 cows (average 7.5, median 6), >2 years of age from each herd, except in two herds where all cows, 32 and 34, respectively, were bled. In almost all herds (61/70) samples from both cows with clinical signs (cases) and cows with normal pregnancies and parturitions (controls) were taken, and in the other nine herds only cows with clinical signs were sampled. A total of 525 animals were blood sampled: 286 cases and 239 controls.

Citation: Ann-Charlotte Godin, Camilla Björkman, Stina Englund, Karl-Erik Johansson, Rauni Niskanen and Stefan Alenius, Investigation of Chlamydophila spp. in dairy cows with reproductive disorders, DOI: 10.1186/1751-0147-50-39.

Of the 286 cases, 179 had aborted (two-thirds during the last trimester). They were bled on the same day or up to 10 months after abortion (mostly within the first 3 months after abortion). The other cases had premature parturition or parturition at full term resulting in death, stillbirth or weak neonate, repeat breeding or vaginitis. The blood samples were centrifuged at 1000 × *g* for 10 minutes and sera collected and stored at -20°C until analysis.

Vaginal swabs (Cytobrush Plus, Medscand Medical AB), milk samples, placentas and organs from aborted foetuses were also collected from some of the herds. In total 107 specimens were submitted: 43 vaginal swabs (from 31 cases and 12 controls in 12 herds), 54 milk samples (37 cases and 17 controls, in 10 herds), organs from 5 aborted foetuses in 3 herds and 5 placentas from abortions in 5 herds. Samples were stored at -70°C prior to preparation and analysis.

Detection of antibodies to *Chlamydophila abortus*

Two commercially available *Cp. abortus* antibody detection kits were used.

The Pourquier ELISA *Chlamydophila abortus* serum verification test (Institut Pourquier) uses a recombinant fragment of an 80–90 kDa polymorphic outer membrane protein as antigen. The kit was used according to the manufacturer›s instructions, where S/P% values equal or more than 100 are considered as positive for cattle.

The CHEKIT-Chlamydia enzyme immunoassay (Dr. Bommeli AG-Idexx) is based on an inactivated antigen originally isolated from a case of abortion in sheep. The test was performed according to the instructions of the manufacturer, considering corrected optical density (OD%) values > 40 as positive.

Detection of *Chlamydiaceae* by Polymerase Chain Reaction (PCR)

DNA was extracted from vaginal swabs for PCR analysis according to the protocol by Sachse and Hotzel [22]. For tissue specimens and milk the High Pure Template Preparation kit (Roche Diagnostics) was applied, following the manual provided by the manufacturer, with a slight modification for milk samples [16].

Analyses were made by a real-time PCR, developed by Everett et al. [23] which targets the 23S ribosomal DNA and detects the family *Chlamydiaceae*. The sensitivity of the test was estimated by spiking samples prior to DNA extraction with 10-fold dilutions of *Cp. abortus* (inactivated strain S26/3 in original concentration of 3×10^8 IFU/ml, kindly provided by D. Longbottom, Moredun Research Institute, UK). The sensitivity was estimated to 1 IFU/PCR for all specimens except milk where the sensitivity was 10 IFU/PCR.

Positive samples by the real-time PCR were further analysed for species identification by a nested PCR as described by Kaltenboeck et al. [24] and modified by Sachse and Hotzel [22]. The nested PCR targets the *omp1*gene and identifies the four species *C. trachomatis, C. psittaci, C. pecorum* and *C. pneumoniae*, according to the old classification.

DNA sequence analysis of the PCR products

Amplicons from the nested PCR were purified prior to sequencing by the GFX PCR DNA and Gel Band Purification Kit (Amersham Bioscience Europe). The PCR products were then sequenced with primers 204 pecor and chomp 336 [22] and with the BigDye Terminator v3.1 Cycle Sequencing Kit (Applied Biosystems) in combination with ethanol/EDTA/sodium acetate precipitation according to the protocol of the manufacturer. Thermocycling was performed in a GeneAmp 2700 Thermocycler (Applied Biosystems). The sequencing products were subjected to electrophoretic separation and on-line detection on an ABI PRISM 3100 Genetic Analyzer (Applied Biosystems), followed by computerized sequence evaluation (BLAST search).

Statistics

The chi-square test was used for Chekit ELISA results to calculate significance (Minitab® Release 14.2, Minitab Inc.).

RESULTS

Antibody assays

Of 525 blood sampled cows, only two (0.4%) were seropositive in the Pourquier *Cp. abortus* ELISA (S/P% values 154 and 114, respectively). They originated from two different herds. One cow had aborted in the last trimester and the other had experienced premature parturition. Most of the samples were well clustered far below the cut-off value 100%; only 6 samples (4 cases and 2 controls) had S/P% values above 60, the recommended cut-off value for sheep sera (Figure 1).

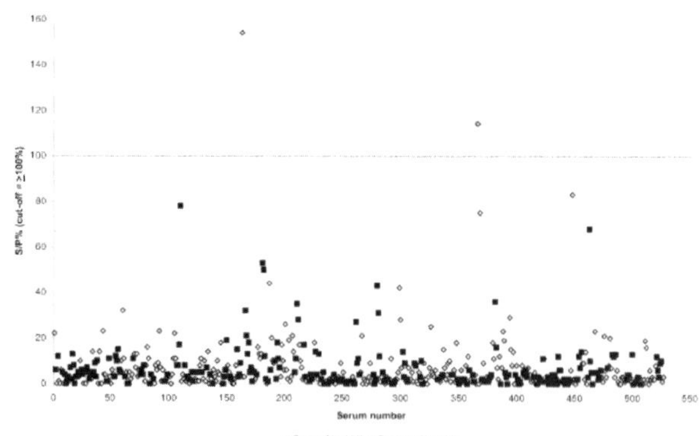

Figure 1: Results of Pourquier® *Cp. abortus* ELISA serology in 525 Swedish dairy cows from 70 herds with reproductive disorders, sampled during January 2000 to December 2005. The dotted line shows the cut-off value. The seroprevalence among cases was 0.4% (2/286) and among controls 0%.

The seroprevalence with the Chekit ELISA was 28% (148/525) and the prevalence did not differ between cases (81/286) and controls (67/239). OD% values for positives ranged between 41–369% (Figure 2). In 81% (57/70) of the herds at least one sampled cow was positive. Of the 179 cases of abortion, antibodies were detected in 55 cows (31%). The two cows seropositive in the Pourquier *Cp. abortus* ELISA were both seronegative in the Chekit assay (OD% value 3 and 21, respectively).

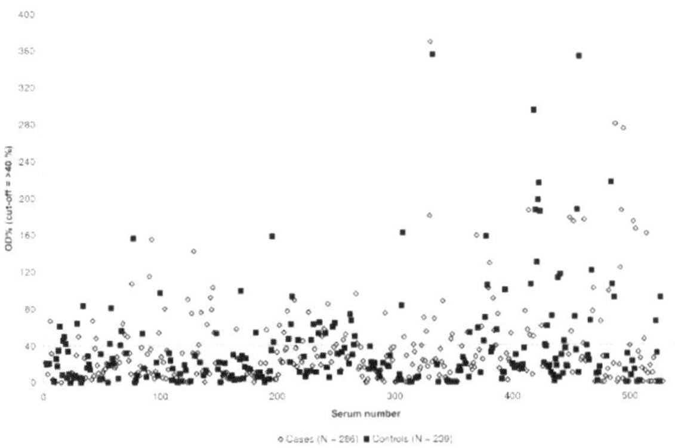

Figure 2: Results of CHEKIT ® -Chlamydia enzyme immunoassay serology in 525 Swedish dairy cows from 70 herds with reproductive disorders, sampled during January 2000 to December 2005. The dotted line shows the cut-off value. The seroprevalence among cases was 28% (81/286) and among controls 28% (67/239).

PCR

Chlamydiaceae was detected by real-time PCR in vaginal swabs from 2 out of 12 control cows but not from any of the 31 cases. *Cp. pecorum* was detected in both swabs by nested PCR and further confirmed by partial *omp1* DNA sequencing of the PCR product. The two cows came from different herds and were both negative in the Pourquier *Cp. abortus* ELISA and positive in the Chekit ELISA (OD% values 100 and 295).

Three more *Chlamydiaceae* positive samples were identified: a placenta from an aborting cow that was not serologically tested, and two milk samples from cows that had aborted and were negative in both antibody tests. These samples were all negative in the nested PCR, probably due to lower sensitivity of this test, and could not be sequenced. The placenta was collected in one of the herds that had a *Cp. pecorum* positive vaginal swab and the milk samples came from two other herds.

DISCUSSION

The results of this first investigation of *Chlamydophila* spp. infection in Swedish dairy cows suggest that *Cp. abortus* infection is absent or rare in Sweden. Only two samples were positive in the Pourquier ELISA. These might well be false positive results because both samples were negative in the Chekit assay, which is based on an antigen containing lipopolysaccharide shared by several *Chlamydiaceae*, including *Cp. abortus*. Even if we had applied the lower cut-off value used for sheep sera, only six samples would have been positive in the Pourquier ELISA, of which all except one, were negative in the Chekit ELISA. The specificity of the Pourquier ELISA has been reported to be 100% when analysed Scottish sheep documented free of OEA [25] and 90% when sera from New Zealand, a country free from *Cp. abortus*, were analysed [26].

The seroprevalence obtained in our study with Chekit ELISA probably represents antibodies against *Cp. pecorum* because it is known to infect cattle and we identified *Cp. pecorum* in vaginal swabs from two Chekit ELISA positive cows. In a recent Austrian investigation, the majority of blood sampled cows from which vaginal and cervical swabs also were taken and found *Cp. pecorum* positive by PCR, were seropositive by Chekit ELISA [27]. Further, the Chekit ELISA reacted with positive results in 26% out of 15 sera from SPF lambs immunized with *Cp. pecorum* [25]. We found no difference in Chekit ELISA seroprevalences between cows with reproductive problems, including abortion, and healthy control cows. This is in concordance with the Austrian study where no correlations between reproductive problems and Chekit ELISA or PCR positivities were found [27]. However, significantly higher seroprevalences among aborting versus healthy cows have been reported in some other studies applying the Chekit ELISA test [28, 29]. Additionally, in an investigation of German herds with diverse fertility disorders, no difference in seropositivity was observed between the group of apparently healthy cows and the group of cows with abnormal reproductive performance. However, a significantly higher proportion of the cows that had aborted were seropositive [11].

The absence, or very low prevalence, of *Cp. abortus* in Swedish dairy cows could be due to the small mean herd size of 44 animals (year 2005) and that most are kept tethered during a nine-month stable period, with little contact within the herd. Further, the tradition of self-contained herds, the sparsely populated Swedish countryside with few external contacts and little movement of animals across country, give few animals a chance to get infected. The absence or very low prevalence could also be due to a generally lower infection pressure owing to lack of other infections, e.g. BVDV. Another explanation could be that *Cp. abortus* infection seems to be very low in Swedish sheep. In a recent investigation, including 800 sheep sera from different parts of Sweden, only 3 sera were positive with the Pourquier *Cp. abortus* ELISA (unpublished data).

CONCLUSION

This investigation suggests that infections with *Cp. abortus* are absent or rare in Swedish cows whereas *Cp. pecorum* are probably more spread. It also suggests that *Chlamydophila* spp. is not related to reproduction disorders in Swedish cattle.

DECLARATIONS

Acknowledgements

We thank Maj Hjort for technical assistance with the serological analyses. The study was supported by the Swedish Farmer's Foundation for Agricultural Research and the Programme for Infection Biology at the Veterinary Faculty, Swedish University of Agricultural Sciences. It was part of the EU research collaboration COST 855.

Authors' contributions

ACG drafted and rewrote the manuscript, carried out the PCR and serology analysis, interpreted the results and performed the statistical analysis. CB and SA conceived and designed the study, and participated in its coordination. SE implemented the PCR systems and carried out the sequencing analysis. KEJ participated in the sequencing analysis. All authors participated in the design of the study and have been involved in revising the manuscript.

REFERENCES

1. Everett KDE: *Chlamydia* and *Chlamydiales*: more than meets the eye. Vet Microbiol. 2000, 75: 109-126. 10.1016/S0378-1135(00)00213-3.
2. Cox HU, Hoyt PG, Poston RP, Snider TG, Lemarchand TX, O'Reilly KL: Isolation of an avian serovar of *Chlamydia psittaci*from a case of bovine abortion. J Vet Diagn Invest. 1998, 10: 280-282.
3. Borel N, Thoma R, Spaeni P, Weilenmann R, Teankum K, Brugnera E, Zimmermann DR, Vaughan L, Pospischil A: Chlamydia-related abortions in cattle from Graubunden, Switzerland. Vet Pathol. 2006, 43: 702-708. 10.1354/vp.43-5-702.
4. Kauffold J, Henning K, Bachmann R, Hotzel H, Melzer F: The prevalence of *chlamydiae* of bulls from six bull studs in Germany. Anim Reprod Sci. 2007, 102: 111-121. 10.1016/j.anireprosci.2006.10.013.
5. Aitken ID: Chlamydial abortion. Diseases of Sheep. Edited by: Martin WB, Aitken ID. 2000, Edinburgh: Blackwell, 81-86. 3
6. Longbottom D, Coulter LJ: Animal chlamydioses and zoonotic implications. J Comp Pathol. 2003, 128: 217-244. 10.1053/jcpa.2002.0629.
7. Storz J: Over of animal diseases induced by chlamydial infections. Microbiology of Chlamydia. Edited by: Barron AL. 1988, Florida: CRC Press, Inc, 167-192.
8. Daniel RG, Holliman A, David GP, Kirby FD, Simpson VR, Cranwell MP, Dawson M, Griffiths PC, Bevan BJ: Bovine chlamydiosis in the United Kingdom. Vet Rec. 1993, 133: 351-352.
9. Wittenbrink MM, Schoon HA, Bisping W, Binder A: Infection of the bovine female genital tract with *Chlamydia psittaci* as a possible cause of infertility. Reprod Dom Anim. 1993, 28: 129-136.
10. Kaltenboeck B, Hehnen HR, Vaglenov A: Bovine *Chlamydophila* spp. infection: do we underestimate the impact on fertility?. Vet Res Comm. 2005, 29: 1-15. 10.1007/s11259-005-0832-4.
11. Wehrend A, Failing K, Hauser B, Jager C, Bostedt H: Production, reproductive, and metabolic factors associated with chlamydial seropositivity and reproductive tract antigens in dairy herds with fertility disorders. Theriogenology. 2005, 63: 923-930. 10.1016/j.theriogenology.2004.05.009.
12. Piercy DW, Griffiths PC, Teale CJ: Encephalitis related to *Chlamydia psittaci* infection in a 14-week-old calf. Vet Rec. 1999, 144: 126-128.
13. Otter A, Twomey DF, Rowe NS, Tipp JW, McElligott WS, Griffiths PC, O'Neill P: Suspected chlamydial keratoconjunctivitis in British cattle. Vet Rec. 2003, 152: 787-788.
14. Twomey DF, Griffiths PC, Hignett BC, Martin TP: Suspected chlamydial polyarthritis in a calf in the UK. Vet Rec. 2003, 152: 340-
15. De Graves FJ, Gao D, Hehnen HR, Schlapp T, Kaltenboeck B: Quantitative detection of *Chlamydia psittaci* and *C. pecorum*by high-sensitivity real-time PCR reveals high prevalence of vaginal infection in cattle. J Clin Microbiol. 2003, 41: 1726-1729. 10.1128/JCM.41.4.1726-1729.2003.
16. Jee J, De Graves FJ, Kim T, Kaltenboeck B: High prevalence of natural *Chlamydophila* species infection in calves. J Clin Microbiol. 2004, 42: 5664-5672. 10.1128/JCM.42.12.5664-5672.2004.
17. Alves D, McEwen B, Hazlett M, Maxie G, Anderson N: Trends in bovine abortions submitted to the Ontario Ministry of Agriculture, Food and Rural Affairs, 1993–1995. Can Vet J. 1996, 37: 287-288.
18. Cabell E: Bovine abortion: aetiology and investigations. In Practice. 2007, 29: 455-463.
19. Hult L, Lindberg A: Experiences from BVDV control in Sweden. Prev Vet Med. 2005, 72: 143-148. 215–219.
20. Björkman C, Alenius S, Emanuelsson U, Uggla A: *Neospora caninum* and bovine virus diarrhoea virus infections in Swedish dairy cows in relation to abortion. Vet J. 2000, 159: 201-206. 10.1053/tvjl.1999.0446.
21. De Verdier K, Persson Waller K: [Abortion in cows – a warning signal that should be investigated (author's transl)]. Svensk Veterinärtidning. 2003, 12: 17-24.
22. Sachse K, Hotzel H: Detection and differentiation of *Chlamydiae* by nested PCR. Methods Mol Biol. 2003, 216: 123-136.
23. Everett KDE, Hornung LJ, Andersen AA: Rapid detection of the *Chlamydiaceae* and other families in the order Chlamydiales: Three PCR tests. J Clin Microbiol. 1999, 37: 575-580.
24. Kaltenboeck B, Schmeer N, Schneider R: Evidence for numerous *omp1* alleles of porcine *Chlamydia trachomatis* and novel chlamydial species obtained by PCR. J Clin Microbiol. 1997, 35: 1835-1841.
25. Vretou E, Radouani F, Psarrou E, Kritikos I, Xylouri E, Mangana O: Evaluation of two commercial assays for the detection of *Chlamydophila abortus* antibodies. Vet Microbiol. 2007, 123: 153-161. 10.1016/j.vetmic.2007.02.023.
26. McCauley LM, Lancaster MJ, Young P, Butler KL, Ainsworth CG: Comparison of ELISA and CFT assays for *Chlamydophila abortus* antibodies in ovine sera. Aust Vet J. 2007, 85: 325-328. 10.1111/j.1751-0813.2007.00189.x.
27. Petit T, Spergser J, Aurich J, Rosengarten R: Prevalence of *Chlamydiaceae* and *Mollicutes* on the genital mucosa and serological findings in dairy cattle. Vet Microbiol. 2008, 127: 325-333. 10.1016/j.vetmic.2007.08.022.
28. Cavirani S, Cabassi CS, Donofrio G, De Iaco B, Taddei S, Flammini CF: Association between *Chlamydia psittaci*seropositivity and abortion in Italian dairy cows. Prev Vet Med. 2001, 50: 145-151. 10.1016/S0167-5877(01)00197-0.
29. Wang FI, Shieh H, Liao YK: Prevalence of *Chlamydophila abortus* infection in domesticated ruminants in Taiwan. J Vet Med Sci. 2001, 63: 1215-1220. 10.1292/jvms.63.1215.

CHAPTER 9

CHLAMYDOPHILA SPP. INFECTION IN HORSES WITH RECURRENT AIRWAY OBSTRUCTION: SIMILARITIES TO HUMAN CHRONIC OBSTRUCTIVE DISEASE

Dirk Theegarten, Konrad Sachse, Britta Mentrup, Kerstin Fey, Helmut Hotzel and Olaf Anhenn

BACKGROUND

Recurrent Airway Obstruction (RAO) in horses, formerly called equine chronic obstructive pulmonary disease (COPD), is a very common illness [1]. Pathology is characterized by bronchiolitis [2, 3], which is similar to findings in human COPD and advanced human pulmonary emphysema [4]. Organic dust exposure and endotoxin are relevant factors for chronic impairment of lung function in horses and are used in experimental animal studies to cause exacerbations [5, 6].

Our own group detected *Chlamydophila psittaci (CPP)* infection by PCR in 38% of human patients with COPD [7, 8], who were suffering from advanced pulmonary emphysema and underwent lung volume reduction surgery. Chlamydial antigens were shown in alveolar parenchyma and bronchioles. *CPP* and also *Chlamydophila abortus (CPA)* was detected in sputum samples from patients with exacerbations of COPD as well [9]. Up to now, *Chlamydophila* spp. have been rarely detected in horses with acute respiratory infections [10, 11]. Mair and Wills [12] found culturable chlamydiae in 5% of equine nasal and conjunctival swabs in a prevalence study, but no association between isolation and clinical diseases was seen. However, these low detection rates in the pre-PCR era may have been due to the known difficulties of culturing these obligate intracellular bacteria. Serologically antibody titres ≥ 32 against *Chlamydophila pneumoniae (CPPN)* were detected in 26.5% of Italian light horses. Some sera with high titres reacted weakly with *CPP* as well [13]. But within aborted equine fetuses *CPP* has been found in high prevalence [14, 15]

In the present study lung tissue samples from horses with RAO as well as a group of clinically healthy horses were examined by immunohistochemistry, immunofluorescence and PCR to assess the extent of chlamydial infection and its association with RAO. PCR positive samples were additionally evaluated by DNA sequencing to define exactly the chlamydial species involved.

METHODS

Samples

Out of 948 horses, which were slaughtered or euthanized in the period between November 2002 and October 2004 in three western districts of Westphalia, 26 horses were identified as possibly suffering from RAO by questioning veterinarians and/or horse owners about reasons for slaughter or euthanasia. Slaughter was done according to federal law in authorized slaughterhouses and under control of a veterinarian. Euthanasia was practised by veterinarians following internationally recognized guidelines. If the horses had shown respiratory disease history, symptoms and therapy as well as conditions of housing were evaluated in detail by using a standardized questionnaire, which is available as online addendum. Possible RAO and control horses were clinically examined before slaughter or euthanasia. The horses had to meet the following criteria: (1) chronic cough for at least 3 months duration; (2) exercise intolerance; (3) worsening of the symptoms due to dust; (4) obvious biphasic expiratory dyspnoea with

Citation: Dirk Theegarten, Konrad Sachse, Britta Mentrup, Kerstin Fey, Helmut Hotzel and Olaf Anhenn, Chlamydophila spp. infection in horses with recurrent airway obstruction: similarities to human chronic obstructive disease, DOI: 10.1186/1465-9921-9-14.

hypertrophy of Mm. recti abdomini, inflated nostrils and nasal discharge; (5) breathing frequency > 20/min; and (6) pathologic findings in lung auscultation. As respiratory healthy controls served 20 horses which completely lacked these clinical criteria. Immediately after death, tissue was taken from 8 different lung regions of each horse and preserved for the following examinations.

Light Microscopic Histology

Formalin-fixed lung tissue was embedded in paraffin wax (Tissuewax™; Medite GmbH, Burgdorf, Germany), slices of 3–7 µm thickness were cut using a rotatory microtome (Microm GmbH, Walldorf, Germany), and stained with haematoxylin and eosin. Slices from the 8 tissue samples of each horse were evaluated for histological changes using a semi-quantitative score (0–4) in a blinded study. No signs of bronchiolitis were scored with 0 points. Minimal infiltration of the bronchioli with lymphocytes was scored with 1, slight inflammation with 2, moderate bronchiolitis with some neutrophils with 3, and severe changes with intraluminal aggregates of neutrophils with 4 points. Results from all 8 regions of each horse were added. Therefore a minimal score of 0 and a maximal score of 32 was possible.

One horse with RAO-like respiratory symptoms and history revealed parasitic lung disease after histological investigation and was excluded therefore.

According to anamnesis, clinical findings and light microscopy, the remaining 45 horses were classified into four subgroups:

- Clinically healthy horses without histological changes of RAO (n = 15),
- Clinically healthy horses with a low inflammation score of 4–6 (n = 5),
- Horses with clinical signs of RAO, but without or with only slight histological changes and a score of 0–5 (n = 16), and
- Horses with symptoms and histological changes of RAO with a score > 10 (n = 9).

Immunohistochemistry and Immunofluorescence

For immunohistochemistry, dewaxed slices were stained with a mouse anti-*CP* primary antibody (Biotrend, Germany; clone 73/0200, dilution 1:60) for 2 hours at room temperature, followed by a peroxidase-based detection system (Histostain®-Bulk-Kit, Zymed Laboratories Inc., San Francisco, USA) according to the instructions of the manufacturer). Three high-power fields showing bronchioli were selected for counting all detectable vs. all *CP*-positive stained bronchiolar epithelial cells (BEC), type II pneumocytes (PII) and macrophages (MP) separately, using a Zeiss Axiophot microscope (Carl Zeiss, Oberkochen, Germany) with a 40-fold objective magnification and a digital imaging system (Diskus Software, Koenigswinter, Germany). For immunofluorescence, triple staining on dewaxed sections was done with a primary mouse monoclonal IgG_{2b}-antibody against *CP* (Biotrend, Germany; clone 73/0200, dilution 1:100) and a primary mouse monoclonal IgG_1-antibody mix against pan-cytokeratin (BioCarta, USA; clones AE1, AE3, 5D3, dilution 1:50), as well as 4',6-diamidino-2-phenylindol-hydrochloride (DAPI, Sigma, Germany, working concentration 0.1 µg/ml). Alexa Fluor 488-conjugates of goat anti-mouse-IgG_1 (dilution 1:400), and Alexa Fluor 594-conjugates of goat anti-mouse-IgG_{2b} (dilution 1:400) were used as secondary antibodies (Molecular Probes Europe, Leiden, The Netherlands). Results were documented with a CCD-camera (Kappa, Gleichen, Germany) attached to an Olympus IX-70 microscope (Olympus Europe, Hamburg, Germany) with 40-fold objective magnification.

Polymerase Chain Reaction (PCR)

Lung tissue was collected immediately after slaughtering/euthanizing of the horses and stored at -80°C. DNA was isolated from lung tissue using the High Pure PCR Template Preparation Kit (Roche Diagnostics, Mannheim, Germany) according to the instructions of the manufacturer. 5 µl of the DNA extract were used as template in PCR. Samples were tested for *CPP/CPA* and *CPPN* by a modified version of the nested PCR procedure described by Kaltenboeck et al. [16] which targets the *omp*A gene. The first step was genus-specific amplification using primers 191CHOMP (5'-GCI YTI TGG GAR TGY GGI TGY GCI AC-3') and CHOMP371 (5'-TTA GAA ICK GAA TTG IGC RTT IAY GTG IGC IGC-3'). For the second amplification, we used 1 µl of the genus-specific product and primer combination 218PSITT (5›-GTA ATT TCI AGC CCA GCA CAA TTY GTG-3›)/CHOMP336s (5›-CCR CAA GMT TTT CTR GAY TTC AWY TTG TTR AT-3›) for *CP*, or 201CHOMP (5'-GGI GCW GMI TTC CAA TAY GCI CAR TC-3')/PNEUM268 (5'-GTA CTC CAA TGT ATG GCA CTA AAG A-3'), for *CPPN*, respectively. The sizes of specific amplicons are: 576–597 bp (genus-specific product), and 389–404 bp for *CP*, or 244 bp for *CPPN* after nested PCR. A detailed protocol of the procedure was previously published by Sachse and Hotzel [17] and is given here:

A. Genus-Specific Detection of Chlamydiae

Prepare a master mix of reagents for all amplification reactions of the series. It should contain the following ingredients per 50-µl reaction:

1 µl dNTP mix (2 mM each), 1 µl primer 191CHOMP (20 pmol/µl), 1 µl primer CHOMP371 (20 pmol/µl), 5 µl reaction buffer (10×), 0.2 µl *Taq* DNA polymerase (5 U/µl), 40.8 µl H_2O. Add template to each reaction vessel: 1 µl of DNA extract from infected tissue or 5 µl of extract from swab samples. Include amplification controls: DNA of a chlamydial reference strain (positive control) and water (negative control 1) instead of sample extract. Run PCR according to the following temperature-time profile: Initial denaturation at 95°C for 30 s, 35 cycles of denaturation (95°C for 30 s), primer annealing (50°C for 30 s) and primer extension (72°C for 30 s). Correct amplification leads to the formation of a 576–597-bp product specific for the genus *Chlamydia*(according to the new taxonomy: *Chlamydia* and *Chlamydophila*).

B. Species-Specific Detection of Chlamydiae

Prepare a master mix of reagents for all amplification reactions of the series. It should contain the following ingredients per 50-µl reaction:

1 µl dNTP mix (2 mM each), 1 µl forward primer 201CHOMP

+ 1 μl reverse primer TRACH269 or PNEUM268 (20 pmol/μl each) OR 1 μl forward primer 204PECOR or 218PSITT + 1 μl reverse primer CHOMP336s (20 pmol/μl each), 5 μl reaction buffer (10×), 0.2 μl *Taq* DNA polymerase (5 U/μl), 40.8 μl H_2O. Add 1 μl of the product from genus-specific PCR as template to each reaction vessel.

Subject the products of positive control and negative control 1 (1 μl of each) from the previous amplification to the second round of nested PCR. Additionally include a fresh reagent control (negative control 2). Run PCR according to the following temperature-time profile: Initial denaturation at 95°C for 30 s, 20 cycles of denaturation (95°C for 30 s), primer annealing (60°C for 30 s) and primer extension (72°C for 30 s). The correct sizes of species-specific amplicons are 250 bp for *C. trachomatis*, 244 bp for *C. pneumoniae*, 389–404 bp for *C. psittaci*, and 426–441 bp for *C. pecorum*.

DNA sequencing

For species identification, products of the first PCR round were amplified using primers 201CHOMP and CHOMP336s. Specific bands from PCR products were cut out of the agarose gel (1%) and DNA was extracted using the QIAquick Gel Extraction Kit (QIAGEN, Hilden, Germany). Prior to processing on the ABI PRISM 310 Genetic Analyzer (Applied Biosystems), these extracts were subjected to cycle sequencing using the same primers as above and the BigDye™ Terminator Cycle Sequencing Ready Reaction Kit (Applied Biosystems, Darmstadt, Germany). The average length of the sequences determined was 400 nucleotides. The species identity was established through BLAST search [18]. Sequence alignments and analysis were conducted using the Vector NTI Suite 8.0 software package (Informax Inc., Oxford, UK).

Statistical analysis

Statistical analysis was done using SPSS, version 12 (SPSS Inc., Chicago, USA). The data were statistically evaluated using Mann-Whitney-U-test, Pearson Chi Square test and Spearman-Rho correlation (2-sided). A test value below 0.05 was considered to be statistically significant.

RESULTS

Clinical data

As a result of the standardized questionnaire and histology 45 out of a total of 948 horses were recruited for the present study. 43 animals were slaughtered and 2 euthanized. The median age was 16.11 years (span: 9–25), among these were 23 mares, 20 geldings and 2 stallions. Concerning the respiratory system, 20 animals were considered clinically as healthy, whereas 25 showed clinical symptoms of RAO (Table 1). Lameness was the main cause to kill the horses (40% in both groups). In horses with RAO, this disease was the reason for killing the animal in 36%; a respective therapy was applied in 56%. Therapeutic regimens differed widely, thus not allowing further statistically evaluation. The majority of horses both in the clinically healthy and the RAO groups were housed in stables with straw bedding (healthy controls: 75%, RAO: 68%). Outdoor housing was reported in 20% of the controls and none of the histologically approved RAO cases. Stable housing with wood shavings or linen straw was reported in 32% of cases with RAO and 5% of controls, respectively.

Table 1: Findings in clinically healthy versus clinically sick horses

	n	Histological score: median (span)	IHC (MP): median (span)	IHC (PII): median (span)	IHC (BE): median (span)	IHC (percentage): median (span)	PCR: positive cases (percentage)
Clinically healthy(Subgroups I + II)	20	0 (0–6)	0 (0–1)	0 (0–4)	17 (0–119)	1.108 (0–8.92)	9 (45)
Clinically sick(Subgroups III + IV)	25	3 (0–29)	0 (0–4)	0 (0–63)	113 (4–535)	7.304 (0.20–37.1)	15 (60)
Mann-Whitney-U *Pearson Chi Square		p = 0.010	p = 0.079	p = 0.127	p < 0.001	p < 0.001	*p = 0.316

Immunohistochemistry (IHC): Number of CP antigen-positive cells in 3 high power fields

MP: macrophages, PII: type II pneumocytes, BE: bronchiolar epithelial cells

IHC (percentage): Number of all CP antigen-positive cells in 3 high power fields in relation to all cells

Light microscopy, immunohistochemistry and Immunofluorescence

Comparing RAO and healthy horses (Table 1) a significantly different histological score (p = 0.010), number of *Chlamydia psittaci (CP)* antigen-positive bronchiolar epithelial cells (p < 0.001), and percentage of all *CP*antigen-positive cells (p < 0.001) were found.

In subgroups II and III the distribution of inclusions and antigens was typical for persistent chlamydial infections in IHC: inclusion bodies were only sparsely seen, but antigens were much more frequently found. This was also true for subgroup 1, but on a much lower level.

Animals which were killed specifically because of RAO (n = 9) were significantly different in the median number of *CP* antigen-positive bronchiolar epithelial cells (83 vs. 42, p = 0.037) compared to horses which were put down due to other reasons (n = 36).

Results of clinical data and histological evaluation of the 45 horses led to the classification shown in Table 2. The four subgroups were significantly different from each other in their light microscopy histological score (Mann-Whitney U-test, $p < 0.05$). Age was not significantly correlated to the histological score (Spearman-Rho, $p = 0.425$).

Table 2: Comparison of results after subgrouping horses due to clinical and light microscopic findings

	n	Histological score: median (span)	IHC (MP): median (span)	IHC (PII): median (span)	IHC (BE): median (span)	IHC (percentage): median (span)	PCR: positive cases (percentage)
Subgroup I	15	0 (0–2)	0 (0–1)	0 (—4)	6 (—63)	0.359 (0–4,79)	5 (33.3)
Subgroup II	5	5 (4–6)	0 (0–1)	0 (0–2)	76 (11–119)	4.853 (0.88–8.92)	4 (80)
Subgroup III	16	1 (0–5)	0 (0–1)	0 (0–2)	81.5 (4–474)	6.065 (0.20–25.4)	13 (81.2)
Subgroup IV	9	22 (12–29)	1 (0–4)	22 (0–63)	246 (20–535)	21.024 (1.37–37.1)	2 (22.2)
Mann-Whitney-U *exact Fisher test		I vs. II: p < 0.001 I vs. III: p = 0.033 I vs. IV: p < 0.001 II vs. III: p = 0.003 II vs. IV: p = 0.001 III vs. IV: p < 0.001	I vs. II: p = n. s. I vs. III: p = n. s. I vs. IV: p = 0.041 II vs. III: p = n. s. II vs. IV: p = n. s. III vs. IV: p = 0.037	I vs. II: p = n. s. I vs. III: p = n. s. I vs. IV: p < 0.001 II vs. III: p = n. s. II vs. IV: p = 0.007 III vs. IV: p < 0.001	I vs. II: p = 0.033 I vs. III: p < 0.001 I vs. IV: p < 0.001 II vs. III: p = n. s. II vs. IV: p = 0.042 III vs. IV: p = 0.023	I vs. II: p = 0.015 I vs. III: p < 0.001 I vs. IV: p < 0.001 II vs. III: p = n. s. II vs. IV: p = 0.042 III vs. IV: p = 0.020	I vs. II: p = n. s.* I vs. III: p = 0.019* I vs. IV: p = n. s.* II vs. III: p = n. s.* II vs. IV: p = n. s.* III vs. IV: p = 0.009*

Subgroup I: Clinically healthy horses without histological changes of RAO

Subgroup II: Clinically healthy horses with a low inflammation score of 4–6

Subgroup III: Horses with clinical signs of RAO, but without or only slight histological changes and a score of 0–5

Subgroup IV: Horses with symptoms and histological changes of RAO with a score > 10

IHC: Number of CP antigen-positive cells in 3 high power fields

MP: macrophages, PII: type II pneumocytes, BE: bronchiolar epithelial cells

IHC (percentage): number of all CP antigen-positive cells in 3 high power fields in relation to all cells

The clinically healthy horses in subgroup I showed no (Figure 1) and in subgroup II only slight bronchiolitis. *CP*antigens were shown in bronchiolar epithelial cells (Figures 2, 3 and 4) as well as occasionally in type 2 pneumocytes and macrophages (Figures 4 and 5). Type II pneumocytes were positive in 12 cases (3 in subgroup I, 1 in subgroup III, 8 in subgroup IV), and in 6 cases positive staining was also seen in macrophages (1 in subgroup I, 5 in subgroup IV). Data and significant differences are shown in detail in Table 2. With increased severity of disease there was a significant rise in antigen-positive cells. Age was not significantly correlated with immunohistological parameters (Spearman Rho, $p > 0.05$). Positive and significant Spearman-Rho correlations were found between all of the following parameters: light microscopy score, the number of *CP* antigen-positive macrophages, type II pneumocytes and bronchiolar epithelial cells. However, the highest correlation coefficient ($r = 0.612$) was found between the number of *CP* antigen-positive type II pneumocytes and the number of *CP* antigen-positive macrophages, the lowest correlation coefficient found was $r = 0.41$ between the number of *CP* antigen-positive macrophages and the histological score (Table 3).

Table 3: Correlations between histological score and immunohistochemical findings

Correlation coefficients (Spearman-Rho, 2-sided)	Histological score	IHC (MP)	IHC (PII)
IHC (MP)	0.410 p = 0.005		
IHC (PII)	0.459 p = 0.002	0.612 p < 0.001	
IHC (BE)	0.493 p = 0.001	0.448 p = 0.002	0.495 p = 0.001

IHC: Number of CP antigen-positive cells in 3 high power fields

MP: macrophages, PII: type II pneumocytes, BE: bronchiolar epithelial cells

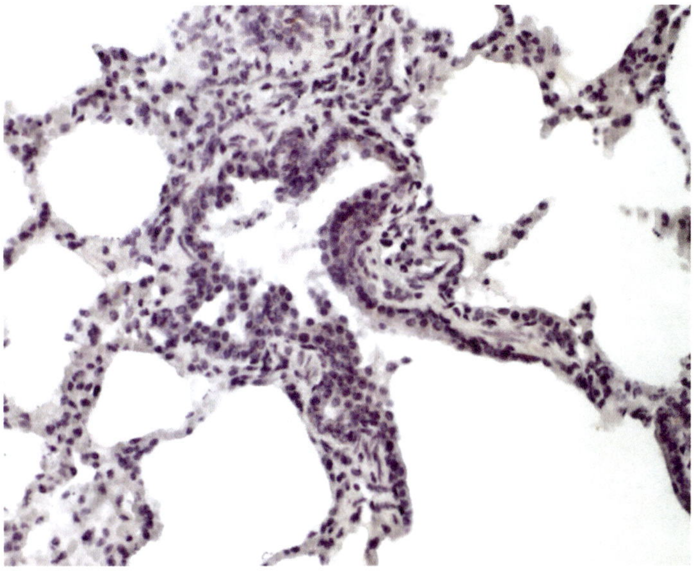

Figure 1: Immunohistochemistry of equine lung tissue in healthy horses. Animal showing no bronchiolitis (original magnification 10×).

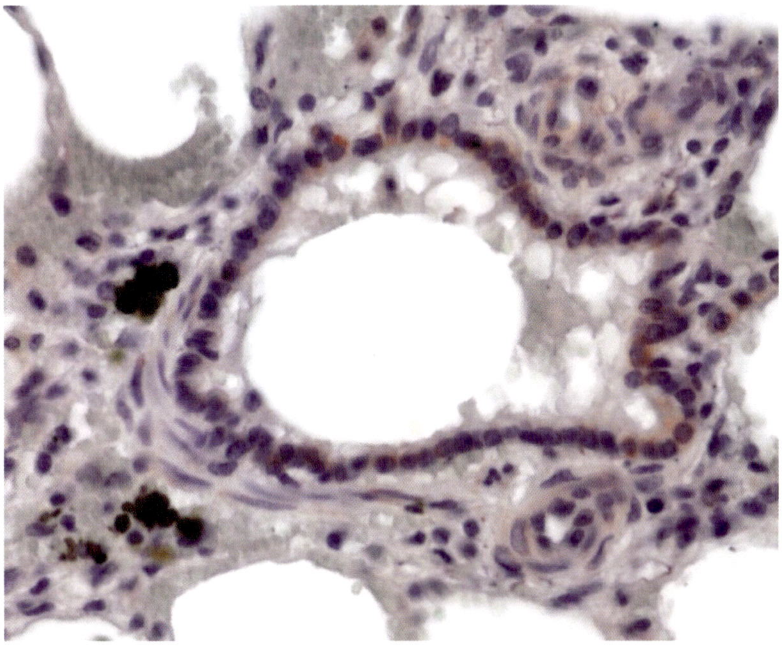

Figure 2: Immunohistochemistry of equine lung tissue in healthy horses. Only occasionally some epithelial cells positive for *Chlamydia psittaci* antigens are detectable (brown staining, original magnification 40×).

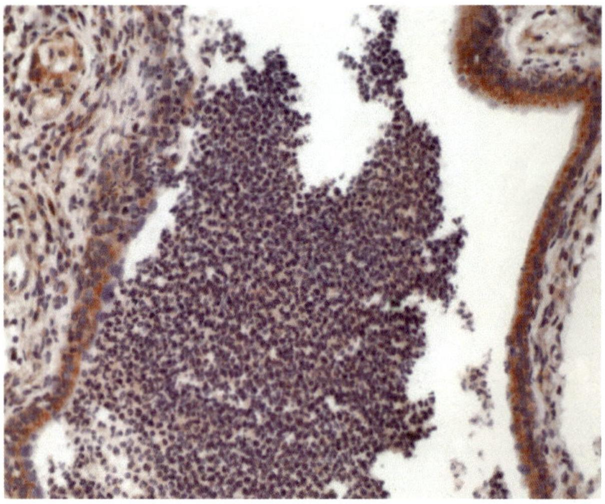

Figure 3: Immunohistochemistry of equine lung tissue in RAO. In RAO, animals with severe bronchiolitis (note the striking intraluminal accumulation of neutrophils and macrophages) most of the bronchiolar epithelial cells carry *CP*antigens (brown staining, original magnification 20×).

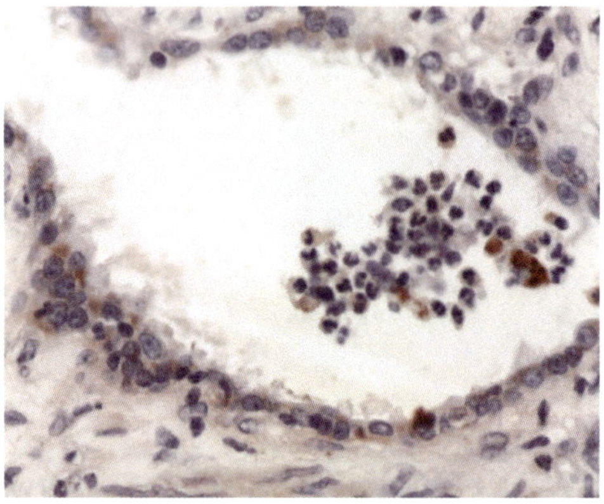

Figure 4: Immunohistochemistry of equine lung tissue in RAO. Also in the respiratory bronchioli inflammation is found, chlamydial antigens (brown staining) are detectable in epithelial cells and macrophages (original magnification 40×).

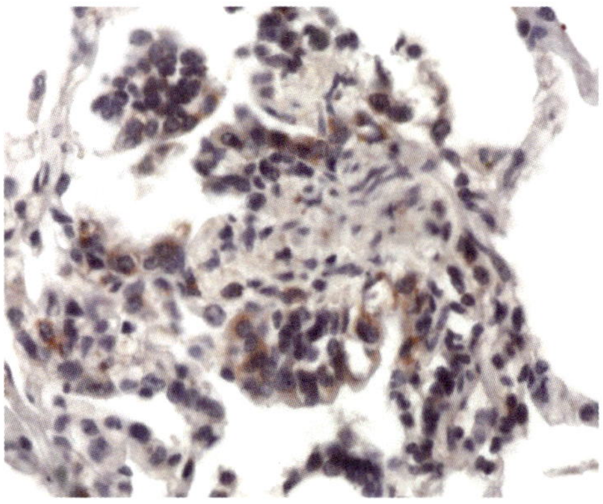

Figure 5: Immunohistochemistry of equine lung tissue in RAO. Proliferating type II pneumocytes show chlamydial antigens as well (brown staining, original magnification 40×).

To obtain further information about localization of chlamydial antigens, immunofluorescence testing was performed in three horses. Multiple typical perinuclear spots in bronchiolar epithelial cells, macrophages and granulocytes were seen in 2 horses of subgroup IV (Figures 6 and 7). In horses with RAO, the abundance of chlamydial inclusion bodies (red spots) in bronchiolar epithelial cells (stained green with an anti-cytokeratin pan antibody) and macrophages varies from high (Figure 6) to low (Figure 7).

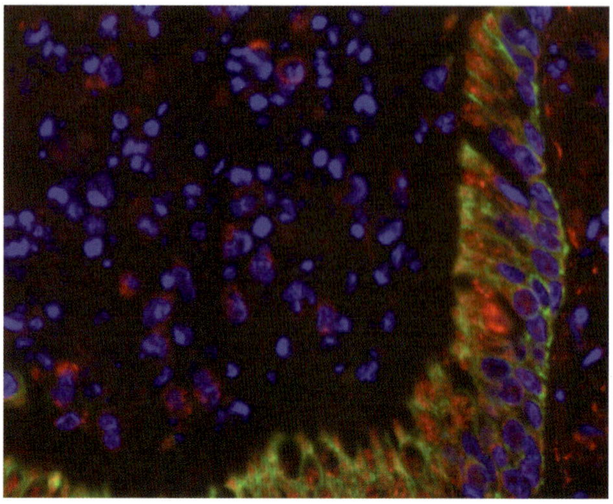

Figure 6: Immunofluorescence of equine lung tissue in RAO. In horses with RAO, the abundance of chlamydial inclusion bodies (red spots) in bronchiolar epithelial cells (stained green with an anti-cytokeratin pan antibody) and macrophages varies from high to low (compare Figure 7) (original magnification 40×).

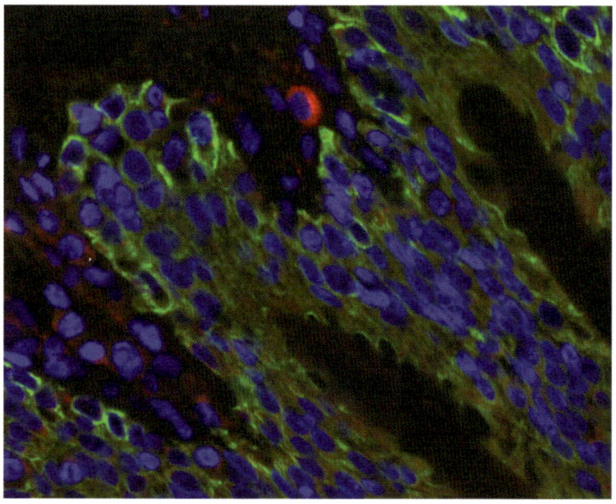

Figure 7: Immunofluorescence of equine lung tissue in RAO. In horses with RAO, the abundance of chlamydial inclusion bodies (red spots) in bronchiolar epithelial cells (stained green with an anti-cytokeratin pan antibody) and macrophages varies from high (compare Figure 6) to low (original magnification 40×).

Housing with straw contact vs. other bedding or RAO with therapy vs. without therapy and all combinations of the parameters histological score, results of immunohistochemistry or PCR, lacked any correlations (Mann-Whitney U-test, $p > 0.05$).

Polymerase Chain Reaction (PCR) and DNA sequencing

No significant differences were seen between clinically healthy and sick horses (Table 1). PCR revealed *CP* DNA in 5 of 15 (= 33.3%) horses in subgroup I, 4 of 5 (= 80%) in subgroup II, 13 of 16 (= 81.2%) in subgroup III and 2 of 9 (= 22.2%)

in subgroup IV. Significant differences in PCR positivity are shown between subgroups I and III as well as between subgroups III and IV (Table 2).

To confirm the identity of the chlamydial species, DNA from 22 of the 24 positive samples was sequenced in the *omp*A gene region (approximately 400 bp). A BLAST search of these sequences revealed close to 100% homology to the species *CPP* in 9 and *CPA* in 13 cases. No significant differences were found between the four subgroups (Pearson Chi Square test, p = 0.309).

DISCUSSION

One principal characteristic of RAO is the excessive production of mucus containing high amounts of neutrophils [19]. In human COPD, mucus hypersecretion is a key event as well, but neutrophils are only dominant in exacerbations [20]. These exacerbations are mainly associated with viral and/or bacterial infections [21]. In equine RAO, high levels of collagenolytic activity [22] and matrix metalloproteinases (MMPs) 8, 9 and 13 [22, 23, 24, 25] were found to be useful markers for ongoing disease. The release of matrix metalloproteinases (MMP-9) is shown to be stimulated by chlamydial heat shock protein 60 [26]. Release of MMPs is also crucial for tissue destruction by macrophages in human emphysema [27] and increased activities of MMP-8 and MMP-9 are found in induced sputum of humans with COPD [28]. Elevated IL-8 and tumor necrosis factor-alpha production are seen in horses with RAO exacerbation [19, 29] and in humans with COPD [30]. The proinflammatory granulocyte-attracting chemokine IL-8 is produced by epithelial cells in the course of infection with *CPP* [31]. Decreased phagocytic activity of alveolar macrophages (MP) is found in RAO after 24 h stimulation with LPS or PMA and ionomycin [19]. In current non-smokers with COPD MP show reduced capacity to ingest apoptotic airway epithelial cells as well [32].

Both RAO and COPD have to be regarded as multicausal diseases with abiotic and biotic factors. The main etiologically relevant factor in both RAO and COPD is an external event (abiotic factor), i.e. environmental dust exposure in horses and cigarette smoking in human beings. Optimal housing can certainly prevent equine RAO in many cases as well as avoidance of smoking will prevent COPD. Some authors even regard human COPD as a dust-induced disease and emphasize the role of kaolinite [33]. Genetic (biotic) factors are relevant in RAO [34] and COPD as well [35].

According to the findings of the present study the predominant location for chlamydial antigens in horse lungs are the bronchial epithelial cells, followed to a much lesser extent by type II pneumocytes and macrophages. For bronchiolar epithelial cells as well as for the total percentage of *CP* antigen-positive cells, there is a highly significant higher antigen load in RAO horses in comparison to healthy controls. Since the first step in the inflammation cascade is caused by inhalation of dust particles, the bronchiolar epithelium represents most likely the "key structure" in establishing and maintaining the disease. Concurrent infection of these cells with chlamydial organisms might lead to chronicity and persistence of the exaggerated inflammatory and tissue destructing response to dust particles.

Distribution of *CP* antigens in the lungs of clinically healthy horses (subgroups I and II) was typical for persisting infection and in those with RAO and histological severe disease (subgroup IV) for acute chlamydial infection. The subgroup with slight inflammation and higher *CP* antigen load within the group of healthy horses could be an indicator of preclinical disease. The same questions come around according to the subgroups within RAO animals. Although no significant morphological differences were seen between healthy horses with slight inflammation (subgroup II) and those with RAO and low histological score (subgroup III) there are severe clinical differences, which can be interpreted only functionally, probably on a genetic background.

PCR positivity shows significant differences between subgroups I and III as well as between subgroups III and IV. This means that there is a significant difference also by PCR between healthy horses and horses that already present with clinical signs of RAO, but show no or only slight signs of inflammation and also between ill horses with only slight inflammation compared with those with marked inflammation. Furthermore, it is known that farmers more often suffer from respiratory symptoms than the average population [36]. Dust exposure and higher endotoxin concentrations in stables are supposed to be the main factors [37]. The possible importance of *Chlamydiaceae* as a source of human infections in animal housings requires further evaluation.

CONCLUSION

For the first time persistence of *CPP* and *CPA* in the lungs of clinically healthy horses and acute (possibly reactivated) chlamydial infections in those with obvious disease is demonstrated. Respiratory chlamydial infection probably becomes clinically relevant only in animals affected by additional pathogenic factors. In this context, inflammation seems to be associated with the activation of chlamydiae. Furthermore, the high prevalence of these chlamydial agents in horse lungs deserves further attention as a reservoir, especially in the light of recent studies, showing an association of *CPP* with cases of equine abortion [14, 15]. The possible risk to acquire *CPP* or *CPA* infections for the staff in animal housings has to be evaluated.

Corresponding pathophysiological aspects (target cell types, cytokine/chemokine release, tissue degrading enzymes like MMPs) between chlamydial infections on the one hand and RAO/COPD on the other hand are shown. The precise role of chlamydial organisms in the pathogenesis of RAO/COPD needs further investigations.

Because of the pathophysiological similarities between both diseases and the detection of *Chlamydiaceae*, RAO could be a model for human COPD and should be studied under these aspects.

DECLARATIONS

Acknowledgements

We thank all the horse owners and veterinarians for giving sufficient information about their animals as well as the staff of the slaughterhouses for supporting this study.

Authors' contributions

Dirk Theegarten (DT) has designed and organized this study, done light microscopy, written most of the manuscript and participitated in its statistical analysis. Konrad Sachse (KS) has done the sequence alignments and written the parts of the manuscript concerning molecular biology and veterinary aspects, and also participated in PCR analysis. Britta Mentrup (BM) has done the clinical parts, collected specimens and did the immunohistochemistry. Kerstin Fey (KF) has designed the clinical parts. Helmut Hotzel (HH) carried out PCR analysis and DNA sequencing. Olaf Anhenn (OA) participated in designing the study, established the immunohistochemistry protocols, collected the data, performed statistical analysis and reviewed the manuscript. All authors have discussed and approved the final manuscript.

REFERENCES

1. Robinson NE, Derksen FE, Olszewski MA, Büchner-Maxwell VA: The pathogenesis of chronic obstructive pulmonary disease of horses. *Brit Vet J* 1996, 152:283–306.
2. Thurlbeck WM, Lowell FC: Heaves in horses. *Am Rev Respir Dis* 1964, 89:82–88.
3. Kaup FJ, Drommer W, Damsch S, Deegen E: Ultrastructural findings in horses with chronic obstructive pulmonary disease (COPD). II: Pathomorphological changes of the terminal airways and the alveolar region. *Equine Vet J* 1990, 22:349–355.
4. Theegarten D, Teschler H, Stamatis G, Konietzko N, Morgenroth K: Pathologisch-anatomische Befunde bei der chirurgischen Lungenvolumenreduktion des fortgeschrittenen Emphysems. *Pneumologie* 1998, 52:702–706.
5. Pirie RS, Collie DDS, Dixon PM, McGorum BC: Inhaled endotoxin and organic dust particulates have synergistic proinflammatory effects in equine heaves (organic dust-induced asthma). *Clin Exp Allergy* 2003, 33:676–683.
6. Simonen-Jokinen T, Pirie RS, McGorum BC, Maisi P: Effect of composition and different fractions of hay dust suspension on inflammation in lungs of heaves-affected horses: MMP-9 and MMP-2 as indicators of tissue destruction. *Equine Vet J* 2005, 37:412–417.
7. Theegarten D, Mogilevski G, Anhenn O, Stamatis G, Jaeschock R, Morgenroth K: The role of Chlamydia in the pathogenesis of pulmonary emphysema. Electron microscopy and immunofluorescence reveal corresponding findings as in atherosclerosis. *Virchows Arch* 2000, 437:190–193.
8. Theegarten D, Anhenn O, Hotzel H, Wagner M, Marra A, Stamatis G, Mogilevski G, Sachse K: A comparative ultrastructural and molecular biological study on *Chlamydia psittaci* infection in alpha-1 antitrypsin deficiency and non-alpha-1 antitrypsin deficiency emphysema versus lung tissue of patients with hamartochondroma. *BMC Infect Dis* 2004, 4:38.
9. Anhenn O, Theegarten D, Hotzel H, Sachse K, Rohde H: Detection of *Chlamydophila psittaci* and *Chlamydophila abortus* in induced sputum of patients with exacerbated or stable chronic obstructive pulmonary disease. In *Proceedings Fifth Meeting of the European Society for Chlamydia Research*. Edited by: Deák J. Budapest: Pauker Nyomdaipari Kft; 2004:245. Google
10. Moorthy AR, Spradbrow PB: *Chlamydia psittaci* infection of horses with respiratory disease. *Equine Vet J* 1978, 10:38–42.
11. McChesney SL, England JJ, McChesney AE: *Chlamydia psittaci* induced pneumonia in a horse. *Cornell Veterinarian* 1982, 72:92–97.
12. Mair TS, Wills JM: *Chlamydia psittaci* infection in horses: results of a prevalence survey and experimental challenge. *Vet Rec* 1992, 130:417–419.
13. Di Francesco A, Donati M, Mattioli L, Naldi M, Salvatore D, Poglayen G, Cevenini R, Baldelli R: *Chlamydophila pneumoniae* in horses: a seroepidemiological survey in Italy. *New Microbiol* 2006, 29:303–305.
14. Henning K, Sachse K, Sting R: Nachweis von Chlamydien bei einem Stutenabort. *Dtsch tierärztl Wschr* 2000, 107:49–52.Google
15. Szeredi L, Hotzel H, Sachse K: High prevalence of chlamydial (*Chlamydophila psittaci*) infection in fetal membranes of aborted equine fetuses. *Vet Res Commun* 2005, 29:37–49.
16. Kaltenboeck B, Schmeer N, Schneider R: Evidence for numerous *omp* 1 alleles of porcine *Chlamydia trachomatis* and novel chlamydial species obtained by PCR. *J Clin Microbiol* 35:1835–1841.
17. Sachse K, Hotzel H: Detection and differentiation of chlamydiae by nested PCR. In *Methods Mol Biol* Edited by: Sachse K, Frey J. 2002, 216:123–136.
18. Blast search [http://www.ncbi.nlm.nih.gov/blast/]
19. Franchini M, Gilli U, Akens MK, Fellenberg RV, Bracher V: The role of neutrophil chemotactic cytokines in the pathogenesis of equine chronic obstructive pulmonary disease (COPD). *Vet Immunol Immunopathol* 1998, 66:53–65.
20. Barnes P: Chronic obstructive pulmonary disease. *New Engl J Med* 2000, 343:269–280.
21. Rohde G, Wiethege A, Borg I, Kauth M, Bauer TT, Gillissen A, Bufe A, Schultze-Werninghaus G: Respiratory viruses in exacerbations of chronic obstructive pulmonary disease requiring hospitalisation: a case control study. *Thorax* 2003, 58:37–42.
22. von Fellenberg R: Proteasen und Proteaseinhibitoren von möglicher klinischer Relevanz bei der COPD des Pferdes. *Tierärztl Prax* 1987, 15:399–407.
23. Raulo SM, Sorsa TA, Kiili MT, Maisi PS: Evaluation of collagenase activity, matrix metalloproteinase-8, and matrix metalloproteinase-13 in horses with chronic obstructive pulmonary disease. *Am J Vet Res* 2001, 62:1142–1148.
24. Raulo SM, Sorsa T, Tervahartiala T, Pirila E, Maisi P: MMP-9 as a marker of inflammation in tracheal epithelial lining fluid (TELF) and in bronchoalveolar fluid (BALF) of COPD horses. *Equine Vet J* 2001, 33:128–136.
25. Nevalainen M, Raulo SM, Brazil TJ, Pirie RS, Sorsa T, McGorum BC, Maisi P: Inhalation of organic dusts

and lipopolysaccharide increases gelatinolytic matrix metalloproteinases (MMPs) in the lungs of heaves horses. *Equine Vet J* 2002, 34:150–155.

26. Kol A, Sukhova GK, Lichtman AH, Libby P: Chlamydial heat shock protein 60 localizes in human atheroma and regulates macrophage tumor necrosis factor-α and matrix metalloproteinase expression. *Circulation* 1998, 98:300–307.
27. Shapiro SD: The macrophage in chronic obstructive pulmonary disease. *Am J Respir Crit Care Med* 1999, 160:S29–32.
28. Vernooy JHJ, Lindeman JHN, Jacobs JA, Hanemaaijer R, Wouters EFM: Increased activity of matrix metalloproteinase-8 and matrix metalloproteinase-9 in induced sputum from patients with COPD. *Chest* 2004, 126:1802–1810.
29. Giguere S, Viel L, Lee E, MacKay RJ, Hernandez J, Franchini M: Cytokine induction in pulmonary airways of horses with heaves and effect of therapy with inhaled fluticasone propionate. *Vet Immunol Immunopathol* 2002, 85:147–158.
30. Keatings VM, Collins PD, Scott DM, Barnes PJ: Differences in interleukin-8 and tumor necrosis factor-alpha in induced sputum from patients with chronic obstructive pulmonary disease or asthma. *Am J Respir Crit Care Med* 1996, 153:530–534.
31. Rasmussen SJ, Eckmann L, Quayle AJ, Shen L, Zhang Y-X, Anderson DJ, Fierer J, Stephens RS, Kagnoff MF: Secretion of proinflammatory cytokines by epithelial cells in response to Chlamydia infection suggests a central role for epithelial cells in Chlamydial pathogenesis. *J Clin Invest* 1997, 99:77–87.
32. Hodge S, Hodge G, Scicchitano R, Reynolds PN, Holmes M: Alveolar macrophages from subjects with chronic obstructive pulmonary disease are deficient in their ability to phagocytose apoptotic airway epithelial cells.*Immunol Cell Biol* 2003, 81:289–296.
33. Girod CE, King TE: COPD: a dust-induced disease? *Chest* 2005, 128:3055–3064.
34. Marti E, Gerber H, Essich G, Oulehla J, Lazary S: The genetic basis of equine allergic diseases. 1. chronic hypersensivity bronchitis. *Equine Vet J* 1991, 23:457–460.
35. Molfino NA: Genetics of COPD. *Chest* 2004, 125:1929–1940.
36. Radon K, Monso E, Weber C, Danuser B, Iversen M, Opravil U, Donham K, Hartung J, Pdersen S, Garz S, Blainey D, Rabe U, Nowak D: Prevalence and risk factors for airway diseases in farmers – summary of results of the European farmers› project. *Ann Agric Environ Med* 2002, 9:207–213.
37. Vogelzang PFJ, van der Gulden JWJ, Folgering H, Kolk JJ, Heederik D, Preller L, Tielen MJM, van Schayck CP: Endotoxin exposure as a major determinat of lung function decline in pig farmers. *Am J Respir Crit Care Med* 1998, 157:15–18.

SECTION III: MYCOPLASMA SPP. - INTRACELLULAR BACTERIA

CHAPTER 10

MICROSCOPY AND GENOMIC ANALYSIS OF MYCOPLASMA PARVUMSTRAIN INDIANA

Naíla C do Nascimento, Andrea P dos Santos, Yuefeng Chu, Ana MS Guimaraes, Aubrey N Baird, Ann B Weil and Joanne B Messick

INTRODUCTION

Hemotrophic mycoplasmas (class *Mollicutes*), trivially known as hemoplasmas, are small cell-wall-less bacteria with a unique tropism for the red blood cells (RBC) of a variety of vertebrate hosts. The genome of ten hemoplasmas, eight different species and two strains each of *Mycoplasma suis* and *M. haemofelis*, had their genomes sequenced to date; seven of these were completed by our research group [1]–[10]. Their genomes have a small core of essential genes; however, they rely on the acquisition of most nutrients from their environment to survive. This feature likely plays a key role in the lack of an established in vitro cultivation of these organisms.

Mycoplasma parvum [*Eperythrozoon parvum*] was first reported in 1950 as a nonpathogenic bacterium of the pig [11]. Unlike *M. suis*, its closest relative, *M. parvum* often accumulates on a single RBC but only a few RBC are infected. Rod and coccoid forms are common in *M. parvum* infection, ranging in size from 0.2 to 0.5 μm, whereas ring forms are frequent in *M. suis*. The latter form is larger and may be up to 2.5 μm in diameter [11]. Infection by *M. parvum* is usually characterized by the absence of clinical signs even in splenectomized pigs; on the contrary, *M. suis* bacteremia, characterized by fever and icteroanemia, may result in death. In addition, cross-inoculation studies differentiate these two hemoplasmas as separate species as well as from other species of red cell bacteria that infect cattle, sheep, goats, and mice [11],[12].

More than 50 years have passed since its first description, and yet less than 10 publications can be found when searching for "*Mycoplasma parvum*" or "*Eperythrozoon parvum*" keywords in scientific databases. The two previous reports documenting *M. parvum* infection in pigs were based solely on the amplification and sequencing of its 16S rRNA or ribonuclease P RNA genes [13],[14]. The sequences of these genes were divergent from those of *M. suis*, sharing only 96% and 88% identity, respectively. These molecular studies corroborated previous morphology, pathogenicity, and cross-inoculation studies, suggesting that *M. parvum*and *M. suis* were distinct hemoplasma species. Nevertheless, new molecular tools for species circumscription are likely to provide a better resolution for this complex definition, especially when dealing with these uncultivable bacteria. The average nucleotide identity (ANI) analysis of conserved and shared genes between bacterial strains and supporting calculation of tetranucleotide signature correlation index (TETRA), has recently been proposed as a reliable substitute for DNA-DNA hybridization (DDH) [15]. A value for species delineation based on ANI is currently set at 95%-96%. The TETRA signature is an alignment-free parameter and generally correlates with ANI.

We report herein the course of infection with *M. parvum* in a naturally infected, splenectomized 6-month-old pig, and the complete genome of *M. parvum* strain Indiana. Furthermore, comparative genomic analyses of *M. parvum* with other hemotrophic mycoplasmas were performed, as well as a gene-by-gene comparison between *M. parvum* strain Indiana and *M. suis* strain Illinois to better understand their contrasting pathogenicity.

Citation: Naíla C do Nascimento, Andrea P dos Santos, Yuefeng Chu, Ana MS Guimaraes, Aubrey N Baird, Ann B Weil and Joanne B Messick, Microscopy and genomic analysis of Mycoplasma parvum-strain Indiana, DOI: 10.1186/s13567-014-0086-7.

MATERIAL AND METHODS

Animal and *Mycoplasma parvum* DNA isolation

A male domestic 6-month-old pig (*Sus scrofa domesticus*, mixed breed) was purchased from the Animal Sciences Research and Education Center-ASREC (West Lafayette, IN, USA). While at the farm, this animal was kept in close contact with other pigs fed a commercial feed containing chlortetracycline (100 grams/ton) during growing and finishing stages (from 7–8 weeks to 6 months old), and vaccinated against *Mycoplasma hyopneumoniae* (RespiSure®/ER Bac Plus®, Pfizer), *Erysipelothrix rhusiopathiae*, and circovirus. The animal was tested for hemotrophic mycoplasma infection [16] on two separate occasions prior to its arrival at the Purdue Animal Housing Facilities (Purdue University, West Lafayette, IN, USA). A conventional PCR (cPCR) developed in our laboratory, which amplifies a larger product (~840 bp) of the 16S rRNA gene of swine hemoplasmas, was also performed [17]. The identity of both qPCR and cPCR products was confirmed by Sanger sequencing. The animal was treated according to the Purdue Animal Care and Use Committee (PACUC) protocol number 1111000223. The pig was fed antibiotic-free commercial feed, as well as water (via a self-controlled nipple waterer) *ad libitum* during the entire study. Eleven days after its arrival, the animal was splenectomized according to the PACUC protocol. The pig was monitored daily (minimum twice a day) for clinical signs (e.g. elevated body temperature, and direct observation of behavior- BAR *status*), and blood was collected into EDTA tubes before and following splenectomy (every 2–8 days depending on clinical signs and blood smear evaluation) for monitoring *M. parvum* infection by qPCR [16].

M. parvum strain Indiana was harvested from the blood of the pig at the peak of bacteremia; EDTA-whole blood was centrifuged at 4000*g* for 10 min and the buffy coat was removed. The remaining red blood cells with *M. parvum* organisms attached were used for the subsequent DNA extraction. Genomic DNA was extracted using Quick-gDNA™ MidiPrep kit according to the manufacturer's instructions (Zymo Research, Irvine, CA, USA).

Light and scanning electron microscopy (SEM) of *M. parvum*

Blood smears were prepared from fresh EDTA-blood every 2 days after splenectomy to follow *M. parvum*infection and stained with Giemsa. Photomicrographs were taken using a total magnification of 100 X.

For SEM, aliquots of 1.0 mL of blood infected with *M. parvum* were centrifuged and pellet was resuspended in 1.0 mL of glutaraldehyde 2.5% in 0.1 M sodium cacodylate buffer, pH 7.4, for fixation. Samples were prepared for scanning electron microscopy using standard procedures at Purdue University's Biological Electron Microscopy Facility, and visualized using FEI Titan Krios microscope.

Sequencing and assembly of *M. parvum* strain Indiana genome

The whole genome was sequenced from paired-end libraries (TruSeq DNA sample preparation kit, Illumina, San Diego, CA, USA) using Illumina HiSeq 2000 (Illumina, Inc., San Diego, CA, USA) at Purdue University Genomics Core Facility. Average reads of about 100 bases were assembled using ABySS 1.2.7 [18]. After assembly resulting from 1000 × genome coverage of the Illumina reads, a single remaining gap was closed using conventional PCR followed by Sanger sequencing in both directions.

Annotation and analyses of the complete genome of *M. parvum* strain Indiana

NCBI's prokaryotic Genomes Annotation Pipeline 2.0 provided the first pass annotation of *M. parvum* genome. The annotation tool Manatee (Institute for Genome Sciences (IGS), School of Medicine, University of Maryland) was used to perform manual annotation of the genome and comparative analysis between the genomes of *M. parvum* and *M. suis* strain Illinois (described below). Genomic data of other mycoplasmas available in the NCBI database (NCBI, Bethesda, MD, USA) were also used for comparative analyses.

Metabolic pathways were predicted based on the KEGG pathway database [19] and the study reported by Yus et al. [20]. BLASTclust tool, by Max-Planck Institute for Developmental Biology [21], was used to assign the paralogous gene families with thresholds of 70% covered length and 30% sequence identity.

Analyses for species differentiation

JSpecies software was used to calculate the average nucleotide identity (ANI; MUMmer algorithm) and tetranucleotide signature correlation indexes between selected genomes as previously described [15]. The following genome sequences were used in the analyses: *M. parvum* strain Indiana [CP006771.1], *M. suis* strain Illinois [CP002525.1], *M. suis* strain KI3806 [FQ790233.1], *M. haemofelis* strain Ohio2 [CP002808.1], *M. haemofelis* strain Langford 1 [FR773153.2], *M. haemocanis* strain Illinois [NC_016638.1], *M. wenyonii* strain Massachusetts [NC_018149.1], "*Candidatus* M. haemominutum" strain Birmingham 1 [HE613254.1], and "*Candidatus* M. haemolamae" strain Purdue [NC_018219]. The thresholds for species circumscription are 94% and 0.99 for ANIm and tetranucleotide indexes, respectively [15].

Comparative genomics of *M. parvum* and *M. suis* strain Illinois

Comparative analyses of the whole genome of *M. parvum* and *M. suis* strain Illinois were performed using BLASTp and/or BLASTn of each CDS or gene of one genome against the other and *vice versa*. BLASTp was applied to identify unique CDS of *M. parvum* or *M. suis*; a CDS was considered unique when there were no matching sequences with $\geq$80% coverage and $\geq$40% or $\geq$90% coverage and $\geq$30% identity to the query sequence.

Each unique CDS of *M. parvum* and *M. suis* was analyzed for the identification of the following parameters: subcellular localization and protein sorting signals using PSORTb v3.0.2 [22],[23]; signal peptide cleavage sites using SignalP 4.1 [24]; and the presence of lipoproteins using LipoP version 1.0 software [25].

Whole genome synteny (gene order) was compared between *M. parvum* strain Indiana and *M. suis* strain Illinois using SynMap from CoGe [26]. SynMap generates two-dimensional dot-plot synteny maps using a DAGchainer algorithm coupled with BLAST to identify syntenic homologous genes; each dot represents putative homologous genes between any two genomes [27].

RESULTS

Mycoplasma parvum infection in a splenectomized pig: bacterial loads and clinical signs

A 6-month-old barrow, domestic pig naturally infected with *M. parvum* was used in this study. The dynamics of its *M. parvum* blood load is shown in Figure 1. Briefly, this animal was initially identified as positive using a specific TaqMan qPCR for swine hemoplasmas [16] while still at the farm (ASREC) (days 1 and 3, Figure 1). In addition, a cPCR employed for amplification of ~840 bp fragment of the 16S rRNA gene of swine hemoplasmas was also positive [17]. Sequencing of the qPCR (157 bp) and cPCR (840 bp) products showed 100% and 99% identity, respectively, to the 16S rRNA sequence described for *M. parvum* (GenBank: JX489599.1), in contrast to 97% identity when compared to the 16S rRNA sequence of *M. suis* strain Illinois (NCBI: NR_103930.1). Moreover, the sequencing chromatograms showed single peaks along the entire length of the amplicons indicating the presence of a single sequence. These results confirmed that the animal was infected with *M. parvum* and free of *M. suis*. At day 22, this pig was transferred to the Purdue Animal Housing Facilities, where it remained for 48 days, from April 11th (day 22) to May 29th (day 70) 2013 (Figure 1). The animal was then splenectomized 11 days after its arrival (day 33, Figure 1) according to the Purdue Animal Care and Use Committee protocol (1111000223). Bacterial loads varied from 10^5 to 10^{10} organisms/mL of blood throughout the course of infection with a peak of bacteremia (10^{10} organisms/mL of blood) occurring 12–14 days after its splenectomy (days 45–47, Figure 1). Organisms were only detected on the peripheral blood smears at peak and for 24 h thereafter. While the pig's body temperature minimally elevated to 103.7 °F (reference range 101.6-103.6 °F) [28] at the peak, no overt clinical signs of infection were observed. The pig's hematocrit varied from 30% (only on one occasion, not at the peak of bacteremia; Figure 1) to 43%, but otherwise remained within the reference interval (32-50%) throughout the course of infection [29].

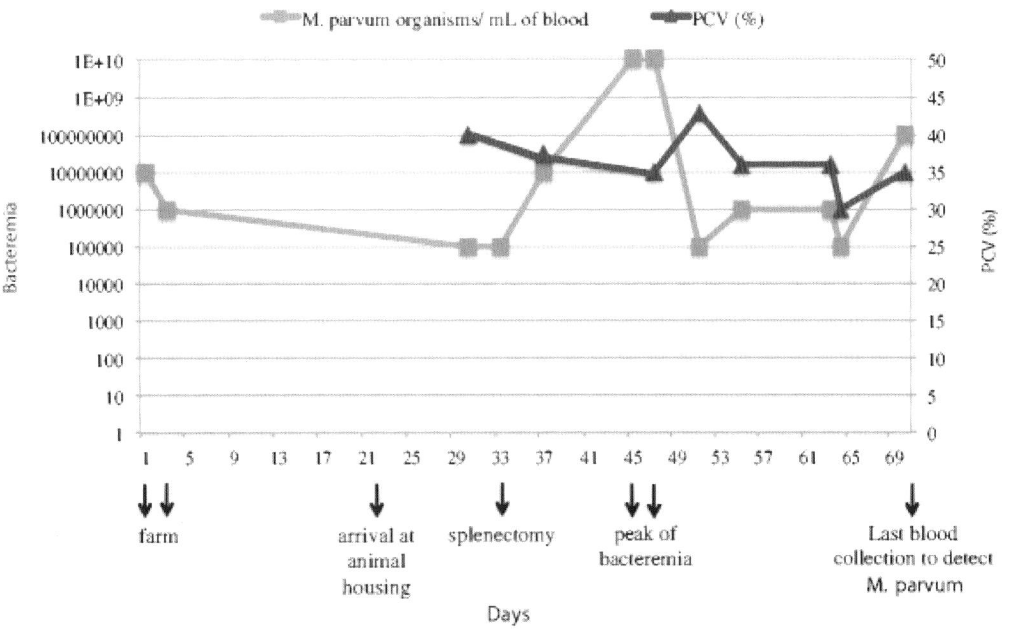

Figure 1: *M. parvum* loads and PCV of a naturally infected pig before and after splenectomy. The loads of *M. parvum* strain Indiana organisms were detected by TaqMan qPCR on blood samples and the (packed cell volume) PCV was determined before and after splenectomy in the naturally infected pig.

Light and Scanning Electron Microscopy (SEM) of *M. parvum* organisms

A photomicrograph of the peripheral blood smear obtained at the peak of bacteremia with *M. parvum* (day 45, Figure 1) shows the shape and distribution of these bacteria (Figure 2A). As described previously [11], the organisms are small (approximately 0.2-0.5 μm in diameter), and often infect a few RBC with large numbers of organisms on a single RBC (Figure 2). The SEM shows three *M. parvum* organisms on the surface of a red blood cell; their size varied from 0.2-0.5 μm in diameter (Figure 2B).

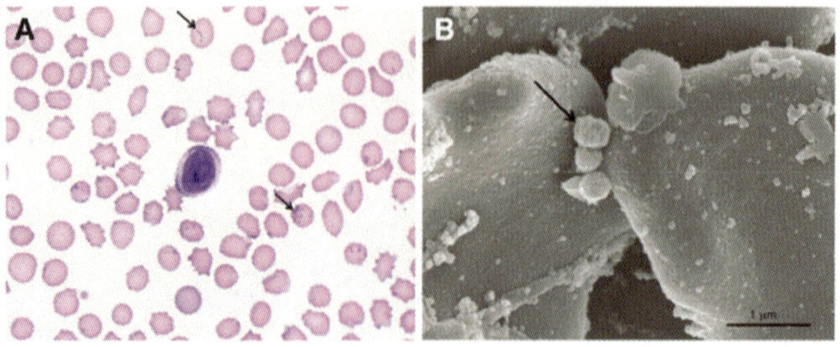

Figure 2: Light microscopy and SEM of *M. parvum* strain Indiana organisms. **A)** Photomicrograph of a blood smear stained with Giemsa obtained from a pig infected with *Mycoplasma parvum* (black arrows) at the peak of bacteremia (100X magnification). **B)** Scanning electron micrograph (SEM) showing red blood cells (RBC) of the pig with *M. parvum*organisms (black arrow) on the RBC surface. Scale bar, 1.0 μm.

General features of the genome of *M. parvum* strain Indiana

The general features of the genome of *M. parvum* strain Indiana regarding size, G + C content, percentage of coding sequences and paralogous genes were within the range of those described for all hemoplasmas sequenced to date [1],[4]–[8],[10] (Table 1). *M. parvum*'s single circular chromosome of 564.395 Kb, the second smallest genome amongst all hemoplasmas, and even smaller than that of *M. genitalium*, which was previously considered the tiniest member of the *Mollicutes* (Table 1). It has a G + C content of 27%, and like other mycoplasmas, it appears to use the opal stop codon (UGA) for tryptophan. The 16S, 23S, and 5S rRNA genes are represented as single copies; however, like that of *Mycoplasma suis*, the 16S rRNA gene is separated from the 5S-23S rRNA in a different operon [1],[2]. Thirty-two tRNA were identified covering all amino acids.

Table 1: General features of the genome of *Mycoplasma parvum* strain Indiana compared to other *Mycoplasma* species of the pneumoniae group

Mollicutes												
	Pneumoniae Group											
	Hemothrophic mycoplasmas								**Mucosal mycoplasmas**			
Genomic feature	***M. parvum* strain Indiana**	***M. suis* strain Illinois**	***M. haemofelis* strain Ohio2**	**'*Candidatus M.* haemominutum' strain Birmingham 1**	***M. haemocanis* strain Illinois**	***M. wenyonii* strain Massachusetts**	**'*Candidatus M.* haemolamae' str. Purdue**	***M. ovis* strain Michigan**	***M. pneumoniae***	***M. gallisepticum***	***M. genitalium***	***M. penetrans***
Size (base pairs)	564 395	742 431	1 155 937	513 880	919 992	650 228	756 845	702 511	816 394	1 012 800	580 076	1 358 633
G + C content	27	31.1	38.8	35.5	35.3	33.9	39.3	31.7	40	31	31.7	25.7
Number of genes	616	884	1584	582	1207	687	961	886	733	817	524	1069
Number of Coding sequences (CDS)	581	844	1549	547	1173	652	925	840	689	763	475	1037
CDS with assigned functions	287 (49.4%)	293 (34.7%)	299 (19.3%)	219 (40%)	286 (24.3%)	309 (47.4%)	280 (30.3%)	323 (38.4%)	333 (48.3%)	469 (61.5%)	323 (68%)	585 (56.4%)
Number of rRNA												
16S	1	1	1	1	1	1	1	2	1	2	1	1
23S	1	1	1	1	1	1	1	1	1	2	1	1
5S	1	1	1	1	1	1	1	1	1	3	1	1
Number of tRNA	32	32	31	32	31	32	33	32	37	32	36	29
Number of CDS in paralogous families	141 (24.3%)	361 (42.8%)	1103 (71.2%)	134 (24.5%)	748 (63.8%)	371 (56.9%)	454 (49.1%)	265 (31.5%)	132 (19.1%)	110 (14.4%)	25 (5.2%)	245 (23.6%)

Data was obtained from GenBank database using the following accession numbers: *M. parvum* strain Indiana [CP006771.1], *M. suis* strain Illinois [CP002525.1], *M. haemofelis* strain Ohio2 [CP002808.1], "*Candidatus* M. haemominutum" strain Birmingham 1 [HE613254.1], *M. haemocanis* strain Illinois [NC_016638.1], *M. wenyonii* strain Massachusetts [NC_018149.1], and "*Candidatus* M. haemolamae" strain Purdue [NC_018219], *M. ovis* strain Michigan [CP006935], *M. pneumoniae* [U00089], *M. gallisepticum* [AE015450], *M. genitalium* [L43967], and *M. penetrans* [BA000026]. Paralogous gene families were assigned using BLASTclust, with 70% coverage and 30% sequence identity thresholds.

A total of 581 protein-coding sequences (CDS) were predicted and putative functions were assigned and manually verified using the Manatee annotation pipeline: 287 CDS have putative functional identities, representing almost 50% of the CDS, while the other 50% were represented by hypothetical proteins. Further, 24.3% of the genome is dedicated to duplicated genes organized in paralogous families, mostly composed of hypothetical CDS (Table 1).

Hemoplasmas and their phylogenomic relationship based on ANI and Tetranucleotide signature indexes

A phylogenomic comparison based on average nucleotide identity (ANI) and tetranucleotide signature correlation indexes (tetra) was performed amongst selected hemoplasmas with sequenced genomes (Table 2). *M. parvum* had an ANI varying from 83.6% to 89.5% when compared to other hemoplasma genomes, including *M. suis*. The tetra correlation indexes of *M. parvum* with other genomes had a range of 0.47 to 0.88. Both ANI and tetra correlation indexes were below the cutoff values of 94% and 0.99, respectively, for species circumscription.

Table 2: Average nucleotide identity* (ANI) and tetranucleotide signature (Tetra) correlation indexes of selected hemotrophic mycoplasmas

	M. suis str. Illinois		*M. suis* str. KI3806		*M. haemofelis* str. Ohio2		*M. haemofelis* str. Langford		*M. haemocanis* str. Illinois		*M. wenyonii* str. Massachusetts		"*Candidatus* M. haemominutum" str. Birmingham 1		"*Candidatus* M. haemolamae" str. Purdue	
	ANI	Tetra	ANI	Tetra	ANI	Tetra	ANI	Tetra	ANI	Tetra	ANI	Tetra	ANI	Tetra	ANI	Tetra
M. parvum str. Indiana	83.94	0.87987	83.65	0.88079	84.66	0.47545	84.3	0.47625	84.04	0.57312	87.33	0.75006	88.45	0.59954	89.48	0.59873
M. suis str. Illinois			97.74	0.997	85.41	0.365	84.83	0.366	85.59	0.452	85.24	0.75777	89.48	0.54917	89.34	0.54636
M. suis str. KI3806					85.3	0.372	87.74	0.372	85.5	0.453	85.5	0.7632	89.57	0.56269	88.6	0.55492
M. haemofelis str. Ohio2							97.3	0.999	85.11	0.959	85.75	0.45892	84.84	0.4172	85.73	0.60193
M. haemofelis str. Langford									85.21	0.962	85.84	0.45953	84.99	0.41409	85.74	0.59729
M. haemocanis str. Illinois											85.71	0.51169	85.58	0.45207	86.32	0.62344
M. wenyonii str. Massachusetts													90.25	0.52911	88.21	0.62571
"*Candidatus* M. haemominutum" str. Birmingham 1															89.83	0.63665

The genomes used for the analyses are available in GenBank under the following accession numbers: *M. parvum* strain Indiana [CP006771.1], *M. suis* strain Illinois [CP002525.1], *M. suis* strain KI3806 [FQ790233.1], *M. haemofelis* strain Ohio2 [CP002808.1], *M. haemofelis* strain Langford [FR773153.2], *M. haemocanis* strain Illinois [NC_016638.1], *M. wenyonii* strain Massachusetts [NC_018149.1], "*Candidatus* M. haemominutum" strain Birmingham 1 [HE613254.1], and "*Candidatus* M. haemolamae" strain Purdue [NC_018219].

*ANI was calculated using MUMmer algorithm in JSpecies software.

Comparing all these species of hemoplasmas, ANI and tetra correlation indexes were between 83.6%-90.25% and 0.36-0.96, respectively, correctly separating these organisms as different species of mycoplasmas. On the contrary, strains of the same species (*M. suis* Illinois and KI3806; *M. haemofelis* Ohio2 and Langford1) showed ANI and tetranucleotide correlation indexes above the proposed thresholds for species definition, as expected.

M. parvum versus *M. suis*: similarities and differences at the genomic level

A complete comparison at the genomic level was performed between the genomes of *M. parvum* strain Indiana and *M. suis* strain Illinois (Figure 3). The genome of *M. suis* is 178 Kb bigger than that of *M. parvum*. SynMap analysis indicated a lack of overall gene synteny between *M. suis* and *M. parvum*. Although some conserved blocks of genes, mostly corresponding to operons (e.g. PTS system), were observed, they do not necessarily occur at the same relative position of the genomes. A more detailed, manual analysis shows that the 16S rRNA gene and 5S-23S rRNA operon of *M. parvum* are located in the first half of its genome (dnaA at position zero), while *M. suis* copies are in the second half of its genome. Moreover, most of the CDS classified by TIGR role category are organized in a different fashion when comparing both genomes (Figure 3). Despite these rearrangements, both genomes share all CDS with known assigned metabolic or other functions, such as transporters and putative virulence factors; this represents 49.4% and 34.7% of the *M. parvum* and *M. suis* genomes, respectively. The remainder of both genomes consisted in hypothetical CDS, most of which are dedicated to paralogous gene families: *M. parvum* has 141 CDS (24.3%) distributed into 38 paralogous gene families, while *M. suis* has 361 CDS (42.8%) in 68 paralogous gene families (Table 1). Twenty-three out of the 38 paralog families of *M. parvum* are represented in the genome of *M. suis* (with a variable number of members per family between the genomes). In contrast, *M. suis* has 40 out of 68 families that are found exclusively in its genome. This difference in paralogous genes is represented by 188 exclusive CDS in the genome of *M. suis* and 64 CDS unique of *M. parvum*. Considering the hypothetical CDS that are not in paralogous families, both genomes share 74 of these, whereas 63 CDS are found only in *M. parvum* and 153 CDS only in *M. suis*. In total, *M. parvum* has a set of 127 unique CDS, while *M. suis* has 341 CDS found exclusively in its genome.

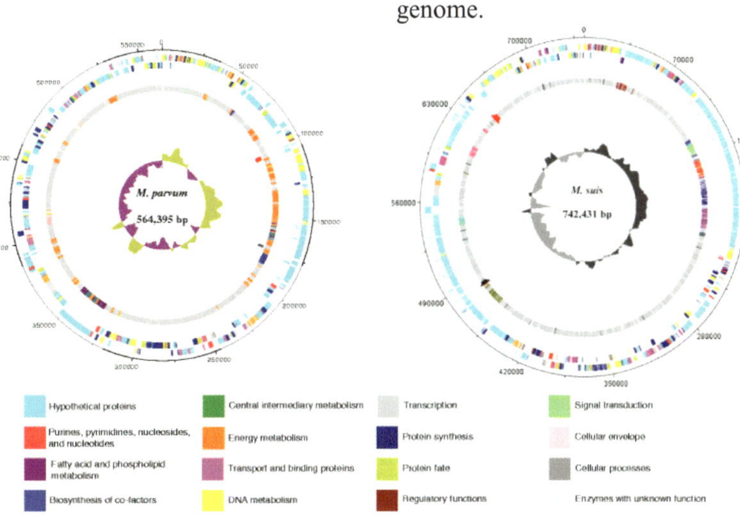

Figure 3: Circular representation of the genomes of *M. parvum* strain Indiana and *M. suis* strain Illinois showing the organization of the coding sequences (CDS). The dnaA gene is at position zero in both genome plots. Outer to inner circles: circle 1: predicted CDS on the positive strand;

circle 2: predicted CDS on the negative strand. Each CDS is classified by TIGR role category according to the color designation in the legend below the plots; circle 3: CDS in the largest paralogous gene families with each family represented by a different color in each genome, non-paralogous CDS are light grey. Paralogous families of *M. parvum* with less than 5 CDS are represented in orange. Black and red marks represent the 16S rRNA gene and the 23S/5S rRNA gene operon, respectively. Circle 4: GC skew. The diagrams were generated using Artemis 12.0 - DNAPlotter version 1.4, Sanger Institute. (*M. suis* plot was extracted from Guimaraes AM, Santos AP, SanMiguel P, Walter T, Timenetsky J, Messick JB: Complete genome sequence of *Mycoplasma suis* and insights into its biology and adaption to an erythrocyte niche. *PLoS One* 2011, 6:e19574 [1], with permission from the copyright holder).

The set of unique CDS of *M. parvum* and *M. suis* were analyzed for subcellular localization and protein sorting signals [22],[23], and the presence of signal peptide cleavage sites [24]. Moreover, the presence of lipoproteins was predicted [25] (Table 3). The majority (54.0-66.5%) of the unique CDS either in paralogous families or not from both *M. parvum* and *M. suis* have an unknown subcellular localization. The remaining CDS are distributed into cytoplasmic membrane, cytoplasmic, and extracellular localization. The unique CDS not in paralogous families from both bacteria are divided mainly into cytoplasmic membrane and cytoplasmic localization, with a smaller number of CDS having a predicted extracellular localization. In contrast, the unique CDS in paralogous families are mostly located in the cytosol, and just a few CDS have cytoplasmic membrane or extracellular localization. The most frequent protein sorting signal amongst all unique CDS is the presence of 1 internal helix, followed by a signal peptide. Analyses of the CDS in paralogous families show that a higher number of CDS of *M. suis* (16.5% by PSORTb, and 4.25% by SignalP) have signal peptides compared to *M. parvum* (1.6% bt PSORTb, and 0% by SignalP). Only three lipoproteins (SpII) were identified using LipoP: one unique CDS not paralog of *M. parvum*, one unique CDS not paralog of *M. suis*, and one unique CDS paralog of *M. suis*.

Table 3: Unique CDS of *M. parvum* strain Indiana and *M. suis* strain Illinois: subcellular localization and protein sorting signals (PSORTb v3.0.2), presence of signal peptide cleavage sites (SignalP), and presence of lipoproteins (LipoP)

Software & parameters	*M. parvum* - unique CDS not in paralogous families	*M. parvum* - unique CDS in paralogous families	*M. suis* - unique CDS not in paralogous families	*M. suis* - unique CDS in paralogous families
PSORTb				
Subcellular localization:				
Unknown	34 (54.0%)	37 (57.8%)	83 (54.2%)	125 (66.5%)
Cytoplasmic Membrane	13 (20.6%)	3 (4.7%)	31 (20.3%)	12 (6.4%)
Cytoplasmic	11 (17.5%)	23 (35.9%)	29 (18.97%)	43 (22.9%)
Extracellular	5 (7.9%)	1 (1.6%)	10 (6.53%)	8 (4.2%)
Features:				
1 internal helix found	30 (47.6%)	20 (31.25%)	77 (50.3%)	153 (81.4%)
2 internal helices found	0	0	7 (4.6%)	0
3 internal helices found	0	0	2 (1.3%)	0
Signal peptide detected	3 (4.8%)	1 (1.6%)	18 (11.8%)	31 (16.5%)
None	30 (47.6%)	43 (67.15%)	49 (32%)	4 (2.1%)
SignalP				
YES	3 (4.8%)	0	11 (7.2%)	8 (4.2%)
NO	60 (95.2%)	64 (100%)	142 (92.8%)	180 (95.8%)
LipoP				
SpI	8 (12.7%)	9 (14.0%)	36 (23.5%)	65 (34.6%)
SpII	0	1 (1.6%)	1 (0.65%)	1 (0.53%)
TMH	2 (3.2%)	3 (4.7%)	18 (11.8%)	29 (15.4%)
None	53 (84.1%)	51 (79.7%)	98 (64.05%)	93 (49.47%)
Total	**63**	**64**	**153**	**188**

PSORTb: results were obtained using the output for Gram-negative bacteria without outer membrane.
SignalP: YES: signal peptide present, NO: signal peptide absent.
LipoP: SpI: signal peptide (signal peptidase I), SpII: lipoprotein signal peptide (signal peptidase II), TMH: n-terminal transmembrane helix. Note from the software: TMH is generally not a very reliable prediction and should be tested. This part of the model is mainly there to avoid transmembrane helices being falsely predicted as signal peptide.

DISCUSSION

The course of infection with *M. parvum* strain Indiana in the single splenectomized pig evaluated was distinguished from what is commonly seen in *M. suis* infection by the absence of clinical signs, even at the peak of bacteremia. While the bacteremia was apparently fleeting with organisms detected on peripheral blood smears for only a few days after the peak, its persistence at low levels were shown by qPCR. However, these observations are limited to the strain of *M. parvum* described herein and to the animal selected for this study. Further studies should be conducted to evaluate the actual virulence of this isolate, including possible variation among strains and individual pigs. Since the prevalence of *M. parvum* by age is unknown, it is not possible to speculate when this animal got infected with this organism. It is likely, however, that an immune response had developed, which effectively controlled the infection, reducing the bacterial loads. Another possibility is that the use of subtherapeutic doses of antibiotics in the feed at the farm may have controlled the infection. However, the bacteria were not completely eliminated and the animal developed a chronic infection, as is often observed with other hemoplasma species [30]. In contrast, the fever and bacteremia in a splenectomized pig that is infected with *M. suis* is unrelenting and without antibiotics the animal may die [31]–[33], which was not observed after splenectomy in the animal herein. The impact of acute and chronic hemoplasma infection on the immune system of the host has been poorly explored [34], and is an ongoing area of investigation in our laboratory.

In this report, *M. parvum* strain Indiana was described morphologically by light and scanning electron microscopy and its genome was completely sequenced, analyzed and compared to the genome of *M. suis*strain Illinois. A transient bacteremia was demonstrated by light microscopy, whereas SEM confirmed the rod and coccoid morphology, epicellular location, and small size of *M. parvum* (Figure 2B) [11]. Its size, 0.2 to 0.5 μm, was similar to that reported for other hemoplasmas [35], but remarkably smaller than that reported for *M. suis* with ring forms approaching 1.0 to 2.5 μm in diameter [11],[36]–[38]. The level of bacteremia for *M. parvum* at its peak as shown by qPCR was considerably less (one log) than that previously reported for *M. suis*[16].

M. parvum has the smallest single, circular chromosome of all the *Mycoplasma* genomes sequenced to date. The characteristics of the *M. parvum* genome, including its small size, low G + C content, use of UGA codon to encode tryptophan, and number of tRNA and rRNA were in agreement with those reported for the genomes of other hemoplasmas and are typical of mycoplasmas [1],[4],[6]. In addition, the percentage of CDS dedicated to paralogous genes (24.3%) was similar to that reported for other hemoplasmas [1]–[8],[10]. Our group and others have hypothesized that archived sequences of these genes distributed throughout the chromosome play a role in the ability of mycoplasma organisms to persist despite an active host immune response [39].

Phylogenetic studies of *M. parvum* and *M. suis,* based on sequence analyses of the 16S rRNA and RNase P genes, suggest that these bacteria are closely related [13],[14]. Some authors have reported that *M. parvum* is an immature developmental stage of *M. suis* that is present concurrently with the mature pathogen [33],[37]. A phylogenomic approach based on ANI and tetranucleotide signatures that uses whole genome sequence information to compare different organisms provides a better resolution than single gene sequence approaches. It is comparable to the method considered as the gold standard for prokaryotic species definition, the DDH [15]. ANI and tetranucleotide results in this study were below the cut-off values for species definition separating all the organisms included in the analyses as distinct species of hemotrophic mycoplasmas. *M. parvum* is, indeed, a distinct species infecting the pig. Further, strains of the same species were clearly distinguished by ANI and tetra scores above the proposed threshold.

M. parvum and *M. suis*, share the same host, the pig; the same environment, the blood; and are phylogenetically, the closest related relatives of one another [13],[14]. However, the interaction of these bacteria with their host is completely distinct. *M. suis* may cause life threatening hemolytic anemia during acute infection [30],[40], while the strain of *M. parvum* shown in this study, and in agreement with previous reports about this organism [11], caused no clinical signs even at the peak of bacteremia in a young, splenectomized pig. At the genomic level, these bacteria are remarkably similar: they share all CDS with known functions. Their genomic synteny, however, is not well conserved. This loss of conservation in the gene order is expected, as different species of hemoplasmas rarely share large syntenic regions, with the exception of *M. haemofelis* and *M. haemocanis*[41]. Nevertheless, the genome of *M. parvum* has orthologous for all the CDS with metabolic functions identified in the genome of *M. suis*, implying that their metabolic pathways work very similarly and they have the same requirements for many nutrients to be acquired from the blood environment [1]. The putative virulence factors described for the *M. suis* genome are also present in *M. parvum*, which raises the question about what is different between these hemoplasmas that reflects in their contrasting pathogenicity. A gene-by-gene comparison between these organisms revealed that their only difference at the genomic level relies in the hypothetical CDS, mostly dedicated to paralogous gene families. *M. suis* has 40 paralogous families that are exclusive to its genome, while *M. parvum* has 15 families that are not found in *M. suis* . In addition, the largest paralogous family (37 CDS) of *M. suis* is unique. Interestingly, the set of unique paralogous CDS of *M. suis* have a higher percentage of signal peptides detected compared to *M. parvum* CDS; this might indicate that these CDS are secreted or inserted into the membrane and therefore they could play an important role in the pathogenicity of *M. suis* as reported for other bacteria [42],[43]. The differences regarding the percentages of signal peptides detected by all three software (PSORTb, SignalP, and LipoP) are due to their distinct prediction algorithms. PSORTb is the only tool amongst the three applied in this study that provides an output for Gram-negative bacteria with no outer membrane or cell wall. It is presumed more accurate for *Mycoplasma* species, which although more phylogenetically similar to Gram-positive organisms, lack a peptidoglycan cell wall.

The maintenance of paralogous gene families in their genomes appears to be a high priority among the hemoplasmas. A prominent role for paralogous genes in the development of antigenic variation has been reported for bacterial species of the genus *Anaplasma*, *Ehrlichia*, *Borrelia* and *Mycoplasma* and linked to virulence as well as persistence of these infections [44]. It is tempting to speculate that differences in paralogous families between *M. parvum* and *M. suis* may be implicated in their differing pathogenic potential.However, this might also be due to variable expression of core genes, especially genes encoding putative virulence factors or to the presence and variable expression of regulatory RNA. The latter has been previously reported for pathogenic versus non-pathogenic bacteria species of *Listeria*[45], while variable expression of virulence genes was observed for different strains of *Escherichia coli*[46], and *Listeria monocytogenes*[47]. An investigation on the differences at the RNA level between *M. parvum* and *M. suis* is warranted, and it is an ongoing project in our laboratory.

Nucleotide sequence accession number

The genome of *M. parvum* strain Indiana was deposited in GenBank under the accession number [CP006771.1].

DECLARATIONS

Acknowledgements

We are extremely grateful to The Genomic Core Facility at Purdue University for constructing the library, running the HiSeq 2000 and performing the ABySS assembly. We also thank the University of Maryland's Institute of Genomic Sciences, which provided us with the manual annotation pipeline Manatee. This work was kindly supported by the Morris Animal Foundation (grant D10FE-0042), and the Brazilian government through CNPq Fellowship Program (Conselho Nacional de Desenvolvimento Científico e Tecnológico) for Postdoctoral Researcher to Dr do Nascimento.

Authors' contributions

Conceived and designed experiments: NCN, APS, YC, AMSG, JBM. Performed experiments: NCN, APS, YC, AMSG, JBM. Analyzed the data: NCN, APS, YC, AMSG, JBM. Anesthesia and splenectomy: ANB, ABW. Wrote and reed the paper: NCN, APS, YC, AMSG, ANB, ABW, JBM. All authors read and approved the final manuscript.

REFERENCES

1. Guimaraes AM, Santos AP, SanMiguel P, Walter T, Timenetsky J, Messick JB: Complete genome sequence of *Mycoplasma suis* and insights into its biology and adaption to an erythrocyte niche. PLoS One. 2011, 6: e19574-10.1371/journal.pone.0019574.
2. Oehlerking J, Kube M, Felder KM, Matter D, Wittenbrink MM, Schwarzenbach S, Kramer MM, Hoelzle K, Hoelzle LE: Complete genome sequence of the hemotrophic *Mycoplasma suis* strain KI3806. J Bacteriol. 2011, 193: 2369-2370. 10.1128/JB.00187-11.
3. Barker EN, Helps CR, Peters IR, Darby AC, Radford AD, Tasker S: Complete genome sequence of *Mycoplasma haemofelis*, a hemotropic mycoplasma. J Bacteriol. 2011, 193: 2060-2061. 10.1128/JB.00076-11.
4. Santos AP, Guimaraes AMS, Do Nascimento NC, Sanmiguel PJ, Martin SW, Messick JB: Genome of *Mycoplasma haemofelis*, unraveling its strategies for survival and persistence. Vet Res. 2011, 42: 102-10.1186/1297-9716-42-102.
5. Barker EN, Darby AC, Helps CR, Peters IR, Hughes MA, Radford AD, Novacco M, Boretti FS, Hofmann-Lehmann R, Tasker S: Genome sequence for "*Candidatus* Mycoplasma haemominutum," a low-pathogenicity hemoplasma species. J Bacteriol. 2012, 194: 905-906. 10.1128/JB.06560-11.
6. Do Nascimento NC, Santos AP, Guimaraes AM, Sanmiguel PJ, Messick JB:*Mycoplasma haemocanis* - the canine hemoplasma and its feline counterpart in the genomic era. Vet Res. 2012, 43: 66-10.1186/1297-9716-43-66.
7. Dos Santos AP, Guimaraes AM, Do Nascimento NC, SanMiguel PJ, Messick JB: Complete genome sequence of *Mycoplasma wenyonii* strain Massachusetts. J Bacteriol. 2012, 194: 5458-5459. 10.1128/JB.01240-12.
8. Guimaraes AM, Toth B, Santos AP, Do Nascimento NC, Kritchevsky JE, Messick JB: Genome sequence of "*Candidatus*Mycoplasma haemolamae" strain purdue, a red blood cell pathogen of alpacas (*Vicugna pacos*) and llamas (*Lama glama*). J Bacteriol. 2012, 194: 6312-6313. 10.1128/JB.01557-12.
9. Do Nascimento NC, Dos Santos AP, Chu Y, Guimaraes AM, Pagliaro A, Messick JB: Genome sequence of *Mycoplasma parvum* (formerly *Eperythrozoon parvum*), a diminutive hemoplasma of the pig. Genome Announc. 2013, 1: pii:e00986-13. 10.1128/genomeA.00986-13.
10. Deshuillers PL, Santos AP, Do Nascimento NC, Hampel JA, Bergin IL, Dyson MC, Messick JB: Complete genome sequence of *Mycoplasma ovis* strain Michigan, a hemoplasma of sheep with two distinct 16S rRNA genes. Genome Announc. 2014, 2: e01235-13. 10.1128/genomeA.01235-13.
11. Splitter EJ:*Eperythrozoon suis* n. sp. and *Eperythrozoon parvum* n. sp., 2 new blood parasites of swine. Science. 1950, 111: 513-514. 10.1126/science.111.2889.513.
12. Seamer J: Studies with *Eperythrozoon parvum* Splitter, 1950. Parasitology. 1960, 50: 67-80. 10.1017/S0031182000025208.
13. Zhou RQ, Nie K, Huang HC, Hu SJ, Zhou ZY, Luo HL: Phylogenetic analysis of *Mycoplasma suis* isolates based on 16S rRNA gene sequence in China. Vet Res Commun. 2009, 33: 855-863. 10.1007/s11259-009-9234-3.
14. Watanabe Y, Fujihara M, Obara H, Nagai K, Harasawa R: Two genetic clusters in swine hemoplasmas revealed by analyses of the 16S rRNA and RNase P RNA genes. J Vet Med Sci. 2011, 73: 1657-1661. 10.1292/jvms.11-0293.
15. Richter M, Rosselló-Móra R: Shifting the genomic gold standard for the prokaryotic species definition. Proc Natl Acad Sci U S A. 2009, 106: 19126-19131. 10.1073/pnas.0906412106.
16. Guimaraes AMS, Vieira RFC, Polleto R, Vemulapalli R, Santos AP, De Moraes W, Cubas ZS, Santos LC, Marchant-Forde JN, Timenetsky J, Biondo AW, Messick JB: A quantitative TaqMan PCR assay for the detection of *Mycoplasma suis*. J Appl Microbiol. 2011, 111: 417-425. 10.1111/j.1365-2672.2011.05053.x.
17. Messick JB, Cooper SK, Huntley M: Development and evaluation of a polymerase chain reaction assay using the 16S rRNA gene for the detection or *Eperythrozoon suis* infection. J Vet Diagn Invest. 1999, 11: 229-236. 10.1177/104063879901100304.
18. Simpson JT, Wong K, Jackman SD, Schein JE, Jones SJ, Birol I: ABySS: a parallel assembler for short read sequence data. Genome Res. 2009, 19: 1117-1123. 10.1101/gr.089532.108.
19. Ogata H, Goto S, Sato K, Fujibuchi W, Bono H, Kanehisa M: KEGG: Kyoto encyclopedia of genes and genomes. Nucleic Acids Res. 1999, 27: 29-34. 10.1093/nar/27.1.29.
20. Yus E, Maier T, Michalodimitrakis K, Van Noort V, Yamada T, Chen WH, Wodke JA, Güell M, Martínez S, Bourgeois R, Kühner S, Raineri E, Letunic I, Kalinina OV, Rode M, Herrmann R, Gutiérrez-Gallego

R, Russell RB, Gavin AC, Bork P, Serrano L: Impact of genome reduction on bacterial metabolism and its regulation. Science. 2009, 326: 1263-1268. 10.1126/science.1177263.

21. Biegert A, Mayer C, Remmert M, Söding J, Lupas AN: The MPI bioinformatics toolkit for protein sequence analysis. Nucleic Acids Res. 2006, 34: W335-W339. 10.1093/nar/gkl217.

22. Nakai K, Horton P: PSORT: a program for detecting sorting signals in proteins and predicting their subcellular localization. Trends Biochem Sci. 1999, 24: 34-36. 10.1016/S0968-0004(98)01336-X.

23. Yu NY, Wagner JR, Laird MR, Melli G, Rey S, Lo R, Dao P, Sahinalp SC, Ester M, Foster LJ, Brinkman FS: PSORTb 3.0: improved protein subcellular localization prediction with refined localization subcategories and predictive capabilities for all prokaryotes. Bioinformatics. 2010, 26: 1608-1615. 10.1093/bioinformatics/btq249.

24. Petersen TN, Brunak S, Von Heijne G, Nielsen H: SignalP 4.0: discriminating signal peptides from transmembrane regions. Nat Methods. 2011, 8: 785-786. 10.1038/nmeth.1701.

25. Juncker AS, Willenbrock H, Von Heijne G, Brunak S, Nielsen H, Krogh A: Prediction of lipoprotein signal peptides in Gram-negative bacteria. Protein Sci. 2003, 12: 1652-1662. 10.1110/ps.0303703.

26. CoGePedia [https://www.genomevolution.org/wiki/index.php/Main_Page]

27. SynMap whole genome synteny [https://genomevolution.org/CoGe/SynMap.pl]

28. Robertshaw D: Temperature regulation and thermal environment. Dukes' Physiology of Domestic Animals. Edited by: Reece WO. 2004, Cornell University Press, New York, 12

29. Thorn CE: Normal hematology of the pig. Schalm's Veterinary Hematology. Edited by: Feldman BF, Zinkl JG, Jain NC. 2000, Lippincott Williams and Wilkins, Philadelphia, 1089-1095. 5

30. Messick JB: Hemotrophic mycoplasmas (hemoplasmas): a re and new insights into pathogenic potential. Vet Clin Pathol. 2004, 33: 2-13. 10.1111/j.1939-165X.2004.tb00342.x.

31. Heinritzi K, Peteranderl W, Plank G:*Eperythrozoon* infection in swine: effect on the acid–base balance and the glucose, lactate and pyruvate content of venous blood. Dtsch Tierarztl Wochenschr. 1990, 97: 31-34. (in German),

32. Heinritzi K, Plank G: The effect of *Eperythrozoon suis* infection on the osmotic fragility of erythrocytes. Berl Munch Tierarztl Wochenschr. 1992, 105: 380-383.

33. Dent BT, Stevens KA, Korvick DL, Clymer JW:*Mycoplasma suis* infection in pigs after splenectomy. Lab Anim (NY). 2013, 42: 125-128. 10.1038/laban.171. (in German),

34. Novacco M, Boretti FS, Franchini M, Riond B, Meli ML, Hofmann-Lehmann R: Protection from reinfection in "*Candidatus*Mycoplasma turicensis"-infected cats and characterization of the immune response. Vet Res. 2012, 43: 82-10.1186/1297-9716-43-82.

35. Neimark H, Hoff B, Ganter M:*Mycoplasma ovis* comb. nov. (formerly *Eperythrozoon ovis*), an epierythrocytic agent of haemolytic anaemia in sheep and goats. Int J Syst Evol Microbiol. 2004, 54: 365-371. 10.1099/ijs.0.02858-0.

36. Pospischil A, Hoffmann R:*Eperythrozoon suis* in naturally infected pigs: a light and electron microscopic study. Vet Pathol. 1982, 19: 651-657. 10.1177/030098588201900609.

37. Liebich HG, Heinritzi K: Light and electron microscopic studies of *Eperythrozoon suis*. Tierarztl Prax. 1992, 20: 270-274. (in German),

38. Groebel K, Hoelzle K, Wittenbrink MM, Ziegler U, Hoelzle LE:*Mycoplasma suis* invades porcine erythrocytes. Infect Immun. 2009, 77: 576-584. 10.1128/IAI.00773-08.

39. Citti C, Nouvel LX, Baranowski E: Phase and antigenic variation in mycoplasmas. Future Microbiol. 2010, 5: 1073-1085. 10.2217/fmb.10.71.

40. Strait EL, Hawkins PA, Wilson WD: Dysgalactia associated with *Mycoplasma suis* infection in a sow herd. J Am Vet Med Assoc. 2012, 241: 1666-1667. 10.2460/javma.241.12.1666.

41. Guimaraes AM, Santos AP, Do Nascimento NC, Timenetsky J, Messick JB: Comparative genomics and phylogenomics of hemotrophic mycoplasmas. PLoS ONE. 2014, 9: e91445-10.1371/journal.pone.0091445.

42. Saleh MT, Fillon M, Brennan PJ, Belisle JT: Identification of putative exported/secreted proteins in prokaryotic proteomes. Gene. 2001, 269: 195-204. 10.1016/S0378-1119(01)00436-X.

43. Leversen NA, De Souza GA, Målen H, Prasad S, Jonassen I, Wiker HG: Evaluation of signal peptide prediction algorithms for identification of mycobacterial signal peptides using sequence data from proteomic methods. Microbiology. 2009, 155: 2375-2383. 10.1099/mic.0.025270-0.

44. Palmer GH: The highest priority: what microbial genomes are telling us about immunity. Vet Immunol Immunopathol. 2002, 85: 1-8. 10.1016/S0165-2427(01)00415-9.

45. Wurtzel O, Sesto N, Mellin JR, Karunker I, Edelheit S, Bécavin C, Archambaud C, Cossart P, Sorek R: Comparative transcriptomics of pathogenic and non-pathogenic *Listeria* species. Mol Syst Biol. 2012, 8: 583-10.1038/msb.2012.11.

46. Dowd SE, Ishizaki H: Microarray based comparison of two *Escherichia coli* O157:H7 lineages. BMC Microbiol. 2006, 6: 30-10.1186/1471-2180-6-30.

47. Severino P, Dussurget O, Vêncio RZ, Dumas E, Garrido P, Padilla G, Piveteau P, Lemaître JP, Kunst F, Glaser P, Buchrieser C: Comparative transcriptome analysis of *Listeria monocytogenes* strains of the two major lineages reveals differences in virulence, cell wall, and stress response. Appl Environ Microbiol. 2007, 73: 6078-6088. 10.1128/AEM.02730-06.

CHAPTER 11

ANTIBIOTIC SUSCEPTIBILITY PROFILES OF MYCOPLASMA BOVIS STRAINS ISOLATED FROM CATTLE IN HUNGARY, CENTRAL EUROPE

Kinga M Sulyok, Zsuzsa Kreizinger, Lilla Fekete, Veronika Hrivnák, Tibor Magyar, Szilárd Jánosi, Nóra Schweitzer, Ibolya Turcsányi, László Makrai, Károly Erdélyi and Miklós Gyuranecz

Keywords: Antibiotic resistance, MIC, Fluoroquinolones, Microbroth dilution, Mycoplasma bovis

BACKGROUND

Mycoplasma bovis is a widely distributed pathogen, first isolated in the USA in 1961 from a case of severe mastitis in cattle [1]. It is associated with various diseases in cattle including calf pneumonia, mastitis, arthritis, otitis media and genital disorders [2]. *M. bovis* is considered responsible for a quarter to a third of economic losses in the cattle industry caused by respiratory diseases [3].

In Hungary, the average seropositivity rate of individual animals was found to be 11.3%, in certain herds it even exceeded 50.0%. Tested by enzyme-linked immunosorbent assay the overall rate of seropositive herds was 64.7% [4]. With the exception of seroprevalence on individual level, these values are relatively high in a European context [3],[5].

Since no effective vaccine is available against *M. bovis*, adequate housing and appropriate antibiotic treatment are promoted in the control of the diseases caused by this agent. Antibiotic therapy of mastitis has often failed, but antimicrobial treatment of pneumonia has shown some success and it may help reduce economic losses [3],[6]. Mycoplasmas are intrinsically resistant to β-lactam antimicrobials and sulphonamides, because they do not possess a cell wall and do not synthesize folic acid. Mycoplasmas are generally susceptible to antibiotics that affect protein (tetracyclines, macrolides, lincosamides, phenicols) or nucleic acid synthesis (fluoroquinolones) [2]. The decreased effectiveness of certain antimicrobial agents (spectinomycin, oxytetracycline and tilmicosin) traditionally used in the therapy of mycoplasma infections was reported in Europe [7].

The aim of this study was to determine the susceptibility of 35 Hungarian *M. bovis* isolates to eleven antibiotics using the microbroth dilution method.

METHODS

Thirty-five *M. bovis* strains originating from dairy herds located in different parts of Hungary were tested in this study (Table 1, Figure 1). The samples were collected during routine diagnostic examinations or necropsies between 2010 and 2013. Ethical approval was not required for the study as all samples were collected during routine diagnostic examinations or necropsies. Nasal swabs, lung samples and a single lymph node were homogenized in 2 ml of *Mycoplasma* broth medium (pH 7.8) (Thermo Fisher Scientific Inc./Oxoid Inc./, Waltham, MA) supplemented with 0.5% (w/v) sodium pyruvate, 0.5% (w/v) glucose and 0.005% (w/v) phenol red and cultured at 37°C in a 5% CO_2 atmosphere. Following colour change (red to yellow shift) the cultures were inoculated onto solid *Mycoplasma* media (Thermo Fisher Scientific Inc. /Oxoid

Citation: Kinga M Sulyok, Zsuzsa Kreizinger, Lilla Fekete, Veronika Hrivnák, Tibor Magyar, Szilárd Jánosi, Nóra Schweitzer, Ibolya Turcsányi, László Makrai, Károly Erdélyi and Miklós Gyuranecz, Antibiotic susceptibility profiles of Mycoplasma bovis strains isolated from cattle in Hungary, Central Europe, DOI: 10.1186/s12917-014-0256-x.

Inc./) and were incubated at 37°C and 5% CO_2 for 3 days, until visible colonies appeared. Mixed cultures were filter cloned only once to exclude contaminant *Mycoplasma* species and to minimize *in vitro* mutations of the isolates. DNA extraction was performed using the QIAamp DNA Mini Kit (Qiagen Inc., Hilden, Germany) according to the manufacturers' instructions for Gram-negative bacteria. All isolates were identified by polymerase chain reaction (PCR) targeting the *uvr*C gene of *M. bovis*[8]. The purity of the cultures (e.g. to exclude *M. arginini* or other *Mycoplasma* spp. contamination) was confirmed by a universal *Mycoplasma* PCR system targeting the 16S/23S rRNA intergenic spacer region in Mollicutes [9] followed by sequencing on an ABI Prism 3100 automated DNA sequencer (Applied Biosystems, Foster City, CA), sequence analysis and BLAST search. The same once filter cloned passage of each *M. bovis* strain was submitted for a 4 gene based multi-locus sequence typing (MLST) and the sequencing data confirmed the purity of the isolates at strain level (i.e. not more than one *M. bovis* strain in the culture) [10]. Mixed primary cultures which failed to be purified by a single filter cloning were excluded from the study (data not shown). Aliquots of the third passage of purified cultures were stored frozen at −70°C until required. The number of colour changing units (CCU) was calculated by microplate dilution method, from the lowest dilution showing colour change after one week of incubation [11],[12].

Table 1: Background information and MIC data of the 35 Hungarian *M. bovis* isolates included in this study

Sample ID	Origin of herd	Date	Sample source	MIC values (µg/ml)										
				Fluoroquinolones			Aminoglycosides		Tetracyclines		Macrolides		Phenicol	Lincosamide
				Danofloxacin	Enrofloxacin	Marbofloxacin	Gentamicin	Spectinomycin	Oxytetracycline	Tetracycline	Tilmicosin	Tylosn	Florfenicol	Lincomycin
PG45	Connecticut	1961	Lung	0.156	0.156	0.625	4	4	2	0.25	0.5	0.5	4	1
MYC2	Püspökhatvan	2011	Lung	0.156	0.156	0.625	2	2	16	4	128	16	4	1
MYC22	Sümeg	2012	Lung	0.156	0.312	0.625	4	256	64	16	128	128	8	64
MYC30	Bugyi	2012	Lung	0.156	0.156	0.625	4	256	32	8	128	128	4	64
MYC42	Nemti	2012	Lung	0.156	0.156	0.625	8	4	64	8	128	32	8	1
MYC43	Zsana	2012	Lung	0.156	0.156	0.312	4	256	64	16	128	128	8	64
MYC44	Győrszentiván	2012	Lung	10	10	10	2	256	64	8	128	128	8	64
MYC45	Budapest	2012	Lung	10	10	10	2	256	64	8	128	128	4	64
MYC46	Budapest	2012	Lung	10	10	10	4	256	64	8	128	128	8	64
MYC47	Dabas	2012	Lung	0.156	0.156	0.625	8	256	64	8	128	128	8	64
MYC48	Ősi	2012	Nasal swab	0.156	0.156	0.625	8	256	64	16	128	128	4	64
MYC49	Ősi	2012	Nasal swab	0.156	0.156	0.625	8	256	64	16	128	128	4	64
MYC50	Ősi	2012	Lung	0.156	0.156	0.625	4	256	64	8	128	128	4	64
MYC51	Ősi	2012	Nasal swab	0.156	0.08	0.312	4	256	64	8	128	128	4	64
MYC52	Solt	2012	Lung	0.156	0.156	0.312	8	4	2	0.25	0.5	0.5	4	0.5
MYC53	Solt	2012	Lung	0.156	0.156	0.625	16	4	2	0.25	0.5	0.5	4	1
MYC65	Csengersima	2012	Nasal swab	0.156	0.156	0.625	2	2	64	16	128	8	4	0.5
MYC66	Csengersima	2012	Nasal swab	0.156	0.156	0.625	8	4	64	8	128	16	8	1
MYC67	Csengersima	2012	Lung	0.08	0.08	0.312	4	4	16	4	128	16	8	2
MYC68	Csengersima	2012	Lung	0.156	0.156	0.625	4	4	32	4	128	16	4	0.5
MYC69	Komárom	2013	Nasal swab	0.156	0.156	0.625	2	4	32	8	128	32	8	1
MYC70	Komárom	2013	Nasal swab	0.156	0.156	0.625	4	2	32	4	128	32	4	1
MYC71	Komárom	2013	Nasal swab	0.156	0.156	0.625	4	2	32	4	128	32	4	1
MYC72	Komárom	2013	Nasal swab	0.156	0.156	0.625	4	4	32	4	128	32	4	1
MYC73	Komárom	2013	Nasal swab	0.156	0.156	0.625	4	4	32	8	128	32	4	1
MYC74	Komárom	2013	Nasal swab	0.156	0.156	0.625	4	4	32	8	128	16	4	1
MYC75	Komárom	2013	Nasal swab	0.156	0.08	0.312	2	2	32	4	128	32	4	1
MYC76	Komárom	2013	Nasal swab	0.156	0.156	0.625	4	4	64	8	128	16	8	2
MYC77	Kertészsziget	2010	Lung	0.312	0.156	0.625	2	256	64	8	128	128	4	64
MYC78	Hosszúpályi	2011	Lung	0.156	0.156	0.625	4	256	64	8	128	128	4	64
MYC79	Hosszúpályi	2011	Lung	0.156	0.156	0.625	8	256	64	16	128	128	8	64
MYC80	Ebes	2011	Lymph node	0.156	0.156	0.625	4	256	32	4	128	128	4	64
MYC81	Felsőnyárád	2013	Lung	0.156	0.156	0.625	8	256	64	8	128	128	4	64
MYC82	Felsőnyárád	2013	Nasal swab	0.156	0.156	0.625	4	256	64	8	128	128	8	64
MYC83	Alsótold	2013	Lung	0.312	0.156	0.625	4	256	64	8	128	128	8	64
MYC84	Felsőnyárád	2013	Nasal swab	0.156	0.156	0.625	4	256	64	8	128	128	4	64

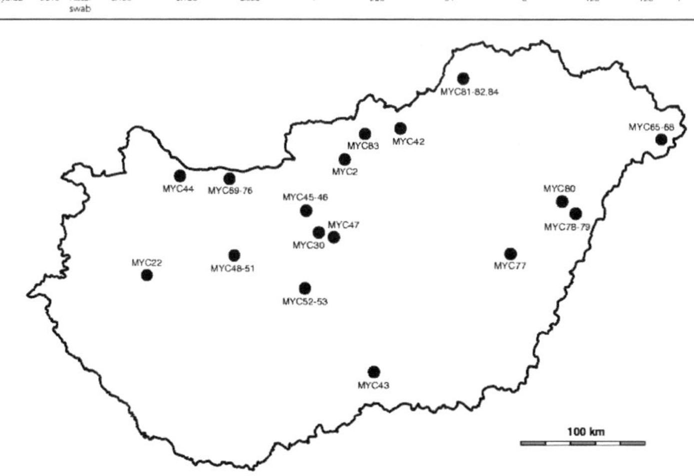

Figure 1: Map of Hungary showing the geographical origins of the 35 *M. bovis* isolates tested.

The following antimicrobial agents were examined during the microbroth dilution tests: three fluoroquinolones: danofloxacin (batch SZBA019XV), enrofloxacin (batch SZBA336XV) and marbofloxacin (batch SZBC248XV); two aminoglycosides: gentamicin (batch 051K17475V) and spectinomycin (batch SZBB166XV); two tetracyclines: oxytetracycline (batch SZBC320XV) and tetracycline (batch SZBA140XV); two macrolides: tilmicosin (batch SZBC345XV) and tylosin (batch SZBB160XV); one phenicol: florfenicol (batch SZBC223XV) and one lincosamide: lincomycin (batch SZBC340XV); all products originated from VETRANAL, Sigma-Aldrich, Germany. They were diluted and stored according to the recommendations of Hannan [11]. Stock solutions of 1 mg/ml enrofloxacin, danofloxacin and marbofloxacin were prepared in 0.1 M NaOH; stock solution of 1 mg/ml florfenicol was prepared in 96% ethanol and in sterile distilled water; and the rest of the stock solutions of 1 mg/ml were prepared in sterile distilled water. All aliquots were stored at −70°C until needed, and dilutions were freshly prepared for each microtest. Twofold dilutions were prepared in the range 0.039-10 μg/ml for fluoroquinolones, 0.125-32 μg/ml for florfenicol, 0.25-64 μg/ml for gentamicin, tetracyclines and lincomycin, 0.5-128 μg/ml for macrolides and 1–256 μg/ml for spectinomycin.

The microbroth dilution test was performed as recommended by Hannan [11] using 10^4-10^5 CCU/ml of each strain. In brief, the 96-wells microtiter plates were designed to contain growth control (broth medium without antibiotic), sterility control (broth medium without antibiotic and *Mycoplasma* inoculum) and pH control (broth medium adjusted to pH 6.8) wells. *Mycoplasma* broth medium (pH 7.8) (Thermo Fisher Scientific Inc./Oxoid Inc./) supplemented with 0.5% (w/v) sodium pyruvate, 0.5% (w/v) glucose and 0.005% (w/v) phenol red was used as a culture medium. The duplicates of three clinical isolates and the duplicate of the type strain (*M. bovis* PG45, NCTC 10131) were tested on each 96-well microtiter plates.

The MIC (minimal inhibitory concentration) value of each isolate was defined as the lowest concentration of the antibiotic that completely inhibits the growth in the broth (no pH and colour change) after a one week incubation period [12]. MIC_{50} and MIC_{90} values were defined as the lowest concentrations that inhibit 50% and 90% of bacterial isolates. The type strain (*M. bovis* PG45, NCTC 10131) was used for the quality control of MIC determination (Table 1).

RESULTS

Our MIC values of *M. bovis* type strain PG45 were identical with values previously obtained for danofloxacin, enrofloxacin, marbofloxacin, spectinomycin, tilmicosin and tylosin using the microbroth dilution method Table 1; [12],[13]. The MIC value of PG45 (2 μg/ml) for oxytetracycline was within the range of previously published studies applying microbroth dilution test (0.1/0.125/0.16/4 μg/ml) [6],[11]-[13]. The MIC value (1 μg/ml) of PG45 for lincomycin was higher than in a previous study (0.25 μg/ml) [13]. For gentamicin, tetracycline, and florfenicol data determined by microbroth dilution test were not available. Our results for type strain PG45 were consistent throughout the study.

The MIC values of the eleven antimicrobial agents obtained from the examinations of the Hungarian *M. bovis*isolates are shown in Figure 2 and listed in Tables 1 and 2. Strains with elevated MIC values were found in the case of all applied antibiotics. Fluoroquinolones were found to be the most active compounds *in vitro*. The antibiotic susceptibility profiles of the Hungarian strains were consistent within the tested group of fluoroquinolones (Figure 2A-C). Three isolates (MYC44, MYC45 and MYC46) had high MIC values (≥10 μg/ml) to danofloxacin, enrofloxacin and marbofloxacin, while the rest of the strains were inhibited by these antimicrobial agents with MICs ≤0.312 or 0.625 μg/ml. The MICs for gentamicin clustered steadily around the MIC_{50} value (4 μg/ml) (Figure 2D). MIC values of spectinomycin divided the strains into two distinct populations, with 48% of isolates yielding MICs of ≤4 μg/ml and the rest clustering with MICs ≥256 μg/ml (Figure 2E). Two *M. bovis* isolates (MYC52 and MYC53) originating from the same herd were inhibited by both tetracyclines and macrolides with low MIC values (Figure 2F-I). Among the macrolides, the MICs of tilmicosin showed bimodal distribution, as two strains yielded MICs ≤0.5 μg/ml, while the rest yielded MICs ≥128 μg/ml. The narrow range of MIC values (4–8 μg/ml) of florfenicol is demonstrated on Figure 2J. MICs for lincomycin also clustered the strains into a group with MICs ≤2 μg/ml and with MICs ≥64 μg/ml (Figure 2K).

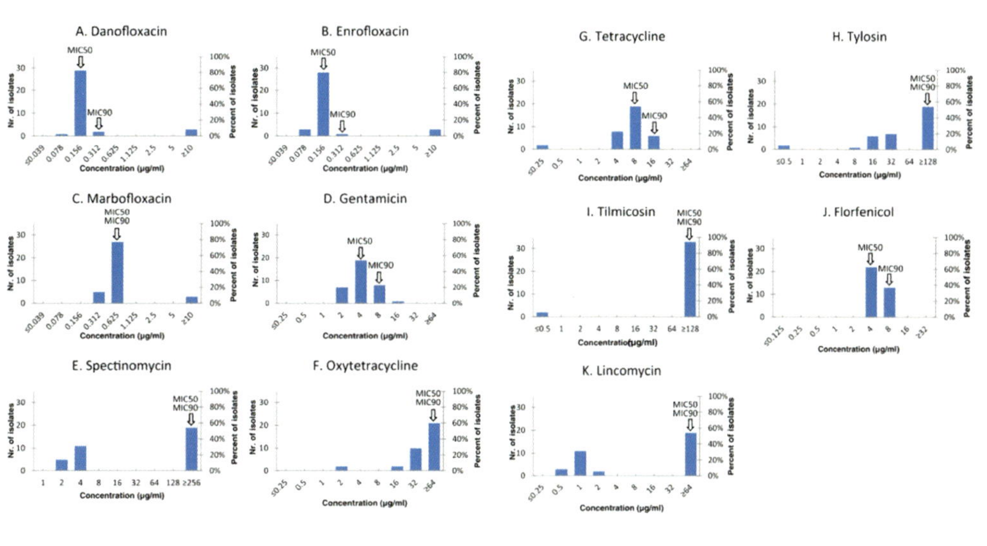

Figure 2: MIC distribution of the Hungarian isolates for each antibiotic tested in this study. Arrows indicate the MIC50 and MIC90 values.

Table 2: Summary of range, mode, MIC_{50} and MIC_{90} values of the 35 *M. bovis* strains isolated from cattle in Hungary

		Range	Mode	MIC_{50}	MIC_{90}
Fluoroquinolones	Danofloxacin	0.078 to ≥10	0.156	0.156	0.312
	Enrofloxacin	0.078 to ≥10	0.156	0.156	0.312
	Marbofloxacin	0.312 to ≥10	0.625	0.625	0.625
Aminoglycosides	Gentamicin	2 to 16	4	4	8
	Spectinomycin	2 to ≥256	≥256	≥256	≥256
Tetracyclines	Oxytetracycline	2 to ≥64	≥64	≥64	≥64
	Tetracycline	≥0.25 to 16	8	8	16
Macrolides	Tylosin	≥0.5 to ≥128	≥128	≥128	≥128
	Tilmicosin	≥0.5 to ≥128	≥128	≥128	≥128
Phenicol	Florfenicol	4 to 8	4	4	8
Lincosamide	Lincomycin	0.5 to ≥64	≥64	≥64	≥64

All values are expressed as μg/ml.

Isolates originating from the same herd showed similar antibiotic susceptibility profiles (Table 1).

DISCUSSION

Gerchman et al. [13] studied 11 *M. bovis* strains isolated from cattle imported from Hungary to Israel between 2005 and 2007. The most active compounds found during *in vitro* examinations were fluoroquinolones (danofloxacin, enrofloxacin and marbofloxacin), which is in accordance with our results, except that the MIC values described before were higher than the ones detected in this study (MIC_{90} 1.25 μg/ml, 1.25 μg/ml, 5 μg/ml versus 0.312 μg/ml, 0.312 μg/ml, 0.625 μg/ml). Decreased spectinomycin susceptibility was detected in the strains from the imported animals (MIC_{90} > 1024 μg/ml obtained with E-test method), which is consistent with our results (MIC_{90}≥256 μg/ml). In contrast to the results obtained by Gerchman et al. [13] (4 μg/ml, 8 μg/ml, 1 μg/ml) the MIC_{90} values of oxytetracycline (≥64 μg/ml), tilmicosin (≥128 μg/ml) and tylosin (≥128 μg/ml) yielded in the present study indicate limited susceptibility to these antibiotics. The comparison of the results of the previous publication and the present study emphasize the importance of the systematic monitoring of antibiotic susceptibility of *M. bovis* strains in the region [13],[14].

Fluoroquinolones inhibited the growth of the majority of the Hungarian *M. bovis* strains at low MIC values (with only 3 exceptions), confirming previous observations that this group of antimicrobial agents is effective against *M. bovis*[6],[7],[13]-[18]. MIC values of marbofloxacin were remarkably higher than that of danofloxacin and enrofloxacin. The observed difference, first noted by Gerchman et al. [13] is probably due to the increased use of marbofloxacin during the past years [13]. Extremely high MIC values for fluoroquinolones (≥10 μg/ml) were found in strains MYC44-46. The similarity in the resistance profile of these three strains is consistent with the results of a previous genetic study in the country, where these strains clustered into a separate subclade by MLST [10].

Most Hungarian *M. bovis* strains included in the present examination showed moderate susceptibility to gentamicin, with similar or lower MIC values (MIC_{90} 8 μg/ml) than isolates from Belgium and Israel (MIC_{90} 6 μg/ml, 32 μg/ml) [13],[19]. Spectinomycin, another member of the aminoglycosides, was used traditionally as an active compound against *M. bovis* and it is still considered effective in Japan [6],[12],[14]. However, high MIC values of spectinomycin (≥256 μg/ml) were observed in more than half of the studied Hungarian isolates, which is in agreement with recent reports from other countries [7],[13],[15]-[17],[19], confirming a globally emerging resistance to spectinomycin.

Heterogenic profiles of *M. bovis* susceptibility to tetracyclines are reported from all over the world [6],[7],[13],[14],[16],[19]. Only two Hungarian isolates showed low MIC value to oxytetracycline and tetracycline, demonstrating the high level of resistance to tetracyclines among the strains. In accordance with our results, increasing resistance to oxytetracycline was reported previously in Britain, Belgium, Japan and France [7],[14],[16],[19].

All but two of the Hungarian *M. bovis* strains showed high level of resistance to macrolides, with MIC_{90} values (≥128 μg/ml) consistent with previously published data, suggesting that macrolides are losing their efficacy on mycoplasmas [6],[7],[13],[14],[16]. For example an earlier clinical study demonstrated the effective use of tilmicosin [20] but another study [21] twelve years later already demonstrated the ineffectiveness of tilmicosin against *M. bovis in vivo* which also emphasizes the spread of antibiotic resistance due to the escalating use of antibiotics in veterinary practice. In the present study MICs of tilmicosin grouped around two distinct values, while the distribution of MICs of tylosin was gradually dispersed (Figure 2H-I). MIC values of tylosin were lower (8-128≥ μg/ml) or similar to MICs of tilmicosin (≥128 μg/ml). Similar observations were reported in the case of *M. bovis* strains by Gerchman et al. [13] and in the case of *M. gallisepticum* isolates by Jordan and Horrocks [22]. The slower development of tylosin resistance is supposed to be the cause of the difference between the MIC values of these antibiotics [23], and our results provide further evidence for this phenomenon.

Outstandingly low MIC values of all tetracyclines and macrolides were observed in two Hungarian isolates originating from the same herd (MYC52-53) and in the case of the reference PG45 strain. These three strains were closely related and they also formed a separate genetic clade in the MLST analysis performed previously [10].

The Hungarian isolates showed high MIC values to florfenicol. The MIC_{90} values (8 μg/ml) were similar to values obtained earlier in the United Kingdom (16 μg/ml), USA (4 μg/ml) and France (16 μg/ml) [6],[7],[16].

MIC_{90} values of lincomycin (≥64 μg/ml) were higher than the ones (1 μg/ml, 8 μg/ml, 64 μg/ml) described elsewhere [12],[14],[19]; and more than half of the strains isolated from cattle in Hungary demonstrated high MIC values to this member of lincosamides.

The results of *in vitro* antibiotic susceptibility tests can only predict the expected *in vivo* efficacy of the antibiotics, thus they only indicate the potential usefulness of a certain antimicrobial agent in the therapy. Standard breakpoints (susceptible, intermedier, resistant categories) have not yet been defined for the interpretation of *M. bovis* susceptibility to antibiotics [24], but several authors derived breakpoints for mycoplasmas from breakpoints of other bovine pathogens, and in some cases values were adopted from other host species [6],[13]-[17]. Taking into account all these criteria, fluoroquinolones seem to be the most active compounds *in vivo* against the *M. bovis* strains existing in Hungary. Although the *in vitro* antibiotic susceptibility tests are promising, the use of fluoroquinolones against *M. bovis* could be controversial *in vivo*. In the United Kingdom Nicholas and Ayling [3] reported on a study where the monthly fluoroquinolone treatment repeated over three months did not prevent the development of respiratory disease caused by *M. bovis*.

CONCLUSIONS

The present study determined the antibiotic susceptibility profiles of 35 *M. bovis* strains isolated from cattle in Hungary and it highlighted the importance of regular testing of antibiotic susceptibility in the region. Our results confirmed the increasing resistance to antibiotics commonly used for the treatment of mycoplasma infections, primarily to tetracyclines and macrolides. Based on the presented *in vitro* examinations, fluoroquinolones could be the most effective in the therapy of *M. bovis* infections in Hungary. However, the identification of three fluoroquinolon resistant isolates lends support for the EU recommendation that prudent antimicrobial use policies have to be strictly observed when members of this antibiotic group are applied [25]. In order to avoid the development of resistance fluoroquinolones should only be used based on the results of susceptibility testing and in cases of severe infections when treatment failed with other classes of antimicrobials.

AUTHORS' CONTRIBUTIONS

KMS and ZK performed the microbroth dilution tests, analysed the data and wrote the manuscript. LF and VH performed the microbroth dilution tests. TM and KE analysed the data and wrote the manuscript. SJ, NS, IT and LM collected the samples and isolated the strains. MG designed the study, analysed the data and wrote the manuscript. All authors read and approved the final manuscript.

DECLARATIONS

Acknowledgements

This work was supported by the Lendület program (LP2012-22) of the Hungarian Academy of Sciences.

REFERENCES

1. Hale HH, Helmboldt CF, Plastridge WN, Stula EF: Bovine mastitis caused by Mycoplasma species. Cornell Vet. 1962, 52: 582-591.
2. Maunsell FP, Woolums AR, Francoz D, Rosenbusch RF, Step DL, Wilson DJ, Janzen ED: *Mycoplasma bovis* infections in cattle. J Vet Intern Med. 2011, 25: 772-783. 10.1111/j.1939-1676.2011.0750.x.
3. Nicholas RAJ, Ayling RD: *Mycoplasma bovis*: disease, diagnosis, and control. Res Vet Sci. 2003, 74: 105-112. 10.1016/S0034-5288(02)00155-8.
4. Tenk M, Stipkovits L, Hufnagel L: Examination of the role of *Mycoplasma bovis* in bovine pneumonia and a mathematical model for its evaluation. Acta Vet Hung. 2004, 52: 445-456. 10.1556/AVet.52.2004.4.7.
5. Nicholas RAJ, Wood E, Baker S, Ayling RD: Mycoplasmas isolated from ruminants in Britain 1995–2000. In Mycoplasmas of Ruminants: Pathogenicity, Diagnostics, Epidemiology and Molecular Genetics, Volume 5. Edited by Poveda JB, Fernandez A, Frey J, Johansson KE. Brussels: European Commission; 2001:116–120.
6. Rosenbusch RF, Kinyon JM, Apley M, Funk ND, Smith SC, Hoffman LJ: In vitro antimicrobial inhibition profiles of *Mycoplasma bovis* isolates recovered from various regions of the United States from 2002 to 2003. J Vet Diagn Invest. 2005, 17: 436-441. 10.1177/104063870501700505.
7. Ayling RD, Baker SE, Peek ML, Simon AJ, Nicholas RA: Comparison of in vitro activity of danofloxacin, florfenicol, oxytetracycline, spectinomycin and tilmicosin against recent field isolates of *Mycoplasma bovis*. Vet Rec. 2000, 146: 745-747. 10.1136/vr.146.26.745.
8. Subramaniam S, Bergonier D, Poumarat F, Capaul S, Schlatter Y, Nicolet J, Frey J: Species identification of *Mycoplasma bovis* and *Mycoplasma agalactiae* based on the *uvrC* genes by PCR. Mol Cell Probes. 1998, 12: 161-169. 10.1006/mcpr.1998.0160.
9. Lauerman LH, Chilina AR, Closser JA, Johansen D: Avian mycoplasma identification using polymerase chain reaction amplicon and restriction fragment length polymorphism analysis. Avian Dis. 1995, 39: 804-811. 10.2307/1592417.
10. Sulyok KM, Kreizinger Z, Fekete L, Jánosi S, Schweitzer N, Turcsányi I, Makrai L, Erdélyi K, Gyuranecz M: Phylogeny of *Mycoplasma bovis* isolates from Hungary based on multi locus sequence typing and multiple-locus variable-number tandem repeat analysis. BMC Vet Res. 2014, 10: 108-10.1186/1746-6148-10-108.
11. Hannan PC: Guidelines and recommendations for antimicrobial minimum inhibitory concentration (MIC)

testing against veterinary mycoplasma species. Vet Res. 2000, 31: 373-395. 10.1051/vetres:2000100.

12. ter Laak EA, Noordergraaf JH, Verschure MH: Susceptibilities of *Mycoplasma bovis*, *Mycoplasma dispar*, and *Ureaplasma diversum* strains to antimicrobial agents in vitro. Antimicrob Agents Chemother. 1993, 37: 317-321. 10.1128/AAC.37.2.317.
13. Gerchman I, Levisohn S, Mikula I, Lysnyansky I: In vitro antimicrobial susceptibility of *Mycoplasma bovis* isolated in Israel from local and imported cattle. Vet Microbiol. 2009, 137: 268-275. 10.1016/j.vetmic.2009.01.028.
14. Uemura R, Sueyoshi M, Nagatomo H: Antimicrobial susceptibilities of four species of Mycoplasma isolated in 2008 and 2009 from cattle in Japan. J Vet Med Sci. 2010, 72: 1661-1663. 10.1292/jvms.10-0165.
15. Francoz D, Fortin M, Fecteau G, Messier S: Determination of *Mycoplasma bovis* susceptibilities against six antimicrobial agents using the E test method. Vet Microbiol. 2005, 105: 57-64. 10.1016/j.vetmic.2004.10.006.
16. Gautier-Bouchardon AV, Ferré S, Le Grand D, Paoli A, Gay E, Poumarat F: Overall decrease in the susceptibility of *Mycoplasma bovis* to antimicrobials over the past 30 years in France. PLoS One. 2014, 9: e87672-10.1371/journal.pone.0087672.
17. Soehnlen MK, Kunze ME, Karunathilake KE, Henwood BM, Kariyawasam S, Wolfgang DR, Jayaro BM: In vitro antimicrobial inhibition of *Mycoplasma bovis* isolates submitted to the Pennsylvania Animal Diagnostic Laboratory using flow cytometry and a broth microdilution method. J Vet Diagn Invest. 2011, 23: 547-551. 10.1177/1040638711404155.
18. Kroemer S, Galland D, Guérin-Faublée V, Giboin H, Woehrlé-Fontaine F: Survey of marbofloxacin susceptibility of bacteria isolated from cattle with respiratory disease and mastitis in Europe. Vet Rec. 2012, 170: 53-53. 10.1136/vr.100246.
19. Gourlay RN, Thomas LH, Wyld SG, Smith CJ: Effect of a new macrolide antibiotic (tilmicosin) on pneumonia experimentally induced in calves by *Mycoplasma bovis* and *Pasteurella haemolytica*. Res Vet Sci. 1989, 47: 84-89.
20. Haines DM, Martin KM, Clark EG, Jim GK, Janzen ED: The immunohistochemical detection of Mycoplasma bovis and bovine viral diarrhea virus in tissues of feedlot cattle with chronic, unresponsive respiratory disease and/or arthritis. Can Vet J. 2001, 42: 857.
21. Thomas A, Nicolas C, Dizier I, Mainil J, Linden A: Antibiotic susceptibilities of recent isolates of *Mycoplasma bovis* in Belgium. Vet Rec. 2003, 153: 428-431. 10.1136/vr.153.14.428.
22. Jordan FTW, Horrocks BK: The minimum inhibitory concentration of tilmicosin and tylosin for *Mycoplasma gallisepticum*and *Mycoplasma synoviae* and a comparison of their efficacy in the control of *Mycoplasma gallisepticum* infection in broiler chicks. Avian Dis. 1996, 40: 326-334. 10.2307/1592228.
23. Wu CM, Wu H, Ning Y, Wang J, Du X, Shen J: Induction of macrolide resistance in *Mycoplasma gallisepticum* in vitro and its resistance-related mutations within domain V of 23S rRNA. FEMS Microbiol Lett. 2005, 247: 199-205. 10.1016/j.femsle.2005.05.012.
24. Performance standards for antimicrobial disk and dilution susceptibility tests for bacteria isolated from animals. 2013, Approved Standard (Fourth Edition) and second informational supplement. NCCLS document VET01-A4 and VET01-S2. NCCLS 2013, Wayne, PA
25. European Medicines Agency, EMA/186029/2010.., [http://www.ema.europa.eu/ema/index.jsp?curl=pages/medicines/veterinary/referrals/Quinolones_containing_medicinal_products/vet_referral_000039.jsp&mid=WC0b01ac05800986a1]

CHAPTER 12

PHYLOGENY OF MYCOPLASMA BOVIS ISOLATES FROM HUNGARY BASED ON MULTI LOCUS SEQUENCE TYPING AND MULTIPLE-LOCUS VARIABLE-NUMBER TANDEM REPEAT ANALYSIS

Kinga M Sulyok, Zsuzsa Kreizinger, Lilla Fekete, Szilárd Jánosi, Nóra Schweitzer, Ibolya Turcsányi, László Makrai, Károly Erdélyi and Miklós Gyuranecz

Keywords: Cattle, Genotyping, MLST, MLVA, *Mycoplasma bovis,* Phylogeny, VNTR

BACKGROUND

Mycoplasma bovis is a worldwide pathogen of intensively farmed cattle which had recently emerged as a significant infectious agent in North America and Europe [1, 2]. *M. bovis* is an important causative agent of respiratory disease, mastitis and arthritis in cattle, and it was occasionally associated with genital infections and abortions as well [2, 3, 4]. This pathogen is estimated to be responsible for up to one third of the economic losses in the cattle industry caused by respiratory diseases [5].

In order to better understand the epidemiology of *M. bovis*, several typing techniques, such as random amplified polymorphic DNA (RAPD) or pulsed-field gel electrophoresis (PFGE) analysis [6, 7, 8, 9], have been used to compare isolates. However, these techniques have their disadvantages, such as the poor reproducibility of results with the RAPD method or the need for special equipment and the time consuming nature of PFGE analysis. Recently, multi locus sequence typing (MLST) and multiple-locus variable-number tandem repeat (VNTR) analysis (MLVA) methods have been developed for the genetic characterization of *M. bovis* isolates [9, 10]. MLST schemes were originally designed to capture the intermediate-level evolutionary relationships between bacterial isolates (e.g. on a country or continent level) while MLVA was proposed to detect the quick mutation events (e.g. during epidemics) within bacterial species [11, 12]. To date, relatively little information is available about the application of these recently introduced assays. MLVA have been used in three *M. bovis* studies during the last years [9, 13, 14], while MLST was successfully applied only in one pilot study [10]. Moreover this latter typing scheme also needs to be tested with a higher number of *M. bovis*isolates.

The aim of the present study was to genetically characterize the Hungarian *M. bovis* population with the MLST and MLVA method in order to evaluate and compare these two typing systems and to better understand the epidemiology of *M. bovis* in Hungary.

METHODS

Nasal swabs, lung samples and a single lymph node were collected through routine diagnostic examinations or necropsies from different parts of Hungary between 2010 and 2013. Ethical approval was not required for the study as all samples were collected during routine diagnostic examinations or necropsies. Swabs and small pieces from the affected parts of lungs and the lymph node were homogenized in 2 ml of *Mycoplasma*broth medium (Thermo Fisher Scientific Inc./

Citation: Kinga M Sulyok, Zsuzsa Kreizinger, Lilla Fekete, Szilárd Jánosi, Nóra Schweitzer, Ibolya Turcsányi, László Makrai, Károly Erdélyi and Miklós Gyuranecz, Phylogeny of Mycoplasma bovis isolates from Hungary based on multi locus sequence typing and multiple-locus variable-number tandem repeat analysis, DOI: 10.1186/1746-6148-10-108.

Oxoid Inc./, Waltham, MA) and cultured at 37°C. On the second day of incubation, when the slight colour change of the broth media occurred, the cultures were inoculated onto solid *Mycoplasma* media (Thermo Fisher Scientific Inc./ Oxoid Inc./) and were incubated at 37°C and 5% CO_2 for 3 days, until visible colonies appeared. *Mycoplasma* strains were filter-cloned only once before DNA extraction from 200 µl of broth culture using the DNeasy blood and tissue kit (Qiagen Inc., Hilden, Germany). In order to identify the isolates, PCR targeting the *uvrC* gene of *M. bovis* was performed on all samples [15]. The thirty-one strains isolated and analyzed in this study are listed in Table 1.

Table 1: Background data for the thirty-one *M. bovis* strains analyzed in this study

Sample ID	Herd of origin	Date	Sample type	GenBank accession numbers				Copy numbers of tandem repeats								
				fusA	*gyrB*	*lepA*	*rpoB*	TR14	TR29	TR30	TR31	TR35	TR40-41	TR49-51	TR52	TR59
PG45	Connecticut	1961	Lung	JQ031392	JQ031411	JQ031435	JQ031493	2.2	4.8	2.3	5.8	4.0	4.0	2.2	4.0	2.4
MYC2	Püspökhatvan	2011	Lung	KF926436	KF926437	KF926438	KF926439	-	-	3.3	-	3.0	-	1.2	-	-
MYC22	Sümeg	2012	Lung	KF926440	KF926441	KF926442	KF926443	-	0.8	3.3	-	3.0	8.0	1.2	3.0	2.4
MYC30	Bugyi	2012	Lung	KJ438237	KJ438174	KJ438195	KJ438216	-	0.8	2.3	5.8	3.0	8.0	1.2	3.0	2.4
MYC42	Nemti	2012	Lung	KJ438238	KJ438175	KJ438196	KJ438217	-	12.8	3.3	5.8	3.0	8.0	1.2	4.0	2.4
MYC43	Zsana	2012	Lung	KF926444	KF926445	KF926446	KF926447	-	2.8	3.3	-	3.0	11.0	1.2	3.0	2.4
MYC44	Győrszentiván	2012	Lung	KJ438239	KJ438176	KJ438197	KJ438218	-	2.8	3.3	-	3.0	-	0.6	3.0	1.4
MYC45	Budapest	2012	Lung	KJ438240	KJ438177	KJ438198	KJ438219	-	2.8	3.3	-	3.0	11.0	0.6	3.0	1.4
MYC46	Budapest	2012	Lung	KF926448	KF926449	KF926450	KF926451	-	2.8	3.3	-	3.0	11.0	0.6	3.0	1.4
MYC47	Dabas	2012	Lung	KJ438241	KJ438178	KJ438199	KJ438220	-	2.8	3.3	-	3.0	11.0	1.2	3.0	-
MYC48	Ősi	2012	Nasal swab	KJ438242	KJ438179	KJ438200	KJ438221	-	-	3.3	-	3.0	-	1.2	-	-
MYC49	Ősi	2012	Nasal swab	KF926452	KF926453	KF926454	KF926455	-	12.8	3.3	-	3.0	8.0	1.2	4.0	2.4
MYC50	Ősi	2012	Lung	KJ438243	KJ438180	KJ438201	KJ438222	-	12.8	3.3	-	3.0	8.0	1.2	4.0	-
MYC51	Ősi	2012	Nasal swab	KJ438244	KJ438181	KJ438202	KJ438223	-	12.8	3.3	-	3.0	8.0	1.2	4.0	2.4
MYC52	Solt	2012	Lung	KJ438245	KJ438182	KJ438203	KJ438224	2.2	4.8	2.3	7.8	4.0	4.0	2.2	4.0	2.4
MYC53	Solt	2012	Lung	KF926456	KF926457	KF926458	KF926459	2.2	4.8	2.3	7.8	4.0	4.0	2.2	4.0	2.4
MYC65	Csengersima	2012	Nasal swab	KJ438246	KJ438183	KJ438204	KJ438225	-	1.8	3.3	5.8	3.0	8.0	1.2	4.0	2.4
MYC66	Csengersima	2012	Nasal swab	KJ438247	KJ438184	KJ438205	KJ438226	-	-	3.3	5.8	3.0	8.0	1.2	6.0	2.4
MYC67	Csengersima	2012	Lung	KF926460	KF926461	KF926462	KF926463	-	-	3.3	5.8	3.0	8.0	1.2	6.0	2.4
MYC68	Csengersima	2012	Lung	KJ438248	KJ438185	KJ438206	KJ438227	-	-	3.3	5.8	3.0	8.0	1.2	6.0	2.4
MYC69	Komárom	2013	Nasal swab	KJ438249	KJ438186	KJ438207	KJ438228	-	1.8	3.3	-	3.0	8.0	1.2	4.0	-
MYC70	Komárom	2013	Nasal swab	KJ438250	KJ438187	KJ438208	KJ438229	-	1.8	3.3	4.8	3.0	8.0	1.2	4.0	-
MYC71	Komárom	2013	Nasal swab	KJ438251	KJ438188	KJ438209	KJ438230	-	1.8	3.3	-	3.0	8.0	1.2	4.0	-
MYC72	Komárom	2013	Nasal swab	KJ438252	KJ438189	KJ438210	KJ438231	-	1.8	3.3	4.8	3.0	8.0	1.2	4.0	-
MYC73	Komárom	2013	Nasal swab	KJ438253	KJ438190	KJ438211	KJ438232	-	1.8	3.3	4.8	3.0	8.0	1.2	4.0	-
MYC74	Komárom	2013	Nasal swab	KF926464	KF926465	KF926466	KF926467	-	1.8	3.3	4.8	-	8.0	1.2	4.0	-
MYC75	Komárom	2013	Nasal swab	KJ438254	KJ438191	KJ438212	KJ438233	-	1.8	3.3	-	3.0	8.0	1.2	4.0	-
MYC76	Komárom	2013	Nasal swab	KJ438255	KJ438192	KJ438213	KJ438234	-	1.8	3.3	4.8	-	8.0	1.2	4.0	-
MYC77	Kertészsziget	2010	Lung	KJ438256	KJ438193	KJ438214	KJ438235	2.2	0.8	3.3	-	3.0	11.0	0.6	3.0	2.4
MYC78	Hosszúpályi	2011	Lung	KF926468	KF926469	KF926470	KF926471	-	0.8	3.3	5.8	3.0	8.0	1.2	4.0	2.4
MYC79	Hosszúpályi	2011	Lung	KJ438257	KJ438194	KJ438215	KJ438236	-	0.8	3.3	5.8	3.0	8.0	1.2	4.0	2.4
MYC80	Ebes	2011	Lymphnode	KF926472	KF926473	KF926474	KF926475	2.2	0.8	3.3	-	-	25.0	1.2	4.0	2.4

Herd of origin, date, sample type, GenBank Accession numbers of locus sequences and number of TRs of the thirty-one *M. bovis* strains analyzed in this study.

The MLST based on four housekeeping genes (*fusA, gyrB, lepA, rpoB*) was performed using the amplification primers and PCR conditions described by Manso-Silván et al. [10] in 25 µl total volume containing 10 to 100 ng of target DNA diluted in nuclease-free water, 5 µl of 5× Green GoTaq Flexi Buffer (Promega, Inc., Madison, WI), 2.5 µl of $MgCl_2$ (25 mM; Promega), 0.75 µl of deoxynucleoside triphosphates (10 mM; Qiagen Inc.), 1 µl of each primer (10 pmol/µl), and 0.25 µl of GoTaq Flexi DNA polymerase (5 U/µl; Promega, Inc.). The PCR were performed in a Biometra – T Personal thermal cycler (Biometra Inc., Göttingen, Germany). PCR products were isolated from agarose gel (QIAquick gel extraction kit; Qiagen Inc.), and direct cycle sequencing was performed with the primers used for amplification on an ABI Prism 3100 automated DNA sequencer (Applied Biosystems, Foster City, CA). The reading errors of the chromatograms were corrected with the SeqMan program (Lasergene package, DNASTAR Inc., Madison, WI). Sequences were trimmed, concatenated and aligned with all published sequences using the BioEdit 7.2.2 software [16].

An MLVA based on nine tandem repeats (TR)s was performed with the amplification primers and PCR conditions described by Pinho et al. [9]. All PCRs were performed in 25 µl total volume as described above. After amplification, 2–5 µl of each reaction mixture was subjected to electrophoresis (8 V/cm) in 2% standard agarose gel (SeaKem LE Agarose, Lonza Inc., Rockland, ME), and the amplified DNA products were visualized with GR Safe nucleic acid gel stain (Lab Supply Malla InnoVita Inc., Gaithersburg, MD). Depending on the length of the tandem repeat units a 100-bp or a 20-bp DNA ladder (GeneRuler 100 bp Plus or O›RangeRuler 20 bp, Thermo Fisher Scientific Inc.) was used as molecular weight marker. Electrophoresis was performed until the yellow dye had run for at least 20 cm. Stained gels were visualized by UV light, photographically documented (Kodak Inc., Rochester, NY) and band sizes were estimated with the help of the Kodak MI SE software package (Kodak Inc.).

Phylogenetic analysis of the concatenated sequences containing the four housekeeping genes was conducted with the neighbour-joining method using pairwise distances and 1000 bootstraps in the MEGA 5.05 software [17]. The average evolutionary divergence of the concatenated sequences was also estimated with MEGA 5.05 [17] both within and between *M. bovis* clades. Analyses were conducted using the Maximum Composite Likelihood model with standard error estimated through 1000 bootstrap replicates. The rate variation among sites was modelled using gamma distribution (shape parameter = 1) including all codon positions. A recombination analysis was performed on the concatenated sequence alignment using the RDP 4 software [18]. The default selection of detection methods (RDP, GeneConv, and MaxChi) and general settings were used to perform the analyses. In MLVA, the band size estimates were converted to numbers of repeat units [9]. The clustering analysis was performed with a neighbour-joining method based on pairwise distances in the MEGA5.05 software [17]. The discriminatory power of the different typing schemes was calculated using Simpson's index of diversity with 95% confidence intervals (CI) [19]. The quantitative level of congruence and respective confidence intervals between the two typing methods was calculated based on the data of the thirty-one isolates and PG45 analyzed with both methods using the adjusted Rand and Wallace coefficients [20]. An online tool was used to perform these calculations [21].

RESULTS

Hungarian *M. bovis* isolates clustered into two clades by MLST (Figure 1). Two strains (MYC52, 53) had the same sequence type (ST) as the reference strain PG45 (NCTC 10131) and were closely related to a strain from Saudi Arabia, while the other Hungarian isolates formed a novel clade with five subclades. Isolates originating from the same herds had the same STs and were assigned to the same subclades by MLST except for one strain (MYC 65). The within-group means of genetic distances between the concatenated sequences were 0.001 (±0.001 standard error, SE) in the Hungarian clade (Clade A) and 0.001 (±0.000 SE) in the PG45 clade (Clade B). The mean values of between clade genetic distances for the concatenated sequences ranged from 0.003 to 0.012 (Table 2). The recombination analyses on the alignment of the concatenated MLST loci did not reveal any recombination events.

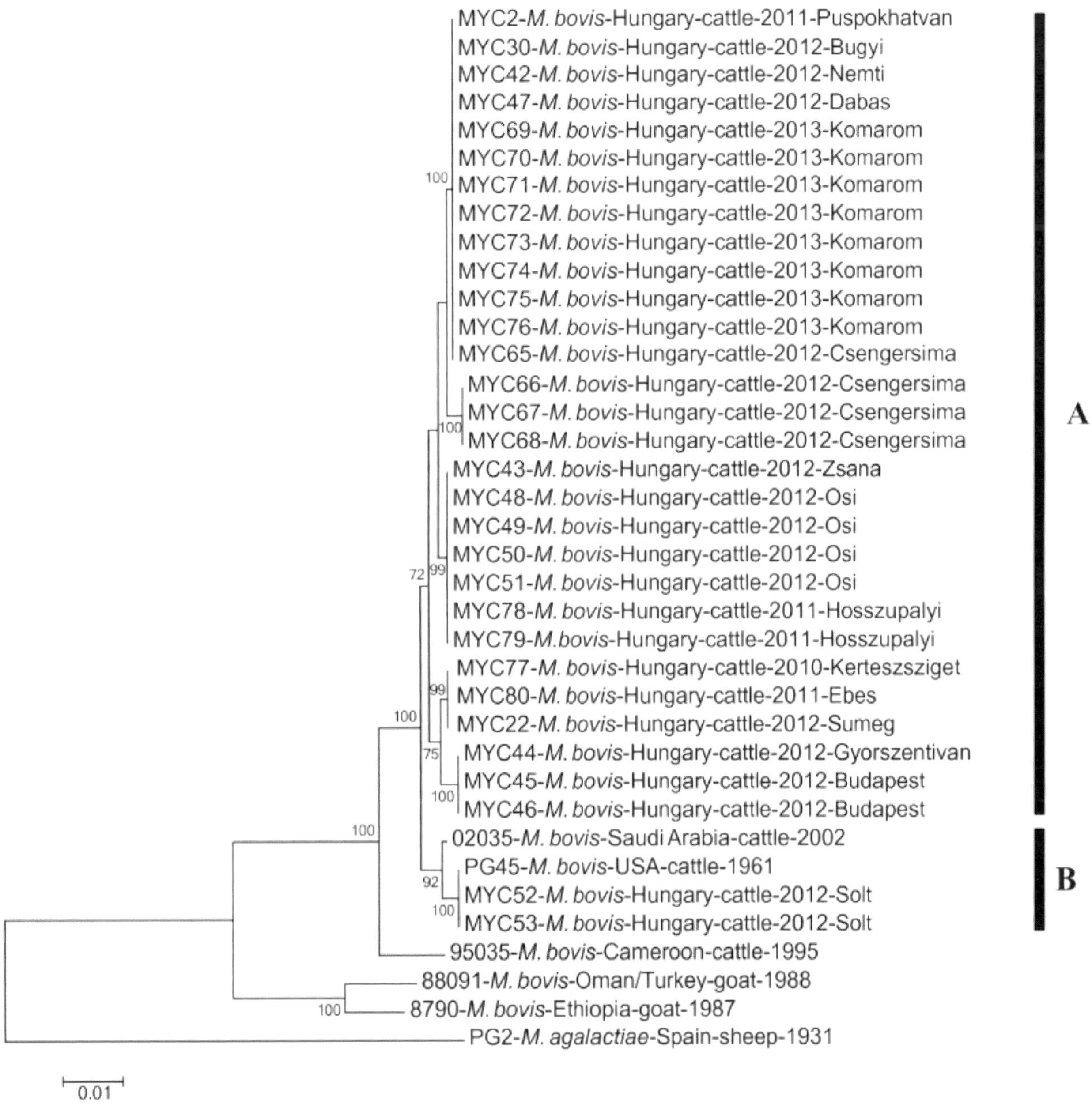

Figure 1: Genetic relationships between *M. bovis* strains based on multi locus sequence typing. Neighbour-joining phylogenetic tree showing relationships between the concatenated partial sequences of four housekeeping genes obtained from *M. bovis* strains characterized in this study (Hungary) and deposited in GenBank. Panels **A** and **B**indicate the major clades. Bootstrap values of neighbour-joining (1000 replicates) of > 70 are shown. The scale bar represents the average number of substitutions per site.

Table 2: Estimates of average evolutionary divergence of concatenated sequence pairs between and within *M. bovis* clades

	Evolutionary divergence					
	Clade A	**Clade B**	**M.b.-Cameroon**	**M.b.-Oman/ Turkey**	**M.b.-Ethiopia**	**Distance (SE)**
Clade A						0.001 (0.001)
Clade B	0.003					0.001 (0.000)
M.b.-Cameroon	0.006	0.005				n/c
M.b.-Oman/ Turkey	0.012	0.012	0.010			n/c
M.b.-Ethiopia	0.012	0.012	0.010	0.003		n/c
M. agalactiae	0.030	0.030	0.029	0.029	0.027	n/c

The numbers of base substitutions per site are shown as calculated from the average substitutions of all sequence pairs between (matrix) and within (column) groups. Standard error estimates are shown in parentheses. n/c: not calculated.

The Hungarian *M. bovis* isolates and the reference strain PG45 formed two major clades with several subclades and branches by MLVA (Figure 2). One main group comprised three strains (MYC 52, 53 and 80) and the reference strain PG45 while the other main branch contained the rest of the strains. Isolates originating from the same herd were generally clustered together or close to each other (MYC 45–46, MYC 52–53, MYC 65–68, MYC 69–76, MYC 78–79), but within herd divergence was also detected (MYC 48–51).

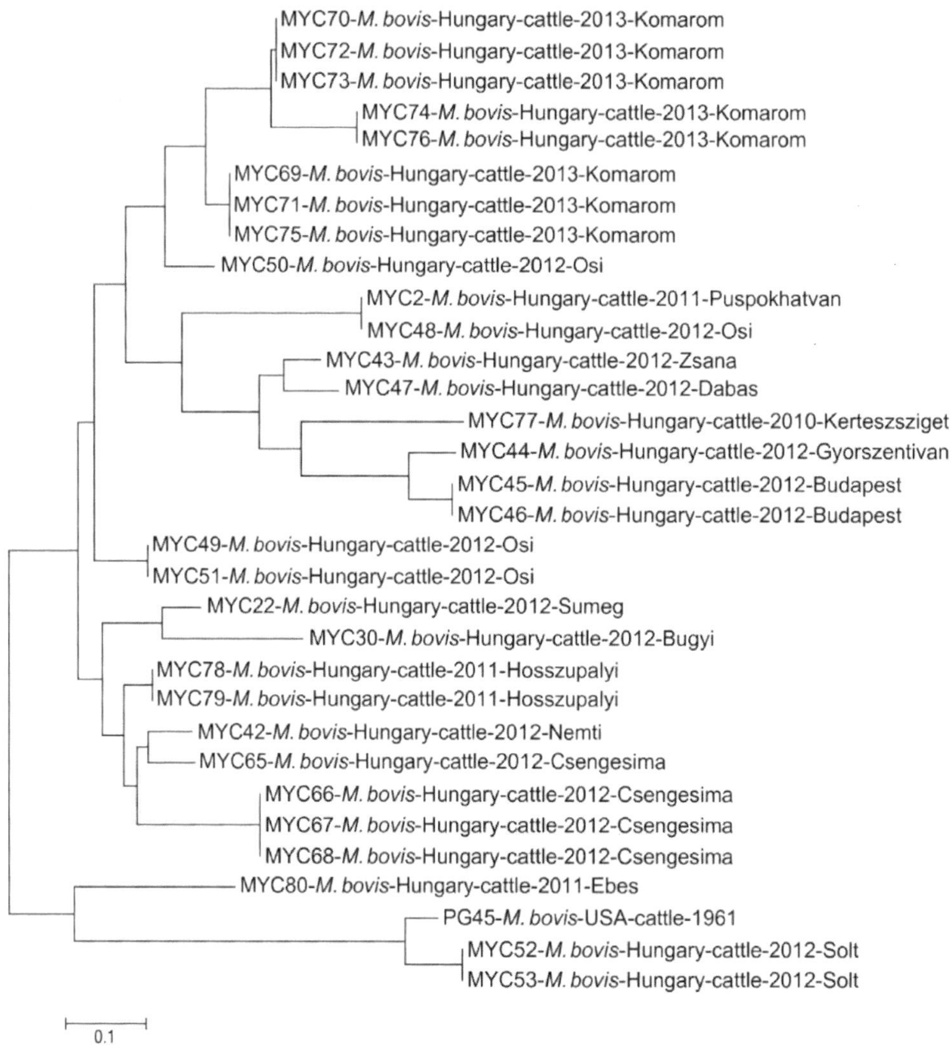

Figure 2: Genetic relationships between *M. bovis* strains based on multiple-locus variable-number tandem repeat analysis. Genetic relationships between thirty-one Hungarian isolates and the reference strain PG45 based on multiple-locus variable-number tandem repeat analysis. Dendrogram was constructed with the neighbour-joining method based on pairwise distances. The scale bar represents the average number of substitutions per site.

Six STs were discriminated by MLST and twenty different MLVA profiles were identified among the analyzed strains and PG45. The Simpson›s index of diversity was 0.776 (CI: 0.678-0.874) in MLST and 0.970 (CI: 0.952-0.987) in MLVA. The value of the Adjusted Rand coefficient was 0.178, the Adjusted Wallance coefficient MLVA→MLST was 0.099 (CI: 0.004-0.194) and the Adjusted Wallance coefficient MLST→MLVA was 0.914 (CI: 0.828-1.000). These values indicate poor concordance between the results of the two typing systems.

Correlation was not found between the genotype and source (lung, nasal swab or lymph node) of the *M. bovis*isolates.

MLST alignment, MLVA data and phylogenetic trees were deposited in Dryad Digital Repository ([22], doi:10.5061/dryad.f4ks8).

DISCUSSION

M. bovis can cause great economic losses in the cattle industry through reduced production, increased costs of treatment and death. The disease is primarily transmitted by direct contact and it is spread through the movement of infected animals; therefore efficient genotyping tools are essential for its monitoring, control and epidemiological investigation. MLST and MLVA of *M. bovis* had been recently developed and they proved to be useful in previous studies [9, 10, 13, 14]. The two methods differ considerably in their applicability. MLST is dedicated to the discovery of intermediate-term evolutionary events while MLVA is a suitable method to perform short-scale epidemiology studies. In the present work we tested these methods on a *M. bovis* strain collection isolated over the last couple of years in Hungary.

MLST results provided an intermediate level genetic resolution among the studied *M. bovis* strains. Isolates originating from the same farms had identical STs except for one case. Strains with distinct origins (e.g. when *M. bovis* infection might have been introduced to the herd through more than one animal of different origin) could explain the case of this exception (Csengersima, MYC 65–68). It is remarkable that the majority of the Hungarian isolates had different STs than the previously examined French, Belgian and German isolates which possessed the same sequence as PG45 [10]. However, it has to be noted, that only one isolate per country was examined in that particular study. Furthermore, unexpectedly high genetic variation was detected among the Hungarian strains by MLST. Similar analyses would be required on strains originating from other countries to explore whether the MLST system really possesses such discriminatory power or whether it is the Hungarian *M. bovis* population that is genetically so diverse. Potentially the high genetic diversity of the Hungarian *M. bovis* population may be partially due to the intensive national and international cattle trade.

It was demonstrated that MLVA has high discriminatory power and is able to distinguish closely related strains. This was best demonstrated during the typing of isolates from the herd from the town of Komárom (MYC 69–76). These strains formed one group with three subgroups. Spergser et al. [13] modified the MLVA typing scheme described by Pinho et al. [9]. With their modification Spergser et al. [13] increased the discriminatory power (Simpson›s index of diversity) of the original MLVA system from 0.952 to 0.981 based on the analysis of their samples. In the present study we analyzed our samples with the original Pinho et al. [9] system resulting a 0.970 Simpson›s index of diversity. This value provides further proof for the high genetic diversity of the Hungarian *M. bovis* population. This finding is consistent with previous data published by Amram et al. [14] who discovered eight different VNTR patterns among the eleven *M. bovis* strains isolated from calves imported to Israel from Hungary. Unfortunately we were unable to compare our isolates with the strains analysed by MLVA in the previous studies [9, 13, 14], as the VNTR patterns of the individual isolates from these studies were not published. Establishing an online database of *M. bovis* VNTR patterns or providing supplementary material with publications would allow the comparison of isolates originating from different parts of the world, necessary for the monitoring of the disease and for performing epidemiological investigations. Furthermore, the availability of a large dataset should also improve the methods for data analysis. Although we think that MLST is a more appropriate method than MLVA for the genetic comparison of weakly related isolates (strains with distant geographic origin, e.g. on a country or continental level), it may also be possible to use the later for this purpose with certain modifications. As MLVA is primarily a fine scale typing tool (e.g. useful in following local epidemics), the different TRs are recommended to be weighted when the method is applied on weakly related isolates in order to avoid homoplasy [23]. However, in order to establish an efficient TR weighting system, it is essential to have access to VNTR profile data of many isolates from different countries.

CONCLUSIONS

This study has compared and evaluated two different molecular epidemiological typing techniques for *M. bovis* characterisation. MLST is a robust and reproducible intermediate scale typing method which proved to be discriminatory among the Hungarian *M. bovis* isolates. MLVA is an appropriate fine-scale typing tool for *M. bovis* strains, as it even allowed the within farm differentiation of certain strains. Based on these results the combined use of the two typing methods is recommended (Figure 3). The isolates have first to be typed by MLST and then the subset of strains sharing the same STs has to be further differentiated by MLVA. In this way information will be gained about both the longer-term evolutionary and the short-term epidemiological relationships of the analysed isolates.

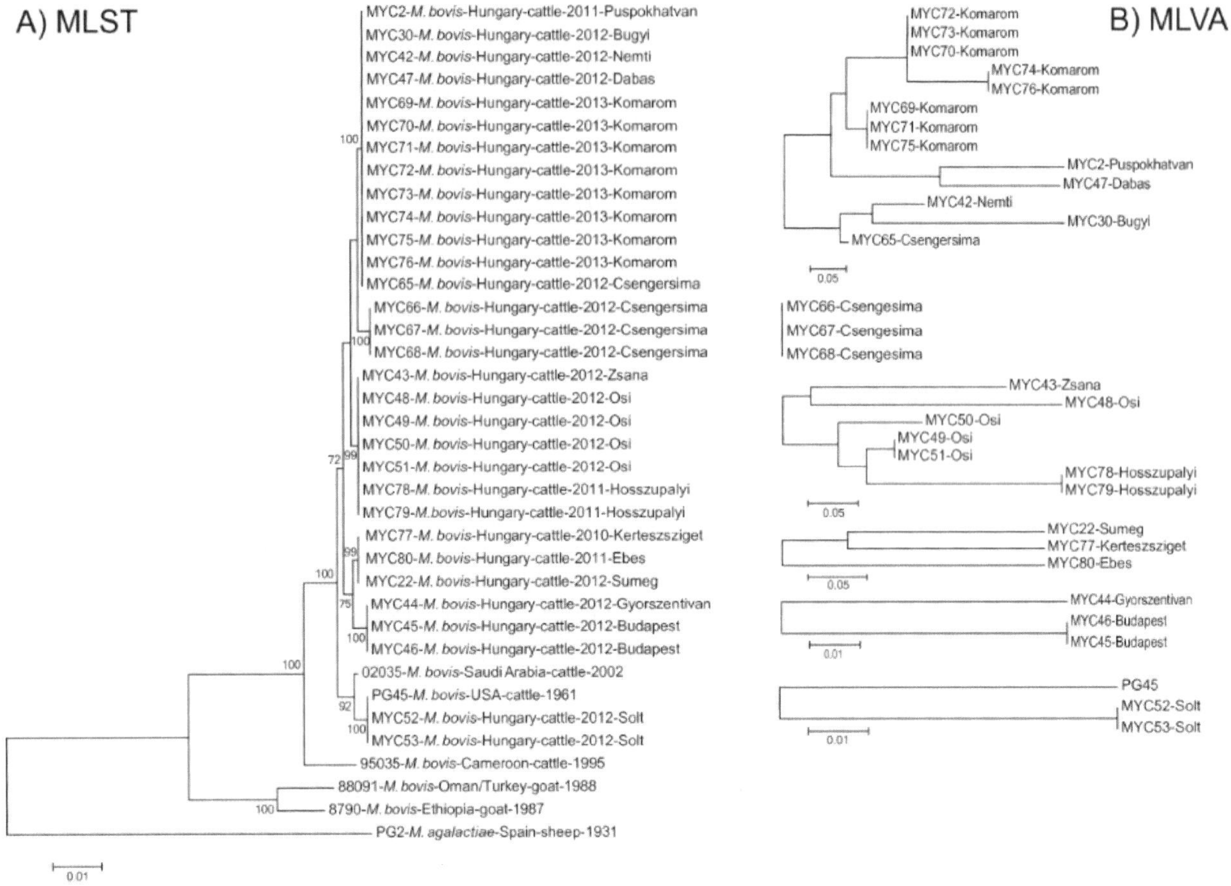

Figure 3: Genetic relationships between *M. bovis* strains based on the combined use of multi locus sequence typing (MLST, A) and multiple-locus variable-number tandem-repeat analysis (MLVA, B). Dendrograms were constructed with neighbour-joining methods. Scale bars represent the average number of substitutions per site.

DECLARATIONS

Acknowledgements

This work was supported by the Lendület program (LP2012-22) of the Hungarian Academy of Sciences.

AUTHORS' CONTRIBUTIONS

KMS and ZK performed MLST and MLVA, analysed the data and wrote the manuscript. LF performed MLST and MLVA. SJ, NS, IT and LM collected the samples and isolated the strains. KE analysed the data and wrote the manuscript. MG designed the study, analysed the data and wrote the manuscript. All authors read and approved the final manuscript.

REFERENCES

1. Caswell JL, Bateman KG, Cai HY, Castillo-Alcala F: *Mycoplasma bovis* in respiratory disease of feedlot cattle. Vet Clin North Am Food Anim Pract. 2010, 26: 365-379. 10.1016/j.cvfa.2010.03.003.
2. Maunsell FP, Donovan GA: *Mycoplasma bovis* infections in young calves. Vet Clin North Am Food Anim Pract. 2009, 25: 139-177. 10.1016/j.cvfa.2008.10.011.
3. Byrne WJ, Ball HJ, Brice N, McCormack R, Baker SE, Ayling RD, Nicholas RA: Application of an indirect ELISA to milk samples to identify cows with *Mycoplasma bovis* mastitis. Vet Rec. 2000, 146: 368-369. 10.1136/vr.146.13.368.
4. Pfützner H, Sachse K: *Mycoplasma bovis* as an agent of mastitis, pneumonia, arthritis and genital disorders in cattle. Rev Sci Tech. 1996, 15: 1477-1494.
5. Nicholas RA, Ayling RD: *Mycoplasma bovis*: disease, diagnosis, and control. Res Vet Sci. 2003, 74: 105-112. 10.1016/S0034-5288(02)00155-8.
6. Citti C, Lischewski A, Siebert-Gulle K, Rosengarten R: Limitations of pulse field gel electrophoresis for the typing of *Mycoplasma bovis*. Mycoplasmas Of Ruminants: Pathogenicity, Diagnostics And Molecular Genetics. Edited by: Poveda JB, Ferandez A, Johansson KE, Frey J. Brussels: European Comission; 2000:46-49.
7. Hotzel H, Schneider B, Sachse K: Investigation of *Mycoplasma bovis* field isolates using PCR fingerprinting. Mycoplasmas Of Ruminants: Pathogenicity, Diagnostics, Epidemiology And Molecular Genetics. Edited by: Leori G, Santini F, Scanziani E, Frey J. Brussels: European Comission; 1998:17-19.
8. McAuliffe L, Kokotovic B, Ayling RD, Nicholas RA: Molecular epidemiological analysis of *Mycoplasma bovis* isolates from the United Kingdom shows two genetically distinct clusters. J Clin Microbiol. 2004, 42: 4556-4565. 10.1128/JCM.42.10.4556-4565.2004.
9. Pinho L, Thompson G, Rosenbusch R, Carvalheira J: Genotyping of *Mycoplasma bovis* isolates using

multiple-locus variable-number tandem-repeat analysis. J Microbiol Methods. 2012, 88: 377-385. 10.1016/j.mimet.2012.01.003.

10. Manso-Silván L, Dupuy V, Lysnyansky I, Ozdemir U, Thiaucourt F: Phylogeny and molecular typing of *Mycoplasma agalactiae* and *Mycoplasma bovis* by multilocus sequencing. Vet Microbiol. 2012, 161: 104-112. 10.1016/j.vetmic.2012.07.015.

11. Keim P, Johansson A, Wagner DM: Molecular epidemiology, evolution, and ecology of *Francisella*. Ann N Y Acad Sci. 2007, 1105: 30-66. 10.1196/annals.1409.011.

12. Margos G, Vollmer SA, Ogden NH, Fish D: Population genetics, taxonomy, phylogeny and evolution of *Borrelia burgdorferi* sensu lato. Infect Genet Evol. 2011, 11: 1545-1563. 10.1016/j.meegid.2011.07.022.

13. Spergser J, Macher K, Kargl M, Lysnyansky I, Rosengaten R: Emergence, re-emergence, spread and host species crossing of *Mycoplasma bovis* in the Austrian Alps caused by a single endemic strain. Vet Microbiol. 2013, 164: 299-306. 10.1016/j.vetmic.2013.02.007.

14. Amram E, Freed M, Khateb N, Mikula I, Blum S, Spergser J, Sharir B, Ozeri R, Harrus S, Lysnyansky I: Multiple locus variable number tandem repeat analysis of *Mycoplasma bovis* isolated from local and imported cattle. Vet J. 2013, 197: 286-290. 10.1016/j.tvjl.2013.03.023.

15. Subramaniam S, Bergonier D, Poumarat F, Capaul S, Schlatter Y, Nicolet J, Frey J: Species identification of *Mycoplasma bovis* and *Mycoplasma agalactiae* based on the uvrC genes by PCR. Mol Cell Probes. 1998, 12: 161-169. 10.1006/mcpr.1998.0160.

16. Hall TA: BioEdit: a user-friendly biological sequence alignment editor and analysis program for Windows 95/98/NT. Nucleic Acids Symp. 1999, 41: 95-98.

17. Tamura K, Peterson D, Peterson N, Stecher G, Nei M, Kumar S: MEGA5: Molecular Evolutionary Genetics Analysis using maximum likelihood, evolutionary distance, and maximum parsimony methods. Mol Biol Evol. 2011, 28: 2731-2739. 10.1093/molbev/msr121.

18. Martin DP, Lemey P, Lott M, Moulton V, Posada D, Lefeuvre P: RDP3: a flexible and fast computer program for analyzing recombination. Bioinformatics. 2010, 26: 2462-2463. 10.1093/bioinformatics/btq467.

19. Hunter PR, Gaston MA: Numerical index of the discriminatory ability of typing systems: an application of Simpson's index of diversity. J Clin Microbiol. 1988, 26: 2465-2466.

20. Carrico JA, Silva-Costa C, Melo-Cristino J, Pinto FR, de Lencastre H, Almeida JS, Ramirez M: Illustration of a common framework for relating multiple typing methods by application to macrolide resistant *Streptococcus pyogenes*. J Clin Microbiol. 2006, 44: 2524-2532. 10.1128/JCM.02536-05.

21. Comparing Partitions Website. http://darwin.phyloviz.net/ComparingPartitions/index.php?link=Home.

22. Dryad. https://datadryad.org/, doi:10.5061/dryad.rc8q4

23. Al Dahouk S, Le Fleche P, Nöckler K, Jacques I, Grayon M, Scholz HC, Tomaso H, Vergnaud G, Neubauer H: Evaluation of *Brucella* MLVA typing for human brucellosis. J Microbiol Methods. 2007, 69: 137-145. 10.1016/j.mimet.2006.12.015.

CHAPTER 13

A SURVEY OF MYCOPLASMA AGALACTIAE IN DAIRY SHEEP FARMS IN SPAIN

Jaime Ariza-Miguel, David Rodríguez-Lázaro and Marta Hernández

Keywords: Mycoplasma agalactiae, Contagious agalactia, Real time PCR, Sheep, Dairy, Spain

BACKGROUND

Contagious Agalactia (CA) is, along with bovine pleuropneumonia and contagious caprine pleuropneumonia, one of the three Mycoplasma-induced diseases affecting small ruminants which are notifiable to the World Organisation for Animal Health due to their economic significance [1]. CA is a syndrome clinically characterized by mastitis, arthritis, keratoconjunctivitis and occasionally abortion [2, 3] and *Mycoplasma agalactiae* is considered its major etiological agent. *M. mycoides* subsp. *capri*, *M. capricolum* subsp. *capricolum* and *M. putrefaciens* cause a clinically similar syndrome, particularly in goats [4, 5]. The syndrome causes major economic losses because of reduction or suppression of milk production, abortion, high morbidity and mortality rates, and costs associated with the diagnosis, treatment and prevention which are estimated to be above 20 million Euros per year in the European countries forming the Mediterranean Basin [3, 4, 6].

CA has its major impact in the Mediterranean countries, where the disease is considered to be endemic. However, it is also widely distributed in west Asian countries, central, north and east African Countries, the USA, and Brazil [1, 2, 7, 8, 9]. Interestingly, the significance of the different *Mycoplasma* species causing CA varies depending on the geographic area. In the United States, *M. mycoides* subsp. *capri* is the most prevalent caprine *Mycoplasma*, although *M. agalactiae* has been recently isolated [9]. In Northern Jordan, *M. agalactiae*and *M. mycoides* subsp. *capri* play the major role in both, sheep and goats [7, 10]. In France, *M. agalactiae* has reemerged in sheep flocks located in the basin of the Western Pyrénées, causing 98 new outbreaks in 2008 [1]. In Spain, which has the second highest number of sheep amongst the 27 European Union member states, research has been focused on caprine CA, and there is a knowledge gap regarding which *Mycoplasma* species are present in sheep flocks from that country.

Consequently, in the present study we aimed to assess for the first time the presence and geographic distribution of the four *Mycoplasma* species causing CA, by analyzing raw milk samples from Spanish dairy sheep farms by classical microbiological methods, and PCR-based methods which have been demonstrated to be specific and sensitive [11, 12, 13]. The knowledge acquired will allow the implementation of appropriate control programs for those pathogens.

RESULTS

Sensitivity of the PCR-based methods and capability to detect coinfected samples

Artificially contaminated milk samples (50 mL) inoculated with from 10^8 cells to 10^2 cells of each *Mycoplasma*gave positive

Citation: Jaime Ariza-Miguel, David Rodríguez-Lázaro and Marta Hernández, A survey of Mycoplasma agalactiae in dairy sheep farms in Spain, DOI: 10.1186/1746-6148-8-171.

results by the three PCR-based systems [11, 12, 13]. Detection failed in the milk samples seeded with 10^1 cells (0.2 cells/mL). Capability to detect samples co-infected with various CA-causing mycoplasmas was demonstrated in samples artificially contaminated with the 4 *Mycoplasma* species analyzed in this study.

Detection of CA-causing mycoplasmas in Spanish sheep farms

All 597 milk samples tested negative for *M. mycoides* subsp. *capri*, *M. capricolum* subsp. *capricolum* and *M. putrefaciens*. On the other hand, 339 out of 922 dairy sheep farms were positive for *M. agalactiae* by real time PCR (36.8%). Furthermore, the pathogen was observed by microscopy identification in samples collected from 85 flocks (9.2%). Thereby, 411 *M. agalactiae* isolates were obtained.

We assessed the level of intermittent excretion of *M. agalactiae* during the sampling period using data obtained from other additional 391 farms sampled repeatedly from 2 to 5 times. In 26.3% of the cases a previously positive farm resulted negative in a later sampling and conversely, 38 farms (9.7%) tested negative in the first sampling but resulted positive in any of the subsequent samplings. Overall, 250 of those sheep farms (63.9%) were positive for *M. agalactiae*.

Geographic distribution of flocks infected with *Mycoplasma agalactiae*

Positive farms for *M. agalactiae* were located in all eleven provinces sampled (Figures 1, 2A). The frequency ranged from 7.7% to 100% of the flocks sampled per province revealing that the microorganism is widely distributed.

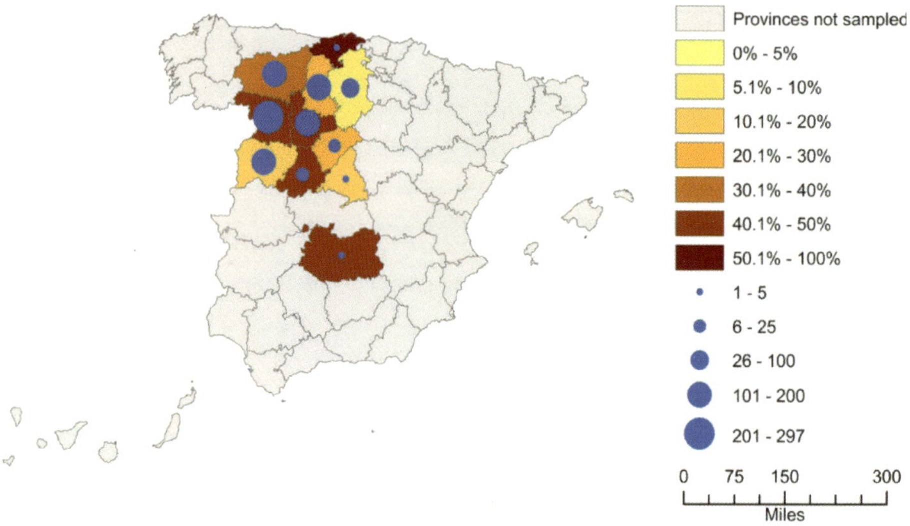

Figure 1: Presence of *Mycoplasma agalactiae* per province over the 2008–2010 period . The color code of each province indicates the presence rate of *M. agalactiae*. The circles indicate the number of dairy sheep farms sampled once in each province over the sampled period.

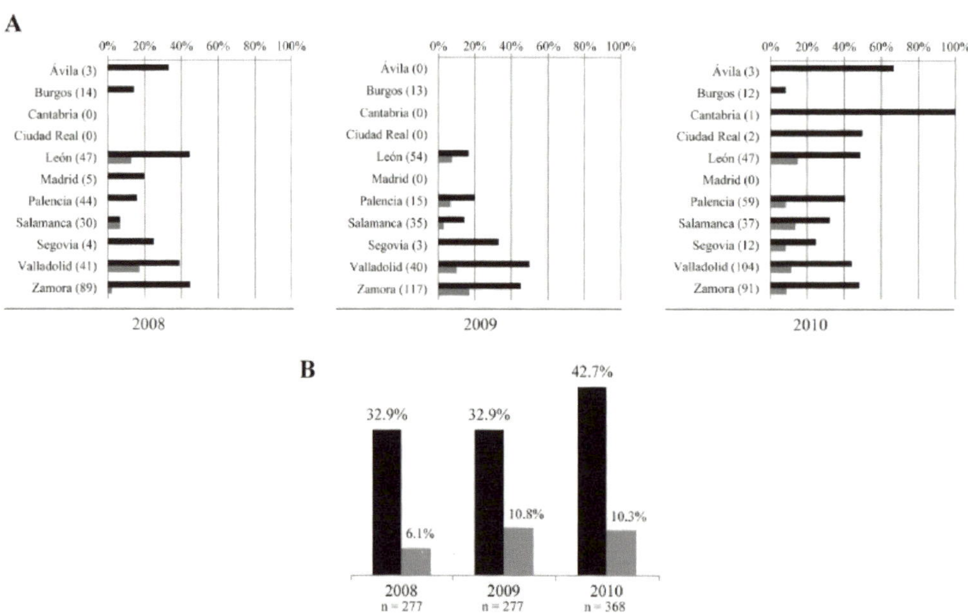

Figure 2: Presence of *Mycoplasma agalactiae* in Spanish sheep farms in 2008, 2009 and 2010 . Black bars represent results by real time PCR and grey bars by microbiological identification. The numbers in brackets represent the number of sampled farms. **A**) Presence per province; **B**) presence per year.

Temporal distribution of *Mycoplasma agalactiae*

The presence of *M. agalactiae* increased between 2008 (32.9%) and 2010 (42.7%) (Figure 2B). The minimum and maximum frequency of detection of *M. agalactiae* ranged from 7.7% in February 2009 to 53.1% in May 2009. The months when the pathogen was most frequently detected were May 2009 (53.1%), July 2010 (51%) and October 2008 (50%). On the contrary, the lowest detection occurred in February 2009 (7.7%), June 2009 (14%) and April 2010 (16.7%). Thereby, 72 out of 194 farms (37.1%) were positive to *M. agalactiae* in Spring (i.e. farms analyzed in March, April and May), 113 out of 286 (39.5%) in Summer (i.e. June, July and August), 110 out of 280 (39.3%) in Autumn (i.e. September, October and November) and 44 out of 162 (27.2%) in Winter (i.e. December, January and February).

DISCUSSION

M. agalactiae was the only CA-causing *Mycoplasma* detected in dairy sheep farms located in the study area, and it was found to be widely distributed as it was detected in all eleven provinces sampled (Figure 1). In contrast, although *M. agalactiae* has been detected with a high prevalence in Spanish goat herds ranging from 40% to 66% [14, 15], it seems that *M. mycoides* subsp. *capri* plays the major role in goat [2, 16]. Interestingly, *M. capricolum* subsp. *capricolum* and *M. putrefaciens* have been recently isolated in goat herds located in the Canary Islands and Extremadura (southwestern Spain) regions [17, 18], and yet those pathogens have not been detected in sheep flocks from the study area suggesting that Spanish dairy sheep are free of their presence or, at least, that their distribution would be restricted outside the sampling area. Furthermore, in this study we have observed that the frequency of detection of *M. agalactiae* increased from 32.9% in 2008 to 42.7% in 2010, suggesting that the pathogen has spread in the sampling area during the study period. On the other hand, we tried to establish relationships between the excretion of the microorganism in milk and the stages in sheep milk production (e.g. period of parturitions, the start of lactation) by analyzing the presence of *M. agalactiae* per month and per season in the different sampling years, but no pattern was found. We hypothesize that this is because the farms from the sampled region frequently had different production systems, and the same production stage may have occurred in a different time between farms.

To our knowledge, few surveys have been carried out internationally to determine which *Mycoplasma* species are circulating in sheep. In Northern Jordan, investigations revealed a seroprevalence in sheep, goat and mixed flocks of 25%, 21% and 30% respectively, for *M. agalactiae,* and 32%, 38% and 34% for *M. mycoides*subsp. *capri*, suggesting that both microorganisms are widely distributed in that country and to the same extent in sheep and goats [7, 10]. This scenario is probably caused because in Jordan more than 93% of sheep and goats are kept together in mixed farms, so both hosts are exposed to the same pathogens. In contrast, the existence of mixed farms in Spain is not common, hindering the dissemination of other *Mycoplasma*species from goat herds to sheep flocks.

Detection of *M. agalactiae* by using microbiological techniques (9.2%) greatly underestimated its presence in comparison to detection by using real time PCR (36.8%). This finding prompts the recommendation that PCR-based methods should be routinely used in *Mycoplasma* detection, as microbiological identification leads to underestimation due to the fastidious growth requirements of mycoplasmas, and serology is not a suitable method in those areas, such as Spain, where systematic vaccination is extended.

The results of this study require careful interpretation. Firstly, this syndrome follows a chronic course in endemic areas and the animals present an intermittent excretion of the microorganism in milk [3, 5]. Therefore, the presence of *M. agalactiae* could have been underestimated, as samples were collected from the milk tanks. In fact, the findings obtained in this study suggest a high level of intermittent excretion, as in more than 26% of the re-sampled farms a previously positive flock tested negative in a later sampling and 63.9% overall tested positive. Considering that *M. agalactiae* is a highly persistent pathogen, remaining in the animals for years [4, 5], and that it is very difficult to eliminate from infected herds, we can assume that in most of those cases infected animals were not excreting the pathogen at the sampling time or that the number of bacteria present was below the limit of detection. Consequently, if monitoring of a herd needs be implemented, the inclusion of other suitable type of samples (e.g. blood, articular, auricular, ear canal, eye and vaginal swabs, nasal secretions, joint fluids) is strongly recommended. Secondly, the lower sensitivity of the conventional-PCR technique in comparison to the real time PCR could have underestimated the presence of the *Mycoplasma* species detected by the first method. Notwithstanding, all CA-causing mycoplasmas were detected after the inoculation of from 10^8 to 10^2 cells of each *Mycoplasma* spp. in 50 mL milk samples. Detection failed in samples containing 10^1 cells (0.2 cells/mL) probably because the initial amount of mycoplasmas was not enough to compete during the enrichment step with all the other microbiota present in the milk samples. This suggests that all the PCR systems can detect the minimum quantity of mycoplasmas needed for growing in the enrichment step, and therefore that the presence of the *Mycoplasma* species as detected by conventional PCR would not be underestimated in detriment of the species detected by real time PCR. In addition, these results confirm that the enrichment step does not favor any species to the detriment to the others, and therefore that we can detect co-infected samples.

CONCLUSIONS

This study provides for the first time an over of the presence of CA-causing mycoplasmas circulating in Spanish dairy sheep farms. *M. agalactiae* was the only species detected in the study area showing a high frequency of presence, and it was found to be widely distributed. The high frequency of detection of the pathogen supports the implementation of control and prevention measures to hinder the dissemination of *M. agalactiae* and to prevent the entrance of other *Mycoplasma* species, such as systematic laboratory detection, isolation or slaughtering of infected flocks and tracing of livestock exchange.

METHODS

Study area and sampling

From August 2008 to July 2009, and from April to December 2010, 1,798 samples were taken from 1,313 dairy sheep farms located in twelve provinces: Ávila, Burgos, Cáceres, Cantabria, Ciudad Real, León, Madrid, Palencia, Salamanca, Segovia, Valladolid and Zamora. Most provinces belong to the Spanish region which presents the highest sheep milk production (60% of total sheep milk) [19]. Selection of the farms was not performed following a formal randomization process, but blind samples were randomly provided by the Regional Interprofessional Dairy Laboratory. As blind sampling was carried out, 922 out of 1,313 farms were sampled once, and the resting 391 farms were sampled from 2 to 5 times. To ensure that no farms contribute more than once in the determination of the frequency of presence of the mycoplasmas, only those results obtained from the 922 farms sampled once have been used to perform the analyses showed in this study. The results obtained from the farms sampled several times have been only used to assess the level of intermittent excretion of the microorganisms in milk.

The sampling represents more than 16% of total dairy sheep farms in Spain and more than 44% of the farms located in the most productive region (Table 1). Location of the farms and overall number of dairy sheep per province is depicted in Figure 3. Each week, twenty raw milk samples of 50 ml were taken from the refrigerated tanks and preserved during transportation at 4°C with 133 μL of a bacteriostatic agent (9.975×10^{-2} μg chloramphenicol, 2.394 μg sodium azide, 1.33 μl ethanol, 5.985 μg trisodium citrate hydrate, 4.655×10^{-2}μg bromophenol blue). The samples were immediately analyzed because freezing considerably reduces the viability of mycoplasmas [20].

Table 1: Geographic distribution of the Spanish dairy sheep farms sampled to detect CA-causing mycoplasmas

Province	No. Farms	No. Sampled Farms	% Sampled Farms
Ávila	91	9	9.9
Burgos	125	65	52.0
Cáceres	130	2	1.5
Cantabria	29	2	6.9
Ciudad Real	829	2	0.2
León	430	205	47.7
Madrid	174	6	3.4
Palencia	414	177	42.8
Salamanca	384	132	34.4
Segovia	79	30	38.0
Valladolid	491	292	59.5
Zamora	902	391	43.3
12 provinces	**4,078**	**1,313**	**32.2**

Study areas for detecting the presence of CA-causing mycoplasmas in Spanish dairy sheep farms. The samples were collected from flocks located in twelve provinces showing highest sheep milk production in Spain.

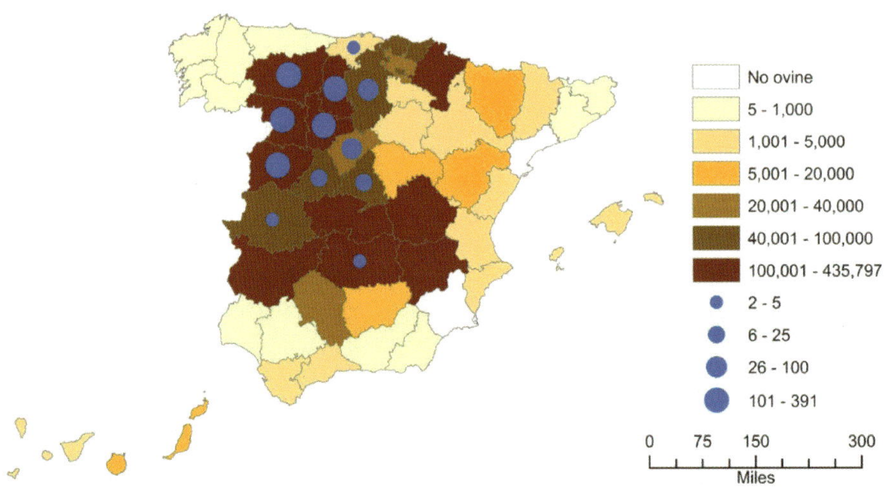

Figure 3: Distribution of dairy sheep in Spain and number of farms sampled per province . The color code of each province indicates the number of dairy sheep present in that province in 2012 (http://www.marm.es/). The circles indicate the number of dairy sheep farms sampled in each province over the 2008–2010 period. Overall, 1,313 farms were sampled.

Culture of milk samples and DNA extraction

One hundred microlitres of the milk samples were cultivated in 9.9 ml of Mycoplasma broth base with Mycoplasma supplement G (Oxoid, Hampshire, UK), at 37°C in 5% CO_2 atmosphere for 3 days. For DNA extraction, 1 ml of culture was centrifuged at $13{,}000 \times g$ for 15 min, and the cell pellet was resuspended in 100 µl of 10 mM Tris–HCl (pH 8.0) for further incubation at 95°C with shaking for 20 min. Then, samples were centrifuged at maximum speed for 3 min, the supernatant was transferred into new tubes, and subsequently analyzed for CA-causing mycoplasmas.

Molecular detection of CA-causing mycoplasmas by PCR-based methods

Since *M. agalactiae* is the main aetiological agent, its presence was assessed in all farms. The presence of *M. mycoides* subsp. *capri*, *M. capricolum* subsp. *capricolum* and *M. putrefaciens* was evaluated in 597 samples taken from 528 sheep farms distributed in the eleven provinces. The latter samples were collected in July 2009 and since April to December 2010. Molecular detection of *M. agalactiae* was conducted by real time PCR as previously described [11] in a 7500 real time PCR system platform (Applied Bios stems, Carlsbad, CA, USA). *M. mycoides* cluster and *M. putrefaciens* detection was carried out by conventional PCR [12, 13]. PCR amplification products were resolved by gel electrophoresis on 1.5% (w/v) agarose gels and visualized after staining with ethidium bromide by using a UV transilluminator (BioRad, Hercules, CA, USA). All samples were analyzed in duplicate and positive, negative extraction and non template controls were included in each run. The limit of detection of the real time PCR system corresponds to approximately 1 genomic equivalent per reaction. Those of the conventional PCR systems have not been reported. Therefore, in order to demonstrate that the PCR methods used in this study could detect the same levels of *Mycoplasma* contamination, and that detection of naturally co-infected samples would be possible, raw milk samples were artificially contaminated with decreasing concentrations of all four mycoplasmas and then processed following the protocol detailed above.

Microbiological detection

Pre-enriched milk samples were cultured in agar plates of the selective medium, which were incubated at 37°C in a 5% CO_2 atmosphere for 3 to 4 days. After incubation, colonies consistent with *Mycoplasma*phenotype were identified using an optical microscope Leica DMLS under 100 × magnifications (LeicaMicrosystems GmbH, Wetzlar, Germany).

Isolation of mycoplasmas

We isolated from 1 to 6 colonies from each positive milk sample and subculture them in specific broth medium at 37°C, in a 5% CO_2 atmosphere for 3 days. The nature of the isolates was reconfirmed by real time PCR [11] and the purity of the culture by checking the morphology of the colonies on agar plates of the selective medium. Finally, the isolates were cryopreserved in glycerol (16% v/v) and stored at −80°C.

DECLARATIONS

Acknowledgements

This study was supported by project RTA 2008–073 of the Spanish Ministry of Education and Science, Government of Spain. We thank Dr. Nigel Cook (FERA, UK) for critical revision of the manuscript.

Authors' contributions

JA carried out the experiments, results analysis and drafted the manuscript. DRL and MH led the project, designed the study and revised the results and manuscript. All authors read and approved the final manuscript.

REFERENCES

1. Chazel M, Tardy F, Le Grand D, Calavas D, Poumarat F: Mycoplasmoses of ruminants in France: recent data from the national surveillance network. BMC Vet Res. 2000, 6: 32.
2. De la Fe C, Assunção P, Antunes T, Rosales RS, Poveda JB: Microbiological survey for Mycoplasma spp. in a contagious agalactia endemic area. Vet J. 2005, 170 (2): 257-259. 10.1016/j.tvjl.2004.05.002.
3. Lambert M: Contagious agalactia of sheep and goats. Rev Sci Tech. 1987, 6 (3): 699-711.
4. Bergonier D, Berthelot X, Poumarat F: Contagious agalactia of small ruminants: current knowledge concerning epidemiology, diagnosis and control. Rev Sci Tech. 1997, 16 (3): 848-873.
5. Corrales JC, Esnal A, De la Fe C, Sánchez A, Assunçao P, Poveda JB, Contreras A: Contagious agalactia in small ruminants. Small Rumin Res. 2007, 68 (1): 154-166. 10.1016/j.smallrumres.2006.09.010.
6. Nicholas RAJ: Improvements in the diagnosis and control of diseases of small ruminants caused by mycoplasmas. Small Rumin Res. 2002, 45: 145-149. 10.1016/S0921-4488(02)00095-0.
7. Al-Momani W, Abo-Shehada MN, Nicholas RAJ: Seroprevalence of and risk factors for Mycoplama mycoides subspecies capri infection in small ruminants in Northern Jordan. Trop Anim Health Prod. 2011, 43 (2): 463-469. 10.1007/s11250-010-9717-9.
8. De Azevedo EO, De Alcântara MDB, Do Nascimento ER, Tabosa IM, Barreto ML, De Almeida JF, Araújo MD, Rodrigues ARO, Riet-Correa F, De Castro RS: Contagious Agalactia by Mycoplasma agalactiae in small ruminants in Brazil: first report. Braz J Microbiol. 2006, 37 (4): 576-581. 10.1590/S1517-83822006000400033.
9. Kinde H, DaMassa AJ, Wakenell PS, Petty R: Mycoplasma infection in a commercial goat dairy caused by Mycoplasma agalactiae and Mycoplasma mycoides subsp. mycoides (caprine biotype). J Vet Diagn Invest. 1994, 6 (4): 423-427. 10.1177/104063879400600404.
10. Al-Momani W, Nicholas RAJ, Abo-Shehada MN: Risk factors associated with Mycoplasma agalactiae infection of small ruminants in northern Jordan. Prev Vet Med. 2008, 83: 1-10. 10.1016/j.prevetmed.2007.08.003.

11. Oravcová K, López-Enríquez L, Rodríguez-Lázaro D, Hernández M: Mycoplasma agalactiae p40 Gene, a novel marker for diagnosis of Contagious Agalactia in sheep by Real-Time PCR: assessment of analytical performance and in-house validation using naturally contaminated milk samples. J Clin Microbiol. 2009, 47 (2): 445-450. 10.1128/JCM.01442-08.
12. Peyraud A, Woubit S, Poveda JB, De la Fe C, Mercier P, Thiaucourt F: A specific PCR for the detection of Mycoplasma putrefaciens, one of the agents of the contagious agalactia syndrome in goats. Mol Cell Probes. 2003, 17 (6): 289-294. 10.1016/j.mcp.2003.07.006.
13. Woubit S, Manso-Silván L, Lorenzon S, Gaurivaud P, Poumarat F, Pellet M-P, Singh VP, Thiaucourt F: A PCR for the detection of mycoplasmas belonging to the Mycoplasma mycoides cluster: Application to the diagnosis of contagious agalactia. Mol Cell Probes. 2007, 21 (5–6): 391-399.
14. Andrada M, Déniz S, González M, Rodríguez F, Poveda JB: Epidemiology of Mycoplasma mycoides subsp. mycoides LC in caprine herds by indirect ELISA in Gran Canaria: preliminary results. COST 826. Agriculture and Biotechnology: Mycoplasmas of Ruminants: Pathogenicity, Diagnostics. Edited by: Poveda J, Fernandez A, Frey J, Johansson KE. Brussels: Epidemiology and Molecular Genetics, vol.5. European Communities; 2000:126-129.
15. Assunçao P, De la Fe C, Ramirez AS, Andrada M, Poveda JB: Serological study of contagious agalactia in herds of goats in the Canary Islands. Vet Rec. 2004, 154: 684-687. 10.1136/vr.154.22.684.
16. Amores J, Gómez-Martín A, Corrales JC, Sánchez A, Contreras A, De la Fe C: Presence of contagious agalactia causing mycoplasmas in Spanish goat artificial insemination centres. Theriogenology. 2011, 75 (7): 1265-1270. 10.1016/j.theriogenology.2010.11.040.
17. De la Fe C, Gutierrez A, Poveda JB, Assunsao P, Ramírez AS, Fabelo F: First isolation of Mycoplasma capricolum subsp. capricolum, one of the causal agents of caprine contagious agalactia, on the island of Lanzarote (Spain). Vet J. 2007, 173 (2): 440-442. 10.1016/j.tvjl.2005.09.011.
18. Gil MC, Peña FJ, Hermoso De Mendoza J, Gomez L: Genital Lesions in an Outbreak of Caprine Contagious Agalactia Caused by Mycoplasma agalactiae and Mycoplasma putrefaciens. J Vet Med. 2003, 50 (10): 484-487.
19. The Spanish Ministry of Agriculture: Food and Environment (MARM). database [http://www.marm.es/app/vocwai/Inicio.aspx?sec=SOC].
20. Amores J, Sánchez A, Martín ÁG, Corrales JC, Contreras A, De La Fe C: Viability of Mycoplasma agalactiae and Mycoplasma mycoides subsp. capri in goat milk samples stored under different conditions. Vet Microbiol. 2010, 145 (3–4): 347-350.

CHAPTER 14

MYCOPLASMA GALLISEPTICUM INFECTION IN THE GREY PARTRIDGE PERDIX PERDIX: OUTBREAK DESCRIPTION, HISTOPATHOLOGY, BIOCHEMISTRY AND ANTIOXIDANT PARAMETERS

Frantisek Vitula, Lucie Peckova, Hana Bandouchova, Miroslav Pohanka, Ladislav Novotny, David Jira, Jiri Kral, Karel Ondracek, Jitka Osickova, Dagmar Zendulkova, Katerina Rosenbergova, Frantisek Treml and Jiri Pikula

BACKGROUND

The grey partridge *Perdix perdix*, a famous bird native to Europe and introduced to many parts of the world, has shown a marked population decline throughout Europe since the second half of the 20th century [1]. Factors driving this decline include a sharp decrease in chick survival due to pesticide use, habitat loss due to agricultural intensification and mechanisation, lower hatching success, and increased predation [2]. As this avian species is both of conservation and commercial game management concern, captive-bred grey partridges are widely used for repopulation purposes [3, 4]. The release of farm-bred birds presents some risks that can combine and result in high mortality rate in the reintroduced population [5]. Game bird reintroductions have been reported to fail because of behavioural deficiencies, post-release predation, lower disease resistance, disease outbreaks, and genetic differences between the released and the wild birds [3, 5, 6, 7]. Birds originating from infected captive flocks may introduce new agents into the wild populations or suffer from adverse effects of the parasite burdens they carry [8, 9]. The release of other game birds, such as *Phasianus colchicus* pheasants and *Alectoris rufa* red-legged partridge, can also prove harmful for grey partridges due to competition and shared pathogens [2].

An outbreak of mycoplasmosis occurred at a game bird farm (Moravia, Czech Republic) producing birds for release and affected a flock of breeding grey partridges in 2010. Laboratory diagnosis confirmed *Mycoplasma gallisepticum*, the most economically significant mycoplasma pathogen of poultry [10, 11]. This organism has already been reported to cause disease in game birds including pheasants, chukar and red-legged partridges, bobwhite quail, Japanese quail and peafowl [11, 12, 13, 14, 15]. Recent isolations of the agent from passerines with conjunctivitis and the spread of the infection throughout eastern USA and Canada have warranted its classification among emerging infectious diseases in wildlife [16, 17].

Mycoplasma infections are known to be associated with oxidative damage of host cells and tissues due to reactive oxygen species generated by both the immune system of the host and the bacterium as its primary virulence factor [18, 19, 20, 21, 22, 23, 24]. Resistance to oxidative stress, therefore, seems to be crucial for mycoplasmas to survive within the host [21]. Responses of the host cell antioxidant defence systems to the human pathogen *Mycoplasma pneumoniae* have been studied extensively *in vitro* using human cell cultures [18, 19, 20, 23, 24]. *M. gallisepticum* infection of cultured chicken embryo fibroblasts has also demonstrated that attachment of viable mycoplasmas to cells is crucial to

Citation: Frantisek Vitula, Lucie Peckova, Hana Bandouchova, Miroslav Pohanka, Ladislav Novotny, David Jira, Jiri Kral, Karel Ondracek, Jitka Osickova, Dagmar Zendulkova, Katerina Rosenbergova, Frantisek Treml and Jiri Pikula, Mycoplasma gallisepticum infection in the grey partridge Perdix perdix: outbreak description, histopathology, biochemistry and antioxidant parameters, DOI: 10.1186/1746-6148-7-34.

decrease catalase activity and that this lower enzyme activity may be important for the development of cytopathic effects [22].

With the exception of one study on the oxidative stress and alterations of antioxidant status in blood samples from goats infected with *Mycoplasma agalactiae* [25], there are no *in vivo* reports concerning other animal species and birds in particular. While clinical signs, lesions, pathogenicity, epizootiology, laboratory diagnosis and control of the *M. gallisepticum* infection in game birds are well described [11, 12, 13, 14, 15], little is known about the effect of the pathogen on the avian host regarding oxidative stress and biochemistry in association with histopathological findings. The molecular and cellular events that lead to the development of lesions and clinical disease are still obscure [10]. Thus, the objective of this study was to describe the outbreak and evaluate normal blood and tissue biochemical parameters as well as biochemical responses and pathology in a flock of grey partridges naturally infected with *M. gallisepticum*.

METHODS

Experimental birds and samples collected

One-year-old captive-bred adult grey partridges were used in the study. The birds were kept at a game bird farm (Moravia, Czech Republic). Control healthy birds (44 males and 44 females) were blood sampled for normal biochemistry and evaluation of gender differences. A total of 5 suspected *Mycoplasma*-infected pairs of birds showing pronounced clinical signs of respiratory disease were blood sampled and then sacrificed by decapitation in order to collect samples for bacterial laboratory diagnosis and organs including the heart, eye and the associated infraorbital sinus, nervous system, lungs, kidney, spleen, liver and gonads for histopathology and measurements of antioxidant parameters. A control group of 5 healthy pairs were also sampled in this way. The study was performed in compliance with the laws for the protection of animals against cruelty as approved by the Ethical Committee of the University of Veterinary and Pharmaceutical Sciences Brno, Czech Republic.

Bacterial diagnosis (*Mycoplasma* culture and identification)

Clinical specimens were collected and cultured as previously recommended [26]. Swabs from the trachea, nares and conjunctival sacs, the inflammatory content of infraorbital sinuses and a piece of lung tissue were plated onto the mycoplasma agar and inoculated into the broth for the isolation of avian mycoplasmas [27], as modified by Bradbury [28]. Samples were incubated at 37°C in an atmosphere of 5% CO_2. Broths were examined daily for colour change in the pH indicator and plates every 2-3 day for colony growth. The *Mycoplasma* spp. isolates were further identified using the nested polymerase chain reaction (PCR). The presence of *M. gallisepticum* DNA was detected using a nested PCR based on the amplification of the 16S rRNA gene sequence specific for *M. gallisepticum* (accession number M22441). Primers for the 1st and 2nd PCR were selected using the Vector NTI Suite 5.5 (INFORMAX) and synthesised on a commercial basis by the Generi Biotech company (Czech Republic). Sequence of primers for the 1st PCR reaction are Sn: 5'ATG CTG AGA GGT AGA ATA ACC 3' and Asn: 5›CCA CCT TAC GGA TTT GC 3›; for the 2nd PCR Sn: 5'GGC GAA GGC GAG GAC TTG GG 3' and Asn: 5›GCA CCG AAG TAT TCG CTC CGA CAC 3›. The NucleoSpin Tissue Kit (Machery - Nagel, Germany) was used to isolate the total DNA from the sample as described by the producer. Both PCR reactions were performed in 20 μl of the reaction mixture in a Biometra *T*-personal thermocycler (Germany). The reaction mixture contained PPP Master Mix (i.e., 200 μM of each dNTP, 2.5 mM $MgCl_2$, 2U Taq Purple DNA polymerase; Top Bio, Czech Republic) and primers in the concentration of 25 pmol/μl. Amplification in both reactions included 30 cycles of denaturation at 94°C for 35 s, annealing at 49°C (the 1st PCR) or 66°C (the 2nd PCR) for 25 s and elongation at 72°C for 90 s. The PCR product (volume 10 μl) gained in the 2nd PCR was analysed by electrophoresis in the 2% agarose gel stained with ethidium bromide and visualised using an UV transilluminator. The specific PCR product of 130 bp was compared with the molecular weight marker O›GeneRuler DNA Ladder Mix (Fermentas International Inc., USA).

Apart from the mycoplasma culture, routine bacteriological examination was performed. Samples collected from the liver, spleen, kidneys, lungs, infraorbital sinuses and air sacs were aerobically incubated at 37°C for 48 hours on blood agar and MacConkey agar. The bacterial growths were then identified by standard methods.

Serological tests

Control healthy birds and partridges suspected from *Mycoplasma* infection were serologically examined for avian respiratory infections including 1) Newcastle disease (haemagglutination inhibition test with VLDIA039 HAG-NDL live antigen for use in the HI test and VLDIA053 HAR-NDL monospecific antiserum for use as a positive control in the HI test; GD-Animal Health Service, Deventer, the Netherlands), 2) avian influenza (AI Ab enzyme-linked immunosorbent assay ELISA; IDEXX Laboratories, Inc., Westbrook, Maine, USA), 3) infectious bronchitis (IBV Ab ELISA; IDEXX Laboratories, Inc., Westbrook, Maine, USA), 4) infectious laryngotracheitis (agar gel immunodiffusion with VLDIA014 AGA-ILT live antigen for use in the AGID test for infectious laryngotracheitis and VLDIA022 AGP-ILT monospecific infectious laryngotracheitis antiserum for use as a positive control in the AGID test and VLDIA030 SPF-CH chicken negative control serum for use as a negative control in most poultry assays; GD-Animal Health Service, Deventer, the Netherlands), 5) avian rhinotracheitis (APV Ab ELISA; IDEXX Laboratories, Inc., Westbrook, Maine, USA), 6) avian chlamydiosis (Chlamydia complement fixation test; Institute Virion Ltd., Zurich, Switzerland) as well as antibodies against 7) *M. gallisepticum* (MG Ab ELISA; IDEXX Laboratories, Inc., Westbrook, Maine, USA).

Histopathology

Specimens of heart, eye and the associated infraorbital sinus, nervous system, lungs, kidney, spleen, liver and gonads (ovaries and testes) were collected and placed in 10% buffered formalin during autopsy, and were treated using a routine histological technique and embedded in paraffin. Sections of 5 μm thicknesses were made from the paraffin blocks and these were stained with haematoxylin and eosin.

Plasma biochemistry

Blood (1 ml) was collected from the right jugular vein using the Omnican® 40 (Braun, Germany). Whole blood was placed in heparinised tubes (Leciva inj., Prague), centrifuged immediately, and plasma was removed and frozen (-20°C). Within a few days, plasma was analysed using an automated analyser (SPOTCHEM™ EZ SP-4430, ARKRAY, Japan) for aspartate aminotransferase (μkat/l), alkaline phosphatase (μkat/l), lactate dehydrogenase (μkat/l), creatine kinase (μkat/l), alanine aminotransferase (μkat/l), total protein (g/l), total cholesterol (mmol/l), high-density lipoprotein cholesterol (mmol/l), triglycerides (mmol/l), glucose (mmol/l), amylase (μkat/l), uric acid (mmol/l), calcium (mmol/l) and phosphorus (mmol/l).

Antioxidant parameters

The antioxidant parameters were assayed in tissues (heart, eye and the associated infraorbital sinus, nervous system, lungs, kidney, spleen, liver, ovaries and testes) and plasma samples were collected at the time of autopsy and kept at -80°C until use. Biochemicals, enzymes and other chemicals used in the study were purchased from Sigma-Aldrich (Prague, Czech Republic) and were of the highest available commercial grade. The tissues were homogenised on ice using a mechanical homogeniser (100 mg of tissue in 1 ml) in 50 mM potassium phosphate buffer (KH_2PO_4 with 1 mM EDTA, pH 7.4) for assessment of catalase (CAT) activity and in phosphate buffered saline (PBS, pH 7.2) for other parameters. The postmitochondrial supernatant was collected after centrifugation (30 min at 30,000 *g* at 4°C for CAT and 15 min at 10,000 *g* at 4°C for the other parameters) and stored frozen at -80°C until biochemical analyses. The methods for the assessment of most of the biochemical markers measured are described in our previous article [29]. Briefly, glutathione-*S*-transferase (GST) activity was measured spectrophotometrically using 1-chloro-2,4-dinitrobenzene. The concentration of reduced glutathione (GSH) was determined using 5,5'-dithiobis-2-nitrobenzoic acid (DTNB) as a chromogen. Activity of glutathione reductase (GR) was determined from the rate of NADPH oxidation. The level of lipid peroxidation in avian tissues was assessed as total thiobarbituric acid reactive species (TBARS). Activity of CAT was evaluated spectrophotometrically at 240 nm in cuvettes as the rate of hydrogen peroxide breakdown in the mixture containing 0.09% hydrogen peroxide in 50 mM TRIS/0.1 mM EDTA buffer [30]. The protein concentrations were determined by the method using the Folin-Ciocalteu phenol reagent. The GENios spectrophotometric microplate reader (Tecan Group, Switzerland) was used to measure the absorbance in all assays and the VARIAN CARY 50 Bio spectrophotometer (Varian, USA) was used for measuring absorbance of solutions in cuvettes. The total antioxidant capacity was measured using the ferric reducing antioxidant power assay (FRAP). The FRAP assay was performed as described previously [31], with minor modifications. In the first round, the FRAP reagent was prepared as a mixture of 2.5 ml of 10 mM 2,4,6-tris(2-pyridyl)-*s*-triazine (TPTZ) in 40 mM HCl and 2.5 ml of 20 mM $FeCl_3$ in 25 ml of 0.1 M acetate buffer pH 3.6. The freshly prepared FRAP reagent was incubated at 37°C for 10 minutes. The volume of 30 μl of the tissue or plasma sample was mixed with 200 μl of the FRAP reagent and then with distilled water up to 1 ml. After 10 min of incubation, the mixture was centrifuged at 10,000 *g*. A blank sample was prepared in the same way as described above but saline solution was used instead of the tissue or plasma sample. Absorbance of the supernatant was measured at 593 nm against the blank.

Statistical analysis

Statistica for Windows® 7.0 (StatSoft, Tulsa, OK, USA) was used to compare different groups by one-way analysis of variance (ANOVA) and post-hoc analysis of means by the LSD test. The homogeneity of variances was tested by Levene›s test. Non-homogenous parameters, as determined by Levene›s test, were log-transformed prior to analysis. In these cases, the non-parametric Kruskal-Wallis test was used for comparing the groups. A *post-hoc* power analysis was conducted to show that the sample size of 10 healthy and 10 infected birds in this study provided sufficient statistical power for comparing tissue biochemical parameters. Values of $p < 0.05$ and $p < 0.01$ were considered statistically significant and highly significant, respectively, for all tests. Spearman rank order correlations were used to assess the relationships among the measured parameters.

RESULTS

Outbreak description

An outbreak of respiratory disease occurred in a flock of adult grey partridges kept at a game bird farm (Moravia, Czech Republic). The infection developed gradually in April to May 2010, culminated by morbidity of 100% and 60% (i.e., a total of 68 partridges) died within three to four weeks of appearance of clinical signs. Clinical signs included nasal and ocular discharge and dyspnoea with laboured open-mouth breathing, eyelid and infraorbital sinus swelling, lethargy, poor intake of feed and weight loss. There was a marked drop in egg production. Culture revealed *Mycoplasma* spp. in tracheal swabs only. A slight colour change (acidity) appeared in the broth medium on the 4th day and first centered mycoplasma colonies were recognized on plates on the 5th day of incubation. The isolated strain was further identified as *M. gallisepticum* using the nested PCR methods (Figure 1). Bacteriological culture of the liver, spleen, kidneys, lungs, small intestinal content, infraorbital sinuses and air sacs yielded *Escherichia coli* from infraorbital sinuses, lungs and air sacs. Serological tests for Newcastle disease, avian influenza, infectious bronchitis, infectious laryngotracheitis, avian rhinotracheitis and avian chlamydiosis were negative in birds included in the control healthy and *Mycoplasma*-infected groups of partridges. The titre of antibodies against *M. gallisepticum* ranged from 1404 to 5884 in the *Mycoplasma*-infected group. Necropsy revealed an accumulation of caseous exudate within the infraorbital sinuses, tracheitis, pneumonia and airsacculitis. Histopathological findings can be summarised as severe purulent infraorbital sinusitis, moderate purulent tracheitis with marked epithelial hyperplasia, moderate to severe purulent bronchitis and extensive purulent and necrotic pneumonia with secondary bacterial colonisation of necrotic areas. Figures 2A and 2B show the comparison of the normal tracheal tissue and tracheitis with inflammatory cell infiltration in *M. gallisepticum*-infected birds. Likewise, Figures 3A and 3Bof normal and mycoplasmal infraorbital sinus, respectively, demonstrate the serious nature of pathology in this tissue and Figures 4A and 4B show the comparison of normal and necrotic lung tissues.

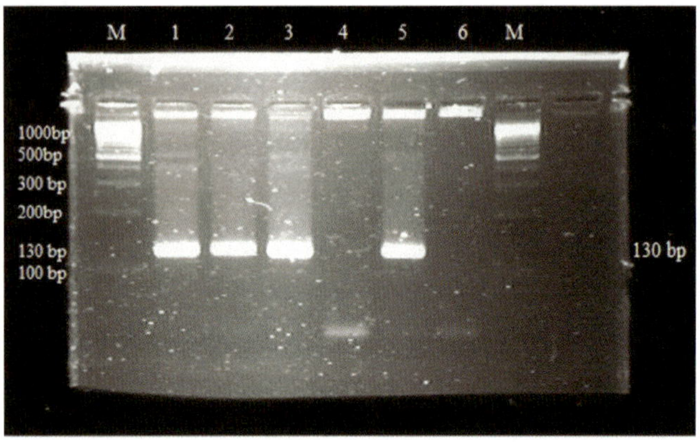

Figure 1: Detection of *M. gallisepticum* by nested PCR. M = Molecular size marker, 100 bp DNA ladder (O›GeneRuler™ DNA Ladder Mix, Fermentas International Inc., USA). 1 to 3 - positive samples, 4 - a negative sample, 5 - positive control, 6 - negative control.

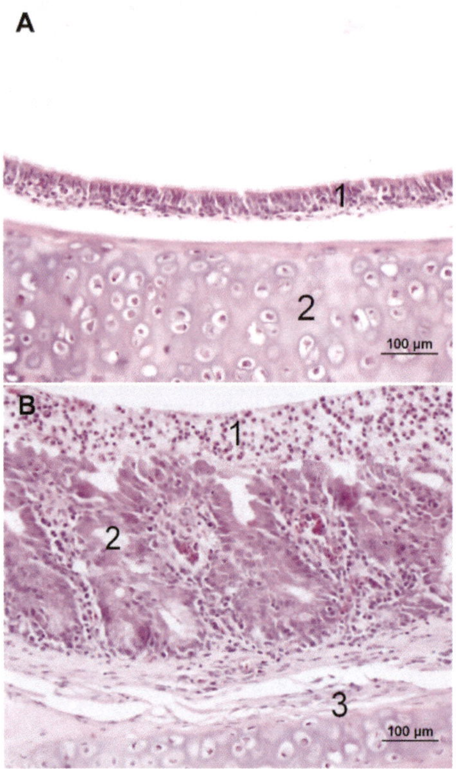

Figure 2: Comparison of normal tracheal tissue and tracheitis with inflammatory cell infiltration in *M. gallisepticum* -infected birds. Figure 2A: Trachea of a partridge from the control group. Normal mucosa lined with a pseudo-stratified columnar epithelium with kinocilia (1) and a fibrocartilaginous layer (2) are presented. No signs of inflammation were observed in any of the tracheal layers. Epithelial detachment is artificial due to sample processing. H&E stain.

Figure 2B: Trachea of a partridge infected with *M. gallisepticum*. The inflammatory exudate, composed mostly of heterophils, is adhered to the epithelium (1). The epithelium is moderately hyperplastic with loss of the kinocilia and lamina propria is moderately infiltrated by lymphocytes and plasma cells (2). The fibrocartilaginous layer (3) is composed of the dense connective tissue mildly infiltrated by lymphocytes and plasma cells, and the perichondrium and hyaline cartilage. H&E stain.

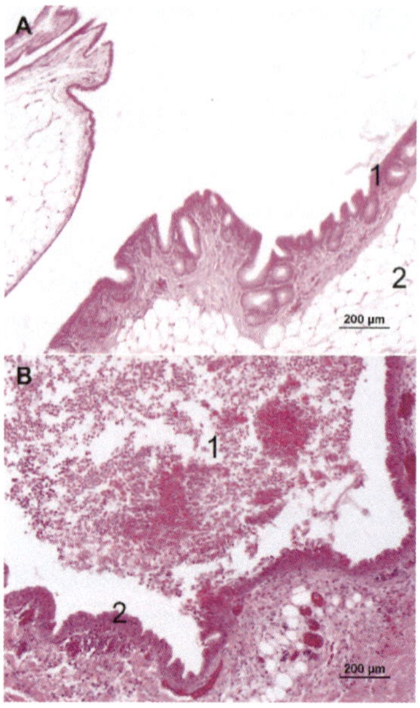

Figure 3: Comparison of normal and mycoplasmal infraorbital sinus demonstrating the serious nature of pathology in *M. gallisepticum* -infected birds. Figure 3A: The infraorbital sinus of a partridge from the control group. The sinus is lined with a simple columnar epithelium (1). The sinus is surrounded by adipose tissue (2). H&E stain.

Figure 3B: The infraorbital sinus of a partridge infected with *M. gallisepticum*. The sinus is richly filled with a dense purulent exudate (1). The epithelium is mildly hyperplastic and the lamina propria is focally infiltrated by lymphocytes and plasma cells (2). H&E stain.

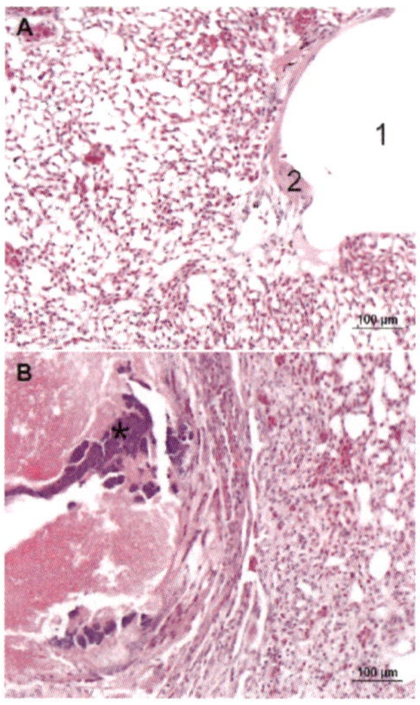

Figure 4: Comparison of normal lungs and pneumonia with necrotic areas and bacterial colonies in *M. gallisepticum* -infected birds. Figure 4A: The lung parenchyma of a partridge from the control group. Parabronchial lumen (1) and wall with bundles of smooth muscle tissue (2) is surrounded by air and blood capillaries. H&E stain.

Figure 4B: A focus of necrotic pneumonia with secondary bacterial colonisation (*) surrounded by a thin layer of heterophils and lymphocytes in a partridge infected with *M. gallisepticum*. H&E stain.

Biochemistry and antioxidant parameters

Table 1 presents normal plasma chemical profiles in healthy adult grey partridges as well as values measured in *Mycoplasma*-infected birds. Comparison of healthy males and females revealed gender differences in creatine kinase, total protein and high-density lipoprotein cholesterol. Significant increases in the biochemical parameters of *Mycoplasma*-infected birds, when compared to controls, included activities of lactate dehydrogenase, creatine kinase and amylase, and levels of total protein and glucose.

Table 1: Differences in biochemical parameters between healthy control and *Mycoplasma*-infected partridges

Parameters	Groups of birds	
	Healthy control birds	***Mycoplasma*-infected birds**
AST (μkat/l)	4.88 ± 1.93	4.84 ± 1.35
ALP (μkat/l)	3.79 ± 1.64	3.42 ± 1.75
LDH (μkat/l)	2.55 ± 1.35	8.20 ± 3.47**
CK (μkat/l)	11.58 ± 13.30 (M 17.21 ± 15.60; F 5.94 ± 7.05**)	28.88 ± 18.13**
ALT (μkat/l)	0.69 ± 0.13	0.62 ± 0.26
TP (g/l)	38.62 ± 7.99 (M 36.52 ± 5.36; F 40.76 ± 9.59*)	54.16 ± 9.64**
T-CHOL (mmol/l)	3.17 ± 1.00	3.70 ± 0.83
HDL-CHOL (mmol/l)	2.30 ± 0.75 (M 2.54 ± 0.80; F 2.06 ± 0.63**)	1.95 ± 0.40
TG (mmol/l)	1.31 ± 0.65	1.02 ± 0.80
GLU (mmol/l)	18.90 ± 2.60	21.68 ± 4.91*
AMY (μkat/l)	3.50 ± 1.47	5.98 ± 1.52**
UAC (μmol/l)	608.46 ± 418.91	918.66 ± 445.45
Ca (mmol/l)	2.63 ± 0.25	2.84 ± 0.22
P (mmol/l)	0.98 ± 0.41	1.09 ± 0.50

Values represent mean ± SD; n = 88 in healthy control birds (44 males and 44 females), n = 10 in *Mycoplasma*-infected birds; * = $p < 0.05$, ** = $p < 0.01$; significant gender differences shown where appropriate. AST = aspartate aminotransferase, ALP = alkaline phosphatase, LDH = lactate dehydrogenase, CK = creatine kinase, ALT = alanine aminotransferase, TP = total protein, T-CHOL = total cholesterol, HDL-CHOL = high-density lipoprotein cholesterol, TG = triglycerides, GLU = glucose, AMY = amylase, UAC = uric acid, Ca = calcium, P = phosphorus, M = male, and F = female.

Differences in antioxidant parameters between healthy control and *Mycoplasma*-infected grey partridges are shown in Table 2. While catalase showed significantly lower activity in the heart, lungs, liver and gonads of *Mycoplasma*-infected birds, glutathione-S-transferase was elevated in the eye and the associated infraorbital sinus and kidney, and decreased in the liver. Decreased levels of reduced glutathione were found in the heart, kidney, liver and gonads of birds affected by mycoplasmosis and the activity of glutathione reductase was lower only in the lungs. Compared to healthy birds, mycoplasmosis in the grey partridge caused significant differences in the level of lipid peroxidation measured as the total thiobarbituric acid reactive species in avian lungs and plasma. The ferric reducing antioxidant power was lower in the heart and kidneys.

Table 2: Differences in antioxidant parameters between healthy control and *Mycoplasma*-infected partridges

Parameters	Tissues	Groups of birds	
		Healthy control birds	***Mycoplasma*-infected birds**
CAT	Eye + infraorbital sinus	61.80 ± 23.37	48.91 ± 16.63
	Heart	66.90 ± 25.95	39.28 ± 4.40*
	nervous system	41.57 ± 9.09	44.18 ± 20.07
	Lungs	61.33 ± 16.16	38.34 ± 11.34*
	Kidney	48.18 ± 14.89	50.75 ± 21.54
	Spleen	57.19 ± 20.00	40.19 ± 8.81
	Liver	63.15 ± 14.38	43.36 ± 6.43*
	Gonads (ovaries/testes)	62.62 ± 22.30	36.95 ± 11.37*
	Plasma	59.67 ± 12.88	47.72 ± 24.24
GST	Eye + infraorbital sinus	19.49 ± 12.55	46.06 ± 19.41*
	Heart	134.16 ± 43.02	215.66 ± 98.39

	nervous system	53.21 ± 34.50	80.41 ± 32.21
	Lungs	67.70 ± 35.61	69.44 ± 34.74
	Kidney	236.40 ± 72.85	362.33 ± 64.05*
	Spleen	25.08 ± 18.82	71.66 ± 67.29
	Liver	389.80 ± 92.82	254.33 ± 98.20*
	Gonads (ovaries/testes)	134.16 ± 43.02	215.68 ± 98.37
	Plasma	645.83 ± 90.52	461.80 ± 157.78
GSH	Eye + infraorbital sinus	2.00 ± 0.04	1.929 ± 0.15
	Heart	1.78 ± 0.04	1.33 ± 0.03**
	nervous system	2.03 ± 0.17	1.91 ± 0.10
	Lungs	1.76 ± 0.05	1.73 ± 0.17
	Kidney	1.82 ± 0.20	1.44 ± 0.17**
	Spleen	1.79 ± 0.06	1.83 ± 0.05
	Liver	2.35 ± 0.30	1.59 ± 0.12**
	Gonads (ovaries/testes)	1.91 ± 0.17	1.49 ± 0.32*
	Plasma	212.52 ± 4.04	232.93 ± 17.27*
GR	Eye + infraorbital sinus	2.46 ± 0.87	3.48 ± 1.51
	Heart	28.45 ± 25.82	7.27 ± 2.34
	nervous system	7.82 ± 3.49	5.49 ± 2.73
	Lungs	57.55 ± 13.07	26.34 ± 9.31**
	Kidney	36.44 ± 8.84	39.03 ± 9.00
	Spleen	28.99 ± 12.22	24.16 ± 16.51
	Liver	53.32 ± 15.68	36.70 ± 9.55
	Gonads (ovaries/testes)	10.93 ± 6.74	8.57 ± 3.58
	Plasma	529.20 ± 392.81	321.54 ± 84.73
TBARS	Eye + infraorbital sinus	0.14 ± 0.03	0.15 ± 0.03
	Heart	0.14 ± 0.01	0.17 ± 0.04
	nervous system	0.19 ± 0.04	0.18 ± 0.03
	Lungs	0.09 ± 0.02	0.14 ± 0.02*
	Kidney	0.20 ± 0.04	0.18 ± 0.04
	Spleen	0.14 ± 0.01	0.17 ± 0.04
	Liver	0.14 ± 0.01	0.17 ± 0.04
	Gonads (ovaries/testes)	0.14 ± 0.01	0.17 ± 0.04
	Plasma	216.46 ± 47.06	133.32 ± 59.80*
FRAP	Eye + infraorbital sinus	4.52 ± 1.31	2.76 ± 1.27
	Heart	1.96 ± 0.27	1.52 ± 0.12**
	nervous system	2.09 ± 0.31	2.00 ± 0.11
	Lungs	1.72 ± 0.44	1.77 ± 0.43
	Kidney	6.84 ± 0.93	3.77 ± 1.62**
	Spleen	4.52 ± 1.31	2.76 ± 1.27
	Liver	1.72 ± 0.44	1.77 ± 0.43
	Gonads (ovaries/testes)	2.47 ± 0.63	3.11 ± 1.01
	Plasma (mmol/g)	1.72 ± 0.44	1.77 ± 0.43

Values represent mean ± SD; n = 10 in healthy control birds (5 males and 5 females), n = 10 in *Mycoplasma*-infected birds (5 males and 5 females); * = $p < 0.05$, ** = $p < 0.01$. CAT = catalase (μmol H_2O_2/min/mg protein), GST = glutathione-*S*-transferase (μkat/g), GSH = reduced glutathione (μmol/g), GR = glutathione reductase (μkat/g), TBARS = total thiobarbituric acid reactive species (μmol/g), FRAP = ferric reducing antioxidant power assay (μmol/g).

As shown in Table 3, significant correlations among responses of the antioxidant parameters were found namely in the heart, lungs, spleen, liver and plasma. Reduced glutathione positively correlated with ferric reducing antioxidant power, glutathione reductase and catalase in the heart and with glutathione reductase, glutathione-S-transferase and catalase in the liver. There was also a positive correlation between glutathione reductase and catalase and ferric reducing antioxidant power in lungs and spleen, respectively, while glutathione-S-transferase and ferric reducing antioxidant power were in a close positive relationship with catalase both in the liver and plasma. Table 3 also presents numerous significant inter-tissue correlations of all the studied antioxidant parameters. Apart from glutathione-S-transferase in lungs and plasma and reduced glutathione in heart and plasma, all other inter-tissue correlations were positive.

Table 3: Spearman rank order correlations of antioxidant parameters in tissues and plasma

Tissue	**Correlated parameters**	**+/- correlation**	**P-level**
Heart	GSH&FRAP	+	< 0.01
	GSH&GR	+	< 0.05
	GSH&CAT	+	< 0.05
Lungs	GR&CAT	+	< 0.05
Spleen	GR&FRAP	+	< 0.01
Liver	GSH&GR	+	< 0.05
	GSH&GST	+	< 0.01
	GSH&CAT	+	< 0.01
	GST&CAT	+	< 0.05
Plasma	FRAP&CAT	+	< 0.05
Parameters	**Correlated tissues**	**+/- correlation**	**P-level**
CAT	Heart & gonads	+	< 0.01
	Heart & liver	+	< 0.05
	Eye & lungs	+	< 0.05
	CNS & kidney	+	< 0.05
	Lungs & liver	+	< 0.05
	Lungs & plasma	+	< 0.05
	Kidney & plasma	+	< 0.05
	Gonads & liver	+	< 0.01
GST	Heart & eye	+	< 0.05
	Heart & gonads	+	< 0.001
	Heart & spleen	+	< 0.05
	Eye & gonads	+	< 0.01
	Eye & spleen	+	< 0.01
	Lungs & plasma	-	< 0.05
	Gonads & spleen	+	< 0.05
GSH	Heart & kidney	+	< 0.01
	Heart & gonads	+	< 0.05
	Heart & liver	+	< 0.001
	Heart & plasma	-	< 0.01
	Eye & gonads	+	< 0.05
	Kidney & liver	+	< 0.01
	Gonads & liver	+	< 0.05
GR	Heart & plasma	+	< 0.05
TBARS	Heart & lungs	+	< 0.05
	Heart & gonads	+	< 0.001
	Heart & spleen	+	< 0.001
	Heart & liver	+	< 0.001
	Lungs & gonads	+	< 0.05
	Lungs & spleen	+	< 0.05
	Lungs & liver	+	< 0.05
FRAP	Eye & spleen	+	< 0.001

	Lungs & plasma	+	< 0.001
	Liver & plasma	+	< 0.001

CAT = catalase, GST = glutathione-*S*-transferase, GSH = reduced glutathione, GR = glutathione reductase, TBARS = total thiobarbituric acid reactive species, FRAP = ferric reducing antioxidant power assay, eye = eye + the associated infraorbital sinus, CNS = nervous system, gonads = ovaries or testes, n = 20.

DISCUSSION

The outbreak of respiratory disease occurred at the peak of the laying period four months after the introduction of new partridges, i.e., the supposed source of infection in the game bird farm. The long incubation period is in agreement with reports on birds remaining asymptomatic until they are stressed [11]. The disease broke out long after removing the birds from the one-month quarantine and the stress of the laying period was probably the factor triggering clinical manifestation. Pheasants and partridges are known to harbour many fast-growing mycoplasmas, making the isolation of the slower-growing *M. gallisepticum* difficult [13]. In the present study, however, the isolation and identification of this mycoplasma species was straightforward. The high titres against *M. gallisepticum* together with its cultural and PCR identification witness for an ongoing systemic *M. gallisepticum* infection. While the high morbidity in the grey partridge flock corresponds with rates observed both in poultry and other avian species infected by *M. gallisepticum* as the sole pathogen, the high mortality is rather typical for mycoplasmosis complicated by some other infectious agent [11, 12, 13, 14, 15, 32]. Indeed, *E. coli* was cultured from infraorbital sinuses, lungs and air sacs of some mycoplasmal birds and there were bacterial colonies in the lungs upon investigation by histopathology. It has been experimentally shown that combined stressors exert enhanced effects in birds [33], and, apart from *E. coli*, other bacteria and viruses such as *Pasteurella multocida* and infectious bronchitis virus, respectively, may be implicated in synergistic respiratory infections with *M. gallisepticum* [13, 14, 15]. Serology, however, excluded other common respiratory infections in birds included in the control healthy and *Mycoplasma*-infected groups of partridges.

Mycoplasmosis affecting birds in the laying period results in reduced egg production and quality [11]. The quantity of eggs laid by the grey partridge breeding flock decreased abruptly following the disease outbreak and eggs produced were not incubated to prevent contamination of the hatching device. It was, therefore, not possible to evaluate the biological quality of the clutch using such characteristics as viability and hatchability. Since an immune challenge decreases the reproductive allocation to the egg in the grey partridge [34], mycoplasmas are egg transmitted [11], and mycoplasmosis can also induce salpingitis in birds [35], the total effect of hatching (i.e., the percentage of chicks hatching from all eggs set) would certainly be very poor if the eggs were incubated.

Gross and microscopic pathology was specifically used to demonstrate the severity of the disease in grey partridges affected by *M. gallisepticum* in this biochemical study. Previous papers have reported sinusitis and bilateral swelling of the infraorbital sinuses as the most outstanding feature, airsacculitis in 46%, and tracheitis and lung lesions in 36 and 21% of cases, respectively [11, 14, 15]. Comparing the effects of experimental intranasal infection with *M. gallisepticum* and *Mycoplasma imitans* in red-legged partridges, nasal and sinus exudates were found in both groups, while tracheal exudates and airsacculitis were only seen in the *M. gallisepticum* infection [14]. As the culture revealed *M. gallisepticum* in tracheal swabs and changes in the grey partridge were very similar to those mentioned above, pathological findings of the present study were in agreement with those observed by other authors [11, 14, 15].

As shown in Table 1, gender differences in healthy control birds do not interfere with the interpretation of significant responses in plasma chemical profiles of *Mycoplasma*-infected partridges. The results indicate that diagnosis of avian mycoplasmosis solely based on clinical biochemical parameters is not possible. They can, nevertheless, be used for the evaluation of the general health status in mycoplasmal birds [36]. One would expect lower total protein and glucose due to starvation and weight loss in the *Mycoplasma*-infected group. Contrary to this, there was an increase in total plasma protein and glucose levels, probably as a consequence of inflammation or dehydration in the former parameter and stress in the latter. A response somewhat different from that in partridges was seen in caprine mycoplasmal pneumonia because total protein level was found to be lower, while the glucose level was increased [37]. Amylase catalyses the hydrolysis of polysaccharides, it is associated with glycaemia and its increase corresponds with the observed higher levels of glucose [38]. Both enzymes activities of which were significantly increased in mycoplasmal partridges, i.e., lactate dehydrogenase and creatine kinase, are closely associated. Lactate dehydrogenase is found in skeletal and cardiac muscle, liver, kidney, bone and erythrocytes and elevations can be observed with disruption of any of these. Distinguishing the source of lactate dehydrogenase elevation is based on measuring creatine kinase that originates mainly in skeletal and cardiac muscle. Elevated lactate dehydrogenase levels (three-fold) with concurrent elevation in creatine kinase (two-fold) in the present study are thus suggestive of skeletal or cardiac muscle damage [36].

The research presented here showed modulations of antioxidant parameters, the total antioxidant capacity and oxidative damage in the form of lipid peroxidation associated with the respiratory disease caused by a natural infection with *M. gallisepticum* of grey partridges. Oxidative stress is an unspecific biochemical process involved in the adverse action of many stressors. There is a clear association between oxidative stress and immune responses of birds to infectious agents [39]. Endogenous antioxidant defences of an enzymatic and non-enzymatic nature are essential for the control of reactive-molecular-species-mediated oxidative damage of biomolecules [40]. Interestingly, changes in oxidative stress parameters were not restricted to the respiratory apparatus of mycoplasmal birds, but also occurred in non-respiratory organs and plasma. Similarly, extrapulmonary complications were recognised in humans with *M. pneumoniae* infection [41]. Statistical analysis also revealed significant correlations among responses of the oxidative stress parameters in the heart, lungs, spleen, liver and plasma, and numerous inter-tissue correlations of all the studied oxidative stress parameters. Correlations among the oxidative stress parameters illustrate the complex character of the response and interdependence of parameters. Significant correlations among the studied parameters observed in the liver confirm the major metabolic role of this organ in birds. It would be an interesting issue for future studies to evaluate the relationship between the tissue mycoplasmal burden and oxidative stress parameters, as has been done in other bacterial infections [42].

Hydrogen peroxide and superoxide radicals produced by mycoplasmas are coupled with endogenous toxic oxygen molecules generated by the host cells to induce oxidative stress that then results in host cell damage [24, 41]. It has been suggested that the pathogenesis of mycoplasmosis comprises the following sequence of events: (a) adherence of mycoplasmas to host cells; (b) generation of superoxide and hydrogen peroxide by the microorganisms and their introduction into host cells; (c) irreversible inhibition of host cell catalase by intracellular reactive-oxygen-species accumulation; and (d) oxidative damage to vital cell constituents [18, 19, 22]. In agreement with the above mentioned *in vitro* findings, catalase showed significantly lower activity in the heart, lungs, liver and gonads of *Mycoplasma*-infected partridges.

Significant changes were found for the glutathione-related parameters. Glutathione-S-transferase was elevated in the eye and the associated infraorbital sinus and kidney, and decreased in the liver. Decreased levels of reduced glutathione were in the heart, kidney, liver and gonads and the activity of glutathione reductase was lower only in the lungs of birds affected by mycoplasmosis. These results correspond basically with data on the protective role of the glutathione redox cycle and its adaptive responses observed in cultured fibroblasts and mice infected with *M. pneumoniae*, respectively [20, 23]. Similarly, decreases in plasma glutathione concentrations and glutathione peroxidase activity were reported in goats naturally infected with *M. agalactiae* [25].

It is possible to evaluate the total antioxidant capacity of biological fluids using the ferric reducing antioxidant power assay as a clinical marker of oxidative stress. Non-enzymatic antioxidants such as ascorbic acid, uric acid, bilirubin, vitamin E, α-tocopherol and albumin contribute to the ferric reducing antioxidant power, the reaction is linearly related to their molar concentrations, and uric acid is estimated to make around 60% of the contribution to the plasma value [31]. Importantly, the primary route of excretion of nitrogenous waste in birds is via the formation of uric acid in the liver and its elimination by renal tubular secretion [36]. As shown in Table 1, uric acid levels were increased in the blood of mycoplasmal birds, but not significantly owing to the greater variability of data. Despite it, the total antioxidant capacity of plasma was nearly the same in both groups of birds and agreed with normal plasma values already published for the grey partridge [43]. The ferric reducing antioxidant power values were significantly lower only in the heart and kidneys of *Mycoplasma*-infected birds.

While ingested carotenoids are both ornamental pigments and antioxidants in birds, *M. gallisepticum*infection can disrupt their utilisation and result in a trade-off between immune system activation, oxidative stress and the health or sexual quality traits [44, 45]. These and other diet-derived antioxidants can therefore be supplemented to feeds for *Mycoplasma*-infected captive birds as a means of supportive therapy.

Compared to healthy birds, mycoplasmosis in the grey partridge caused significant differences in the level of lipid peroxidation, i.e., a parameter of damage to membrane lipids, measured as the total thiobarbituric acid reactive species in avian lungs and plasma. Contrary to the situation in goats naturally infected with *M. agalactiae* [25], lipid peroxidation was decreased in plasma samples collected from mycoplasmal partridges. This is, however, understandable in light of the birds from the group infected by *M. gallisepticum* being able to maintain normal blood antioxidant capacity and induction of higher levels of the non-enzymatic antioxidant glutathione. As expected, avian mycoplasmosis was associated with increased lipid peroxidation in the lungs.

Mycoplasmas are considered to be extracellular pathogens. It has, however, been demonstrated recently that *M. gallisepticum* has the capability of entering nonphagocytic host cells, where it resists host defences and antibiotic therapy. This is also a mechanism of establishing chronic infections, while passage through the respiratory mucosal barrier is responsible for the ability to cause systemic infections [46]. As eradication is very difficult or even impossible once *M. gallisepticum* has been introduced, the breeding flock of grey partridges should be depopulated rather than used for repopulation [11].

CONCLUSIONS

The present study demonstrated the high susceptibility of grey partridges to a natural infection with *M. gallisepticum*, the severity of the disease based on histopathology and the biochemical responses to mycoplasmosis in this avian host. While the reported data make a contribution to the understanding of the pathogenic mechanisms of mycoplasmal respiratory disease in birds, the normal biochemistry and antioxidant parameters of tissues and plasma may also prove useful as future references in experimental studies, and clinical or laboratory tests using grey partridges.

DECLARATIONS

Acknowledgements

This study was supported by the Ministry of Education, Youth and Sports of the Czech Republic and the Internal Grant Agency of the University of Veterinary and Pharmaceutical Sciences Brno (Projects MSM 6215712402 and 80/2010/ FVHE, respectively).

Authors' contributions

FV carried out the whole study and drafted the manuscript. LP, HB, DJ, JK, KO and JO planned the study design, sampled the birds and performed biochemical evaluations. MP analysed plasma and tissue samples for antioxidant parameters and lipid peroxidation. LN evaluated histopathological findings. DZ performed mycoplasmal culture. KR examined the isolated mycoplasmas using the nested PCR. FT evaluated the outbreak of avian mycoplasmosis in the breeding flock of partridges.

JP supervised the whole study, performed data analyses and drafted the manuscript. All authors read and approved the final manuscript.

REFERENCES

1. BirdLife International (2011) Species factsheet: *Perdix perdix*. [http://www.birdlife.org]
2. Kuijper DPJ, Oosterveld E, Wymenga E: Decline and potential recovery of the European grey partridge (Perdix perdix) population - a re. Eur J Wildl Res. 2009, 55 (5): 455-463. 10.1007/s10344-009-0311-2.
3. Rantanen EM, Buner F, Riordan P, Sotherton N, Macdonald DW: Habitat preferences and survival in wildlife reintroductions: an ecological trap in reintroduced grey partridges. J Appl Ecol. 2010, 47 (6): 1357-1364. 10.1111/j.1365-2664.2010.01867.x.
4. Wiberg S, Gunnarsson S: Health and welfare in Swedish game bird rearing. Sustainable Animal Production - the Challenges and Potential Developments for Professional Farming. Edited by: Aland A, Madec F. 2009, Wageningen: Wageningen Academic Publishers, 395-407.
5. Meriggi A, Brangi A, Cuccus P, Della Stella RM: High mortality rate in a re-introduced grey partridge population in Italy. Ital J Zool. 2002, 69 (1): 19-24. 10.1080/11250000209356433.
6. Gortazar C, Acevedo P, Ruiz-Fons F, Vicente J: Disease risks and overabundance of game species. Eur J Wildl Res. 2006, 52 (2): 81-87. 10.1007/s10344-005-0022-2.
7. Liukkonen T: Finnish native grey partridge (Perdix perdix) population differs clearly in mitochondrial DNA from the farm stock used for releases. Ann Zool Fenn. 2006, 43 (3): 271-279.
8. Millan J, Gortazar C, Villafuerte R: A comparison of the helminth faunas of wild and farm-reared red-legged partridge. J Wildl Manage. 2004, 68 (3): 701-707. 10.2193/0022-541X(2004)068[0701:ACOTHF]2.0.CO;2.
9. Villanua D, Perez-Rodriguez L, Casas F, Alzaga V, Acevedo P, Vinuela J, Gortazar C: Sanitary risks of red-legged partridge releases: introduction of parasites. Eur J Wildl Res. 2008, 54 (2): 199-204. 10.1007/s10344-007-0130-2.
10. Bradbury JM: Poultry mycoplasmas: sophisticated pathogens in simple guise. Br Poult Sci. 2005, 46 (2): 125-136. 10.1080/00071660500066282.
11. Levisohn S, Kleven SH: Avian mycoplasmosis (Mycoplasma gallisepticum). Rev Sci Tech Off Int Epizoot. 2000, 19 (2): 425-442.
12. Bencina D, Mrzel I, Rojs OZ, Bidovec A, Dovc A: Characterisation of Mycoplasma gallisepticum strains involved in respiratory disease in pheasants and peafowl. Vet Rec. 2003, 152 (8): 230-234. 10.1136/vr.152.8.230.
13. Bradbury JM, Yavari CA, Dare CM: Mycoplasmas and respiratory disease in pheasants and partridges. Avian Pathol. 2001, 30 (4): 391-396. 10.1080/03079450120066395.
14. Ganapathy K, Bradbury JM: Pathogenicity of Mycoplasma gallisepticum and Mycoplasma imitans in red-legged partridges (Alectoris rufa). Avian Pathol. 1998, 27 (5): 455-463. 10.1080/03079459808419369.
15. Welchman DD, Bradbury JM, Cavanagh D, Aebischer NJ: Infectious agents associated with respiratory disease in pheasants. Vet Rec. 2002, 150 (21): 658-664. 10.1136/vr.150.21.658.
16. Benskin CMH, Wilson K, Jones K, Hartley IR: Bacterial pathogens in wild birds: a re of the frequency and effects of infection. Biol Rev. 2009, 84 (3): 349-373. 10.1111/j.1469-185X.2008.00076.x.
17. Williams ES, Yuill T, Artois M, Fischer J, Haigh SA: Emerging infectious diseases in wildlife. Rev Sci Tech Off Int Epizoot. 2002, 21 (1): 139-157.
18. Almagor M, Yatziv S, Kahane I: Inhibition of host-cell catalase by Mycoplasma pneumoniae - a possible mechanism for cell injury. Infect Immun. 1983, 41 (1): 251-256.
19. Almagor M, Kahane I, Yatziv S: Role of superoxide anion in host-cell injury induced by Mycoplasma pneumoniae infection - a study in normal and trisomy 21 cells. J Clin Invest. 1984, 73 (3): 842-847. 10.1172/JCI111279.
20. Almagor M, Kahane I, Gilon C, Yatziv S: Protective effects of the glutathione redox cycle and vitamin E on cultured fibroblasts infected by Mycoplasma pneumoniae. Infect Immun. 1986, 52 (1): 240-244.
21. Jenkins C, Samudrala R, Geary SJ, Djordjevic SP: Structural and functional characterization of an organic hydroperoxide resistance protein from Mycoplasma gallisepticum. J Bacteriol. 2008, 190 (6): 2206-2216. 10.1128/JB.01685-07.
22. Nunoya T, Tajima M, Yagihashi T: Decrease in catalase activity of cultured cells by Mycoplasma gallisepticum infection. Vet Microbiol. 1987, 13 (4): 343-351. 10.1016/0378-1135(87)90065-4.
23. Kariya C, Chu HW, Huang J, Leitner H, Martin RJ, Day BJ: Mycoplasma pneumoniae infection and environmental tobacco smoke inhibit lung glutathione adaptive responses and increase oxidative stress. Infect Immun. 2008, 76 (10): 4455-4462. 10.1128/IAI.00136-08.
24. Sun GP, Xu XF, Wang YS, Shen XY, Chen ZM, Yang J: Mycoplasma pneumoniae infection induces reactive oxygen species and DNA damage in A549 human lung carcinoma cells. Infect Immun. 2008, 76 (10): 4405-4413. 10.1128/IAI.00575-08.
25. Kizil O, Ozdemir H, Karahan M, Kizil M: Oxidative stress and alterations of antioxidant status in goats naturally infected with Mycoplasma agalactiae. Rev Med Vet. 2007, 158 (6): 326-330.
26. Bradbury JB: Recovery of Mycoplasmas from birds. In Methods in Molecular Biology. Volume 104. Edited by: Miles RJ, Nicholas RAJ. New Jersey: Humana Press Inc; 1998:45-51.
27. Edward DG: A selective medium for pleuropneumonia-like organisms. J Gen Microbiol. 1947, 1: 238-243.
28. Bradbury JM: Rapid biochemical tests for characterization of the *Mycoplasmatales*. J Clin Microbiol. 1977, 5: 531-534.

29. Paskova V, Adamovsky O, Pikula J, Skocovska B, Band'ouchova H, Horakova J, Babica P, Marsalek B, Hilcherova K: Detoxification and oxidative stress responses along with microcystins accumulation in Japanese quail exposed to cyanobacterial biomass. Sci Total Environ. 2008, 398 (1-3): 34-47. 10.1016/j.scitotenv.2008.03.001.

30. Aebi H: Catalase in vitro. Method Enzymol. 1984, 105: 121-126.

31. Benzie IFF, Strain JJ: The ferric reducing ability of plasma (FRAP) as a measure of ''antioxidant power'': the FRAP assay. Anal Biochem. 1996, 239 (1): 70-76. 10.1006/abio.1996.0292.

32. Nunoya T, Yagihashi T, Tajima M, Nagasawa Y: Occurrence of keratoconjunctivitis apparently caused by Mycoplasma gallisepticum in layer chickens. Vet Pathol. 1995, 32 (1): 11-18. 10.1177/030098589503200102.

33. Pikula J, Bandouchova H, Hilscherova K, Paskova V, Sedlackova J, Adamovsky O, Knotkova Z, Lany P, Machat J, Marsalek B, Novotny L, Pohanka M, Vitula F: Combined exposure to cyanobacterial biomass, lead and the Newcastle virus enhances avian toxicity. Sci Total Environ. 2010, 408 (21): 4984-4992. 10.1016/j.scitotenv.2010.07.050.

34. Cucco M, Guasco B, Malacarne G, Ottonelli R: Effects of beta-carotene on adult immune condition and antibacterial activity in the eggs of the Grey Partridge, Perdix perdix. Comp Biochem Physiol A Mol Integr Physiol. 2007, 147 (4): 1038-1046. 10.1016/j.cbpa.2007.03.014.

35. Domermut CH, Gross WB, Dubose RT: Mycoplasmal salpingitis of chickens and turkeys. Avian Dis. 1967, 11 (3): 393-398. 10.2307/1588185.

36. Fudge AM: Avian clinical pathology - hematology and chemistry. Avian Medicine and Surgery. Edited by: Altman RB, Clubb SL, Dorrestein GM, Quesenberry K. 1997, Philadelphia: W.B. Saunders Company, 142-157. 1

37. Mondal D, Pramanik AK, Basak DK: Clinico-haematology and pathology of caprine mycoplasmal pneumonia in rain fed tropics of West Bengal. Small Ruminant Res. 2004, 51 (3): 285-295. 10.1016/S0921-4488(02)00177-3.

38. Place AR: Birds and lipids: living off the fat of the earth. Poult Avian Biol Rev. 1996, 7 (2-3): 127-141.

39. Costantini D, Moller AP: Does immune response cause oxidative stress in birds? A meta-analysis. Comp Biochem Physiol A Mol Integr Physiol. 2009, 153 (3): 339-344. 10.1016/j.cbpa.2009.03.010.

40. Halliwell B, Gutteridge JMC: Free Radicals in Biology and Medicine.Oxford: Oxford University Press; 1999.

41. Waites KB, Talkington DF: Mycoplasma pneumoniae and its role as a human pathogen. Clin Microbiol Rev. 2004, 17 (4): 697-728. 10.1128/CMR.17.4.697-728.2004.

42. Bandouchova H, Sedlackova J, Pohanka M, Novotny L, Hubalek M, Treml F, Vitula F, Pikula J: Tularemia induces different biochemical responses in BALB/c mice and common voles. BMC Infect Dis. 2009, 9: 9-10.1186/1471-2334-9-9.

43. Pohanka M, Bandouchova H, Vlckova K, Zdarova Karasova J, Kuca K, Damkova V, Peckova L, Vitula F, Pikula J: Square wave voltammetry on screen printed electrodes: comparison to ferric reducing antioxidant power in plasma from model laboratory animal (Grey Partridge) and comparison to standard antioxidants. J Appl Biomed. 2011, 9: 103-109. 10.2478/v10136-009-0032-6.

44. Blount JD: Carotenoids and life-history evolution in animals. Arch Biochem Biophys. 2004, 430 (1): 10-15. 10.1016/j.abb.2004.03.039.

45. Hill GE, Farmer KL, Beck ML: The effect of mycoplasmosis on carotenoid plumage coloration in male house finches. J Exp Biol. 2004, 207 (12): 2095-2099. 10.1242/jeb.00998.

46. Winner F, Rosengarten R, Citti C: In vitro cell invasion of Mycoplasma gallisepticum. Infect Immun. 2000, 68: 4238-4244. 10.1128/IAI.68.7.4238-4244.2000.

CHAPTER 15

MYCOPLASMA ALKALESCENS DEMONSTRATED IN BRONCHOALVEOLAR LAVAGE OF CATTLE IN DENMARK

Branko Kokotovic, Niels F Friis and Peter Ahrens

FINDINGS

Mycoplasma alkalescens is a bovine mycoplasma species, which was originally isolated from the nasal cavity of cattle in Australia [1]. Like many other mycoplasmas, *M. alkalescens* is a normal inhabitant of the upper respiratory tract, but it has also been associated with disease. *M. alkalescens* has mostly been implicated in mastitis in cattle. It has been isolated from bulk tank milk samples, as well as from outbreaks and sporadic cases of clinical mastitis [2, 3, 4, 5]. Furthermore, *M. alkalescens* has been isolated from cases of severe arthritis, and its ability to induce joint lesions has been confirmed under experimental conditions [6, 7]. Rosenfeld & Hill [8] isolated *M. alkalescens* in pure culture from abomasum and lung of an aborted bovine foetus, while Lamm et al. [9] found *M. alkalescens* in association with otitis in calves. Finally, *M. alkalescens*has occasionally been found in association with disorders of the respiratory tract [10, 11].

Recently, 17 bronchoalveolar lavage samples from calves suffering from pneumonia in a single herd in Denmark were submitted, on two occasions, to the National Veterinary Institute for laboratory examinations. The samples were examined for the presence of bacterial pathogens, bovine respiratory mycoplasmas, as well as for the presence of bovine respiratory syncytial virus (BRSV), bovine coronavirus and parainfluenza-3 virus (PI-3). The samples were not examined for infectious bovine rhinotracheitis virus, as Denmark is considered free of this infection. Thereby, eight arginine-metabolizing mycoplasmas were isolated. In the present study the identification of the isolates as *M. alkalescens* is presented. This is the first report of isolation of this species in Denmark.

Bacteriological examination was performed according to standard laboratory procedures. Examination for BRSV, bovine coronavirus and PI-3 was performed using an indirect sandwich-ELISA assay [12]. Isolation of mycoplasmas was performed according to standard laboratory procedures using a Hayflick›s type of medium enriched with arginine [13], with and without addition of 5% of rabbit hyperimmune antiserum against *Mycoplasma bovirhinis*. The isolates were filtered through 0.45 μm membrane filters (Millipore), cloned and submitted to serologic identification, which was performed by the disc growth inhibition test (DGI) with 6 mm filter paper discs prepared with rabbit hyperimmune antisera against *M. alkalescens* PG51^T (ATCC 29103; NCTC 10135), *Mycoplasma arginini* G230^T (ATCC 23838; NCTC 10129) and *Mycoplasma canadense* 275C^T(ATCC 29418; NCTC 10152), as well as by the indirect epi-immunofluorescence test (IF) on colonies on solid medium. Molecular identification of the isolates was performed by amplification and sequencing of their 16S rRNA genes by using universal primers [14].

Laboratory examinations revealed the presence of several bacterial pathogens in 15 of the 17 bronchoalveolar lavage samples, while no pathogenic bacteria were detected in the two remaining samples. *Pasteurella multocida*, *Mannheimia haemolytica*, *Histophilus somni* and *Salmonella* Dublin were found in three, three, one and one samples, respectively. *Mycoplasma bovirhinis* was found in five samples, while arginin-metabolizing mycoplasmas were found in eight samples. Two *P. multocida*, three *M. bovirhinis* and five arginin-metabolizing mycoplasma isolates were found as sole bacteriological findings in 10 respective samples. From

Citation: Branko Kokotovic, Niels F Friis and Peter Ahrens, Mycoplasma alkalescens demonstrated in bronchoalveolar lavage of cattle in Denmark, DOI: 10.1186/1751-0147-49-2.

five samples multiple bacterial species were isolated: *M. bovirhinis* was found once in combination with *P. multocida* and once in combination with *M. haemolytica*, while arginin-metabolizing mycoplasmas were found once in combination with *M. haemolytica*, once in combination with *S.* Dublin and once in combination with *M. haemolytica* and *H. somni*. No viral pathogens were detected in any of the analysed samples.

Further examinations on arginin-metabolizing mycoplasmas showed that all eight isolates could be serologically identified as *M. alkalescens* and that they were clearly different from the two other arginine-degrading species that are commonly found in cattle, *M. canadense* and *M. arginini* (Table 1). The reactions were clear-cut for the DGI tests showing approximately 3–5 mm broad zones of total or nearly total inhibition around the disc. In the IF test some minor cross reactions were noted when three of the isolates and the type strain of *M. alkalescens* PG51^T were tested with anti-*M. canadense* 275C^T hyperimmune serum. The 16S rDNA sequences of the analysed isolates were identical to each other and to the 16S rDNA sequence of the type strain *M. alkalescens* PG51^T (GenBank accession no. U44764; [15]), which corroborated the serological identification of the isolates as *M. alkalescens*.

Table 1: Serological identification of eight mycoplasma field isolates from cattle by DGI and IF test using type strain antisera against *Mycoplasma alkalescens, Mycoplasma arginini and Mycoplasma canadense*

	Antiserum					
	M. alkalescens PG51^T		*M. arginini* G230^T		*M. canadense* 275C^T	
Mycoplasma strains	DGI[a]	IF[b]	DGI[a]	IF[b]	DGI[a]	IF[b]
M. alkalescens PG51^T	5	+	0	-	0	?
Field strain MK19/02	≥ 3	+	0	-	0	-
Field strain MK20/02	≥ 3	+	0	-	0	?
Field strain MK21/02	≥ 3	+	0	-	0	-
Field strain MK49/02*	≥ 3	+	0	-	0	?
Field strain MK51/02	≥ 3	+	0	-	0	-
Field strain MK52/02*	≥ 3	+	0	-	0	-
Field strain MK53/02	≥ 3	+	0	-	0	-
Field strain MK56/02*	≥ 3	+	0	-	0	?
M. arginini G230^T	0	-	5	+	0	-
M. canadense 275C^T	0	-	0	-	5	+

[a] zone of inhibition in mm; [b] distinct FITC colour of stained colonies; ? inconclusive results; * examined by 16S rDNA sequencing.

Previous studies have shown that *H. somni*, *M. haemolytica* and *P. multocida* are the bacteria that are most commonly associated with bronchopneumonia in calves in Denmark, although they are also part of the normal bacterial flora of the respiratory tract [16, 17]. Also, *S.* Dublin, which is predominantly found in cattle, is capable of causing pneumonia in calves. Isolation of these bacterial species in the submitted samples most likely indicate their role as the primary cause of respiratory disease in the herd, probably in combination with unidentified environmental factors. In addition to the bacteria, *M. bovirhinis* and *M. alkalescens* were also isolated. *M. bovirhinis* is commonly found as a part of the normal respiratory tract microflora of cattle and is not considered to be pathogenic. *M. alkalescens*, however, has been found in association with disorders of the respiratory tract but its role as a respiratory pathogen remains equivocal. Experimental infections have demonstrated that *M. alkalescens* has the ability to colonize lung tissue [18], but the two strains used in the study apparently failed to produce pneumonia [18]. In the present study, we found *M. alkalescens* in pure culture in five of the analysed bronchoalveolar lavage samples. This finding is, however, not sufficient to warrant a role of *M. alkalescens* as a cause of bronchopneumonia, since we also found two samples containing only a non-pathogenic *M. bovirhinis*, and two samples without any bacterial or viral pathogens, despite the fact that they derived from calves with clinical signs of a respiratory disease. The failure to detect respiratory tract pathogens in these samples may be due to i.e., their absence in a particular disease stadium when sampling took a place or due to antibiotic treatment. Taking into the consideration the overall bacteriological findings of this study, it seems likely that *M. alkalescens* may have had a role either as a secondary invader or as an opportunistic pathogen rather than suggesting a causal role of the organism in the pneumonia complex.

M. alkalescens is regarded as one of the most common causative agents of mastitis [19]. So, with demonstration of the organism in a Danish cattle herd, a further member of *Mycoplasma* is added to the group of bovine mastitis-inducing microorganisms in Denmark. The only mycoplasma species isolated from clinical outbreaks of mastitis in Denmark so far has been *Mycoplasma bovis* [20], while other mastitis-inducing species, *Mycoplasma bovigenitalium* and *M. canadense*, have been isolated only from the respiratory and the genital tract and semen samples [21]. Further investigations are needed in order to determine the prevalence of *M. alkalescens* in the Danish cattle population and, indeed, to draw a firm conclusions on its importance in disease conditions other than mastitis.

DECLARATIONS

Acknowledgements

Authors thank Ulla Amtoft for skilful technical assistance.

Authors' contributions

BK carried out bacteriological examination of samples, isolation and cloning of mycoplasmas and drafted the manuscript.

NFF carried out identification of mycoplasma isolates by DGI test and epi-immunofluorescence.

PA carried out molecular identification of mycoplasma isolates.

All authors read and approved the final manuscript.

REFERENCES

1. Hudson JR, Etheridge JR: A new type of pleuropneumonia-like microorganism (PPLO) from the nose of cattle. Aust Vet J. 1963, 39: 1-5.
2. Brookbanks EO, Carter ME, Holland JTS: Mycoplasma mastitis. NZ Vet J. 1969, 17: 179-180.
3. Dellinger JD, Jasper DE, Ilic M: Characterization studies on mycoplasmas isolated from bovine mastitis and the bovine respiratory tract. Cornell Vet. 1977, 67: 351-360.
4. Jasper DE: Prevalence of mycoplasmal mastitis in the Western States. California Vet. 1980, 34: 24-26.
5. Jasper DE: The role of *Mycoplasma* in bovine mastitis. J Amer Vet Med Assoc. 1982, 181: 158-162.
6. Bennett RH, Jasper DE: *Mycoplasma alkalescens*-induced arthritis in dairy calves. J Amer Vet Med Assoc. 1978, 172: 484-488.
7. Whithear KG: Isolation of *Mycoplasma alkalescens* from cases of polyarthritis in embryo-transplant calves. Aust Vet J. 1983, 60: 191-192.
8. Rosenfeld LE, Hill MWM: The isolation of *Mycoplasma alkalescens* from an aborted bovine foetus. Aust Vet J. 1980, 56: 350-
9. Lamm CG, Munson L, Thurmond MC, Barr BC, George LW: Mycoplasma otitis in California calves. J Vet Diagn Invest. 2004, 16: 397-402.
10. Hewicker-Trautwein M, Feldmann M, Kehler W, Schmidt R, Thiede S, Seeliger F, Wohlsein P, Ball HJ, Buchenau I, Spergser J, Rosengarten R: Outbreak of pneumonia and arthritis in beef calves associated with *Mycoplasma bovis* and *Mycoplasma californicum*. Vet Rec. 2002, 151: 699-703.
11. Ayling RD, Bashiruddin SE, Nicholas RAJ: Mycoplasma species and related organisms isolated from ruminants in Britain between 1990 and 2000. Vet Rec. 2004, 155: 413-416.
12. Uttenthal A, Jensen NPB, Blom JY: Viral aetiology of enzootic pneumonia in Danish dairy herds: Diagnostic tools and epidemiology. Vet Rec. 1996, 139: 114-117.
13. Kobisch M, Friis NF: Swine mycoplasmosis. Rev Sci Tech Off Int Epiz. 1996, 15: 1569-1605.
14. Weisburg WG, Barns SM, Pelletier DA, Lane DJ: 16S ribosomal DNA amplification for phylogenetic study. J Bacteriol. 1991, 173: 697-703.
15. Pettersson B, Uhlen M, Johansson K-E: Phylogeny of some mycoplasmas from ruminants based on 16S rRNA sequences and definition of a new cluster within the hominis group. Int J Syst Bacteriol. 1996, 46: 1093-1098.
16. Tegtmeier C, Uttenthal A, Friis NF, Jensen NE, Jensen HE: Pathological and microbiological studies on pneumonic lungs from Danish calves. J Vet Med. 1999, 46: 693-700. 10.1046/j.1439-0450.1999.00301.x.
17. Watts JL, Yancey RJ, Sarah JR, Salmon SA, Case CA: A 4-year survey of antimicrobial susceptibility trends for isolates from cattle with bovine respiratory disease in North America. J Clin Microbiol. 1994, 32: 725-731.
18. Gourlay RN, Howard CJ, Thomas LH, Wyld SG: Pathogenicity of some *Mycoplasma* and *Acholeplasma* species in the lungs of gnotobiotic calves. Res Vet Sci. 1979, 27: 233-237.
19. Gonzalez RN, Wilson DJ: Mycoplasma mastitis in dairy herds. Vet Clin North Am Food Anim Pract. 2003, 19: 199-221. 10.1016/S0749-0720(02)00076-2.
20. Friis NF: *Mycoplasma bovis*-induced mastitis in cattle in Denmark. Nord Vet Med. 1984, 36: 324-325.
21. Friis NF, Blom E: Isolation of *Mycoplasma canadense* from bull semen. Acta Vet Scand. 1983, 24: 315-317.

SECTION IV: STAPHYLOCOCCUS AUREUS - RESPIRATORY DISEASE

CHAPTER 16

ALARMING PROPORTIONS OF METHICILLIN-RESISTANT STAPHYLOCOCCUS AUREUS (MRSA) IN WOUND SAMPLES FROM COMPANION ANIMALS, GERMANY 2010–2012

Szilvia Vincze, Ivonne Stamm, Peter A. Kopp, Julia Hermes, Cornelia Adlhoch, Torsten Semmler, Lothar H. Wieler, Antina Lu¨bke-Becker, Birgit Walther

INTRODUCTION

Staphylococcus (S.) aureus is an important pathogen in human and veterinary medicine that is capable of causing purulent and toxin-mediated infections. An uptake of the *mec*A gene, which is encoded on the Staphylococcal cassette chromosome *mec*, enables the expression of an additional penicillin-binding protein (PBP)2a which substitutes an essential cross-linking step of the native PBP2 in the presence of ß-lactams, leading to resistance against antibiotics of this group [1]. In addition, methicillin-resistant *S. aureus* (MRSA) are often resistant against further antimicrobial classes [2].

MRSA raised attention in companion animal medicine during the last decades, especially with regard to transmission from humans to dogs and cats and vice versa [3]–[5]. Further, MRSA are known as important nosocomial pathogens in both human and veterinary medicine [6].

Data concerning the proportion and impact of *S. aureus* and MRSA infections in clinical samples of companion animals are variable but give evidence of an increased infection rate in horses [7] as well as dogs and cats [8] during the last years. Wound infections in particular are described to be frequently caused by *S. aureus* [9], [10].

Genotypic characterization of MRSA from several infection sites of dogs and cats revealed the predominant occurrence of well-known regional hospital associated (HA-) MRSA [5], [11]–[13]. Within Germany, clonal complex (CC) 22-MRSA was reported as the most common lineage in small animals in 2003 and 2004 [9], [13]. Only recently, CC398-MRSA was reported as a cause of canine infections in Germany, as well [14], [15].

In contrast, CC8-MRSA were mainly identified in equine infections, leading to suggestions of adaptation of this lineage to horses [16]. In the recent past, studies revealed the occurrence of LA-MRSA CC398 in horses, as well [7], [16]–[18].

Suspected transmission events between humans and small animals or horses were reported several times in the past [3]–[5], [19] and strains of these lineages with the ability to infect different hosts were denominated as Extended Host Spectrum Genotypes (EHSGs) [17].

The predominance of infections with regularly occurring regional human lineages in companion animals raised the question whether dogs and cats might be an important source of human infection and colonization [20]. Therefore, continuous *S. aureus*-screening in specimens of companion animal origin with further molecular characterization is important to determine changes in frequency or possible adaptation of specific lineages to different hosts.

Hence, we conducted a Germany-wide survey to investigate the frequency of *S. aureus* among samples from clinical wound infections of dog, cat and horse origin. The MRSA-proportion was identified for *S. aureus*-positive samples. Each phenotypically methicillin-resistant *S. aureus*was verified by PCR detection of either the *mec*A or *mec*C gene and characterised by *spa*typing as well as screening for the Panton-Valentine leukocidin (PVL).

Citation: Vincze S, Stamm I, Kopp PA, Hermes J, Adlhoch C, Semmler T, et al. (2014) Alarming Proportions of Methicillin-Resistant Staphylococcus aureus (MRSA) in Wound Samples from Companion Animals, Germany 2010–2012. PLoS ONE 9(1): e85656. doi:10.1371/journal.pone.0085656.

MATERIALS AND METHODS

Sampling and Case Definition

We included all swabs from dogs, cats and horses suffering from wound infections, which were sent from 1,170 veterinarians within Germany to Vet Med Labor GmbH (Ludwigsburg, Germany) for bacteriological analysis between November 2010 and March 2012. Vet Med Labor GmbH is one of the largest veterinary microbiological laboratories, covering most areas within Germany. The samples originated from either veterinarian clinicians or practitioners working at mixed or specialized practices in 1,018 different areas with regard to the postal code throughout Germany. TargetMap (www.targetmap.com) was used to visualize the geographic origin of wound samples (figure 1). *S. aureus* positive wound swabs were phenotypically investigated towards methicillin-resistance based on susceptibility testing for oxacillin and cefoxitin (VITEK®2, bioMérieux, Germany). All MRSA were sent to the Institute of Microbiology and Epizootics, FU Berlin for genotypic characterization.

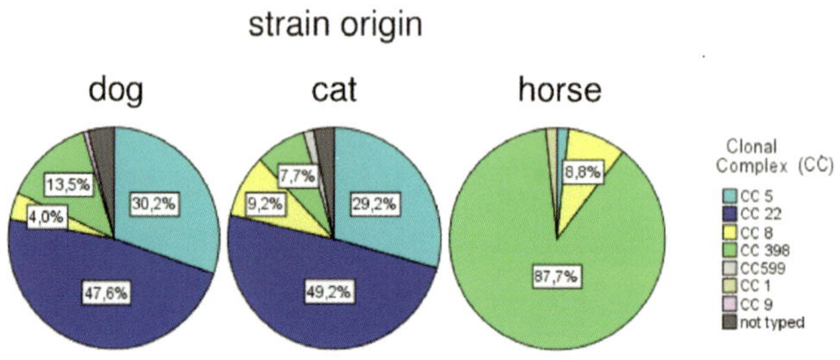

Figure 1: Sample origin.

Figure 1 shows the Germany-wide origin of the 5,229 wound swabs from dogs, cats and horses. Areas are shaped in color with regard to the sample frequency. Black dots represent the sample origin with regard to the postal code. The dot size displays the submission frequency of each veterinary practice/ clinic.

Screening Procedure and Bacterial Characterization

All wound samples were streaked onto tryptic soy agar plates supplemented with 5% sheep blood (Becton Dickinson, Heidelberg, Germany) and the plates were investigated after 24 and 48 hours. Colonies suspected to be staphylococci were identified using the bioMérieux VITEK®2 system (Germany) according to the manufactureŕs instructions. Automated antimicrobial susceptibility testing of *S. aureus* was performed using the bioMerieux VITEK®2 system (Germany) according to the manufacturer's instructions, including penicillin, ampicillin-sulbactam, oxacillin, cefoxitin, gentamicin, kanamycin, enrofloxacin, marbofloxacin, erythromycin, clindamycin, tetracycline, nitrofurantoin, chloramphenicol and trimethoprim- sulfamethoxazole, following the approved standards of the Clinical and Laboratory Standards Institute (CLSI) [21], [22].

MRSA isolates were stored in glycerol stocks at −80°C at the Institute of Microbiology and Epizootics (IMT). Species verification and detection of the *mec*A or *mec*C gene by PCR was performed for all MRSA as described before [23], [24]. Further, 121 MRSA were characterized by *spa* typing [25]. Associations of *spa* types with corresponding clonal complexes (CC) were determined according to Ridom (http://spaserver.ridom.de/).

Multilocus sequence typing (MLST) was performed for one to seven representatives of each detected *spa* type as described elsewhere [26].

Detection of the genes encoding the Panton-Valentine leukocidin (PVL)-factor was carried out as described before [27].

RESULTS

Within a 17-month sampling period, veterinarians from 15 German Federal States sent 3,479 swabs declared as "wound swabs" from dogs, 1,146 samples from cats and 604 samples from horses to Vet Med Labor GmbH (Ludwigsburg, Germany) (table 1). *S. aureus* was identified in 5.8% of canine, 12.2% of feline and 22.8% of equine samples, respectively. MRSA accounted for 62.7% of canine, 46.4% of feline and 41.3% of equine *S. aureus* isolates. In total, 121 MRSA strains obtained from dogs, 63 from cats and all isolates from horses were further characterized by *spa* typing while five of the canine and two feline MRSA were not available for the typing procedure. A detailed overview of all detected *spa* types and corresponding CCs is given in table 2. Most of the canine isolates belonged to clonal complexes CC22 (47.6%; n=60) and CC5 (30.2%; n=38), followed by CC398 (13.5%; n=17), CC8 (4.0%; n=5) and CC9 (0.8%; n=1). Comparable results were obtained for feline strains with CC22 (49.2%; n=32), CC5 (29.2%; n=19), CC398 (7.7%; n=5) and CC8 (9.2%; n=6). In addition, a CC599-MRSA was identified in one feline sample. The majority of MRSA isolates of equine origin possessed *spa* types associated with CC398 (87.7%; n=50). The remaining equine isolates belonged to CC8 (8.8%; n=5) as well as CC5 and CC1 (each: one isolate) (figure 2).

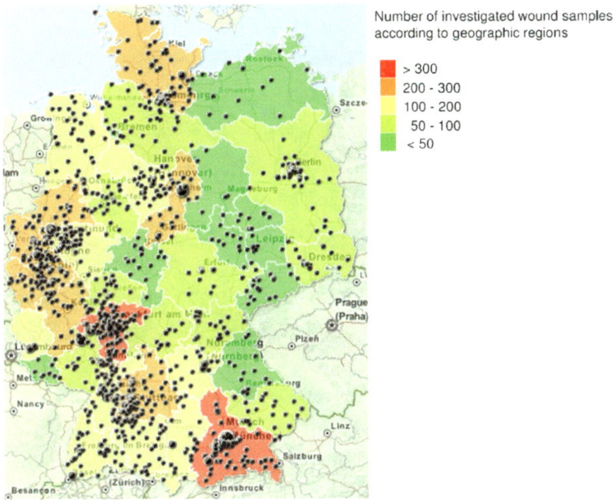

Figure 2: Overview of lineage-diversity among MRSA from dogs, cats and horses.

Table 1: *S. aureus* **proportion in wound** samples from companion animals

	total	%	dog	%	cat	%	horse	%
wound swabs	5,229	100	3,479	66.5	1,146	21.9	604	11.6
S. aureus	479	100	201	5.8	140	12.2	138	22.8
MSSA	231	48.2	75	2.2	75	6.5	81	13.4
MRSA	248	51.8	126	3.6	65	5.7	57	9.4

doi:10.1371/journal.pone.0085656.t001

http://dx.doi.org/10.1371/journal.pone.0085656.t001

Table 2: *Spa* **type frequency and predicted clonal complexes based on** *spa* **typing and MLST for representative MRSA from wound infections of canine, feline and equine orig**in in Germany

		MRSA		
CC	***spa* type**	**dog (n = 121)**	**cat (n = 62)**	**horse (57)**
1	t127	0	0	1
5	t002	1	1	0
	t003	31	17	1
	t045	4	1	0
	t1007	1	0	0
	t264	1	0	0
8	t008	2	6	0
	t009	1	0	4
	t024	1	0	0
	t12131	0	0	1
	t036	1	0	0
9	t1430	1	0	0
22	t016	0	1	0
	t020	0	4	0
	t022	11	6	0
	t032	43	17	0
	t3846	0	1	0
	t294	1	0	0
	t557	1	0	0
	t613	0	1	0
	t1292	1	0	0
	t747	2	0	0
	t7982	0	2	0
	t910	1	0	0
599	t278	0	1	0
398	t011	10	5	24
	t034	2	0	0
	t108	1	0	0
	t6867	4	0	24
	t10643	0	0	2

doi:10.1371/journal.pone.0085656.t002

http://dx.doi.org/10.1371/journal.pone.0085656.t002

MLST analysis, performed for at least one representative isolate of each distinct *spa* type, revealed common sequence types (ST) for isolates of CC1 (ST1), CC5 (ST5, ST225), CC8 (ST8, ST254), CC9 (ST9) and CC398 (ST398). Representatives of CC22 showed sequence types ST22, ST1117 as well as two new sequence types (ST2743 and ST2745). The feline CC599-MRSA belonged to ST599. All MRSA were *mec*A-positive except for the ST599-MRSA, which yielded a positive signal for *mec*C [28]. Screening for PVL revealed one positive canine CC8-MRSA (t008) as well as one positive feline CC22-MRSA (t016).

Antimicrobial susceptibility testing was performed for all MRSA. A detailed overview of all phenotypic resistance profiles is given in table 3.

Table 3: Phenotypic resistance for 241 MRSA grouped according to their clonal complexes

CC	CC22	CC5	CC398	CC8	CC1	CC9	ST599
total number	**n = 92**	**n = 58**	**n = 72**	**n = 16**	**n = 1**	**n = 1**	**n = 1**
GEN	3 (3.3%)	2 (3.4%)	57 (79.2%)	7 (43.8%)	0	0	0
KAN	3 (3.3%)	35 (60.3%)	58 (80.6%)	14 (87.5%)	1	0	0
ENR	90 (97.8%)	57 (98.2%)	28 (38.9%)	14 (87.5%)	0	1	0
MAR	90 (97.8%)	57 (98.2%)	30 (41.7%)	14 (87.5%)	0	1	0
ERY	32 (34.8%)	57 (98.2%)	7 (9.7%)	3 (18.8%)	1	1	0
CLI	34 (37.0%)	57 (98.2%)	8 (11.1%)	2 (12.5%)	1	1	0
TET	7 (7.6%)	1 (1.7%)	68 (94.4%)	7 (43.8%)	1	1	0
NIT	0	0	0	2 (12.5%)	0	0	0
CHL	1 (1.1%)	0	0	0	0	0	0
SXT	1 (1.1%)	1 (1.7%)	25 (34.7%)	6 (37.5%)	0	1	0

Number (n) and percentage (%) of resistant strains according to VITEK®2 system (bioMérieux, Germany).
Abbreviations: GEN: gentamicin, KAN: kanamycin, ENR: enrofloxacin, MAR: marbofloxacin, ERY: erythromycin, CLI: clindamycin, TET: tetracycline, NIT: nitrofurantoin, CHL: chloramphenicol and SXT: trimethoprim- sulfamethoxazole.
doi:10.1371/journal.pone.0085656.t003

http://dx.doi.org/10.1371/journal.pone.0085656.t003

DISCUSSION

This survey describes for the first time the Germany-wide occurrence of MRSA and methicillin-susceptible *S. aureus* (MSSA) in wound samples of companion animal origin. The considerable high proportion of *S. aureus*-positive wound swabs from horses, cats and dogs clearly shows the prominent clinical importance of this pathogen in companion animal medicine. In view of MRSA being a zoonotic pathogen, proportions of 9.4% (horses), 5.7% (cats) and 3.6% (dogs) among wound swabs are alarming and provide a significant source for the spread in both veterinary clinics and the community.

The genotypic characterization of MRSA in this study provides comprehensive insights into the clonal background of MRSA in wound infection samples of companion animal origin (figure 2) and confirms the previous finding of CC22 and CC5 as predominant lineages in dogs and cats [14], [20] for Germany. The predominance of these lineages in dogs and cats is in accordance with findings in human medicine within Germany, where most wound infections are caused by CC22- and CC5-MRSA as well [29]. These findings lead to the suggestion that humans might be a likely infection source for dogs and cats. In addition, dogs and cats should be considered as (re-)infection and/or colonization source for humans as well.

However, a recent study by Holden et al. demonstrated the genetic changes that accompanied the emergence of EMRSA-15, a typical hospital associated CC22-MRSA. A series of gene acquisition events and mutations seemed to promote the success of this clone in (human) hospitals. Accordingly, further comparative genomic studies on MRSA obtained from veterinary and human health care settings are warranted to evaluate factors influencing success in veterinary environments (e.g. prescription of certain antibiotics, acquisition of phages encoding virulence-enhancing factors) [30].

Reports about LA-MRSA in pet animals [15], [31], [32] raised the question whether these results represent incidental findings from screening studies in companion animals [33]. As shown in this study, the frequent finding of LA-MRSA CC398 among canine and feline MRSA isolates demonstrates that CC398-MRSA is an important lineage for canine and feline infections in Germany at present. Further investigation is needed to determine whether this genotype has the capacity to replace other common MRSA-lineages in dogs and cats. However, the characterization of different CC398 clades among humans in comparison to livestock already demonstrated the adaptability of this genetic lineage [34]. Based on this knowledge and the regular appearance of CC398-MRSA in pet animals, dogs and cats should be considered as a potential source for human CC398-MRSA colonization and infection, especially if contact to livestock or horses can be excluded.

The CC398 proportion among equine MRSA identified in this study is in concordance with previous reports of high CC398-MRSA infection- and colonization rates in horses [7], [18] and gives evidence that MRSA of CC8 are almost completely replaced by CC398 in equine wound infections within Germany. The predominance of CC398-MRSA in wound swabs of horse origin leads to the assumption that this lineage might have developed some mechanisms for adaptation to the equine host.

Host adaptation has been described for several *S. aureus*-lineages in the past. The emergence of a poultry-specific ST5-clade for example was probably caused by a single human-to-poultry host jump. Further acquisition of mobile genetic elements (MGE) from avian specific lineages and the inactivation of several proteins with importance in human infection led to the occurrence of a poultry-specific clade [35]. Another example was given for CC97-*S. aureus,* a lineage that has been predominantly identified in samples from ruminants in the past. Only recently, CC97-MRSA were identified as a cause of human infections as well. The emergence of two new CC97 clones in the human population seems to be associated with the acquisition of MGE which encode factors that enhance the capacity to adapt to the human host [36].

In accordance with findings for CC5- and CC97-*S. aureus,* different studies revealed the capacity of CC398 to adapt to specific hosts including humans and livestock. The recent analysis of 89 diverse CC398-*S. aureus* from Price et al. strongly suggests an initial jump from humans to livestock, followed by adaptive processes like the loss of phage-carried human-associated virulence genes and the acquisition of tetracycline and methicillin resistance [37]. Besides, a recent study showed the emergence of an animal-independent ST398-MSSA with relevance in human infections in northern Manhattan. In addition to a different subset of MGE, these strains varied according to the set of intact adhesins, resulting in enhanced adhesion to human keratinocytes and keratin and demonstrated the adaptive capacity of ST398 strains to humans [38]. Further investigation is required to see if CC398-MRSA of equine origin harbour similar adaptive features.

Only one of the 243 MRSA yielded a positive signal for the *mec*A-homologue *mec*C, indicating a sporadic occurrence of *mec*C-MRSA in companion animals in Germany, as previously reported [28]. A rather sporadic occurrence of PVL-carriage among companion animal MRSA strains (two positives) is in accordance with previous findings [39], [40].

Phenotypic resistance profiles of all MRSA revealed a high number of multi-resistant strains, in particular for CC5- and CC398-MRSA, highlighting the limited therapeutic options to treat most of these MRSA infections (table 3). Resistance profiles from isolates of human origin associated with epidemic MRSA lineages like CC22, CC5 and CC8 within German hospitals were regularly reported by the national reference laboratory Robert Koch-Institute (RKI) [29]. For ST22, the "Barnim epidemic strain" (*spa* types t005, t002 and t032), resistance against fluoroquinolones (ciprofloxacin, moxifloxacin) was frequently observed. While care should be taken before comparing study results (CC22-MRSA reported on here comprise more than these three *spa* types), the frequent resistance (97.8%) against fluoroquinolones (enrofloxacin, marbofloxacin) is also present in CC22-MRSA of companion animal origin. CC5-MRSA, human as well as companion animal strains, seem to express resistance against fluoroquinolones, clindamycin and erythromycin on a regular basis. For CC8-MRSA, a diverse phenotypic resistance pattern was observed. These results are in accordance with findings for CC8-MRSA of human origin [41].

The study was biased to some degree due to inhomogeneity of the case definition "wound infection" which was dependent on veterinarians who sent their samples to Vet Med Labor GmbH (Ludwigsburg, Germany). This survey focused on wound infections which have been sent to a diagnostic lab for microbiological examination but does not take empirically treated wound infections into account. Thus, calculated MRSA proportions might not reflect the MRSA and MSSA rates in the general companion animal population.

Another limitation is the lack of information for seven strains (five canine and two feline MRSA), which were not available for genotypic characterization.

CONCLUSION

This study provides evidence for the importance and impact of *S. aureus* in general, and MRSA in particular, as a cause of wound infections in dogs, cats and horses. The emergence of CC398-MRSA as predominant genotype in equine wound infections demonstrates the adaptive capacity of this lineage to other hosts than livestock and humans. Since CC398-MRSA can be also regularly identified in samples from dogs and cats, each of these animals should be considered as potential infection and/or colonization source for humans as well. Our findings clearly demonstrate the need for on-going screening studies to gain information about the replacement and emergence of certain genetic lineages among these animals. Further investigation including whole genome sequencing, phenotypic appearance and functional studies are needed to unveil factors and structures influencing the host adaptation processes like it has been successfully demonstrated for adaptation of CC398 to humans [38] and a CC5-clade to poultry [35]. Further attempts to reduce the total burden of MRSA, in each field afflicted with this pathogen, are clearly needed. Transmission of MRSA between different hosts (humans, animals) as well as between different ecological niches (hospital, community, veterinarian hospitals) should be regarded as a major "One Health" problem.

ACKNOWLEDGMENTS

We thank E. Antao for critical reading of the manuscript.

AUTHOR CONTRIBUTIONS

Conceived and designed the experiments: BW JH SV ALB. Performed the experiments: SV IS PAK. Analyzed the data: SV IS CA TS. Contributed reagents/materials/analysis tools: PAK IS LHW ALB. Wrote the paper: SV BW ALB.

REFERENCES

1. Pinho MG, de Lencastre H, Tomasz A (2001) An acquired and a native penicillin-binding protein cooperate in building the cell wall of drug-resistant staphylococci. Proc Natl Acad Sci U S A 98: 10886–10891. doi: 10.1073/pnas.191260798
2. Otto M (2012) MRSA virulence and spread. Cell Microbiol 14: 1513–1521. doi: 10.1111/j.1462-5822.2012.01832.x
3. Manian FA (2003) Asymptomatic nasal carriage of mupirocin-resistant, methicillin-resistant Staphylococcus aureus (MRSA) in a pet dog associated with MRSA infection in household contacts. Clin Infect Dis 36: e26–28. doi: 10.1086/344772
4. van Duijkeren E, Wolfhagen MJ, Box AT, Heck ME, Wannet WJ, et al. (2004) Human-to-dog transmission of methicillin-resistant Staphylococcus aureus. Emerg Infect Dis 10: 2235–2237. doi: 10.3201/eid1012.040387
5. Weese JS, Dick H, Willey BM, McGeer A, Kreiswirth BN, et al. (2006) Suspected transmission of methicillin-resistant Staphylococcus aureus between domestic pets and humans in veterinary clinics and in the household. Vet Microbiol 115: 148–155. doi: 10.1016/j.vetmic.2006.01.004
6. Wieler LH, Ewers C, Guenther S, Walther B, Lubke-Becker A (2011) Methicillin-resistant staphylococci (MRS) and extended-spectrum beta-lactamases (ESBL)-producing Enterobacteriaceae in companion animals: nosocomial infections as one reason for the rising prevalence of these potential zoonotic pathogens in clinical samples. Int J Med Microbiol 301: 635–641. doi: 10.1016/j.ijmm.2011.09.009
7. van Duijkeren E, Moleman M, Sloet van Oldruitenborgh-Oosterbaan MM, Multem J, Troelstra A, et al. (2010) Methicillin-resistant Staphylococcus aureus in horses and horse personnel: an investigation of several outbreaks. Vet Microbiol 141: 96–102. doi: 10.1016/j.vetmic.2009.08.009
8. Leonard FC, Markey BK (2008) Meticillin-resistant Staphylococcus aureus in animals: a review. Vet J 175: 27–36. doi: 10.1016/j.tvjl.2006.11.008
9. Walther B, Wieler LH, Friedrich AW, Hanssen AM, Kohn B, et al. (2008) Methicillin-resistant Staphylococcus aureus (MRSA) isolated from small and exotic animals at a university hospital during routine microbiological examinations. Vet Microbiol 127: 171–178. doi: 10.1016/j.vetmic.2007.07.018
10. Axon JE, Carrick JB, Barton MD, Collins NM, Russell CM, et al. (2011) Methicillin-resistant Staphylococcus aureus in a population of horses in Australia. Aust Vet J 89: 221–225. doi: 10.1111/j.1751-0813.2011.00711.x
11. Malik S, Coombs GW, O'Brien FG, Peng H, Barton MD (2006) Molecular typing of methicillin-resistant staphylococci isolated from cats and dogs. J Antimicrob Chemother 58: 428–431. doi: 10.1093/jac/dkl253
12. Moodley A, Stegger M, Bagcigil AF, Baptiste KE, Loeffler A, et al. (2006) spa typing of methicillin-resistant Staphylococcus aureus isolated from domestic animals and veterinary staff in the UK and Ireland. J Antimicrob Chemother 58: 1118–1123. doi: 10.1093/jac/dkl394
13. Strommenger B, Kehrenberg C, Kettlitz C, Cuny C, Verspohl J, et al. (2006) Molecular characterization of methicillin-resistant Staphylococcus aureus strains from pet animals and their relationship to human isolates. J Antimicrob Chemother 57: 461–465. doi: 10.1093/jac/dki471
14. Vincze S, Stamm I, Monecke S, Kopp PA, Semmler T, et al. (2013) Molecular Analysis of Human and Canine Staphylococcus aureus Strains Reveals Distinct Extended-Host-Spectrum Genotypes Independent of Their Methicillin Resistance. Appl Environ Microbiol 79: 655–662. doi: 10.1128/aem.02704-12
15. Witte W, Strommenger B, Stanek C, Cuny C (2007) Methicillin-resistant Staphylococcus aureus ST398 in humans and animals, Central Europe. Emerg Infect Dis 13: 255–258. doi: 10.3201/eid1302.060924
16. Weese JS, van Duijkeren E (2010) Methicillin-resistant Staphylococcus aureus and Staphylococcus pseudintermedius in veterinary medicine. Vet Microbiol 140: 418–429. doi: 10.1016/j.vetmic.2009.01.039
17. Walther B, Monecke S, Ruscher C, Friedrich AW, Ehricht R, et al. (2009) Comparative molecular analysis substantiates zoonotic potential of equine methicillin-resistant Staphylococcus aureus. J Clin Microbiol 47: 704–710. doi: 10.1128/jcm.01626-08
18. Van den Eede A, Martens A, Lipinska U, Struelens M, Deplano A, et al. (2009) High occurrence of methicillin-resistant Staphylococcus aureus ST398 in equine nasal samples. Vet Microbiol 133: 138–144. doi: 10.1016/j.vetmic.2008.06.021
19. Weese JS, Caldwell F, Willey BM, Kreiswirth BN, McGeer A, et al. (2006) An outbreak of methicillin-resistant Staphylococcus aureus skin infections resulting from horse to human transmission in a veterinary hospital. Vet Microbiol 114: 160–164. doi: 10.1016/j.vetmic.2005.11.054
20. Loeffler A, Lloyd DH (2010) Companion animals: a reservoir for methicillin-resistant Staphylococcus aureus in the community? Epidemiol Infect 138: 595–605. doi: 10.1017/s0950268809991476
21. Wayne P (2008) Performance Standards for Antimicrobial Disk and Dilution Susceptibility Tests for Bacteria Isolated from Animals; Approved Standard – Third Edition. CLSI document M31-A3.Vol. 28 No.

8 ed. Pennsylvania: Clinical and Laboratory Standards Institute (CLSI).

22. Wayne P (2010) Performance Standards for Antimicrobial Susceptibility Testing; Twentieth Informational Supplement. CLSI document M100-S20. Pennsylvania: Clinical and Laboratory Standards Institute (CLSI).
23. Cuny C, Layer F, Strommenger B, Witte W (2011) Rare occurrence of methicillin-resistant Staphylococcus aureus CC130 with a novel mecA homologue in humans in Germany. PLoS One 6: e24360. doi: 10.1371/journal.pone.0024360
24. Merlino J, Watson J, Rose B, Beard-Pegler M, Gottlieb T, et al. (2002) Detection and expression of methicillin/oxacillin resistance in multidrug-resistant and non-multidrug-resistant Staphylococcus aureus in Central Sydney, Australia. J Antimicrob Chemother 49: 793–801. doi: 10.1093/jac/dkf021
25. Harmsen D, Claus H, Witte W, Rothganger J, Turnwald D, et al. (2003) Typing of methicillin-resistant Staphylococcus aureus in a university hospital setting by using novel software for spa repeat determination and database management. J Clin Microbiol 41: 5442–5448. doi: 10.1128/jcm.41.12.5442-5448.2003
26. Enright MC, Day NP, Davies CE, Peacock SJ, Spratt BG (2000) Multilocus sequence typing for characterization of methicillin-resistant and methicillin-susceptible clones of Staphylococcus aureus. J Clin Microbiol 38: 1008–1015.
27. Lina G, Piemont Y, Godail-Gamot F, Bes M, Peter MO, et al. (1999) Involvement of Panton-Valentine leukocidin-producing Staphylococcus aureus in primary skin infections and pneumonia. Clin Infect Dis 29: 1128–1132. doi: 10.1086/313461
28. Walther B, Wieler LH, Vincze S, Antao EM, Brandenburg A, et al. (2012) MRSA variant in companion animals. Emerg Infect Dis 18: 2017–2020. doi: 10.3201/eid1812.120238
29. Robert-Koch-Institut (2011) Epidemiologic Bulletin Nr. 26: 12.
30. Holden MT, Hsu LY, Kurt K, Weinert LA, Mather AE, et al. (2013) A genomic portrait of the emergence, evolution, and global spread of a methicillin-resistant Staphylococcus aureus pandemic. Genome Res 23: 653–664. doi: 10.1101/gr.147710.112
31. Zhang W, Hao Z, Wang Y, Cao X, Logue CM, et al. (2011) Molecular characterization of methicillin-resistant Staphylococcus aureus strains from pet animals and veterinary staff in China. Vet J 190: e125–129. doi: 10.1016/j.tvjl.2011.02.006
32. Nienhoff U, Kadlec K, Chaberny IF, Verspohl J, Gerlach GF, et al. (2009) Transmission of methicillin-resistant Staphylococcus aureus strains between humans and dogs: two case reports. J Antimicrob Chemother 64: 660–662. doi: 10.1093/jac/dkp243
33. McCarthy AJ, Lindsay JA, Loeffler A (2012) Are all meticillin-resistant Staphylococcus aureus (MRSA) equal in all hosts? Epidemiological and genetic comparison between animal and human MRSA. Vet Dermatol 23: 267–e254. doi: 10.1111/j.1365-3164.2012.01072.x
34. McCarthy AJ, van Wamel W, Vandendriessche S, Larsen J, Denis O, et al. (2012) Staphylococcus aureus CC398 clade associated with human-to-human transmission. Appl Environ Microbiol 78: 8845–8848. doi: 10.1128/aem.02398-12
35. Lowder BV, Guinane CM, Ben Zakour NL, Weinert LA, Conway-Morris A, et al. (2009) Recent human-to-poultry host jump, adaptation, and pandemic spread of Staphylococcus aureus. Proc Natl Acad Sci U S A 106: 19545–19550. doi: 10.1073/pnas.0909285106
36. Spoor LE, McAdam PR, Weinert LA, Rambaut A, Hasman H, et al.. (2013) Livestock Origin for a Human Pandemic Clone of Community-Associated Methicillin-Resistant Staphylococcus aureus. MBio 4.
37. Price LB, Stegger M, Hasman H, Aziz M, Larsen J, et al.. (2012) Staphylococcus aureus CC398: Host Adaptation and Emergence of Methicillin Resistance in Livestock. MBio 3.
38. Uhlemann AC, Porcella SF, Trivedi S, Sullivan SB, Hafer C, et al.. (2012) Identification of a Highly Transmissible Animal-Independent Staphylococcus aureus ST398 Clone with Distinct Genomic and Cell Adhesion Properties. MBio 3.
39. Rankin S, Roberts S, O'Shea K, Maloney D, Lorenzo M, et al. (2005) Panton valentine leukocidin (PVL) toxin positive MRSA strains isolated from companion animals. Vet Microbiol 108: 145–148. doi: 10.1016/j.vetmic.2005.02.013
40. Sing A, Tuschak C, Hormansdorfer S (2008) Methicillin-resistant Staphylococcus aureus in a family and its pet cat. N Engl J Med 358: 1200–1201. doi: 10.1056/nejmc0706805
41. Strommenger B, Bartels MD, Kurt K, Layer F, Rohde SM, et al.. (2013) Evolution of methicillin-resistant Staphylococcus aureus towards increasing resistance. J Antimicrob Chemother.

CHAPTER 17 METHICILLIN-RESISTANT STAPHYLOCOCCUS AUREUS IN PIGS AND FARM WORKERS ON CONVENTIONAL AND ANTIBIOTIC-FREE SWINE FARMS IN THE USA

Tara C. Smith, Wondwossen A. Gebreyes, Melanie J. Abley, Abby L. Harper, Brett M. Forshey, Michael J. Male, H. Wayne Martin, Bayleyegn Z. Molla, Srinand Sreevatsan, Siddhartha Thakur, Madhumathi Thiruvengadam, Peter R. Davies

INTRODUCTION

Staphylococcus aureus is a commensal and opportunistic pathogen of man and many homeothermic species. In humans, the clinical manifestations of S. aureus infections vary broadly from minor superficial skin lesions to severe and sometimes fatal invasive disease. Approximately 20–30% of people are colonized with S. aureus, with the most common site for colonization being the anterior nares [1], [2]. While colonization itself does not harm the host, it has been associated with increased risk of developing infections [3]. Both asymptomatic carriers and infected individuals may transmit S. aureus directly or indirectly to others.

Throughout the antimicrobial era, *S. aureus* has displayed great capacity to respond to novel antibiotics by acquisition of resistance determinants, including the rapid emergence of methicillin-resistant strains (MRSA) following the introduction of that drug for medical use in 1961 [4]. On the basis of data from the 2001–2004 National Health and Nutrition Examination Survey (NHANES), it was estimated that 1.5% of the U.S. population (~4.1 million persons) is colonized with MRSA [1]. Antimicrobial resistance in S. aureus is a major concern in human clinical medicine, and case fatality rates for bacteremic cases remain of the order of 20–40%, with mortality risk in MRSA cases approximately twofold that of cases of methicillin-susceptible S. aureus bacteremia (MSSA) [5], [6].

Before 1995, human MRSA infections occurred predominantly in hospitalized patients who acquired the infections nosocomially. Subsequently, MRSA infections have been reported increasingly in people who had not been hospitalized nor had underlying illnesses. Furthermore, the predominant strains causing healthcare-associated MRSA infections (HA-MRSA) have been distinct from those isolated from community-associated MRSA infections (CA-MRSA) [7].

Although S. aureus is a commensal of several mammalian species, until recently animals were considered of negligible significance as reservoirs for human S. aureus infections. Since 2004 multiple reports of MRSA in animals worldwide, and apparent animal-to-human transmission, have heightened concerns about the risks of animal populations as potential reservoirs of zoonotic MRSA infections [8], [9]. Of particular concern is the high prevalence of ST398 clonal complex strains (termed 'livestock associated MRSA', or LA-MRSA) detected from nasal swabs from livestock (particularly pigs and cattle) and livestock workers in several countries [10], [11], [12]. Much uncertainty remains about the origin and public health implications of LA-MRSA, including the use of antibiotics as drivers of resistance development. Given the paucity of information available about these organisms in the US swine industry, we sampled pigs and farm workers on conventional and antibiotic-free swine farms in several US states.

MATERIALS AND METHODS

Farm selection and enrollment

We collected samples from weaned pigs between 6 and 18 weeks of age (target of 24 per farm) and all workers willing

Citation: Smith TC, Gebreyes WA, Abley MJ, Harper AL, Forshey BM, Male MJ, et al. (2013) Methicillin-Resistant Staphylococcus aureus in Pigs and Farm Workers on Conventional and Antibiotic-Free Swine Farms in the USA. PLoS ONE 8(5): e63704. doi:10.1371/journal.pone.0063704.

to participate on 45 farms in five major swine producing states in the USA that were readily accessible to collaborating groups: Iowa and Illinois (University of Iowa); Ohio and North Carolina (The Ohio State University); and Minnesota (University of Minnesota). Samples were collected between April 2008 and July 2010. The sample size was adequate to detect a positive herd with more than 99% confidence at an expected prevalence of 20% assuming a population size of 1000 animals. The study was designed so that half of the farms sampled by each collaborating group would be conventional confinement farms and half would be farms raising pigs without use of antibiotics (antibiotic-free, "ABF"). Farms were selected by convenience based on willingness of owners to participate. Due to difficulty in recruiting eligible farms, ultimately 45 farms were included in the study: 18 farms in Minnesota (9 conventional, 9 ABF); 18 farms in Iowa-Illinois (9 conventional, 9 ABF); and 9 farms in Ohio-North Carolina (6 conventional; 3 ABF). Where possible, swine selected were not comingled prior to sampling. This was not always possible on the smaller ABF farms. Twenty-four pigs were sampled on 42 of the farms; 22 on one; 25 on one; and 30 on another.

All swine farm workers at each study farm were invited to participate in the study. After giving written informed consent, participants completed a questionnaire providing demographic data and provided swab samples from the nares and oropharynx to determine MRSA colonization status. The survey recorded data on potential risk factors for MRSA colonization, including information about contact with swine and use of personal protective equipment.

Ethics Statement

The Institutional Review Boards and the Institutional Animal Care and Use Committees of the three participating universities approved the protocols prior to the initiation of the study.

Sample collection and bacteriology

Using sterile swabs, nasal samples were collected from both nares of weaned pigs. Swab samples were collected from both nares and the oropharynx of farm workers, apart from in Minnesota where only nasal swabbing was conducted. Swabs were transported in Stuart's medium at 4°C to the respective laboratories. Samples were inoculated into 2 mL enrichment broth containing 10 g tryptone/L, 75 g NaCl/L, 10 g mannitol/L and 2.5 g yeast extract/L. After 24 h incubation at 35°C, a loopful of broth was inoculated onto selective MRSA agar plates (BBL CHROMagar MRSA, Becton, Dickinson and Company). These plates were incubated 24–48 hours at 35°C and examined for MRSA. Isolates were confirmed to be S. aureus by examining their appearance on Gram stain, by catalase test, tube coagulase test and a S. aureus latex agglutination assay (Pastorex Staph-plus, Bio-Rad). Presumptive Methicillin resistant strains were identified by testing for the presence of penicillin binding protein 2 (PBP2′) (MRSA latex agglutination test, Oxoid Ltd., Hants, UK). MRSA isolates were stored at −80°C.

spa typing

All MRSA isolates were typed by partial sequencing of the Staphylococcus protein A (spa) gene [13], [14]. PCR amplicons of the spa gene were obtained using SpAF (5′-GAACAACGTAACGGCTTCATCC-3′) and 1517R (5′-GCTTTTGCAATGTCATTTACTG-3′).»). spa types were assigned using both the eGenomics, Inc (www.egenomics.com) and Ridom (http://spaserver.ridom.de) spa servers.

Statistical analysis

Risk factors were compared for MRSA-positive and MRSA-negative workers on farms with MRSA-positive herds using Fisher's exact test for categorical variables and the Wilcoxon rank sum test for continuous variables. Swine MRSA-positive prevalence rates and associated 95% confidence intervals were adjusted for clustering within herds using generalized linear mixed models in PROC GLIMMIX to better reflect the uncertainty around the point estimates. For evaluating risk factors for MRSA carriage among swine workers, a multivariable logistic regression model was developed using generalized estimating equations in PROC GENMOD with an exchangeable correlation matrix to adjust for correlation within farms. Specifically, we evaluated the effect of length of swine contact (i.e., daily hours of contact) on MRSA carriage along with potential confounders (including age, race, and gender). A final model was selected based on the minimized Quasilikelihood under the Independence model Criterion statistic. Statistical significance was assessed at $\alpha=0.05$. All analyses were conducted using SAS version 9.3 (Cary, NC).

RESULTS

Weaned pigs

The number of pigs sampled per farm ranged from 22 to 30, but was within one pig of the target sample size (i.e., 23 to 25 pigs) on 43 farms. On one ABF farm, only 22 pigs were present. A total of 50 of the 1085 pigs sampled in the study were culture positive for MRSA (4.6%; adjusted for clustering: 4.1%, 95% CI 1.2%–14.3%), with culture positive pigs clustered on 4 (9%) conventional farms in Iowa and Illinois. No positive herds were detected among the 27 farms sampled in Minnesota, North Carolina, or Ohio, and all pigs sampled on the 21 ABF herds were negative for MRSA. The MRSA prevalence among pigs on conventional farms overall was 8.5% (50/588; adjusted for clustering: 7.9%, 95% CI 2.2%–28.6%). On MRSA-positive farms, the prevalence of positive cultures ranged from 17% (4 of 24) to 100% (30 of 30) of weaned pigs sampled.

Farm workers

The number of participating workers per farm ranged from zero to 28. Between one and three workers were sampled on the majority of farms (31/45; 69%). The median age of participants was 38 years (range 17–73 years). The majority of participants were male (122; 82.4%), white (121; 81.7%), and recruited from farms in Iowa or Illinois (87; 58.8%). Four (2.7%) reported a skin or soft tissue infection within the prior year, whereas none reported previous diagnosis with a MRSA infection. A total of 31 of 148 farm workers (20.9%) were culture positive for MRSA. Of these, 27 (87%) worked on farms where MRSA was detected among the sampled swine. The vast majority of positive samples (24/31; 77%) were from 40 workers sampled on the two farms with the highest prevalence of MRSA in pigs. As working on a farm with a MRSA-positive herd was by far the greatest risk factor for worker colonization (53% [27/51] positive vs 4% [4/97]; p-value <0.0001), we restricted our analysis of other potential risk factors to workers from MRSA-positive farms (Table 1). The majority of participants (85%; 41/48 [3 missing data]) reported contact with swine within the three days prior to sample collection. In univariate analysis, no significant association was observed between MRSA carriage and demographic characteristics, various indicators of swine exposure intensity, or use of personal protective gear (Table 1), although there was a general trend of lower MRSA carriage among those using personal protective gear. In a multivariable logistic regression model, white race (OR 5.5 [95% CI 2.0 – 15.2]; reference: Hispanic) and more than 7 hours of swine exposure per day (OR 5.2 [95% CI 4.2 – 6.5]; reference: ≤7 hours of swine exposure per day) were associated with increased risk for MRSA carriage.

Table 1: Demographic and occupational characteristics of participating workers from farms with MRSA-positive swine

Variable	MRSA negative N = 24*	MRSA positive N = 27*	p-value[1]
Sex			0.232
Female	5 (21%)	2 (7%)	
Male	19 (79%)	24 (93%)	
Race			0.144
White	12 (50%)	20 (65%)	
Hispanic	11 (46%)	7 (35%)	
American Indian	1 (4%)	0 (0%)	
Median years worked with swine (IQR[2])	3 (1–13)	5 (1–20)	0.378
Median number of swine (IQR)	2400 (2000–5000)	3200 (1000–5000)	0.679
Median hours of exposure per day (IQR)	7 (3.5–8)	8 (4–9)	0.226
Use eye protection			
Rarely or never	11 (46%)	19 (70%)	0.094
At least sometimes	13 (54%)	8 (30%)	
Use protective mask			
Rarely or never	12 (52%)	17 (65%)	0.394
At least sometimes	11 (48%)	9 (35%)	
Use coveralls			
Rarely or never	2 (10%)	8 (33%)	0.083
At least sometimes	18 (90%)	16 (67%)	
Use washable boots			
Rarely or never	0 (0%)	2 (9%)	0.223
At least sometimes	24 (100%)	20 (91%)	
Use gloves			
Rarely or never	1 (4%)	0 (0%)	0.469
At least sometimes	22 (96%)	26 (100%)	

*Not all categories sum to the column total because of missing data for some participants.
[1]p-values are based on Fisher's exact test (for categorical data) or the Wilcoxon rank sum test (for continuous data).
[2]Interquartile range (IQR), represented by the values of the 25th and 75th percentiles.
doi:10.1371/journal.pone.0063704.t001

http://dx.doi.org/10.1371/journal.pone.0063704.t001

spa typing

A total of 11 spa types were detected from 68 isolates tested (Table 2). t034, a common spa type within the ST398 lineage of LA-MRSA, was the predominant spa type detected among humans and swine (50 of 68 tested; 74%). One farm accounted for 6 of 7 isolates belonging to spa type t002, including 4 isolates from humans and 2 from pigs. On three farms (one each from Iowa [t034], Minnesota [t021], and Ohio [t034]), single human samples were positive for MRSA where all pigs tested culture negative. The Iowa worker was a truck driver who worked on multiple farms; such information is not known regarding the t034-positive worker from Ohio.

Table 2: Distribution of *spa* **types among h**uman and swine isolates of MRSA

spa type*	Human	Swine	Total
t002	5	2	7
t011#	1	0	1
t021	1	0	1
t034#	20	41	61
t084	1	0	1
t179	1	0	1
t330	1	0	1
t337	0	1	1
t571#	0	1	1
t688	1	0	1
t3446	0	3	3
Non-typeable	0	2	2
Total	31	50	81

*Ridom *spa* type.
#*spa* types of ST398 lineage.
doi:10.1371/journal.pone.0063704.t002

http://dx.doi.org/10.1371/journal.pone.0063704.t002

DISCUSSION

The emergence of LA-MRSA in major food animal species has raised numerous questions and concerns for public health and livestock industries. First identified in The Netherlands around 2004, these organisms have since been found in swine herds in many European countries and also in North America [10], [11], [15]. Based on screening using farm dust samples, the prevalence of positive swine herds varied widely among European countries, from 0% in England, Ireland and Sweden, to over 41% in Germany and 51% in Spain [16]. As found in our study, within positive herds, prevalence of culture positive pigs is typically high (17% to 100% of pigs positive). Initial studies in North America indicated that the prevalence of LA-MRSA in swine may be similar to that reported in Europe. In a convenience sample of 20 herds in Ontario, Khanna et al (2008) found 25% of 285 pigs and 20% (5 of 25) of swine farm workers were culture positive, with spa type t034 predominant [11]. Smith et al (2009) first documented the presence of LA-MRSA in the USA in one of two swine production systems studied, and found a high within-herd prevalence (70% of pigs) in the positive system [10]. Davies et al (in preparation) found LA-MRSA occurring in US swine veterinarians (5%) and in 25% of 539 market hogs from 45 herds slaughtered at major US packing plants, with t034 again being the most common spa type. Given the narrow scope of the study of Smith et al (2009) and the difficulty in interpreting data from market hogs due to the possibility of exposure during transport and lairage, further studies are required to obtain more reliable estimates of the prevalence of MRSA in US livestock industries.

The prevalence found for both farms and pigs in the current study was lower than anticipated from the North American studies, but are very similar to recent data from Canada on market age hogs sampled on farms. Weese et al (2011) found MRSA in 4.6% of pigs on 5 of 46 (11%) of farms. Limited data comparing age groups of pigs suggests that prevalence may be higher in weaned pigs [10], [17], which was why we selected this age group for the current study. Both studies suggest that the prevalence of MRSA in North American pigs may be toward the lower end of the range reported across European countries. Important caveats to this study, like preceding studies, are the limited scope and use of convenience sampling rather than formal random sampling to select herds. For this reason, considerable uncertainty remains about the prevalence of LA-MRSA in the US swine industry. The current study was also deliberately biased by the inclusion of a relatively large proportion of antibiotic-free herds (21/45 herds, 46.7% of the tested farms), and a larger herd level study of pigs on farms across the USA may be warranted.

A substantial obstacle to conducting this study was difficulty in recruiting farms. We attribute this to the unfortunate coincidence of conducting the study in the wake of the 2009 HIN1 influenza pandemic, and the alarmist nature of journalistic coverage of both “swine flu” and LA-MRSA, which together contributed to understandable reluctance by producers to participate. This difficulty may complicate efforts to obtain a random sample of herds in the future.

The observation that LA-MRSA isolated from animals are almost uniformly resistant to tetracyclines (relatively uncommon among common human isolates) focused attention on the role that antimicrobial use, particularly of tetracyclines, in food animals may have had in the emergence of LA-MRSA [17], [18], [19]. Our decision to purposively include both ABF and conventional herds was to obtain preliminary data on MRSA prevalence in these different groups of farms in the USA. It is important to point out that the two groups of farms differ in many respects other than use of antimicrobials, including herd size, sources of genetic stock, and general housing systems. The relatively low prevalence of MRSA we observed among conventional herds confirms that routine antimicrobial use in pigs is not a sufficient cause for emergence of LA-MRSA. Also, the high prevalence of MRSA reported on an ABF herd in Canada suggests that exposure to antimicrobials is also not a necessary condition for the occurrence of LA-MRSA in pigs [17].

LA-MRSA was first detected in Europe in 2004 after several decades of widespread use of tetracyclines and other antimicrobials in food animals, but paradoxically in the aftermath of increased restrictions on in-feed antimicrobial use in several EU countries. Recent studies showing that both MRSA and MSSA isolates of ST398 S. aureus from pigs are resistant to tetracyclines is consistent with the hypothesis that widespread tetracycline use may have resulted in tetracycline resistance in S. aureus in pigs [20], [21], [22], [23]. However it is inconsistent with the suggestion that tetracycline use has been an influential factor in the emergence of LA-MRSA, as MSSA isolates are equally resistant (Aarestrup et al., 2010; Cavaco et al., 2011). In contrast, the concurrent finding of high levels of zinc tolerance in LA-MRSA, but not in LA-MSSA presents an alternative selective factor given the widespread use of zinc as a feed additive to control enteric disease in weaned pigs [22]. However, it is optimistic to expect simple explanations for such complex ecological events.

Our observations on farm workers are consistent with numerous studies demonstrating that people working in close contact with animals colonized with MRSA have a high risk of culture positive nasal swabs [9], [10], [12], [24]. Further confirmation of this phenomenon is unlikely to provide new insight unless accompanied by efforts to understand its biological nature and implications for occupational health. The extent to which culture positive nasal swabs represent transient contamination (as workers are typically sampled in the farm environment) versus ‘true’ colonization (where the organisms are an established component of the human nasopharyngeal microbiota) is unknown. As S. aureus appear be a predominant organism in bioaerosols of swine barns [25] discriminating between transient contamination of airways and true colonization of humans working daily in barns is problematic. In our study, the majority of participants reported swine exposure within three days prior to swab sampling, preventing analysis of longer-term ST398 carriage. It is likely that both contamination and colonization can occur, and recent studies of both research workers and workers on veal farms in The Netherlands indicate the transient contamination may be more common and that regular and continuing exposure to livestock is the major determinant of culture positivity for LA-MRSA [26], [27], [28], [29].

Community based studies in The Netherlands and Germany in regions with high prevalence of LA-MRSA in swine found that risk of culture positivity was largely confined to groups with regular occupational exposure to livestock (farmers and veterinarians) and their immediate families but did not occur in unexposed groups in the communities [8], [24]. Furthermore, although very high prevalence has been described in cross-sectional studies of farm workers, the routine use of multiple enrichment methods to culture samples is likely to result in detection of samples with low numbers. Quantification of LA-MRSA organisms in culture positive farm workers may provide a more meaningful context for evaluating contamination versus colonization events and informing assessment of associated health risks.

Several reports of severe or fatal systemic infections indicate that S. aureus strains of the ST398 lineage have the potential to be serious human pathogens. [30], [31], [32]. Unfortunately, many European reports have not clearly distinguished clinical infections from culture positive swabs from screening [33], and the actual clinical risks associated with livestock exposures and colonization with LA- MRSA are uncertain. Some spa types of ST398 appear to be represented more commonly among human clinical isolates than livestock isolates [34], [35], [36], [37], raising the possibility that different ST398 subtypes may vary in their abilities to colonize and cause disease in humans. Further studies should address the lack of quantitative information about the actual clinical risks associated with livestock exposures and colonization with LA-MRSA.

ACKNOWLEDGMENTS

We thank Raymond P. Scheibel, Blake M. Hanson, Shylo E. Wardyn, Lisa K. Roberts, and Sheila Berrios-Nazario for their assistance in executing this study.

AUTHOR CONTRIBUTIONS

Conceived and designed the experiments: WG PD TS. Performed the experiments: TS MA AH MM HWM BMF SS ST MT. Analyzed the data: TS WG SS BZ BF. Wrote the paper: TS WG MA AH BF MM HWM BMF SS ST MT PD.

REFERENCES

1. Graham PL 3rd, Lin SX, Larson EL (2006) A U.S. population-based survey of Staphylococcus aureus colonization. Ann Intern Med 144: 318–325. doi: 10.7326/0003-4819-144-5-200603070-00006

2. Kluytmans J, van Belkum A, Verbrugh H (1997) Nasal carriage of Staphylococcus aureus: epidemiology, underlying mechanisms, and associated risks. Clin Microbiol Rev 10: 505–520.

3. Wertheim HF, Melles DC, Vos MC, van Leeuwen W, van Belkum A, et al. (2005) The role of nasal carriage in Staphylococcus aureus infections. Lancet Infect Dis 5: 751–762. doi: 10.1016/s1473-3099(05)70295-4

4. Stefani S, Goglio A (2010) Methicillin-resistant Staphylococcus aureus: related infections and antibiotic resistance. Int J Infect Dis 14 Suppl 4S19–22. doi: 10.1016/j.ijid.2010.05.009

5. Cosgrove SE, Sakoulas G, Perencevich EN, Schwaber MJ, Karchmer AW, et al. (2003) Comparison of mortality associated with methicillin-resistant and methicillin-susceptible Staphylococcus aureus bacteremia: a meta-analysis. Clin Infect Dis 36: 53–59. doi: 10.1086/345476

6. Laupland KB, Ross T, Gregson DB (2008) Staphylococcus aureus bloodstream infections: risk factors, outcomes, and the influence of methicillin resistance in Calgary, Canada, 2000–2006. J Infect Dis 198: 336–343. doi: 10.1086/589717

7. David MZ, Daum RS (2010) Community-associated methicillin-resistant Staphylococcus aureus: epidemiology and clinical consequences of an emerging epidemic. Clin Microbiol Rev 23: 616–687. doi: 10.1128/cmr.00081-09

8. Cuny C, Friedrich A, Kozytska S, Layer F, Nubel U, et al. (2010) Emergence of methicillin–resistant Staphylococcus aureus (MRSA) in different animal species. Int J Med Microbiol 300: 109–117. doi: 10.1016/j.ijmm.2009.11.002

9. Weese JS (2010) Methicillin-resistant Staphylococcus aureus in animals. ILAR J 51: 233–244. doi: 10.1093/ilar.51.3.233

10. Smith TC, Male MJ, Harper AL, Kroeger JS, Tinkler GP, et al. (2009) Methicillin-resistant Staphylococcus aureus (MRSA) strain ST398 is present in midwestern U.S. swine and swine workers. PLoS ONE 4: e4258. doi: 10.1371/journal.pone.0004258

11. Khanna T, Friendship R, Dewey C, Weese JS (2008) Methicillin resistant Staphylococcus aureus colonization in pigs and pig farmers. Vet Microbiol 128: 298–303. doi: 10.1016/j.vetmic.2007.10.006

12. Wulf MW, Sorum M, van Nes A, Skov R, Melchers WJ, et al. (2008) Prevalence of methicillin-resistant Staphylococcus aureus among veterinarians: an international study. Clin Microbiol Infect 14: 29–34. doi: 10.1111/j.1469-0691.2007.01873.x

13. Shopsin B, Gomez M, Montgomery SO, Smith DH, Waddington M, et al. (1999) Evaluation of protein A gene polymorphic region DNA sequencing for typing of Staphylococcus aureus strains. J Clin Microbiol 37: 3556–3563.

14. Koreen L, Ramaswamy SV, Graviss EA, Naidich S, Musser JM, et al. (2004) spa typing method for discriminating among Staphylococcus aureus isolates: implications for use of a single marker to detect genetic micro- and macrovariation. J Clin Microbiol 42: 792–799. doi: 10.1128/jcm.42.2.792-799.2004

15. Voss A, Loeffen F, Bakker J, Klaassen C, Wulf M (2005) Methicillin-resistant Staphylococcus aureus in pig farming. Emerg Infect Dis 11: 1965–1966. doi: 10.3201/eid1112.050428

16. EFSA (2009) Assessment of the Public Health significance of meticillin resistant Staphylococcus aureus (MRSA) in animals and foods: Scientific Opinion of the Panel on Biological Hazards. The EFSA Journal 993: 1–73.

17. Weese JS, Zwambag A, Rosendal T, Reid-Smith R, Friendship R (2011) Longitudinal investigation of methicillin-resistant Staphylococcus aureus in piglets. Zoonoses Public Health 58: 238–243. doi: 10.1111/j.1863-2378.2010.01340.x

18. van Duijkeren E, Ikawaty R, Broekhuizen-Stins MJ, Jansen MD, Spalburg EC, et al. (2008) Transmission of methicillin-resistant Staphylococcus aureus strains between different kinds of pig farms. Vet Microbiol 126: 383–389. doi: 10.1016/j.vetmic.2007.07.021

19. de Neeling AJ, van den Broek MJ, Spalburg EC, van Santen-Verheuvel MG, Dam-Deisz WD, et al. (2007) High prevalence of methicillin resistant Staphylococcus aureus in pigs. Vet Microbiol 122: 366–372. doi: 10.1016/j.vetmic.2007.01.027

20. Cavaco LM, Hasman H, Aarestrup FM (2011) Zinc resistance of Staphylococcus aureus of animal origin is strongly associated with methicillin resistance. Vet Microbiol 150: 344–348. doi: 10.1016/j.vetmic.2011.02.014

21. Cavaco LM, Hasman H, Stegger M, Andersen PS, Skov R, et al. (2010) Cloning and occurrence of czrC, a gene conferring cadmium and zinc resistance in methicillin-resistant Staphylococcus aureus CC398 isolates. Antimicrob Agents Chemother 54: 3605–3608. doi: 10.1128/aac.00058-10

22. Aarestrup FM, Cavaco L, Hasman H (2010) Decreased susceptibility to zinc chloride is associated with methicillin resistant Staphylococcus aureus CC398 in Danish swine. Vet Microbiol 142: 455–457. doi: 10.1016/j.vetmic.2009.10.021

23. Price LB, Stegger M, Hasman H, Aziz M, Larsen J, et al.. (2012) Staphylococcus aureus CC398: host adaptation and emergence of methicillin resistance in livestock. mBio 3.

24. Van Cleef BA, Broens EM, Voss A, Huijsdens XW, Zuchner L, et al. (2010) High prevalence of nasal MRSA carriage in slaughterhouse workers in contact with live pigs in The Netherlands. Epidemiol Infect 138: 756–763. doi: 10.1017/s0950268810000245

25. Gibbs SG, Green CF, Tarwater PM, Mota LC, Mena KD, et al. (2006) Isolation of antibiotic-resistant bacteria from the air plume downwind of a swine confined or concentrated animal feeding operation. Environ Health Perspect 114: 1032–1037. doi: 10.1289/ehp.8910

26. van Cleef BA, Monnet DL, Voss A, Krziwanek K, Allerberger F, et al. (2011) Livestock-associated methicillin-resistant Staphylococcus aureus in humans, Europe. Emerg Infect Dis 17: 502–505. doi: 10.3201/eid1703.101036

27. van Cleef BA, Graveland H, Haenen AP, van de Giessen AW, Heederik D, et al. (2011) Persistence of livestock-associated methicillin-resistant Staphylococcus aureus in field workers after short-term occupational exposure to pigs and veal calves. J Clin Microbiol 49: 1030–1033. doi: 10.1128/jcm.00493-10

28. Graveland H, Duim B, van Duijkeren E, Heederik D, Wagenaar JA (2011) Livestock-associated methicillin-resistant Staphylococcus aureus in animals and humans. Int J Med Microbiol 301: 630–634. doi: 10.1016/j.ijmm.2011.09.004

29. Graveland H, Wagenaar JA, Bergs K, Heesterbeek H, Heederik D (2011) Persistence of livestock associated MRSA CC398 in humans is dependent on intensity of animal contact. PLoS One 6: e16830. doi: 10.1371/journal.pone.0016830

30. Ekkelenkamp MB, Sekkat M, Carpaij N, Troelstra A, Bonten MJ (2006) [Endocarditis due to meticillin-resistant Staphylococcus aureus originating from pigs]. Ned Tijdschr Geneeskd 150: 2442–2447.

31. Hartmeyer GN, Gahrn-Hansen B, Skov RL, Kolmos HJ (2010) Pig-associated methicillin-resistant Staphylococcus aureus: family transmission and severe pneumonia in a newborn. Scand J Infect Dis 42: 318–320. doi: 10.3109/00365540903510708

32. Mammina C, Bonura C, di Carlo P, Cala C, Aleo A, et al. (2010) Daptomycin non-susceptible, vancomycin intermediate methicillin-resistant Staphylococcus aureus ST398 from a chronic leg ulcer, Italy. Scand J Infect Dis 42: 955–957. doi: 10.3109/00365548.2010.524662

33. Huijsdens XW, Bosch T, van Santen-Verheuvel MG, Spalburg E, Pluister GN, et al.. (2009) Molecular characterisation of PFGE non-typable methicillin-resistant Staphylococcus aureus in The Netherlands, 2007. Euro Surveill 14.

34. Davies PR, Wagstrom EA, Bender JB (2011) Lethal necrotizing pneumonia caused by an ST398 Staphylococcus aureus strain. Emerg Infect Dis 17: 1152–1153 author reply 1153. doi: 10.3201/eid1706.101394

35. Vandendriessche S, Kadlec K, Schwarz S, Denis O (2011) Methicillin-susceptible Staphylococcus aureus ST398-t571 harbouring the macrolide-lincosamide-streptogramin B resistance gene erm(T) in Belgian hospitals. J Antimicrob Chemother 66: 2455–2459. doi: 10.1093/jac/dkr348

36. van der Mee-Marquet N, Francois P, Domelier-Valentin AS, Coulomb F, Decreux C, et al. (2011) Emergence of unusual bloodstream infections associated with pig-borne-like —Staphylococcus aureus ST398 in France. Clin Infect Dis 52: 152–153. doi: 10.1093/cid/ciq053

37. Wulf MW, Verduin CM, van Nes A, Huijsdens X, Voss A (2012) Infection and colonization with methicillin resistant Staphylococcus aureus ST398 versus other MRSA in an area with a high density of pig farms. Eur J Clin Microbiol Infect Dis 31: 61–65. doi: 10.1007/s10096-011-1269-z

CHAPTER 18

PRESENCE OF METHICILLIN-RESISTANT STAPHYLOCOCCUS AUREUS IN PIGS IN PERU

Carmen S. Arriola, Mariella E. Gu¨ere, Jesper Larsen, Robert L. Skov, Robert H. Gilman, Armando E. Gonzalez, Ellen K. Silbergeld

INTRODUCTION

Recent reports of methicillin-resistant *Staphylococcus aureus* (MRSA) in livestock, particularly pigs, and in individuals with contact to livestock provided the first evidence of the existence of a true livestock-associated MRSA (LA-MRSA) reservoir throughout Europe [1], [2]. Subsequently, LA-MRSA has been identified in Canada [3] and in the United States [4]. LA-MRSA isolates have important genotypic and phenotypic characteristics (reviewed in [5]): (1) they are nontypeable by pulsed-field gel electrophoresis (PFGE) using *Sma*I [6]; (2) many of them belong to clonal complex (CC)398 by multi-locus sequence typing (MLST); (3) the staphylococcal chromosomal cassette (SCC)*mec* elements encoding β-lactam resistance are different from those carried by other MRSA genotypes commonly found in the community and healthcare settings [7]; (4) they often exhibit co-resistance to many non-β-lactam antimicrobials (e.g., antibiotics and metals) including those commonly used in animal production [7], [8]; and (5) the majority of isolates lacks toxins such as Panton-Valentine leukocidin (PVL) and other enterotoxins [8], [9].

With a population of about 80 million pigs (http://faostat.fao.org), Latin America has a large potential reservoir for LA-MRSA. In Peru, a variety of different pig production systems exists, including scavenging pigs, semi-intensive backyard production, small-scale intensive production, and large-scale confined production, which are characterized by specific management practices and biosecurity risks. We undertook this study to investigate whether MRSA is present in different production systems in Peru.

METHODS

From February through November 2009, nasal swabs were taken from a total of 240 ready-to-market pigs (143–150 days old), including 20 pigs from each of 6 large-scale confined production holdings located in agricultural areas of the Department of Lima and 20 scavenging pigs from each of 6 rural communities in the Department of Tumbes. The Johns Hopkins University Animal Care and Use (ACUC) Committee approved the research protocol (SW08H111). The different pig production systems were categorized based on the definitions of the Food and Agriculture Organization of the United Nations [10]. Samples were stored in Stuart transport medium (Eurotubo, Deltalab, Barcelona, Spain) and streaked on mannitol salt agar (MSA, Merck, Darmstadt, Germany) supplemented with cefoxitin (4 μg/ml) within 24 h. Presumptive MRSA isolates were subcultured after 24 h onto oxacillin resistance screening agar base (ORSAB, Oxoid, Basingstoke, United Kingdom) and identified by coagulase test and multiplex PCR for 16S rRNA, *mecA,* and *nuc* genes as described elsewhere [11]. All MRSA isolates were characterized by staphylococcal protein A *(spa)* typing using the Ridom Staph Type standard protocol (http://www.ridom.com) and the Ridom SpaServer (http://spa.ridom.de/index.shtml) and were typed for SCC*mec* using a multiplex PCR assay described by Kondo et al. [12].

Citation: Arriola CS, Güere ME, Larsen J, Skov RL, Gilman RH, Gonzalez AE, et al. (2011) Presence of Methicillin-Resistant Staphylococcus aureus in Pigs in Peru. PLoS ONE 6(12): e28529. doi:10.1371/journal.pone.0028529.

RESULTS

Eight (40%) of 20 pigs from 1 of 6 sampled large-scale holdings carried MRSA; all isolates belonged to *spa* type t571 and carried SCC*mec* type V. In comparison, only 1 (5%) of 20 scavenging pigs from 1 of 6 sampled communities carried MRSA; this isolate belonged to *spa*type t008 and carried SCC*mec* type IVc.

A representative t571 isolate and the single t008 isolate were selected for further analyses. MLST types were determined (http://www.mlst.net), and the presence of 6 virulence-associated genes (*lukF-PV*, *lukF-PV*, *arcA*, *sek*, *seq*, and *bsaA*) was investigated, using PCR assays and primers that have been described elsewhere [13]. The USA300-0114 strain was used as a positive control for the PCR amplifications. The antimicrobial susceptibility profiles (spectinomycin, gentamicin, kanamycin, tobramycin, rifampin, trimethoprim-sulfamethoxazole, clindamycin, erythromycin, linezolid, chloramphenicol, mupirocin, ciprofloxacin, minocycline, tetracycline, and fusidic acid) were determined by the agar dilution method using Neo-Sensitabs (Rosco, Taastrup, Denmark), in accordance with the Clinical Laboratory Standards Institute guidelines [14]. Screening for reduced susceptibility to glycopeptides was performed on brain-heart infusion agar supplemented with 5 µg/ml teicoplanin followed by testing of positive MRSA isolates using Etest glycopeptide-resistance detection strips (vancomycin, 32–0.5 µg/ml; teicoplanin, 32–0.5 µg/ml) (bioMérieux, Marcy l'Etoil, France) as described by Fitzgibbon et al. [15].

The t571 isolate had genotypic and phenotypic characteristics of LA-MRSA: it belonged to ST398, was resistant to 6 of 16 non-β-lactam antibiotics (clindamycin, erythromycin, chloramphenicol, ciprofloxacin, minocycline, and tetracycline), and lacked all investigated virulence-associated genes. In contrast, the t008 isolate showed genotypic and phenotypic characteristics related to a USA300-like ST8-IV variant, which is the predominant community-associated MRSA (CA-MRSA) lineage in Latin America [13], [16], [17]; it belonged to ST8, was susceptible to all 16 non-β-lactam antibiotics, and carried *lukF-lukS* genes encoding PVL as well as genes encoding enterotoxins (*sek* and *seq*) and bacteriocin (*bsaA*) but lacked *arcA* (an indicator of the arginine catabolic mobile element).

DISCUSSION

This study provides the first evidence of a porcine reservoir of LA-MRSA-ST398-V in Latin America and the presence of a highly virulent USA300-like CA-MRSA lineage, ST8-IV, in Peru. However, the extent of the MRSA reservoir in animals remains speculative because of limitations in sample size and sampling locations.

The origin of LA-MRSA-ST398-V in Latin America is not known. Methicillin-susceptible *S. aureus* (MSSA) ST398 strains characterized by *spa* type t571 and lack of the *lukF-lukS* genes encoding PVL have been reported in non-hospitalized and hospitalized community-dwelling individuals with no livestock-associated risk factors in Latin America [18], [19], [20], which may suggest that LA-MRSA-ST398-V is a derivative of a progenitor CA-like MSSA ST398 strain. On the other hand, the emergence of LA-MRSA in Latin America could also be due to animal importation from other countries with established LA-MRSA reservoirs, as previously reported in Europe [21], but not yet extensively studied in Peru.

While high rates of MRSA isolation have been reported among hospitalized patients in the Andean region of Latin America [13], LA-MRSA carriage and disease in individuals have not been reported. However, we hypothesize that the proportion of LA-MRSA in humans will be higher in areas where LA-MRSA has been successfully established in the pig population, as previously reported in The Netherlands [22].

Of note, a single MRSA isolate from a scavenging pig was determined to be of the highly virulent USA300-like ST8-IV lineage, which is the predominant and almost exclusive CA-MRSA clone in the Andean region of South America, including Peru [13], [16], [17]. Such scavenging pig production systems are characterized by little confinement of the animals or lack thereof, such that pigs have access to human feces and greater likelihood of exposure to human strains of MRSA. Consequently, our finding is likely to reflect infrequent human-to-animal transmission, rather than the existence of a true animal reservoir.

In conclusion, our findings demonstrate that LA-MRSA is present in large-scale pig production systems in Peru. However, the extent of the porcine MRSA reservoir and their implications for MRSA colonization and disease in humans in Peru and other Latin American countries have still to be determined.

ACKNOWLEDGMENTS

Special acknowledgements to Dr. Sonia Calle at San Marcos University for her invaluable support in this study's implementation and to Daniel Ehlman for reviewing the manuscript.

AUTHOR CONTRIBUTIONS

Conceived and designed the experiments: CA MG JL RS RG AG ES. Performed the experiments: CA MG JL. Analyzed the data: CA MG JL. Contributed reagents/materials/analysis tools: CA JL RS RG AG ES. Wrote the paper: CA JL. Drafting the article or revising it critically for important intellectual content: CA MG JL RS RG AG ES. Final approval of the version to be published: CA MG JL RS RG AG ES.

REFERENCES

1. Armand-Lefevre L, Ruimy R, Andremont A (2005) Clonal comparison of Staphylococcus aureus isolates healthy pig farmers, human controls, and pigs. Emerg Infect Dis 11: 711–714.
2. Voss A, Loeffen F, Bakker J, Klaassen C, Wulf M (2005) Methicillin-resistant Staphylococcus aureus in pig farming. Emerg Infect Dis 11: 1965–1966.
3. Khanna T, Friendship R, Dewey C, Weese JS (2008) Methicillin resistant Staphylococcus aureus colonization in pigs and pig farm workers. Vet Microbiol 128: 298–303.
4. Smith TC, Male MJ, Harper AL, Kroeger AS, Tinkler GP, et al. (2008) Methicillin-resistant Staphylococcus aureus strain ST398 is present in midwestern U.S. swine

and swine workers. PloS One 4: e4258.

5. Smith TC, Pearson N (2010) The emergence of Staphylococcus aureus ST398. Vector Borne Zoonotic Dis 11: 327–339.
6. Bens CC, Voss A, Klaassen CH (2006) Presence of a novel DNA methylation enzyme in methicillin-resistant Staphylococcus aureus isolates. J Clin Microbiol 44: 1875–1876.
7. Li S, Skov RL, Han X, Larsen AR, Larsen J, et al. (2011) T.Novel types of staphylococcal cassette chromosome mec elements identified in clonal complex 398 methicillin-resistant Staphylococcus aureus strains. Antimicrob Agents Chemother 55: 3046–3050.
8. Argudín MA, Tenhagen BA, Fetsch A, Sachsenröder J, Käsbohrer A, et al. (2011) Virulence and resistance determinants of German Staphylococcus aureus ST398 isolates from nonhuman. Appl Environ Microbiol 77: 3052–3060.
9. Hallin M, De Mendonça R, Denis O, Lefort A, El Garch F, et al. (2011) Diversity of accessory genome of human and livestock-associated ST398 methicillin resistant Staphylococcus aureus strains. Infect Genet Evol 11: 290–299.
10. Food and Agriculture Organization of the United Nations/World Organisation for Animal Health/World Bank (2010) Good practices for biosecurity in the pig sector: issues and options in developing and transition countries. Rome: FAO Animal Production and Health Paper No. 169. 74 p.
11. Maes N, Magdalena J, Rottiers S, De Gheldre Y, Struelens MJ (2002) Evaluation of a triplex PCR to discriminate Staphylococcus aureus from coagulase negative staphylococci and determine methicillin resistance from blood cultures. J Clin Microbiol 40: 1514–1517.
12. Kondo Y, Ito T, Ma XX, Watanabe S, Kreiswirth BN, et al. (2007) Combination of multiplex PCRs for staphylococcal cassette chromosome mec type assignment: rapid identification system for mec, ccr, and major differences in junkyard regions. Antimicrob Agents Chemother 51: 264–274.
13. Reyes J, Rincon S, Díaz L, Panesso D, Contreras GE, et al. (2009) Dissemination of methicillin-resistant Staphylococcus aureus USA300 sequence type 8 lineage in Latin America. J Infect Dis 49: 1861–1867.
14. Clinical and Laboratory Standards Institute (2011) Performance standards for antimicrobial susceptibility testing: Twenty-First Informational Supplement M100-S21. Wayne (PA): The Institute.
15. Fitzgibbon MM, Rossney AS, O'Connell B (2007) Investigation of reduced susceptibility to glycopeptides among Staphylococcus aureus isolates from patients in Ireland and evaluation of agar screening methods for detection of heterogeneously glycopeptide-intermediate S. aureus. J Clin Microbiol 45: 3263–3269.
16. Arias CA, Rincon S, Chowdhury S, Martínez E, Coronell W, et al. (2008) MRSA USA300 clone and VREF: a U.S.-Colombian connection? N Engl J Med 359: 2177–2179.
17. García C, Deplano A, Denis O, León M, Siu H, et al. Spread of community-associated methicillin-resistant Staphylococcus aureus to Peru. J Infect. In press.
18. Bhat M, Dumortier C, Taylor BS, Miller M, Vasquez G, et al. (2009) Staphylococcus aureus ST398, New York City and Dominican Republic. Emerg Infect Dis 15: 285–287.
19. Ruimy R, Angebault C, Djossou F, Dupont C, Epelboin L, et al. (2010) Are host genetics the predominant determinant of persistent nasal Staphylococcus aureus carriage in humans? J Infect Dis 202: 924–34.
20. Jiménez JN, Vélez LA, Mediavilla JR, Ocampo AM, Vanegas JM, et al. (2011 Oct [cited 2011 Oct 27]) Livestock-associated methicillin-susceptible Staphylococcus aureus ST398 infection in woman, Colombia [letter]. Emerg Infect Dis. http://dx.doi.org/10.3201/eid1710.110638.
21. European Food Safety Authority (2010) Analysis of the baseline survey on the prevalence of methicillin-resistant Staphylococcus aureus (MRSA) in holdings with breeding pigs, in the EU, 2008, Part B: factors associated with MRSA contamination of holdings; on request from the European Commission. EFSA J 8: 1597.
22. van Rijen MML, Van Keulen PH, Kluytmans JA (2008) Increase in a Dutch hospital of methicillin-resistant Staphylococcus aureus related to animal farming. Clin Infect Dis 46: 261–263.

CHAPTER 19

METHICILLIN RESISTANT STAPHYLOCOCCUS AUREUS ST398 IN VEAL CALF FARMING: HUMAN MRSA CARRIAGE RELATED WITH ANIMAL ANTIMICROBIAL USAGE AND FARM HYGIENE

Haitske Graveland, Jaap A. Wagenaar, Hans Heesterbeek, Dik Mevius, Engeline van Duijkeren, Dick Heederik

INTRODUCTION

The continuing emergence of pathogenic organisms resistant to antimicrobials is a global concern. Infections with antibiotic resistant bacteria have been associated with frequent treatment failure and increased severity of disease [1],[2],[3]. Both human and non-human antimicrobial usage may result in increased occurrence of bacterial resistance [4]. Transfer of antimicrobial resistance (genes) from animals to humans may occur through transmission of zoonotic pathogens or commensals through food or direct contact [3]. Methicillin Resistant *Staphylococcus aureus* (MRSA) has traditionally been considered a nosocomial pathogen. More recently MRSA emerged in the community [5] and since 2003 a specific sequence type of MRSA emerged, which was observed in food producing animals and farmers and is referred to as livestock associated MRSA (LA-MRSA) [6]–[11]. This MRSA sequence type is characterized by being non-typable by use of Pulsed Field Gel Electrophoresis with *Sma*I, and was therefore previously called non-typable MRSA (NT-MRSA). All NT-MRSA belong to one clonal complex, in particular multilocus sequence type 398 (ST398) [5]. A high prevalence of ST398 was found among farm animals, predominantly pigs and veal calves, and people occupationally in contact with these animals [5],[6]. Carriers of MRSA may develop an MRSA (wound) infection after disruption of the skin (scarification) or after surgery and are therefore at risk. Additionally, the impact of this MRSA sequence type on farming communities has been considerable because carriers have been treated in isolation in the health care system as part of the infection control measures: the search and destroy policy, common in low prevalence countries [12]. Many case studies show parallel occurrence of MRSA ST398 in both animals and humans [8], [10], [13]–[15]. Risk factors for carrying MRSA ST398 in both animals and humans have not been fully evaluated. Evidence for animal to human transmission of MRSA is often indirect and based on parallel observations in genetic [16],[17] or resistance patterns [18]among isolates or else indications obtained by *in vitro* experiments [19].

This study focussed on the presence of MRSA among veal farmers, their family members and their animals. Specific attention has been given to associations between the presence of MRSA among animals and humans as well as identification of

Citation: Graveland H, Wagenaar JA, Heesterbeek H, Mevius D, van Duijkeren E, Heederik D (2010) Methicillin Resistant Staphylococcus aureus ST398 in Veal Calf Farming: Human MRSA Carriage Related with Animal Antimicrobial Usage and Farm Hygiene. PLoS ONE 5(6): e10990. doi:10.1371/journal.pone.0010990.

potential determinants of MRSA occurrence such as antibiotic use, hygiene practices at the farm and farm characteristics.

MATERIALS AND METHODS

Study design

We conducted a cross-sectional study on 102 randomly selected veal calf farms. All farms have been visited from October 2007 to March 2008. Nasal swabs (from both anterior nares) were taken from veal calf growers, family members and employees. All participants were asked to fill in a questionnaire containing items about activities on the farm, intensity and duration of animal contact and MRSA history. Questions on potential confounders such as age, sex and smoking were included. In addition questions on farm structure, antibiotic intake (group- and individual treatments, timing and duration of treatment and kind of antibiotics administered) of the calves and farm hygiene were incorporated. The study protocol was approved by the Medical Ethical Committee of Utrecht University. All participants completed an informed consent.

On each farm the square root of the number of veal calves (a minimum of 10 and a maximum of 25 calves for each farm) was randomly selected and sampled using a sterile cotton-wool swab (Cultiplast®). From each calf, one nasal swab was taken from both nares by rubbing the swab in each nostril. Collecting animal samples was in accordance with the Dutch Law on Animal Health and Welfare. The swabs were immediately transported to the laboratory and processed within four hours after collection.

Laboratory analysis

The nasal swabs were analysed individually using a pre-enrichment containing Mueller Hinton broth with 6.5% NaCl [20]. After overnight incubation at 37°C, 1 mL of the pre-enrichment was transferred into 9 mL selective enrichment of phenyl red mannitol broth (bioMérieux, France) with 75 mg/L aztreonam and 5 mg/L ceftizoxime followed. Ten µL of the selective enrichment broth was inoculated onto sheep blood agar (Biotrading, The Netherlands) and a MRSA Brilliance™ agar (Oxoid, The Netherlands). All suspected colonies were identified as *S. aureus*using standard techniques: colony morphology and slide coagulase assay with rabbit serum [20]. In addition, the presence of the *mecA* gene was confirmed by PCR as described previously [21]. A random selection of the *mecA*-positive colonies (n=208) was confirmed to be MRSA by PCR of the *S. aureus* specific DNA-fragment Martineau [22].

For all MRSA human isolates (n=62), and a random selection of MRSA strains isolated from veal calves with a maximum of three per farm (n=207), *spa* types were determined. The strains were *spa* typed by sequencing of the repetitive region of the protein A gene *spa* [23]. Data were analyzed by using the Ridom Staphtype software version 1.4 (www.ridom.de/staphtype). A random selection of three strains per *spa* type was tested with ST398 specific PCR [24]. Non-ST398 strains were analysed by multilocus sequence typing (MLST) [25] (www.saureus.mlst.net).

Data analysis

Statistical analysis was performed using SAS software 9.1. Descriptive analyses were undertaken followed by logistic regression analysis (GLIMMIX procedure) to identify determinants of MRSA carriage on individual level (human/calf). Risk factors for MRSA carriage were first identified by univariate logistic regression analysis. Thereafter, multivariate analysis was done by stepwise, forward entry including factors associated with MRSA positivity in humans and calves ($P<0.2$). Hierarchical structure of the data was taken into account to adjust for the fact that observations of human and calves on the same farm may not be independent. Relationships between MRSA carriage in humans and veal calves were further studied by assessing the shape of these relationships by means of nonparametric regression modelling (smoothing) using generalized additive models (PROC GAM). A P-value<0.05 was considered statistically significant.

RESULTS

Humans

Nasal swabs of 390 individuals, working or living on 102 veal calf farms were tested for the presence of MRSA. The response rate was 81%: 97 farmers, 259 family members and 34 employees were included. Reasons for non-participation were no interest, lack of time, or retirement from farming. MRSA prevalence in farmers was 33% and 8% in family members (Table 1). This large difference in MRSA prevalence could be explained by the difference in time spent in the stables, even after adjustment for smoking, age and gender (Table 1). The risk for being MRSA carrier increased with increasing number of working hours spent per week in stables (Odds Ratio (OR)=1.4, expressed per 10 hours/week). The shape of this relationship was investigated, showing a strong increase in prevalence with increasing time spent with animals (Figure 1A). In addition, those who spent more time on feeding calves (OR=1.5), veterinary care (OR=1.6) and stable management (OR=2.0) were more often MRSA carrier (Table 2).

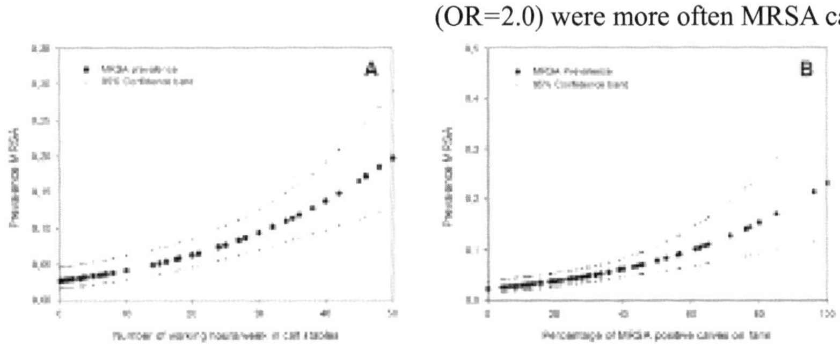

Figure 1: Human MRSA prevalence, working hours in calf stables per week and MRSA positive calves on the farm.

Figure 1 A shows the relationship between MRSA carrier prevalence in humans and the number of working hours / week in the calf stable, adjusted for gender, age, smoking habits and percentage of positive calves on the farm. Figure 1 B shows the relationship between MRSA carrier prevalence in humans and the percentage of positive calves on the farm, adjusted for gender, age, smoking habits and number of hours working/ week in calf stables. In both figures smoothed plots are given with 95% confidence bands.

Table 1: Characteristics of 390 farmers, family members, employees and determinants for MRSA carriage in human (multiple logistic regression analysis)

	No. (Prevalence %)	
Total	390 (16)	
General charcteristics		
Farmers	97 (33)	
Family members	259 (8)	
Employees	34 (26)	
OR (95% Confidence interval) multiple regression model		
Gender		
Female	177 (7)	1
Male	213 (24)	3.0 (1.4–6.8)*
Age (yr)		
0–18	130 (6)	
19–65	248 (21)	
66–85	12 (25)	
Per 10 years		1.3 (1.1–1.5)*
Smoking habits		
No smoking	334 (17)	1
Smoking	55 (11)	0.5 (0.2–1.4)
Level of animal contact / # working hours in veal calf stable/week		
<20 hours a week	250 (7)	
20–40 hours a week	56 (23)	
>40 hours a week	72 (42)	
Per 10 hours/week		1.4 (1.2–1.7)*
Percentage of positive calves on farm		
<28% (below mean)	232 (12)	
>28% (above mean)	158 (22)	
Difference between 0–28%		2.1 (1.4–3.0)*

P<0.05.
doi:10.1371/journal.pone.0010990.t001

http://dx.doi.org/10.1371/journal.pone.0010990.t001

Table 2: Associations between human MRSA carriage and specific tasks on the farm

Task	MRSA carriage
	OR (95% Confidence interval)[1▲]
Feeding calves	1.5 (1.2–1.8)*
Veterinary care	1.6 (1.0–2.5)**
Stable management; sorting calves	2.0 (1.3–3.4)*

*P<0.05.
**P 0.10–0.05.
[1]OR expressed per hour/week difference.
▲adjusted for gender, age, smoking and percentage of positive calves on farm.
doi:10.1371/journal.pone.0010990.t002

http://dx.doi.org/10.1371/journal.pone.0010990.t002

MRSA carriage in humans was associated with the prevalence of MRSA in calves. Farmers were more often MRSA carrier when they had more MRSA positive calves. The estimated prevalence in humans was approximately 1% when less than 20% of the calves were carrier. On farms with a higher carrier prevalence in calves MRSA prevalence in humans was above 10%. (Figure 1B). We adjusted for potential confounding variables, like age, gender and smoking habits; age was positively associated (OR=1.2 per 10 years) and males were significantly more often MRSA colonized compared to females (OR=3.0). Smoking was negatively associated (OR=0.5), however not statistically significant. The associations between human MRSA carriage and any of the described determinants (task, duration animal contact, prevalence among animals) did not change when potential confounders were included in the model.

Calves

Nasal swabs were taken from 2151 veal calves of 102 farms (Table 3) and MRSA prevalence was 28%. On 88% of the farms MRSA could be detected in one or more calves. MRSA carriers were more often seen in calves treated with antibiotics (group treatment) (OR=1.8), compared to calves not treated. Since veal calves were frequently treated with different kinds of antibiotics, even during one treatment, it was not possible to unravel the effect of individual antibiotics or antibiotic classes. Besides this, older calves were more often MRSA positive than calves of younger age (OR=1.3 (per 10 weeks). The shape of the relationship with age is shown in Figure 2. MRSA carriage with age is higher ($p<0.05$) in calves treated with antibiotics compared to untreated calves. Calves from large farms (farms with many animals) were significantly more often colonized compared to calves from smaller farms (OR=2.7 per 500 calves/farm. Moreover, a negative association was found between MRSA carriage and farm hygiene (OR=0.3). i.e. cleaning of stables before entrance of new calf populations to the farm. Disinfection was applied in less than 20% of the farms and was not associated with MRSA carriage in calves. No associations were found with other possible determinates like country of origin of calves, drinking- or feeding systems and numbers of animals used.

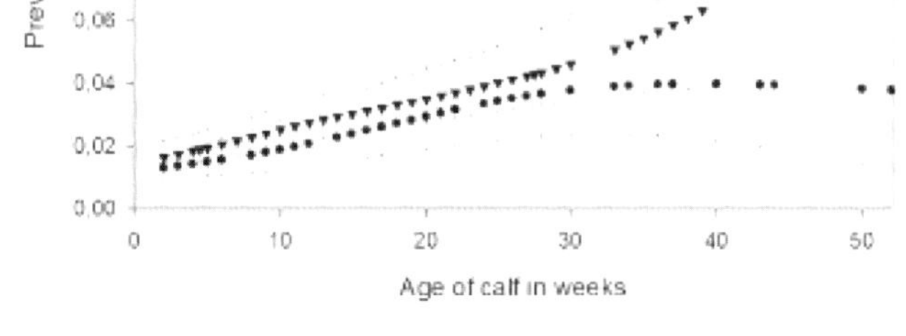

Figure 2: MRSA carriage in veal calves, age and antibiotic treatment.

The relationship between MRSA carriage in veal calves and age for calves treated and not treated with antibiotics as group treatment (adjusted for age, number of calves per farm, farm hygiene, calf category (white versus rose veal), number of stables on farm, number of calves per pen, presence of other animals on the farm and rodent control). Smoothed plots are presented with 95% confidence bands.

Table 3: Characteristics of 2151 veal calves from 102 veal farms and associations between MRSA carriage and some determinants (logistic multiple regression analysis)

	No. (Prevalence %)	
Total		
General characteristics		
Farms	102 (88)	
Veal calves	2151 (28) (range 0–100%)	
OR (95% Confidence interval) multiple regression model▲		
Antibiotic (group) treatment		
No	570 (21)	1
Yes	1581 (30)	1.8 (1.1–3.0)*
Age calf (wk)		
0–6	301 (12)	
7–12	458 (36)	
>12	1392 (28)	
Per 10 weeks		1.3 (1.1–1.5)*
Number of calves on the farm		
<500	985 (22)	
>500	1166 (32)	
Per 100 calves		1.1 (1.0–1.2)*
Farm hygiene		
No	375 (35)	1
yes	1776 (26)	0.3 (0.1–0.7)*

*P<0.05.

▲adjusted for calf category (white versus rose veal), number of stables on farm, number of calves per pen, presence of other animals on the farm and rodent control.

doi:10.1371/journal.pone.0010990.t003

http://dx.doi.org/10.1371/journal.pone.0010990.t003

Genotyping isolates

In total 16 different *spa* types were identified; 9 different *spa* types in human isolates and 12 different types in veal calves (Table 4). In humans, all identified *spa* types belonged to ST398, except four. These four non ST398 strains were identified as t002, t015, t084 and t166), respectively belonging to ST5, ST45, ST15 and CC34.

Table 4: Spa typing and MLST typing results (non ST398 sequence types in bold)

Spa type	*No. (Prevalence %)*	MLST
Human isolates n = 62		
t002	**1**	**ST5**
t011	51	ST398
t015	**1**	**ST45**
t084	**1**	**ST15**
t108	2	ST398
t166	**1**	**CC34**
t899	3	ST398
t1457	1	ST398
t2383	1	ST398
Calve isolates n = 207		
t011	166	ST398
t034	17	ST398
t108	7	ST398
t421	**2**	**ST239**
t899	5	ST398
t1197	1	ST398
t1236	**2**	**ST97**
t1451	1	ST398
t1457	1	ST398
t1580	1	ST398
t1685	**1**	**ST1159**
t2383	2	ST398
t3856	**1**	**CC425**

doi:10.1371/journal.pone.0010990.t004

http://dx.doi.org/10.1371/journal.pone.0010990.t004

In calves, the predominant *spa* type found was t011 (80%); also *spa* type t034 was frequently found (8%). Among calves, also four non ST398 strains were found, t421, t1236, t1685, t3856, respectively, ST239, ST97, ST1159 and CC425. All *spa* types found in humans matched with the types found in calves on the same farm except for the non ST398.

DISCUSSION

This study shows that people in close contact with veal calves have a highly elevated risk of MRSA carriage. Human carriers came more often from farms where veal calves appeared carriers as well. Overall the prevalence of MRSA was 15.9% in persons living and working on a veal calf farm which is a strong elevation compared to the general population. The prevalence of MRSA in the Dutch community is estimated to be below 1%. Moreover, strong associations with duration of animal contact and specific tasks on the farm were found. Furthermore, veal calves carrying MRSA were more often treated with antibiotics. This is the strongest evidence of a direct relationship between antibiotic use in animals and transfer of antimicrobial resistant organisms to humans at present. In addition, this evidence is strengthened by the similarity of *spa* types and antimicrobial susceptibility patterns (data not shown) of the isolates found in both humans and animals.

The presence of LA-MRSA in farmers forms a potential threat for public health, for individuals carrying MRSA and for the health care system. The carriers are at risk for (wound) infections with LA-MRSA. For the health care system, the frequent occurrence of ST398 especially in countries with low and moderate MRSA prevalence put the infection control policy under pressure. In addition, a possible change in virulence (*e.g.* introduction of toxin genes) will change the public health perspective considerably and further challenges the Search and Destroy Strategy. The unexpected and sudden increase of LA-MRSA incidence in hospitals which occurred since 2007, resulted in a shortage of isolation facilities. An additional problem is the treatment of carriers, which is also part of this strategy [26]. Decolonisation of patients who are constantly exposed to MRSA in their work and home settings is not effective: at present the 'destroy' element is impossible to execute.

The observation that MRSA carriage in humans is associated with MRSA prevalence among their calves is remarkable. This might indicate that the prevalence in humans in close contact with animals follows the prevalence of MRSA among animals over time. Evidence for an association between the use of antimicrobials in animals and increase in occurrence of resistant bacteria in humans is often not as direct as observed in this study. Parallel occurrence of resistant bacteria in humans and animals is observed in ecological studies. The risk of transfer of resistance from animals to humans is seldom observed directly. For instance, vancomycin-resistant *enterococci* (VRE) acquired their resistance gene (*vanA*) after glycopeptide use as growth promoter in animals and later emerged in hospitals. However, detailed genetic analysis demonstrated that the isolates in animals and humans were not genetically related, and a direct association has never been demonstrated [27]. Similarly, use of fluoroquinolones in poultry co-incided with an increased occurrence of food borne infections in humans with fluoroquinolone resistant *Campylobacter jejuni* [28].

Our results suggest that occurrence of ST398 in humans is transient and varies over time within individuals, because of the correlation with the prevalence in animals. The number of positive calves on the farm is a characteristic that changes over time as shown in this study. Veal calves live between 7–10 months before being slaughtered and new animals are brought in from many different dairy farms, from across the European Union. The prevalence in a new herd of animals is likely to differ from herd to herd. Also the results from fieldworkers who took nasal swabs directly after the farm visits and two days thereafter suggest transient carriage. They were rarely tested MRSA positive during several hundred days of fieldwork but few appeared colonized and when this occurred the duration of colonization was never more than one day (data not shown).

Few studies investigated risk factors for the occurrence of ST398 in humans. High animal to human transmission of ST398 has been reported in pig farming [6], [29]–[32]. In these studies also a large difference in MRSA prevalence is observed between the farmer and family members, which is indicative of a comparable role for intensive animal contact as risk factor for ST398 occurrence [29], [31].

A major finding is that the prevalence of ST398 in veal calves appeared associated with antimicrobial (group) treatments. Also hygiene and some other farm characteristics, such as herd size, were associated with ST398 prevalence. These associations may give further direction to preventive strategies and indicate that is a potential to influence the occurrence of ST398 MRSA in humans and animals.

The large difference in MRSA prevalence between farmers (33%) and family members (8%) may indicate infrequent human to human transmission of ST398. This was also suggested in studies where comparisons were made of ST398 and non-ST398 MRSA regarding the occurrence of secondary cases in hospitals [26], [33]. However, in our study, we did not investigate contact patterns between humans as an explanatory variable. Our observation of a likely low human to human transmission needs further exploration.

MRSA was more frequently observed on veal calf farms as on pig farms [6]. However a larger variety in *spa* types appears present in veal farming, not only in veal calves but also in human isolates. The large number of dairy farms supplying young calves for veal production and their distribution across Europe, and thereby the large variety in origin of veal calves compared to pigs, may play a role in this finding. A limitation of our study is the cross-sectional design in which both cause and effect are measured at the same time. For that reason, results from this study need to be confirmed in a longitudinal study in which occurrence of MRSA carriage over time is associated with the use of antibiotics and other determinants. A longitudinal design may also provide valuable information about dynamics and persistence of MRSA carriage in both animals and humans. Nevertheless, results of this study indicate that prudent use of antibiotics is warranted. This is recognised by all parties responsible for use of antimicrobials in veterinary practice; the Dutch calf producers and the Dutch Government therefore recently agreed on a covenant to reduce antibiotic resistance.

In conclusion, this is the first study showing direct associations between animal and human carriage of ST398. MRSA carriage in calves was positively associated with use of antibiotics while farm hygiene was associated with a lower prevalence of MRSA. For optimal design and implementation of infection control strategies in both animals and humans, detailed combined human-animal studies exploring direct associations are essential. These not only refers to MRSA, but to all (resistant) pathogens in general, where direct associations between animals and humans may be expected.

ACKNOWLEDGMENTS

We thank all farmers for their participation. We are grateful to Isabella Oosting-Schothorst, Marian Broekhuizen-Stins Anky Schoormans, Koen Verstappen for fieldwork and laboratory assistance, Lützen Portengen for his assistance with data analysis, Birgitta Duim for her help with interpretation of the information on genotyping. We thank Xander Huijsdens for *spa* typing.

AUTHOR CONTRIBUTIONS

Conceived and designed the experiments: HG JAW DH. Performed the experiments: HG DM. Analyzed the data: HG HH DH. Wrote the paper: HG JAW HH DM EvD DH.

REFERENCES

1. Finch R, Hunter PA (2006) Antibiotic resistance–action to promote new technologies: report of an EU Intergovernmental Conference held in Birmingham, UK. J Antimicrob Chemother 1: i3–i22.
2. Swartz MN (2004) Human diseases caused by foodborne pathogens of animal origin. Clin Infect Dis 3: 111–122.
3. Angulo FJ, Nargund VN, Chiller TC (2004) Evidence of an association between use of anti-microbial agents in food animals and anti-microbial resistance among bacteria isolated from humans and the human health consequences of such resistance. J Vet Med B Infect Dis Vet Public Health 51: 374–379.
4. Anderson AD, Nelson JM, Rossiter S, Angulo FJ (2003) Public health consequences of use of antimicrobial agents in food animals in the United States. Microb Drug Resist 9: 373–379.
5. van Loo I, Huijsdens X, Tiemersma E, de Neeling A, van de Sande-Bruinsma N, et al. (2007) Emergence of methicillin-resistant Staphylococcus aureus of animal origin in humans. Emerg Infect Dis 13: 1834–1839.
6. Smith TC, Male MJ, Harper AL, Kroeger JS, Tinkler GP, et al. (2009) Methicillin-resistant Staphylococcus aureus (MRSA) Strain ST398 is Present in Midwestern U.S. Swine and Swine workers. Plos one 4:
7. Tiemersma EW, Bronzwaer SL, Lyytikainen O, Degener JE, Schrijnemakers P, et al. (2004) Methicillin-resistant Staphylococcus aureus in Europe, 1999–2002. Emerg Infect Dis 10: 1627–1634.
8. Guardabassi L, Schwarz S, Lloyd DH (2004) Pet animals as reservoirs of antimicrobial-resistant bacteria. J Antimicrob Chemother 54: 321–332.
9. de Neeling AJ, van den Broek MJ, Spalburg EC, van Santen-Verheuvel MG, Dam-Deisz WD, et al. (2007) High prevalence of methicillin resistant Staphylococcus aureus in pigs. Vet Microbiol 21: 366–372.

10. Huijsdens XW, van Dijke BJ, Spalburg E, van Santen-Verheuvel MG, Heck ME, et al. (2006) Community-acquired MRSA and pig-farming. Ann Clin Microbiol Antimicrob 5: 26.

11. van Duijkeren E, Box AT, Heck ME, Wannet WJ, Fluit AC (2004) Methicillin-resistant staphylococci isolated from animals. Vet Microbiol 5: 91–97.

12. Vandenbroucke-Grauls CM (1996) Methicillin-resistant Staphylococcus aureus control in hospitals: the Dutch experience. Infect Control Hosp Epidemiol 17: 512–513.

13. Juhász-Kaszanyitzky E, Jánosi S, Somogyi P, Dán A, van der Graaf-van Bloois L, et al. (2007) MRSA transmission between cows and humans. Emerg Infect Dis 13: 630–632.

14. Simoons-Smit AM, Savelkoul PH, Stoof J, Starink TM, Vandenbroucke-Grauls CM (2000) Transmission of Staphylococcus aureus between humans and domestic animals in a household. Eur J Clin Microbiol Infect Dis 19: 150–152.

15. van Duijkeren E, Wolfhagen MJ, Box AT, Heck ME, Wannet WJ, et al. (2004) Human-to-dog transmission of methicillin-resistant Staphylococcus aureus. Emerg Infect Dis 10: 2235–2237.

16. Lee JH (2003) Methicillin (Oxacillin)-resistant Staphylococcus aureus strains isolated from major food animals and their potential transmission to humans. Appl Environ Microbiol 69: 6489–6494.

17. Strommenger B, Kehrenberg C, Kettlitz C, Cuny C, Verspohl J, et al. (2006) Molecular characterization of methicillin-resistant Staphylococcus aureus strains from pet animals and their relationship to human isolates. J Antimicrob Chemother 57: 461–465.

18. Fessler A, Scott C, Kadlec K, Ehricht R, Monecke S, et al. (2010) Characterization of methicillin-resistant Staphylococcus aureus ST398 from cases of bovine mastitis. J Antimicrob Chemother 65: 619–625.

19. Dancer SJ (2008) The effect of antibiotics on methicillin-resistant Staphylococcus aureus. J Antimicrob Chemother 61: 246–253.

20. Graveland H, van Duijkeren E, van Nes A, Schoormans A, Broekhuizen-Stins M, et al. (2009) Evaluation of isolation procedures and chromogenic agar media for the detection of MRSA in nasal swabs from pigs and veal calves. Vet Microbiol 20: 121–125.

21. Fluit AC, Wielders CL, Verhoef J, Schmitz FJ (2001) Epidemiology and susceptibility of 3,051 Staphylococcus aureus isolates from 25 university hospitals participating in the European SENTRY study. J Clin Microbiol 39: 3727–3732.

22. Martineau F, Picard FJ, Roy PH, Ouellette M, Bergeron MG (1998) Species-specific and ubiquitous-DNA-based assays for rapid identification of Staphylococcus aureus. J Clin Microbiol 36: 618–623.

23. Harmsen D, Claus H, Witte W, Rothganger J, Turnwald D, et al. (2003) Typing of methicillin-resistant Staphylococcus aureus in a university hospital setting by using novel software for spa repeat determination and database management. J Clin Microbiol 41: 5442–5448.

24. van Wamel WJ, Hansenová Manásková S, Fluit AC, Verbrugh H, de Neeling AJ, et al. (2010) Short term micro-evolution and PCR-detection of methicillin-resistant and -susceptible Staphylococcus aureus sequence type 398. Eur J Clin Microbiol Infect 29: 119–122.

25. Enright MC, Day NP, Davies CE, Peacock SJ, Spratt BG (2000) Multilocus sequence typing for characterization of methicillin-resistant and methicillin-susceptible clones of Staphylococcus aureus. J Clin Microbiol 38: 1008–1015.

26. van Rijen MM, Van Keulen PH, Kluytmans JA (2008) Increase in a Dutch hospital of methicillin-resistant Staphylococcus aureus related to animal farming. Clin Infect Dis 46: 261–263.

27. Willems RJ, Top J, van den Braak N, van Belkum A, Mevius DJ, et al. (1999) Molecular diversity and evolutionary relationships of Tn1546-like elements in enterococci from humans and animals. Antimicrob Agents Chemother 43: 483–491.

28. Nelson JM, Chiller TM, Powers JH, Angulo FJ (2007) Fluoroquinolone-resistant Campylobacter species and the withdrawal of fluoroquinolones from use in poultry: a public health success story. Clin Infect Dis 7: 977–980.

29. Lewis HC, Molbak K, Reese C, Aarestrup FM, Selchau M, et al. (2008) Pigs as source of methicillin-resistant Staphylococcus aureus CC398 infections in humans, Denmark. Emerg Infect Dis 14: 1383–1389.

30. Khanna T, Friendship R, Dewey C, Weese JS (2008) Methicillin resistant Staphylococcus aureus colonization in pigs and pig farmers. Vet Microbiol 30: 298–303.

31. van den Broek IV, van Cleef BA, Haenen A, Broens EM, van der Wolf PJ, et al. (2008) Methicillin-resistant Staphylococcus aureus in people living and working in pig farms. Epidemiol Infect 24: 1–9.

32. Denis O, Suetens C, Hallin M, Catry B, Ramboer I, et al. (2009) Methicillin-resistant Staphylococcus aureus ST398 in swine farm personnel, Belgium. Emerg Infect Dis 15: 1098–1101.

33. Wassenberg MW, Hopmans TE, Troelstra A, Kluytmans JA, Bonten MJ (2008) Methicillin-resistant Staphylococcus aureus of livestock origin in Dutch hospitals: high-risk patients need only to be investigated if admitted to hospital. Ned Tijdschr Geneeskd 152: 2681–2688.

CHAPTER 20

ANTIBIOTIC RESISTANCE IN STAPHYLOCOCCUS AUREUS AND COAGULASE NEGATIVE STAPHYLOCOCCI ISOLATED FROM GOATS WITH SUBCLINICAL MASTITIS

Salvatore Virdis, Christian Scarano, Francesca Cossu, Vincenzo Spanu, Carlo Spanu, and Enrico Pietro Luigi De Santis

INTRODUCTION

Raw goat's milk can be a potential source of antibioticresistant pathogens of animal, human, and environmental origin. The microorganisms which contaminate raw milk may originate from the farm environment or from the goats and include the etiological agents responsible for clinical and Subclinical Mastitis (SCM). In dairy goats with SCM, Coagulase Negative Staphylococci (CNS) make up 44.7% to 95.9% of the isolated pathogens from milk samples, and S. aureus, which is usually considered to have the greater pathogenicity, accounts from 4.1% to 18.0% of SCM agents [1]. The average prevalence of SCM in dairy goat's farms is between 20.0%–35.0% and results in significant economic losses due to reduction in milk production and poor milk quality [1].

The intramammary administration of antibiotics used on farms has increased, as it was proved to be effective for treating SCM in dry small ruminants [2, 3]. The efficacy of intramammary antibiotic treatment could be compromised by staphylococci that produce biofilms in the udder. The widespread use of antibiotics on dairy farms, could lead to the selection and to the emergence of antibioticresistant bacterial strains [4].

Most published scientific research papers had for object the antimicrobial resistance of intramammary infection pathogens isolated from raw bovine milk. The detection in raw milk of multiple resistant strains, and especially methicillin resistant S. aureus (MRSA) and CNS (MRCNS) strains, is regarded as an issue of great concern for their potential spread through the dairy food chain. In small ruminants, the spread of MRSA strains is controversial. MRSA strains are characterized by the presence of the mecA gene encoding low-affinity penicillin binding protein (PBP2), which mediates resistance to all classes of β-lactam antibiotics [5]. Few studies have reported that S. aureus strains, isolated from ewes milk affected by SCM, did not carry the mecA gene [6], or that, the few strains that were resistant to methicillin (oxacillin), probably were of human origin [7]. Instead, other studies showed how MRCNS strains can be isolated from goats milk with SCM [8]. Antibiotic resistance pattern for staphylococci isolated from SCM refers mainly to cattle, and little is known about dairy goats [8–12]. Studies on antimicrobials susceptibility of these pathogens [13] have been mainly conducted using the agar disc diffusion method of Bauer et al. The broth microdilution and the agar dilution methods [14] instead allow the evaluation of the minimum inhibitory concentrations (MIC).

The evaluation of the antimicrobial susceptibility of Staphylococcus spp. isolated from goats with SCM is of great interest for clinical purposes in order to decide which antibiotics should be administered, as well as, for monitoring the spread of multiple resistant strains on farms. The current study seeks to support the sparse literature on antibiotic resistance of S. aureus and CNS isolated from goats with SCM. MICs and in

Citation: Salvatore Virdis, Christian Scarano, Francesca Cossu, Vincenzo Spanu, Carlo Spanu, and Enrico Pietro Luigi De Santis, "Antibiotic Resistance in Staphylococcus aureus and Coagulase Negative Staphylococci Isolated from Goats with Subclinical Mastitis," Veterinary Medicine International, vol. 2010, Article ID 517060, 6 pages, 2010. doi:10.4061/2010/517060.

vitro susceptibilities to ten antibiotics used in the medical and veterinary fields were determined against 25 S. aureus and 75 CNS strains. On these strains, the frequencies of single and multiple antibiotic-resistance were also evaluated.

MATERIALS AND METHODS

Dairy Farms.

The milk samples were collected from eight goats flocks in the island of Sardinia (Italy) where mainly Sarda and Sarda-Maltese breeds were reared. The rearing system was extensive and the animals were handmilked. The goats, fed on bushes and grass, occasionally were supplemented with concentrates. The mean flock size was 187.5 ± 25.2 (mean ± SD) with a range from 160 to 234. Goats were not treated with systemic or intramammary antimicrobial agents during the lactation previous to the enrollment in this study nor during the dry period.

Sampling

A clinical examination of half-udders was conducted in order to exclude animals with signs of clinical mastitis [15]. A total of 3,000 half-udder milk samples (1,500 goats) were collected in a single sampling time in each of the eight flocks during the early lactation period (from January to April of 2006). The first few streams of foremilk were discarded, and duplicate half-udder milk samples were aseptically collected into sterile tubes after cleaning and disinfection of each teat end. One sample (10 mL) was used for bacteriological analysis and the other one (50 mL) was added with bronopol (2-bromo-2-nitropropane-1,3-diol) and analysed for Somatic Cell Count (SCC). The milk samples were stored at +4°C, and bacteriological and SCC examinations were carried out within 6 and 72 hours after sampling.

Bacteriological Analysis and Isolation Procedures.

Each half-udders milk sample was mixed by inversion and 10 µL were then inoculated onto 5.0% Sheep Blood Agar (SBA) plates. The SBA plates were then incubated aerobically at +37°C and examined after 48 and 72 hours. A significant bacterial count was considered when a growth of ≥500 identical cfu/mL was detected. Bacterial strains were isolated on Brain Heart Infusion agar (BHI, Oxoid, Basingstoke, UK), and identified using routinary microbiological procedures such as colony morphology, microscopic characteristics and Gram staining, hemolysis pattern on SBA, catalase and oxidase reactions. The strains were identified using API ID32 STAPH system (bioMerieux, Lyon, France) and the ′ strips were read by the mini API instrument and associated software V 1.5.2 (bioMerieux, Lyon, France). The strains ′ were then frozen at −80°C in BHI broth (Oxoid, Basingstoke, UK) with 15.0% glycerol.

Bacterial Characterization.

Among the isolated microorganisms 100 Staphylococcus spp. strains were selected, 25 S. aureus (all isolates) and 75 CNS (randomly). Each strain was analysed for: haemolysis pattern on SBA at 5.0%, lecithinase activity on Baird Parker Medium (BPM, Oxoid, Basingstoke, UK), supplemented with Egg Yolk Tellurite Emulsion (EYTE) at 5.0% (Oxoid, Basingstoke, UK); thermostable DNase (TDNase, Biolife, MI, Italy) tested on toluidine blue-DNA agar plates [16], free coagulase (Coagulase plasma - EDTA, bioMerieux, Lyon, France) and bound coagulase (clump- ′ ing factor) production (Staphylase test, bioMerieux, Lyon, ′ France), following the manufacturer's instructions.

Somatic Cell Count (SCC).

The SCC was determined by the fluoro-opto-electronic cell counting method according to the FIL-IDF no. 148 (1995) method C [17], using a Fossomatic 5000 (Foss Electric, Hillerød, Denmark).

Definition of Subclinical Mastitis.

For the purpose of this work, a mammary gland was considered as affected by subclinical mastitis when having no clinical signs or abnormal milk, in which ≥500 cfu/mL were isolated and a somatic cell count was ≥300,000 cells/mL [18].

Antimicrobial Agents and Minimal Inhibitory Concentration (MIC).

On each strain the MICs of ten antibiotics used in human and veterinary medicines were determined. The antibiotics tested were ampicillin (AMP), cephalothin (KF), cefoperazone (CFP), ceftriaxone (CRO), cloxacillin (OB), kanamycin (K), novobiocin (NV), ofloxacin (OFX), oxytetracycline (OT), and vancomycin (VA). The MICs were determined by the broth microdilution method [14, 22] using cation-adjusted Mueller-Hinton broth (CAMHB, Oxoid, Basingstoke, UK). Each antimicrobial agent, in powder form (Sigma-Aldrich-Fluka, MI, Italy), was weighed and dissolved in an appropriate solvent [14, 22], thus obtaining a stock solution (2,560 µg/mL). Stock solutions were stored at −80°C until used. From each stock solution, 12 serial twofold working dilutions in deionized water (only for AMP, the diluents were phosphate buffer, pH 6.0, 0.1 mol/L) was prepared according to CLSI standard protocols, and the antimicrobial agent final concentrations in each microplate ranged between 0.06 and 128 µg/mL. Each strain stored at −80°C until testing were subcultured twice on BHI agar (Oxoid, Basingstoke, UK) before inoculum preparation.

Two or more identical colonies were picked from BHI plates after overnight incubation and suspended in saline solution (0.85% w/v) to match a McFarland 0.5 turbidity standard, using an inoculum reader (portable photometer Densimat, bioMerieux, Lyon, France). Each suspension was ′ further diluted 1 : 100 in CAMHB in order to achieve the adequate inoculum concentration ($\simeq 10^6$ cfu/mL). Fifty microliters of the final suspension were inoculated into the wells of microtiter plates, which also contained 50 µL of the antimicrobial agent, so that the final inoculum density on test plates contained $\simeq 5 \times 10^5$ cfu/mL in each well. Reference strains, Staphylococcus aureus ATCC 29213 and Enterococcus faecalis ATCC 29212, were used for quality control. Each microplate was then incubated at 35 ± 2°C under aerobic environment for 20 hours. The susceptibility of each strain to the antimicrobial agents was then defined by comparing the results to those of the breakpoint values [19–21]. The MICs range and mode, MIC_{50} and MIC_{90} of each antimicrobial agent were also determined.

Detection of mecA Gene.

Genomic DNA used as target for polymerase chain reaction (PCR) assay was extracted using the following procedure: strains grown in BHI broth at +37°C overnight were centrifuged (10 minutes at 3,000 × g) and resuspended in 500 μL of Tris-EDTA buffer saline (Tris base 10 mM + EDTA 1 mM). The suspension was added with 10 μL of a 1.5 mg/mL lysostaphin solution (SigmaAldirich, MI, Italy) and incubated for 1 hour at +37°C. Then, 5 μL of a 20 mg/mL proteinase K solution (Eurobio, Sarreguemines, France) were added and the incubation was continued at +50°C for 60 minutes. An equal volume of phenol/chloroform/isoamyl alcohol (25 : 24 : 1) was added and mixed by inversion. After centrifuging (15 minutes at 10,000 × g), the upper layer was collected and 500 μL of chloroformisoamyl alcohol (24 : 1) solution were added. The mixture was centrifuged again (15 minutes at 10,000 × g) and the upper aqueous phase was transferred into a new tube. A volume of 800–1,000 μL of refrigerated absolute ethanol was added and gently mixed until DNA precipitation. DNA was resuspended in 100 μL of sterile deionized water. The DNA concentration was estimated spectrophotometrically. The mecA gene coding for methicillin resistance was detected by PCR as previously described [23]. The primers used for the detection of the mecA gene were AAAATCGATGGTAAAGGTTGGC (forward) and AGTTCTGCAGTACCGGATTTGC (reverse). S. aureus HT 2004 0874 reference strain was used as positive control [24].

RESULTS

Isolates

Bacteriological cultures were positive in 469 (15.6%) out of 3,000 half-udder milk samples. The intramammary infection rates in the eight flocks were, respectively, of 16.7% (range 15.0%–18.6%) and 14.6% (range 12.6%–17.4%) for the left and right half-udders. Bacterial strains isolated from milk samples were 415 CNS (88.5%), 25 S. aureus (5.3%), 4 Micrococcus spp. (0.9%), while 21 (4.5%) were identified as belonging to other species (Bacillus spp, Enterococcus spp. and Gram-Negative Bacilli), and 4 (0.9%) could not be identified by API system. The CNS strains were identified as follows: 187 S. caprae (45.1%), 64 S. warneri (15.4%), 41 S. simulans (9.9%), 31 S. chromogenes (7.5%), 16 S. epidermidis (3.9%), 9 S. xylosus (2.2%), 8 S. haemolyticus (1.9%), 7 S. capitis(1.7%), 6 S. cohnii(1.4%), 6 S. lugdunensis (1.4%), 5 S. equorum (1.2%), 5 S. hominis (1.2%), and 30 Staphylococcus spp. (7.2%). The mean SCC of bacteriological positive samples was 6.3 Log10 cells/mL, while in the negative ones it was 5.7 Log_{10} cells/mL. The mean SCC was greater in milk samples positive for S. aureus (6.8 Log_{10} cells/mL) when compared to those positive for CNS (6.4 Log_{10} cells/mL).

Selected Isolates

A total of 100 isolates were selected for antimicrobial agent susceptibility testing as follows: S. aureus (25), S. caprae (25), S. warneri (16), S. simulans (15), S. chromogenes (7), S. epidermidis (6), S. equorum (2), S. cohnii (1), S. haemolyticus (1), S. lugdunensis (1), and S. xylosus (1). The S. aureus strains were isolated from five out of eight flocks ranging between 2 and 8 for each one. Fifteen (60.0%) of the S. aureus strains showed hemolytic activity and among these, 5 (20.0%) produced α-hemolysin, 8 (32.0%) β- hemolysin and 2 (8.0%) were α and β-hemolytic. Thirteen (17.3%) of the CNS strains showed a weak hemolytic activity on SBA. Free coagulase was produced by all the S. aureus strains tested, while three of these (12.0%) were negative to the bound coagulase test. All the CNS strains were found to be negative for the free coagulase and only one S. lugdunensis strain (1.3%) was clumping factor positive. TDNase was produced by all the S. aureus strains and by 17 (22.7%) of the CNS strains. Lecithinase was produced by 12 S. aureus (48.0%) and 27 CNS strains (36.0%).

Antimicrobials Susceptibility.

The MICs of antibiotics and the susceptibility of S. aureus and CNS strains isolated from goats with SCM are shown Tables 1-2. Fourteen (56.0%) of 25 S. aureus and thirty-one (41.3%) out of 75 CNS strains were resistant to one or more antimicrobials. The susceptibility of S. aureus was 92.0% or greater for seven out of ten antibiotics tested but was lower for kanamycin (60.0%), oxytetracycline (84.0%), and ampicillin (88.0%). The susceptibility of CNS was between 94.0%– 100.0% for eight antimicrobials, but was somewhat lower for ampicillin (64.0%) and kanamycin (78.7%). Staphylococcus spp. isolates showed a poor susceptibility to AMP. The MIC_{90} (1–4 μg/mL) of this antibiotic was higher than the breakpoint value for susceptibility. Among CNS resistant to AMP, the most prevalent species were S. caprae (37.0%) and S. chromogenes (22.2%), while only 12.0% of the S. aureus strains were resistant. On the other hand, almost all staphylococci (98.0%) were susceptible to OB and only 2 out of 75 (2.7%) of the CNS were resistant. Cephalosporins showed high activity against Staphylococcus spp. isolates. The percentages of susceptible staphylococci were 98.0%, 99.0% and 96.0% for KF, CFP, and CRO, respectively. The mecA gene was not found in any of the tested isolates. For K a low susceptibility of the isolates (74.0%) was recorded. The MIC_{90} of K against the CNS and S. aureus strains (32– ≥128 μg/mL) was higher than the reference breakpoint for antimicrobial susceptibility. A different susceptibility to OT was observed in CNS isolates (94.7%) when compared to that of S. aureus (84.0%). The MIC_{90} of OFX for both S. aureus and CNS was comparable with the reference breakpoint for antimicrobial susceptibility (≤1 μg/mL). All the tested staphylococci were susceptible to VA (100.0%), and 98.0% of these to NV. The NV resistant strains belonged to the S. chonii (n = 1) and S. xylosus (n = 1) species. The isolates which were resistant to two or more antimicrobial agents are shown in Table 3. It is remarkable that one S. epidermidis strain was resistant to six different antibiotics (AMP, CRO, K, OB, OFX, and OT).

Table 1: MIC (µg/mL) of antimicrobials against S. aureus and CNS strains isolated from goats subclinical mastitis

	S. aureus				*CNS*			
Antimicrobial agents	MIC_{50}	MIC_{90}	mode	range	MIC_{50}	MIC_{90}	mode	range
Ampicillin[(a)]	0.12	1.0	≤0.06	≤0.06–16.0	0.12	4.0	≤0.06	≤0.06–16.0
Cefoperazone[(b)]	2.0	8.0	1.0	1.0–8.0	2.0	4.0	2.0	≤0.06–32.0
Ceftriaxone[(b)]	4.0	8.0	4.0	1.0–16.0	2.0	8.0	2.0	≤0.06–≥128
Cephalothin[(a)]	0.25	0.25	0.25	≤0.06–≥128	0.25	0.25	0.25	≤0.06–16.0
Cloxacillin[(a)]	0.25	0.5	0.25	1.0–0.12	0.5	1.0	0.5	≤0.06–≥128
Kanamycin[(a)]	16.0	≥128	32.0	1.0–≥128	8.0	32.0	16.0	≤0.06–≥128
Novobiocin[(c)]	0.12	0.5	≤0.06	≤0.06–0.5	0.12	0.5	≤0.06	≤0.06–32.0
Ofloxacin[(b)]	0.5	1.0	0.5	0.25–2.0	0.5	1.0	0.5	≤0.06–32.0
Oxytetracycline[(a)]	0.25	64.0	0.25	0.12–≥128	0.25	1.0	0.25	≤0.06–≥128
Vancomycin[(a)]	2.0	4.0	2.0	0.5–4.0	2.0	4.0	2.0	≤0.06–4.0

[(a)]Breakpoints NCCLS, [19]; [(b)]= breakpoints CLSI, [20]; [(c)]= breakpoint [21].

Table 2: Antimicrobial susceptibility of S. aureus and CNS strains isolated from goats subclinical mastitis

		S. aureus						*CNS*					
Antimicrobial	MIC (µg/mL)	Susceptible		Intermediate		Resistant		Susceptible		Intermediate		Resistant	
agents	breakpoints	*n*	%	*n*	%	*n*	%	*n*	%	*n*	%	*n*	%
Ampicillin[(a)]	≤0.25–≥0.5	22	*88.0*	–	–	3	12.0	48	*64.0*	–	–	27	*36.0*
Cefoperazone[(b)]	≤16.0–≥64.0	25	*100.0*	–	–	–	–	74	*98.7*	1	*1.3*	–	–
Ceftriaxone[(b)]	≤8.0–≥64.0	23	*92.0*	2	*8.0*	–	–	73	*97.3*	1	*1.3*	1	*1.3*
Cephalothin[(a)]	≤8.0–≥32.0	24	*96.0*	–	–	1	4.0	74	*98.7*	1	*1.3*	–	–
Cloxacillin[(a)]	≤2.0–≥4.0	25	*100.0*	—	—	–	–	73	*97.3*	—	—	2	*2.7*
Kanamycin[(a)]	≤16.0–≥64.0	15	*60.0*	3	*12.0*	7	28.0	59	*78.7*	11	*14.7*	5	*6.7*
Novobiocin[(c)]	≤4.0	25	*100.0*	—	—	–	–	73	*97.3*	—	—	2	*2.7*
Ofloxacin[(b)]	≤1.0–≥4.0	23	*92.0*	2	*8.0*	–	–	71	*94.7*	1	*1.3*	3	*4.0*
Oxytetracycline[(a)]	≤4.0–≥16.0	21	*84.0*	–	–	4	16.0	71	*94.7*	–	–	4	*5.3*
Vancomycin[(a)]	≤4.0–≥32.0	25	*100.0*	–	–	–	–	75	*100.0*	–	–	–	–

[(a)]Breakpoints NCCLS, [19]; [(b)]= breakpoints CLSI, [20]; [(c)]= breakpoint [21].

DISCUSSION

In the present study, the average prevalence of SCM was 15.6%, which is within the range (6.5%–67.0%) reported in previous studies carried out on dairy goat farms [1].

Staphylococci, which made up 88.5% of the isolated microorganisms in this study, are the most common pathogens associated with SCM in dairy goats [25].

AMP was less effective than the other β-lactam antimicrobial agents. The susceptibility of the isolates against AMP was within the range reported by other authors [9, 26], even if Moroni et al. [27], have found a markedly greater prevalence of AMP resistant S. aureus (67.9%). These findings are consistent with AMP sensitivity to the penicillinases, frequently produced by Staphyloccus spp. and particularly by CNS strains. OB, a penicilinase-resistant penicillin (PRP), was very effective in vitro. Two CNS resistant to OB were simultaneously resistant to other β-lactamic antimicrobials, such as AMP (n = 1) and AMP-CRO (n = 1). The Cephalosporins showed a strong activity with regard to staphylococci. The MIC90 values of CFP ranged between 0.25 and 8 µg/mL, that were comparable (1.87–3.75 µg/mL) to those found by Moroni et al [12]. Nevertheless, a low susceptibility to CFP was previously found in some CNS strains isolated from goats with SCM, particularly with regard to S. chromogenes, S. warneri, S. simulans, and S. kloosii [11]. Other authors found that the susceptibility to KF of CNS isolated in goats with SCM was between 86.0% and 100.0% [10, 28], that is, comparable with the results (98.7%) obtained in this study. The mecA gene was not found in any of the strains tested, in agreement with the results of a previous study carried out on S. aureus strains isolated from sheep with SCM [6]. The results of the present study confirm that methicillin-resistant staphylococci prevalence is still low in ruminants as observed in previous research [29]. The finding of some mecA-negative isolates which were phenotipically resistant to β-lactam antimicrobial agents could be related to a less common type of resistance due to either overproduction of β-lactamase or the presence of altered Penicillin Binding Protein (PBP) not related to 2a or 2 [30]. The susceptibility to OT was lower in S. aureus (84.0%) than in CNS (94.7%). In previous studies, a number of authors have observed a marked variability in the susceptibility of both these microorganisms to tetracycline, as it ranged between 10.0% and 100.0% [8, 10, 12, 28]. The susceptibility of CNS against NV was 97.3% and this peculiarity is of interest in the taxonomy for bacterial typing since it is also well related with pathogenic activity [31]. All staphylococci were sensitive to VA, thus confirming the results of other authors [10, 32]. The VA breakpoint value was recently reduced from ≤4 µg/mL to ≤2 µg/mL in testing the susceptibility of bacterial strains isolated from humans [20]. Some staphylococci isolated from milk samples taken from goats with SCM showed MIC values of 4 µg/mL. When these strains are transferred from animals to humans, they could increase the spreading of vancomycin-intermediate S. aureus (VISA) strains. Indeed, comparing the MIC values of VA that we found with the breakpoint actually used for human origin strains, a relevant percentage of S. aureus (16.0%) and CNS (13.3%) would be classified as intermediate.

Table 3: Staphylococcus spp. with multiple resistance to antibiotics (μg/mL)

	n (%)	AMP[a]	CRO[b]	K[a]	OB[a]	OFX[b]	OT[a]
S. aureus	1 (4)	—	—	≥128	—	—	≥128.0
S. caprae	3 (12)	0.25–2–8	—	—	—	4	≥128.0
S. epidermidis	2 (33)	8.0	≥128.0	≥128.0–64.0	≥128.0	8.0–32.0	≥128.0
S. simulans	1 (7)	0.5	—	—	16.0	—	—
S. warneri	1 (6)	1.0	—	—	—	—	≥128.0

AMP = Ampicillin; CFP = Cefoperazone; CRO = Ceftriaxone; KF = Cephalothin; K = Kanamycin; NV = Novobiocina; OB = Cloxacillin; OFX = Ofloxacin; OT = oxytetracycline; VA = Vancomycin. [a]breakpoints NCCLS, [19]; [b]breakpoints CLSI, [20].

CONCLUSION

This study confirms that staphylococci are the most common pathogens associated with SCM in dairy goats. As expected, the bacteriological positive milk samples had a SCC greater than the negative ones. Over 40.0% of the tested staphylococci were resistant to at least one antimicrobial agent. Single resistance against β-lactamics or aminoglicosides is the most common trait observed. Multiple antibiotic resistance was found in few of the tested Staphylococci strains, mainly in CNS. Although the methicillin-resistant staphylococci represent the most important pathogens responsible of humans severe hospital-acquired infections, the absence of mecA gene and the low prevalence of single and multiple antibiotic resistance suggest that SCM in goats does not play a significant role in the spreading of multiresistant staphylococci and it does not represent a great public health concern.

ACKNOWLEDGMENTS

The authors express their gratitude to the goat farmers and the Regional Farmers Association of Sardinia for their cooperation in completing the surveys. The research was carried out with the help of FAR funds from the University of Sassari.

REFERENCES

1. A. Contreras, C. Luengo, A. Sanchez, and J. C. Corrales, "The role of intramammary pathogens in dairy goats," Livestock Production Science, vol. 79, no. 2-3, pp. 273–283, 2003.
2. B. Poutrel, R. De Cremoux, M. Ducelliez, and D. Verneau, ´ "Control of intramammary infections in goats: impact on somatic cell counts," Journal of Animal Science, vol. 75, no. 2, pp. 566–570, 1997.
3. E. P. L. De Santis, A. Mencarelli, M. P. Nieddu, et al., "Effi- cacia della somministrazione endomammaria di cloxacillina benzatina per il trattamento delle infezioni intramammarie dell'ovino nel corso dell'asciutta," Large Animals Review, vol. 7, pp. 39–47, 2001.
4. B. Walther, A. W. Friedrich, L. Brunnberg, L. H. Wieler, and A. Lubke-Becker, "Methicillin-resistant ¨ Staphylococcus aureus (MRSA) in veterinary medicine: a "new emerging pathogen"?" Berliner und Munchener Tierarztliche Wochenschrift, vol. 119, no. 5-6, pp. 222–232, 2006.
5. C. Schnellmann, V. Gerber, A. Rossano, et al., "Presence of new mecA and mph(C) variants conferring antibiotic resistance in Staphylococcus spp. isolated from the skin of horses before and after clinic admission," Journal of Clinical Microbiology, vol. 44, no. 12, pp. 4444–4454, 2006.
6. E. P. L. De Santis, A. Mureddu, R. Mazzette, C. Scarano, and M. Bes, "Detection of enterotoxins and TSST-1 genes in S. aureus isolates from sheep subclinical mastitis," in Proceedings of the 4th IDF International Mastitis Conference, pp. 410–504, Maastricht, The Netherlands, June 2005.
7. E. Vautor, H. Carsenti-Dellamonica, M. Sabah, G. Mancini, M. Pepin, and P. Dellamonica, "Characterization of´ Staphylococcus aureus isolates recovered from dairy sheep farms (agr group, adherence, slime, resistance to antibiotics)," Small Ruminant Research, vol. 72, no. 2-3, pp. 197–199, 2007.
8. I. Bochev and N. Russenova, "Resistance of Staphylococcus spp strains isolated from goat with sub clinical mastitis," Bulgarian Journal of Veterinary Medicine, vol. 8, pp. 109–118, 2005.
9. G. O. Adegoke and M. O. Ojo, "Biochemical characterization of staphylococci isolated from goats," Veterinary Microbiology, vol. 7, no. 5, pp. 463–470, 1982.
10. N. Bedidi-Madani, Y. Richard, E. Borges, and C. Lerondelle, "Identification and susceptibility to antibiotics of coagulase negative staphylococci isolated from goat milk," Revue de M´edecine V´et´erinaire, vol. 143, pp. 539–545, 1992.
11. P. Moroni, F. Vellere, M. Antonini, G. Pisoni, G. Ruffo, and S. Carli, "Antibiotic susceptibility of coagulase-negative staphylococci isolated from goats' milk," International Journal of Antimicrobial Agents, vol. 23, no. 6, pp. 637–640, 2004.
12. P. Moroni, G. Pisoni, M. Antonini, et al., "Subclinical mastitis and antimicrobial susceptibility of Staphylococcus caprae and Staphylococcus epidermidis isolated from two Italian goat herds," Journal of Dairy Science, vol. 88, no. 5, pp. 1694–1704, 2005.
13. C. Wray and J.-C. Gnanou, "Antibiotic resistance monitoring in bacteria of animal origin: analysis of national monitoring programmes," International Journal of Antimicrobial Agents, vol. 14, no. 4, pp. 291–294, 2000.
14. Clinical and Laboratory Standards Institute, Methods for Dilution Antimicrobial Susceptibility Tests for Bacteria That Grow Aerobically; Approved Standard, Clinical and Laboratory Standards Institute, Wayne, Pa, USA, 7th edition, 2006, Document M7-A7.

15. G. A. Donovan, C. A. Risco, and J. K. Shearer, "Assessment of the mammary system," The Veterinary Clinics of North America, vol. 8, no. 2, pp. 361–372, 1992.

16. R. V. Lachica, C. Genigeorgis, and P. D. Hoeprich, "Metachromatic agar-diffusion methods for detecting staphylococcal nuclease activity," Applied Microbiology, vol. 21, no. 4, pp. 585– 587, 1971.

17. FIL-IDF, Enumeration of Somatic Cells, Standard, no. 148A, FIL-IDF International Dairy Federation, Brussels, Belgium, 1995.

18. M. G. Ribeiro, J. Megid, D. R. Meira, V. M. Lara, and A. Cortez, "Mastite caprina. Estudo microbiologico, f ′ ′ısico-qu′ımico e do diagnostico atrav ′ es de provas indiretas," ′ Biologico ′ , vol. 61, pp. 27–33, 1999.

19. National Committee for Clinical Laboratory Standards, Performance Standards for Antimicrobial Disk and Dilution Susceptibility Tests for Bacteria Isolated from Animals; Approved Standard, National Committee for Clinical Laboratory Standards, Wayne, Pa, USA, 2nd edition, 2002, Document M31- A2.

20. Clinical and Laboratory Standards Institute, Performance Standards for Antimicrobial Susceptibility Testing; Sixteenth Informational Supplement, Clinical and Laboratory Standards Institute, Wayne, Pa, USA, 2006, Document M100-S16.

21. C. Thornsberry, P. J. Burton, Y. C. Yee, J. L. Watts, and R. J. Yancey Jr., "The activity of a combination of penicillin and novobiocin against bovine mastitis pathogens: development of a disk diffusion test," Journal of Dairy Science, vol. 80, no. 2, pp. 413–421, 1997.

22. National Committee for Clinical Laboratory Standards, Development of in Vitro Susceptibility Testing Criteria and Quality Control Parameters for Veterinary Antimicrobial Agents; Approved Guideline, National Committee for Clinical Laboratory Standards, Wayne, Pa, USA, 2nd edition, 2002, Document M37-A2.

23. K. Murakami, W. Minamide, K. Wada, E. Nakamura, H. Teraoka, and S. Watanabe, "Identification of methicillinresistant strains of staphylococci by polymerase chain reaction," Journal of Clinical Microbiology, vol. 29, no. 10, pp. 2240–2244, 1991.

24. F. Vandenesch, T. Naimi, M. C. Enright, et al., "Communityacquired methicillin-resistant Staphylococcus aureus carrying Panton-Valentine leukocidin genes: worldwide emergence," Emerging Infectious Diseases, vol. 9, no. 8, pp. 978–984, 2003.

25. B. Poutrel, R. De Cremoux, R. Pillet, V. Heuchel, and M. ′ Ducelliez, "Relations entre statut infectieux des mamelles et numerations cellulaires du lait de ch ` evre," in ` Somatic Cells and Milk of Small Ruminants, R. Rubino, Ed., pp. 61–64, Wageningen Academic, Wageningen, The Netherlands, 1996.

26. A. Ebrahimi, S. Lotfalian, and S. Karimi, "Drug resistance in isolated bacteria from milk of sheep and goats with subclinical mastitis in Shahrekord district," Iranian Journal of Veterinary Research, vol. 8, pp. 76–79, 2007.

27. P. Moroni, G. Pisoni, C. Vimercati, et al., "Characterization of Staphylococcus aureus isolated from chronically infected dairy goats," Journal of Dairy Science, vol. 88, no. 10, pp. 3500–3509, 2005.

28. E. R. da Silva, A. P. Siqueira, J. C. D. Martins, W. P. B. Ferreira, and N. da Silva, "Identification and in vitro antimicrobial susceptibility of Staphylococcus species isolated from goat mastitis in the Northeast of Brazil," Small Ruminant Research, vol. 55, no. 1–3, pp. 45–49, 2004.

29. P. D. D. Alves, J. A. McCulloch, S. Even, et al., "Molecular characterisation of Staphylococcus aureus strains isolated from small and large ruminants reveals a host rather than tissue specificity," Veterinary Microbiology, vol. 137, no. 1-2, pp. 190– 195, 2009.

30. N. H. Georgopapadakou, "Penicillin-binding proteins and bacterial resistance to β-lactams," Antimicrobial Agents and Chemotherapy, vol. 37, no. 10, pp. 2045–2053, 1993.

31. M. Deinhofer and A. Pernthaner, "Staphylococcus spp. as mastitis-related pathogens in goat milk," Veterinary Microbiology, vol. 43, no. 2-3, pp. 161–166, 1995.

32. E. P. L. De Santis, S. Virdis, R. Mazzette, M. P. Nieddu, S. Farina, and A. Corona, "Sensibilita nei confronti degli ` antibiotici di stafilococchi coagulasi negativi isolati in mastiti subcliniche dell'ovino," in Proceedings of the 14th S.I.P.A.O.C. National Congress, vol. 14, pp. 79–82, Vietri sul Mare, Italy, 2000.

CHAPTER 21

PREVALENCE AND MOLECULAR CHARACTERISTICS OF METHICILLIN-RESISTANT STAPHYLOCOCCUS AUREUS (MRSA) AMONG PIGS ON GERMAN FARMS AND IMPORT OF LIVESTOCK-RELATED MRSA INTO HOSPITALS

R. Köck, J. Harlizius, N. Bressan, R. Laerberg, L. H. Wieler, W. Witte, R. H. Deurenberg, A. Voss, K. Becker, A. W. Friedrich

INTRODUCTION

During recent decades methicillin-resistant *Staphylococcus aureus* (MRSA) have emerged as human nosocomial pathogens throughout the world [1]. More recently, several reports described their importance in veterinary medicine. MRSA were found to colonize and infect various animal species comprising horses [2–4], cows [5], dogs and cats [6, 7], rabbits [7] and other companion animals [8]. A special focus was put on the isolation of MRSA from pigs in several countries including The Netherlands, Denmark, France, Canada, the USA and Singapore [9–15]. Although in the majority of reports pigs were colonized, but not infected by MRSA, some studies also described the development of mastitis or urinary tract infections in the animals [16]. Molecular typing showed that the porcine MRSA isolates were mostly associated with clonal complex (CC) 398 by multilocus sequence typing (MLST), corresponding to *S. aureus* protein A (*spa*) types t011, t034, t108, t1451 and relatives [9, 13].

Consecutively, several reports suggested transmission between pigs and humans causing MRSA colonization in 23–45% of pig-farmers [14, 17, 18] and 4.6% of pig-care veterinarians [19]. A porcine MRSA reservoir therefore might exert manifold influence on human healthcare. Since MRSA CC398 will potentially cause severe infections in humans [20, 21], contact to pig-farming might represent a risk-factor for the development of MRSA-associated illness. Moreover, as studies indicated the entrance of MRSA in the food chain, e.g. via contamination of carcasses during the slaughtering process [22] or via secondary contamination by slaughterhouse staff [23], the potential of these MRSA to cause foodborne disease has to be evaluated. Apart from a direct pathogenic impact for carriers, patients colonized with MRSA originating from the livestock-reservoir might introduce antibiotic-resistant pathogens into the hospitals. As MRSA screening strategies in hospitals are usually based upon on-admission swabbing of patients who are attached to classical nosocomial risk factors for MRSA carriage, the established "search" policies might fail to detect patients with a livestock-related MRSA-acquisition.

Currently, there is growing concern about MRSA colonization of livestock in Germany, but, besides a first pilot study [24], no further data are available. In order to elucidate this issue, we performed a prevalence study on MRSA colonization among pigs at randomly selected farms in Germany in an area with a high density of pig production. The MRSA isolates were characterized using *spa* typing, MLST, SCCmec typing and detection of important *S. aureus*toxin-encoding genes.

Furthermore, the importance of an import of livestock-related MRSA into hospitals in countries with medium or high MRSA prevalence, as described for Germany [25], is currently unknown. In consequence, we performed a retrospective case control study among patients admitted to a tertiary-care

Citation: R. Köck, J. Harlizius, N. Bressan, R. Laerberg, L. H. Wieler, W. Witte, R. H. Deurenberg, A. Voss, K. Becker, A. W. Friedrich, Prevalence and molecular characteristics of methicillin-resistant Staphylococcus aureus (MRSA) among pigs on German farms and import of livestock-related MRSA into hospitals, DOI: 10.1007/s10096-009-0795-4.

hospital situated in the region in which the prevalence study was carried out. In this case control study, we included patients carrying such MRSA *spa* types identified among regional pigs at admission to the hospital. As a control group, we chose patients colonized with other MRSA *spa* types hitherto not associated with livestock. For both groups we assessed classical nosocomial risk factors for MRSA carriage [26] and asked for a status of contact to pigs, cattle, horses, sheep or other animals. The comparison of risk factors among patients in the case group and the control group shall clarify whether patients carrying presumptive livestock-related MRSA types are likely to be colonized via transmission from animals.

METHODS

MRSA screening on pig farms

From April 2007 to November 2007 we collected nasal swabs from weaned pigs living on 40 different randomly chosen pig farms (25 farrowing farms, 4 rearing farms and 11 farrow-to-finishing farms) on the German side of the Euregio, situated in the central Dutch-German border area. The farms were situated in the following districts according to the nomenclature of territorial units for statistics (NUTS) (http://ec.europa.eu/comm/eurostat/ramon/nuts): DEA34, DEA37, DEA35, DEA29, DEA1B, DEA14, DEA15, DEA1D, DEA1E, DEA1F. The average animal density was 1,277 pigs (range 375–3400 pigs) in the farrowing and farrow-to-finish units and 1,900 pigs (range 1800–2000 pigs) on the rearing farms.

On each farm we derived 40 swabs from weaned piglets. For microbiological analysis the 40 swabs were pooled into eight culture samples. After 24-h enrichment culture in selective broth [27], all cultures were streaked onto Columbia-blood agar and a chromogenic medium for the detection of MRSA (bioMérieux, Marcy l'Etoile, France). Presumptive *S. aureus* colonies were confirmed by coagulase tube test, by use of VITEK2 automated systems (bioMérieux) and by *S. aureus*-specific PCR [28]. Strains with ambiguous results in phenotypic tests were analyzed by 16 S rRNA gene sequencing. Methicillin-resistance was tested by cefoxitin disc agar diffusion and was confirmed by *mecA*-specific polymerase chain reaction as described [29]. Susceptibility to antimicrobial agents was tested by VITEK2 automated systems according to recommendations of the manufacturer. The presence of the Panton-Valentine leukocidin (PVL) encoding genes (*lukS*-PV, *lukF*-PV) was determined as described elsewhere [30]. Genes of other members of the staphylococcal bicomponent leukotoxin family (*lukM*, *lukE*, *lukD*) were tested as published [31]. Detection of genes of the members of the staphylococcal pyrogenic toxin superantigen (PTSAg) family including the toxic shock syndrome 1 gene (*tst*), classical and newly described enterotoxin and enterotoxin-like genes (*sea*, *seb*, sec_{1-3}, *sed*, *seg*, *seh*, *sei*, *sej*, *sem*, *sen* and *seo*), exfoliative toxin genes (*eta*, *etb* and *etd*) as well as of genes of the epidermal cell differentiation inhibitor family (*edinA*, *edinB* and *edinC*) and the accessory gene regulatory loci (*agr*I, *agr*II, *agr*III and *agr*IV) was carried out using previously reported methods [31, 32]. All MRSA isolates were typed by *S. aureus* protein A (*spa*) sequence-based typing as described [33]. Multilocus sequence typing (MLST) was performed on one isolate of each different *spa* type [34]. Typing of SCCmec elements of types I to IV was carried out for one isolate of every *spa* type from every farm using a PCR approach, including a combination of different PCRs [35]. To demonstrate SCCmec-elements of type V, we used primers type VF/type VR, as described by Zhang et al. [36], and primer pair ccrC9f 5′-CACTTAATCCATGTACACAG-3′ and ccrC-R [36].

MRSA *spa* types found on regional pig farms among patients in a tertiary-care university hospital: a case control study

The University Hospital Münster (UHM) is a 1300-bed maximum care teaching hospital in the central part of the Dutch-German border area. Its referral area mostly comprises the regions involved in the screening at pig farms. The MRSA database (Ridom StaphType, Würzburg, Germany) of the UHM includes *spa* typing results of every first MRSA isolate of each patient for isolates obtained from January 2005 to December 2008. The isolates were obtained from admission screening cultures from the nasopharynx and non-infected skin of patients at the UHM. Screening was performed by swabbing of defined risk patients according to the national German guideline (www.rki.de, version 1.12.99 and comment 12.11.04) between January 2005 and June 2006 and was then replaced by a general nasal screening of all patients at admission. Microbiological diagnostics were performed as described previously [29]. We searched the UHM database for MRSA isolates which were derived from screening samples and which were characterized by *spa* types which were identified on regional pig farms in this study (t011, t034, t108, t1451, t2510). Using a standardized questionnaire, we interviewed randomly selected patients from whom such presumptive livestock-related MRSA *spa* types were isolated ($n = 100$ patients, case group). As a control group, we randomly chose a corresponding group of patients ($n = 100$) from whom MRSA with other than known livestock-associated *spa* types were isolated from screening specimens. Randomization was performed using an internet tool (http://www.wesleyan.edu/spn/random/form.htm). The patients were asked whether they shared one or more of the following classical nosocomial risk factors for MRSA acquisition at the time when the MRSA was detected for the first time: contact to another person with MRSA carriage or infection, prescribing of any antibiotics during the previous 6 months, hospitalization for >24 h within the past 6 months, direct transfer of the patient from long-term care facilities to the admitting hospital, need for long-term care, presence of indwelling devices (urinary catheters, intravenous catheters, percutaneous gastrostomies, postsurgical drains), presence of skin lesions (ulcers, eczema, other wounds), need for haemodialysis. Furthermore, the age of the patient, contact to horses, sheep, cattle, pigs and pets (e.g. cats, dogs) were assessed. For statistical analysis with SPSS Statistics 17.0 (SPSS, Chicago, IL, USA), data were entered into an Excel database (Microsoft, Redmond, WA, USA). Univariate analysis was performed using Chi-square test or Fisher exact test for ordinal variables and Student's *t*-test for continuous variables. All risk factors associated with a different distribution among the case and control groups with a *P*-value <0.2 were included in the initial logistic regression model. The backward stepwise method was used to create the models. Choice of the optimal regression model was based on comparison of likelihood ratios and Hosmer-Lemshow goodness-of-fit statistics. A *P* value <0.05 was considered significant.

RESULTS

Screening on pig-farms

Screening of 1,600 weaned piglets at 40 pig farms in the Dutch-German border area identified nasal MRSA colonization in animals on a total of 28 farms (70%). Among these, two were rearing farms (50% of all rearing farms), seven were farrow-to-finish farms (64% of all farrow-to-finish farms) and 19 were farrowing farms (76% of all farrowing farms). On these farms, MRSA were isolated from all eight culture pools in 16 cases (57%). On four farms MRSA were isolated from 5–7 pools, on three farms from 3–4 pools and on five farms from 1–2 pools. Overall, we isolated 169 MRSA. The isolates were associated with *spa* types t011 (75%, $n=127$), t034 (5.3%, $n=9$), t108 (0.6%, $n=1$), t1451 (3.6%, $n=6$) and t2510 (15.4%, $n=26$). MLST results showed that every *spa* type was associated with ST398. We typed SCCmec elements of one isolate per different *spa* type found on each farm (in total: $n=33$ isolates; t011 ($n=24$), t034 ($n=2$), t108 ($n=1$), t1451 ($n=1$), t2510 ($n=5$)). All isolates were associated with SCCmec type V with one exception which was an MRSA t011 harbouring SCCmec type IV. None of the MRSA harboured the genes encoding PVL and other leukocidins tested. All isolates were negative for the genes encoding enterotoxins, exfoliative toxins, toxic shock toxin 1 and epidermal cell differentiation inhibitors. All isolates were associated with *agr* type I. All porcine MRSA strains were resistant to tetracycline, 8 (52%) to erythromycin and clindamycin, 4 (26%) to gentamicin, and 4 (8%) to trimethoprim-sulfomethoxazole. All isolates were susceptible to ciprofloxacin, rifampin, fusidic acid and vancomycin.

Case control study

In the UHM database, we identified 249 different patients from whom MRSA with *spa* types identified on regional pig farms (t011, t034, t108, t1451, t2510) were isolated from screening samples between January 2005 and December 2008. The MRSA shared *spa* types t011 ($n=139$, 56%), t034 ($n=98$, 39%), t108 ($n=8$, 3%) and t1451 ($n=4$, 2%); *spa* type t2510 was not detected among patients. These isolates accounted for 13% of all MRSA isolated from screening samples at the UHM in 2005 ($n=16$ of 121 isolates), increasing to 15% in 2006 ($n=43$ of 286 isolates), 21.9% in 2007 ($n=96$ of 438 isolates) and 22.4% in 2008 ($n=94$ of 419 isolates). Among the patients colonized by presumptive livestock-related MRSA, 100 were available for telephone interviews and were included in the case group. The 100 patients within the control group were randomly selected out of 1,015 MRSA isolates obtained from screening between January 2005 and December 2008 and exhibiting *spa* types which were not found on regional pig farms. These 1,015 isolates were associated with a total of 136 (predominantly classical nosocomial) *spa* types among which nine *spa* types were outstanding: t003 (34%), t032 (28%), t004 (4%), t001, t008, t014 (each 2%), t002, t015, and t065 (each 1%). All other *spa* types were found in less than 1% of the isolates.

Isolates within the case group exhibited *spa* types t011 ($n=57$), t034 ($n=39$), t108 ($n=3$) and t1451 ($n=1$). Those within the control group were associated with 26 *spa* types including t003 ($n=39$), t032 ($n=29$), t004 ($n=5$), t002, t008, t014, t061 (each $n=2$), t001, t012, t018, t020, t022, t024, t038, t045, t065 t068, t069, t091, t256, t284, t578, t660, t1329, t1996, and t4111 (each $n=1$).

Since the age of the patients differed between the case and control groups ($P=0.06$; case group mean/median age: 48.2/48 years; control group mean/median age 53.7/56 years), age categories were built and included in the statistical analysis (Table 1). At least one of the classical nosocomial risk factors for MRSA acquisition was identified among $n=64$ (64%) of patients in the case group and among $n=91$ (91%) of patients in the control group ($P<0.001$). Table 1 shows in detail the distribution of risk factors in the case and control groups as well as the results of univariate analysis. The final logistic regression model included the variables: age 3–18 years, contact to pigs, to cattle and to horses, chronic need for nursing care, presence of indwelling devices and chronic skin lesions. In this model, the risk factors contact with pigs (OR=20.455; 95% confidence interval (CI) 7.831–64.386), contact with cattle (OR=8.607; 95% CI 1.729–42.854) and age between 3 and 18 years (OR=9.629; 95% CI 1.374–67.476) were independently associated with the case group (Table 1). The risk factor chronic need for nursing care (OR=0.065; 95% CI 0.008–0.524) was less frequent among patients in the case group.

Table 1: Results of univariate analysis and results of logistic regression. Number of patients in the case group (presumptive livestock-related MRSA *spa* types) and the control group (other than livestock-related MRSA *spa* types) sharing several potential risk factors for MRSA carriage

Risk factor	Number of patients				Univariate analysis	Final logistic regression model	
	Case group		Control group		*P* value[a]	Odds ratio (CI 95%)[b]	*P*value[b]
	Yes	No	Yes	No			
Residence in a nursing home	0	100	2	98	0.497	NA	NA
Prescribing of antibiotics[c]	35	65	39	61	0.7	NA	NA
Haemodialysis	0	100	2	98	0.3	NA	NA
Male gender	77	23	62	38	0.03	NA	NA
Age 0–2 years	3	97	2	98	1.0	NA	NA

Age 3–18 years	9	91	2	98	0.0588	9.629 (1.374–67.476)	0.023
Age 19–65 years	61	39	60	40	0.885	NA	NA
Age 66–80 years	24	76	33	67	0.159	NA	NA
Age>81 years	3	97	3	97	1.0	NA	NA
Indwelling devices	12	88	28	72	0.008	0.327 (0.105–1.024)	0.055
Hospitalization[c]	46	54	70	30	<0.001	NA	NA
Contact with human MRSA carriers	8	92	13	87	0.356	NA	NA
Chronic need for nursing care	3	97	23	77	<0.001	0.065 (0.008–0.524)	0.010
Skin lesions	5	95	23	77	0.001	0.247 (0.060–1.009)	0.052
Contact with pets	78	22	48	52	<0.001	NA	NA
Contact with horses	19	81	5	95	0.005	2.955 (0.834–10.473)	0.093
Contact with cattle	25	75	3	97	<0.001	8.607 (1.729–42.854)	0.009
Contact with pigs	62	38	6	94	<0.001	20.455 (7.831–64.386)	<0.001
Contact with sheep	2	98	2	98	0.689	NA	NA

NA not available

[a]*P* value resulting from univariate (Chi-square or Fisher Exact test) analysis; all factors with $P<0.2$ were included in the initial regression model

[b]Odds ratio (95% confidence interval, CI) and *P* value of variables included in the final logistic regression model

[c] During the previous 6 months

DISCUSSION

In 2003, a new MRSA clone exhibiting MLST CC398 (*spa* types t108, t011 and relatives) emerged among patients in Dutch hospitals. Since the occurrence of this MRSA type was shown to be epidemiologically linked to regions with a high density of pig farming [37], and as screening of pigs yielded high colonization rates [9], it was assumed that pigs might be a potential zoonotic source for MRSA transmissions.

It is unknown how often pigs at German farms, which are major European pig producers (Eurostat yearbook 2008, http://epp.eurostat.ec.europa.eu), are colonized with MRSA. In this study, we identified MRSA colonization in pigs on 70% of the regional farms. This corresponds to data from The Netherlands where 23–80% of the pig farms were affected [9, 38], and it clearly reflects that porcine MRSA colonization is a common phenomenon on farms in Germany, at least in the study area. However, genotypic investigations on MRSA isolates from pigs with acute diseases (urinary tract infection, skin infection, metritis mastitis agalactia syndrome) [16] and screening of clinical specimens and cadavers [24] recently indicated that other German geographic regions may also be involved.

Molecular typing revealed that the regional pigs' isolates were associated with a subset of *spa*types associated with MLST CC398, *agr* type I and SCCmec types V and IV, as observed in other countries [9, 18]. All isolates derived from pigs in this study did not harbour genes encoding exfoliative toxin, the toxic shock syndrome toxin 1 and enterotoxins. Moreover, the porcine isolates lacked leukocidal toxin genes *lukE/lukD*, *lukM* and the PVL-encoding *lukS/lukF*. These results confirm previous investigations [38] and suggest a low capacity of regionally disseminated porcine MRSA subtypes to induce toxin-mediated diseases among humans. The importance of these findings is highlighted against the background that MRSA CC398 have entered the food chain [22] and an outbreak of foodborne disease caused by enterotoxin-producing MRSA exhibiting a different (non-CC398) molecular type has been described previously [39]. Hence, a close surveillance of *S. aureus* from different species and from food samples should reveal the potential emergence of toxin-producing MRSA isolates.

Logistic regression modelling in our case control study yielded that, in addition to contact with pigs, contact with cattle was also independently associated with an increased risk for MRSA CC398 colonization. This finding confirms recent observations by van Loo et al. who also found a correlation of human MRSA CC398 carriage and contact to cattle [37]. Since no data on the prevalence of MRSA among cattle on German farms are published, further studies are warranted to investigate this issue.

It has previously been observed that rates of antimicrobial resistance in the commensal flora of (pig) farmers are significantly higher than in the general population [40]. The recent emergence of MRSA among farmers [17] therefore might reflect another facet of a long-known phenomenon. Nevertheless, we showed that the proportion of MRSA with presumptively livestock-associated *spa* types among all MRSA isolated from admission screenings at the UHM increased from 13% in 2005 to 22.4% in 2008. This proportion is higher than suggested by national German surveillance data [20, 41]. It has been confirmed that MRSA CC398 are not only found locally at the UHM, but are frequently isolated from admission screenings in an entire region of Northwestern Germany [42, 43]. The high burden of this MRSA subtype might therefore primarily reflect a regional situation, which could be explainable by the fact that the region involved is the area with the highest pig density (number of pigs/km^2) in Germany (information.medien.agrar e.V., Agraratlas Jan 2005, http://www.ima-agrar.de).

In this retrospective case control study, we showed a significant association of the *spa* types t011 and relatives with contact to pigs and cattle. We recognize the limitations (recall bias) inherent within this study type and state that our findings, which represent correlation data, are not suitable for proving a direct transmission of MRSA between animals and humans. However, we demonstrated that 36% of presumptive livestock-related MRSA carriers lacked classical risk factors hitherto used for admission screening of patients. Moreover, carriers of MRSA CC398 in this study comprised younger patient groups who are usually less frequent carriers of MRSA [42] and less frequently associated with classical MRSA risk factors. This raises the question of whether commonly used recommendations for admission screening are convenient to detect patients harbouring livestock-associated strains. Therefore, we favour considering adding “contact to livestock” as a risk factor to the admission screening schedule for hospitals, at least in regions with a high density of farming. Otherwise the floodgates for a clonal spread of MRSA CC398 could be opened in these regions. Furthermore, efforts of molecular MRSA surveillance and reports on prevalence will fail to reflect the actual epidemiological situation. In The Netherlands, current reports show that an adaptation of the on-admission MRSA screening protocol in this manner revealed that 32% of pig-exposed patients admitted to a Dutch hospital were colonized by MRSA. This led to a three-fold increase in the local MRSA incidence in a predominantly agriculturally structured region [44]. Moreover, our observation that the increase of MRSA CC398 at the UHM was related to the introduction of a new local MRSA “search policy” performing screening in all patients, irrespective of risk factors, emphasizes the importance of the risk patient definition for the identification of these isolates. This is highlighted by the threat that continuous introduction of MRSA CC398 to the hospital setting, might cause nosocomial spread to patient groups with underlying comorbidities and thereby facilitate infections. This threat has recently been increased by the first nosocomial outbreak of MRSA ST398 in a Dutch hospital [45].

Apart from giving impetus to antimicrobial resistance import to hospitals, colonization with MRSA CC398 might set livestock-exposed persons under risk of developing severe *S. aureus*CC398-associated infections [21, 46]. First, this highlights the special need to consider MRSA as causative agents when treating such patient groups. Second, it raises the question as to whether the implementation of preventive measures (consequent alcoholic hand disinfection, wearing of gloves and prevention of dust inhalation) could forestall MRSA colonization of livestock-exposed workers.

In conclusion, our findings confirm that MRSA associated with *spa* type t011 and relatives can be found on German pig farms and indicate that livestock might represent a relevant source for MRSA imports to hospitals.

ACKNOWLEDGMENTS

This study was partly performed within the framework of the INTERREG-IIIa project “EUREGIO MRSA-net Twente/Münsterland” (reference no. 2-EUR-V-1=96) and the INTERREG-IVa Euregio-project Safeguard MRSA VetMed-net (reference no. 34-INTERREG IV A-II-2-05=025).

We are especially grateful to M.G. Ron Hendrix (MD, PhD), Laboratorium Microbiologie, Enschede, for fruitful discussion, and we thank Monique Henderikx, Isabell Ramminger and Ursula Keckevoet for their skilled technical assistance.

REFERENCES

1. Deurenberg RH, Vink C, Kalenic S, Friedrich AW, Bruggeman CA, Stobberingh EE (2007) The molecular evolution of methicillin-resistant *Staphylococcus aureus*. Clin Microbiol Infect 13:222–235
2. Walther B, Monecke S, Ruscher C, Friedrich AW, Ehricht R, Slickers P, Soba A, Wleklinski CG, Wieler LH, Lubke-Becker A (2009) Comparative molecular analysis substantiates a zoonotic potential of equine methicillin-resistant *Staphylococcus aureus* (MRSA). J Clin Microbiol 47(3):704–710
3. Weese JS, Lefebvre SL (2007) Risk factors for methicillin-resistant *Staphylococcus aureus*colonization in horses admitted to a veterinary teaching hospital. Can Vet J 48:921–926
4. Cuny C, Kuemmerle J, Stanek C, Willey B, Strommenger B, Witte W (2006) Emergence of MRSA infections in horses in a veterinary hospital: strain characterisation and comparison with MRSA from humans. Euro Surveill 11:44–47
5. Juhasz-Kaszanyitzky E, Janosi S, Somogyi P, Dan A, van der Graaf-van Bloois L, van Duijkeren E, Wagenaar JA (2007) MRSA transmission between cows and humans. Emerg Infect Dis 13:630–632
6. Moodley A, Stegger M, Bagcigil AF, Baptiste KE, Loeffler A, Lloyd DH, Williams NJ, Leonard N, Abbott Y, Skov R, Guardabassi L (2006) spa typing of methicillin-resistant *Staphylococcus aureus* isolated from domestic animals and veterinary staff in the UK and Ireland. J Antimicrob Chemother 58:1118–1123
7. Walther B, Wieler LH, Friedrich AW, Hanssen AM, Kohn B, Brunnberg L, Lubke-Becker A (2007) Methicillin-resistant *Staphylococcus aureus* (MRSA) isolated from small and exotic animals at a university hospital during routine microbiological examinations. Vet Microbiol

127:171–178

8. Rich M, Roberts L (2006) MRSA in companion animals. Vet Rec 159:535–536
9. De Neeling AJ, van den Broek MJ, Spalburg EC, van Santen-Verheuvel MG, Dam-Deisz WD, Boshuizen HC, van de Giessen AW, van Duijkeren E, Huijsdens XW (2007) High prevalence of methicillin resistant *Staphylococcus aureus* in pigs. Vet Microbiol 122:366–372
10. Guardabassi L, Stegger M, Skov R (2007) Retrospective detection of methicillin resistant and susceptible *Staphylococcus aureus* ST398 in Danish slaughter pigs. Vet Microbiol 122:384–386
11. Lewis HC, Molbak K, Reese C, Aarestrup FM, Selchau M, Sorum M, Skov RL (2008) Pigs as source of Methicillin-resistant *Staphylococcus aureus* CC398 infections in humans, Denmark. Emerg Infect Dis 14:1383–1389
12. Armand-Lefevre L, Ruimy R, Andremont A (2005) Clonal comparison of *Staphylococcus aureus* isolates from healthy pig farmers, human controls, and pigs. Emerg Infect Dis 11:711–714
13. Khanna T, Friendship R, Dewey C, Weese JS (2007) Methicillin resistant *Staphylococcus aureus* colonization in pigs and pig farmers. Vet Microbiol 128:298–303
14. Smith TC, Male MJ, Harper AL, Kroeger JS, Tinkler GP, Moritz ED, Capuano AW, Herwaldt LA, Diekema DJ (2008) Methicillin-resistant *Staphylococcus aureus* (MRSA) strain ST398 is present in midwestern U.S. swine and swine workers. PLoS ONE 4:e4258
15. Sergio DMB, Koh TH, Hsu L, Ogden BE, Goh ALH, Chow PKH (2007) Investigation of methicillin-resistant *Staphylococcus aureus* in pigs used for research. J Med Microbiol 56:1107–1109
16. Schwarz S, Kadlec K, Strommenger B (2008) Methicillin-resistant *Staphylococcus aureus*and *Staphylococcus pseudintermedius* detected in the BfT-GermVet monitoring programme 2004–2006 in Germany. J Antimicrob Chemother 61:282–285
17. Voss A, Loeffen F, Bakker J, Klaassen C, Wulf M (2005) Methicillin-resistant *Staphylococcus aureus* in pig farming. Emerg Infect Dis 11:1965–1966
18. Huijsdens XW, van Dijke BJ, Spalburg E, van Santen-Verheuvel MG, Heck MEOC, Pluister GN, Voss A, Wannet WJB, de Neeling AJ (2006) Community-acquired MRSA and pig-farming. Ann Clin Microbiol Antimicrob 5:26
19. Wulf M, van Nes A, Eikelenboom-Boskamp A, de Vries J, Melchers W, Klaassen C, Voss A (2006) Methicillin-resistant *Staphylococcus aureus* in veterinary doctors and students, the Netherlands. Emerg Infect Dis 12:1939–1941
20. Witte W, Strommenger B, Stanek C, Cuny C (2007) Methicillin-resistant *Staphylococcus aureus* ST398 in humans and animals, Central Europe. Emerg Infect Dis 13:255–258
21. Ekkelenkamp MB, Sekkat M, Carpaij N, Troelstra A, Bonten MJM (2006) Endocarditis due to methicillin-resistant *Staphylococcus aureus* originating from pigs. Ned Tijdschr Geneeskd 150:2442–2447
22. van Loo IHM, Diederen BMW, Savelkoul PHM, Woudenberg JHC, Roosendaal R, van Belkum A, Lemmens-den Toom N, Verhulst C, van Keulen PHJ, Kluytmans JAJW (2007) Methicillin-resistant *Staphylococcus aureus* in meat products, the Netherlands. Emerg Infect Dis 13:1753–1755
23. Pu S, Han F, Ge B (2009) Isolation and characterization of methicillin-resistant *Staphylococcus aureus* strains from Louisiana retail meats. Appl Environ Microbiol 75:265–267
24. Meemken D, Cuny C, Witte W, Eichler U, Staudt R, Blaha T (2008) Occurrence of MRSA in pigs and in humans involved in pig production–preliminary results of a study in the northwest of Germany. Dtsch Tierarztl Wochenschr 115:132–139
25. Tiemersma EW, Bronzwaer SLAM, Lyytikainen O, Degener JE, Schrijnemakers P, Bruinsma N, Monen J, Witte W, Grundman H (2004) Methicillin-resistant *Staphylococcus aureus* in Europe, 1999–2002. Emerg Infect Dis 10:1627–1634
26. Harbarth S, Sax H, Fankhauser-Rodriguez C, Schrenzel J, Agostinho A, Pittet D (2006) Evaluating the probability of previously unknown carriage of MRSA at hospital admission. Am J Med 119(275):e15–e23
27. Wertheim H, Verbrugh HA, van Pelt C, de Man P, van Belkum A, Vos MC (2001) Improved detection of methicillin-resistant *Staphylococcus aureus* using phenyl mannitol broth containing aztreonam and ceftizoxime. J Clin Microbiol 39:2660–2662
28. Martineau F, Picard FJ, Roy PH, Ouellette M, Bergeron MG (1998) Species-specific and ubiquitous-DNA-based assays for rapid identification of *Staphylococcus aureus*. J Clin Microbiol 36:618–623
29. Becker K, Pagnier I, Schuhen B, Wenzelburger F, Friedrich AW, Kipp F, Peters G, von Eiff C (2006) Does nasal cocolonization by methicillin-resistant coagulase-negative staphylococci and methicillin-susceptible *Staphylococcus aureus* strains occur frequently enough to represent a risk of false-positive methicillin-resistant *S. aureus* determinations by molecular methods? J Clin Microbiol 44:229–231
30. Lina G, Piemont Y, Godail-Gamot F, Bes M, Peter MO, Gauduchon V, Vandenesch F, Etienne J (1999) Involvement of Panton-Valentine leukocidin-producing *Staphylococcus aureus* in primary skin infections and pneumonia. Clin Infect Dis 29:1128–1132
31. von Eiff C, Friedrich AW, Peters G, Becker K (2004) Prevalence of genes encoding for members of the staphylococcal leukotoxin family among clinical isolates of *Staphylococcus aureus*. Diagn Microbiol Infect Dis 49:157–162
32. Becker K, Friedrich AW, Lubritz G, Weilert M, Peters G, von Eiff C (2003) Prevalence of genes encoding pyrogenic toxin superantigens and exfoliative toxins among strains of *Staphylococcus aureus* isolated from blood and nasal specimens. J Clin Microbiol 41:1434–1439

33. Mellmann A, Friedrich AW, Rosenkotter N, Rothganger J, Karch H, Reintjes R, Harmsen D (2006) Automated DNA sequence-based early warning system for the detection of methicillin-resistant *Staphylococcus aureus* outbreaks. PLoS Med 3:e33

34. Enright MC, Day NP, Davies CE, Peacock SJ, Spratt BG (2000) Multilocus sequence typing for characterization of methicillin-resistant and methicillin-susceptible clones of *Staphylococcus aureus*. J Clin Microbiol 38:1008–1015

35. Strommenger B, Kehrenberg C, Kettlitz C, Cuny C, Verspohl J, Witte W, Schwarz S (2006) Molecular characterization of methicillin-resistant *Staphylococcus aureus* strains from pet animals and their relationship to human isolates. J Antimicrob Chemother 57:461–465

36. Zhang K, McClure JA, Elsayed S, Louie T, Conley JM (2005) Novel multiplex PCR assay for characterization and concomitant subtyping of staphylococcal cassette chromosome mec types I to V in methicillin-resistant *Staphylococcus aureus*. J Clin Microbiol 43:5026–5033

37. van Loo I, Huijsdens X, Tiemersma E, de Neeling A, van de Sande-Bruinsma N, Beaujean D, Voss A, Kluytmans J (2007) Emergence of methicillin-resistant *Staphylococcus aureus*of animal origin in humans. Emerg Infect Dis 13:1834–1839

38. van Duijkeren E, Ikawaty R, Broekhuizen-Stins MJ, Jansen MD, Spalburg EC, de Neeling AJ, Allaart JG, van Nes A, Wagenaar JA, Fluit AC (2008) Transmission of methicillin-resistant *Staphylococcus aureus* strains between different kinds of pig farms. Vet Microbiol 126:383–389

39. Jones TF, Kellum ME, Porter SS, Bell M, Schaffner W (2002) An outbreak of community-acquired foodborne illness caused by methicillin-resistant *Staphylococcus aureus*. Emerg Infect Dis 8:82–84

40. Aubry-Damon H, Grenet K, Sall-Ndiaye P, Che D, Cordeiro E, Bougnoux M, Rigaud E, Le Strat Y, Lemanissier V, Armand-Lefevre L, Delzescaux D, Desenclos J, Lienard M (2004) Antimicrobial resistance in commensal flora of pig farmers. Emerg Infect Dis 10:873–839

41. Strommenger B, Braulke C, Heuck D, Schmidt C, Pasemann B, Nubel U, Witte W (2008) spa Typing of *Staphylococcus aureus* as a frontline tool in epidemiological typing. J Clin Microbiol 46:574–581

42. Köck R, Brakensiek L, Mellmann A, Kipp F, Henderikx M, Harmsen D, Daniels-Haardt I, von Eiff C, Becker K, Hendrix MG, Friedrich AW (2009) Cross-border comparison of the admission prevalence and clonal structure of methicillin-resistant *Staphylococcus aureus*. J Hosp Infect 71:320–326

43. Friedrich AW, Daniels-Haardt I, Köck R, Verhoeven F, Mellmann A, Harmsen D, van Gemert-Pijnen JE, Becker K, Hendrix MGR (2008) EUREGIO MRSA-net Twente/Munsterland—a Dutch-German cross-border network for the prevention and control of infections caused by methicillin-resistant *Staphylococcus aureus*. Euro Surveill 13(pii):18965

44. van Rijen MML, Van Keulen PH, Kluytmans JA (2008) Increase in a Dutch hospital of methicillin-resistant *Staphylococcus aureus* related to animal farming. Clin Infect Dis 46:261–263

45. Wulf MWH, Markestein A, van der Linden FT, Voss A, Klaassen C, Verduin CM (2008) First outbreak of methicillin-resistant *Staphylococcus aureus* ST398 in a Dutch hospital, June 2007. Euro Surveill 28(13)pii:8051

46. van Belkum A, Melles DC, Peeters JK, van Leeuwen WB, van Duijkeren E, Huijsdens XW, Spalburg E, de Neeling AJ, Verbrugh HA, On Behalf Of The Dutch Working Party On Surveillance And Research (2008) Methicillin-resistant and -susceptible *Staphylococcus aureus* sequence type 398 in pigs and humans. Emerg Infect Dis 14:479–483

CHAPTER 22 METHICILLIN-RESISTANT STAPHYLOCOCCUS AUREUS (MRSA) STRAIN ST398 IS PRESENT IN MIDWESTERN U.S. SWINE AND SWINE WORKERS

Tara C. Smith, Michael J. Male, Abby L. Harper, Jennifer S. Kroeger, Gregory P. Tinkler, Erin D. Moritz, Ana W. Capuano, Loreen A. Herwaldt, Daniel J. Diekema

INTRODUCTION

Staphylococcus aureus is one of the most common and devastating human pathogens [1]. Though approximately a third of the population is colonized with *S. aureus* [2], [3], colonization by strains of *S. aureus* that are resistant to methicillin (methicillin-resistant *S. aureus*, MRSA) is less common. A recent publication estimated that 1.5% of the United States (U.S.) population (~4.1 million persons) is colonized with MRSA [4]. Klevens et al. recently showed that deaths from MRSA infections in the U.S. have eclipsed those from many other infectious diseases, including HIV/AIDS. On the basis of data from several major metropolitan areas in the U.S., these investigators estimated that MRSA caused 94,000 infections and over 18,000 deaths in the U.S. in 2005 [5].

Moreover, MRSA has been found in a variety of animals, including horses [6], [7], cattle [8], dogs, cats [9], and swine [10], [11], [12]. Voss et al. reported that the prevalence of MRSA among pig farmers was >760 times higher than that among patients admitted to Dutch hospitals [13]. Multi locus sequence typing (MLST) suggested that these MRSA isolates belonged to sequence type 398 (ST398), and had been transmitted from pigs to pig farmers, among pig farmers and their family members, and from the colonized son of a swine veterinarian to a hospital nurse. A subsequent study found that 4.6% of veterinarians and veterinary students were colonized with MRSA compared with a population-based estimate of 1% [14].

Additional studies in swine have shown that isolates obtained from swine and their human caretakers are frequently indistinguishable, suggesting transmission between the two animal species [11], [12]. Indeed, investigations in the Netherlands demonstrated that ST398 now accounts for 20% of all MRSA detected in that country, documenting the importance of considering livestock and other animals when examining the epidemiology of MRSA [15]. However, despite research examining swine-associated MRSA in the Netherlands and Canada [10], [12], currently the prevalence of MRSA in swine or their caretakers is unknown in the U.S. In a rural state such as Iowa, which produces 25% of the swine raised in the U.S., transmission of MRSA on swine farms or in veterinary facilities could complicate efforts to reduce MRSA transmission statewide and beyond. Therefore, we conducted a pilot culture survey to examine the prevalence of MRSA in swine and swine workers in two swine farming production systems in Iowa and Illinois.

MATERIALS AND METHODS

Description of farms and swine sampled

Production system A (PSA) is a conventional commercial confinement operation consisting of a 5200 head breed-to-wean

Citation: Smith TC, Male MJ, Harper AL, Kroeger JS, Tinkler GP, Moritz ED, et al. (2009) Methicillin-Resistant Staphylococcus aureus (MRSA) Strain ST398 Is Present in Midwestern U.S. Swine and Swine Workers. PLoS ONE 4(1): e4258. doi:10.1371/journal.pone.0004258.

sow farm with multiple age-segregated nurseries, finishing, and wean-to-finish sites scattered throughout northern Illinois and eastern Iowa. Collectively, approximately 60,000 swine are present at any one time. Sows in this herd originated from both Canada (Manitoba, Ontario and Quebec) and the U.S. (Minnesota and Illinois). The crossbred sows are from a major swine genetic supplier. The sow herd is relatively young, having been repopulated in 2006. Samples (n=210) were taken from swine housed at 7 geographically distinct farms within this closed system. The nares of adult sows and swine ages 9, 12, 15, 18, 21, and 24 weeks were swabbed (30 per age group). Animals were not co-mingled prior to sampling. One sample was eliminated because it became contaminated. Nine weeks after the first visit, 20 additional cultures were obtained from swine that were initially 12 and 15 weeks old (10 from each age group). Sixteen weeks after the first visit, 20 samples were obtained from randomly selected dam-piglet pairs.

Production system B (PSB) is also a relatively young herd sow herd comprising approximately 2600 sows at the single sow farm location and 27,000 total animals housed at multiple, age-segregated nursery, finisher and wean-to-finish sites throughout eastern Iowa. The sow farm was populated in 2006 with crossbred females originating solely in the United States (Michigan). The breeding stock females in this herd are also from a major swine genetic supplier, but different than those of PSA. Thirty samples were taken from swine in each of 3 age groups: adult sows, and pigs at 11 and 20 weeks of age (n=90). Animals were not co-mingled prior to sampling.

Human participants

Human caretakers (n=20) provided nasal and oropharyngeal swabs. Employees filled out a questionnaire providing demographic data, potential risk factors for MRSA infection, information about contact with swine, and use of personal protective equipment. The institutional review board (IRB) and the institutional animal care and use committee (IACUC) approved the protocols. All human participants gave written informed consent prior to enrollment.

Sample collection and bacterial isolation

One naris from each animal and both nares from caretakers were sampled with sterile swabs. Cultures were done as described previously [12]. Briefly, samples were collected using sterile swabs and inserted into Stuart's medium at 4°C for transportation. Samples were inoculated into 2 mL enrichment broth containing 10 g tryptone/L, 75 g NaCl/L, 10 g mannitol/L and 2.5 g yeast extract/L. After 24 h incubation at 35°C, a loopful of broth was inoculated onto selective MRSA agar plates (BBL CHROMagar MRSA, Becton, Dickinson and Company). These plates were incubated 24–48 hours at 35°C and examined for MRSA. Isolates were confirmed to be *S. aureus* by examining their appearance on Gram stain, and by doing the catalase test, the tube coagulase test and the *S. aureus* latex agglutination assay (Pastorex Staph-plus, Bio-Rad). Methicillin resistance was confirmed by testing for the presence of penicillin binding protein 2 (PBP2′) (MRSA latex agglutination test, Oxoid Ltd., Hants, UK). MRSA isolates were stored at −80°C.

Molecular testing

All human isolates and 15 isolates from swine (representing all age groups) were selected for molecular typing. Pulsed field gel electrophoresis (PFGE) was performed as previously described [16]. Isolates that were non-typeable after *Sma*I digestion were examined after digestion with *Eag*I. Isolates from this study were compared with the type strains for USA100, USA300, and USA400 [17]. For SCC*mec* typing and *pvl* PCR, genomic DNA was extracted using the Wizard Genomic DNA preparation kit (Promega). The multiplex SCC*mec* PCR included ten primer sets: CIF2 F2/R2, mecI P2/P3, RIF5 F10/R13, dcs F2/R1, mecA P4/P7, kdp F1/R1, SCCmec III J1 F/J1 R, ccrB2 F2/R2, SCCmec V J1 F/J1 R, and ccrC F2/R2 [18]. The presence of *pvl* was determined by an additional PCR [19]. Multi locus sequence typing (MLST) was performed on a subset of isolates which were identical by PFGE and analyzed as previously described [20]. All molecular procedures employed known positive and negative controls.

Antimicrobial susceptibility testing

All human MRSA isolates and the 15 swine isolates evaluated by molecular typing were tested for antimicrobial susceptibility by the broth dilution method described by the Clinical and Laboratory Standards Institute [21]. Isolates were tested for susceptibility to penicillin, oxacillin, tetracycline, erythromycin, clindamycin, trimethoprim-sulfamethoxazole, quinupristin/dalfopristin, gentamicin, levofloxacin, moxifloxacin, linezolid, daptomycin, vancomycin, and rifampin.

Survey/data analysis

Questionnaire and laboratory data were linked by a unique specimen number. Initially, potential risk factor associations were assessed with Fisher's exact test. Bivariate and multivariate modeling of risk factors were performed by exact logistic regression. A trend in prevalence of MRSA in swine by age group was tested with the Cochran-Armitage trend test. A significance level of 0.05 was used in the analyses. Analyses were performed using SAS software version 9.1 (SAS Institute Inc., Cary, NC).

RESULTS

MRSA prevalence in swine

Nasal swabs were taken from 209 swine representing 7 different age groups at PSA. The overall prevalence of MRSA was 70% (147/209). Figure 1 illustrates the significant decreasing trend in prevalence found with the increase in age group (Cochran-Armitage trend test, p-value <0.01). Swine 15 weeks or younger had higher odds of MRSA colonization (OR: 2.17, 95% confidence interval=1.6 to infinity) when compared to adult swine.

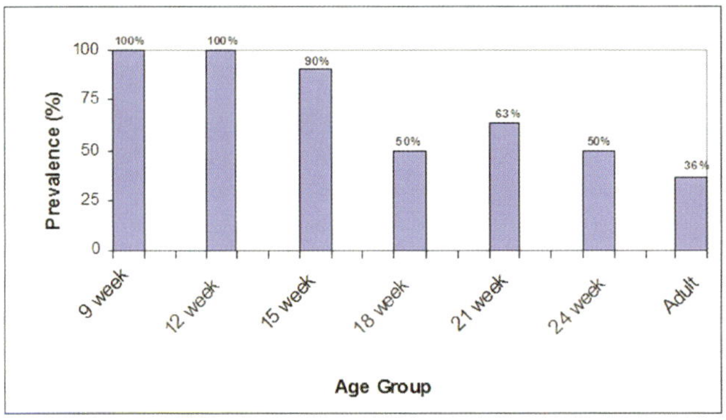

Figure 1: Prevalence of MRSA in swine from production system A by age aroup.

At a follow-up visit 9 weeks later, 20 of 20 samples obtained from the youngest animals were positive. Twelve of 20 (60%) samples obtained 16 weeks after the first visit from 10 randomly selected piglet-dam pairs were positive. Results were concordant for 4 pairs (in 1 pair both dam and piglet had negative nares cultures; in 3 pairs both animals had positive nares cultures) and discordant for 6 pairs (in 2 pairs the dam›s nares culture grew MRSA and the piglet›s culture did not; in 4 pairs the piglet›s nares culture grew MRSA and the dam›s culture did not).

Swine from a second production system (PSB) were also tested. Because the prevalence of MRSA carriage was high among younger pigs at PSA, we sampled fewer age groups at PSB. We collected 90 samples from 3 age groups (11 weeks, 20 weeks, and adult). We did not detect MRSA in any of these swabs.

MRSA prevalence in humans and risk factors for MRSA carriage

Persons working in these swine facilities were invited to participate in the study. PSA employed 18 staff who had contact with swine at the sow farm; 14 (77%) volunteered to provide swabs and respond to a questionnaire. PSB employed 7 staff in contact with swine at the sow farm; 6 (86%) participated in our study. Overall, 9/20 (49%) carried MRSA, all of whom were employed at PSA (9/14 persons sampled at PSA, 64% prevalence). Seven persons were colonized in the nares only and 2 were colonized in both the nares and throat. As all swine and human samples obtained at PSB were negative for MRSA, only PSA was included in the risk factor analyses. Age, gender, use of tobacco products, underlying medical conditions, respiratory illness in the prior 12 months, use of antimicrobial agents in the prior 3 months, exposure to healthcare facilities (including long-term-care facilities), a history of skin and soft tissue infections or of having MRSA in the prior 12 months, duration of employment, the number of swine contacted per day, eating pork products, and exposure to raw pork were not associated with nasal carriage of MRSA (see Table 1). All14 PSA subjects work with breeding swine. Persons who do not obtain blood or other specimens from swine (separate analyses) were at higher risk of carrying MRSA than staff that did do these chores.

Table 1: Characteristics of Production System A swine workers and MRSA prevalence

Variable	Response	N	MRSA positive (%)
Gender			
	Female	1	0 (0.0)
	Male	13	8 (61.5)
Age group			
	<31	6	3 (50.0)
	31–43	3	3 (100)
	>=44	5	2 (40.0)
Tobacco			
	No	6	4 (66.7)
	Yes	8	4 (50.0)
Lung problems			
	No	12	6 (50.0)
	Yes	2	2 (100)
Heart problems			
	No	13	8 (61.5)
	Yes	1	0 (0.0)
Chronic medical problem			
	No	11	7 (63.6)
	Yes	3	1 (33.3)
Respiratory illness with fever in last 12 months			
	No	10	7 (70.0)
	Yes	4	1 (25.0)
Missed work because of respiratory illness in last 12 months			
	No	10	7 (70.0)
	Yes	4	1 (25.0)
Taken antibiotics in the past 3 months			
	No	11	7 (63.6)
	Yes	3	1 (33.3)
Visited hospital in past 12 months			
	No	9	7 (77.8)
	Yes	5	1 (20.0)
Visited long-term care facility in past 12 months			
	No	11	6 (54.6)
	Yes	3	2 (66.7)
You or family member work in hospital or long-term care facility			
	No	10	7 (70.0)
	Yes	4	1 (25.0)
Diagnosed with skin of soft tissue infection in past 12 months			
	No	14	8 (57.1)
	Yes	0	0 (0.0)
Diagnosed with MRSA in past 12 months			
	No	14	8 (57.1)
	Yes	0	0 (0.0)
Length of employment (years)			
	<=3	5	4 (80.0)
	4–14	6	3 (50.0)
	>=14	3	1 (33.3)
Perform cleaning in the swine farm*			
	No	5	5 (100)
	Yes	9	3 (33.3)
Obtain blood or other specimens from swine*			
	No	10	8 (80.0)
	Yes	4	0 (0.0)
Average number of swine you are exposed in a typical day			
	<=2400	3	2 (66.7)
	2401–5000	8	3 (37.5)
	>=5000	3	3 (100)
Consume pork products			
	No	1	0 (0.0)
	Yes	13	8 (61.5)
Frequency of consuming pork products			
	2–3 times per week	4	2 (50.0)
	Approximately once per week	6	4 (66.7)
	Less than once per week	2	2 (100)
	More than 4 times per week	1	0 (0.0)
Frequency of handling raw pork products			
	2–3 times per week	3	0 (0.0)
	Approximately once per week	3	3 (100)
	Less than once per week	7	5 (71.4)

*Significant at 95% confidence level using Fisher exact.

doi:10.1371/journal.pone.0004258.t001

http://dx.doi.org/10.1371/journal.pone.0004258.t001

Molecular typing

As previously described [22], the isolates from swine and caretakers were not typeable when the DNA was digested with *Sma*I (Fig. 2a) but were typeable when *Eag*I was used (Fig. 2b). All isolates from swine and from swine workers were closely related by the Tenover criteria [23]and they were distinct from common human strains (USA100, USA300, and USA400, not shown).

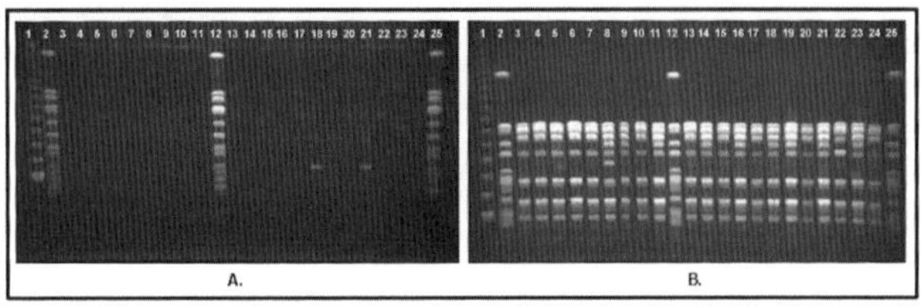

Figure 2: A: PFGE of MRSA isolates from swine and swine workers; DNA digested with *Sma*I. B: PFGE of MRSA isolates from swine and swine workers; DNA digested with *Eag*I. Lane 1: molecular weight ladder. Lanes 2, 12, 25: NCTC 8325 (control strain). Lanes 3–11: isolates from swine workers. Lanes 13–24: isolates from swine.

All isolates were SCC*mec* type V and *pvl*-negative (data not shown). MLST analysis of a subset of isolates confirmed that these isolates were ST398.

Antibiotic resistance

All isolates from swine and from humans were resistant to penicillin, oxacillin and tetracycline, and all were susceptible to trimethoprim-sulfamethoxazole, gentamicin, levofloxacin, moxifloxacin, linezolid, daptomycin, vancomycin, and rifampin. Three of 15 (20%) swine isolates were resistant to erythromycin, 2 (13%) were resistant to quinupristin-dalfopristin, and 13 (87%) were resistant to clindamycin. None of the 9 human isolates tested were resistant to erythromycin or quinupristin-dalfopristin, but 1 (11%) was resistant to clindamycin. The unusual pattern of erythromycin susceptibility and clindamycin resistance among 11 of the isolates was confirmed with repeat testing.

DISCUSSION

This study is the first to document MRSA in U.S. swine and swine workers, and to our knowledge, the first to report the presence of ST398 (also reported as non-typeable MRSA, NT-MRSA) [15] in the U.S. Like previous studies in Canada, Denmark, and the Netherlands [11], [12], [24], ST398 was found in both animals and humans, suggesting transmission between the two. The prevalence of MRSA colonization among swine and swine workers was high at one farm system that we examined in the Midwestern U.S., suggesting that agricultural animals could become an important reservoir for this bacterium. Strain ST398 was the only MRSA identified among the swine and swine workers. This strain has been the predominant strain among swine in the Netherlands and Canada. However, Khanna et al. in Canada recently found both ST398 and ST5/USA100 colonizing the nares of swine and swine workers [12]. This difference may indicate that the epidemiology of MRSA on Canadian swine farms is different than on the affected farm system in Iowa and Illinois. On the other hand, the difference may have resulted from differing sampling methodologies. Khanna et al. sampled a small number of humans and swine on 20 farms whereas we took a larger number of samples from a smaller number of farms in two corporate systems. Furthermore, because we did not type all isolates in this pilot study, additional strain types may be present that we did not detect.

The rate of MRSA colonization in both humans and swine on the farms in one of the corporate systems in our study was high, suggesting that once MRSA is introduced, it may spread broadly among both swine and their caretakers. Other investigators have postulated that this spread may be facilitated by use of tetracycline in swine farming [10]. The ST398 isolates identified in our study were resistant to tetracycline, and thus, could have been selected by antimicrobial pressure on this farm. However, both production systems that we sampled employ similar protocols for prophylactic and therapeutic use of antimicrobial agents, including tetracycline. Therefore, our data do not allow us to speculate on the relationship between antimicrobial use and MRSA carriage. In addition to tetracycline resistance, we found an unusual macrolide-lincosamide resistance phenotype among a subset of isolates (erythromycin susceptible, clindamycin resistant), one which is not explained by the commonly-recognized mechanisms of macrolide-lincosamide resistance [25].

At present, we do not know why one farm system had a high prevalence rate of MRSA among its swine and its swine handlers. The two production systems did have several differences. First, they raised different breeds of swine. Second, PSA was an older, more established operation that had approximately twice the number of animals as PSB. Additionally, a portion of the sows at PSA were imported from Canada, while those from PSB originated in Michigan. Canada is the most important exporter of live hogs to the U.S. [26]. Thus, it is possible that ST398 may have been brought into the U.S. via live swine or pork products. However, this study was not designed to identify the source of the MRSA and additional research should further examine this question.

In addition, our survey did not help us understand why a high proportion of PSA staff carried MRSA. Most of the potential risk factors examined were not statistically different between the carriers and the non-carriers. We cannot explain the observation that staff who do not obtain blood and other samples from the animals were more likely to be carriers than were staff who obtained such samples. Additional studies in larger populations will be needed to identify risk factors and to assess whether this association is real.

Investigators in other countries have documented that ST398 causes infections in humans [11], [13], [15] and Wulf et al. have recently described a hospital-based outbreak in the Netherlands [27]. Iowa ranks first in the nation in swine production, with over 19 million hogs at any time point distributed over more than 10,000 farms [28], [29]. Therefore, one would expect that Iowa would be a good state in which to assess the prevalence of infections caused by ST398 among humans. None of the swine workers in this small study reported prior MRSA infections. In addition, we have not identified this strain among the hundreds of human MRSA isolates examined in several ongoing studies of MRSA (including invasive infections) in Iowa [30], [31].

Our study had several limitations. We demonstrated that MRSA can remain in a population of swine for up to 6 months. However, we did not re-test the same animals over time. Thus, we cannot comment about duration of carriage in particular animals and we could not determine whether the lower rate of colonization in older animals observed at PSA was a true difference related to biological mechanisms or an incidental finding. The latter observation contrasts with prior research that found no significant difference in the rates of MRSA carriage by age group [12]. In addition, we did not evaluate whether the environment was contaminated and could have been a source of transmission for swine or for humans, or whether transmission occurred through direct contact with a colonized animal or human. Moreover, we studied only 9 farms in 2 production systems. Thus, our results may not be generalizable to other swine farms in Iowa and Illinois or to other areas of the U.S.

In summary, we report the first isolation of MRSA from swine and swine workers in the U.S. Although the extent of this problem in the U.S. is currently unknown, our findings may have important implications for the epidemiology of MRSA disease. For example, Van Loo et al. identified MRSA in meat products in the Netherlands [32], suggesting that persons who handle raw pork products might be at risk for acquiring MRSA. Future studies should assess the risk of MRSA disease among swine workers and their contacts, survey retail meat products for MRSA contamination, study larger populations of swine and humans to define the epidemiology of MRSA within swine operations, and assess MRSA carriage rates in other livestock.

ACKNOWLEDGMENTS

We thank the production systems that allowed us to study their swine and employees. Portions of this research were presented at the 2008 International Conference for Emerging Infectious Diseases and the 2008 American Society for Microbiology General Meeting (abstract Y-036). The authors report no conflicts of interest. Research was approved by the University of Iowa Institutional Review Board (#200802740) and University Animal Care and Use Committee (#0804064).

AUTHOR CONTRIBUTIONS

Conceived and designed the experiments: TCS MJM LAH DJD. Performed the experiments: TCS MJM ALH JSK GPT EDMK. Analyzed the data: TCS AC. Contributed reagents/materials/analysis tools: TCS DJD. Wrote the paper: TCS MJM LAH DJD. Critically revised the manuscript: TCS MJM JSK GPT EDMK LAH DJD.

REFERENCES

1. Lowy FD (1998) Staphylococcus aureus infections. N Engl J Med 339: 520–532.
2. Shorr AF (2007) Epidemiology of staphylococcal resistance. Clin Infect Dis 45: Suppl 3S171–176.
3. Graham PL 3rd, Lin SX, Larson EL (2006) A U.S. population-based survey of Staphylococcus aureus colonization. Ann Intern Med 144: 318–325.
4. Gorwitz RJ, Kruszon-Moran D, McAllister SK, McQuillan G, McDougal LK, et al. (2008) Changes in the prevalence of nasal colonization with Staphylococcus aureus in the United States, 2001–2004. J Infect Dis 197: 1226–1234.
5. Klevens RM, Morrison MA, Nadle J, Petit S, Gershman K, et al. (2007) Invasive methicillin-resistant Staphylococcus aureus infections in the United States. JAMA 298: 1763–1771.
6. Weese JS, Archambault M, Willey BM, Hearn P, Kreiswirth BN, et al. (2005) Methicillin-resistant Staphylococcus aureus in horses and horse personnel, 2000–2002. Emerg Infect Dis 11: 430–435.
7. Weese JS, Caldwell F, Willey BM, Kreiswirth BN, McGeer A, et al. (2006) An outbreak of methicillin-resistant Staphylococcus aureus skin infections resulting from horse to human transmission in a veterinary hospital. Vet Microbiol 114: 160–164.
8. Juhasz-Kaszanyitzky E, Janosi S, Somogyi P, Dan A, van der Graaf-van Bloois L, et al. (2007) MRSA transmission between cows and humans. Emerg Infect Dis 13: 630–632.
9. Baptiste KE, Williams K, Willams NJ, Wattret A, Clegg PD, et al. (2005) Methicillin-resistant staphylococci in companion animals. Emerg Infect Dis 11: 1942–1944.
10. de Neeling AJ, van den Broek MJ, Spalburg EC, van Santen-Verheuvel MG, Dam-Deisz WD, et al. (2007) High prevalence of methicillin resistant Staphylococcus aureus in pigs. Vet Microbiol 122: 366–372.
11. Huijsdens XW, van Dijke BJ, Spalburg E, van Santen-Verheuvel MG, Heck ME, et al. (2006) Community-acquired MRSA and pig-farming. Ann Clin Microbiol Antimicrob 5: 26.
12. Khanna T, Friendship R, Dewey C, Weese JS (2008) Methicillin resistant Staphylococcus aureus colonization in pigs and pig farmers. Vet Microbiol 128: 298–303.
13. Voss A, Loeffen F, Bakker J, Klaassen C, Wulf M (2005) Methicillin-resistant Staphylococcus aureus in pig farming. Emerg Infect Dis 11: 1965–1966.
14. Wulf M, van Nes A, Eikelenboom-Boskamp A, de Vries J, Melchers W, et al. (2006) Methicillin-resistant Staphylococcus aureus in veterinary doctors and students, the Netherlands. Emerg Infect Dis 12: 1939–1941.
15. van Loo I, Huijsdens X, Tiemersma E, de Neeling A, van de Sande-Bruinsma N, et al. (2007) Emergence of methicillin-resistant Staphylococcus aureus of animal origin in humans. Emerg Infect Dis 13: 1834–1839.
16. Pfaller MA, Hollis R, Sader H (1994) Chromosomal restriction fragment analysis by pulsed field gel electrophoresis. In: Isenberg H, editor. Clinical Microbiology Procedures Handbook, Supplement 1. Washington, DC: American Society for Microbiology.
17. McDougal LK, Steward CD, Killgore GE, Chaitram JM, McAllister SK, et al. (2003) Pulsed-field gel electrophoresis typing of oxacillin-resistant Staphylococcus aureus isolates from the United States: establishing a national database. J Clin Microbiol 41: 5113–5120.
18. Milheirico C, Oliveira DC, de Lencastre H (2007) Update to the multiplex PCR strategy for assignment of

mec element types in Staphylococcus aureus. Antimicrob Agents Chemother 51: 3374–3377.

19. Lina G, Piemont Y, Godail-Gamot F, Bes M, Peter MO, et al. (1999) Involvement of Panton-Valentine leukocidin-producing Staphylococcus aureus in primary skin infections and pneumonia. Clin Infect Dis 29: 1128–1132.
20. Enright MC, Day NP, Davies CE, Peacock SJ, Spratt BG (2000) Multilocus sequence typing for characterization of methicillin-resistant and methicillin-susceptible clones of Staphylococcus aureus. J Clin Microbiol 38: 1008–1015.
21. Institute CaLS (2006) Methods for Dilution Antimicrobial Susceptibility Tests for Bacteria that Grow Aerobically. Approved standard M07-A7. Villanova, PA: Clinical and Laboratory Standards Institute.
22. Bens CC, Voss A, Klaassen CH (2006) Presence of a novel DNA methylation enzyme in methicillin-resistant Staphylococcus aureus isolates associated with pig farming leads to uninterpretable results in standard pulsed-field gel electrophoresis analysis. J Clin Microbiol 44: 1875–1876.
23. Tenover FC, Arbeit RD, Goering RV, Mickelsen PA, Murray BE, et al. (1995) Interpreting chromosomal DNA restriction patterns produced by pulsed-field gel electrophoresis: criteria for bacterial strain typing. J Clin Microbiol 33: 2233–2239.
24. Guardabassi L, Stegger M, Skov R (2007) Retrospective detection of methicillin resistant and susceptible Staphylococcus aureus ST398 in Danish slaughter pigs. Vet Microbiol 122: 384–386.
25. Leclercq R (2002) Mechanisms of resistance to macrolides and lincosamides: nature of the resistance elements and their clinical implications. Clin Infect Dis 34: 482–492.
26. Economic Research Service UDoAER (2006) Hogs: Trade. http://www.ers.usda.gov/Briefing/Hogs/Trade.htm.
27. Wulf M, Markenstein A, van der Linden F, Voss A, Klaassen C, et al. (2008) First outbreak of MRSA ST398 in a Dutch hospital. 18th European Congress of Clinical Microbiology and Infectious Diseases, April 19–22, Barcelona, Spain.
28. USDA National Agriculture Statistics Service
29. Honeyman M, Duffy M (2006) Iowa's Changing Swine Industry. http://www.econ.iastate.edu/research/webpapers/paper_12581.pdf.
30. Ince D, Winokur P, Beekmann S, Herwaldt L, Pfaller M, et al. (2005) Prevalence of Panton Valentine Leukocidin genes among methicillin-resistant Staphylococcus aureus in Iowa. Society for Healthcare Epidemiology of America 15th Annual Scientific Meeting, April 9–12, Los Angeles, CA.
31. Van de Griend P, Herwaldt LA, Alvis B, Demartino M, Heilmann K, et al. (2007) Community-associated methicillin-resistant Staphylococcus aureus (CA-MRSA): an emerging cause of bloodstream infection (BSI) in Iowa. 47th Interscience Conference on Antimicrobial Agents and Chemotherapy, September 17–20, Chicago, IL.
32. van Loo IH, Diederen BM, Savelkoul PH, Woudenberg JH, Roosendaal R, et al. (2007) Methicillin-resistant Staphylococcus aureus in meat products, the Netherlands. Emerg Infect Dis 13: 1753–1755.

SECTION V: LISTERIA MONOCYTOGENES – FOODBORNE BACTERIA

CHAPTER 23 LISTERIA MONOCYTOGENES ASSOCIATED KERATO-CONJUNCTIVITIS IN FOUR HORSES IN NORWAY

Tobias Revold, Takele Abayneh, Hege BrunHansen, Signe L. Kleppe, ErnstOtto Ropstad, Robert A. Hellings and Henning Sørum

Keywords: Equine, Cornea, Bacterial keratitis, Conjunctivitis, *Listeria monocytogenes,* Antimicrobial susceptibility

BACKGROUND

Listeria monocytogenes is an aerobic, Gram positive rod that can be found ubiquitously in nature, but is also capable of causing severe disease [1, 2]. Sheep, cattle, goats and chickens are considered to be the most susceptible species [3], but all animals including humans can be infected [1]. The bacterium is also recognized as an important foodborne pathogen [4]. Septicemia, encephalitis or abortions are the most common clinical manifestations of infection [2], but ocular symptoms may also be seen. In food animal species ocular symptoms are most commonly associated with infections affecting the nervous system [5]. The term "silage eye" refers to listerial kerato-conjunctivitis, and may involve uveitis with hypopyon and miosis [6, 7]. In a questionnaire survey in England, "silage eye" was recognized as the most common clinical manifestation of listerial infection in dairy cattle, but the study did not include bacteriological data [6].

In humans, conjunctivitis is the most common ocular presentation of *L. monocytogenes* infection. Listerial conjunctivitis may either be endogenous in patients with meningitis, or exogenous [8]. Human cases of listerial keratitis and endophthalmitis have also been reported [8, 9, 10, 11, 12]. Human listerial endophthalmitis has been associated with a characteristic pigmented hypopyon and elevated intraocular pressure [8, 13].

Citation: Tobias Revold, Takele Abayneh, Hege Brun-Hansen, Signe L. Kleppe, Ernst-Otto Ropstad, Robert A. Hellings and Henning Sørum, Listeria monocytogenes associated kerato-conjunctivitis in four horses in Norway, DOI: 10.1186/s13028-015-0167-2.

Although listeriosis is less common in horses than in ruminants, there have been reports on abortions [2, 14, 15], intra-uterine infection [16, 17], meningo-encephalitis [18, 19, 20] and septicaemia [17, 18, 21, 22, 23, 24]. The authors are only aware of two previously reported cases of equine kerato-conjunctivitis associated with *L. monocytogenes* [25, 26]. This report describes four cases of equine kerato-conjunctivis in Norway. The clinical course of the disease, as well as microbiological features and antimicrobial susceptibility (both in vitro *and* in vivo) of *L. monocytogenes* isolated from all 4 cases are described.

CASE PRESENTATIONS

Case 1

A 12-year-old brown Standardbred mare with a 12 months history of unilateral recurrent kerato-conjunctivitis was presented to the field practice of the Norwegian School of Veterinary Science (NSVS). The horse was fed plastic wrapped silage and a commercial concentrate mix. Two previous attempts to treat the horse with topical fucidic acid eyedrops (Fucithalmic[1]) and oxytetracyclin/polymyxin B (Terramycin-Polymyxin B[2]) eye ointment were unsuccessful.

The ophthalmic examination was performed using a focal light source and revealed mild blepharospasm of the right eye with a mild mucopurulent discharge. The palpebral conjunctivae were moderately hyperaemic and chemotic. Direct and consensual pupillary light reflexes were normal, and no sign of miosis or aqueous flare were seen. Multiple grayish-white sub-epithelial opacities were observed in the part of the cornea, with an irregular overlying epithelial surface in an area of approximately 5 × 5 mm. This area was surrounded by a diffuse stromal edema covering approximately half of the cornea. A bacterial swab was collected from the corneal lesion, and transferred to a sterile transport medium. The fluorescein dye test was negative.

The preliminary diagnosis was bacterial kerato-conjunctivitis, and treatment with chloramphenicol eye ointment (Chloramphenicol[3]) 3–4 times daily was initiated. *L. monocytogenes* and *Micrococcus* sp. were cultured from the bacterial swab. The *L. monocytogenes* was considered to be of potential clinical relevance, and was found to be sensitive to chloramphenicol. However, no improvement was observed upon re-examination 15 days later. A new bacterial swab confirmed the continuous presence of *L. monocytogenes*. Treatment was altered to topical ampicillin (Pentrexyl 500 mg[4] in 5 ml sterile water), gentamicin eyedrops (Garamycin[5]) and diclofenac eye drops (Voltaren Ophtha[6]); all four times daily. In addition, the horse was treated with systemic procaine penicillin (Penovet vet[7]; 20 000 IU i.m.) twice daily and gentamicin (Genta-Kél[8]; 6.6 mg/kg i.v.) once daily; both for 5 days. A continuous gradual improvement was seen until the horse was deemed sound by the owner around day 55, and all treatment was discontinued.

At day 69, however, symptoms similar to those described at day 1 recurred, and again, *L. monocytogenes* and *Micrococcus* sp. were cultured. Treatment with topical ciprofloxacin eyedrops (Cilox[9]) and diclofenac eye drops [Voltaren Ophtha (see footnote 6)]; both four times daily, was initiated. At day 114 the horse was hospitalized at the NSVS equine clinic.

Ophthalmic examination at the NSVS confirmed abnormal findings restricted to the cornea and the conjunctiva. The fluorescein dye test was still negative. Bacterial swabs were collected both prior to and after epithelial scrapings for cytology, which resulted in considerable epithelial detachment. *L. monocytogenes* was cultured from both bacterial swabs, but the highest numbers were found prior to scraping. No fungi were cultured. Cytology revealed a high number of rods associated with the squamous epithelial cells that were seen both as aggregates and isolated. No neutrophils or fungi were seen.

A sub-palpebral lavage system attached to a continuous infusion pump system[10] was inserted through the upper eyelid. Benzylpenicillin sodium (Penicillin 600 mg[11] in 5 ml sterile water) and gentamicin [Garamycin (see footnote 5)] eye drops were mixed daily and used in the infusion pump. In addition, the horse was given systemic procaine penicillin [Penovet vet (see footnote 7); 20,000 IU i.m.] twice daily for 10 days, and systemic vedaprofen [Quadrisol vet (see footnote 2); 1 mg/kg after an initial dose of 2 mg/kg] once daily for 15 days.

At day 118, the footplate of the lavage system was noted to have caused a superficial ulceration in the dorsal cornea. The infusion set was therefore removed, and a new set was inserted in the nasal part of the lower eye lid, thereby protected by the membrana nictitans. The corneal lesion created by the lavage system healed uneventfully within a week, indicating a normal corneal healing ability.

At day 128, at which no bacteria were identified in a follow-up cytological evaluation, the apparently irritating topical benzylpenicillin sodium treatment was discontinued. Topical treatment with gentamicin [Garamycin (see footnote 5)] eye drops via the lavage system was maintained. The following days the inflammation was gradually reduced. At day 140, severe kerato-conjunctivitis recurred. Slides for cytological examination were prepared, of which one contained a high number of bacteria morphologically identical to *L.monocytogenes*associated with squamous epithelial cells. Interestingly, such bacteria were not seen on three further slides. The combined treatment with benzylpenicillin sodium [Penicillin 600 mg (see footnote 11) in 5 ml sterile water] and gentamicin [Garamycin (see footnote 5)] eye drops via continuous flow was restarted, but financial constraints made further treatment at the clinic impossible. Due to the nervous disposition of the horse, enucleation was not considered to be an option.

The horse was therefore released from the clinic against medical advice on day 150, and treated by the owner with oxytetracyclin/polymyxin B [Terramycin-Polymyxin B (see footnote 2)] eye ointment three times daily in an attempt to control the infection. Four weeks later, the horse was involved in a car accident and had to be euthanized due to its injuries.

Case 2

A 7-year-old grey Connemara gelding with a history of recurrent unilateral kerato-conjunctivitis the last 6 months was referred to the NSVS. The pony was fed hay and a commercial concentrate mix, but was also fed plastic wrapped haylage from the ground of the paddocks at daytime. Although treatment with chloramphenicol eye ointment [Chloramphenicol (see footnote 3)] and diclofenac eye drops [Voltaren Ophtha (see footnote 6)] appeared to be effective, clinical signs recurred repeatedly after treatment withdrawal. The pony exhibited a marked blepharospasm of the left eye, a moderate periorbital edema with moderately hyperemic and chemotic palpebral conjunctivae, combined with a mild serous discharge. Slightly nasal to the centre of the cornea, there was a faint, diffusely outlined greyish-white epithelial and sub-epithelial opacity of approximately 2–3 mm diameter. There were no signs of uveitis. A bacterial swab was collected prior to the fluorescein dye test, which revealed a strong dye uptake in the centre of the lesion. There were no signs of neovascularisation. A corneal scraping for cytological evaluation resulted in epithelial detachment in an area of approximately 4 × 4 mm. The preliminary diagnosis was kerato-conjunctivitis of possible viral aetiology. Treatment with idoxuridine eye ointment (Iducher[12]) four times daily, fucidic acid eye drops [Fucithalmic (see footnote 1)] twice daily and diclofenac eye drops [Voltaren Ophtha (see footnote 6)] three times daily was initiated. The cytological findings indicated possible listeria keratitis. This was confirmed by culturing of *L. monocytogenes*. Based on the results of the sensitivity testing, topical antibiotics were changed to oxytetracyclin/polymyxin B [Terramycin-Polymyxin B (see footnote 2] three times daily, and antiviral and anti-inflammatory treatment was continued.

On day 12, the opacities were hardly visible, and there was no discharge or signs of conjunctivitis. Treatment with oxytetracyclin/polymyxin B [Terramycin-Polymyxin B (see footnote 2)] and idoxuridine eye ointment [Iducher (see footnote 12)] was continued for another 7 days, while diclofenac was discontinued.

On day 29, the pony was re-examined. The symptoms had gradually returned, and the owner had restarted treatment with oxytetracyclin/polymyxin B [Terramycin-Polymyxin B (see footnote 2)]. There was a diffuse stromal edema in the ventronasal cornea, surrounding several white "spots" of approximately 1 mm diameter. The left pupil was slightly miotic consistent with mild anterior uveitis, but successfully dilated after 1 drop of 1 % atropine eye drops (Atropin Minims[13]). Treatment with oxytetracyclin/polymyxin B [Terramycin-Polymyxin B (see footnote 2)], idoxuridine eye ointment [Iducher (see footmote 12)] and diclofenac eyedrops [Voltaren Ophtha (see footnote 6)] as described above was restarted. Again, *L. monocytogenes* was cultured from a bacterial swab from the corneal lesions. Around day 45, the horse was judged sound by the owner, and all medication was discontinued.

On day 76, the same symptoms recurred. Treatment with ciprofloxacin eye drops [Cilox (see footnote 9)] QID was started, and maintained for 4 weeks. In a telephone interview 6 years later, the owner reported that the pony had shown no symptoms of ocular disease since this treatment. They had, however, also stopped using haylage in the paddocks.

Case 3

A 10-year-old Icelandic horse, which was kept in a group and fed plastic wrapped silage, was referred to the NSVS for evaluation of kerato-conjunctivitis in the right eye of 1 month duration. Despite initial improvement after treatment with fucidic acid eye drops [Fucithalmic (see footnote 1)] twice daily for 10 days, the symptoms recurred when treatment was stopped. The same treatment was re-initiated, this time without noticeable effect.

The horse was presented with a mild blepharospasm of the right eye, a moderate periorbital edema with moderately hyperaemic and chemotic palpebral conjunctivae. Slightly nasal to the centre of the cornea, there was a very faint grayish epithelial opacity, only visible with a focal light source. No further pathology was seen. A bacterial swab was collected as previously described. The fluorescein dye test was negative. Treatment with chloramphenicol eye ointment [Chloramphenicol (see footnote 3)] three to four times daily and diclofenac eye drops [Voltaren Ophtha (see footnote 6)] two to three times daily was initiated awaiting sampling results.

At day 6, *L. monocytogenes* was cultured from a bacterial swab. The topical antibiotic treatment was changed to ciprofloxacin eyedrops [Cilox (see footnote 9)] four times daily for 4 weeks. At day 30, the owner reported that the symptoms were reduced, but that a mild epiphora was still present. The treatment was therefore prolonged for another 14 days.

A few days after discontinuation of treatment, the symptoms recurred. At re-examination on day 48, the clinical findings were identical to those described at day 1. A new bacterial swab revealed continuous growth of *L. monocytogenes* without changes to the sensitivity pattern. Due to the poor clinical effect of ciprofloxacin, treatment was changed back to chloramphenicol [Chloramphenicol (see footnote 3)] eyedrops 5 times daily (ointment at night) for 6 weeks. Around day 90, the owner discontinued the treatment without further veterinary consultation. The following days symptoms as originally described recurred. On day 104 the horse was hospitalized at the NSVS.

The diffusely outlined epithelial opacity was still faint, but now covering more than 50 % of the corneal surface. A few superficial stromal, very thin blood vessels were now seen progressing approximately 7 mm from the dorsal limbus. Mild uptake of fluorescein dye was found in a 5 mm diameter area located 5–10 mm from the ventronasal limbus.

The horse was treated with a continuous flow of chloramphenicol eyedrops [Chloramphenicol (see footnote 3)] via a superior subpalpebral lavage system attached to a continuous infusion pump system (see footnote 10) for 14 days and systemic procaine penicillin [Penovet vet (see footnote 7); 20,000 IU i.m.] twice daily for 10 days. At day 118 there were no signs of conjunctivitis, but still a faint epithelial opacity. The horse was sent home on another 14 days of chloramphenicol eye ointment [Chloramphenicol (see footnote 3)] four times daily.

According to a telephone interview with the owner at day 191 the horse had not showed signs of ocular disease after termination of treatment at day 132. Around day 280, the horse was presented to a field practitioner with bilateral conjunctivitis. Bacterial swabs were collected from both eyes and submitted to the NSVS for culturing. A mixed flora was cultured, dominated by *Staphylococcus aureus* in the right eye and *Pasturella sp* in the left eye; both sensitive to chloramphenicol. *L. monocytogenes* was not found at this stage.

Case 4

An 8-year-old Icelandic pony with a six month history of unilateral recurrent kerato-conjunctivitis, affecting the left eye was presented to the horse clinic at Bjerke Equine Hospital, Oslo. The owner had first noticed a problem approximately 5 months earlier whilst the horse was at pasture and described symptoms of recurrent blepharospasm with ocular discharge. The eye was treated topically on several occasions with no lasting improvement, however the examination findings and medications used are not known. Three months after the symptoms were first noticed, a superficial corneal ulcer associated with a corneal foreign body was observed by the attending veterinary surgeon. During the past 2 months, the horse had been fed plastic wrapped haylage from the ground. The foreign body was removed and the loose corneal epithelium surrounding the ulcer was debrided. The eye was medicated with topical chloramphenicol eye ointment [Chloramphenicol (see footnote 3)] three times daily for 1 week.

Two months after removal of the foreign body the horse was presented to Bjerke Equine Hospital due to persistent problems with the eye. On examination the eye showed moderate blepharospasm with slight epiphora. No sign of anterior uveitis was evident. The cornea had a dull appearance and there was a small area of epithelium, approximately 1 cm in diameter, in the cornea which had an uneven, stippled appearance. Fluorescein and Rose Bengal staining was negative. No further abnormalities were found.

The cornea was treated topically with neomycin sulphate, polymyxin B sulphate and dexamethasone [Maxitrol (see footnote 9)] three times daily. The owner noticed an immediate improvement and on re-examination 1 week later the horse exhibited no blepharospasm or ocular discharge. The corneal surface was shiny and smooth. The only abnormality noticed was several very small, <1 mm, white sub-epithelial opacities in the cornea. Medication was continued for one week.

Two to three days after treatment was discontinued, the owner noticed that the horse was showing signs of ocular discomfort once more. Treatment with topical 0.1 % dexamethasone disodium phosphate (Spersadex[14]) three times daily was instigated. The eye showed no improvement and was presented for re-examination 2 weeks later.

At re-examination the horse showed obvious blepharospasm and significant epiphora. The ventral palpebral conjunctiva was chemotic. A superficial corneal ulcer was present in the corneal area, approximately 8 × 5 mm, which was associated with a very mild, diffuse edema. The pupil was moderately miotic, indicating mild anterior uveitis. No corneal neovascularization was evident. Fluorescein testing resulted in a faint staining of the ulcer margins.

The epithelial surface was carefully scraped and slides prepared for cytology, thereby removing loosely adherent epithelium in an area of approximately 15 × 15 mm. A swab for bacterial and fungal culture was collected from the affected area of the cornea.

Whilst awaiting the results for the samples taken, the horse was hospitalized and the eye treated topically with oxytetracyclin/polymyxin B [Terramycin-Polymyxin B (see footnote 2)] three times daily. A 1 % atropine eyedrop [Atropin Minims (see footnote 13)] was applied on one occasion which resulted in a profound mydriasis. In addition the horse was treated with systemic flunixin meglumine (Finadyne Vet[15]; 1,1 mg/kg iv) once daily for a period of 5 days. After 5 days the horse showed no ocular discomfort or inflammation; the ulcer had healed and fluorescein staining was negative. At this point the horse was discharged and the owner continued with the antibiotic treatment for a further 7 days. Cytology revealed the presence of many rod-shaped bacteria in short chains indicative of *L. monocytogenes*. The bacteria were associated with squamous epithelial cells (Fig. 1). From the corneal swab it was cultured a sparse, mixed bacterial growth dominated by *L. monocytogenes*.

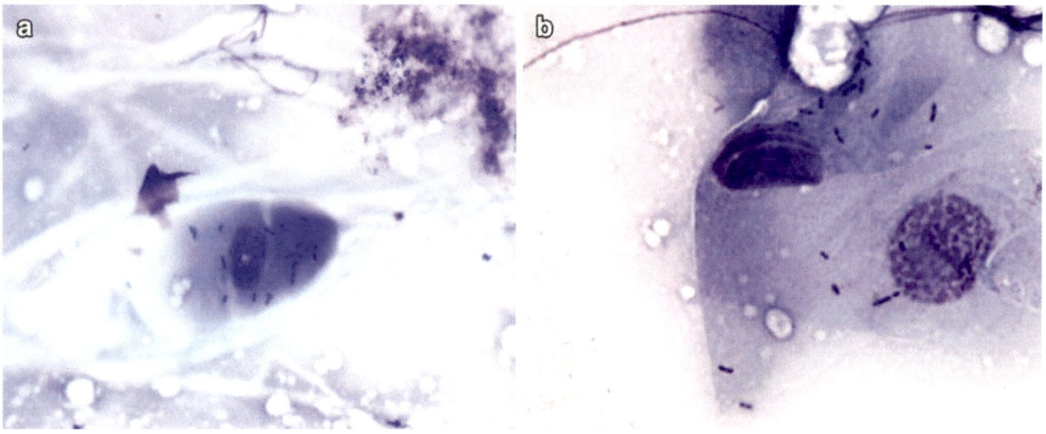

Figure 1: a. Squamous epithelial cell with typical rod-shaped bacteria on the surface. Note the absence of inflammatory cells. ×600 Modified Wright stain. **b** The rod-shaped bacteria are suggestive of *L. monocytogenes*. ×1000 Modified Wright stain.

The horse was re-examined 5 days after cessation of antibiotic treatment, 12 days after discharge from the hospital. On examination the horse showed no blepharospasm or ocular discharge. The conjunctivae were not inflamed and the cornea was smooth with a healthy, shiny corneal surface. No corneal ulcer, edema or neovascularisation was evident. Fluorescein and Rose Bengal staining was negative. Three small, <1 mm, white, sub-epithelial opacities in the area of previous ulceration were still visible with magnification. No bacterial growth was cultured from a corneal swab. Four months after discharge, the owner reported no sign of recurrence.

A brief overview of key clinical observations, culturing results and treatments in all four cases is given in Table 1.

Table 1: Key clinical observations, culturing results, topical and systemic treatments in four cases of equine keratitis

Case No	Day after initial examination	Clinical diagnoses	Bacterial growth after culturing[a]	Topical medication (frequency)[b]	Systemic medication (days)
1	1	Conjunctivitis, moderate superficial keratitis[1]	*Micrococcus* spp.—moderate *L. monocytogenes*—sparse	*Chloramphenicol (TID – QID)*	–
	15	Unchanged[1]	*L. monocytogenes*—sparse	*Ampicillin, Gentamicin (QID)Diclofenac (QID)*	*Procaine penicillin, Gentamicin (5 days)*
	55	No symptoms[2]		–	–
	69	Conjunctivitis, moderate superficial keratitis[1]	Normal flora dominated by *Micrococcus* spp. and *L. monocytogenes*	*Ciprofloxacin (QID)Diclofenac (QID)*	–
	114	Unchanged[1]	*L. monocytogenes*abundant before scraping/ very sparse after	Penicillin-Na, Gentamicin (CF)	Procaine penicillin (10 days) Vedaprofen (X days)
	128	superficial keratitis improved[1]	No listerial growth (selective enrichment)	Gentamicin (CF)	–
	140	Conjunctivitis, moderate superficial keratitis[1]		Penicillin-Na, Gentamicin (CF)	–
	150 (*released against medical advice)*	superficial keratitis improved[1]		*Oxytetracyclin - PolymyxinB (TID)*	–
	178 (*euthanized—unrelated reason)*	Unchanged[2]			
2	1	Conjunctivitis, mild–moderate superficial keratitis[1]	*L. monocytogenes*—sparse	*Oxytetracyclin - PolymyxinB (QID), Idoxuridine (QID), Diclofenac (TID)*	–
	12	Mild keratitis[1]		*Oxytetracyclin - PolymyxinB (QID 7 days), Idoxuridine (QID–7 days)*	–
	29	Conjunctivitis, mild–moderate superficial keratitis, mild anterior uveitis[1]	*L. monocytogenes*—moderate (pure culture)	*Oxytetracyclin - PolymyxinB (QID), Atropin (1 single drop), Idoxuridine QID, Diclofenac TID*	–
	45	No symptoms[2]		–	–
	76	Conjunctivitis, mild–moderate superficial keratitis[1]		*Ciprofloxacin (QID* 28 days *)*	–
	2200	No further symptoms[2]			–

3	1	Conjunctivitis, mild superficial keratitis[1]	*L. monocytogenes*—moderate (pure culture)	*Ciprofloxacin (QID)Diclofenac (BID-TID)*	–
	30	Conjunctivitis[2]		*Ciprofloxacin (QID)*	–
	44	None[2]		–	–
	48	Conjunctivitis, mild superficial keratitis[1]	*L. monocytogenes*—sparse (pure culture)	*Chloramphenicol (Eyedrops 5x/day* *Ointment at night 42 days)*	–
	90	None[2]			
	104	Conjunctivitis, mild–moderate superficial keratitis[1]	*L. monocytogenes*—very sparse (pure culture)	Chloramphenicol (CF)	Procaine penicillin (10 days)
	118	Mild keratitis[1]		*Chloramphenicol (QID – ointment 14 days)*	–
	162	No symptoms[2]			
4	1	Mild superficial keratitis[1]		*Neomycin - Polymyxin B-Dexamethasone (TID 14 days)*	–
	16	Conjunctivitis[2]		*Dexamethasone (TID)*	–
	28	Conjunctivitis, mild–moderate superficial keratitis (ulcerative), mild anterior uveitis[1]	Sparse, mixed bacterial growth dominated by *L. monocytogenes*	Oxytetracyclin-PolymyxinB (TID 5 days) Atropin (1 single drop) *Oxytetracyclin - PolymyxinB (TID 7 days)*	Flunixin (5 days)
	45	None[1]	No bacterial growth		
	160	No symptoms[2]			

Treatment prior to referral and short term medications awaiting culture results not included in the table. [1] Veterinary diagnoses, [2] Owner observation

italic treatment outside clinic, *BID* treatment twice daily, *TID* treatment 3 times daily, *QID* treatment 4 times daily, *CF*continuous flow via subpalpebral lavage system, underlined: antibiotic treatments

[a]Typically 3–5 days after sampling

[b]Topical antibiotics initiated after received culture report

Bacteriological examination and findings

In all cases, samples for microbiology were collected during the initial examination and for follow-up and evaluation of treatment response. Sterile cotton swabs in Amies transport medium without charcoal (Copan M40 Transystem[16]) were used for transporting swab specimens to the bacteriological and mycological diagnostic laboratory at the NSVS, where culturing was started within a few hours after sampling.

Media and cultivation

The samples were in all cases incubated on parallel agar plates (blood agar base no 1)[17] with 5 % cattle blood of which one was incubated at 37 °C in 5 % CO_2 atmosphere for 24 h while the other was incubated anaerobically for 48 h. The samples were also inoculated in serum broth (see footnote 17) and incubated at 37 °C in 5 % CO_2 atmosphere for 24 h for enrichment of growth for secondary plating on blood agar in case of no visual growth on primary blood agar after 24 h.

In addition, the samples were routinely incubated on bromothymol blue agar used for detection of bacteria in the *Enterobacteriaceae* family and other Gram-negative rods.

Materials from samples were also directly Gram stained to detect any bacteria in the sample before cultivation.

Culture examination and biochemical tests

Growth on the plates was examined followed by recording of morphological and other features of the colonies such as occurrence of any haemolytic zones. Gram stained colony material was examined and cell morphology recorded. Potential *Listeria*-like colonies were secondarily streaked on blood agar plates at right angles close to simultaneously streaked cultures of *Staphylococcus pseudintermedius* and *Rhodococcus equi*to detect any CAMP phenomenon.

Biochemical tests of *Listeria*-like colonies included the catalase test, fermentation of glucose, degradation of aesculin, hippurat and H_2S. The methyl red, Voges Proskauer and motility tests (in semi-liquid agar grown at 22 and 37 °C) were also performed.

Bacteriological findings from all eye swab samples collected during the course of the disease in all cases are summarized in Table 1. Colonies suspected to be *L. monocytogenes* were 1.0 mm in diameter, convex and grey to white in colour with a clear zone of β-haemolysis extending barely (about 0.5 mm) outside the colony edge. There was no growth on bromothymol blue agar from any of the corneal swabs. There was no evidence of any antibacterial agent in the material from initial corneal swabs as seen from the control growth of *S. pseudintermedius* on the blood agar incubated in CO_2 atmosphere. The same type of colony was detected on blood agar after cultivation from the LB enrichment broth after one, two and 3 days. In all four cases culturing revealed a low to moderate number of colonies in pure culture with similar cultural characteristics to *L. monocytogenes* (Table 1).

Phenotypical and biochemical features of β-hemolytic colonies

The β-hemolytic colonies from the corneal swabs contained bacteria that were Gram positive, short coccoid and regular sized rods. The isolates were catalase positive, fermented glucose, did not metabolise aesculin or hippurate, produced H_2S, and were negative on methyl red and Voges Proskauer tests. They were non-motile on semi-solid agar at 37 °C, but motile at 22 °C. They showed weak CAMP reaction with β-toxic *S. pseudintermedius* but were CAMP negative with *R. equi.* The biochemical profile and phenotypic features suggest that the colonies were *L. monocytogenes*.

Serotyping and antimicrobial susceptibility testing

Incubation of the test samples and cultures of *L. monocytogenes* reference strains CCUG 15527 (serotype 1) and CCUG 7995 (serotype 4) for 24 h at 37 °C demonstrated that the isolated *L. monocytogenes* of all cases belonged to the O serotype 1 judged by the phenotypical similarity of the colonies and their haemolytic zones.

Agglutination tests performed on glass slides with antisera against *Listeria* O type 1 (see footnote 17) and *Listeria* O type 4 (see footnote 17) also showed the same result. Antimicrobial susceptibility tests were carried out using the tablet diffusion method with twelve different antibacterial drugs including penicillin, ampicillin, cefalexin, amoxycillin, amoxycillin with clavulanic acid, sulphadiazine/trimethoprim, tetracycline, gentamicin, lincomycin, chloramphenicol, fucidic acid, enrofloxacin, and colicin. Agar diffusion on Müller-Hinton (MH) agar (see footnote 17) was used with tablets containing antibiotics (Neo-Sensitabs)[18] for the susceptibility tests. The tests showed that isolates of *L. monocytogenes* from all four cases were found to be either moderately susceptible or in some cases resistant towards fucidic acid. The isolates of *L. monocytogenes* from case 3 and 4 (both from the initial and follow-up isolations) were found to be intermediate susceptible towards enrofloxacin. The isolates were found to be susceptible to all other antimicrobial drugs tested.

General discussion

The four cases of kerato-conjunctivitis in horses associated with *L. monocytogenes* reported in this study represent the first reported cases in Scandinavia.

L. monocytogenes is a facultative intracellular pathogen widely distributed in the environment where most animals are exposed to the organism during their lifetime. The bacterium causes disease either when the host's immune system is compromised or when the bacterium occurs in numbers high enough to overwhelm the host's defence mechanisms [2, 9, 11]. Although the common route of infection is oral, the bacterium may also enter the body through the nasal mucosa or open wounds. The conjunctiva has also been mentioned as a possible entrance [24, 34]. In contrast to the high frequency of ocular signs of listeriosis described in cattle [2], ocular listerial infections seem to be rare in horses with only two cases reported so far [25, 26].

All cases reported here had symptoms of corneal disease for an extended time period prior to referral. Hence, it is not possible to determine the pathogenesis in these cases with certainty. *L. monocytogenes* serotype O type 1, a common strain found in the environment, in silage and in systemically infected animals [22], was cultured from all cases reported here. This is in agreement with the theory of silage as the most likely source of infection, and with the findings of Evans et al. [26] that ocular listerial infections seem to be caused by common strains of the bacterium that are also found in systemic infection.

The intact and healthy cornea is highly resistant to bacterial infection, due to a continuous flow of a tear film with antimicrobial properties, as well as the physical barrier of a healthy epithelium [27]. It has, however, been shown that *L. monocytogenes* may penetrate into undamaged corneal epithelial cells of guinea pigs [28]. Further, conjunctivitis and/or kerato-conjunctivitis has been induced experimentally in guinea pigs and rabbits simply by direct inoculation of *L. monocytogenes*, while similar direct inoculation of a variety of other bacteria did not cause infection [29]. In fact, this characteristic ability to cause conjunctivitis and keratitis was in 1939 even proposed as a method to identify an infectious culture as *L. monocytogenes* [30]. It has also been shown that the infectivity of listerial cultures after direct inoculation in rabbits is dose dependent [9]. Whether direct inoculation would cause kerato-conjunctivitis in a horse remains speculative, not least given the more than 3 times thicker corneal epithelium in horses [31, 32] compared to rabbits [33].

There is a well-known general association between silage feeding and listeriosis [5, 34, 35, 36, 37]. In horses, systemic *L. monocytogenes* infections have been associated with silage feeding [22, 26], feeding on poor quality hay [17] or grazing on spray and flood-irrigated grass clover pasture [14]. Plastic wrapped forage (silage or haylage) is commonly used to feed horses in Norway, especially during the winter season, and appears to be the most likely source of *L. monocytogenes* in the cases described here. Grass silage produced in cool, wet climates tends to have lower sugar levels and higher moisture contents than silage produced in warmer climates. This may result in a poorer and slower fermentation, which provides better conditions for the proliferation of *L. monocytogenes* in the silage [38]. Poor quality hay or soil-contaminated forage represent other possible sources of infection in these cases.

In several studies, feeding of animals with silage placed at or above head height in such a way that silage material could fall into the eyes of the animals has been incriminated as a possible predisposing factor of listerial eye infection [35, 37, 39]. Such feeding routines are not common in horses. Still, frozen forage or forage made into a hard bale as in silage or haylage may be difficult to pretend, and horses may pull forage out of the bale and throw it up in the air, increasing the likelihood of ocular exposure to contaminated material. Hence, it appears possible that feeding routines, although not further investigated, may have played a role in these cases.

Corticosteroid treatment is known to increase the infectivity of *L. monocytogenes* in laboratory animals [1]. The case of equine listerial keratitis reported by Sanchez et al. [25] had been treated with topical steroids prior to referral. Only one of the horses included in this report (case 4) had been treated with topical steroids prior to the identification of *L. monocytogenes,* and no other signs of immunosuppression were identified in any of these cases.

L. monocytogenes is often detected in low numbers by cultivation, sometimes together with other bacteria. This observation is important for the bacteriologist when cultivating samples from cases of keratitis, and may be related to the intracellular growth of *L. monocytogenes.* The low number of *Listeria* bacteria seen on culturing may have contributed to the low number of reported cases in the literature. Also, as noted by other authors there may be lacking awareness among clinicians as well as bacteriologists regarding the potential role of *L. monocytogenes* in ocular infections [9, 11, 26]. A thorough cytologic evaluation of corneal scrapings was found to be of great help in these cases, but comprehensive sampling is crucial as indicated by positive findings in only one out of several slides at the last recurrence in case 1.

Listerial infections are commonly treated with penicillins or tetracylines, which may be effective in early stages of systemic disease. However, if severe symptoms have developed prior to initiation of intensive antibiotic treatment, the outcome is commonly fatal [2].

Combined use of gentamycin and penicillin was found to be more effective than either of the antibiotics used alone in treatment of experimental listerial keratitis in rabbits [9]. The same combination of antibiotics was used systemically as well as topically for successful treatment of a severe case of human listerial keratitis [9].

Based on these findings, penicillins (ampicillin or penicillin G) and gentamicin were used systemically and topically in case 1. Some comments need to be made regarding this combined treatment: The low lipophilicity of Penicillin G likely restricts its ability to penetrate the barrier of the lipophilic corneal epithelium. Although topical penicillin treatment has been recommended for use in humans with ocular surface disease [40], the poor penetration of the epithelium may well limit the efficacy of the drug against intracellularly located strains of *Listeria.* Notable in this context is the fact that the horses in this study on many occasions had intact epithelium covering the corneal lesions, as demonstrated by negative Fluorescein dye tests. Further, aminoglycosids may be inactivated in plasma in approximately 8–48 h in the presence of ß-lactams [41]. In order to minimize inactivation, a fresh mixture for continuous flow treatment was prepared daily in case 1. The extent of potential aminoglycoside inactivation was not investigated. Despite these factors, this combined treatment appeared to be effective, but was probably stopped too early.

Various other recommendations have been published with regards to treatment of ocular listerial infections. Both the previously reported cases of listerial kerato-conjunctivitis in horses were treated successfully with kinolones (alone or in combination) [25, 26]. Based on these reports, the kinolone Ciprofloxacin was used in cases 1–3, but this treatment was only successful in case 2. These treatments were carried out by the horse owners, and it is possible that the lack of success may have been related to owners' compliance. On the other hand, failure of listerial keratitis to respond to treatment with the kinolone Ofloxacin despite in vitro susceptibility has been reported in a human patient [10]. Interestingly, the isolates from cases 3 and 4 were found to be intermediate susceptible towards enrofloxacin, which was the only kinolone available for susceptibility testing.

The isolates described here were found to be susceptible to most of the antibiotics tested, but intermediately susceptible or in some cases resistant to fucidic acid. Fucidic acid is commonly used as a "first choice" antibiotic to treat suspected bacterial keratitis or conjunctivitis in Norway, and had been used prior to referral at least in cases 1 and 3.

Despite extremely prolonged unsuccessful treatment with chloramphenicol in case 3, hospitalization and intensified treatment with continuous flush using the same antibiotic led to final resolution of the symptoms, although this final treatment was supplemented by systemic penicillin for 10 days. Although the possibility of re-infections cannot be completely ruled out, we believe recurrences of symptoms in these horses after termination of treatment were related to lack of successful elimination of the infective agent, not least due to the consistent unilaterality of the clinical signs. In summary, we believe that several antibiotics may be used successfully for treatment, but that extra attention must be paid to intensity and duration of treatment once *L. monocytogenes* has been identified in cases of equine kerato-conjunctivitis. Cases should also be monitored closely after termination of antibiotic treatment. Difficulties in treatment similar to those described here have also been reported in human ophthalmology [9, 10, 11, 42].

CONCLUSIONS

L. monocytogenes should be considered a potential pathogen in cases of indolent bacterial kerato-conjunctivitis in horses, especially in animals fed with silage or haylage.

Special attention may be required from clinicians as well as bacteriologists and clinical pathologists in order to identify the bacteria. The generally poor response to treatment and frequent recurrences in the cases described here indicate that clinicians should pay extra attention to the choice of antimicrobial drugs, and to the intensity and duration of the treatment regimen if *L. monocytogenes* is identified from equine keratitic lesions. Further research is needed to determine whether *L. monocytogenes* may act as a primary pathogen, or rather as a secondary invader in cases of pre-existing corneal lesions.

Footnotes

[1]Dechra Veterinary Products A/S, Uldum, Denmark.

[2]Pfizer Inc, New York, USA.

[3]Nycomed Pharma A/S, Asker, Norway.

[4]Bristol-Myers Squibb Company, New York, USA.

[5]Schering-Plough International, Kenilworth, New Jersey, USA.

[6]Novartis Healthcare A/S, København, Denmark.

[7]Boehringer Ingelheim Danmark A/S, København, Denmark.

[8]Kela N.V., Hoogstraten, Belgium.

[9]Alcon Laboratories, Inc., Fort Worth Texas, USA.

[10]Mila International, http://milainternational.com/.

[11]Actavis Group, Hafnarfjordur, Iceland.

[12]Farmigea S.p.A., Pisa, Italy.

[13]Bausch & Lomb U.K. Ltd., Surrey, England.

[14]OmniVison AB, Danderyd, Sweden.

[15]Intervet International B.V, Boxmeer, The Netherlands.

[16]Copan Italia S.p.A., Brescia, Italy.

[17]Difco Laboratories Inc., Detroit, Michigan, USA.

[18]Rosco, Taastrup, Denmark.

DECLARATIONS

Authors' contributions

SLK was largely involved in the description of case 1, and had the initial idea of reporting it together with HBH and HS. EOR was largely involved in treatment and description of cases 2 and 3, TR of cases 1-3, RAH treated and described case 4, HBH was responsible for cytological evaluations and descriptions, TA and HS were responsible for the bacteriology. TR and TA drafted the manuscript. All authors were involved in continuous discussions regarding the manuscript. All authors read and approved the final manuscript.

REFERENCES

1. Gray ML, Killinger AH. *Listeria monocytogenes* and listeric infections. Bacteriol Rev. 1966;30:309–74.
2. Radostits OM, Blood DC, Gay CC. Diseases caused by *Listeria* spp. In: Veterinary medicine. 8th edition. London: Bailliere Tindall; 1994, p. 660-6.
3. Wesley IV. Listeriosis in animals. In: Ryser ET, Marth EH, editors. Listeria, listeriosis, and food safety. New York: Marcel Dekker; 1999. p. 39–40.
4. Schlech WF. Listeriosis: epidemiology, virulence and the significance of contaminated foodstuffs. J Hosp Infect. 1991;19:211–24.
5. Cullen CL, Webb AA. Ocular manifestations of systemic disease. Part 4: food animals. In: Gelatt KN, Gilger BC, Kern TJ, Ames IA (editors) Veterinary Ophthalmology. Volume 2. 5th edition. : Wiley-Blackwell; 2013. p. 2071–101.
6. Erdogan HM, Cetinkaya B, Green LE, Cripps PJ, Morgan KL. Prevalence, incidence, signs and treatment of clinical listeriosis in dairy cattle in England. Vet Rec. 2001;149:289–93.
7. Pearce JW, Moore CP. Food animal ophthalmology. In: Gelatt KN, Gilger BC, Kern TJ, Ames IA, editors. Veterinary ophthalmology. Volume 2. 5th edition. Wiley-Blackwell; 2013. p. 1610–74.
8. Eliott D, O'Brien TP, Green WR, Jampel HD, Goldberg MF. Elevated intraocular pressure, pigment dispersion and dark hypopyon in endogenous endophthalmitis from *Listeria monocytogenes*. Surv Ophthalmol. 1992;37:117–24.
9. Zaidman GW, Coudron P, Piros J. *Listeria monocytogenes* keratitis. Am J Ophthalmol. 1990;109:334–9.
10. Altaie R, Fahy GT, Cormican M. Failure of *Listeria monocytogenes* keratitis to respond to topical ofloxacin. Cornea. 2006;25:849–50.
11. Eiferman RA, Flaherty KT, Rivard AK. Persistent corneal defect caused by *Listeria monocytogenes*. Am J Ophthalmol. 1990;109:97–8.
12. Duch ST, Quintana MC, Pujol OG. *Listeria monocytogenes* endophthalmitis. Acta Ophthalmol. 1991;69:108–10.
13. Alkatan HM, Al-Dhibi HA, Edward DP, Al-Rajhi AA. Pigmented hypopyon in association with *Listeria monocytogenes*endophthalmitis: An interesting case report following refractive surgery procedure with literature review. Middle East Afr J Ophthalmol. 2014;21:40–3.
14. Mason RW, Brennan RG, Corbould A. *Listeria monocytogenes* abortion in a mare. Austr Vet J. 1980;56:613.
15. Welsh RD. Equine abortion caused by *Listeria monocytogenes* serotype 4. J Am Vet Med Assoc. 1983;183:291.
16. Mayer H, Kinler M, Sickel E. Listeriose in einem Reitpferdebestand. Berl Münch Tierärztl Wochenschr. 1976;89:209–11.
17. Higgins R, Goyette G, Sauvageau R, Lemaire T. Septicemia due to *Listeria monocytogenes* in a newborn foal. Can Vet J. 1987;28:1–2.
18. Pirs T, Zdovc I, Gombac M, Svara T, Juntes P, Vengust M. *Listeria monocytogenes* septicaemia in a foal. Slov Vet Res. 2005;42:49–53.
19. Clark EG, Turner ES, Boysen BG, Rouse BT. Listeriosis in an Arabian foal with combined immunodeficiency. J Am Vet Med Assoc. 1978;172:363–6.
20. Rütten M, Lehner A, Pospischil A, Sydler T. Cerebral listeriosis in an Adult Freiberger Gelding. J Comp Path. 2006;134:249–53.
21. Monteiro F, Wong D, Scarratt WK, Buechner-Maxwell V, Crisman M. *Listeria monocytogenes* septicaemia in two neonatal foals. Equine Vet Educ. 2006;18:27–31.

22. Gudmundsdottir KB, Svansson V, Aalbæk B, Gunnarsson E, Sigurdarson S. *Listeria monocytogenes* in horses in Iceland. Vet Rec. 2004;155:456–9.
23. Jose-Cunilleras E, Hinchcliff KW. *Listeria monocytogenes* septicaemia in foals. Equine Vet J. 2001;33:519–22.
24. Wilkins PA, Marsh PS, Acland H, Piero FD. *Listeria monocytogenes* septicemia in a Thoroughbred foal. J Vet Diagn Invest. 2000;12:173–6.
25. Sanchez S, Struder M, Currin P, Barell P, Bounous D. Listeria keratitis in a horse. Vet Ophthalmol. 2001;4:129–217.
26. Evans K, Smith M, McDonough P, Wiedmann M. Eye infections due to *Listeria monocytogenes* in three cows and one horse. J Vet Diagn Invest. 2004;16:464–9.
27. English R, Gilger BC. Ocular immunology. In: Gelatt KN, Gilger BC, Kern TJ, Ames IA, editors. Veterinary Ophthalmology. Volume 1. 5th edition. Wiley-Blackwell; 2013. p. 273–299.
28. Rácz P, Tenner K, Szivessy K. Electron microscopic studies in experimental keratoconjunctivitis listeriosa. I: Penetration of *Listeria monocytogenes* into corneal epithelial cells. Acta microbiol Acad Sci Hung. 1970;17:221–36.
29. Morris MC, Julianelle LA. A study of an infection induced experimentally with bacterium monocytogenes. Am J Ophthalmol. 1935;18:535–41.
30. Julianelle LA, Pons CA. Identification of *Listerella monocytogenes*. Proc Soc Exp Biol Med. 1939;40:362–3.
31. Ledbetter EC, Scarlett JM. In *vivo* confocal microscopy of the normal equine cornea and limbus. Vet Ophthalmol. 2009;12(Supplement 1):57–64.
32. Pirie CG, Alario AF, Barysauskas CM, Gradil C, Uricchio CK. Manual corneal thickness measurements of healthy equine eyes using a portable spectral-domain optical coherence tomography device. Equine Vet J. 2014;46:631–4.
33. Reiser BJ, Ignacio TS, Wang Y, Taban M, Graff JM, Sweet P, et al. *In vitro* measurement of rabbit corneal epithelial thickness using ultrahigh resolution optical coherence tomography. Vet Ophthalmol. 2005;8:85–8.
34. Braun U, Stehle C, Ehrensperger F. Clinical findings and treatment of listeriosis in 67 sheep and goats. Vet Rec. 2002;150:38–42.
35. Morgan JH. Infectious keratoconjunctivitis in cattle associated with *Listeria monocytogenes*. Vet Rec. 1977;100:113–4.
36. Kummeneje K, Mikkelsen T. Isolation of *Listeria monocytogenes* Type 04 from cases of keratoconjunctivitis in cattle and sheep. Nord Vet Med. 1975;27:144–9.
37. Welchman D, Hooton JK, Low JC. Ocular disease assosiated with silage feeding and *Listeria monocytogenes* in fallow deer. Vet Rec. 1997;140:684–5.
38. Fenlon DR. *Listeria monocytogenes* in the natural environment. In: Ryser ET, Marth EH, editors. *Listeria*, listeriosis and food safety. 2nd edition. New York: Marcel Dekker; 1999. p. 21–37.
39. Walker JK, Morgan JH. Ovine ophthalmitis associated with *Listeria monocytogenes*. Vet Rec. 1993;132:636.
40. Regnier A. Antimicrobials, Antiinfalmmatory Agents, and Antiglaucoma Drugs. In: Gelatt KN, Ames IA, editors. Veterinary ophthalmology. Volume 1. 4th edition. Blackwell Publishing; 2007. p. 288–331.
41. Riff LJ, Thomason JL. Comparative aminoglycoside inactivation by ß-lactam antibiotics. Effect of a cephalosporin and six penicillins on five aminoglycosides. J Antibiot. 1982;35:850–7.
42. Tay E, Rajan M, Tuft S. *Listeria Monocytogenes* sclerokeratitis. A case report and literature review. Cornea. 2008;27:947–9.

CHAPTER 24

OUTBREAK OF LISTERIA MONOCYTOGENES IN AN URBAN POULTRY FLOCK

Rocio Crespo, Michael M Garner, Sharon G Hopkins and Devendra H Shah

BACKGROUND

Listeriosis is caused by the bacterium *Listeria monocytogenes* and has a worldwide distribution. Although many species of birds are susceptible to infection, clinical disease in birds is rare. Young birds are most susceptible. *L. monocytogenes* infections in chickens occur in two forms: encephalitic or septicemic form. The encephalitic form is characterized by neurologic signs such as depression, incoordination and torticollis; whereas the septicemic form is characterized by diarrhea and emaciation.

L. monocytogenes has been isolated from poultry, poultry products, and ready-to-eat poultry meat [1, 2, 3]. One study showed that *L. monocytogenes* was isolated from >40% of the organic as well as non-organic commercial chicken meat in Maryland [4]. The vast majority of serotypes included 1/2a, 1/2b and 4b. Interestingly, out of more than 14 reported serotypes of *L. monocytogenes,* these three serotypes cause most of the clinical cases [5]. Several studies have reported that handling and consumption of contaminated raw broiler meat is an important risk factor for human infection. Because of the epidemiological importance of certain serotypes of *L. monocytogenes* to human health and potential transmission of the pathogen from poultry to humans, accurate detection of *L. monocytogenes* followed by subtyping methods to identify the specific serotype or genotype involved in outbreaks is essential.

Citation: Rocio Crespo, Michael M Garner, Sharon G Hopkins and Devendra H Shah, Outbreak of Listeria monocytogenes in an urban poultry flock, DOI: 10.1186/1746-6148-9-204.

This report describes an unusual presentation of listeriosis in adult chickens and the systematic use of molecular tests performed to diagnose listeriosis in this backyard poultry flock. Also, it stresses the importance of being aware of potentially zoonotic diseases.

CASE PRESENTATION

Clinical history

Several chickens from a backyard flock (Seattle, WA) were presented to a private veterinarian. The affected flock consisted of 20 chickens that were approximately 8 months of age at the time of presentation. During the course of the previous five months, a total of 7 birds had died and other 5 had shown clinical signs of illness. Most birds stopped producing eggs. The clinical signs included depression, anorexia and panting. The owner medicated the flock with sulfadimethoxine sodium in the water (1 fl oz of 12.5% Sulmet per gallon of drinking water; Fort Dodge Animal Health, Fort Dodge, IA) for 5 days. Despite this treatment, no improvement in clinical signs or egg production was noticed. The owner provided commercial layer feed (Payback®, CHS Inc., Sioux Falls, SD) purchased from the local feed store in Issaquah, WA. The owner also reported occasionally feeding some fresh garden produce grown on the premises, but no processed foods (e.g., cold cuts, hot dogs, cheese) were offered to birds.

Pathology

The owner submitted a dead chicken (the 6th one that died) to a local veterinarian for necropsy. The veterinarian collected several tissues (including heart, lung, air sac, intestine, pancreas, and liver) and submitted them for histologic examination to a private veterinary diagnostic laboratory. Two weeks later, another bird, an 8-month-old female chicken, died (the 7th death in the flock) and was submitted to the Avian Health and Food Safety Laboratory (AHFSL) for necropsy. The bird submitted to AHFSL had small comb fecal pasting around the cloaca. The bird was in good body condition and weighed 2,065 grams. The gross findings were 1-2 cc serous fibrinous pericardial effusion, thickening and opacity of pericardium with multiple pale foci throughout the myocardium. Pulmonary congestion, fibrinous exudate on the pleura, and thickening of air sacs were noted. The liver and spleen were enlarged and mottled.

Portions of the heart, liver, lung, kidney, gizzard, proventriculus, intestine, pancreas, ovary, oviduct, thyroid, parathyroid skeletal muscle, peripheral nerve, and brain were collected for histopathology. Tissues were fixed in 10% buffered neutral formalin, routinely processed, embedded in paraffin, sectioned at 4 µm, stained with hematoxylin and eosin, and examined by light microscopy. Additionally, sections of heart, liver and spleen were stained with modified Brown-Hopps tissue Gram stain [6].

Histologic findings were similar in the two birds submitted separately. The most prominent lesion was extensive inflammation of the heart (Figure 1), consisted of lymphocytes, macrophages, numerous multinucleated giant cells, and occasional heterophils. The lumen of larger blood vessels contained numerous large lymphocytes and scattered heterophils. In the liver there were random, small necrotic foci and accumulation of heterophils and macrophages (Figure 2). Lung sections revealed interstitial pneumonia, with infiltration of heterophils in the air capillaries and edema accumulating in the interparabronchial spaces. Lesions in the pancreas consisted of mild lymphocytic inflammation around the ducts. Spleen sections revealed severe lymphoid depletion, random accumulation of fibrin in the white pulp, and several macrophages contained intracytoplasmic cellular debris. Rod-shaped, Gram-positive bacteria were noted in the heart (Figure 3) and spleen.

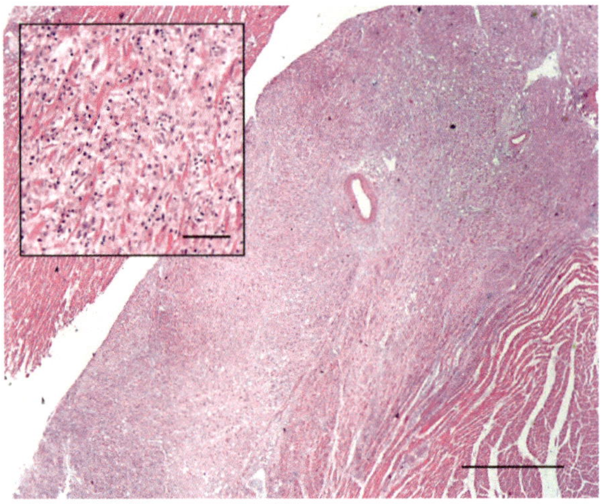

Figure 1: Extensive chronic-active myocardial inflammation. Histologic section of the heart showing extensive inflammation. H&E. Bar = 1 mm. Insert: higher magnification of the heart showing the inflammatory cell infiltration and disruption of myofibers. Inflammatory cells consisted mostly of lymphocytes and macrophages with scattered heterophils. H&E. Bar = 50 µm.

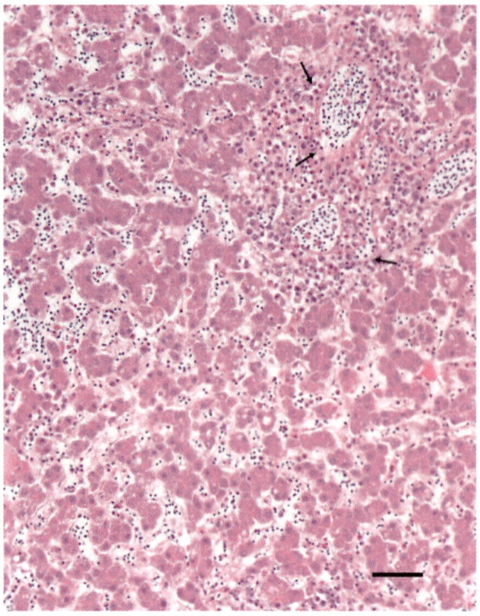

Figure 2: Periportal hepatic inflammation. Histologic section of the liver showing accumulation of heterophils and macrophages mostly around portal areas (arrows). H&E. Bar = 50 µm.

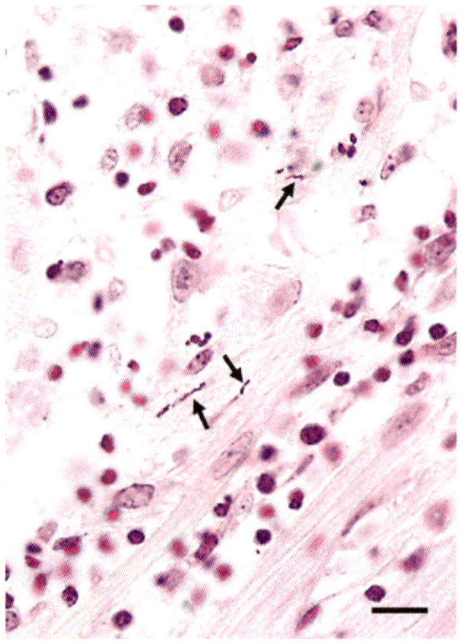

Figure 3: Gram positive bacteria in the heart. Histologic section of the heart showing inflammation and presence of Gram-positive rod-shaped bacteria (arrows) between the myofibers. Modified Brown-Hopps gram stain. Bar = 10 µm.

Bacteriology

Heart, liver, spleen and lung specimens were inoculated on blood and McConkey's agar (Remel, Lenaxa, KS) plates and incubated aerobically at 37°C for a minimum of up to 48 h. Cultures were examined for bacterial growth at approximately 24 and 48 h post-inoculation. Additionally, multiple sections of intestine were collected and cultured for *Salmonella spp*. The intestinal contents were selectively enriched in tetrathionate (TT) Hajna (BD Worlwide, Franklin Lakes, NJ) broth at 40°C for 20-24 hr. After enrichment, TT broth was plated on brilliant green with novobiocin and xylose-lysine-tergitol agar 4 agars (Remel) and the plates were incubated at 35°C for an additional 24 h.

Identical small round colonies with a narrow zone of β-hemolysis on the blood agar were isolated in pure form from liver, spleen, and lung. The bacteria were identified as Gram-positive rods, catalase-positive and oxidase-negative. The liver isolate was biochemically characterized as *L. monocytogenes* by testing with the API Coryne kit (bioMérieux, Inc., Hazelwood, MO) and Christie–Atkins–Munch–Peterson (CAMP) test.

Molecular characterization

The isolate was confirmed to be *L. monocytogenes* by the real-time polymerase chain reaction (RT-PCR) using iQ-Check Listeria monocytogenes II kit (BioRad, Hercules, CA) according to the manufacturer's instructions. In addition, the genomic DNA was extracted from paraffin sections of heart from both birds, and the liver and the spleen from the bird submitted at AHFSL using a QIAamp® DNA Mini Kit (Qiagen, Valencia, CA) and tested by RT-PCR. *L. monocytogenes* was detected from both fixed sections of heart (Ct = 28.35 and 38.45) and the single fixed section of spleen (Ct = 32.48). No bacteria were isolated from the heart. None of the samples were positive for *Salmonella* sp.

A complete ORF of 16S rDNA (~1500 bp) was PCR amplified, cloned in pGEM-T Easy vector system (Promega, Madison, WI) and sequenced using protocols described previously [7]. The sequences were edited, aligned and phyologenetic analysis (data not shown) was performed as described previously [7]. The 16S rRNA gene sequence from *L. monocytogenes* strain showed 99.9% similarity with several *L. monocytogenes* strains in the GenBank database, but serotype of this isolate could not be determined based on the 16S rDNA sequence similarity. Consequently, PCR based serotyping was performed following the procedures described previously using following sets of primers that amplify variable regions of *L. monocytogenes* genome: D1, D2, FlaA, GLT and MAMA-C [8]. These primer pairs can accurately classify *L. monocytogenes* into specific serotype. The *L. monocytogenes* isolate in this study tested PCR positive only by one primer set (D1), but negative for all the other primer pairs tested (Figure 4). These results suggested that the isolate belonged to *L. monocytogenes*serotype 4b.

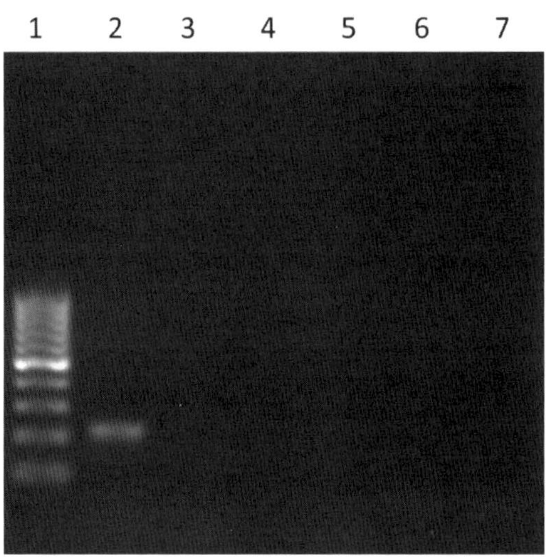

Figure 4: Molecular serotyping of L. monocytogenes. Results of PCR-based serotyping of *L. monocytogenes*. Lane 1: 100-bp ladder; lane 2: D1 primers; lane 3: D2 primers; lane 4: FlaA primers; lane 5: GLT primers; lane 6: MAMA-C primers; lane 7: no template control. Positive amplification with D1 primer pair only. This suggests that the *L. monocytogenes* isolate is serotype 4b [8].

DISCUSSION

In animals and humans the most common *Listeria* infections are caused by three serotypes: 1/2a, 1/2b, and 4b. PCR-based serotyping of the *L. monocytogenes* isolate in the current study identified this as serotype 4b, one of the most pathogenic serovars that is known to cause majority of human infections [9]. Experimental studies have shown that serotype 4b strains may have increased virulence compared with other serotypes [9] and are often responsible for invasive disease outbreaks in mammals. This serotype is also found in poultry meat [4]. In addition, serotype 4b has been isolated from a chicken flock with encephalitis [10]. However, no signs of nervous system disease were observed in the current outbreak.

In the current case, *L. monocytogens* were isolated from the lung, liver and spleen, but not from the heart. On the other hand the bacteria were detected by RT-PCR from fixed heart and spleen. Molecular techniques have been used to detect *L. monocytogenes* in enriched samples or pure cultures. The limit of detection for the commercial real time PCR kit used in this study is 1,000 coliform forming units. The Ct value for qPCR for this bird was 38.45 which indicated that this bird likely had low numbers of *L. monocytogenes* in heart and that could have led to failure of isolation. It is possible that cold-enrichment might have helped recovering the bacteria from the heart. However cold-enrichment was not conducted because all other samples were positive.

The exact source of infection for this flock is unknown. Possible sources of the *Listeria* infection include feces, soil, decaying plant material, feed, and water. Neither the environment where the chickens were housed nor the commercial ration or drinking water were collected or tested. Furthermore, various species of mammals and birds may be infected with *Listeria* and may serve as asymptomatic carriers [11].

The first clinical signs in the flock appeared when investigation from a multistate outbreak of listeriosis linked to whole cantaloupes was ongoing [12]. The number of outbreak-associated deaths in the mentioned outbreak was 33 people. According to the history and confirmed by the King's County Public Health investigation, the chicken flock was fed a commercial layer's ration and occasional fresh produce grown in the owner's garden. The birds did not have access to compost or kitchen leftovers that may be contaminated with listeria (e.g. like cold cuts, hot dogs, soft cheeses, or cantaloupes). Conjunctivitis due to *L. monocytogenes* has been reported in individuals handling apparently healthy but infected chickens [13]. Human infections have also resulted from the consumption of contaminated poultry or ready-to-eat poultry products. Although the family continued to consume the eggs produced by the flock during the outbreak, no family member was ever sick during the outbreak or diagnosed with Listeriosis.

The sick birds were treated intramuscularly with 25 mg/kg of enrofloxacin (Bayer Corp., Pittsburgh, PA) for 5 days. All the birds recovered. Enrofloxacin is a fluoroquinolone antibiotic used for the treatment of a wide variety of bacterial infections in companion animals and horses. In 2005, the Food and Drug Adminstraton withdrew approval of enrofloxacin for use in water to treat flocks of poultry, as this practice was noted to promote the evolution of fluoroquinolone-resistant strains of the bacterium Campylobacter, a human pathogen [14]. Unlike commercial poultry, these birds or their eggs were not sold for food. The veterinarian educated the clients regarding the potential of contamination of eggs with the antibiotic and recommended not to consume the eggs laid by treated hens.

CONCLUSION

This is the first report of outbreak of listeriosis in the backyard poultry flock in Washington State. In addition, this paper describes the use of real time PCR, for the first time, to confirm *L. monocytogenes* infection from formalin fixed tissues. Because most of human infections are caused by three major serotypes (serotyping must be performed to identify the specific serotypes of *Listeria* (1/2a, 1/2b and 4b), serotyping must be undertaken to determine potential public health risk associated with exposure to infected birds. It is important to note that most reported outbreaks of listeriosis in poultry involve relatively very young birds. Systemic listeriosis in birds older than 5 months of age described in this report is relatively rare, but the current outbreak suggests that veterinarians and public health officials must be vigilant and should raise suspicion for listeriosis irrespective of age of the chickens. Finally, because antibiotics may remain in meat and other animal products, it is essential to educate the owners of urban poultry on these potential risks.

DECLARATIONS

Acknowledgements

The authors gratefully acknowledge Dennis Schaberg, Sylvia Weber, and Gail Deckert for their technical support. The authors also thank Elaine Lively and Chandra Miller of Phoenix Laboratory, Mukilteo, WA, for data retrieval. This work was partially funded by the Agricultural Animal Health Program, College of Veterinary Medicine, Washington State University.

Authors' contributions

RC performed the necropsy, the histologic examination, isolation, and PCR from fixed tissues, reviewed the literature and prepared the manuscript. MG performed the histologic examination and prepared the photos. SH performed the field investigation and interviewed the owner. DS performed the molecular characterization and serotype-specific identification of *Listeria* isolate. All authors read and approved the final manuscript.

REFERENCES

1. Berrang ME, Meinersmann RJ, Frank JF, Smith DP, Genzlinger LL: Distribution of Listeria monocytogenes subtypes within a poultry further processing plant. J Food Prot. 2005, 68: 980-985.
2. Berrang ME, Meinersmann RJ, Frank JF, Ladely SR: Colonization of a newly constructed commercial chicken further processing plant with *Listeria monocytogenes*. J Food Prot. 2010, 73: 286-291.
3. Loura CAC, Almeida RCC, Almeida PF: The incidence and level of Listeria spp. and *Listeria monocytogenes*contamination in processed poultry at a poultry processing plant. J Food Prot. 2005, 25: 19-29.
4. Yeh ET: Characterization of Listeria monocytogenes isolated from retail organic chicken. University of Maryland, MD, USA: Food Science: 2004.
5. Tappero JW, Schuchat A, Deaver KA, Mascola L, Wenger JD: Reduction in the incidence of human listeriosis in the United States: effectiveness of prevention efforts?. JAMA. 1995, 273: 1118-1122. 10.1001/jama.1995.03520380054035.
6. Carson FL, Hladik C: Brown-Hopps modification of the gram strain. In Histotechnology: a self instructional text. 3rd edition. Hong Kong: American Society for Clinical Pathology Press; 2009:231–233.
7. Burbank DR, Shah DH, LaPatra SE, Fornshell G, Cain KD: Enhanced resistance to coldwater disease following feeding of probiotic bacterial strains to rainbow trout (*Oncorhynchus mykiss*). Aquaculture. 2011, 321: 185-190. 10.1016/j.aquaculture.2011.09.004.
8. Borucki MK, Call DR: Listeria monocytogenes serotype identification by PCR. J Clin Microbiol. 2003, 41: 5537-5540. 10.1128/JCM.41.12.5537-5540.2003.
9. Czuprynski CJ, Faith NG, Steinberg H: Ability of the *Listeria monocytogenes* strain Scot A to cause systemic infection in mice infected by the intragastric route. Appl Environ Microbiol. 2002, 68: 2893-2900. 10.1128/AEM.68.6.2893-2900.2002.
10. Kurazono M, Nakamura K, Yamada M, Yonemaru T, Sakoda T: Pathology of listerial encephalitis in chickens in Japan. Avian Dis. 2003, 47: 1496-1502. 10.1637/7066.
11. Barnes HJ: Miscellaneous and sporadic bacterial infections. Diseases of poultry. Edited by: Saif YM, Fadly AA, Glisson JR, McDougald LR, Nolan L, Swayne DE. 2008, Ames, IA: ISU Press, 952-970. 12
12. Centers for Disease Control and Prevention: Multistate outbreak of listeriosis linked to whole cantaloupes from Jensen Farms, Colorado. 2012, http://www.cdc.gov/listeria/outbreaks/cantaloupes-jensen-farms/index.html; (accessed on March 29, 2013)
13. Morishita TY: Listeriosis. The merck veterinary manual. Edited by: Kahn CM, Allen DG, Constable PD, Davies PR, Quesenberry KE, Reeves PT, Sharma JM, Smith RKW, Treadwell T. 2010, Kendallville, IN: Merck & Co., Inc, 2441-10
14. U. S. Food and Drug Administration: Enrofloxacin for poultry. 2012, http://www.fda.gov/AnimalVeterinary/SafetyHealth/RecallsWithdrawals/ucm042004.htm; (accessed on March 29, 2013)

CHAPTER 25 A CASE OF BOVINE RAW MILK CONTAMINATION WITH LISTERIA MONOCYTOGENES

Karen Hunt, Niall Drummond, Mary Murphy, Francis Butler, Jim Buckley and Kieran Jordan

Keywords: *Listeria monocytogenes,* Raw milk, Subclinical mastitis, Milk quality

BACKGROUND

Listeria monocytogenes is a pathogenic bacterium that can cause Listeriosis in humans and various animal species. In humans, foodborne *L. monocytogenes* causes large outbreaks of Listeriosis, with a mortality rate of 9% to 44%[1]. In a wide variety of host animals *Listeria* infection has been confirmed in more than 40 species of domestic and wild animals including birds. The most susceptible domestic species are sheep, goats and cattle. Listeriosis manifests itself clinically in ruminants as encephalitis, neo-natal mortality (abortion) and septicaemia. The most common clinical form in cattle is encephalitis, in general, small numbers being affected (8-10% of the herd) with the animals surviving from 4–14 days. In animals, susceptibility to infection with *L. monocytogenes* has been attributed to decreased cell-mediated immunity associated with advanced pregnancy[2]. *L. monocytogenes* has the ability to invade both phagocytic and non-phagocytic cells, to survive and replicate intra cellularly, and to transfer from cell to cell without exposure to humeral defence mechanisms.

In raw milk and the dairy environment, the source of *L. monocytogenes* contamination is mainly from poor silage and bedding[3, 4]. On the farm, contamination of *L. monocytogenes* can spread from the environment to the animals and also from animal to animal[2, 5, 6, 7]. Contamination of milking equipment with bovine faeces can also occur[8]. During storage of raw milk on the farm, *L. monocytogenes* can grow and multiply, even at refrigerated conditions[9].

Udder infection with *L. monocytogenes* is most commonly reported in sheep and goats[10]; *L. monocytogenes*bovine mastitis is less commonly reported where sub-clinical mastitis in cows can go undetected[11, 12, 13, 14, 15, 16], where their milk remains visually unchanged, and with no clinical signs contamination can normally persist even after treatment[14]. Most cases of human listeriosis are foodborne related[17]. The occurrence of *L. monocytogenes* in raw milk was reported as 4.8%, 6%, 3.4% and 6%, respectively[6, 18, 19, 20]. Raw milk can be contaminated from the environment or by direct excretion into the milk, therefore, consumption of raw milk is associated with increased risk factors. None of the above studies indicated the source of milk contamination, but it was most likely from the environment.

The aim of this study was to identify the source of *L. monocytogenes* that was contaminating bulk milk at farm level.

MATERIALS AND METHODS

Environmental swabbing of the dairy environment

Environmental samples were collected from non-milk contact sampling sites including pipes, tanks, drains, floors, and walls. Environmental samples from milk contact points were collected from bulk milk filters and from a milk spill area on the floor of the dairy beside the bulk tank. All swab samples and milk filters were collected as previously described[6].

Citation: Karen Hunt, Niall Drummond, Mary Murphy, Francis Butler, Jim Buckley and Kieran Jordan, A case of bovine raw milk contamination with Listeria monocytogenes, DOI: 10.1186/2046-0481-65-13.

Milk sampling

To investigate *L. monocytogenes* contamination of milk, the herd of 180 individual cows was divided into 9 groups with 20 cows in each group. A composite sample was taken aseptically, in sterile containers, from each group and analysed. Within each positive sample from the groups, each of the 20 individual cow's milk was sampled and analysed. Where milk from a cow was positive, milk from the four quarters of the mammary gland was sampled and analysed.

L. monocytogenes analysis

The presence/absence of *L. monocytogenes* in all milk and environmental samples was analysed using an AFNOR validated "One step enrichment broth" method (Oxoid FT0401). This AFNOR validated method has been shown to give equivalent results to ISO (11290–1:1997). Milk samples were enumerated for *L. monocytogenes* by direct plating of the milk onto selective agar (Brilliance™ Listeria Agar; Oxoid CM1080). Typical *L. monocytogenes* colonies (which are blue-green with a surrounding precipitate) were isolated and purified by re-streaking on ALOA agar (Agosti & Ottaviani *Listeria* Agar; LabM, Lancashire, UK, HAL010), followed by streaking on tryptone soy agar (TSA). Single pure isolated colonies were grown overnight in tryptone soy broth (TSB) and frozen in cryovials in a glycerol/TSB mixture at −20°C.

Milk quality analysis

Bulk milk and *L. monocytogenes* contaminated milk samples were tested for quality parameters. The pH was measured using BS770:5:1975 with an Orion pH meter model 420A. Enumeration of total bacterial counts using ISO 6610:1992 method with Milk Plate Count Agar (Oxoid CM0681), coliforms using method ISO 4831:2006 on VRBL agar (Oxoid CM0968) and *S. aureus* using method ISO 6888–2 with Baird Parker Rabbit Plasma Fibrinogen agar (Oxoid CM0961). The fat, protein, lactose, casein and Somatic Cell Count (SCC) were measured by infrared analysis (Milkoscan 605, Foss Electric, Denmark).

Molecular characterisation of *L. monocytogenes* isolates

All purified isolates were confirmed as *L. monocytogenes* using Real-Time polymerase chain reaction (RT-PCR)[21, 22]. Pulsed-Field Gel Electrophoresis (PFGE) of all *L. monocytogenes* isolates was performed with the restriction enzymes *Asc* I and *Apa* I, in two separate experiments, using the standard PulseNet protocol[23]. Serotyping of the isolates was performed using a combination of antibodies and serotype-specific PCR[24].

Examination of cows

The infected cow under examination was physically examined and medically treated by a veterinary surgeon. The treatment included intra-mammary injection of 4 tubes of Sinulux, at 12 hour intervals. This was followed by a five day treatment with Tylosil and a subsequent five day treatment with Oxytetracycline. After antibiotic treatment the infected animal's milk continued to test positive for *L. monocytogenes.*

RESULTS

Environment sampling

All environmental swabs were negative for *L. monocytogenes,* except the milk filters from the bulk tank and the floor of the dairy beside the bulk tank. The isolates obtained had indistinguishable PFGE profiles from the original milk isolate.

L. monocytogenes microbiological analysis

Once the cow that was excreting *L. monocytogenes* into the milk was identified, the milk from individual quarters was examined (Table1). *L. monocytogenes* was excreted from only one quarter, and this quarter also had a higher Somatic Cell Count (SCC) than the other quarters, although it was still within acceptable limits. Detailed analysis of the milk was undertaken on several days (Table2). The milk was positive for *L. monocytogenes* on all dates tested. In addition, TBC and SCC were elevated. Fat, protein and lactose concentrations were generally within accepted limits.

Table 1: Milk analysis results from the four quarters of the mammary gland, from the Listeria infected cow

Sample	*Listeria* Enrichment	*Listeria* cfu/ml	SCCx 10^3/ml
Front right	pos	280	207
Front left	neg	<10	79
Back left	neg	<10	9
Back right	neg	<10	4

Table 2: Milk analysis results from the Listeria infected milk and the bulk milk (without the infected cow)

Date	Milk source	ListeriaEnrich-ment	Listeriacfu/ml	Total counts(cfu/ml)	SCCX 10^3/ml	Fat(%)	Pro-tein(%)	Lac-tose(%)
18/07/11	In-fected cow	pos	<10	ND	387	3.19	3.11	4.71

26/07/11	In-fected cow	pos	20	98000	459	2.81	2.98	4.60
28/07/11	In-fected cow	pos	307	16000	469	3.26	2.97	4.66
02/08/11	In-fected cow	pos	50	77000	427	3.52	2.97	4.65
03/08/11	In-fected cow	pos	520	140000	727	4.10	2.81	4.49
03/08/11	In-fected cow	pos	520	140000	727	4.10	2.81	4.49
22/07/11	Bulk milk	neg	neg	ND	125	3.71	3.27	4.80
16/08/11	Bulk milk	neg	neg	ND	183	4.13	3.31	4.67

ND not determined.

Milk quality

The average pH of infected bulk milk was pH 6.81(n=5). *L. monocytogenes* contaminated milk samples tested had enumeration results of <10 cfu/ml for *coliforms* and *S aureus*. Table2 shows total bacteria count values for *L. monocytogenes* infected milk and the fat, protein lactose, casein and SSC results for both the infected milk and the non infected bulk milk.

L. monocytogenes characterisation

All *L. monocytogenes* strains isolated in this study had indistinguishable PFGE profiles (Figure1) and were all serotype 1/2a.

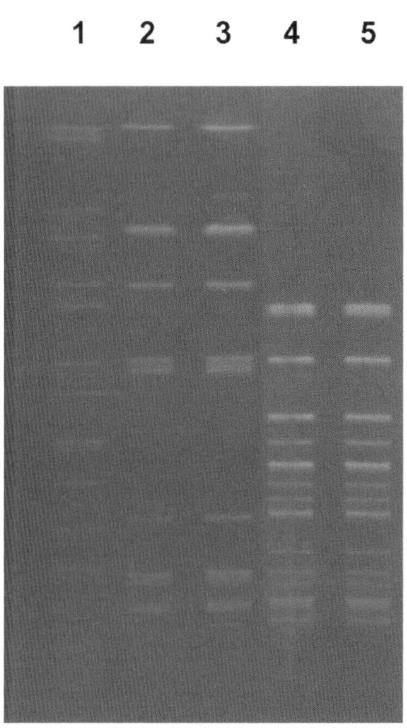

Figure 1: PFGE profiles of *L. monocytogenes* from bulk tank milk.

DISCUSSION

L. monocytogenes has been described as a "*less common cause*" of bovine environmental mastitis and may often be associated with the accidental introduction of the organism during intramammary infusion[25]. Mild persistent, antibiotic resistant, low grade infections have been documented in cattle and may result in decreased production from infected mammary tissue over time. In addition, *L. monocytogenes* infection and secretion may have potential public health implications for susceptible consumers[2], if raw milk is consumed. *L. monocytogenes* has been isolated from different species and from soil, plants, mud, pasture, waste water and streams. Cattle and many other animal species excrete *L. monocytogenes* in their faeces. Controls to reduce the level of contamination and infection include such measures as the pasteurisation of milk, rodent control and common practices of dairy husbandry, personal hygiene and environmental management. Animals with encephalitis or those that have aborted should be isolated and all in contact material including placenta and foetuses aseptically removed and destroyed[13].

In cases of *L. monocytogenes* contamination of milk, the most likely source of the *listeria* is from the environment post-milking. Direct excretion of *L. monocytogenes* into the milk, i.e., clinical or sub-clinical mastitis is rare.

In this case, *L. monocytogenes* contamination of a bulk raw milk sample led to an investigation of the source of contamination. Environmental swabs from the dairy environment were negative, except for milk contact surfaces. It is possible that the contamination from the dairy floor led to contamination of the milk, but with milk contamination lasting for several months, this is unlikely. Previous studies of *L. monocytogenes*contamination of raw milk found that animal faeces, poor quality of feed and general lack of hygiene on the dairy farm are factors associated with contamination[3, 26, 27]. Biofilms formation has been known to cause adhesion and persistence of *L. monocytogenes* onto equipment[28]. Levels of hygiene on the farm involved in this study were visually very good, and all non-milk contact dairy environmental swabs were negative, indicating the source of contamination was direct excretion into the milk. Following a visual inspection, none of the cows in the herd had any physical signs of infection.

The *L. monocytogenes* contamination in the bulk milk was further investigated in herd milk testing. Using segregated composite bulk milk sampling (20 cows per sample), one mammary quarter from one cow infected, without any clinical or sub-clinical signs of mastitis was eventually identified[29]. This infected cow was segregated from the herd; the bulk milk was then *L. monocytogenes* negative. After the cow was segregated from the herd, the SCC results of the contaminated milk samples increased (Table2), indicating sub clinical mastitis, although the stress of separation could also result in increased SCC counts. In dairy cattle herds with mastitis it is found that in almost all cases where Listeria occurred, only one quarter is infected, and 95% of cases yielded a pure culture[30], similar to the results of this study.

The quality of the infected milk was variable with regards to TBC, fat, protein and lactose levels (Table2). When the SCC was measured initially, the values were elevated slightly in the contaminated quarter, but when diluted with the 3 non-contaminated quarters the average ~50,000 cells/ml, is well within expected limits for good quality milk. Even the contaminated quarter was acceptable at 207,000 cells/ml. When the cow was isolated from the herd and in a new environment, this could have imposed an additional stress where the SCC was raised to sub-clinical levels of >400,000 cells/ml (current EU limit as Annex III, Section IX, Chapter I,

Part III, to Regulation (EC) No 853/2004.) However, no visual defects in the milk, nor clinical signs of infection were seen in the infected cow during this study.

Testing of the infected cow and the remaining bulk milk was carried out for a further 2 months (6 months from initial identification of the problem). Over the 6 months of testing, all the strains of *L. monocytogenes*from the infected milk were indistinguishable when characterised by PFGE (Figure1) and serotyping, indicating that the same strain of *L. monocytogenes* was persistently present in the infected milk. The persistence of infection was also reported by Bourry 1995[16] with sub-clinical mastitis. With sub-clinical listeria mastitis, cows not showing any clinical signs go undetected where they may produce milk with normal appearance containing large numbers of pathogenic *L. monocytogenes*[15, 16]. Clinical mastitis is, by definition, abnormal milk and no reference to SCC is required[31]. The presence of flakes, clots, or other gross alterations in appearance of quarter milk is evidence of clinical mastitis and is by definition, abnormal milk.

CONCLUSIONS

In this study we find bulk raw milk to be directly contaminated from a case of *L. monocytogenes* infection in a dairy cow. The SCC was slightly elevated from the infective quarter with no visual defects in the milk, or clinical signs seen of infection in the cow. This *L. monocytogenes* strain was isolated from all milk samples and by molecular characterisation, found to be a pure and persistent isolate over a 6 month period, even after antibiotic treatment.

DECLARATIONS

Acknowledgements

Karen Hunt was in receipt of a Teagasc Walsh Fellowship. The authors gratefully acknowledge funding support from the Irish Government under the Food Institutional Research Measure Irish Microbial Risk Assessment Network project, and the EU 6th Framework Programme under the project BIOTRACER.

Author' contributions

KH, KJ and ND carried out sampling and molecular genetic studies. KJ, MM, JB and FB planned the work and drafted the manuscript. All authors read and approved the final manuscript.

REFERENCES

1. Clark CG, Farber J, Pagotto F, Ciampa N, Dore K, Nadon C, Bernard K, Ng LK: Surveillance *for Listeria monocytogenes* and listeriosis, 1995–2004. Epidemiol Infect. 2010, 138: 559-72. 10.1017/S0950268809990914.
2. Quinn PJ, Markey BK, Carter ME, Donnelly WJ, Leonard FC: Veterinary Microbiology & Microbial Disease. Blackwell Science Ltd. 2002, 72–73: 468-469.
3. Sanaa M, Poutrel B, Menard JL, Serieys F: Risk Factors Associated with Contamination of Raw Milk by *Listeria monocytogenes* in Dairy Farms. J. Dairy Sci. 1993, 76: 2891-2898. 10.3168/jds.S0022-0302(93)77628-6.
4. Wagner M, Melzner D, Bago Z, Winter P, Egerbacher M, Schilcher F, Zangana A, Schoder D: Outbreak of clinical listeriosis in sheep: evaluation from possible contamination routes from feed to raw produce and humans. J Vet Med B. 2005, 52: 278-83. 10.1111/j.1439-0450.2005.00866.x.
5. Ho AJ, Lappi VR, Wiedmann M: Longitudinal monitoring of *Listeria monocytogenes* contamination patterns in a farmstead dairy processing facility. J Dairy Sci. 2007, 90: 2517-2524. 10.3168/jds.2006-392.
6. Fox E, Hunt K, O'Brien M, Jordan K: *Listeria monocytogenes* in Irish Farmhouse cheese processing environments. Int J Food Microbiol. 2011, 145 (Suppl 1): S39-45.
7. Barrett DJ, Healy AM, Leonard FC, Doherty ML: Prevalence of pathogens causing subclinical mastitis in 15 dairy herds in the Republic of Ireland. Irish Veterinary Journal. 2005, 58: 333-337. 10.1186/2046-0481-58-6-333.
8. Mohammed HO, Stipetic K, McDonough PL, Gonzalez RN, Nydam DV, Atwill ER: Identification of potential on-farm sources of *Listeria monocytogenes* in herds of dairy cattle. Am J Vet Res. 2009, 70: 383-8. 10.2460/ajvr.70.3.383.
9. Yilmaz T, Moyer B, MacDonell RE, Cordero-Coma M, Gallagher MJ: Outbreaks associated with unpasteurized milk and soft cheese: an over of consumer safety. Food Protection Trends. 2009, 29: 211-222.
10. Low JC, Donachie W: A re of *Listeria monocytogenes* and listeriosis. Vet J. 1997, 153 (1): 9-29. 10.1016/S1090-0233(97)80005-6.

11. Schoder D, Winter P, Kareem A, Baumgartner W, Wagner M: A case of sporadic ovine mastitis caused by *Listeria monocytogenes* and its effect on contamination of raw milk and raw-milk cheeses produced in the on-farm dairy. J Dairy Res. 2003, 70: 395-401. 10.1017/S0022029903006277.

12. van Daelen AM, Jaartsveld FH: Listeria mastitis in cattle. Tijdschr Diergeneeskd. 1988, 113: 380-3.

13. Gitter M, Bradley R, Blampied PH: *Listeria monocytogenes* infection in bovine mastitis. Vet Rec. 1980, 107: 390-3. 10.1136/vr.107.17.390.

14. Fedio WM, Schoonderwoerd M, Shute RH, Jackson H: A case of bovine mastitis caused by *Listeria monocytogenes*. Can Vet J. 1990, 31: 773-5.

15. Winter P, Schilcher F, Bagò Z, Schoder D, Egerbacher M, Baumgartner W, Wagner M: Clinical and Histopathological Aspects of Naturally Occurring Mastitis Caused by *Listeria monocytogenes* in Cattle and Ewes. J Vet Med B. 2004, 51: 176-179. 10.1111/j.1439-0450.2004.00751.x.

16. Bourry A, Poutrel B, Rocourt J: Bovine mastitis caused by *Listeria monocytogenes*: characteristics of natural and experimental infections. J Med Microbiol. 1995, 43: 125-32. 10.1099/00222615-43-2-125.

17. Chakraborty T, Wehland J: The host cell infected with *Listeria monocytogenes*. Host response through intra celleur pathogens. Edited by: Kaufmann SHE. 1997, New York: Springer, 271-290.

18. D'Amico DJ, Donnelly CW: Microbiological quality of raw milk used for small-scale artisan cheese production in Vermont: effect of farm characteristics and practices. J Dairy Sci. 2010, 93: 134-47. 10.3168/jds.2009-2426.

19. Oliver SP, Boor KJ, Murphy SC, Murinda SE: Food safety hazards associated with consumption of raw milk. Foodborne Pathog Dis. 2009, 6: 793-806. 10.1089/fpd.2009.0302.

20. Rea MC, Cogan TM, Tobin S: Incidence of pathogenic bacteria in raw milk in Ireland. J Appl Bacteriol. 1992, 73: 331-6. 10.1111/j.1365-2672.1992.tb04985.x.

21. Rodriguez-Lazaro D, Hernandez M, Scortti M, Esteve T, Vazquez-Boland JA, Pla M: Quantitative detection of *Listeria monocytogenes* and *Listeria innocua* by real-time PCR: assessment of hly, iap, and lin02483 targets and AmpliFluor technology. Appl Environ Microbiol. 2004, 70: 1366-1377. 10.1128/AEM.70.3.1366-1377.2004.

22. O'Brien M, Hunt K, McSweeney S, Jordan K: Occurrence of foodborne pathogens in Irish farmhouse cheese. Food Microbiol. 2009, 26: 910-914. 10.1016/j.fm.2009.06.009.

23. Graves LM, Swaminathan B: PulseNet standardized protocol for subtyping *Listeria monocytogenes* by macrorestriction and pulsed-field gel electrophoresis. Int J Food Microbiol. 2001, 65: 55-62. 10.1016/S0168-1605(00)00501-8.

24. Doumith M, Buchrieser C, Glaser P, Jacquet C, Martin P: Differentiation of the Major *Listeria monocytogenes* Serovars by Multiplex PCR. J Clin Microbiol. 2004, 42: 3819-3822. 10.1128/JCM.42.8.3819-3822.2004.

25. Menzies FD, McBride SH, McDowell SWJ, McCoy MA, McConnell W, Bell C: Clinical and laboratory findings in cases of toxic mastitis in cows in Northern Ireland. Veterinary Record. 2000, 147: 123-128. 10.1136/vr.147.5.123.

26. Nightingale KK, Fortes ED, Ho AJ, Schukken YH, Grohn YT, Wiedmann M: Evaluation of farm management practices as risk factors for clinical listeriosis and fecal shedding of *Listeria monocytogenes* in ruminants. J Am Vet Med Assoc. 2005, 227: 1808-14. 10.2460/javma.2005.227.1808.

27. Schoder D, Melzner D, Schmalwieser A, Zangana A, Winter P, Wagner M: Important vectors for *Listeria monocytogenes*transmission at farm dairies manufacturing fresh sheep and goat cheese from raw milk. J Food Prot. 2011, 74: 919-24. 10.4315/0362-028X.JFP-10-534.

28. Latorre AA, Van Kessel JS, Karns JS, Zurakowski MJ, Pradhan AK, Boor KJ, Jayarao BM, Houser BA, Daugherty CS, Schukken YH: Biofilm in milking equipment on a dairy farm as a potential source of bulk tank milk contamination with *Listeria monocytogenes*. J. Dairy Sci. 2010, 93: 2792-2802. 10.3168/jds.2009-2717.

29. Le Maréchal C, Thiery R, Vautor R, Le Loir Y: Mastitis impact on technological properties of milk and quality of milk products - a re. Dairy Sci. & Technol. 2011, 91: 247-282. 10.1007/s13594-011-0009-6.

30. Jensen NE, Aarestrup FM, Jensen J, Wegener HC: *Listeria monocytogenes* in bovine mastitis. Possible implication for human health. Int J Food Microbiol. 1996, 32: 209-216. 10.1016/0168-1605(96)01105-1.

31. Kitchen BJ: Bovine mastitis: milk compositional changes and related diagnostic tests. J Dairy Res. 1981, 48: 167-188. 10.1017/S0022029900021580.

SECTION VI: STREPTOCOCCUS SPP.

CHAPTER 26

GENOME CHARACTERIZATION AND POPULATION GENETIC STRUCTURE OF THE ZOONOTIC PATHOGEN, STREPTOCOCCUS CANIS

Vincent P Richards, Ruth N Zadoks, Paulina D Pavinski Bitar, Tristan Lefébure, Ping Lang, Brenda Werner, Linda Tikofsky, Paolo Moroni and Michael J Stanhope

Keywords: Streptococcus canis, Comparative genomics, Pathogen, Zoonotic, Mastitis, Lateral gene transfer, Host adaptation, Bovine Canine

BACKGROUND

Originally described as β-hemolytic streptococci isolated from dogs and cows that possessed the Lancefield group G antigen [1], Streptococcus canis has subsequently been isolated from a variety of animal sources including cats, rats, rabbits, minks, foxes, a Japanese raccoon dog, and humans [2, 3, 4]. The species is an important opportunistic pathogen of cats and dogs infecting a wide range of tissues such as the nervous system, respiratory tract, genitourinary system, blood, skin, bones, cardiovascular system, and abdomen [1, 4, 5, 6]. Infection can cause serious invasive disease, such as streptococcal toxic shock syndrome (STSS), necrotizing fasciitis (NF), septicemia, pneumonia, and meningitis, with numerous reports of fatal infection [5, 7, 8, 9], whereas in cows S. canis can cause mastitis [10, 11, 12]. Of concern are the accumulating reports of human infection (including numerous cases of dog to human transmission) [13, 14, 15, 16], with clinical manifestations similar to those seen in cats and dogs. For example, descriptions of human cases include soft tissue infection, bacteremia, urinary infection, bone infection, pneumonia, and two reports of death from sepsis [13].

Although the phylogeny of the species is not completely resolved, a general consensus from the literature shows S. canis to be closely related to Streptococcus dysgalactiae subsp. dysgalactiae, Streptococcus dysgalactiae subsp. equisimilis, and Streptococcus pyogenes[2, 17, 18, 19, 20, 21]. S. canis and S. dysgalactiaesubsp. equisimilis are both β-hemolytic streptococci that share the same Lancefield group G antigen. Consequently, by the Lancefield system they are indistinguishable, and have traditionally only been classified as group G streptococci (GGS) from either animal (S. canis) or human (S. dysgalactiae subsp. equisimilis) origin. Therefore, it's possible that human S. canis infection has been underestimated [13, 15]. Investigating this problem, Broyles et al. [22] performed a survey of human invasive infection using techniques capable of distinguishing S. canis from S. dysgalactiae subsp. equisimilis. Results showed a low frequency of S. canis in blood samples. However, their study was biased towards the characterization of isolates from blood samples (isolates from other body sites were less likely to be characterized).

In humans, STSS and NF are serious diseases typically caused by S. pyogenes infection. The emergence of strikingly similar STSS and NF in cats and dogs coupled with the close relationship between the causal species prompted preliminary investigation and subsequent discovery of two shared virulence factors between these species [23]. To shed light on the molecular basis of S. canis virulence and further investigate the role S. pyogenes and other species of Streptococcus may have played in its evolution we determined the first genome sequence for this pathogen and compared it to an extensive range of streptococcal genomes (40 species, 213 strains). In addition, we explored population structure among canine, feline, and bovine isolates.

Our findings reveal a diverse array of genes within the S. canis genome homologous to known virulence factors, including several established virulence factors from S. pyogenes,

Citation: Vincent P Richards, Ruth N Zadoks, Paulina D Pavinski Bitar, Tristan Lefébure, Ping Lang, Brenda Werner, Linda Tikofsky, Paolo Moroni and Michael J Stanhope, Genome characterization and population genetic structure of the zoonotic pathogen, Streptococcus canis, DOI: 10.1186/1471-2180-12-293.

Streptococcus agalactiae, and Streptococcus pneumoniae. We found evidence for multiple LGT events between S. canis and (i) other bovine mastitis causing pathogens, and (ii) the human pathogen Streptococcus urinalis, suggesting LGT in both shared bovine and human environments. This LGT was mediated by a variety of mobile genetic elements [plasmid, phage, integrative conjugative element] that carried many of the virulence factors, highlighting the importance of LGT in the evolution of this pathogen and the potential for its emergence as a zoonotic pathogen.

RESULT AND DISCUSSION

Assembly and general features of the genome

Roche/454 pyrosequencing produced 128,749 single-end reads and 140,788 paired-end reads that were assembled into 91 contigs (>200 bp) and eight scaffolds, representing an average 23X site coverage. Utilizing additional Illumina/Sanger sequencing and alignment to an optical map, the eight scaffolds were assembled into a single 2,267,856 bp contig. Unfortunately, we were unable to obtain sequence for one small section of the genome (Figure 1). The gap was within a collagen-like surface protein. The best BLAST hit at the NCBI nr database for each gene fragment (SCAZ3_06900 and SCAZ3_06785) was to an identically annotated gene within S. agalactiae (A909), (each fragment shared approximately 75% sequence identity). Alignment of the S. canis fragments to this gene suggested that we were missing approximately 1.6 kb. For S. agalactiae (A909), this gene contained 75 repeats of a 9 bp imperfect repeat (DCCRTCTTT). The majority of these repeats (70) were contained within a 2.5 kb region that spanned the S. canis gap and flanking regions. S. canis contained 26 repeats in the regions that flanked the gap. Consequently it seems likely that these repeats were also present within the un-sequenced section of the collagen gene for S. canis and that their presence confounded our sequencing attempts. Inclusion of this small gap made the total length of the genome approximately 2,269,456 bp. In comparison to 53 genome sequences representing 19 additional Streptococcus species, the S. canis genome was among the largest with regard to sequence length, ranking fourth (with one exception S. agalactiae-FSL S3-026], sequences were obtained from the manually curated RefSeq database at NCBI. S. canis had a relatively high number of CDS (2,212), ranking fifth, an intermediate number of tRNAs (67; range 41–80) and an average GC content of 39.7%. A 5,871 bp section of the genome appeared to have been perfectly duplicated (locus tags SCAZ3_r06686 through SCAZ3_t06810 plus 126 bp of non-coding DNA that preceded SCAZ3_r06686). The section contained an rRNA operon (16S-23S-5S) and 10 tRNAs that were immediately down stream (Val, Asp, Lys, Leu, Thr, Gly, Leu, Arg, and Pro). The entire section was perfectly duplicated immediately upstream (one nucleotide separated the two duplicated sections). Similar rRNA operon duplications are present in the genomes of Streptococcus thermophilus (LMD-9) and Streptococcus salivarius (CCHSS3). The number of rRNA operons in publicly available Streptococcus genomes ranges from one to seven, and the number within the S. canis genome was again relatively high, with six. It is possible that this reflects selection for rapid growth. For example, during rapid growth genes are likely to be expressed at high levels, and this is often associated with codon usage bias [24], which in turn, has been shown to be positively correlated with the number of rRNA operons within a bacterial genome [25].

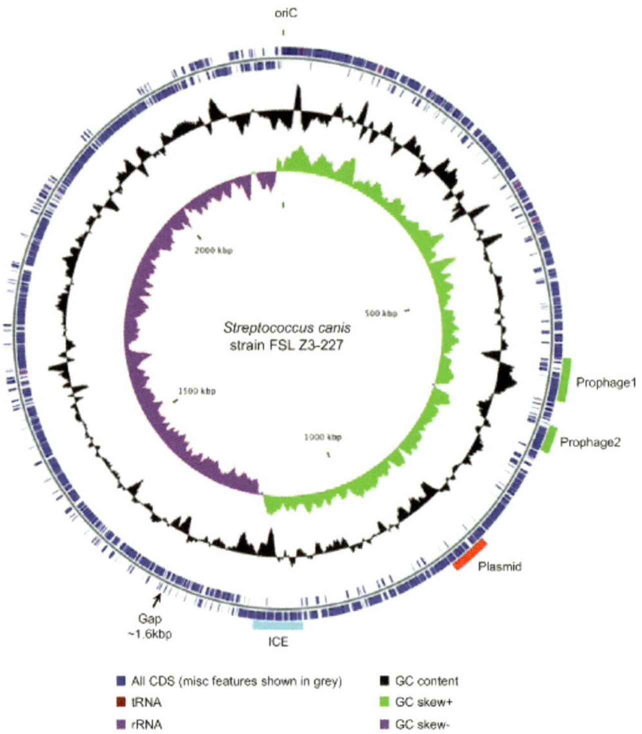

Figure 1: Genome map of Streptococcus canis strain FSL Z3-227. Starting from the outermost ring and moving inwards, rings show the location of: (1) four mobile genetic elements (see text for detailed description), (2) all annotated CDS on the leading strand, and (3) all annotated CDS on the lagging strand. Two innermost rings show GC content and GC skew. Map was created using the software CG [26].

Virulence factors

A total of 291 CDS within the S. canis genome were homologous with established virulence factors in the Virulence Factor of Pathogenic Bacteria database (VFDB) (available at http://www.mgc.ac.cn/VFs/main.htm. Throughout the manuscript, two genes (query and subject) are considered homologous if they can be locally aligned using BLAST with an E value of 1e-5 or less. A refined search, focusing only on established Streptococcus virulence factors, detected 34 CDS homologous to three other species of streptococci: S. pyogenes (17), S. agalactiae (9), and S. pneumoniae (8). Of these, the majority (50%) was homologous with S. pyogenes, likely reflecting the close relationship between these two species. More specifically, 9 of the 17S. pyogenes virulence factors homologous to S. canis were categorized as either exoenzymes or complement proteases. These gene products damage tissue, and may contribute to necrotizing fasciitis. When considering all 291 of the virulence factors homologous to S. canis, there were only three additional genes with similar categorization, two of these homologous to S. pneumoniae. Consequently, it appears that several genes possibly involved in necrotizing fasciitis are shared between S. canis and S. pyogenes. In contrast, S. canis CDSs were not homologous with genes producing pyrogenic exotoxins associated with toxic shock syndrome. However, S. canis possessed two other streptoccocal toxin-producing genes: streptolysin O (SLO) (S. pyogenes) and

CAMP factor (S. agalactiae) [27, 28]. Two S. canis genes were homologous to a well-characterized S. pyogenes virulence factor, the M protein (emm18), which aids in antiphagocytosis, adherence, and cellular invasion [29]. However, unlike S. pyogenes, these genes were not located within a contiguous 35-gene pathogenicity island that is found in all currently genome sequenced strains of S. pyogenes[30]. A BLASTn search of the NCBI nr database showed SCAZ3_01465 to be homologous with the gene SPASc from S. canis[31] (accession number: FJ594772). Global nucleotide sequence alignment showed these sequences to have 87.7% identity. Yang et al.[31] showed experimentally that SPASc was a new protective antigen, however they did not report the strain ID or isolation source. For SCAZ3_11010, a BLASTn search of the NCBI nr database returned no hits. However, a BLASTp search returned numerous hits and the gene with the most sequence similarity was an emm-like cell surface protein CspZ.2 of Streptococcus equisubsp. zooepidemicus ATCC 35246 (31% identity, 48% coverage). Neither SCAZ3_01465 nor SCAZ3_11010 were homologous with the S. canis emm gene type stG1389 (accession number EU195120) reported from one human and two canine sources [22]. These findings confirm previous studies showing that some S. canisisolates can possess M like proteins [18, 22, 23] and additionally show that a diversity of M like proteins is possible for S. canis strains.

S. canis also possessed the nine gene sag operon (sagABCDEFGHI) responsible for the production of streptolysin S (SLS) [32]. Both SLS and SLO are toxins that lyse mammalian erythrocytes [33], and the toxicity of SLS has been shown to contribute to necrotizing fasciitis [34, 35]. Furthermore, it has been suggested that SLS interacts with numerous additional virulence factors to accelerate necrosis [36]. These factors include SLO, the M protein, and proteases. Genes for all these factors can be present in the S. canis genome. Utilizing a BLASTn search of the NCBI nr database and subsequent global nucleotide sequence alignment, we detected the sag operon in four additional Streptococcus species (strain and percent sequence identity with S. canis are given in parentheses): S. dysgalactiae subsp. equisimilis (ATCC 12394; 81.1%), Streptococcus pseudoporcinus(LQ940-04 T; 78.8%), S. pyogenes (MGAS10270; 76.5%), and Streptococcus iniae (9117; 74.4%). The likely presence of the sag operon in S. dysgalactiae subsp. equisimilis was first shown by Humar et al. [34] who detected a functional sagA homolog in strains capable of producing SLS. S. canis and S. iniae are somewhat distinctive in that the other species are predominately human pathogens, whereas the former are predominately animal pathogens (S. iniae is a common fish pathogen), although occasionally are associated with zoonotic disease [37, 38, 39]. S. dysgalactiae subsp. dysgalactiae, which is predominantly associated with disease in animals but not in humans, lacks an intact sag operon, possessing only sagA and sagI. The occurrence of the complete operon in the other close relatives of S. canis (S. dysgalactiae subsp. equisimilisand S. pyogenes) suggests that S. dysgalactiae subsp. dysgalactiae may have lost the remainder of the genes from the operon. However, the occurrence of the operon in two species more distantly related to S. canis, that are themselves likely not sister species (S. pseudoporcinus and S. iniae) [40], is suggestive in this case of lateral gene transfer of the operon. Fish handling and close association with domestic dogs may have facilitated lateral gene transfer between species occupying human and animal hosts [14, 16, 41].

Genes specific to *S. canis*(FSL Z3-227)

To identify genes that are likely S. canis species specific from genes present in multiple species of the genus, we performed a clustering analysis among 214 Streptococcus genomes representing 41 species including S. canis . The analysis identified 97 genes that were not homologous to any other gene in the analysis and were unique to S. canis . Unfortunately, all were annotated as hypothetical proteins, highlighting the need for future studies exploring functional genomics for this species. S. canis belongs to the pyogenic 16S rRNA phylogenetic group [42]. Limiting the comparison to pyogenic genomes (14 species and 40 genomes, excluding S. canis), we identified an additional 14 genes unique to the S. canis genome. Two of these genes were homologous to two established virulence factors in the VFDB. The first gene (neuraminidase C, SCAZ3_10275) was homologous with neuraminidase B (nanB) from S. pneumoniae (TIGR4). The product of nanB is a glycosidase that, by damaging surface glycans and exposing the cell surface, aids in the adhesion to host cells and is therefore likely important in host invasion [43]. The second gene (Gfo/Idh/MocA family oxidoreductase, SCAZ3_10270) was homologous with bplA from Bordetella pertussis (Tohama I). In Bordetella, bpl genes are involved in the synthesis of the LPS, which has been shown to be essential for the expression of complete virulence in mice [44]. Given that the additional 14 genes unique to the S. canis genome were absent in the other pyogenic genomes, it is possible that these loci were gained via LGT. The two genes homologous to the virulence factors discussed above, were contiguous in the genome suggesting they were gained in a single evolutionary event.

Integrative plasmid

With the exception of two loci, S. canis shared a contiguous section of 53 CDS with S. agalactiae (NEM316) (Figure 2). Sequence identity between the shared 53 CDS was very high: 99.2%. First described in S. agalactiae (NEM316) [45], this section of DNA (designated pNEM316-1) was proposed to be a putative integrative plasmid (it could exist in circular form and was present as three copies within the genome). Here we designate the S. canis copy of the putative plasmid as FSL Z3-227-p. The last 24 bp at the terminal ends of pNEM316-1 were imperfect repeats of themselves. Alignment of pNEM316-1 with FSL Z3-227-p revealed identical terminal sequence for FSL Z3-227-p. Putative recombination attL and attR sites were also identified. As for pNEM316-1, these sites were 9 bp direct repeats.

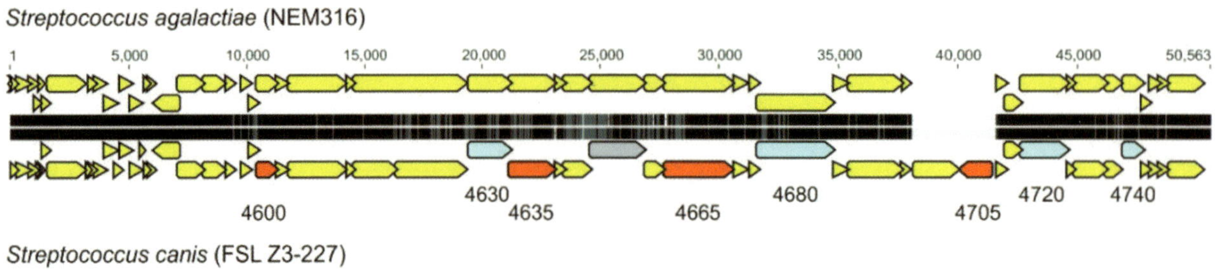

Figure 2: Gene organization within putative integrative plasmids for S. agalactiae strain NEM316 (plasmid designated pNEM316-1) and S. canis strain FSL Z3-227 (plasmid designated FSL Z3-227-p). Locus IDs for (i) CDS with putative plasmid functional role (blue arrows), and (ii) CDS homologous with established virulence factors (red arrows) are shown for S. canis (see text for detailed description). Grey arrow shows a miscellaneous feature that is a common BLAST hit with the M protein from S. pyogenes. Two horizontal black/grey bars are a generalized representation of the aligned nucleotide sequences, with black shading representing 100% identity. Figure created using Geneious v5.1.2 and Adobe Illustrator.

Annotation of several S. canis CDS within this 50 kb region suggest a plasmid functional role. For example, DNA topoisomerase (SCAZ3_04630), conjugation protein (SCAZ3_04680, SCAZ3_04720), and plasmid partition protein (SCAZ3_04740) were identified. In addition, four CDS were homologous with established virulence factors, locus tags are highlighted in red in the annotations worksheet). Specifically, SCAZ3_04635 (ATP-dependent clp protease) was homologous with clpE, an ATP-dependent protease from Listeria monocytogenes; clp genes have been shown to play a role in competence, development, and stress survival (thermotolerance) in S. pneumoniae[46]. SCAZ3_04705 (DNA-cytosine methyltransferase) was homologous with a putative DNA methylase from Escherichia coli (strain 536), which is located within a pathogenicity island [47] that included MGEs as an integral part of its evolutionary history [48]. Likewise, SCAZ3_04705 is located within a MGE and its specific function may involve plasmid defense. For example, the conjugative plasmid Tn5252, which infects streptococci, contains DNA methyltransferases that may methylate the plasmid DNA, thereby providing protection from host restriction nucleases [49]. SCAZ3_04600 (DNA-entry nuclease) was homologous with a putative deoxyribonuclease (DNase) from S. pyogenes. DNA-entry nuclease facilitates entry of DNA into competent bacterial cells and may aid plasmid cell-to-cell transmission [50]. Although the role of DNase in S. pyogenes is not fully understood, Sumby et al. [51] provided strong evidence that it may enhance host evasion. SCAZ3_04665 (cell wall surface anchor family protein) was homologous with a gene from Enterococcus faecalis producing a putative aggregation substance that was categorized as an adherence factor. SCAZ3_04665 was contiguous with two additional sequences with similar function. The first (SCAZ3_04660) contained an LPXTG-motif (a cell wall anchor domain). The second, according to the PGAAP annotation, was a common BLAST hit with the M protein from S. pyogenes (MGAS10270), and subsequent global nucleotide alignment showed 56.3% sequence identity between the sequences. However, the S. canis sequence contained a C insertion (site 746) that had shifted the reading frame. Although the insertion had disrupted the gene sequence in this strain, it does not preclude the presence of functional copies in other strains of S. canis. Together, these last three genes may play an important role in cell adherence possibly producing enhanced virulence of S. canis strains containing the plasmid.

Recently, Richards et al. [52] detected multiple copies of this plasmid (exact repeats) in a second strain of S. agalactiae: the bovine strain FSL S3-026. Designated FSL S3-026-S20, this copy of the plasmid showed 60.9% sequence identity (global alignment) with S. canis. There is strong differentiation between human and bovine S. agalactiae populations [52] and the S. canis strain studied here was isolated from bovine milk. Consequently, it seems plausible that the plasmid was exchanged between these species in the bovine environment. Indeed, out of the ten S. agalactiae genome sequences available, nine are human isolates and eight lack the plasmid. The ninth (NEM316), however, shows very high sequence identity for the plasmid when compared to S. canis (92.4%, global alignment), suggesting, on first consideration, that the plasmid may have been exchanged recently in the human environment. However, although NEM316 is usually listed as a human sourced isolate, Sørensen et al. [53] determined its origin to be unknown, and the observations that it can ferment lactose (human sourced isolates typically cannot) [53], and compared to other human sourced isolates, it grows well in milk (PD Pavinski Bitar unpublished data), suggest that the strain may have had a close association with the bovine environment. In addition, the strain is MLST sequence type 23, which occurs in both bovine and human environments [53, 54, 55].

Phages

S. canis contained a 59 CDS prophage (Prophage 1, Figure 1). In general, the prophage had the distinctive modular arrangement of tailed phage structural genes described for lactic acid bacteria [56]. Putative att sites (a 12 bp direct repeat) were identified 776 bp upstream of SCAZ3_03020 (hypothetical cytosolic protein) and 133 bp downstream of SCAZ3_03310 (site-specific recombinase). Upstream of the site-specific recombinase were two genes characteristic of the lysis module (holin and lysin) and upstream of this were genes characteristic of the tail modules. Consequently, this end of the prophage likely contained the attR site. However, site-specific recombinase (present as two contiguous copies) belongs to the resolvase family of enzymes, and these enzymes usually occur in the lysogeny module [57], which typically occurs at the other end of the phage. In addition to phage structural genes, the prophage also contained five CDS that were homologous with virulence factors in the VFDB. SCAZ3_03175 (DNA-cytosine methyltransferase) was homologous with the same DNA methylase from E. coli as the methyltransferase gene within the integrative plasmid and therefore may provide the phage with similar protection from host restriction nucleases. Similarly, both the phage (SCAZ3_03220: ATP-dependent clp proteolytic subunit) and plasmid contained CDS that were homologous with clp genes from L. monocytogenes, which play a role in competence, development, and stress survival in S. pneumoniae[46]. SCAZ3_03045 (serine/threonine rich platelet-type antigen) was homologous with C protein alpha antigen (bca) from S. agalactiae (A909), which is important in the initial stages of mice infection [58]. Gene ontology (GO) terms for this CDS also suggest virulence, indicating that the gene product is a cell surface component that binds to calcium ions, and this molecular function can be linked to pathogenesis. The remaining two CDS homologous with virulence factors (SCAZ3_03050 and SCAZ3_03060) were insertion sequences (transposases) homologous to the E. coli virulence plasmid pB171. These findings indicate several similarities between phage and the integrative plasmid genes; possibly reflecting shared infection and survival characteristics between these two types of mobile genetic element.

Using BLASTn we detected the presence of the prophage in three additional Streptococcus species: S. agalactiae (strains S3-026 [bovine isolate] and A909 [human isolate]), S. urinalis, and Streptococcus porcinus. Subsequent global nucleotide alignment revealed high sequence identity with S. agalactiae (S3-026) (97.3%) and particularly with S. urinalis (99.4%) suggesting very recent exchange between S. canis and S. urinalis. Sequence identities for S. agalactiae (A909) and S. porcinus were 63.1% and 64.1% respectively, suggesting older exchanges. To the knowledge of the authors, S. urinalis has only been reported as being isolated from humans [59, 60]. S. canis however, is typically found in animal hosts such as dogs and cats, but there are reports of human infection, usually ulcer or wound infection in patients who own domestic dogs [14, 15, 16]. Therefore, it's possible that S. canis and S. urinalis exchanged the phage within a shared human environment. However, it's also possible, that since S. urinalis is rare in humans, that a different, as yet unknown niche, is its principal habitat and that S. canis may be present in that same niche.

We also found evidence for a second prophage (~63 CDS) (Prophage 2, Figure 1). Although putative attL/R sites could not be found, the putative attL end was a site-specific recombinase (SCAZ3_03510), typical of the lysogeny module. BLASTn detected the phage in three additional Streptococcus species: S. dysgalactiae subsp. equisimilis, S. pyogenes, and S. dysgalactiae subsp. dysgalactiae. However, global nucleotide alignment revealed only moderate sequence identity to S. canis: 65.7%, 62.9%, and 58.0% respectively. Being the last of a generally contiguous sequence of phage genes for S. canis, S. pyogenes, and S. dysgalactiae subsp. equisimilis, and typical of the lysis module, a phage holin gene (SCAZ3_03820) was assumed to represent the attR end of the phage.

Integrative conjugative element

S. canis also contained a contiguous section of 54 CDS (SCAZ3_05800 - SCAZ3_06105) (62,915 bp) that was characteristic of an ICE. The section contained an integrase, three CDS homologous to the conjugative transposon Tn5252 (one of which was relaxase), Type IV secretory pathway genes belonging to the VirB4 family (implicated in conjugation) [61], and was flanked by putative attL/R sites (a 41 bp imperfect direct repeat that differed by 2 bp). However, unlike the ICE reported for numerous other Streptococcusspecies [62], the 5' end was not inserted at the 3' end of a tRNA or ribosomal gene, rather its 3' end was inserted at the 5' end of a ribosomal gene (ribosomal biogenesis GTPase). The ICE also possessed numerous additional genes characteristic of a mobile genetic element; for example, excisionase, helicase, abortive infection (Abi) system genes, and a zeta toxin gene characteristic of toxin-anti toxin (TA) systems, as well as a group II intron reverse transcriptase/maturase (SCAZ3_05875). In addition, the ICE contained three CDS that were homologous with virulence factors. Two of these CDS (agglutinin receptors, SCAZ3_05915 and SCAZ3_05930) were homologous with aggregation substance (AS) genes from Enterococcus faecalis plasmids. These genes (i) facilitate conjugative exchange by mediating cell binding, (ii) contribute to pathogenicity by enhancing cell adhesion and internalization, and (iii) favor intracellular survival within macrophages [63]. The third CDS (methyl transferase, SCAZ3_05815) was homologous with the same DNA methylase of E. coli, as for both the plasmid and phage, and therefore may provide the ICE with similar protection from host restriction nucleases.

A BLASTn search detected the ICE in two additional Streptococcus species: S. agalactiae (strains S3-026 and NEM316) and S. dysgalactiae subsp. dysgalactiae. Global nucleotide alignment showed these ICE to have only moderate identity with the S. canis ICE: 58.2%, 55.0%, and 60.1% respectively. In addition to the genes described, the S. canis ICE also contained the lactose operon Lac.2 [52, 64], suggesting that the ability to ferment lactose may have been acquired via lateral gene transfer. Furthermore, Lac.2 is also contained within the S. agalactiae (NEM316) and S. dysgalactiae subsp. dysgalactiae ICE, suggesting that these strains may have also acquired the ability to ferment lactose via lateral gene transfer.

Given S. canis strain FSL S3-227's association with the bovine environment, it is notable that there is a putative nisin resistance CDS (SCAZ3_06155) within the genome. Nisin is a lantibiotic produced by some strains of the mastitis causing pathogen Streptococcus uberis, and has been shown to provide these strains with a competitive advantage during intramammary infection when compared to non-producer strains [65]. The gene operon required for nisin production is also present in bovine isolates of S. agalactiae[52]. Although S. canis strain FSL S3-227 lacked this operon, the presence of a nisin resistance CDS might assist S. canis during intramammary infection.

Population genetics

To assess the population genetic structure of S. canis we ribotyped an additional 82 isolates obtained from bovine, canine, and feline hosts (see Methods). Of these, a subset of 46 isolates was selected for multi locus sequence typing (see Methods). The ribotyping revealed a total of 17 ribotypes for all 83 isolates (Table 1). With one exception, isolates from multiple cows within each dairy herd belonged to a single ribotype per herd. This supports previous observations, which found that mastitis outbreaks due to S. canis were generally caused by a single strain within a herd [10, 12], suggesting contagious transmission, exposure to a point-source, or host-adaptation of specific S. canis strains [66]. Among the 46 isolates selected for the MLST scheme, we identified 16 sequence types (STs). Diversity among canine isolates was substantially higher than among bovine isolates (Table 2). For example, there were 14 canine STs (diversity: 0.90) compared to 3 bovine STs (diversity: 0.49). For the ribotypes, there were 13 canine ribotypes (diversity: 0.88) compared to 4 bovine ribotypes (diversity: 0.67). Nucleotide diversity showed a different pattern. Although values were similar, bovine diversity was slightly higher (canine: 0.0094, bovine: 0.0127). The distinctiveness of the canine and bovine isolates was confirmed by the Fisher exact test, which showed the frequency distribution of ribotypes and STs between canine and bovine isolates to be significantly different (P=0.0000 [ribotypes], P=0.0030 [STs]). An analysis of molecular variance (AMOVA) [67], however, did not detect any significant differentiation between these isolates (Φ_{ST}=0.082, P=0.052).

Table 1: Isolate screening data

ID	Host/Tissue	Herd/State/Country	N1	N2	Ribotype	ST	CC
FSL Z3-022	Bovine	Not available, Belgium	1		116-1000-4	1	3
IT-SCA-35	Bovine	I-1, Italy	3		116-679-1	1	3
IT-SCA-65	Bovine	I-2, Italy	3		116-679-1	1	3
IT-SCA-73	Bovine	I-3, Italy	1		116-679-1	1	3
IT-SCA-31	Bovine	I-4, Italy	1		116-1000-4	1	3
IT-SCA-92	Bovine	I-5, Italy	3		116-1000-4	1	3
IT-SCA-80	Bovine	I-6, Italy	2		116-1000-4	2	3
IT-SCA-24	Bovine	I-7, Italy	3		116-679-1	1	3
FSL Z3-012*	Bovine	U-1, NY, USA	4		116-679-1	1	3
FSL Z3-006*	Bovine	U-2, NY, USA	4		116-679-1	1	3
R2-766	Bovine	U-3, NY, USA	5		116-679-1	1	3
FSL Z3-227*	Bovine	U-4, NY, USA	11		116-679-1	1	3
FSL Z3-316	Bovine	U-5, NY, USA	3	2[1]	116-1180-4	14	
FSL Z3-010	Bovine	U-6, NY, USA	4		116-975-3	14	
FSL Z3-346	Bovine	U-7, NY, USA	2		116-679-1	1	3
FSL Z3-013*	Bovine	U-8, NY, USA	2		116-975-3	14	
FSL Z3-015*	Bovine	U-9, NY, USA	1	1[2]	116-975-3	14	
FSL Z3-011*	Bovine	U-10, NY, USA	1		116-679-1	1	3
FSL Z3-234*	Bovine	U-10, NY, USA	2		116-975-3	14	
FSL Z3-023*	Canine, wound exudate	Not available, Belgium			1000-5	11	2
FSL Z3-046*	Canine, lip	NY, USA			1168-1	9	
FSL Z3-048	Canine, ear swab	NY, USA			1000-5	11	2
FSL Z3-049	Canine, ear swab	NY, USA			1000-4	1	3
FSL Z3-050	Canine, vaginal swab	NY, USA			1000-4	1	3
FSL Z3-053	Canine, vaginal swab	NY, USA			679-1	1	3
FSL Z3-054	Canine, vaginal swab	NY, USA			679-1	1	3
FSL Z3-057	Canine, hock abscess	NY, USA			975-3	15	
FSL Z3-058	Canine, ear swab	NY, USA			1171-2	6	
FSL Z3-116	Canine, pharyngeal swab	NY, USA			1168-5	8	
FSL Z3-117	Canine, ear swab	NY, USA			1000-5	12	2
FSL Z3-118	Canine, ear swab	NY, USA			697-1	1	3
FSL Z3-119	Canine, ear swab	NY, USA			1000-4	9	4
FSL Z3-120	Canine, vaginal swab	NY, USA			679-1	1	3

FSL Z3-121*	Canine, vaginal swab	NY, USA			1173-7	4	1
FSL Z3-154*	Canine, vaginal swab	NY, USA			1173-8	10	4
FSL Z3-155	Canine, urine	NY, USA			679-1	1	3
FSL Z3-156	Canine, throat	NY, USA			1168-1	10	4
FSL Z3-157*	Canine, pharyngeal swab	NY, USA			1174-4	16	1
FSL Z3-158	Canine, pharyngeal swab	NY, USA			1174-4	5	1
FSL Z3-159	Canine, eye	NY, USA			679-1	3	3
FSL Z3-160	Canine, vaginal swab	NY, USA			679-1	3	3
FSL Z3-162*	Canine, ear swab	NY, USA			1174-7	13	2
FSL Z3-163	Canine, dermis	NY, USA			679-1	1	3
FSL Z3-165	Canine, vaginal swab	NY, USA			1000-5	11	2
FSL Z3-166*	Canine, pharyngeal swab	NY, USA			1170-7	7	
FSL Z3-007*	Feline	U-4, NY, USA			679-1	1	3

N1 = Number of isolates from each herd ribotyped (either individual cow or quarter milk sample). For each herd, only one isolate representing a distinct ribotype was typed using MLST.

N2 = Number of isolates from milking machine rubber liners or bulk tank milk.

ST = sequence type.

CC = clonal complex.

[1] Isolated from milking machine rubber liners.

[2] Isolated from bulk tank milk.

* Isolate contains plasmid (see text).

Table 2: Isolate diversity indices and summary statistics

	***n*-RT**	**RT**	**RT-*h***	***n*-ST**	**ST**	**ST-*h***	**θ**	**π**	**plasmid**
All	83	17	0.90	46	16	0.76	0.0127	0.0111	15
Bovine*	56	4	0.67	19	3	0.49	0.0089	0.0127	7
Canine	26	13	0.88	26	14	0.90	0.0139	0.0094	7
Feline	1	1		1	1				1

n-RT = number of isolates ribotyped.

n-ST = number of isolates sequence typed.

RT = number of ribotypes.

RT-h = ribotype (gene) diversity.

ST = number of STs.

ST-h = ST (gene) diversity.

θ = population parameter theta (per site).

π = nucleotide diversity.

plasmid = number of strains containing the plasmid.

*The bovine isolates represent 18 distinct herds (farms). With one exception a single ST was obtained from each herd (two STs were obtained from one herd) (see Methods).

Examination of evolutionary relationships among STs using a Bayesian phylogenetic approach (ClonalFrame, [68]) produced a well-supported phylogeny (Figure 3), with three independent runs of the Markov chain all producing congruent topologies. Repeating the runs without the recombination model (we assume no recombination) had no affect on the topology, but branch lengths did vary (Figure 4). The average total branch length for the three phylogenies, not accounting for recombination (15.9 coalescent time units), was slightly larger than the average length of the three phylogenies that did account for recombination (14.2 coalescent time units).

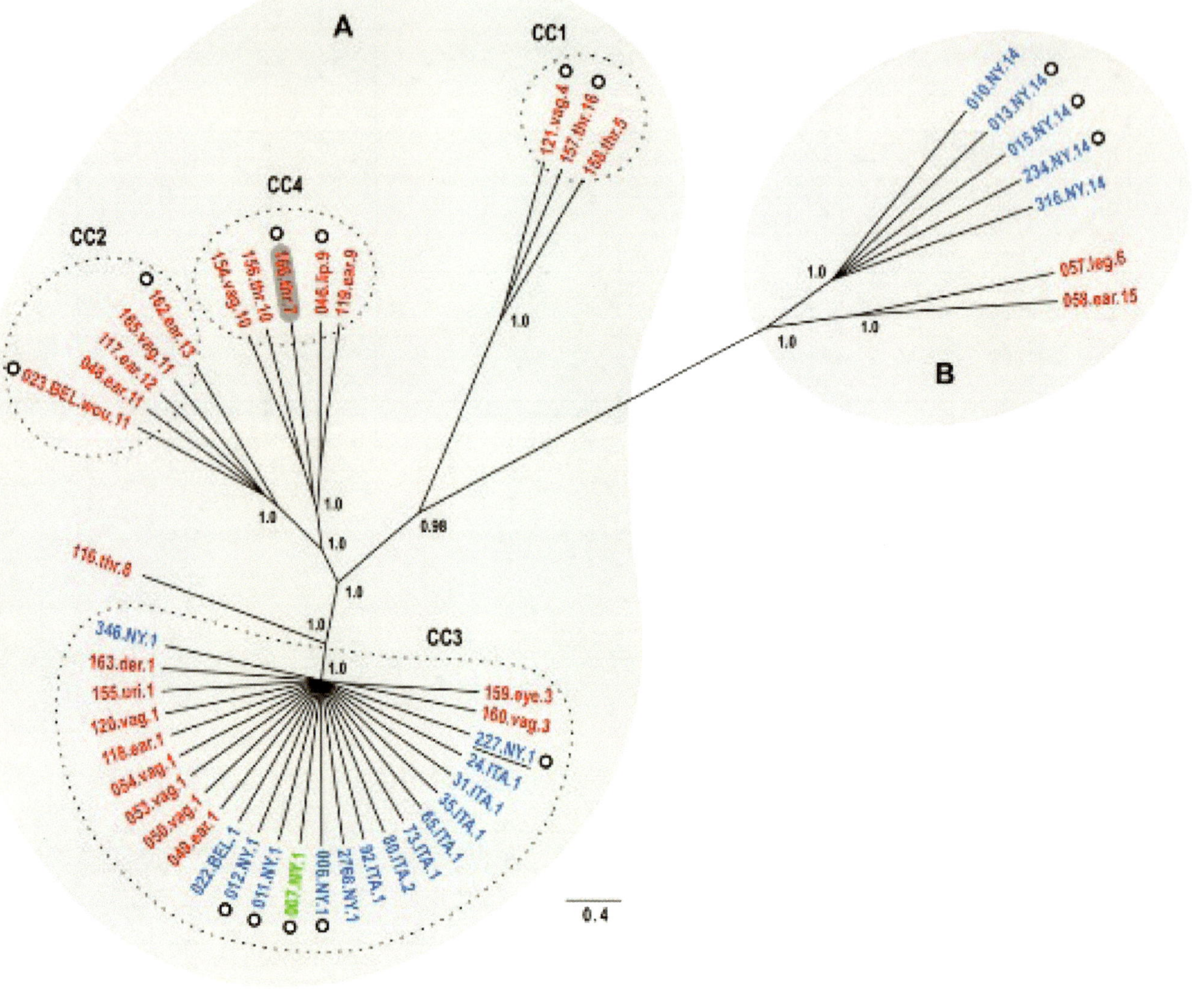

Figure 3: ClonalFrame 75% majority-rule consensus phylogeny (node posterior probabilities are at least 0.75). Posterior probabilities for major lineages are shown at nodes. Dashed circles show each clonal complex (CC) and grey shading shows isolates assigned to the two clusters (**A** and **B**) determined by the Structure analysis. Taxa labels are colored as follows: red = canine isolate, blue = bovine isolate, green = feline isolate. The first number in the label shows isolate ID. For canine isolates, tissue source follows the isolate ID, which is followed by the ST. Tissue source abbreviations are as follows: thr = throat, vag = vaginal, uri = urine, der = dermis, wou = wound exudate. For bovine and feline isolates, the ID is followed by the geographic location of collection (ITA = Italy, BEL = Belgium, NY = New York state, USA). Strain 227.NY.1 (underlined) is the strain who's genome was sequenced in this study. Circles with white centers indicate those strains that contained the plasmid discussed in the text. The strain shaded in dark grey (166.thr.7) was grouped with CC4 members based on ClonalFrame analysis but it was not contained within CC4 based on eBURST.

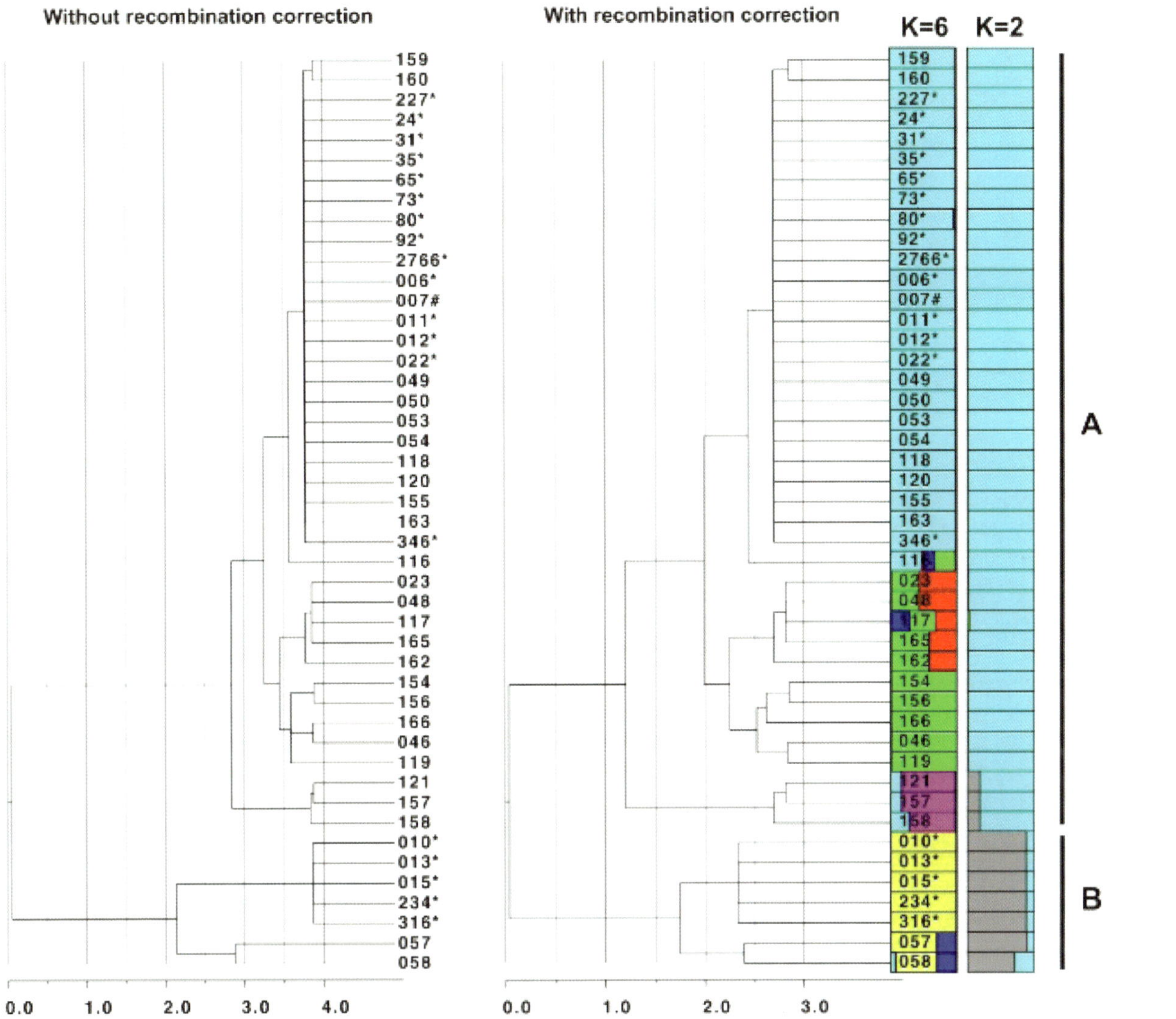

Figure 4: ClonalFrame 75% majority-rule consensus phylogenies with and without correction for recombination. The scale shows time in coalescent units. The phylogeny with recombination correction also shows for each isolate its proportion of ancestry for each genetic cluster determined by the Structure analyses. For K=2 and K=6, the different colors represent each cluster. The proportion of color shading for each bar represents the proportion of ancestry for the respective cluster. Vertical bars show the isolates assigned to clusters **A** and **B** when K=2. Asterisk refers to bovine isolates; # refers to feline isolate.

The amount of recombination in bacteria can be quantified using two ratios: (i) the ratio of the frequency at which recombination occurs relative to mutation (ρ/θ), and (ii) the ratio of the rates at which nucleotides become substituted as a result of recombination and mutation (r/m). The latter ratio accounts for length and nucleotide diversity of imported fragments and therefore contains more information regarding the evolutionary impact of recombination [69]. Using ClonalFrame, we calculated these ratios to be: $\rho/\theta = 0.1$ and $r/m = 1.5$, with the latter ratio indicating that recombination exceeded point mutation. Vos and Didelot [70] calculated r/m for 48 diverse species of bacteria, and their results revealed a wide range of values (63.6 – 0.02). r/m for S. canis ranked 25th in this distribution (approximately in the middle). However, the average of the 48 rates was 7.7, suggesting a below average rate of recombination for S. canis when compared to these species of bacteria. When compared to the two Streptococcus species in the distribution, S. canis was much lower: S. pneumoniae=23.1 (6th), S. pyogenes=17.2 (8th). Similar results were obtained when ρ/θ for S. caniswas compared to other Streptococcus species: S. uberis=17.2 [71], S. pneumoniae=23.1 [72].

We expanded the evolutionary analysis by also applying the parsimony-based approach e-BURST [73], which explores fine scale evolutionary relationships among STs. The ClonalFrame phylogeny and e-BURST results were generally concordant regarding the grouping of STs (Figure 3). The only discrepancy was ST7, which showed an intermediate relationship between STs 9 and 10 in the phylogeny, but was not grouped within the same clonal complex (CC) as STs 9 and 10 (ST7 was not grouped into any of the four clonal complexes).

Population structure was further examined using the Bayesian clustering approach implemented in the program Structure [74, 75]. The number of clusters K was estimated by calculating the ad hoc statistic ΔK, which is a measure of the second order rate of change of the probability of the data L(K) for each value of K[76] (see Methods for a full explanation of the approach). The analysis showed the optimum number of genetic clusters (K) to be two (A and B) (Figure 3). All four clonal complexes and ST8 were grouped into cluster A, whereas cluster B contained STs 6, 14, and 15. The ClonalFrame phylogeny showed CC1 to be the most closely related lineage to cluster B; concordantly, this lineage shared a small proportion (~12%) of its ancestry with cluster B (Figure 4). Although ΔK indicated that K was two and the Ln P(D) scores plateaued for K values of two, three, and four, the Ln P(D) scores rose slightly after K=4 and again plateaued starting with K=6. This suggests a pattern of hierarchal differentiation among isolates, with further subdivision present within clusters. Assuming K=6 for this additional subdivision, the assignment of individuals (proportion of ancestry) into these clusters delineated isolates into groups concordant with the six major lineages seen in the ClonalFrame phylogeny (Figure 4).

Only three (1, 2, and 14) of the 16 STs were found in bovines, and one of these (ST2) was a single locus variant of the predominant ST in cattle (ST1). Consequently, there was a much higher diversity of STs found in canine, producing a significant differentiation in the frequency of STs between the two hosts. Previous studies have shown the incidence of S. canis isolation from bovine to be rare [77, 78, 79, 80, 81, 82]. This observation coupled with the relatively low diversity of bovine STs suggests a recent adaptation to the bovine environment. Thus, the MLST data, the genomic features shared between S. canis and other bovine adapted Streptococcus species discussed earlier, and the epidemiological information associated with the original study regarding this strain [12], suggest that ST1 could be bovine adapted. The AMOVA, however, did not detect any significant differentiation between hosts. This is likely due to the fact that this analysis incorporates genetic distance and the strongest signal of differentiation (as detected by the Structure analysis) was between clusters A and B (Figure 3), both of which contain a bovine-associated ST (ST1 and ST14, respectively). This result does not necessarily preclude a very recent adaptation to the bovine environment for specific STs/lineages. If the adaptation were very recent, any phylogenetic signal recovered from the ST sequence data resulting from host partitioning would be very weak. Examination of the phylogeny (Figure 3) shows STs 1 and 2 to be closely related and contained within CC3, whereas ST14 is one of the most divergent ST from CC3. Given the above reasoning, this observation suggests that recent adaptation to the bovine environment must have occurred independently in these two lineages. A similar scenario was recently proposed for S. agalactiaewhere virulent lineages independently evolved from an ancestral core that were specific to human or bovine hosts [53].

There is, however, a possible alternative interpretation, that is contrary to the recent bovine adaptation argument. The most frequent ST was clearly ST1 (n=22, 48% of isolates). This ST was also seen in all three hosts (canine, bovine, feline), including a wide range of canine tissue types (vaginal, ear, skin, urine, eye), and also all three sampling locations (USA, Italy, and Belgium). In contrast, with one exception, no other ST was seen in more than one host or geographic location. The exception was ST11, which was seen in both USA and Belgium. These observations suggest that ST1 is the most ancestral ST in the data set [83, 84], and also possibly a generalist, with the ability to infect different hosts and tissue types. Genomic comparisons showed that strain FSL S3-227 shared multiple mobile genetic elements with S. agalactiae and S. dysgalactiae subsp. dysgalactiae strains isolated from the bovine environment, with one of these elements (the ICE) showing high sequence divergence. Although the ICE contained the Lac.2 operon, suggesting that this LGT may have contributed to bovine adaptation, the high divergence and multiple additional LGTs suggest that S. canis ST1 may have had an extended association with the bovine environment, arguing against more recent adaptation. Consequently, if ST1's lineage has possessed the ability to infect cows for an extended period of time, and is also the most ancestral with all lineages having descended from it, in order for the ST14 lineage to have recently acquired the ability to infect cows, all lineages intermediate between ST1 and ST14 must have previously lost this ability. This might have occurred as a single event on the branch connecting CC3 to ST8. Alternatively, all strains are generalist and the more recent lineages have simply had insufficient time to encounter the bovine environment and/or that our sample size was too low to detect their presence.

The distribution of the plasmid provides yet another perspective. The plasmid has only been observed in one additional species: S. agalactiae (strain FSL-S3026 [isolated from a bovine host], and strain NEM316 [potential association with the bovine environment]). Therefore, it is possible that the plasmid was exchanged between S. canis and S. agalactiae in the bovine environment, however, the plasmid appears randomly distributed among S. canis isolates, regardless of host species or ST. For example, (i) a Fisher exact test showed no significant difference in its distribution between bovine and canine isolates (P=1.0), (ii) it was present in all clonal complexes and clusters, and (iii) it was present in all three hosts including a wide range of canine tissue types (vaginal, ear, throat, lip). Consequently, the plasmid appears to have moved freely between bovine and canine environments, supporting the generalist argument. An alternative explanation is that S. canis may have obtained the plasmid on independent occasions from one or more different hosts. A similar process involving various mobile genetic elements has been observed for various Streptococcus species [17, 85, 86].

CONCLUSION

Characterization of the genome sequence for S. canis strain FSL S3-227 detected a high diversity of virulence factors. Approximately three quarters of the genes that were homologous to known Streptococcus virulence factors are involved in invasion, evasion, and colonization, perhaps explaining S. canis's ability to infect a wide range of tissue types. Furthermore, the putative ancestral clonal complex (accounting for more than half of collected isolates) occurred in a wide range of tissue types, all hosts, and all geographic locations suggesting a wide and diverse niche. It has been demonstrated that the source of bovine S. canis infection can be other farm-yard animals such as domestic cats [12]. Our results, revealed high genetic similarity among bovine, feline, and canine sourced isolates further supporting domestic farm-yard animals as infection sources. Despite the modest level of recombination for S. canis when compared to other Streptococcus species, LGT is still clearly an important evolutionary phenomenon in this species as evidenced by the multiple MGE present within its genome (i.e. plasmid, phage, and ICE) and the occurrence of an integrative plasmid in approximately half of the collected isolates. Furthermore, the evidence for LGT between S. canis and two additional bovine mastitis causing pathogens (S. agalactiae, and S. dysgalactiae subsp. dysgalactiae) suggests a close association with the bovine environment for S. canis, with this LGT possibly contributing to adaptation to this environment. Many virulence factors are also carried within these MGE, further highlighting the importance of these mobile elements in the evolution of this pathogen. Furthermore, the high frequency of virulence factors within multiple MGE, coupled with LGT between S. canis and a human sourced bacteria (S. urinalis), suggests the possibility for additional transport of virulence factors into the human environment.

METHODS

Strain selection, sequencing, and assembly

S. canis strain FSL Z3-227 was isolated from a composite milk sample obtained from a cow with an intra-mammary infection. The sample was collected on the 6th of April 1999 from a cow located in New York State within a dairy herd experiencing an outbreak of S. canis induced mastitis. Bacterial culture and ribotyping results indicated that a farm cat with chronic sinusitus was the likely source of the outbreak [12]. Utilizing a seven-gene MLST scheme developed here (see below), strain FSL Z3-227 was determined to be ST1. This ST was associated with multiple host species (bovine, canine, feline). In addition, it was the most common ST among bovine isolates and the only ST to be found in all three countries represented in the study. Therefore, it was thought to have the potential to have a broad complement of virulence factors, including those potentially associated with niche adaptation in cattle, and was consequently selected for genome sequencing.

Roche/454 pyrosequencing was used to determine the genome sequence, and Newbler v1.1 (454 Life Sciences Corporation) was used to assemble the reads. Using restriction enzyme BgIII, an optical map of the genome was built by OpGen Technologies, Inc. (Madison, WI). Scaffold order and orientation was determined by alignment to the optical map using Opgen Maper. Small inter and intra-scaffold gaps were closed by PCR and Sanger sequencing. Seven larger gaps were closed using long range PCR and Illumina sequencing. Illumina reads were assembled using Velvet [87], and the optimum assembly was determined using the N50 statistic. Annotation of the genome assembly was performed using the NCBI Prokaryotic Genomes Automatic Annotation Pipeline (PGAAP) and Blast2GO v.2.5.0 (E value cut-off=1e-6 and minimum amino acid alignment length cut-off [hsp-length]=33) [88]. This Whole Genome Shotgun project has been deposited at DDBJ/EMBL/GenBank under the accession AIDX00000000. The version described in this paper is the first version, AIDX01000000.

Homologous gene clustering

The MCL algorithm [89] as implemented in the MCLBLASTLINE pipeline (available at http://micans.org/mcl) was used to delineate homologous protein sequences among 214 Streptococcus genomes including S. canis. Based on sequence similarity, the pipeline uses Markov clustering (MCL) to assign genes to homologous clusters. Similarity was obtained from a reciprocal BLASTp within and between all genome pairs using an E value cut-off of 1e-5. The MCL algorithm was implemented using an inflation parameter of 1.8. Simulations have shown this value to be generally robust to false positives and negatives [90].

Virulence factors

Amino acid sequences for all S. canis CDS were searched against the VFDB using BLASTp. We used an E value cut-off of 1e-5 and retained the single best hit. The search was refined by repeating the BLASTp search against a database that contained only Streptococcus virulence factors (88 genes).

Population genetics

Including the strain genome sequenced here, a total of 83 S. canis isolates were obtained from bovine (n=56), canine (n=26), and feline (n=1) hosts (Table 1). Isolates of canine/feline origin included 25 canine isolates from patients of Cornell University's College of Veterinary Medicine, Ithaca, NY, USA, one canine isolate from Belgium, and one isolate from a cat living on a dairy farm in upstate New York. The feline isolate was the likely source of a mastitis outbreak at the same farm. Canine isolates from NY originated from dermis (n=1), ear swabs (n=7), eye (n=1), hock abscess (n=1), lip (n=1), pharyngeal swabs (n=5), urine (n=1), and vaginal swabs (n=8), and were collected from December 2003 to May 2004. The canine isolate from Belgium originated from wound exudate [1] and the feline isolate originated from a nasal swab taken from a cat with chronic sinusitis [12]. Bovine isolates originated from one herd in Belgium (from mastitic milk; [1], seven dairy herds in Italy (16 isolates from bovine milk; collected in 2003 and 2004), and 10 dairy herds in NY (two isolates from milking machine liners, one isolate from bulk tank milk, and 34 cow milk isolates; collected from 1999 to 2005). In addition to strain FSL Z3-227, all 82 isolates were ribotyped using the commercial RiboPrinter system with EcoRI.

Single isolates representing the ribotypes seen in each herd (two isolates from the herd U-10 and a single isolate from each of the remaining herds) (n = 19) were combined with all canine/feline isolates (n=27) and further screened using a seven housekeeping MLST scheme with PCR primers previously used for characterization of S. pyogenes, S. pneumoniae, or S. uberis[91, 92, 93, 94, 95]. MLST allele sequences were aligned using MAFFT v6.814b [96] as implemented in Geneious v5.1.2. Isolate genetic diversity indices were calculated using the program DNASP version 4.0 [97]. Diversity indices among STs were obtained by concatenating the seven alleles (4,014 bp). Diversity among ribotypes and STs was calculated using the formula for haplotype (gene) diversity [97]. Again using the concatenated allele sequences, population differentiation between bovine and canine groupings of isolates (bovine=19 canine=26) was determined by assessing the frequency distribution of STs (Fisher exact test) between the groups. Differentiation was also determined by an AMOVA as implemented in Arlequin v3.11 [98]. The AMOVA differs from the exact test because in addition to assessing ST frequency distribution, it also considers genetic divergence among isolate sequences in its determination of differentiation.

With the exception of strain FSL Z3-227 (our genome sequence), all isolates typed using the MLST scheme (n=45) were also PCR screened for the presence of a 55 CDS plasmid (see Results and discussion). Presence/absence of the plasmid was determined using 25 primer pairs that were contiguous along the length of the plasmid.

Evolutionary relationships among STs were examined using eBURSTv3 [73]. STs were grouped into clonal complexes and support for complex founders was estimated using 1000 bootstrap replicates. We used the most stringent (default) eBURST setting for grouping STs into a complex, where STs within the same complex shared identical alleles at $\geq$ six of the seven loci with at least one other member of the complex.

Deeper evolutionary relationships (among clonal complexes for example) were inferred using the Bayesian phylogenetic approach implemented in ClonalFrame v1.1 [68]. This approach incorporates a model that attempts to account for recombination. The Markov chain was run with 1,000,000 iterations after an initial burn-in of 50,000 iterations. Three independent runs were used to assess topological convergence. To assess the effect of recombination, all runs were repeated with the recombination rate parameter (R) held at zero (i.e. the effect of recombination on the topology was not accounted for). We used ClonalFrame to calculate the recombination ratios ρ/θ and r/m (average of the three runs).

Isolates were clustered using the Bayesian approach implemented in Structure v2.3.2 [74]. The number of clusters K was estimated by calculating the ad hoc statistic ΔK[76]. ΔK was calculated for K=1 through 10 using 5 Markov chains for each value of K. The simulations of Evanno et al. [76] showed that the highest value for ΔK reliably identified the optimum value of K. Chains were run for 500,000 steps following an initial burn-in of 100,000 steps, using the admixture ancestry and correlated allele frequency models. Once the optimum value of K was identified, strains were assigned to clusters using assignment coefficients (proportion of cluster membership) generated from an additional run utilizing the linkage ancestry and correlated allele frequency models. A study of recombinant bacterial populations showed the linkage model of ancestry to produce the most accurate assignment scores in situations where there are multiple linked loci along contiguous sections of DNA [75]. The model assumes these sections, which could be recombinant, to be discrete units of inheritance. Markov chains were run for 2,000,000 steps following an initial burn-in of 500,000 steps.

DECLARATIONS

Acknowledgements

We would like to thank staff from Cornell University's Quality Milk Production Services and Animal Health Diagnostic Centre for their contribution to sample and isolate collection. This study made use of PathogenTracker 2.0 (http://www.microbtracker.net), developed by Martin Wiedmann. This work was supported by the National Institute of Allergy and Infectious Disease, U.S. National Institutes of Health, under Grant No. AI073368 awarded to M.J.S.

Authors' contributions

VPR conducted data analysis and wrote the manuscript; MJS provided the conceptual framework, experimental design, and helped write the manuscript; PDPB and PL conducted laboratory work associated with genome sequencing; TL conducted data analysis and genome assembly; BW conducted laboratory work associated with the survey of plasmid distribution across canine and bovine isolates; LT, and PM conducted field work associated with population genetics; RNZ conceived of the field and laboratory work for population genetics, conducted MLST and ribotyping, and was involved in manuscript preparation. All authors read and approved the final manuscript.

REFERENCES

1. Devriese LA, Hommez J, Kilpper-Balz R, Schleifer KH: Streptococcus canis sp. nov.: a species of group G streptococci from animals. Int J Syst Bacteriol. 1986, 36 (3): 422-425. 10.1099/00207713-36-3-422.
2. Vandamme P, Pot B, Falsen E, Kersters K, Devriese LA: Taxonomic study of Lancefield streptococcal groups C, G, and L (Streptococcus dysgalactiae) and proposal of S. dysgalactiae subsp. equisimilis subsp. nov. Int J Syst Bacteriol. 1996, 46 (3): 774-781. 10.1099/00207713-46-3-774.
3. Murase T, Morita T, Sunagawa Y, Sawada M, Shimada A, Sato K, Hikasa Y: Isolation of Streptococcus canis from a Japanese raccoon dog with fibrinous pleuropneumonia. Vet Rec. 2003, 153 (15): 471-472. 10.1136/vr.153.15.471.
4. Iglauer F, Kunstyr I, Morstedt R, Farouq H, Wullenweber M, Damsch S: Streptococcus canis arthritis in a cat breeding colony. J Exp Anim Sci. 1991, 34 (2): 59-65.
5. Pesavento PA, Bannasch MJ, Bachmann R, Byrne BA, Hurley KF: Fatal Streptococcus canis infections in intensively housed shelter cats. Vet Pathol. 2007, 44 (2): 218-221. 10.1354/vp.44-2-218.
6. Kruger EF, Byrne BA, Pesavento P, Hurley KF, Lindsay LL, Sykes JE: Relationship between clinical manifestations and pulsed-field gel profiles of Streptococcus canis isolates from dogs and cats. Vet Microbiol. 2010, 146 (1–2): 167-171.
7. Matsuu A, Kanda T, Sugiyama A, Murase T, Hikasa Y: Mitral stenosis with bacterial myocarditis in a cat. J Vet Med Sci. 2007, 69 (11): 1171-1174. 10.1292/jvms.69.1171.
8. Sura R, Hinckley LS, Risatti GR, Smyth JA: Fatal necrotising fasciitis and myositis in a cat associated with Streptococcus canis. Vet Rec. 2008, 162 (14): 450-453. 10.1136/vr.162.14.450.
9. DeWinter LM, Prescott JF: Relatedness of Streptococcus canis from canine streptococcal toxic shock syndrome and necrotizing fasciitis. Can J Vet Res. 1999, 63 (2): 90-95.
10. Hassan AA, Akineden O, Usleber E: Identification of Streptococcus canis isolated from milk of dairy cows with subclinical mastitis. J Clin Microbiol. 2005, 43 (3): 1234-1238. 10.1128/JCM.43.3.1234-1238.2005.
11. Chaffer M, Friedman S, Saran A, Younis A: An outbreak of Streptococcus canis mastitis in a dairy herd in Israel. N Z Vet J. 2005, 53 (4): 261-264. 10.1080/00480169.2005.36557.
12. Tikofsky LL, Zadoks RN: Cross-infection between cats

and cows: origin and control of Streptococcus canis mastitis in a dairy herd. J Dairy Sci. 2005, 88 (8): 2707-2713. 10.3168/jds.S0022-0302(05)72949-0.

13. Galperine T, Cazorla C, Blanchard E, Boineau F, Ragnaud JM, Neau D: Streptococcus canis infections in humans: retrospective study of 54 patients. J Infect. 2007, 55 (1): 23-26. 10.1016/j.jinf.2006.12.013.
14. Lam MM, Clarridge JE, Young EJ, Mizuki S: The other group G Streptococcus: increased detection of Streptococcus canisulcer infections in dog owners. J Clin Microbiol. 2007, 45 (7): 2327-2329. 10.1128/JCM.01765-06.
15. Whatmore AM, Engler KH, Gudmundsdottir G, Efstratiou A: Identification of isolates of Streptococcus canis infecting humans. J Clin Microbiol. 2001, 39 (11): 4196-4199. 10.1128/JCM.39.1.4196-4199.2001.
16. Bert F, Lambert-Zechovsky N: Septicemia caused by Streptococcus canis in a human. J Clin Microbiol. 1997, 35 (3): 777-779.
17. Lefebure T, Richards VP, Lang P, Pavinski-Bitar P, Stanhope MJ: Gene repertoire evolution of Streptococcus pyogenesinferred from phylogenomic analysis with Streptococcus canis and Streptococcus dysgalactiae. PLoS One. 2012, 7 (5): e37607-10.1371/journal.pone.0037607.
18. Jensen A, Kilian M: Delineation of Streptococcus dysgalactiae, its subspecies, and its clinical and phylogenetic relationship to Streptococcus pyogenes. J Clin Microbiol. 2012, 50 (1): 113-126. 10.1128/JCM.05900-11.
19. Shinozaki-Kuwahara N, Takada K, Hirasawa M: Streptococcus ursoris sp. nov., isolated from the oral cavities of bears. Int J Syst Evol Microbiol. 2011, 61 (Pt 1): 40-44.
20. Tapp J, Thollesson M, Herrmann B: Phylogenetic relationships and genotyping of the genus Streptococcus by sequence determination of the RNase P RNA gene, rnpB. Int J Syst Evol Microbiol. 2003, 53 (Pt 6): 1861-1871.
21. Suzuki H, Lefebure T, Hubisz MJ, Pavinski Bitar P, Lang P, Siepel A, Stanhope MJ: Comparative genomic analysis of the Streptococcus dysgalactiae species group: gene content, molecular adaptation, and promoter evolution. Genome Biol Evol. 2011, 3: 168-185. 10.1093/gbe/evr006.
22. Broyles LN, Van Beneden C, Beall B, Facklam R, Shewmaker PL, Malpiedi P, Daily P, Reingold A, Farley MM: Population-based study of invasive disease due to beta-hemolytic streptococci of groups other than A and B. Clin Infect Dis. 2009, 48 (6): 706-712. 10.1086/597035.
23. DeWinter LM, Low DE, Prescott JF: Virulence of Streptococcus canis from canine streptococcal toxic shock syndrome and necrotizing fasciitis. Vet Microbiol. 1999, 70 (1–2): 95-110.
24. Kanaya S, Yamada Y, Kudo Y, Ikemura T: Studies of codon usage and tRNA genes of 18 unicellular organisms and quantification of Bacillus subtilis tRNAs: gene expression level and species-specific diversity of codon usage based on multivariate analysis. Gene. 1999, 238 (1): 143-155. 10.1016/S0378-1119(99)00225-5.
25. Sharp PM, Bailes E, Grocock RJ, Peden JF, Sockett RE: Variation in the strength of selected codon usage bias among bacteria. Nucleic Acids Res. 2005, 33 (4): 1141-1153. 10.1093/nar/gki242.
26. Stothard P, Wishart DS: Circular genome visualization and exploration using CG. Bioinformatics. 2005, 21 (4): 537-539. 10.1093/bioinformatics/bti054.
27. Bhakdi S, Tranum-Jensen J, Sziegoleit A: Mechanism of membrane damage by streptolysin-O. Infect Immun. 1985, 47 (1): 52-60.
28. Lang SH, Palmer M: Characterization of Streptococcus agalactiae CAMP factor as a pore-forming toxin. J Biol Chem. 2003, 278 (40): 38167-38173. 10.1074/jbc.M303544200.
29. Bisno AL, Brito MO, Collins CM: Molecular basis of group A streptococcal virulence. Lancet Infect Dis. 2003, 3 (4): 191-200. 10.1016/S1473-3099(03)00576-0.
30. Panchaud A, Guy L, Collyn F, Haenni M, Nakata M, Podbielski A, Moreillon P, Roten CA: M-protein and other intrinsic virulence factors of Streptococcus pyogenes are encoded on an ancient pathogenicity island. BMC Genomics. 2009, 10: 198-10.1186/1471-2164-10-198.
31. Yang J, Liu Y, Xu J, Li B: Characterization of a new protective antigen of Streptococcus canis. Vet Res Commun. 2010, 34 (5): 413-421. 10.1007/s11259-010-9414-1.
32. Nizet V, Beall B, Bast DJ, Datta V, Kilburn L, Low DE, De Azavedo JC: Genetic locus for streptolysin S production by group A Streptococcus. Infect Immun. 2000, 68 (7): 4245-4254. 10.1128/IAI.68.7.4245-4254.2000.
33. Todd E: The differentiation of two distinct serologic varieties of streptolysin, streptolysin O and streptolysin S. J Pathol Bacteriol. 1938, 47: 423-445. 10.1002/path.1700470307.
34. Humar D, Datta V, Bast DJ, Beall B, De Azavedo JC, Nizet V: Streptolysin S and necrotising infections produced by group G Streptococcus. Lancet. 2002, 359 (9301): 124-129. 10.1016/S0140-6736(02)07371-3.
35. Fuller JD, Camus AC, Duncan CL, Nizet V, Bast DJ, Thune RL, Low DE, De Azavedo JC: Identification of a streptolysin S-associated gene cluster and its role in the pathogenesis of Streptococcus iniae disease. Infect Immun. 2002, 70 (10): 5730-5739. 10.1128/IAI.70.10.5730-5739.2002.
36. Molloy EM, Cotter PD, Hill C, Mitchell DA, Ross RP: Streptolysin S-like virulence factors: the continuing sagA. Nat Rev Microbiol. 2011, 9 (9): 670-681. 10.1038/nrmicro2624.
37. Koh TH, Sng LH, Yuen SM, Thomas CK, Tan PL, Tan SH, Wong NS: Streptococcal cellulitis following preparation of fresh raw seafood. Zoonoses Public Health. 2009, 56 (4): 206-208. 10.1111/j.1863-2378.2008.01213.x.
38. Sun JR, Yan JC, Yeh CY, Lee SY, Lu JJ: Invasive infection with Streptococcus iniae in Taiwan. J Med Microbiol. 2007, 56 (Pt 9): 1246-1249.

39. Facklam R, Elliott J, Shewmaker L, Reingold A: Identification and characterization of sporadic isolates of Streptococcus iniae isolated from humans. J Clin Microbiol. 2005, 43 (2): 933-937. 10.1128/JCM.43.2.933-937.2005.

40. Bekal S, Gaudreau C, Laurence RA, Simoneau E, Raynal L: Streptococcus pseudoporcinus sp. nov., a novel species isolated from the genitourinary tract of women. J Clin Microbiol. 2006, 44 (7): 2584-2586. 10.1128/JCM.02707-05.

41. Weinstein MR, Litt M, Kertesz DA, Wyper P, Rose D, Coulter M, McGeer A, Facklam R, Ostach C, Willey BM, et al: Invasive infections due to a fish pathogen, Streptococcus iniae. S. iniae Study Group. N Engl J Med. 1997, 337 (9): 589-594. 10.1056/NEJM199708283370902.

42. Kawamura Y, Hou XG, Sultana F, Miura H, Ezaki T: Determination of 16S rRNA sequences of Streptococcus mitis and Streptococcus gordonii and phylogenetic relationships among members of the genus Streptococcus. Int J Syst Bacteriol. 1995, 45 (2): 406-408. 10.1099/00207713-45-2-406.

43. Jedrzejas MJ: Pneumococcal virulence factors: structure and function. Microbiol Mol Biol Rev. 2001, 65 (2): 187-207. 10.1128/MMBR.65.2.187-207.2001. first page, table of contents

44. Harvill ET, Preston A, Cotter PA, Allen AG, Maskell DJ, Miller JF: Multiple roles for Bordetella lipopolysaccharide molecules during respiratory tract infection. Infect Immun. 2000, 68 (12): 6720-6728. 10.1128/IAI.68.12.6720-6728.2000.

45. Glaser P, Rusniok C, Buchrieser C, Chevalier F, Frangeul L, Msadek T, Zouine M, Couve E, Lalioui L, Poyart C, et al: Genome sequence of Streptococcus agalactiae, a pathogen causing invasive neonatal disease. Mol Microbiol. 2002, 45 (6): 1499-1513. 10.1046/j.1365-2958.2002.03126.x.

46. Chastanet A, Prudhomme M, Claverys JP, Msadek T: Regulation of Streptococcus pneumoniae clp genes and their role in competence development and stress survival. J Bacteriol. 2001, 183 (24): 7295-7307. 10.1128/JB.183.24.7295-7307.2001.

47. Blum G, Ott M, Lischewski A, Ritter A, Imrich H, Tschape H, Hacker J: Excision of large DNA regions termed pathogenicity islands from tRNA-specific loci in the chromosome of an Escherichia coli wild-type pathogen. Infect Immun. 1994, 62 (2): 606-614.

48. Dobrindt U, Blum-Oehler G, Nagy G, Schneider G, Johann A, Gottschalk G, Hacker J: Genetic structure and distribution of four pathogenicity islands (PAI I(536) to PAI IV(536)) of uropathogenic Escherichia coli strain 536. Infect Immun. 2002, 70 (11): 6365-6372. 10.1128/IAI.70.11.6365-6372.2002.

49. Sampath J, Vijayakumar MN: Identification of a DNA cytosine methyltransferase gene in conjugative transposon Tn5252. Plasmid. 1998, 39 (1): 63-76. 10.1006/plas.1997.1316.

50. Saunders J, Saunders V: Bacterial transformation with plasmid DNA. Methods in Microbiology Volume 21. Edited by: Grinsted J, Bennett P. 1988, London: Academic Press,

51. Sumby P, Barbian KD, Gardner DJ, Whitney AR, Welty DM, Long RD, Bailey JR, Parnell MJ, Hoe NP, Adams GG, et al: Extracellular deoxyribonuclease made by group A Streptococcus assists pathogenesis by enhancing evasion of the innate immune response. Proc Natl Acad Sci U S A. 2005, 102 (5): 1679-1684. 10.1073/pnas.0406641102.

52. Richards VP, Lang P, Bitar PD, Lefebure T, Schukken YH, Zadoks RN, Stanhope MJ: Comparative genomics and the role of lateral gene transfer in the evolution of bovine adapted Streptococcus agalactiae. Infect Genet Evol. 2011, 11 (6): 1263-1275. 10.1016/j.meegid.2011.04.019.

53. Sørensen UB, Poulsen K, Ghezzo C, Margarit I, Kilian M: Emergence and Global Dissemination of Host-Specific Streptococcus agalactiae Clones. MBio. 2010, 1 (3):

54. Brochet M, Couve E, Zouine M, Vallaeys T, Rusniok C, Lamy MC, Buchrieser C, Trieu-Cuot P, Kunst F, Poyart C, et al: Genomic diversity and evolution within the species Streptococcus agalactiae. Microbes Infect. 2006, 8 (5): 1227-1243. 10.1016/j.micinf.2005.11.010.

55. Bisharat N, Crook DW, Leigh J, Harding RM, Ward PN, Coffey TJ, Maiden MC, Peto T, Jones N: Hyperinvasive neonatal group B Streptococcus has arisen from a bovine ancestor. J Clin Microbiol. 2004, 42 (5): 2161-2167. 10.1128/JCM.42.5.2161-2167.2004.

56. Canchaya C, Proux C, Fournous G, Bruttin A, Brussow H: Prophage genomics. Microbiol Mol Biol Rev. 2003, 67 (2): 238-276. 10.1128/MMBR.67.2.238-276.2003.

57. Lucchini S, Desiere F, Brussow H: Similarly organized lysogeny modules in temperate Siphoviridae from low GC content gram-positive bacteria. Virology. 1999, 263 (2): 427-435. 10.1006/viro.1999.9959.

58. Li J, Kasper DL, Ausubel FM, Rosner B, Michel JL: Inactivation of the alpha C protein antigen gene, bca, by a novel shuttle/suicide vector results in attenuation of virulence and immunity in group B Streptococcus. Proc Natl Acad Sci U S A. 1997, 94 (24): 13251-13256. 10.1073/pnas.94.24.13251.

59. Peltroche-Llacsahuanga H, Frye B, Haase G: Isolation of Streptococcus urinalis from a human blood culture. J Med Microbiol. 2012, 61 (Pt 5): 740-742.

60. Collins MD, Hutson RA, Falsen E, Nikolaitchouk N, LaClaire L, Facklam RR: An unusual Streptococcus from human urine, Streptococcus urinalis sp. nov. Int J Syst Evol Microbiol. 2000, 50 Pt 3: 1173-1178.

61. Rabel C, Grahn AM, Lurz R, Lanka E: The VirB4 family of proposed traffic nucleoside triphosphatases: common motifs in plasmid RP4 TrbE are essential for conjugation and phage adsorption. J Bacteriol. 2003, 185 (3): 1045-1058. 10.1128/JB.185.3.1045-1058.2003.

62. Haenni M, Saras E, Bertin S, Leblond P, Madec JY, Payot S: Diversity and mobility of integrative and conjugative elements in bovine isolates of Streptococcus agalactiae,S. dysgalactiaesubsp. dysgalactiae, and S. uberis. Appl Environ Microbiol. 2010, 76 (24): 7957-7965. 10.1128/AEM.00805-10.

63. Paoletti C, Foglia G, Princivalli MS, Magi G, Guaglianone E, Donelli G, Pruzzo C, Biavasco F, Facinelli B: Co-transfer of vanA and aggregation substance genes from Enterococcus faecalis isolates in intra- and interspecies matings. J Antimicrob Chemother. 2007, 59 (5): 1005-1009. 10.1093/jac/dkm057.

64. Ferretti JJ, McShan WM, Ajdic D, Savic DJ, Savic G, Lyon K, Primeaux C, Sezate S, Suvorov AN, Kenton S, et al: Complete genome sequence of an M1 strain of Streptococcus pyogenes. Proc Natl Acad Sci U S A. 2001, 98 (8): 4658-4663. 10.1073/pnas.071559398.

65. Pryor SM, Cursons RT, Williamson JH, Lacy-Hulbert SJ: Experimentally induced intramammary infection with multiple strains of Streptococcus uberis. J Dairy Sci. 2009, 92 (11): 5467-5475. 10.3168/jds.2009-2223.

66. Zadoks RN, Schukken YH: Use of molecular epidemiology in veterinary practice. Vet Clin North Am Food Anim Pract. 2006, 22 (1): 229-261. 10.1016/j.cvfa.2005.11.005.

67. Excoffier L, Smouse PE, Quattro JM: Analysis of molecular variance inferred from metric distances among DNA haplotypes: Application to human mitochondrial DNA restriction data. Genetics. 1992, 131: 479-491.

68. Didelot X, Falush D: Inference of bacterial microevolution using multilocus sequence data. Genetics. 2007, 175 (3): 1251-1266.

69. Guttman DS, Dykhuizen DE: Clonal divergence in Escherichia coli as a result of recombination, not mutation. Science. 1994, 266 (5189): 1380-1383. 10.1126/science.7973728.

70. Vos M, Didelot X: A comparison of homologous recombination rates in bacteria and archaea. ISME J. 2009, 3 (2): 199-208. 10.1038/ismej.2008.93.

71. Lang P, Lefebure T, Wang W, Zadoks RN, Schukken Y, Stanhope MJ: Gene content differences across strains of Streptococcus uberis identified using oligonucleotide microarray comparative genomic hybridization. Infect Genet Evol. 2009, 9 (2): 179-188. 10.1016/j.meegid.2008.10.015.

72. Fraser C, Hanage WP, Spratt BG: Neutral microepidemic evolution of bacterial pathogens. Proc Natl Acad Sci U S A. 2005, 102 (6): 1968-1973. 10.1073/pnas.0406993102.

73. Feil EJ, Li BC, Aanensen DM, Hanage WP, Spratt BG: eBURST: inferring patterns of evolutionary descent among clusters of related bacterial genotypes from multilocus sequence typing data. J Bacteriol. 2004, 186 (5): 1518-1530. 10.1128/JB.186.5.1518-1530.2004.

74. Pritchard JK, Stephens M, Donnelly P: Inference of population structure using multilocus genotype data. Genetics. 2000, 155 (2): 945-959.

75. Falush D, Stephens M, Pritchard JK: Inference of population structure using multilocus genotype data: linked loci and correlated allele frequencies. Genetics. 2003, 164 (4): 1567-1587.

76. Evanno G, Regnaut S, Goudet J: Detecting the number of clusters of individuals using the software STRUCTURE: a simulation study. Mol Ecol. 2005, 14 (8): 2611-2620. 10.1111/j.1365-294X.2005.02553.x.

77. Persson Y, Nyman AK, Gronlund-Andersson U: Etiology and antimicrobial susceptibility of udder pathogens from cases of subclinical mastitis in dairy cows in Sweden. Acta Vet Scand. 2011, 53: 36-10.1186/1751-0147-53-36.

78. Piepers S, De Meulemeester L, de Kruif A, Opsomer G, Barkema HW, De Vliegher S: Prevalence and distribution of mastitis pathogens in subclinically infected dairy cows in Flanders, Belgium. J Dairy Res. 2007, 74 (4): 478-483.

79. Sampimon O, Barkema HW, Berends I, Sol J, Lam T: Prevalence of intramammary infection in Dutch dairy herds. J Dairy Res. 2009, 76 (2): 129-136. 10.1017/S0022029908003762.

80. Petrovski KR, Heuer C, Parkinson TJ, Williamson NB: The incidence and aetiology of clinical bovine mastitis on 14 farms in Northland, New Zealand. N Z Vet J. 2009, 57 (2): 109-115. 10.1080/00480169.2009.36887.

81. Guelat-Brechbuehl M, Thomann A, Albini S, Moret-Stalder S, Reist M, Bodmer M, Michel A, Niederberger MD, Kaufmann T: Cross-sectional study of Streptococcus species in quarter milk samples of dairy cows in the canton of Bern, Switzerland. Vet Rec. 2010, 167 (6): 211-215. 10.1136/vr.167.6.211.

82. Bengtsson B, Unnerstad HE, Ekman T, Artursson K, Nilsson-Ost M, Waller KP: Antimicrobial susceptibility of udder pathogens from cases of acute clinical mastitis in dairy cows. Vet Microbiol. 2009, 136 (1–2): 142-149.

83. Avise JC: Phylogeography. The history and formation of species. 2000, Cambridge,MA: Harvard University Press,

84. Templeton AR: Population genetics and microevolutionary theory. 2006, New Jersey:Wiley,

85. Delorme C, Poyart C, Ehrlich SD, Renault P: Extent of horizontal gene transfer in evolution of Streptococci of the salivarius group. J Bacteriol. 2007, 189 (4): 1330-1341. 10.1128/JB.01058-06.

86. Davies MR, Tran TN, McMillan DJ, Gardiner DL, Currie BJ, Sriprakash KS: Inter-species genetic movement may blur the epidemiology of streptococcal diseases in endemic regions. Microbes Infect. 2005, 7 (9–10): 1128-1138.

87. Zerbino DR, Birney E: Velvet: algorithms for de novo short read assembly using de Bruijn graphs. Genome Res. 2008, 18 (5): 821-829. 10.1101/gr.074492.107.

88. Gotz S, Garcia-Gomez JM, Terol J, Williams TD, Nagaraj SH, Nueda MJ, Robles M, Talon M, Dopazo J, Conesa A: High-throughput functional annotation and data mining with the Blast2GO suite. Nucleic Acids Res. 2008, 36 (10): 3420-3435. 10.1093/nar/gkn176.

89. van Dongen S: University of Utrecht. Graph clustering by flow simulation. 2000

90. Brohee S, van Helden J: Evaluation of clustering algorithms for protein-protein interaction networks. BMC Bioinformatics. 2006, 7: 488-10.1186/1471-2105-7-488.

91. Enright MC, Spratt BG: A multilocus sequence typing scheme for Streptococcus pneumoniae: identification of clones associated with serious invasive disease. Microbiology. 1998, 144 (Pt 11): 3049-3060.

92. Enright MC, Spratt BG, Kalia A, Cross JH, Bessen DE: Multilocus sequence typing of Streptococcus pyogenes and the relationships between emm type and clone. Infect Immun. 2001, 69 (4): 2416-2427. 10.1128/IAI.69.4.2416-2427.2001.

93. Goh SH, Santucci Z, Kloos WE, Faltyn M, George CG, Driedger D, Hemmingsen SM: Identification of Staphylococcusspecies and subspecies by the chaperonin 60 gene identification method and reverse checkerboard hybridization. J Clin Microbiol. 1997, 35 (12): 3116-3121.

94. Ke D, Picard FJ, Martineau F, Menard C, Roy PH, Ouellette M, Bergeron MG: Development of a PCR assay for rapid detection of enterococci. J Clin Microbiol. 1999, 37 (11): 3497-3503.

95. Zadoks RN, Schukken YH, Wiedmann M: Multilocus sequence typing of Streptococcus uberis provides sensitive and epidemiologically relevant subtype information and reveals positive selection in the virulence gene pauA. J Clin Microbiol. 2005, 43 (5): 2407-2417. 10.1128/JCM.43.5.2407-2417.2005.

96. Katoh K, Misawa K, Kuma K, Miyata T: MAFFT: a novel method for rapid multiple sequence alignment based on fast Fourier transform. Nucleic Acids Res. 2002, 30 (14): 3059-3066. 10.1093/nar/gkf436.

97. Rozas J, Sánchez-DelBarrio J, Messegyer X, Rozas R: DNASP, DNA polymorphism analyses by the coalescent and other methods. Bioinformatics. 2003, 19: 2496-2497. 10.1093/bioinformatics/btg359.

98. Excoffier L, Laval G, Schneider S: Arlequin (version 3.0): an integrated software package for population genetics data analysis. Evol Bioinform Online. 2005, 1: 47-50.

CHAPTER 27

EVIDENCE FOR NICHE ADAPTATION IN THE GENOME OF THE BOVINE PATHOGEN STREPTOCOCCUS UBERIS

Philip N Ward, Matthew TG Holden, James A Leigh, Nicola Lennard, Alexandra Bignell, Andy Barron, Louise Clark, Michael A Quail, John Woodward, Bart G Barrell, Sharon A Egan, Terence R Field, Duncan Maskell, Michael Kehoe, Christopher G Dowson, Neil Chanter, Adrian M Whatmore, Stephen D Bentley and Julian Parkhill

BACKGROUND

Streptococcus uberis is a gram positive bacterium belonging to family Streptococcaceae, a diverse family of bacteria that encompasses species capable of commensal and/or pathogenic traits. Pathogenic streptococci cause a variety of disease states across a range of animal hosts as well as man. The zoonotic potential of streptococci normally considered pathogenic for animal species has been recently documented for *Streptococcus suis* [1] and *Streptococcus agalactiae* [2].

Phylogenetic analysis [3] placed *S. uberis* within the pyogenic cluster, a large grouping containing the human pathogens *Streptococcus pyogenes* and *Streptococcus dysgalactiae* subsp. *equisimilis*, the zoonotic *S. agalactiae* and a number of animal pathogens occupying diverse ecological niches including *S. dysgalactiae, Streptococcus equi, Streptococcus canis* and *Streptococcus iniae*.

S. uberis is commensal at many body sites and has been isolated from the skin, gut, tonsils and genital tract of asymptomatic cattle. Furthermore it can infect the bovine mammary gland and act as a major pathogen of the mammary gland causing the inflammatory disease, mastitis. Infection with *S. uberis* is one of the major causes of bovine mastitis worldwide [4, 5, 6] and the most common cause in the UK [7]. Procedures to control bacterial infection of the mammary glands of dairy cattle are based on limiting duration of existing infection and restricting exposure of potentially infectious material from one gland to another. These procedures have resulted in decreased transmission of infections due to certain bacterial species (*Staphylococcus aureus*, *S. agalactiae*) but have had little impact on the incidence of infection due to *S. uberis*. The failure of these measures to control intramammary infection due to *S. uberis* implies transmission from additional/alternate sources [8]. Typing of isolates from cases of mastitis also implies that *S. uberis* is not transmitted from reservoirs containing single outbreak strains as multiple bacterial types are often detected within a single herd. *S. uberis* is often detected in faeces and can also be isolated from the environment (pasture, bedding materials) populated by these animals [9, 10]. However, survival of *S. uberis* in the environment is limited. A recent report from New Zealand, which operates a pasture-based dairy system where cattle are housed rarely if at all, showed that the organism survived in the environment for less than 4 weeks [11]. This implies that persistence in pasture is dependent on constant reintroduction, probably via faecal contamination. It is, therefore reasonable to conclude that a successful clone of *S. uberis* isolated from a mastitic mammary gland is able to colonise and increase in number within the ruminant gut, survive in environmental niches such as pasture or bedding in sufficient numbers to gain access to the mammary gland where it must replicate and avoid a number of host defence mechanisms. In addition to infection of the lactating mammary gland, *S. uberis* is also able to infect the involuted or dry gland [12]. In this niche the secretion in which the organism replicates and the range of host defences encountered differ markedly from those present during lactation [13].

Citation: Philip N Ward, Matthew TG Holden, James A Leigh, Nicola Lennard, Alexandra Bignell, Andy Barron, Louise Clark, Michael A Quail, John Woodward, Bart G Barrell, Sharon A Egan, Terence R Field, Duncan Maskell, Michael Kehoe, Christopher G Dowson, Neil Chanter, Adrian M Whatmore, Stephen D Bentley and Julian Parkhill, Evidence for niche adaptation in the genome of the bovine pathogen Streptococcus uberis, DOI: 10.1186/1471-2164-10-54.

Epidemiologically, *S. uberis* strain 0140J, the strain chosen for sequence determination, was placed within a major UK lineage, the clonal complex based around sequence type 5, of an ongoing MLST scheme [14]. As such, strain 0140J represents a typical UK isolate in terms of its ancestry. It is also among the most thoroughly characterised strains [15] that is pathogenic for both the lactating and non-lactating bovine mammary gland. Therefore it was deemed ideally suited to be the first strain of this species to be sequenced. The complete *S. uberis* genome provides insights into host-cell interactions and pathogenesis.

Since the completion of the first streptococcal genome [16] many comparative projects have centred upon the main species pathogenic for humans, namely *S. agalactiae* [17], *Streptococcus pneumoniae* [18, 19] and *S. pyogenes* [20, 21]. Such studies have indicated the pairing of significant levels of conserved gene content with considerable gene sequence heterogeneity. Additionally, the proportion and content of such genomes that was attributable to a variety of mobile genetic elements appeared considerable. Comparative genomics has recently enabled the scale of both inter and intra-species horizontal gene transfer to be realised, for example within the oral streptococci [22]. Intriguingly, the gene content of some streptococci also appears to have been augmented from non-streptococcal species with which they co-exist in discrete ecological niches [23, 24]. It is against such a backdrop that analysis of pathogenic streptococci of veterinary significance can derive added value. The genome sequences of several other related streptococcal species, with different host ranges and disease associations are available for comparison. We utilized the genomes of *S. equi* subsp. *zooepidemicus* (*S. zooepidemicus*) [25]; a veterinary pathogen causing lower airway disease, foal pneumonia, endometritis, and abortion in horses, and hemorrhagic streptococcal pneumonia in dogs; and *S. pyogenes*(alternatively referred to as group A Streptococcus, GAS) [26]; responsible for a diverse number of diseases in humans, including pharyngitis, toxic shock syndrome (TSS), impetigo and scarlet fever, and the post infection sequelae, acute rheumatic fever (ARF). Comparisons with these related pathogens and their virulence determinants highlighted the components of the genome that distinguish it from these species, and genes that are important for the niche-adaptation and virulence of *S. uberis*.

RESULTS AND DISCUSSION

Comparative genomics

The genome of *S. uberis* 0140J consists of a single circular chromosome of 1,852,352 bp (Figure 1), which places it at the lower end of the 1.8 Mb–2.3 Mb size range of streptococcal genomes sequenced to date. The genome contains 1,825 predicted protein coding sequences (CDSs), 62 of which are pseudogenes or gene fragments. Comparative genomic analysis with other streptococci by reciprocal FASTA revealed a conserved core of orthologous CDSs (Figure 1); comparisons using representatives of each of the sequenced *Streptococcus* species identified that ~40% of *S. uberis* CDSs had orthologous matches in all the streptococcal genomes compared. Supplementing this core were variably distributed orthologues (~48% of the CDSs) that were identified in one or more streptococci, and *S. uberis*-specific CDSs (~11% of the CDSs).

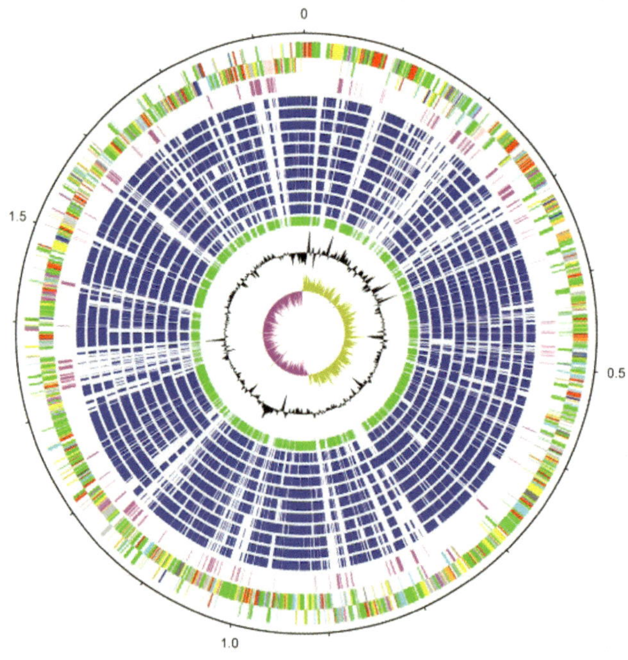

Figure 1: Schematic circular diagram of the *S. uberis* 0140J genome. Key for the circular diagram: scale (in Mb); annotated CDSs coloured according to predicted function represented on a pair of concentric circles, representing both coding strands; *S. uberis* unique CDSs, magenta; CDSs with Streptococcal ortholog matches, blue; ortholog matches shared with the Streptococcal species, *S. pyogenes* Manfredo, *S. zooepidemicus* H70, *S. equi* 4047, *S. mutans* UA159, *S. gordonii* Challis CH1, *S. sanguinis* SK36, *S. pneumoniae* TIGR4, *S. agalactiae* NEM316, *S. suis* P1/7, *S. thermophilus*CNRZ1066; *Lactococcus lactis* subsp. *lactis*, green; G + C% content plot; G + C deviation plot (>0% olive, <0% purple). Colour coding for CDS functions: dark blue; pathogenicity/adaptation, black; energy metabolism, red; information transfer, dark green; surface associated, cyan; degradation of large molecules, magenta; degradation of small molecules, yellow; central/intermediary metabolism, pale green; unknown, pale blue; regulators, orange; conserved hypothetical, brown; pseudogenes, pink; phage and IS elements, grey; miscellaneous.

For any one streptococcal species comparison, between 57% and 72% of the *S. uberis* CDSs had orthologue matches, which compared with 58% for a comparison with *Lactococcus lactis* subsp. *lactis*. The highest numbers of orthologue matches were identified in comparisons with pyogenic streptococci, while more taxonomically divergent species yielded lower numbers of orthologous matches. Comparison of the structure of the *S. uberis* 0140J chromosome with other streptococci revealed the greatest overall conservation with *S. zooepidemicus* and *S. pyogenes* (Figure 2A).

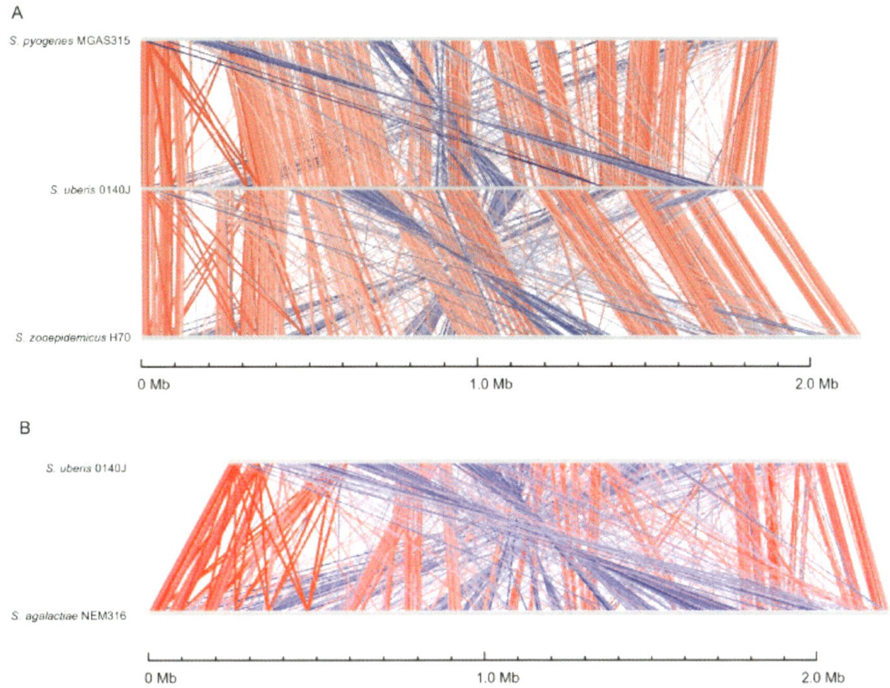

Figure 2: Genome comparison of pyogenic streptococci. Pairwise comparisons of the chromosomes of *S. pyogenes*MGAS315, *S. uberis* 0140J and *S. zooepidemicus* H70 (A), and *S. uberis* 0140J and *agalactiae* NEM316 (B) displayed using the Artemis Comparison Tool (ACT) [89]. The sequences have been aligned from the predicted replication origins (oriC; right). The coloured bars separating each genome (red and blue) represent similarity matches identified by reciprocal TBLASTX analysis [81], with a score cut off of 100. Red lines link matches in the same orientation; blue lines link matches in the reverse orientation.

Most of the conserved regions of these genomes appear to be co-linear, interspersed with regions that appear to be translocated and inverted. Of the currently sequenced streptococci, these two pyogenic species are also the most closely related to *S. uberis* as defined by 16S rDNA phylogeny [27]. A comparison with *S. agalactiae* revealed less conservation of genome structure (Figure 2B), suggesting a more distant genetic relationship.

In addition to the conserved regions identified in these comparisons, discrete regions of difference were identified throughout the genome of *S. uberis* 0140J, suggestive of diverse evolutionary origins for this component of the genome. Three discrete tracts of the sequence were identified as bacteriophage-derived islands, and a putative genomic island. When considered with additional remote CDS that are remnants of mobile genetic elements (MGEs), it was determined that MGEs constitute 1.7% of the genome. The low number of MGEs in the *S. uberis* genome is in marked contrast to other related streptococci [28, 29]. Notably the genome does not contain any CDSs with similarity to insertion sequence (IS) elements.

Whilst the genome comparison of *S. uberis* with other related pyogenic streptococci illustrates the common evolutionary origins of these species, it is apparent from the differences in host associations and pathogenicity that they have become specialized since they diverged from their common ancestor. Insight into the functional specialisations of the *S. uberis* genome can be gleaned from a tripartite comparison with *S. pyogenes* [26] and *S. zooepidemicus* [25] (Figure 3). The relative compositions of the differentially shared versus unique genome components exhibit differences that illustrate niche adaptation between the species. For example, the group of CDSs shared between *S. uberis* and *S. zooepidemicus* encodes functions associated with central metabolism, transport and gene regulation, which are absent in the group shared between *S. uberis* and *S. pyogenes*. In comparison to *S. uberis* and *S. zooepidemicus*, *S. pyogenes* is highly niche-restricted, therefore the spectrum of substrates and stimuli it experiences is narrower. This probably explains why *S. pyogenes* does not share the broader metabolic, transport and regulatory repertoire of the other two species. The *S. uberis*-specific group contains CDSs that differentiate this species from the other two pyogenic streptococci in this three-way comparison, but also distinguish *S. uberis* from other *Streptococcus* species (Figure 3).

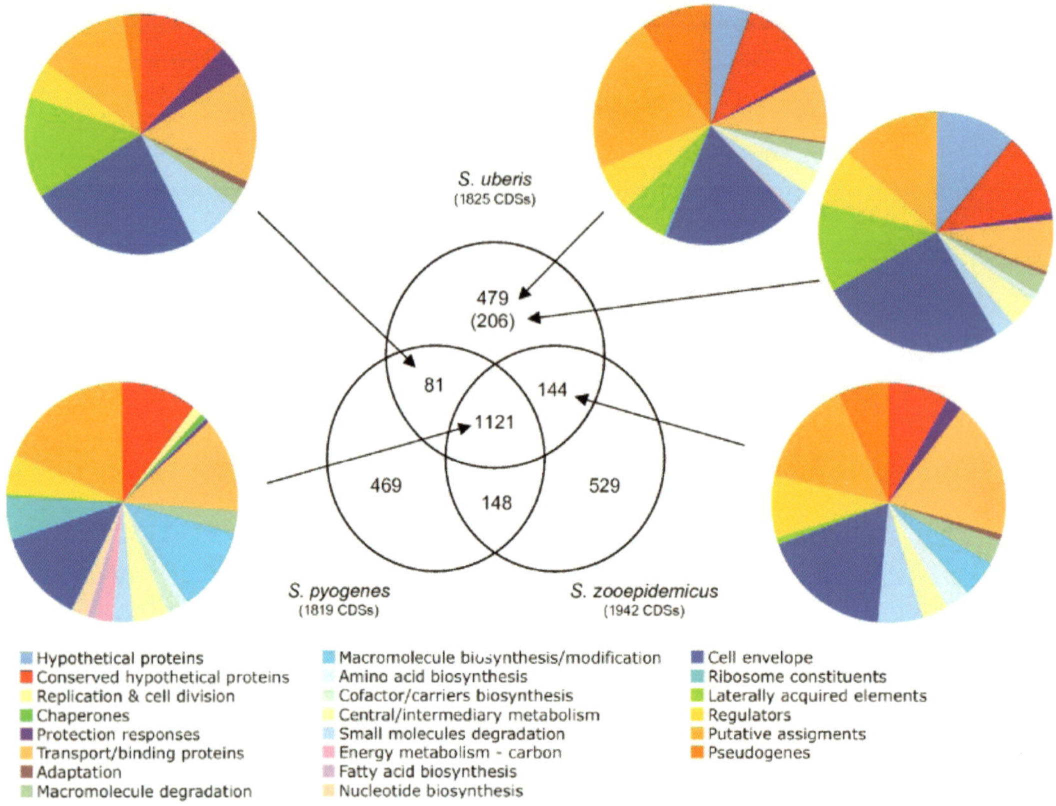

Figure 3: Distribution of orthologous CDSs in *S. uberis* strain 0140J, *S. pyogenes* strain Manfredo and *S. zooepidemicus*strain H70. The Venn diagram shows the number of predicted CDS unique or shared between one or more Streptococcal species. The figure in brackets indicates the number of unique CDSs that do not have ortholog matches in any of the other sequenced *Streptococcus* species. The relative distribution of functional groups of *S. uberis* 0140J CDSs in the various sections is illustrated in the pie charts. Colour legend for the functional classification is below.

Comparison of the relative compositions of the *S. uberis* vs. *S. zooepidemicus-S. pyogenes* unique CDSs (Figure 3) and the *S. uberis* vs. other streptoccoci unique CDSs (Figure 3) shows similar functional makeups to each other. The functions encoded in these groups encompass a diverse range including those associated with growth (central, catabolic and energy metabolism) and host- and environmental-interactions (transport, regulators, protective responses, and cell envelope), and reflect the potential for niche adaptation by *S. uberis*.

Sugar utilization

In comparison to other streptococci, the *S. uberis* genome contains a distinct inventory of CDSs encoding carbohydrate degradation and utilization functions. The diversity of the sugar transport and utilization apparatus in the genome provides *S. uberis* with the capacity to survive in complex host and environmental niches. In particular, *S. uberis* is well equipped to utilize microbial metabolites and products arising from the digestion of plant material found in the rumen.

S. uberis contains an expansion of glycoside hydrolase family 1 proteins [30] that catalyse the hydrolysis of glycosidic bonds between two or more carbohydrates, or between a carbohydrate and a non-carbohydrate moiety. The *S. uberis* 0140J genome contains 12 members of a glycoside hydrolase family 1 (Pfam domain PF00232) in contrast to 4 in *S. pyogenes* Manfredo, 3 in *S. equi* 4047, 4 in *S. zooepidemicus* H70, 4 in *S. suis*P1/7, 6 in *S. pneumoniae* TIGR4, 4 in *S. sanguinis* SK36, 4 in *S. mutans* UA159, 3 in *S. agalactiae* NEM316, 5 in *S. gordonii* CH1, and 6 in *Lactococcus lactis* subsp. *lactis* IL1403. The large number of glycoside hydrolase family 1 proteins suggests that *S. uberis* has the capacity to hydrolyse a wide range of sugars. Protein sequence similarity searches (Table 1) and phylogenetic analysis (Figure 4) demonstrates the diversity of the *S. uberis*proteins. The topology of the phylogenetic tree constructed with the glycoside hydrolase family 1 proteins suggests complex evolutionary origins of the proteins (Figure 4). For example, *S. uberis* SUB0800 is found in a clade containing a group of orthologous proteins from different streptococcal species (*S. pyogenes*SpyM51607, *S. zooepidemicus* SZO15220, *S. suis* SSU0891, *S. pneumoniae* SpT_1100, *S. sanguinis* SSA_1692, *S. mutans* Sm_1351, *S. agalactiae* SaN1329, *S. gordonii* SGO_1512) as well as SUB1448. The branch lengths of this clade suggest that SUB0800 is more closely related to most of the other streptococcal species proteins than to SUB1448, and therefore the likely ortholog. However, comparative genomic analysis examining synteny in the regions of the *S. uberis* loci with the other streptococcal members of this clade, identified SUB1448 as the orthologous protein rather than SUB0800. Analysis of the other glycoside hydrolase family 1 proteins shows that none of them can be identified as orthologues of glycoside hydrolase family 1 proteins in closely related streptococci on the basis of synteny. It is therefore not possible to resolve the complex evolutionary origins of the glycoside hydrolase family 1 proteins in *S. uberis* from the limited genomic datasets currently available. It is likely that expansion in the number of members of this family in *S. uberis* is the result of horizontal gene transfer, possibly from outside the genus. Database searches using the family members showed that for many of the proteins, the highest levels of amino acid identity are to proteins belonging to bacteria outside the genus. The most marked example is SUB0200, where the top Fasta matches are to proteins in Gram-negative enteric bacteria (Table 1).

Table 1: Homologues of the *S. uberis* glycoside hydrolase family 1 proteins

***S. uberis* CDS**	**Protein**	**Organism**	**Identity**
SUB0198	Q3Y0U6_ENTFC	*Enterococcus faecium*	64.1%
	Q2BFH3_9BACI	*Bacillus* sp. NRRL B-14911	60.0%
	Q8ES64_OCEIH	*Oceanobacillus iheyensis*	60.3%
SUB0200	A1JLK3_YERE8	*Yersinia enterocolitica*	58.2%
	A4WDS3_9ENTR	*Enterobacter* sp. 638	56.8%
	Q6D574_ERWCT	*Erwinia carotovora* subsp. *atrosep-tica*	57.9%
SUB0309	A5A692_BACLD	*Bacillus licheniformis*	65.8%
	Q65MN0_BACLD	*Bacillus licheniformis*	65.8%
	Q3XWU5_ENTFC	*Enterococcus faecium*	64.2%
SUB0800	Q300R9_STRSU	*Streptococcus suis*	99.6%
	LACG2_STRPN	*Streptococcus pneumoniae*	92.9%
	A5M4I0_STRPN	*Streptococcus pneumoniae*	92.7%
SUB0834	Q300V6_STRSU	*Streptococcus suis*	80.9%
	O50658_9LACO	*Lactobacillus gasseri*	68.2%
	Q041B2_LACGA	*Lactobacillus gasseri*	68.0%
SUB0837	Q300W6_STRSU	*Streptococcus suis*	78.5%
	Q92F20_LISIN	*Listeria innocua*	61.6%
	Q8YA94_LISMO	*Listeria monocytogenes*	61.2%
SUB0841	Q839A6_ENTFA	*Enterococcus faecalis*	74.6%
	A3CKZ2_STRSV	*Streptococcus sanguinis*	73.6%
	Q8DU50_STRMU	*Streptococcus mutans*	72.2%
SUB0864	Q65D52_BACLD	*Bacillus licheniformis*	65.8%
	Q97TT6_CLOAB	*Clostridium acetobutylicum*	62.8%
	Q6D774_ERWCT	*Erwinia carotovora* subsp. *atrosep-tica*	62.1%
SUB0905	Q3XXU1_ENTFC	*Enterococcus faecium*	60.2%
	Q9CF10_LACLA	*Lactococcus lactis* subsp. *lactis*	59.6%
	Q3K0Z4_STRA1	*Streptococcus agalactiae*	58.6%
SUB1448	LACG_LACLA	*Lactococcus lactis* subsp. *lactis*	77.5%
	Q02V89_LACLS	*Lactococcus lactis* subsp. *cremoris*	77.3%
	LACG_STAHJ	*Staphylococcus haemolyticus*	76.8%
SUB1539	Q02YI9_LACLS	*Lactococcus lactis* subsp. *cremoris*	66.7%
	Q9CFI7_LACLA	*Lactococcus lactis* subsp. *lactis*	63.6%
	Q8XI15_CLOPE	*Clostridium perfringens*	59.0%
SUB1579	A6M0G4_CLOB8	*Clostridium beijerinckii*	68.1%
	A3UPR9_VIBSP	*Vibrio splendidus*	66.2%
	Q0KKN9_STALU	*Staphylococcus lugdunensis*	65.5%

Top 3 UniProt matches identified for each protein using FASTA.

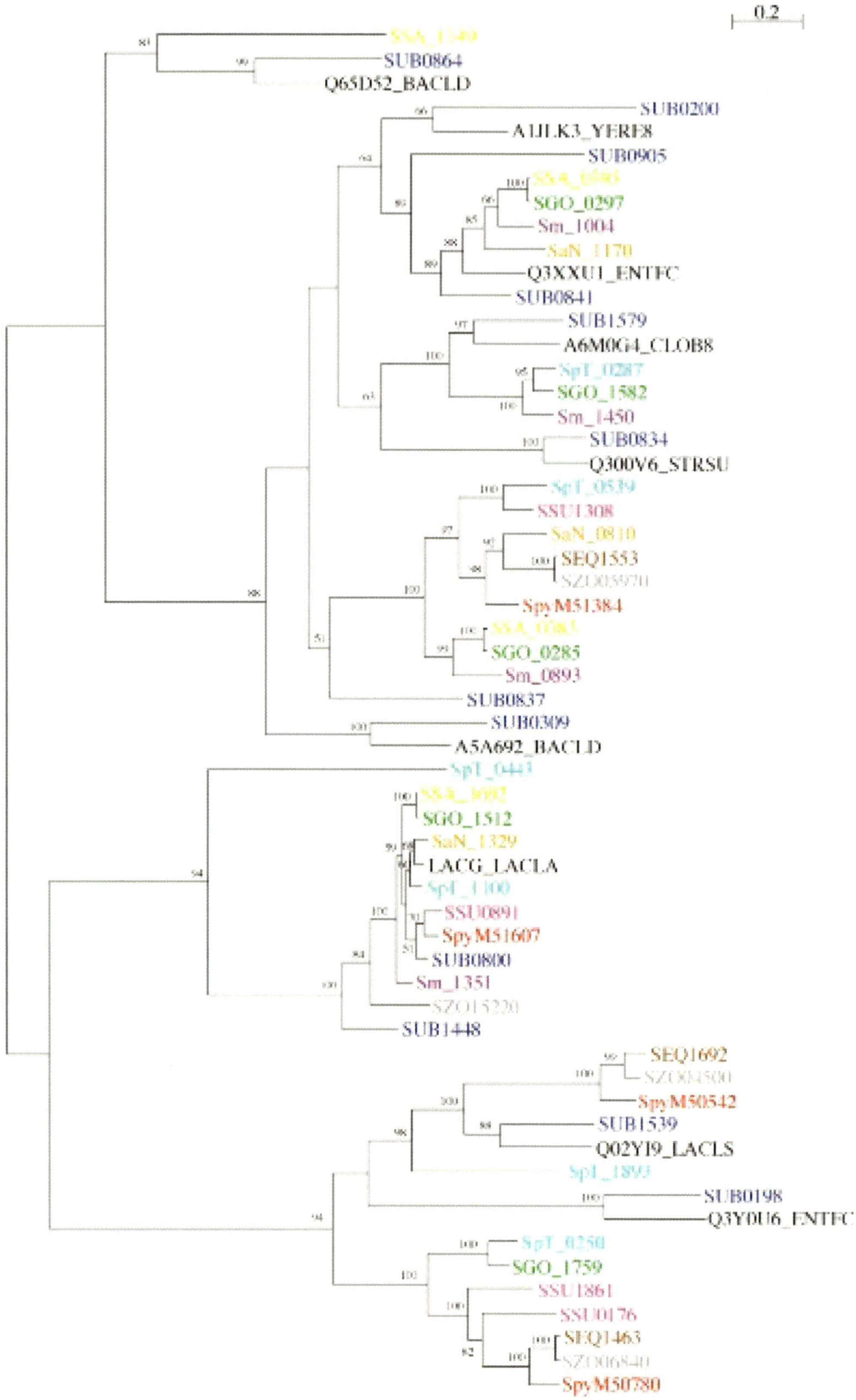

Figure 4: Phylogenetic relationships of streptococcal glycoside hydrolase family 1 proteins. Maximum-likelihood tree of streptococcal glycoside hydrolase family 1 proteins from: *S. uberis*, dark blue; S. *pyogenes* Manfredo, red; *S. equi*4047, brown; *S. zooepidemicus* H70 grey; *S. suis* P1/7, pink; *S. pneumoniae* TIGR4, *S. gordonii* Challis, green; light blue; *S. sanguinis* SK36, yellow; *S. mutans* UA159, purple; *S. algalactiae* NEM316, orange; black. Sequences of Fasta searches 'top match' hits in UniProt (Table 1), outside the streptococcal genomes used above have been included, black: Q3Y0U6_ENTFC, *Enterococcus faecium*; A1JLK3_YERE8, *Yersinia enterocolitica*; A5A692_BACLD, *Bacillus licheniformis*; Q300V6_STRSU, *Streptococcus suis*; Q65D52_BACLD, *Bacillus licheniformis*; Q3XXU1_ENTFC, *Enterococcus faecium*; LACG_LACLA, *Lactococcus lactis* subsp. *lactis*; Q02YI9_LACLS, *Lactococcus lactis* subsp. *cremoris*; A6M0G4_CLOB8, *Clostridium beijerinckii*. The tree was constructed with the WAG model of amino acid substitution, assuming a gamma distribution of among-site substitution rates. The numbers at the tree branches are percentage bootstrap values indicating the confidence levels, values below 50 are not shown.

Bacterial phosphoenolpyruvate-dependent sugar phosphotransferase systems (PTS) bind, phosphorylate, and transport sugar substrates across the bacterial cell membrane. In addition to performing sensing functions with respect to metabolite availability, components of PTS can also regulate metabolic and transcriptional processes [31]. Streptococci appear variously endowed with PTS, enabling uptake and growth on a range of carbohydrate energy sources, thereby equipping the respective species with the ability to survive and grow in a variety of ecological niches. *S. pneumoniae* (TIGR4) displays 21 PTS sugar-specific enzyme II complexes reflecting the utility of nutritional flexibility with respect to its host niche. Similarly, some fourteen PTS were identified in another oral streptococcus, *S. mutans* UA159 [32]. *S. uberis* can call upon an array of at least fifteen PTS to satisfy the requirements of fermentative or glycolytic energy production based upon the sugars available to itwithin the bovine gut and also in mammary gland secretions. Fifteen loci were identified in the 0140J genome that contained complete PTS, with an additional five loci containing components of PTS that may represent partial or divergent systems. In comparison, the non pathogenic dairy-industry bacterium, *S. thermophilus*, was reported to have seven PTS, of which four contain pseudogenes [23].

The *S. uberis* 0140J genome contains a mannitol-specific PTS (SUB0288 and SUB0289) as part of an operon with a ribulose-phosphate 3-epimerase (SUB0285), 6-phospho-3-hexuloisomerase (SUB0286) and a mannitol-1-phosphate 5-dehydrogenase (SUB0287). These five CDSs do not have orthologous matches in the other streptococci. The metabolic genes in this cluster encode functions for conversion of D-ribulose 5-phosphate to D-xylulose 5-phosphate, isomerisation of hexulose-6-phosphate to fructose-6-phosphate and the production of D-fructose 6-phosphate from D-mannitol 1-phosphate.

Concomitant with its ability to colonise the bovine gut, the lumen of the mammary gland in lactating and non-lactating animals, and its ability to survive in pasture, *S. uberis* retains numerous regulatory CDSs. Many of the regulators in the accessory genome are associated with sugar detection and metabolism. These include 6 antiterminator type regulators associated with PTS (SUB0194, SUB0530, SUB0797, SUB0829 (a pseudogene), SUB1452, SUB1704), and 4 RpiR family regulators that contain SIS phospho-sugar binding domains (SUB0170, SUB0904, SUB1541, SUB1582)

Energy metabolism

Within the CDSs unique to *S. uberis* when compared to *S. pyogenes* and *S. zooepidemicus* were two CDSs associated with energy metabolism (SUB0104 and SUB0105), that encode subunits of a cytochrome *d*ubiquinol oxidase. These CDSs are part of an operon (SUB0102 to SUB0107) similar to the respiratory chain operon of *S. agalactiae* (*menA*, *ndh*, *cydA, cydB, cydC*, and *cydD*) [33]. This respiratory chain is incomplete in *S. uberis*, as it is in *S. agalactiae*, as the genome does not encode the biosynthetic pathways for quinone, required for electron transfer, and haem, a cytochrome oxidase cofactor. However respiration in *S. agalactiae*can be stimulated under aerobic conditions if exogenous haem and quinone are supplied [33]. The presence of two distinct metabolic routes for energy production, fermentation and respiration, bestows *S. uberis* with a metabolic versatility that may promote survival in the diverse niches it occupies. *In vitro* experiments with *S. agalactiae* have shown a survival advantage for cells grown under respiratory conditions as opposed to under fermentation conditions [33]. Mutants of cytochrome *d* ubiquinol oxidase demonstrated lower levels of growth in blood under aerobic conditions, and also had reduced virulence in a neonatal rat sepsis model [33]. The ability to respire aerobically may be important for the spread and dissemination of *S. uberis*, although the requirement for exogenous haem and quinone suggest that this is strongly linked to environmental conditions dictated by the host or niche microbiota.

A recent study showed that quinones produced by *Lactococcus lactis* cross-feed *S. agalactiae* and activate respiration when the two organism were co-cultured [34]. Given the complexity of the microbial ecosystems in which *S. uberis* resides, it is not unreasonable to hypothesize that heme and quinone would be available permitting reconstitution of the respiratory chain. Cross-feeding of these key respiratory molecules by resident bacteria in the lower gastrointestinal tract may promote the fecal shedding of *S. uberis*. Whilst the anaerobic conditions of the gut may preclude respiration in this environment, once outside the gut it is possible that a shift in energy metabolism may promote growth and/or survival of *S. uberis* in fecal matter.

Protective responses and environmental survival

The *S. uberis* genome encodes a polyphosphate kinase (SUB0262), a phosphate metabolism enzyme absent in other streptococci. This enzyme catalyzes the reversible transfer of the terminal phosphate of ATP to form a long-chain polyphosphate (polyP). The accumulation of polyP within *E. coli* cells has been shown to be a response to nutritional and osmotic stresses [35], and polyP has been demonstrated to be essential for long-term survival of *Shigella* and *Salmonella* spp. [36]. In *Vibrio cholerae*, polyphosphate stores enhance the ability of to overcome environmental stresses in a low-phosphate environment [37]. The presence of this enzyme in *S. uberis* suggests that this organism is equipped to tolerate comparatively low phosphate-availability environments such as those that might be encountered in faeces and pasture. Recent studies have also demonstrated a role for polyphosphate kinase in the pathogenicity of *Salmonella* and *Camylobacter* species [38, 39].

Quaternary ammonium compound (QAC) disinfectants are used routinely as part of the everyday milking procedure in dairies as a hygiene measure. The *S. uberis* 0140J genome contains a putative quaternary ammonium compound-resistance protein (SUB0162) that has 41% identity with QACH_STASA the quaternary ammonium compound-resistance protein QacH from *Staphylococcus saprophyticus* plasmid pST2H6 [40]. Downstream of this CDS there are two other CDSs that make a putative operon: SUB0163, binding-protein-dependent transport system membrane protein; and SUB0164, a fusion protein pseudogene. This latter CDS consists of an N-terminus similar to ABC transporter permease proteins and a C-terminus similar to fibronectin binding protein, containing an LPXTG motif. It is likely that this CDS arose due to a deletion event that resulted in the fusion of these functionally distinct domains.

The three CDSs make up an operon, however it is not apparent what effect, if any, the mutation in SUB0164 will have upon resistance to QACs.

A distinct feature of the *S. uberis* genome that has emerged from the comparative genomic analysis with other streptococcal species is that there is an abundance of bacteriocins and associated processing, transport and immunity proteins. With the exception of the mammary gland, the niches that *S. uberis* colonize are highly competitive, and are populated by a diverse microbiota. Bacteriocins are proteinaceous antibiotics produced by bacteria that typically kill other bacteria of the same or closely related species. The production of bacteriocins by *S. uberis* is thought to provide a competitive edge and promote colonization.

Uberolysin is a novel cyclic bacteriocin produced by *S. uberis* (SUB0032 to SUB0036) [41]. It has been reported that some strains of *S. uberis* produce nisin U, a lantibiotic, which is similar to nisin A produced by *Lactococcus lactis* [42]. The 16 kb nisin U biosynthesis and resistance locus is absent in *S. uberis* 0140J. The genome also contains a locus (SUB0502 to SUB0516) that encodes an array of bacteriocin structural proteins and immunity proteins. In total there are six CDSs encoding putative bacteriocin proteins (SUB0502, SUB0503, SUB0505, SUB0506, SUB0509 and SUB0512). The presence of multiple structural and immunity CDSs suggests a degree of redundancy. Several of the CDSs at this locus are pseudogenes (two of which are bacteriocin structural CDSs), suggesting that recent mutations have altered the bacteriocin expression repertoire of strain 0140J, and that there may be have been selection for the differential expression of CDSs at this locus. There is evidence of allelic variation at this locus in other strains of *S. uberis*; *S. uberis* strain E, contains a gene encoding (UbaA), a 5.3-kDa class IIa (pediocin-like) bacteriocin at this locus [43], whereas strain 0140J lacks *ubaA*, but contains divergent bacteriocin CDSs. Notably the ubericin A putative immunity protein UbaI is conserved in both strains (SUB0516; 98% identical at the amino acid level).

3.4% of the *S. uberis* 0140J genome encodes pseudogenes. Comparable levels are observed in the genomes of *S. suis* (strain P1/7) (unpublished data) and *S. pyogenes* (Manfredo) [26]; other Gram positive pathogens of similarly low GC content such as *Staphylococcus aureus* have a pseudogene content of between 0.8 and 2.5% [44, 45]. These figures are significantly below the 10% figure reported for two *S. thermophilus* strains (CNRZ1066, LMG18311) for which disruption due to numerous mobile elements and an ongoing depletion of superfluous carbon utilisation CDS were deemed contributory factors [23]. Statistical analysis suggests that pseudogenes are over-represented in genomes of bacteria experiencing either new environmental niches or those becoming equipped to live in a diversity of habitats [45]. Although the relative level of pseudogenes is not high, it is a point of debate that the high representation of regulators and surface-associated proteins within this, is suggestive of an organism engaged in the process of adapting to the challenge of successfully colonising the bovine gut and the mammary gland.

Virulence

The majority of virulence factors in *S. uberis* genome are found in the variable component of the genome (Figure 3) although some are also found in the core gene set, for example fibronectin-binding protein (SUB1111) [46], hemolysin-like protein (SUB1273), and a C5A peptidase-like precursor (SUB1154). Overall there was a lack of what might be considered classical virulence determinants when compared with *S. pyogenes*. For example, genes associated with the production and surface anchoring of M protein in *S. pyogenes* are absent from *S. uberis* 0140J. Orthologs of *emm* and *mga* (a transcriptional activator of *emm*) were not present and none of the CDSs identified previously as putative sortase substrates [47] suggested M-like properties. Other structural proteins that utilise sortase-mediated surface-anchoring such as pilin are also absent from the genome. As a pathogen, *S. zooepidemicus* has been less intensively studied, therefore the paucity of virulence determinants in this species, and consequently identified by comparison with *S. uberis*, reflects this. Detailed analysis of the *S. uberis* genome however identified several CDSs that have potential roles in virulence.

Pathogenic bacteria display an assortment of cell surface-associated proteins that can interact with host cells and tissues and contribute to the pathogenicity of the organism. Bacteria utilise a number of different mechanisms to attach proteins to the cell wall, one of which is through covalent linkage initiated by sortase enzymes. Up to 5 different classes of sortase enzymes have been identified in Gram positive bacteria [48, 49] with one gene identified in the *S. uberis* genome, *srt* A (SUB0881). Anchoring of protein A of *Staphylococcus aureus* via SrtA has been well characterised [50]. Proteins that are destined for anchoring by sortase typically have N-terminal signal sequences for protein secretion and a cell wall sorting signal consisting of an LPXTG, or occasionally an LPX(A/S)G, anchoring motif followed by a C-terminal hydrophobic region with a positively charged tail of amino acids [51].

Seven genes were identified that contained LPXTG sorting motifs; SUB0145, SUB0164, SUB0348, SUB0888, SUB1095, SUB1730 and SUB1739 and a further two (SUB0207 and SUB0241) containing LPXAG motifs. However, two of these, SUB0164 and SUB1739, are highly likely to be pseudogenes and thus unlikely to be translated into fully functional, anchored proteins. A number of these genes have similarity with previously characterised streptococcal proteins; SUB0145, encodes a lactoferrin binding protein (Lbp) [52] which displays homology to fibrinogen-binding/M-like proteins, and SUB1095 shows similarity to an array of SclB collagen-like surface proteins of *S. pyogenes* [53]. Four additional CDSs, SUB0135, a fructan beta-fructosidase precursor and SUB0764, a surface-anchored 5›-nucleotidase (pseudogene), SUB0826, a subtilase family protein, and SUB1154, a C5A peptidase-like precursor, are also putative sortase-processed surface-anchored CDSs, containing the variant motifs LPXTS, LPXTS, LPXTR and LPXTV respectively.

A typical response to intra-mammary infection by the host is an increase in lactoferrin, an iron-binding glycoprotein that acts to restrict the availability of iron for bacterial growth [54, 55]. Streptococci are considered to be resistant to the antibacterial effects of lactoferrin, most likely due to the low requirement for iron for growth [56]. However, the ability to sequester iron from host glycoproteins is considered to be essential for bacterial pathogenesis and bacterial iron-binding proteins have been investigated as potential virulence factors. Within the *S. uberis* genome both Lbp (SUB0145) and *S.*

uberis adhesion molecule or SUAM proteins (SUB1635) have been investigated as potential iron-binding proteins [52, 57, 58]. The SUAM protein has an affinity for lactoferrin and is involved in the adherence of *S. uberis* to a bovine mammary epithelial cell line *in vitro* and therefore may be important during the initial stages of infection and colonisation [57, 59]. Adherence experiments using *lbp* mutants however, suggest that Lbp is not required for attachment of *S. uberis* to host epithelial cells and it is also not essential for growth in iron-limiting conditions. The predicted protein sequence of Lbp is weakly similar (~28% identity) to the streptococcal M proteins, and the genome also contains a partial CDS (SUB0144) with homology to VirR12 and Mry which are positive regulators of M protein genes in group A streptococci [52]. The M protein and C5a peptidase are well characterised virulence determinants of *S. pyogenes* which act on different arms of the complement pathway, inhibiting bacterial opsonisation and inflammation and also phagocyte recruitment to the site of infection [60, 61]. In *S. pyogenes*, these virulence determinants contain LPXTG motifs.

The hyaluronic acid capsule of *S. pyogenes* has been implicated in the pathogenesis of invasive GAS infections [62] and is essential for the maturation of GAS biofilms [63]. Strains of *S. uberis* isolated from cases of bovine mastitis display variable amounts of hyaluronic acid capsule. The complement and arrangement of hyaluronic acid biosynthetic genes in *S. uberis* differs from the *hasABC* arrangement common to GAS [64]. The *has*operon, consisting of *hasA* (SUB1697) encoding hyaluronan synthase and *hasB* (SUB1696) encoding UDP-glucose dehydrogenase, is similarly arranged to that in GAS. However a *hasC* homologue (SUB1691), encoding UDP-glucose pyrophosphorylase, was identified downstream of *hasB* in the reverse orientation and separated from it by some 3 kb containing CDSs apparently unrelated to capsule biosynthesis. The *hasA* gene product is essential for capsule production in both *S. pyogenes* and *S. uberis* [64, 65]. However, capsule production in GAS is dependent only upon functional *hasA* and *hasB*, but not *hasC* [66]. The implication of functional redundancy for UDP-glucose pyrophosphorylase activity in GAS was further supported by the identification of additional homologous CDS in multiple GAS genomes. In contrast, lesions in isogenic acapsular *S. uberis* 0140J mutants were confined to the *hasA* and *hasC* open reading frames suggesting no redundancy existed for these enzymes [64]. Correspondingly, a homologue (SUB1027) of the *S. uberis hasB* gene product (SUB1696) was identified that might account for the apparent inability to isolate a *hasB* mutant using phenotypic screening methods [64].

The lesions identified in non-mucoid mutants of *S. uberis* 0140J are distributed between genetic loci likely to be involved in biosynthesis and also regulation. Three independent acapsular insertion mutants mapped within a putative GntR-like transcriptional regulator SUB0978 (unpublished data) suggestive of a role in upregulation of capsule precursors. The exploitation of an isogenic mutant lacking functional HasA demonstrated that the hyaluronic acid capsule of *S. uberis* plays little role in the early stages of infection of the lactating bovine mammary gland, and resistance to phagocytosis was ascribed to an undefined component unconnected with the capsular phenotype [67]. Activation of host plasminogen to plasmin, a potent serine protease that can bind to the surface of numerous bacterial pathogens, is a mechanism thought likely to augment a variety of streptococcal infections. Many of the streptococci within the pyogenic cluster express one of a variety of plasminogen activators that associate with the respective host›s plasminogen to form an activation complex capable of recruiting and activating further substrate plasminogen to plasmin. The considerable sequence diversity, various substrate specificities and origins of the streptococcal plasminogen activators remain subjects of considerable research interest. The overwhelming majority of *S. uberis* isolates encode PauA (SUB1785) located between the *hexA* and *hexB*genes which display homology to the highly prevalent *mutS* and *mutL* DNA mismatch repair genes [68]. A single *S. uberis* isolate lacking *pauA* encoded an alternative novel plasminogen activator (PauB) [69] also at the *hexAB* locus.

An alternative locus in all human isolates of group A, C and G streptococci is populated by streptokinase (SK) [70]. The genes flanking SK did not appear to encode related functions, being an ATP-binding cassette protein and a leucine rich protein lying upstream of *ska*, while genes encoding a homologue of the *E. coli relA* and *spoT* genes which moderate levels of guanosine 5’,3› polyphosphate during nutritional stress lie downstream [71]. The corresponding SK locus in *S. uberis* 0140J is devoid of plasminogen activator CDS.

Some clues concerning the origins of the diversity of plasminogen activator sequences and the variety of genomic loci within which they appear in pyogenic streptococci are drawn from the observation that in at least three *S. pyogenes* serotypes (M1, M5 and M6) [26, 72, 73], prophage are located between the *hexA* and *hexB* orthologues with the phage attachment site for SF370.4 being mapped to overlie the start of the *mutL*coding sequence [72]. Further evidence of the role that phage play in generating variation at this locus is found in the CDS upstream of *pauA*, which encodes a putative exported protein (SUB1784), and is similar to proteins from *L. lactis* prophage.

Hyaluronidase, has long been considered to be a streptococcal virulence determinant due to its ability to break down the hyaluronic acid component of connective tissue and thereby facilitate spread of the pathogen, but there is little experimental evidence to support this assertion. Hyaluronic acid capsule produced by some streptococci, including *S. uberis*, is somewhat paradoxically also a substrate for hyaluronidase. Recently, it has been suggested that hyaluronidase facilitates the spread of high molecular weight compounds rather than bacterial cells *per se* [74] and also augments the effects of other streptococcal virulence factors such as pneumolysin [75]. In GAS, *hylA* encodes a large secreted hyaluronidase. In addition, numerous ‘phage-associated’ hyaluronidases (*hylP*) are evident. Neither GAS *hylA* or *hylP* homologues were present in the *S. uberis* 0140J sequence. Interestingly the GBS2603 V/R locus encoding a chromosomal hyaluronidase (SAG1197) abuts *mutX* with the equivalent locus in GAS Manfredo being the prophage phiman.3, encoding one of a number of M5 phage hyaluronidase CDS. It appears highly likely that the hyaluronidase complement of streptococci has been and continues to be influenced by bacteriophage.

The CAMP factor [76], a further putative virulence factor homologous to the Fc-binding and haemolytic *cfb*gene product in *S. agalactiae* is absent from numerous strains of *S. uberis* [77]. A CDS encoding CAMP factor was not identified in *S. uberis* 0140J or within 8 of a panel of 9 further pathogenic *S. uberis* strains tested (unpublished data) and can therefore be considered as non-essential to the infection of the bovine mammary gland.

CONCLUSION

Analysis of the whole genome sequence of the bovine mastitis associated *S. uberis* strain 0140J has identified a relative paucity of classical streptococcal virulence determinants. In contrast, a plethora of metabolic options appear available to the bacterium. These endow it with the potential to flourish in a variety of nutritionally constrained habitats including the lumen of the mammary gland and the bovine gut. There are evidently survival advantages for an organism able to occupy multiple environmental niches. Critical to this aspect is nutritional flexibility, and the ability to derive carbon and energy by a variety of means. The genome provides compelling evidence supporting this proposal. Furthermore, *S. uberis* also appears equipped to cope with stresses likely to be encountered when shifting from one environmental niche to another for example through the use of polyphosphate kinase (SUB0262). We present here evidence that suggests *S. uberis* should no longer be regarded merely as a pathogen of the bovine mammary gland, but equally as a commensal microorganism of a wider bovine-based environment. Within this context, it will be of great interest to determine the current distribution of such features within the species and also whether *S. uberis* continues to refine or augment its genetic load along such lines in the future.

METHODS

Strain

Streptococcus uberis 0140J was isolated from milk obtained from a clinical case of bovine mastitis in 1972 within the UK. The strain *S. uberis* 0140J has been deposited under ATCC® Number BAA-854.

Preparation of genomic DNA

Genomic DNA was prepared from *S. uberis* using a modification of the method of Hill and Leigh [78]. Todd Hewitt broth (400 ml) was inoculated with a single colony of *S. uberis* 0140J picked from solid media and incubated for 18 h at 37°C. Bacterial cells were harvested, washed with 180 ml of Tris, 5 mM EDTA (pH 7.8) and the cell walls disrupted by incubation at 37°C for 30 mins in 50 ml of the same buffer, containing 30 u/ml mutanolysin and 10 mg/ml lysozyme. Cells were lysed by addition of 2.67 ml SDS (20% w/v in 50 mM Tris, 20 mM EDTA pH 7.8), 0.4 ml Proteinase K (20 mg/ml) and incubation at 37°C for 1 h. Saturated NaCl (26.7 ml) was added and after 5 min. cell wall material was removed by centrifugation for 20 mins at 16,000 × *g*. The supernatent was extracted twice with an equal volume of Tris-equilibrated (pH 8.0) phenol:chloroform:isoamyl alcohol (25:24:1). RNAase A was added to 20 μg/ml and the mixture incubated for 30 mins at 37°C. Genomic DNA was precipitated by addition of 2 volumes of ice-cold ethanol and incubation at 4°C for 2 h prior to centrifugation at 16,000 × *g* for 15 mins. The pelleted DNA was washed with cold 70% ethanol and air-dried prior to resuspension at 4°C in 2.5 ml of TE buffer.

Whole genome sequencing

Sequence data were obtained from end sequences (giving approximately 8 × coverage) derived from M13 and pUC18 genomic shotgun libraries (with insert sizes of 1.4 to 2 kb and 2.8 to 3.3 kb respectively) using dye terminator chemistry on ABI3700 automated sequencers. End sequences from a large insert BAC library (pBACe3.6, 12 to 48 kb insert size) and Fosmid library (pEpiFos, 30–40 kb) were used as a scaffold. All identified repeats were bridged by read-pairs or end-sequenced polymerase chain reaction (PCR) products. The sequence was assembled and finished as described previously [79].

The sequence was annotated using Artemis software [79]. Initial coding sequence (CDS) predictions were performed using Orpheus [80], Glimmer2 [81], and EasyGene [82] software. These predictions were amalgamated, and codon usage, positional base preference methods and comparisons to the non-redundant protein databases using BLAST [83] and FASTA [84] software were used to refine the predictions. The entire DNA sequence was also compared in all six reading frames against UniProt, using BLASTX [83] to identify any possible coding sequences previously missed. Protein motifs were identified using Pfam [85] and Prosite [86], transmembrane domains were identified with TMHMM [87], and signal sequences were identified with SignalP version 2.0 [88]. rRNAs were identified using BLASTN [83] alignment to defined rRNAs from the EMBL nucleotide database; tRNAs were identified using tRNAscan-SE [89]; non-coding RNA (ncRNA) were identified using Rfam [90]. The sequence and annotation of the *Streptococcus uberis* 0140J genome has been deposited in the EMBL database under accession number AM946015.

Comparative genomics

Comparison of the genome sequences was facilitated by using the Artemis Comparison Tool (ACT) [91] which enabled the visualization of BLASTN and TBLASTX comparisons [83] between the genomes. Orthologous proteins were identified as reciprocal best matches using FASTA [84] with subsequent manual curation. Orthology inferred from positional information was investigated using ACT. Pseudogenes had one or more mutations that would prevent correct translation; each of the inactivating mutations was subsequently checked against the original sequencing data.

Streptococcus sequences used for comparative genomic analysis were: *S. pyogenes* Manfredo (accession number AM295007) [26], *S. pyogenes* MGAS315 (accession number AE014074) [92], *S. equi* 4047 http://www.sanger.ac.uk/Projects/S_equi/[25], *S. zooepidemicus* H70 http://www.sanger.ac.uk/Projects/S_zooepidemicus/[25], *S. thermophilus* CNRZ1066 (accession number CP000024) [23], *S. suis* P1/7 http://www.sanger.ac.uk/Projects/S_suis/[93], *S. pneumoniae* TIGR4 (accession number AE005672) [94], *S. sanguinis* SK36 (accession number CP000387) [95], *S. mutans* UA159 (accession number AE014133) [32], *S. agalactiae* NEM316 (accession number AL732656) [96], and *S. gordonii* str. Challis substr. CH1 (accession number

CP000725) [97], and *Lactococcus lactis* subsp. *lactis* IL1403 (accession number AE005176) [98].

Phylogentic analysis

Unrooted maximum likelihood trees were built using PhyML [99, 100] and drawn using NJplot [101]. Sequences were aligned using ClustalX (Version 1.82) [102]

DECLARATIONS

Acknowledgements

This work was supported by the Wellcome Trust. We would like to acknowledge the support of the Wellcome Trust Sanger Institute's Pathogen Production Group for shotgun sequencing and finishing.

Authors' contributions

PNW and SAE drafted the manuscript, MTGH annotated the genome and drafted the manuscript, JL conceived of the study, participated in the study design, and drafted the manuscript, MAQ and JW carried out the genomic library preparation, NL, ABi, ABa, LC, carried out the genome finishing and closure, DM and AW conceived of the study, participated in the study design and undertook critical re of the manuscript, TRF, MK, CD and NC conceived of the study, participated in the study design, BH, BGB, JP and SDB participated in the study design, managed the project and undertook critical re of the manuscript. All authors have read and approved the final manuscript.

REFERENCES

1. Gottschalk M, Segura M, Xu J: *Streptococcus suis* infections in humans: the Chinese experience and the situation in North America. Anim Health Res Rev. 2007, 8: 29-45. 10.1017/S1466252307001247.
2. Bisharat N, Crook DW, Leigh J, Harding RM, Ward PN, Coffey TJ, Maiden MC, Peto T, Jones N: Hyperinvasive neonatal group B streptococcus has arisen from a bovine ancestor. J Clin Microbiol. 2004, 42: 2161-2167. 10.1128/JCM.42.5.2161-2167.2004.
3. Bentley RW, Leigh JA, Collins MD: Intrageneric structure of *Streptococcus* based on comparative analysis of small-subunit rRNA sequences. Int J Syst Bacteriol. 1991, 41: 487-494.
4. Compton CW, Heuer C, Parker K, McDougall S: Epidemiology of mastitis in pasture-grazed peripartum dairy heifers and its effects on productivity. J Dairy Sci. 2007, 90: 4157-4170. 10.3168/jds.2006-880.
5. Olde Riekerink RG, Barkema HW, Kelton DF, Scholl DT: Incidence rate of clinical mastitis on Canadian dairy farms. J Dairy Sci. 2008, 91: 1366-1377. 10.3168/jds.2007-0757.
6. Sorensen LP, Guldbrandtsen B, Thomasen JR, Lund MS: Pathogen-specific effects of quantitative trait loci affecting clinical mastitis and somatic cell count in Danish Holstein cattle. J Dairy Sci. 2008, 91: 2493-2500. 10.3168/jds.2007-0583.
7. Bradley AJ, Leach KA, Breen JE, Green LE, Green MJ: Survey of the incidence and aetiology of mastitis on dairy farms in England and Wales. Vet Rec. 2007, 160: 253-257.
8. Leigh JA: Streptococcus uberis: a permanent barrier to the control of bovine mastitis?. Vet J. 1999, 157: 225-238. 10.1053/tvjl.1998.0298.
9. Bramley AJ: Sources of *Streptococcus uberis* in the dairy herd. I. Isolation from bovine faeces and from straw bedding of cattle. J Dairy Res. 1982, 49: 369-373.
10. Kruze J, Bramley AJ: Sources of Streptococcus uberis in the dairy herd. II. Evidence of colonization of the bovine intestine by Str. uberis. J Dairy Res. 1982, 49: 375-379.
11. Lopez-Benavides MG, Williamson JH, Pullinger GD, Lacy-Hulbert SJ, Cursons RT, Leigh JA: Field observations on the variation of Streptococcus uberis populations in a pasture-based dairy farm. J Dairy Sci. 2007, 90: 5558-5566. 10.3168/jds.2007-0194.
12. Hill AW: Pathogenicity of two strains of *Streptococcus uberis* infused into lactating and non-lactating bovine mammary glands. Res Vet Sci. 1988, 45: 400-404.
13. Sordillo LM, Shafer-Weaver K, DeRosa D: Immunobiology of the mammary gland. J Dairy Sci. 1997, 80: 1851-1865.
14. Coffey TJ, Pullinger GD, Urwin R, Jolley KA, Wilson SM, Maiden MC, Leigh JA: First insights into the evolution of *Streptococcus uberis*: a multilocus sequence typing scheme that enables investigation of its population biology. Appl Environ Microbiol. 2006, 72: 1420-1428. 10.1128/AEM.72.2.1420-1428.2006.
15. Leigh JA, Ward PN, Field TR: The exploitation of the genome in the search for determinants of virulence in *Streptococcus uberis*. Vet Immunol Immunopathol. 2004, 100: 145-149. 10.1016/j.vetimm.2004.04.004.
16. Ferretti JJ, McShan WM, Ajdic D, Savic DJ, Savic G, Lyon K, Primeaux C, Sezate S, Suvorov AN, Kenton S, Lai HS, Lin SP, Qian Y, Jia HG, Najar FZ, Ren Q, Zhu H, Song L, White J, Yuan X, Clifton SW, Roe BA, McLaughlin R: Complete genome sequence of an M1 strain of *Streptococcus pyogenes*. Proc Natl Acad Sci USA. 2001, 98: 4658-4663. 10.1073/pnas.071559398.
17. Tettelin H, Masignani V, Cieslewicz MJ, Eisen JA, Peterson S, Wessels MR, Paulsen IT, Nelson KE, Margarit I, Read TD, Madoff LC, Wolf AM, Beanan MJ, Brinkac LM, Daugherty SC, DeBoy RT, Durkin AS, Kolonay JF, Madupu R, Lewis MR, Radune D, Fedorova NB, Scanlan D, Khouri H, Mulligan S, Carty HA, Cline RT, Van Aken SE, Gill J, Scarselli M, Mora M, Iacobini ET, Brettoni C, Galli G, Mariani M, Vegni F, Maione D, Rinaudo D, Rappuoli R, Telford JL, Kasper DL, Grandi G, Fraser CM: Complete genome sequence and comparative genomic analysis of an emerging human pathogen, serotype V Streptococcus agalactiae. Proc Natl Acad Sci USA. 2002, 99: 12391-12396. 10.1073/pnas.182380799.
18. Shen K, Gladitz J, Antalis P, Dice B, Janto B, Keefe R, Hayes J, Ahmed A, Dopico R, Ehrlich N, Jocz J, Kropp L, Yu S, Nistico L, Greenberg DP, Barbadora K, Preston RA, Post JC, Ehrlich GD, Hu FZ: Characterization, distribution, and expression of novel genes among eight

clinical isolates of Streptococcus pneumoniae. Infect Immun. 2006, 74: 321-330. 10.1128/IAI.74.1.321-330.2006.

19. Hiller NL, Janto B, Hogg JS, Boissy R, Yu S, Powell E, Keefe R, Ehrlich NE, Shen K, Hayes J, Barbadora K, Klimke W, Dernovoy D, Tatusova T, Parkhill J, Bentley SD, Post JC, Ehrlich GD, Hu FZ: Comparative genomic analyses of seventeen Streptococcus pneumoniae strains: insights into the pneumococcal supragenome. J Bacteriol. 2007, 189: 8186-8195. 10.1128/JB.00690-07.

20. Ferretti JJ, Ajdic D, McShan WM: Comparative genomics of streptococcal species. Indian J Med Res. 2004, 119 (Suppl): 1-6.

21. Marri PR, Hao W, Golding GB: Gene gain and gene loss in streptococcus: is it driven by habitat?. Mol Biol Evol. 2006, 23: 2379-2391. 10.1093/molbev/msl115.

22. Delorme C, Poyart C, Ehrlich SD, Renault P: Extent of horizontal gene transfer in evolution of Streptococci of the salivarius group. J Bacteriol. 2007, 189: 1330-1341. 10.1128/JB.01058-06.

23. Bolotin A, Quinquis B, Renault P, Sorokin A, Ehrlich SD, Kulakauskas S, Lapidus A, Goltsman E, Mazur M, Pusch GD, Fonstein M, Overbeek R, Kyprides N, Purnelle B, Prozzi D, Ngui K, Masuy D, Hancy F, Burteau S, Boutry M, Delcour J, Goffeau A, Hols P: Complete sequence and comparative genome analysis of the dairy bacterium *Streptococcus thermophilus*. Nat Biotechnol. 2004, 22: 1554-1558. 10.1038/nbt1034.

24. Delorme C: Streptococcus thermophilus. International Journal of Food Microbiology. 126: 274-277. 10.1016/j.ijfoodmicro.2007.08.014.

25. Holden MTG, Heather Z, Paillot R, Steward K, Webb K, Ainslie F, Jourdan T, Bason N, Holroyd N, Mungall K, Quail MA, Sanders M, Simmonds M, Willey D, Brooks K, Aanensen DM, Spratt BG, Jolley KA, Maiden MC, Kehoe M, Chanter N, Robinson C, Maskell D, Parkhill J, Waller AS: Genomic evidence for the evolution of *Streptococcus equi*: host restriction, increased virulence and genetic exchange with human pathogens.

26. Holden MT, Scott A, Cherevach I, Chillingworth T, Churcher C, Cronin A, Dowd L, Feltwell T, Hamlin N, Holroyd S, Jagels K, Moule S, Mungall K, Quail MA, Price C, Rabbinowitsch E, Sharp S, Skelton J, Whitehead S, Barrell BG, Kehoe M, Parkhill J: Complete genome of acute rheumatic fever-associated serotype M5 *Streptococcus pyogenes* strain manfredo. J Bacteriol. 2007, 189: 1473-1477. 10.1128/JB.01227-06.

27. Facklam R: What happened to the streptococci: over of taxonomic and nomenclature changes. Clin Microbiol Rev. 2002, 15: 613-630. 10.1128/CMR.15.4.613-630.2002.

28. Beres SB, Musser JM: Contribution of exogenous genetic elements to the group A Streptococcus metagenome. PLoS ONE. 2007, 2: e800-10.1371/journal.pone.0000800.

29. Tettelin H, Masignani V, Cieslewicz MJ, Donati C, Medini D, Ward NL, Angiuoli SV, Crabtree J, Jones AL, Durkin AS, Deboy RT, Davidsen TM, Mora M, Scarselli M, Margarit y Ros I, Peterson JD, Hauser CR, Sundaram JP, Nelson WC, Madupu R, Brinkac LM, Dodson RJ, Rosovitz MJ, Sullivan SA, Daugherty SC, Haft DH, Selengut J, Gwinn ML, Zhou L, Zafar N, Khouri H, Radune D, Dimitrov G, Watkins K, O'Connor KJ, Smith S, Utterback TR, White O, Rubens CE, Grandi G, Madoff LC, Kasper DL, Telford JL, Wessels MR, Rappuoli R, Fraser CM: Genome analysis of multiple pathogenic isolates of Streptococcus agalactiae: implications for the microbial "pan-genome". Proc Natl Acad Sci USA. 2005, 102: 13950-13955. 10.1073/pnas.0506758102.

30. Cantarel BL, Coutinho PM, Rancurel C, Bernard T, Lombard V, Henrissat B: The Carbohydrate-Active EnZymes database (CAZy): an expert resource for Glycogenomics. Nucleic Acids Res. 2008

31. Poolman B: Transporters and their roles in LAB cell physiology. Antonie Van Leeuwenhoek. 2002, 82: 147-164. 10.1023/A:1020658831293.

32. Ajdic D, McShan WM, McLaughlin RE, Savic G, Chang J, Carson MB, Primeaux C, Tian R, Kenton S, Jia H, Lin S, Qian Y, Li S, Zhu H, Najar F, Lai H, White J, Roe BA, Ferretti JJ: Genome sequence of Streptococcus mutans UA159, a cariogenic dental pathogen. Proc Natl Acad Sci USA. 2002, 99: 14434-14439. 10.1073/pnas.172501299.

33. Yamamoto Y, Poyart C, Trieu-Cuot P, Lamberet G, Gruss A, Gaudu P: Respiration metabolism of Group B Streptococcus is activated by environmental haem and quinone and contributes to virulence. Mol Microbiol. 2005, 56: 525-534. 10.1111/j.1365-2958.2005.04555.x.

34. Rezaiki L, Lamberet G, Derre A, Gruss A, Gaudu P: Lactococcus lactis produces short-chain quinones that cross-feed Group B Streptococcus to activate respiration growth. Mol Microbiol. 2008, 67: 947-957. 10.1111/j.1365-2958.2007.06083.x.

35. Ault-Riche D, Fraley CD, Tzeng CM, Kornberg A: Novel assay reveals multiple pathways regulating stress-induced accumulations of inorganic polyphosphate in *Escherichia coli*. J Bacteriol. 1998, 180: 1841-1847.

36. Kim KS, Rao NN, Fraley CD, Kornberg A: Inorganic polyphosphate is essential for long-term survival and virulence factors in Shigella and Salmonella spp. Proc Natl Acad Sci USA. 2002, 99: 7675-7680. 10.1073/pnas.112210499.

37. Jahid IK, Silva AJ, Benitez JA: Polyphosphate stores enhance the ability of Vibrio cholerae to overcome environmental stresses in a low-phosphate environment. Appl Environ Microbiol. 2006, 72: 7043-7049. 10.1128/AEM.00924-06.

38. McMeechan A, Lovell MA, Cogan TA, Marston KL, Humphrey TJ, Barrow PA: Inactivation of ppk differentially affects virulence and disrupts ATP homeostasis in Salmonella enterica serovars Typhimurium and Gallinarum. Res Microbiol. 2007, 158: 79-85. 10.1016/j.resmic.2006.10.008.

39. Candon HL, Allan BJ, Fraley CD, Gaynor EC: Polyphosphate kinase 1 is a pathogenesis determinant in *Campylobacter jejuni*. J Bacteriol. 2007, 189: 8099-8108. 10.1128/JB.01037-07.

40. Heir E, Sundheim G, Holck AL: The Staphylococcus

qacH gene product: a new member of the SMR family encoding multidrug resistance. FEMS Microbiol Lett. 1998, 163: 49-56. 10.1111/j.1574-6968.1998.tb13025.x.

41. Wirawan RE, Swanson KM, Kleffmann T, Jack RW, Tagg JR: Uberolysin: a novel cyclic bacteriocin produced by *Streptococcus uberis*. Microbiology. 2007, 153: 1619-1630. 10.1099/mic.0.2006/005967-0.
42. Wirawan RE, Klesse NA, Jack RW, Tagg JR: Molecular and genetic characterization of a novel nisin variant produced by *Streptococcus uberis*. Appl Environ Microbiol. 2006, 72: 1148-1156. 10.1128/AEM.72.2.1148-1156.2006.
43. Heng NC, Burtenshaw GA, Jack RW, Tagg JR: Ubericin A, a class IIa bacteriocin produced by *Streptococcus uberis*. Appl Environ Microbiol. 2007, 73: 7763-7766. 10.1128/AEM.01818-07.
44. Holden MTG, Feil EJ, Lindsay JA, Peacock SJ, Day NPJ, Enright MC, Foster TJ, Moore CE, Hurst L, Atkin R, Barron A, Bason N, Bentley SD, Chillingworth C, Chillingworth T, Churcher C, Clark L, Corton C, Cronin A, Doggett J, Dowd L, Feltwell T, Hance Z, Harris B, Hauser H, Holroyd S, Jagels K, James KD, Lennard N, Line A, Mayes R, Moule S, Mungall K, Ormond D, Quail MA, Rabbinowitsch E, Rutherford K, Sanders M, Sharp S, Simmonds M, Stevens K, Whitehead S, Barrell BG, Spratt BG, Parkhill J: Complete genomes of two clinical *Staphylococcus aureus* strains: Evidence for the rapid evolution of virulence and drug resistance. Proc Natl Acad Sci USA. 2004, 101: 9786-9791. 10.1073/pnas.0402521101.
45. Lerat E, Ochman H: Recognizing the pseudogenes in bacterial genomes. Nucleic Acids Res. 2005, 33: 3125-3132. 10.1093/nar/gki631.
46. Christie J, McNab R, Jenkinson HF: Expression of fibronectin-binding protein FbpA modulates adhesion in Streptococcus gordonii. Microbiology. 2002, 148: 1615-1625.
47. Comfort D, Clubb RT: A comparative genome analysis identifies distinct sorting pathways in gram-positive bacteria. Infect Immun. 2004, 72: 2710-2722. 10.1128/IAI.72.5.2710-2722.2004.
48. Dramsi S, Trieu-Cuot P, Bierne H: Sorting sortases: a nomenclature proposal for the various sortases of Gram-positive bacteria. Res Microbiol. 2005, 156: 289-297. 10.1016/j.resmic.2004.10.011.
49. Pallen MJ, Lam AC, Antonio M, Dunbar K: An embarrassment of sortases – a richness of substrates?. Trends Microbiol. 2001, 9: 97-102. 10.1016/S0966-842X(01)01956-4.
50. Mazmanian SK, Liu G, Ton-That H, Schneewind O: *Staphylococcus aureus* sortase, an enzyme that anchors surface proteins to the cell wall. Science. 1999, 285: 760-763. 10.1126/science.285.5428.760.
51. Schneewind O, Mihaylova-Petkov D, Model P: Cell wall sorting signals in surface proteins of gram-positive bacteria. Embo J. 1993, 12: 4803-4811.
52. Moshynskyy I, Jiang M, Fontaine MC, Perez-Casal J, Babiuk LA, Potter AA: Characterization of a bovine lactoferrin binding protein of *Streptococcus uberis*. Microb Pathog. 2003, 35: 203-215. 10.1016/S0882-4010(03)00150-5.
53. Whatmore AM: *Streptococcus pyogenes sclB* encodes a putative hypervariable surface protein with a collagen-like repetitive structure. Microbiology. 2001, 147: 419-429.
54. Hagiwara S, Kawai K, Anri A, Nagahata H: Lactoferrin concentrations in milk from normal and subclinical mastitic cows. J Vet Med Sci. 2003, 65: 319-323. 10.1292/jvms.65.319.
55. Harmon RJ, Schanbacher FL, Ferguson LC, Smith KL: Changes in lactoferrin, immunoglobulin G, bovine serum albumin, and alpha-lactalbumin during acute experimental and natural coliform mastitis in cows. Infect Immun. 1976, 13: 533-542.
56. Todhunter DA, Smith KL, Schoenberger PS: *In vitro* growth of mastitis-associated streptococci in bovine mammary secretions. J Dairy Sci. 1985, 68: 2337-2346.
57. Almeida RA, Luther DA, Park HM, Oliver SP: Identification, isolation, and partial characterization of a novel *Streptococcus uberis* adhesion molecule (SUAM). Vet Microbiol. 2006, 115: 183-191. 10.1016/j.vetmic.2006.02.005.
58. Fang W, Oliver SP: Identification of lactoferrin-binding proteins in bovine mastitis-causing *Streptococcus uberis*. FEMS Microbiol Lett. 1999, 176: 91-96. 10.1111/j.1574-6968.1999.tb13647.x.
59. Fang W, Almeida RA, Oliver SP: Effects of lactoferrin and milk on adherence of *Streptococcus uberis* to bovine mammary epithelial cells. Am J Vet Res. 2000, 61: 275-279. 10.2460/ajvr.2000.61.275.
60. Chen CC, Cleary PP: Complete nucleotide sequence of the streptococcal C5a peptidase gene of *Streptococcus pyogenes*. J Biol Chem. 1990, 265: 3161-3167.
61. Hollingshead SK, Fischetti VA, Scott JR: Complete nucleotide sequence of type 6 M protein of the group A *Streptococcus*. Repetitive structure and membrane anchor. J Biol Chem. 1986, 261: 1677-1686.
62. Martin PR, Hoiby EA: Streptococcal serogroup A epidemic in Norway 1987–1988. Scand J Infect Dis. 1990, 22: 421-429. 10.3109/00365549009027073.
63. Cho KH, Caparon MG: Patterns of virulence gene expression differ between biofilm and tissue communities of *Streptococcus pyogenes*. Mol Microbiol. 2005, 57: 1545-1556. 10.1111/j.1365-2958.2005.04786.x.
64. Ward PN, Field TR, Ditcham WG, Maguin E, Leigh JA: Identification and disruption of two discrete loci encoding hyaluronic acid capsule biosynthesis genes *hasA*, *hasB*, and *hasC* in *Streptococcus uberis*. Infect Immun. 2001, 69: 392-399. 10.1128/IAI.69.1.392-399.2001.
65. Dougherty BA, Rijn van de I: Molecular characterization of *hasA* from an operon required for hyaluronic acid synthesis in group A streptococci. J Biol Chem. 1994, 269: 169-175.
66. Ashbaugh CD, Alberti S, Wessels MR: Molecular analysis of the capsule gene region of group A *Streptococcus*: the *hasAB*genes are sufficient for capsule expression. J

Bacteriol. 1998, 180: 4955-4959.

67. Field TR, Ward PN, Pedersen LH, Leigh JA: The hyaluronic acid capsule of *Streptococcus uberis* is not required for the development of infection and clinical mastitis. Infect Immun. 2003, 71: 132-139. 10.1128/IAI.71.1.132-139.2003.

68. Rosey EL, Lincoln RA, Ward PN, Yancey RJ, Leigh JA: PauA: a novel plasminogen activator from *Streptococcus uberis*. FEMS Microbiol Lett. 1999, 178: 27-33. 10.1111/j.1574-6968.1999.tb13755.x.

69. Ward PN, Leigh JA: Characterization of PauB, a novel broad-spectrum plasminogen activator from *Streptococcus uberis*. J Bacteriol. 2002, 184: 119-125. 10.1128/JB.184.1.119-125.2002.

70. Malke H, Steiner K, Gase K, Frank C: Expression and regulation of the streptokinase gene. Methods. 2000, 21: 111-124. 10.1006/meth.2000.0982.

71. Mechold U, Steiner K, Vettermann S, Malke H: Genetic organization of the streptokinase region of the *Streptococcus equisimilis* H46A chromosome. Mol Gen Genet. 1993, 241: 129-140. 10.1007/BF00280210.

72. Canchaya C, Desiere F, McShan WM, Ferretti JJ, Parkhill J, Brussow H: Genome analysis of an inducible prophage and prophage remnants integrated in the *Streptococcus pyogenes* strain SF370. Virology. 2002, 302: 245-258. 10.1006/viro.2002.1570.

73. Banks DJ, Porcella SF, Barbian KD, Beres SB, Philips LE, Voyich JM, DeLeo FR, Martin JM, Somerville GA, Musser JM: Progress toward characterization of the group A *Streptococcus* metagenome: complete genome sequence of a macrolide-resistant serotype M6 strain. J Infect Dis. 2004, 190: 727-738. 10.1086/422697.

74. Starr CR, Engleberg NC: Role of hyaluronidase in subcutaneous spread and growth of group A streptococcus. Infect Immun. 2006, 74: 40-48. 10.1128/IAI.74.1.40-48.2006.

75. Feldman C, Cockeran R, Jedrzejas MJ, Mitchell TJ, Anderson R: Hyaluronidase augments pneumolysin-mediated injury to human ciliated epithelium. Int J Infect Dis. 2007, 11: 11-15. 10.1016/j.ijid.2005.09.002.

76. Christie R, Atkins NE, Munch-Petersen E: A note on a lytic phenomenon shown by group B streptococci. Aust J Exp Biol Med Sci. 1944, 22: 197-200. 10.1038/icb.1944.26. **Article**

77. Jiang M, Babiuk LA, Potter AA: Cloning, sequencing and expression of the CAMP factor gene of *Streptococcus uberis*. Microb Pathog. 1996, 20: 297-307. 10.1006/mpat.1996.0028.

78. Hill AW, Leigh JA: DNA fingerprinting of *Streptococcus uberis*: a useful tool for epidemiology of bovine mastitis. Epidemiol Infect. 1989, 103: 165-171.

79. Rutherford K, Parkhill J, Crook J, Horsnell T, Rice P, Rajandream MA, Barrell B: Artemis: sequence visualization and annotation. Bioinformatics. 2000, 16: 944-945. 10.1093/bioinformatics/16.10.944.

80. Frishman D, Mironov A, Mewes HW, Gelfand M: Combining diverse evidence for gene recognition in completely sequenced bacterial genomes. Nucleic Acids Res. 1998, 26: 2941-2947. 10.1093/nar/26.12.2941.

81. Delcher AL, Harmon D, Kasif S, White O, Salzberg SL: Improved microbial gene identification with GLIMMER. Nucleic Acids Res. 1999, 27: 4636-4641. 10.1093/nar/27.23.4636.

82. Larsen TS, Krogh A: EasyGene–a prokaryotic gene finder that ranks ORFs by statistical significance. BMC Bioinformatics. 2003, 4: 21-10.1186/1471-2105-4-21.

83. Altschul SF, Gish W, Miller W, Myers EW, Lipman DJ: Basic local alignment search tool. J Mol Biol. 1990, 215: 403-410.

84. Pearson WR, Lipman DJ: Improved tools for biological sequence comparison. Proc Natl Acad Sci USA. 1988, 85: 2444-2448. 10.1073/pnas.85.8.2444.

85. Bateman A, Birney E, Cerruti L, Durbin R, Etwiller L, Eddy SR, Griffiths-Jones S, Howe KL, Marshall M, Sonnhammer EL: The Pfam protein families database. Nucleic Acids Res. 2002, 30: 276-280. 10.1093/nar/30.1.276.

86. Falquet L, Pagni M, Bucher P, Hulo N, Sigrist CJ, Hofmann K, Bairoch A: The PROSITE database, its status in 2002. Nucleic Acids Res. 2002, 30: 235-238. 10.1093/nar/30.1.235.

87. Krogh A, Larsson B, von Heijne G, Sonnhammer EL: Predicting transmembrane protein topology with a hidden Markov model: application to complete genomes. J Mol Biol. 2001, 305: 567-580. 10.1006/jmbi.2000.4315.

88. Nielsen H, Engelbrecht J, Brunak S, von Heijne G: Identification of prokaryotic and eukaryotic signal peptides and prediction of their cleavage sites. Protein Eng. 1997, 10: 1-6. 10.1093/protein/10.1.1.

89. Lowe TM, Eddy SR: tRNAscan-SE: a program for improved detection of transfer RNA genes in genomic sequence. Nucleic Acids Res. 1997, 25: 955-964. 10.1093/nar/25.5.955.

90. Griffiths-Jones S, Bateman A, Marshall M, Khanna A, Eddy SR: Rfam: an RNA family database. Nucleic Acids Res. 2003, 31: 439-441. 10.1093/nar/gkg006.

91. Carver TJ, Rutherford KM, Berriman M, Rajandream MA, Barrell BG, Parkhill J: ACT: the Artemis Comparison Tool. Bioinformatics. 2005, 21: 3422-3423. 10.1093/bioinformatics/bti553.

92. Beres SB, Sylva GL, Barbian KD, Lei BF, Hoff JS, Mammarella ND, Liu MY, Smoot JC, Porcella SF, Parkins LD, Campbell DS, Smith TM, McCormick JK, Leung DYM, Schlievert PM, Musser JM: Genome sequence of a serotype M3 strain of group A *Streptococcus*: Phage-encoded toxins, the high-virulence phenotype, and clone emergence. Proc Natl Acad Sci USA. 2002, 99: 10078-10083. 10.1073/pnas.152298499.

93. Holden MTG, Sanders M, Hauser H, Hoa NT, Cherevach I, Chillingworth T, Churcher C, Cronin A, Dowd L, Feltwell T, Hamlin N, Holroyd N, Jagels K, Moule S, Mungall K, Quail MA, Price C, Rabbinowitsch E, Sharp S, Skelton J, Whitehead S, Croucher NJ, Kehoe M, Leigh J, Ward NL, Dowson C, Whatmore AM, Chanter N, Iversen P, Gottschalk M, Slater J, Smith HO, Spratt B, Xe J, Ye C, Bentley SD, Barrell BG, Schultsz C,

Maskell D, Parkhill J: Evidence for the rapid evolution of virulence and drug resistance in the zoonotic pathogen *Streptococcus suis*.

94. Tettelin H, Nelson KE, Paulsen IT, Eisen JA, Read TD, Peterson S, Heidelberg J, DeBoy RT, Haft DH, Dodson RJ, Durkin AS, Gwinn M, Kolonay JF, Nelson WC, Peterson JD, Umayam LA, White O, Salzberg SL, Lewis MR, Radune D, Holtzapple E, Khouri H, Wolf AM, Utterback TR, Hansen CL, McDonald LA, Feldblyum TV, Angiuoli S, Dickinson T, Hickey EK, Holt IE, Loftus BJ, Yang F, Smith HO, Venter JC, Dougherty BA, Morrison DA, Hollingshead SK, Fraser CM: Complete genome sequence of a virulent isolate of *Streptococcus pneumoniae*. Science. 2001, 293: 498-506. 10.1126/science.1061217.

95. Xu P, Alves JM, Kitten T, Brown A, Chen Z, Ozaki LS, Manque P, Ge X, Serrano MG, Puiu D, Hendricks S, Wang Y, Chaplin MD, Akan D, Paik S, Peterson DL, Macrina FL, Buck GA: Genome of the opportunistic pathogen *Streptococcus sanguinis*. J Bacteriol. 2007, 189: 3166-3175. 10.1128/JB.01808-06.

96. Glaser P, Rusniok C, Buchrieser C, Chevalier F, Frangeul L, Msadek T, Zouine M, Couve E, Lalioui L, Poyart C, Trieu-Cuot P, Kunst F: Genome sequence of *Streptococcus agalactiae*, a pathogen causing invasive neonatal disease. Mol Microbiol. 2002, 45: 1499-1513. 10.1046/j.1365-2958.2002.03126.x.

97. Vickerman MM, Iobst S, Jesionowski AM, Gill SR: Genome-wide transcriptional changes in *Streptococcus gordonii* in response to competence signaling peptide. J Bacteriol. 2007, 189: 7799-7807. 10.1128/JB.01023-07.

98. Bolotin A, Wincker P, Mauger S, Jaillon O, Malarme K, Weissenbach J, Ehrlich SD, Sorokin A: The complete genome sequence of the lactic acid bacterium *Lactococcus lactis* ssp. *lactis* IL1403. Genome Res. 2001, 11: 731-753. 10.1101/gr.GR-1697R.

99. Guindon S, Gascuel O: A simple, fast, and accurate algorithm to estimate large phylogenies by maximum likelihood. Syst Biol. 2003, 52: 696-704. 10.1080/10635150390235520.

100. Guindon S, Lethiec F, Duroux P, Gascuel O: PHYML Online–a web server for fast maximum likelihood-based phylogenetic inference. Nucleic Acids Res. 2005, 33: W557-559. 10.1093/nar/gki352.

101. Perriere G, Gouy M: WWW-query: an on-line retrieval system for biological sequence banks. Biochimie. 1996, 78: 364-369. 10.1016/0300-9084(96)84768-7.

102. Thompson JD, Gibson TJ, Plewniak F, Jeanmougin F, Higgins DG: The CLUSTAL_X windows interface: flexible strategies for multiple sequence alignment aided by quality analysis tools. Nucleic Acids Res. 1997, 25: 4876-4882. 10.1093/nar/25.24.4876.

SECTION VII: FRANCISELLA – AGENT OF TULAREMIA

CHAPTER 28

GENOME CHARACTERISATION OF THE GENUS FRANCISELLA REVEALS INSIGHT INTO SIMILAR EVOLUTIONARY PATHS IN PATHOGENS OF MAMMALS AND FISH

Andreas Sjödin, Kerstin Svensson, Caroline Öhrman, Jon Ahlinder, Petter Lindgren, Samuel Duodu, Anders Johansson, Duncan J Colquhoun, Pär Larsson and Mats Forsman

Keywords: *Francisella,* Next-generation sequencing, Recombination, Fish, Genetics, Evolution

BACKGROUND

Tularemia is a zoonotic disease caused by the highly infectious, virulent, Gram-negative bacterium *Francisella tularensis*. Due to its infectious nature, ease of dissemination and associated high fatality rate (especially from respiratory infection), *F. tularensis* has been included in military biological weapons programs and is regarded as one of the top six agents which have a high potential for misuse in bioterrorism[1].

The known diversity of the genus *Francisella* has recently expanded substantially and the boundaries between taxonomic units within the genus is currently under debate[2, 3]. In mammals, including man, the disease tularemia is caused by two *F. tularensis* subspecies: subsp. *tularensis* (type A, endemic in North America) and subsp. *holarctica* (type B, found throughout the Northern hemisphere)[4]. Nearly all fatalities due to tularemia are caused by *F. tularensis* type A infections, for which mortality rates up to 30% have been reported[5]. In contrast, *F. tularensis* type B causes a milder disease, for which fatalities rarely occur. A third accepted subspecies, *F. tularensis* subsp. *mediasiatica* is found in Asia. This subspecies has been found to display level of virulence comparable to strains of subspecies *holarctica* and very rarely cause human infections[6, 7]. Disease in humans has also been presented following opportunistic infection by *F. novicida* (in individuals with a weakened immune system) and *F. philomiragia* (in individuals with a weakened immune system exposed to sea water)[8, 9, 10].

A number of *Francisella* lineages also exist that do not appear to be associated with human disease. Strains closely related to *F. philomiragia*, which have recently been designated as *Francisella noatunensis,* have been identified as etiological agents of Francisellosis in fish[11, 12, 13, 14, 15]. *F. noatunensis* is further divided into two subspecies, subsp. *noatunensis*[16] and subsp. *orientalis*[17, 18]. Recent published studies have also identified several new related and as yet uncultured forms of *Francisella* from soil and water[19, 20, 21, 22, 23], as well as tick endosymbionts with high similarity to *F. tularensis* (*Francisella*-like endosymbionts) [24]. One isolated tick endosymbiont has inaccurately been designated *Wolbachia persica*[25], incorrectly placing it within the *alpha-* proteobacteria[26]. Further, a marine ciliate endosymbiont has been proposed to represent '*Candidatus F. noatunensis* subsp. *endociliophora*'[23] and a bacterium

Citation: Andreas Sjödin, Kerstin Svensson, Caroline Öhrman, Jon Ahlinder, Petter Lindgren, Samuel Duodu, Anders Johansson, Duncan J Colquhoun, Pär Larsson and Mats Forsman, Genome characterisation of the genus Francisella reveals insight into similar evolutionary paths in pathogens of mammals and fish, DOI: 10.1186/1471-2164-13-268.

isolated from an air-conditioning system has been tentatively classified as *Francisella cantonensis*[27]. Thus, in recent years the existence of substantial sub-species diversity within the *Francisella* genus has become increasingly apparent. Members of *Francisella* appear to be associated with a multitude of different ecological niches, ranging from specialised endosymbionts and pathogens with different host spectrums, to generalists believed capable of a free-living existence.

There are several reasons for sequencing *Francisella* strains other than those belonging to *F. tularensis*. Analysis of gene content and genetic relationships may help to improve our understanding of the biology and evolution of these bacteria, including that of the human pathogen *F. tularensis*. Sequencing multiple strains of environmental *Francisella* may also reveal important sequence differences between environmental species and *F. tularensis*. This would allow the design of increasingly specific *F. tularensis* detection assays for use in anti-bioterrorism applications and epidemiological studies, particularly important since current methods frequently falsely detect *F. tularensis* in environmental samples[28].

The genome sequence data generated by the present study represents a considerable advancement of knowledge of the genus *Francisella* and includes genome sequences for 18 environmental *Francisella* strains, four *F. tularensis* and two distant but genetically related species *Fangia hongkongensis*[29] and *Piscirickettsia salmonis*[30]. Here we describe the population structure of the genus *Francisella*, suggest that ancestral *Francisella* strains originated in marine habitats, show that present-day strains can be divided into two main genetic clades occupying continental and aquatic habitats and provide evidence that similar evolutionary paths of host adaptations have occurred independently in *F. tularensis* (infecting mammals) and *F. noatunensis* subsp. *noatunensis* (infecting fish).

RESULTS

Bacterial strains and classifications

Here, we present 24 novel genome sequences representing all major subclades of the *Francisella* genus (Table 1), with the exception of the recently discovered *F. cantonensis*[27]. The data doubles the number of published *Francisella* genomes and significantly extends the known range of genetic diversity. The studied material includes seven previously unsequenced *F. noatunensis* isolates and a single representative from the tick endosymbiont group[31]. In addition, representatives of *Fa. hongkongensis*[29] and *P. salmonis*[32], both of which are related to the genus *Francisella*, were also sequenced. Interestingly, *Francisella* strain 3523[33, 34] appeared to belong to the *F. hispaniensis* clade and not the *F. novicida* clade as reported previously[34].

Table 1: Strains sequenced in this study

Species	FSC ID	Alternate designation	Year isolated	Source	Location	NCBI ID
F. tularensis subsp. holarctica	FSC021	F0014, Tsuchiya	1958	Human lymph node	Fukushima prefecture, Japan	73369
F. tularensis subsp. holarctica	FSC208	3049UBG	1998	Human	Gävleborg county, Sweden	73467
F. tularensis subsp. holarctica	FSC539	2004-32-55	2004	Human blood	Örebro county, Sweden	73393
F. tularensis subsp. mediasiatica	FSC148	F0012, 240, 840	1982	Tick	Jambyl oblast, Kazakhstan	73379
F. tularensis subsp. tularensis	FSC054	F0010, Nevada 14	1953	Hare (*Lepus californicus*)	Nevada state, USA	73375
F. novicida	FSC159	F0052; fx2; 110	1995	Human blood	Texas state, USA	73383
F. novicida	FSC160	fx1; Houston, 2766	1991	Human blood	Texas state, USA	73385
F. novicida	FSC595	F58	2003	Human blood	Brazil/UK/Germany	73395
F. hispaniensis	FSC454	FhSp1	2003	Human blood	Elche, Spain	73391
F. noatunensis subsp. noatunensis	FDC178	NVI 7601, F/134/09A	2009	Atlantic cod (*Gadus morhua*)	Waterford, Ireland	73465

F. noatunensis subsp. noatunensis	FSC769	NVI 2005/50/ F292-6C, NCIMB14265, LMG23800, DSM12596	2005	Atlantic cod (*Gadus morhua*)	Hordaland county, Norway	73397
F. noatunensis subsp. noatunensis	FSC772	NVI 5888, PQ1106	2006	Atlantic salmon (*Salmo salar*)	Lake Llanquihue, Chile	73449
F. noatunensis subsp. noatunensis	FSC774[2]	NVI 5865, GM2212	2004	Atlantic cod (*Gadus morhua*)	Rogaland county, Norway	73457
F. noatunensis subsp. noatunensis	FSC775[2]	DSM18777, GM2212	2004	Atlantic cod (*Gadus morhua*)	Rogaland county, Norway	73459
F. noatunensis subsp. noatunensis	FSC846	NVI 5518, SVA 74/04	2004	Atlantic cod (*Gadus morhua*)	Southern Skagerrak, Sweden	73463
F. noatunensis subsp. orientalis	FSC770	NVI 5409, PQ1104,	2006	Tilapia (*Oreochromis* sp.)	Costa Rica	73389
F. noatunensis subsp. orientalis	FSC771	Ehime-1, PQ1105	2001	Three-line grunt (*Parapristipoma trilineatum*)	Uwajima, Ehime prefecture, Japan	73447
Wolbachia persica	FSC845	ATCC VR - 331	1960	Soft tick (Oken) (*Argas persicus*) from buff-backed heron (*Bubulcus ibis*)	Nile Barrage Park, Cairo, Egypt	73171
F. philomiragia	FSC037	F0047, ATCC 25016	1960	Water	Bear River Refuge, Utah state, USA	73371
F. philomiragia	FSC039	F0049, ATCC 25018	1960	Water	Odgen Bay Refuge, Utah state, USA	73373
F. philomiragia	FSC145	F0046; CCUG 12603	1982	Human abscess	Göteborg, Sweden	73377
F. philomiragia	FSC154	Swiss	1979	Bone marrow, ascitic fluid	Zürich, Switzerland	73381
Fangia hongkongensis	FSC776	JCM14605	2004	Seawater at the outlet of a sand filter	Port Shelter, Hongkong, China	73461
Piscirickettsia salmonis	FSC773	NVI 5692	2006	Atlantic salmon (*Salmo salar*)	Møre & Romsdal county, Norway	73451

1 FDC178 was supplied by the Marine Institute, Oranmore, Ireland.

2 FSC774 was supplied by the National Veterinary Institue (NVI), Norway and FSC775 was requisitioned from the German Microorganism Collection (DSM).

3 FSC 160 (fx1) was supplied by VAMC, Houston, Texas. (Previously published FSC156 (fx1) was supplied by another lab.).

4 FSC539 from same patient as FSC529 in Svensson et al 2009.

Information about isolates sequenced in this study.

Overall, a major bifurcation into two genetic lineages was identified (Figure 1) with clade 1 comprising *F. tularensis, F. novicida, F. hispaniensis* and *W. persica*, and clade 2 containing *F. noatunensis* and *F. philomiragia*.

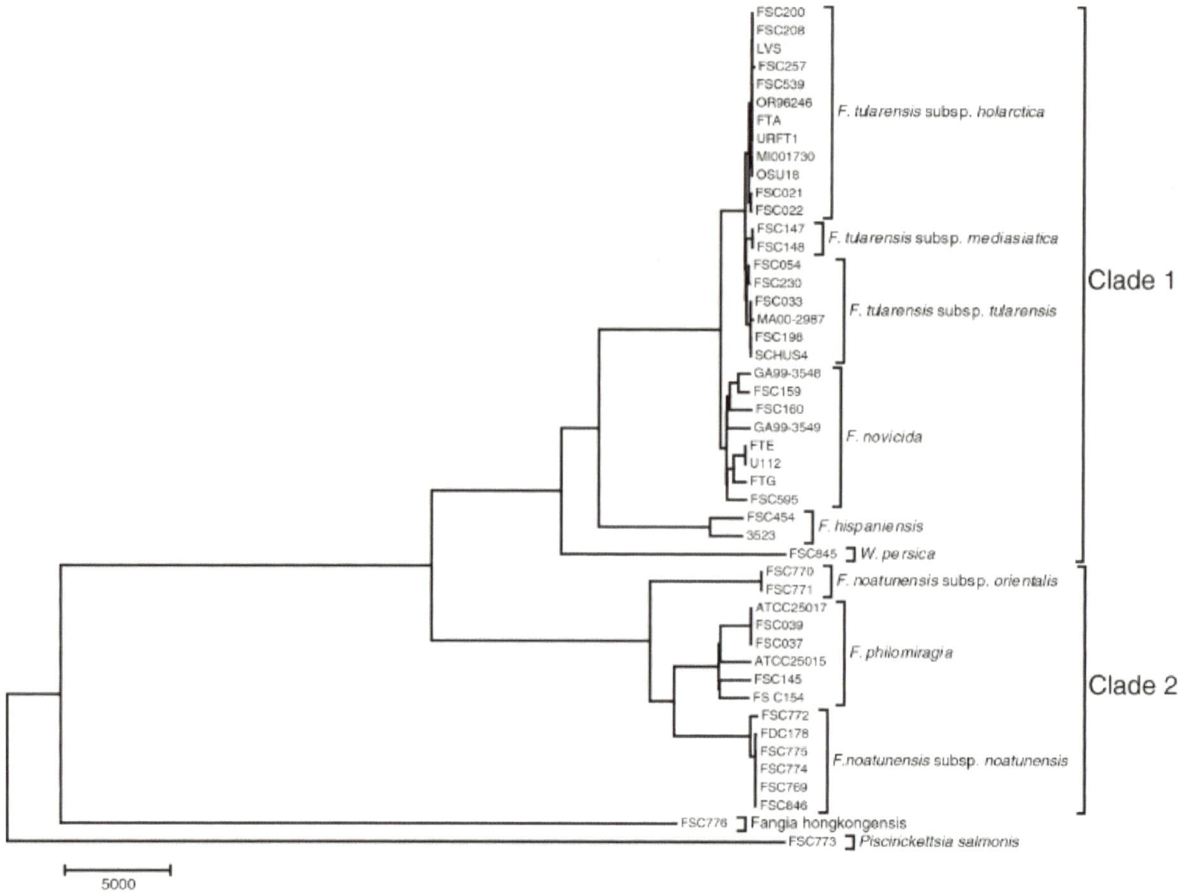

Figure 1: Whole-genome phylogeny. The phylogeny of 45 *Francisella* strains and two genetic relatives, *Fangia hongkongensis*and *Piscirickettsia salmonis,* based on single nucleotide polymorphism in the core genome. The *Francisella* genus is divided into two parts, clade 1 (*F. tularensis* and *F. novicida*) and clade 2 (*F. noatunensis* and *F. philomiragia*).

Francisella whole-genome phylogeny and average nucleotide identities

Whole-genome alignments were produced using progressiveMauve[35]. A phylogeny based on core genome single nucleotide polymorphisms is shown in Figure 1.

Analysis of the whole-genome phylogeny showed that strains of *F. philomiragia* and *F. noatunensis* subsp. *noatunensis* formed sister clades, while strains of *F. noatunensis* subsp. *orientalis* diverged at a more basal position, indicating the newly named species *F. noatunensis* is paraphyletic. This interpretation was supported by an analysis of average nucleotide identities (ANI): ANI for *F. philomiragia* compared to *F. noatunensis*subsp. *noatunensis* is higher (95%) than *F. philomiragia* compared to *F. noatunensis* subsp. *orientalis* (92–93%).

Phylogenetic inference using whole-genome data and 16 S ribosomal RNA genes resulted in incongruent topologies. The phylogenetic position of *F. philomiragia* (Figure 1) was different from previous publications of phylogenies calculated based on 16 S ribosomal RNA genes [13, 14].

Analysis of *Francisella* pan and core genomes

Based on the analysed gene orthologs, the core genome of the genus *Francisella* contained 803 genes (Figure 2A). Clade 1 shared 854 genes, while clade 2 (*F. noatunensis* and *F. philomiragia*) shared 1359 genes (Figure 2B).

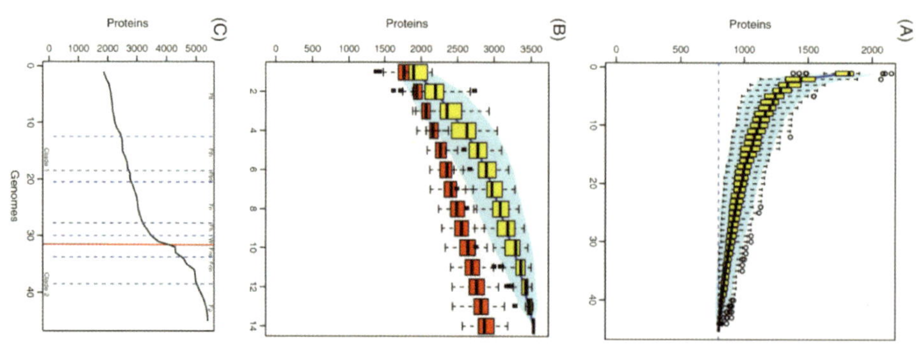

Figure 2: Over of core and pan genome structure for the *Francisella* genus. A. Accumulation curve (core genome) for the number of genes in common as a function of the number of genomes analysed for the *Francisella* genus. **B.** Accumulation curve for the total number of genes (pan genome) as a function of the number of genomes analysed for clade 1 (*F. tularensis, W. persica and F. hispaniensis*)(red) and clade 2 (*F.*

philomiragia and *F. noatunensis*)(yellow). **C.** Cumulative accumulation of total number genes when genomes are added according to the structure in the SNP phylogeny. Ftt – F. tularensis subsp. tularensis, Fth – *F. tularensis subsp. holarctica*, Ftm – F. *tularensis subsp. mediasiatica*, Fn – *F. novicida*, Fh – *F. hispaniensis*, W – *Wolbachia persica*, Fno – *F. noatunensis* subsp. *orientalis*, Fnn – *F. noatunensis* subsp. *noatunensis*, Fp – *F. Philomiragia.*

The pan-genome of the genus *Francisell a* contained a total of 5396 genes (Figure 2C). Separate analysis of the pan-genome size within clade 1, excluding *F. hispaniensis and W. persica*, and clade 2 identified 3222 and 3535 genes, respectively (Figure 2B). The pan-genome of *F. tularensis* contained 2769 genes.

Clade-specific genes

An over of the gene distribution in the genus *Francisella* is depicted in Figure 3 and the clade-specific genes are summarised in Table 2. The human pathogen, *F. tularensis* contained only seven unique genes (FTT0794, FTT0795, FTT0796, FTT1188, FTT1453c, FTT1454c and FTT1458), which grouped at three different locations in the genome. No unique genes were found in *F. novicida* genomes. *F. hispaniensis*, *F. noatunensis*and *F. philomiragia* exhibited seven, nine and ten unique genes, respectively. The complete clade 2 (*F. noatunensis* and *F. philomiragia*) genomes displayed 41 genes that were not present in clade 1. However, the clade 2 species *F. noatunensis* subsp. *noatunensis* and *F. noatunensis* subsp. *orientalis* shared 32 and 114 genes, respectively, which were not present in other genomes.

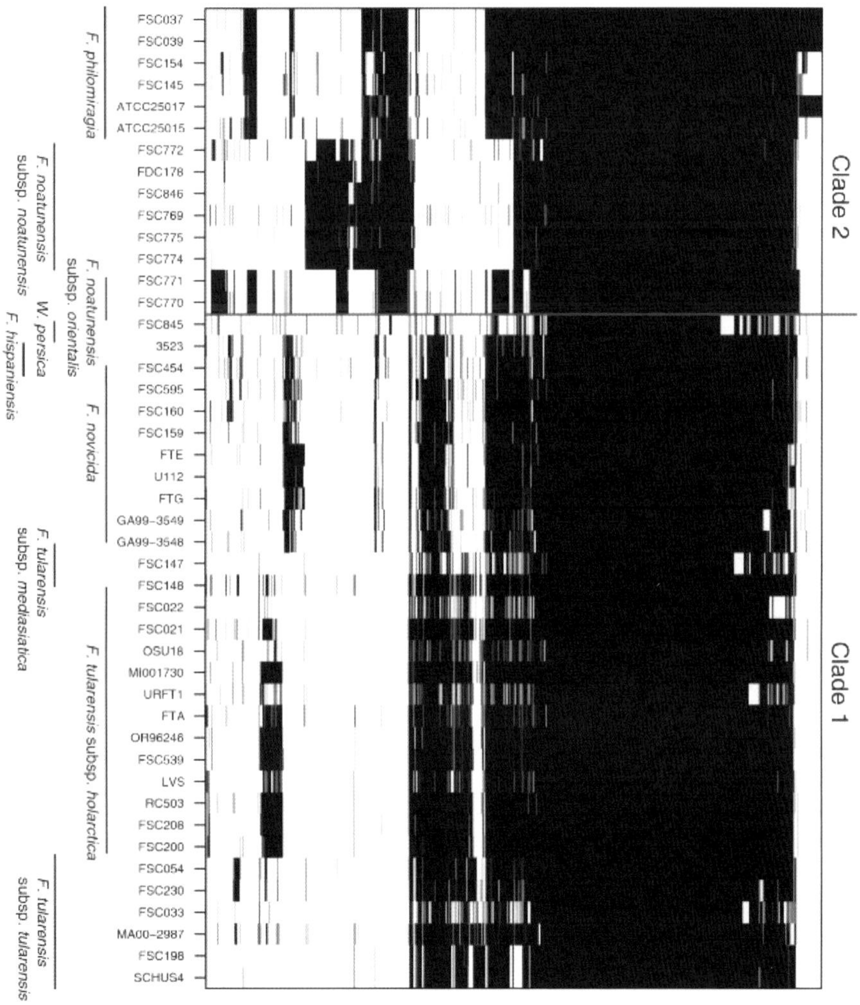

Figure 3: Whole-genome comparison of the pan-genome of 45 *Francisella* strains. Presence of a gene in a genome is indicated in black. The core genome of 803 genes, and the genes unique to clade 1 (*F. tularensis*, *F. novicida, F. hispaniensis and W. persica*) and clade 2 (*F. noatunensis* and *F. philomiragia*) are clustered together in the heat map.

Table 2: Clade-specific genes

Included species/subspecies	Excluded species/subspecies	#unique genes	Reference genome
F. tularensis subsp. tularensis	All other	0	SCHUS4
F. tularensis subsp. holarctica	All other	0	LVS
F. tularensis subsp. mediasiatica	All other	0	FSC147

F. philomiragia	All other	9	ATOC 25017
F. noatunensis subsp. noatunensis	All other	32	FSC769
F. noatunensis subsp. orientalis	All other	114	FSC770
F. novicida	All other	0	U112
F. hispaniensis	All other	7	FSC454
Wolbachia persica	All other	125	FSC845
Fangia hongkongensis	All other	1104	FSC776
Piscirickettsia salmonis	All other	1725	FSC773
F. tularensis subsp. tularensis, F. tularensis subsp. holarctica, F. tularensis subsp. mediasiatica	F. novicida, F. hispaniensis, W. persica F. noatunensis subsp. orientalis, F. noatunensis subsp. noatunensis, P salmonis	7	SCHUS4
F. noatunensis subsp. orientalis, F. noatunensis subsp. noatunensis, F. philomiragia	F. tularensis subsp. tularensis, F. tularensis subsp. holarctica, F. tularensis subsp. mediasiatica, F. novicida, F. hispaniensis, W. persica, F. hongkongensis, P. salmonis	41	FSC769
F. noatunensis subsp. orientalis, F. noatunensis subsp. noatunensis	F. philomiragia, F tularensis subsp. tularensis, F. tularensis subsp. holarctica, F. tularensis subsp. mediasiatica, F. novicida, F. hispaniensis, W. persica, F. hongkongensis, P.	10	FSC769
F. noatunensis subsp. noatunensis, F. philomiragia	F. noatunensis subsp. orientalis, F. tularensis subsp. tularensis, F. tularensis subsp. holarctica, F. tularensis subsp. mediasiatica, F. novicida, F. hispaniensis, P. salmonis	9	FSC769

Summary of clade-specific genes in the *Francisella* genus.

IS elements

Notable differences in IS element content were identified between different species and clades. In clade 1, *F. hispaniensis* contained a few copies of ISFtu2, ISFtu3, ISFtu4, ISFpi1 and IS4502, while *W. persica* contained very few copies of ISFtu2 and ISFtu3. The isolates in clade 2 exhibited a different pattern of IS elements. Whereas *F. noatunensis* subsp. *orientalis* was almost completely lacking IS elements (only a potential trace of ISFpi1 was found), *F. noatunensis* subsp. *noatunensis* exhibited an expansion trend similar to that previously reported for *F. tularensis*[36]. The expansion was within the ISFpi1 group and included a handful of copies of the IS4502 element, and single copies of ISFtu1, ISFtu2 and ISFtu3 elements.

The more distant relatives studied, i.e. *Fa. hongkongensis* and *P. salmonis,* contained completely different sets of IS elements compared with *Francisella*. The genome of *P. salmonis* was enriched with ISPsa1 and ISPsa2[37], whereas only one copy of ISFpi1 was found in *Fa. hongkongensis.* The IS element distributions of *F. tularensis*, *F. novicida* and *F. philomiragia* have been reported previously[36, 38].

Recombination

Results of the recombination analyses are presented in Figure 4. The proportion of genes within the *Francisella* core genome demonstrating evidence of recombination was 32%, although the presence of recombination was highly variable across the different *Francisella* lineages. For some species/subspecies, recombination was entirely absent (i.e. *F. tularensis* subsp. *tularensis, F. tularensis* subsp. *holarctica* and *F. noatunensis* subsp. *noatunensis*), whereas recombination in *F. philomiragia* and *F. novicida*occurred frequently.

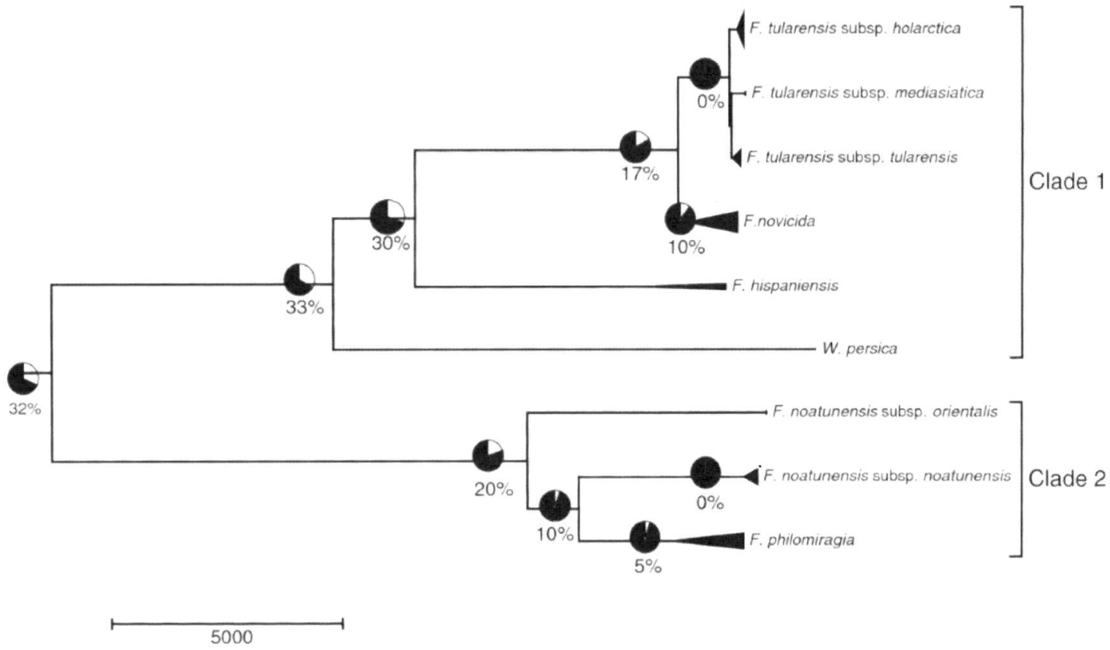

Figure 4: Over of the recombination. The proportion of genes showing evidence of recombination overlaid on the *Francisella* phylogeny. Recombination detection was performed using the PHI method with the number of significant tests ($P<0.01$) reported as a percentage of recombinant genes within the *Francisella* genus.

DISCUSSION

To date, sequenced *Francisella* genomes have mainly been of the human pathogenic species *F. tularensis.*Consequently, conclusions about evolutionary processes within the genus *Francisella* have largely been based on *F. tularensis* genomes[36, 38].

Moreover, a number of identification assays developed on the basis of *F. tularensis* genome sequences have been shown to give false-positive results. These have been attributed to the presence of the same sequence signatures as in other environmental *Francisella* lineages[39].

In the present study, we provide details of the genetic content of nearly all currently known members of the genus *Francisella*, with the exception of the recently published *F. cantonensis*[27]. Despite a generally high sequence similarity within the genus, we found that different genetic clades demonstrated different population structures (recombination frequencies). This suggests differences in lifestyle and host association.

F. tularensis has been found to be a highly clonal species, differentiating it from environmental lineages characterised by moderate recombination rates. We also found evidence that the fish pathogen *F. noatunensis* subsp. *noatunensis* also possesses a highly clonal lineage. The low recombination frequency in *F. noatunensis* subsp. *noatunensis* may indicate that a close host association reduced contact with other *Francisella* species, and thereby, lowered opportunities for gene acquisition by recombination, as previously hypothesised for *F. tularensis*[36]. The data of population structure and variability observed among *F. novicida*opposed to *F. tularensis* subspecies *tularensis*, *holarctica* and *mediasiatica* strains should be taken in consideration for the on-going discussion whether it should be a separate species or included as a subspecies in *F. tularensis*.

Whole genome phylogeny

Our analyses of 45 *Francisella* genomes showed that recognised species could be divided into two main genetic clades (Figure 1) and suggested that the pathogenic species in each clade emerged independently by similar evolutionary paths of host adaptation. *F. tularensis*, which can infect mammals, belonged to clade 1, whereas *F. noatunensis* subsp. *noatunensis,* which infects fish, belonged to clade 2. Our analyses based on the phylogeny of *Francisella* genomes and genetic relatives suggest that the ancestral *Francisella* species originated in a marine habitat.

Using whole-genome analysis, we found evidence that *F. noatunensis* subsp. *noatunensis* and *F. noatunensis*subsp. *orientalis* represent a paraphyletic group. *F. philomiragia* and *F. noatunensis* subsp. *noatunensis*together form a sister clade to *F. noatunensis* subsp. *orientalis* (Figure 1, Table 1). This result was not supported by 16S RNA analysis, which suggested that the two subspecies *F. noatunensis* subsp. *orientalis* and *F. noatunensis* subsp. *noatunensis* form a clade. There are limited nucleotide differences in the 16S region and more comprehensive core genome SNP analysis gives a better of the real relationship. Identification of genetic factors coding for fish pathogenicity may therefore be possible via comparative analyses. Further phenotypic studies and experiments are needed to confirm this hypothesis. Since *F. noatunensis* subsp. *noatunensis* is isolated from cod and salmon, while *F. noatunensis* subsp. *orientalis* isolates are recovered from tilapia and three-line grunt, an alternative hypothesis is that these subspecies evolved their abilities for fish infection independently.

In agreement with other studies[26, 40], our analyses verified the phylogenetic position of the tick endosymbiont *W. persica* within the *Francisella* genus. Several lines of genomic evidence support the that this organism adapted as a primary symbiont; its genome size was found to be significantly less (about 80–85%) than other *Francisella* genomes. Moreover, in *W. persica,* regulatory genes were found to be depleted, while biosynthesis pathways supplying amino acids to their insect host were retained, and there was a low abundance of IS elements. Our results confirm that *W. persica* and other *Francisella*-like endosymbionts (FLE)[19, 24, 41, 42] belong to the genus *Francisella* and that *W. persica* has undergone a significant reduction in its genome.

An important outcome of the present study was reclassification of the isolate 3523 from Australia. It was initially classified as an unusual *F. novicida*[33], a classification which remained despite whole genome sequencing[34]. It was clear from the present analyses that isolate 3523 belongs to the *F. hispaniensis*clade[43]. This result demonstrates the importance of broad-scale intra-genus sequencing for correct classification of new isolates.

Francisella pan- and core- genome

The overall core genome size of 799 genes for the genus *Francisella* was similar to that reported for the genus *Bacillus* (Figure2A)[44]. Bacterial pan-genomes at the genus level have only recently been reported in the literature, and the number of gene families in these genera is expected to grow as more genomes are included. This approach may be valuable in revealing genes specific for niche commonalities between subspecies.

We detected different pan-genome sizes for clade 1 and clade 2 (Figure2B), where clade 2 contain more genes compared to clade 1 and especially *F. tularensis* clade alone. As a result, *F. tularensis* may be fully sampled by sequencing smaller set of representative isolates, whereas more isolates of clade 2 would need to be fully sequenced to give a true pan-genome size.

The contribution of each genome to the complete pan-genome of the genus *Francisella* and related organisms is illustrated in Figure2C. Most genomes contribute to the increase of the pan-genome, although the increase is less pronounced when similar genomes are added.

Clade specific genes

Genomes in the *Francisella* genus have, with the exception of *W. persica*, similar gene composition. *W. persica*has not retained genes included in the COG group 'amino acid transport and metabolism', which it does not require because of its endosymbiotic lifestyle.

An extensive list of 80 potential candidate virulence genes has previously been published, which are specific for the human pathogen *F. tularensis*[45]. Surprisingly, analysis of the more complete collection of *Francisella*genomes in the present study reduced this list to only seven *F. tularensis* specific genes. The general lack of specific genes agrees with previous observations that pathogens exhibit specialisation and host-adaption by gene loss rather than gene gain[46]. Thus, a pathogen such as *F. tularensis* should be defined not only by genes that are present but also by those that are lacking.

The seven specific genes in *F. tularensis* were located in three separate gene clusters. The genes in the first cluster (FTT0794, FTT0795, FTT0796) are organised in an operon and were predicted to be involved in exopolysaccharide synthesis. It has been suggested that an exopolysaccharide capsule plays a role in *F. tularensis* virulence[47].

The second gene cluster (FTT1453c, FTT1454c and FTT1458) is present within the *wbt* locus of *F. tularensis*. Genes in this locus encode proteins involved in lipopolysaccharide O-antigen synthesis. The O-antigens of *F. tularensis* contain an insertion element that differentiates it from *F. novicida*[48]. A similar insertion element structure has been reported to be essential for virulence in *Shigella sonnei*[49]. Finally, the last gene cluster contained a single gene, FTT1188, which encodes for a hypothetical membrane protein. This protein does not exhibit significant homology to other proteins in the NCBI non-redundant database and has not yet been characterised in depth. Identification of virulence genes and their role in the virulence of *Francisella* is not straight-forward. Our data suggest that *F. tularensis* virulence cannot be easily explained by a simplistic model which just considers the presence or absence of specific "virulence genes"[36].

Fa. hongkongensis and *P. salmonis* both contain many genes that are absent from the *Francisella* genus and are therefore likely to occupy distinctly different ecological niches.

IS elements

The two principal clades of the *Francisella* genus exhibit several similarities and differences in IS element content and composition. *F. noatunensis* subsp. *noatunensis* contains an expanded set of IS elements similar to those reported for *F. tularensis*. The expanded IS elements in *F. tularensis* are ISFtu1 and ISFtu2, whereas the expanded IS element in *F. noatunensis* is ISFpil. Interestingly, the two subspecies of *F. noatunensis*exhibited contrasting contents of IS elements. While *F. noatunensis* subsp. *noatunensis* contained the highest number of IS elements of all species in the genus, *F. noatunensis* subsp. *orientalis* contains very few IS elements. This may have arisen because of different evolutionary modes in these subspecies.

Recombination

Recombination is an important process for generating new genetic diversity within bacterial populations and is a known driver of evolution in many bacterial species[50]. The recombination analysis of 45 genomes in the present study confirmed that the level of recombination within the *Francisella* genus is highly variable, ranging from undetectable in *F. tularensis* to moderate in *F. novicida*[36].

We found that the subspecies of *F. noatunensis* exhibited apparently low rates of recombination at levels similar to the human pathogen group of *F. tularensis*. Otherwise, both clade 1 and II displayed moderate recombination rates, largely due to frequent recombination within *F. novicida* (clade 1) and *F. philomiragia*(clade 2). According to our findings, 33% of the core gene set provided evidence of past recombination events, similar in magnitude to estimates for *Campylobacter*[51] and *Neisseria*[52], but higher than previously reported for *Francisella*[36]. It was reported previously that 19.2% of the genes in the core genome of *F. novicida* and *F. philomiragia* have been recombined, but our data suggests that this is could be an underestimate due to a lack of genomic sequences available at that time.

Our findings are similar to reports for other bacterial genera that include highly specialized pathogens. Variable recombination rates have previously been reported for several pathogenic populations, (*Yersina pestis*[53], *Bacillus anthracis*[54] and *Mycobacterium tuberculosis*[55]). It should be noted that if closely related clones of pathogens with low recombination rates are over-represented, this can result in an under-estimation of recombination rates for the entire genus[50, 56]. By ensuring proper representation of all subspecies of the *Francisella* genus in the present work, such effects were minimised.

CONCLUSIONS

This work significantly expands the number of sequenced *Francisella* genomes, and therefore provides an important resource for assessing evolutionary and functional relationships within the genus. We identified the core genome in the *Francisella* genus and single nucleotide polymorphisms within these genes were used to infer a robust phylogeny. A high degree of clonality confirmed for *F. tularensis* type A and B, was also identified in *F. noatunensis* subsp. *noatunensis*. Despite infecting different species, it is apparent that these lineages also share certain important evolutionary properties.

Next-generation sequencing enables rapid generation of high quality data for the fast assembly of novel genomes[57]. Growing databases of genome sequences are of significant interest for improving the designs of specific detection assays, conducting epidemiological and ecological studies, microbial forensics[58] and classification of novel bacterial isolates. Comparative genomic approaches together with functional datasets will be critical for the development of assays that specifically target pathogenic *Francisella* strains.

METHODS

Cultivation and DNA preparation

All strains (Table 1), except FSC845, were cultured on cysteine heart agar plates supplemented with 5–9% chocolatised sheep blood (CHAB) (BD Biosciences, Franklin Lakes, NJ USA), or Modified Thayer-Martin (McLeod) agar plates[59], at 25°C for the eight strains FSC769 to FSC776, and at 37°C for all other strains, in 5% CO_2 for 5 days (*F. tularensis* strains) or up to ~30 days (non-*F. tularensis* strains).

A loopful of bacteria was suspended in 1 x TRIS-EDTA (TE) buffer to 10^9 CFU/ml and heat-killed at 95°C for 15 minutes. The bacteria were lysed using Buffer ATL (Qiagen, Hilden, Germany), or similar non-denaturing lysis buffer. DNA was prepared using phenol extraction (PE), or extraction with Biorobot EZ1 (Qiagen, Hilden, Germany) according to the manufacturer's protocol. Sterility was verified by lack of growth on Modified Thayer-Martin (McLeod) plates[59] after incubation of 10 µl DNA (if PE was used) or lysate (if EZ1 was used) for 10 days.

The strain FSC845 (*Wolbachia persica*) was propagated in cells, and bacteria were collected by differential centrifugation. Bacterial cell pellets were suspended in phosphate-buffered saline (PBS) and DNA was prepared as above. For FSC772 and FDC178, DNA was prepared using the Gentra Puregene Cell kit (Qiagen, Hilden, Germany) and was re-suspended in a hydration solution supplied with the kit. DNA concentrations were measured using Nanodrop (Thermo Scientific, Wilmington, DE, USA).

Genome sequencing and assembly

DNA for genomic sequencing of 24 isolates from the *Francisella* genus and genetic relatives were prepared as described in Table 1. 19 genomes were sequenced at the National Bioforensic Analysis Center using a 454 FLX machine (454 Life Sequencing Inc., Branford, CT, USA) according to the manufacturer's instructions. Additional sequencing was performed using the Illumina GS II sequencing 36 bp or 76 bp SE technology.

Isolates sequenced with both technologies were first assembled using Newbler. Obtained contigs were corrected using the Illumina reads in Nesoni. Isolates sequenced only with the Illumina technology were assembled using Velvet.[60, 61].

All 24 isolates included in this study were submitted to IMG/ER[62] for functional annotation. All sequence reads were deposited in Genbank and are freely downloadable from the Genbank project number listed in Table 1.

16 S rRNA alignment

The *Francisella* 16 S ribosomal RNA data were obtained using the ribosomal database project[63, 64]. The key search words '*Francisella*', '*Fangia hongkongensis*' and '*Piscirickettsia salmonis*' produced 171 hits in the database. After removing duplicates, small sequences and sequences of poor quality, the final dataset consisted of 69 sequences and 1557 bases. To infer the phylogenetic tree of the 16 S data, the software RAxML[65] was used, which is suitable for analysing ribosomal RNA data as covariation patterns are taken into account in the model. The secondary structure was analysed using the substitution model RNA6A by maximising the log-likelihood. The GTR and gamma model was chosen as the standard DNA substitution model. The number of bootstrap replicates was 1000.

Whole-genome alignment

Multiple genome alignments were computed by employing the progressiveMauve algorithm of the Mauve software[35] using default options. Sequences were extracted and concatenated from each of the 45 genomes to build a core genome of multiple alignments. Core genome SNPs were identified from this alignment as the loci where at least one sequence had a mutated base and it had no missing sequences from any genome included in this study. While it is possible that some of the SNP's that were specific to a single sequence could have been incorrect due to sequencing errors, this was unlikely in the case of informative sites. Strain-specific SNP's can have an effect on the estimated value of the mutation rate and the branch length of the phylogenetic tree. However, they do not affect the structure of the tree. The phylogenetic data is deposited in treeBASE[66, 67].

Whole-genome phylogenetic construction

An unrooted neighbour joining tree for the genus *Francisella* with the genetic relatives *Fa. hongkongensis* and *P. salmonis* as an outgroup was constructed using the MEGA5 software[68] based on the numbers of substitutions per nucleotide site in the genome sequences of all strains. The Complete Deletion Method was used for handling alignment gaps.

Estimation of evolutionary distance

Average nucleotide identity (ANI) was calculated by pairwise genome comparisons with the MUMmer and BLAST algorithms using JSpecies v1.2.1[69]. A threshold of >95% identity was used to classify genomes as the same species.

IS element finding

This study focuses on newly sequenced genomes of previously uncharacterized *Francisella* species and subspecies. Potential IS elements were identified using the BLASTN program (no low-complexity filtering), by querying genome sequences using the ISFinder tool[70] in the IS database and querying flanking regions of the draft genome contigs against the NCBI 'nt' database. Altogether, 41 IS elements were found to be present (*e*-value $< 10^{-2}$) in the included genomes. Pairwise BLAST alignments of both left and right flanking regions, and full length IS sequence elements, were constructed for all genomes. The results were evaluated by *e*-value ($<10^{-3}$), identity (90%), bit score (>40) alignment length and proximity to contig ends. Inherently, *de novo* assembly of next-generation sequence data implies problems in resolving repeat structures, resulting in an increased risk of underestimating the IS element copy number.

Protein orthologs

Forty-five genomes of *Francisella* and two genetic relatives were downloaded from IMG/ER (Table 1). Coding sequences were extracted from GenBank files and orthologs were determined using OrthoMCL with a BLAST *e*-value cut-off of 10^{-5} and an inflation parameter of 1.5. We used the OrthoMCL output to construct a table describing genome gene content that were used for all pan- and core gene analysis.

Heat maps showing the presence of genes in the *Francisella* genus were generated using custom code in the statistical software R.

Analysis of recombination

To infer recombination events in the *Francisella* dataset, three recombination detection methods were used: pairwise homoplasy index (Phi)[71], neighbour similarity score (NSS) [72] and maximum chi-square (MaxChi)[73]. These methods are conveniently implemented in the PHI Package[71]. A subset of 742 genes (i.e. the core genome excluding multiple copies of genes) was tested for recombination detection on the entire data as well as on individual lineages in the phylogeny (subspecies populations). It should be mentioned that all recombination methods used here do not correct for multiple testing, which may result in an over-estimation of the presence of recombination, in particular for the full data analysis (comprising 45 isolates in total).

DISCLAIMER

The s and conclusions contained in this document are those of the authors and should not be interpreted as necessarily representing the official policies, either expressed or implied, of the U.S. Department of Homeland Security or the Swedish Civil Contingencies Agency.

DECLARATIONS

Acknowledgments

Research for this publication was funded by the U.S. Department of Homeland Security and the Swedish Civil Contingencies Agency pursuant to the Agreement between the Government of the United States of America and the Government of the Kingdom of Sweden on Cooperation in Science and Technology for Homeland Security Matters.

Authors' contributions

AS assembled all genomes and performed analysis of genome and gene content. JA performed the 16S rRNA alignment, analysis of over-represented COGs and recombination. CO performed the analysis of average nucleotide identity, IS elements and clade specific genes. SD and DJC provided *Francisella* isolates that infect fish and knowledge of fish pathogenic *Francisella*, and contributed to completion of the manuscript. PLA and MF conceived the study. AS, KS, JA, PLI, AJ, PLA, MF drafted the manuscript. All authors read and approved the manuscript.

REFERENCES

1. Darling RG, Catlett CL, Huebner KD, Jarrett DG: Threats in bioterrorism. I: CDC category A agents. Emerg Med Clin North Am. 2002, 20: 273-309. 10.1016/S0733-8627(02)00005-6.
2. Johansson A, Celli J, Conlan W, Elkins KL, Forsman M, Keim PS, Larsson P, Manoil C, Nano FE, Petersen JM, Sjöstedt A: Objections to the transfer of Francisella novicida to the subspecies rank of Francisella tularensis. Int J Syst Evol Microbiol. 2010, 60: 1717-1718. 10.1099/ijs.0.022830-0. author reply 1718–20
3. Busse H-J, Huber B, Anda P, Escudero R, Scholz HC, Seibold E, Splettstoesser WD, Kämpfer P: Objections to the transfer of Francisella novicida to the subspecies rank of Francisella tularensis - response to Johansson et al. Int J Syst Evol Microbiol. 2010, 60: 1718-1720.
4. Keim P, Johansson A, Wagner DM: Molecular epidemiology, evolution, and ecology of Francisella. Ann N Y Acad Sci. 2007, 1105: 30-66. 10.1196/annals.1409.011.
5. Dienst FT: Tularemia: a perusal of three hundred thirty-nine cases. The Journal of the Louisiana State Medical Society: official organ of the Louisiana State Medical Society. 1963, 115: 114-127.
6. Sandström G, Sjöstedt A, Forsman M, Pavlovich NV, Mishankin BN: Characterization and classification of strains of Francisella tularensis isolated in the Asian focus of the Soviet Union and in Japan. J Clin Microbiol. 1992, 30: 172-175.
7. Olsufiev NG, Meshcheriakova IS: Subspecific Taxonomy

of Francisella tularensis McCoy and Chapin 1912. Int J Syst Bacteriol. 1983, 33: 872-874. 10.1099/00207713-33-4-872.

8. Hollis DG, Weaver RE, Steigerwalt AG, Wenger JD, Moss CW, Brenner DJ: Francisella philomiragia comb. nov. (formerly Yersinia philomiragia) and Francisella tularensis biogroup novicida (formerly Francisella novicida) associated with human disease. J Clin Microbiol. 1989, 27: 1601-1608.

9. Wenger JD, Hollis DG, Weaver RE, Baker CN, Brown GR, Brenner DJ, Broome CV: Infection caused by Francisella philomiragia (formerly Yersinia philomiragia). A newly recognized human pathogen. Ann Intern Med. 1989, 110: 888-892.

10. Mailman TL, Schmidt MH: Francisella philomiragia adenitis and pulmonary nodules in a child with chronic granulomatous disease. The Canadian journal of infectious diseases & medical microbiology. Journal canadien des maladies infectieuses et de la microbiologie médicale / AMMI Canada. 2005, 16: 245-248.

11. Brevik ØJ, Ottem KF, Nylund A: Multiple-locus, variable number of tandem repeat analysis (MLVA) of the fish-pathogen Francisella noatunensis. BMC Vet Res. 2011, 7: 5-10.1186/1746-6148-7-5.

12. Ottem KF, Nylund A, Karlsbakk E, Friis-Møller A, Kamaishi T: Elevation of Francisella philomiragia subsp. noatunensis Mikalsen et al. (2007) to Francisella noatunensis comb. nov. [syn. Francisella piscicida Ottem et al. (2008) syn. nov.] and characterization of Francisella noatunensis subsp. orientalis subsp. nov. J Appl Microbiol. 2009, 106: 1231-1243. 10.1111/j.1365-2672.2008.04092.x.

13. Colquhoun DJ, Duodu S: Francisella infections in farmed and wild aquatic organisms. Vet Res. 2011, 42: 47-10.1186/1297-9716-42-47.

14. Birkbeck T, Feist S, Verner-Jeffreys D: Francisella infections in fish and shellfish. J Fish Dis. 2011, 34: 173-187. 10.1111/j.1365-2761.2010.01226.x.

15. Olsen AB, Mikalsen J, Rode M, Alfjorden A, Hoel E, Straum-Lie K, Haldorsen R, Colquhoun DJ: A novel systemic granulomatous inflammatory disease in farmed Atlantic cod, Gadus morhua L., associated with a bacterium belonging to the genus Francisella. J Fish Dis. 2006, 29: 307-311. 10.1111/j.1365-2761.2006.00714.x.

16. Ottem KF, Nylund A, Karlsbakk E, Friis-Møller A, Krossøy B: Characterization of Francisella sp., GM2212, the first Francisella isolate from marine fish, Atlantic cod (Gadus morhua). Arch Microbiol. 2007, 187: 343-350. 10.1007/s00203-006-0198-1.

17. Kamaishi T, Fukuda Y, Nishiyama M, Kawakami H, Matsuyama T, Yoshinaga T, Oseko N: Identification and pathogenicity of intracellular Francisella bacterium in three-line grunt Parapristipoma trilineatum. Fish Pathology. 2005, 40: 67-72. 10.3147/jsfp.40.67.

18. Birkbeck TH, Bordevik M, Frøystad MK, Baklien A: Identification of Francisella sp. from Atlantic salmon, Salmo salar L., in Chile. J Fish Dis. 2007, 30: 505-507. 10.1111/j.1365-2761.2007.00837.x.

19. Barns SM, Grow CC, Okinaka RT, Keim P, Kuske CR: Detection of diverse new Francisella-like bacteria in environmental samples. Appl Environ Microbiol. 2005, 71: 5494-5500. 10.1128/AEM.71.9.5494-5500.2005.

20. Dillon J, McMath L, Trout A: Seasonal changes in bacterial diversity in the Salton Sea. Hydrobiologia. 2009, 632: 49-64. 10.1007/s10750-009-9827-4.

21. Kugeler KJ, Mead PS, McGowan KL, Burnham JM, Hogarty MD, Ruchelli E, Pollard K, Husband B, Conley C, Rivera T, Kelesidis T, Lee WM, Mabey W, Winchell JM, Stang HL, Staples JE, Chalcraft LJ, Petersen JM: Isolation and characterization of a novel Francisella sp. from human cerebrospinal fluid and blood. J Clin Microbiol. 2008, 46: 2428-2431. 10.1128/JCM.00698-08.

22. Petersen JM, Carlson J, Yockey B, Pillai S, Kuske C, Garbalena G, Pottumarthy S, Chalcraft L: Direct isolation of Francisella spp. from environmental samples. Lett Appl Microbiol. 2009, 48: 663-667.

23. Schrallhammer M, Schweikert M, Vallesi A, Verni F, Petroni G: Detection of a novel subspecies of Francisella noatunensis as endosymbiont of the ciliate Euplotes raikovi. Microb Ecol. 2011, 61: 455-464. 10.1007/s00248-010-9772-9.

24. Scoles GA: Phylogenetic analysis of the Francisella-like endosymbionts of Dermacentor ticks. J Med Entomol. 2004, 41: 277-286. 10.1603/0022-2585-41.3.277.

25. Weiss E, Myers WF, Suitor EC, Neptune EM: Respiration of a Rickettsialike Microorganism, Wolbachia Persica. J Infect Dis. 1962, 110: 155-164. 10.1093/infdis/110.2.155.

26. Noda H, Munderloh UG, Kurtti TJ: Endosymbionts of ticks and their relationship to Wolbachia spp. and tick-borne pathogens of humans and animals. Appl Environ Microbiol. 1997, 63: 3926-3932.

27. Qu P, Deng X, Zhang J, Chen J, Zhang J, Zhang Q, Xiao Y, Chen S: Identification and characterization of the Francisella sp. strain 08HL01032 isolated in air condition systems. Wei sheng wu xue bao = Acta microbiologica sinica. 2009, 49: 1003-1110.

28. Kugeler KJ, Gurfield N, Creek JG, Mahoney KS, Versage JL, Petersen JM: Discrimination between Francisella tularensis and Francisella-like endosymbionts when screening ticks by PCR. Appl Environ Microbiol. 2005, 71: 7594-7597. 10.1128/AEM.71.11.7594-7597.2005.

29. Lau KWK, Ren J, Fung M-C, Woo PCY, Yuen K-Y, Chan KKM, Qian P-Y, Wong P-K, Wu M: Fangia hongkongensis gen. nov., sp. nov., a novel gammaproteobacterium of the order Thiotrichales isolated from coastal seawater of Hong Kong. Int J Syst Evol Microbiol. 2007, 57: 2665-2669. 10.1099/ijs.0.65156-0.

30. Fryer JL, Lannan CN, Giovannoni SJ, Wood ND: Piscirickettsia salmonis gen. nov., sp. nov., the causative agent of an epizootic disease in salmonid fishes. Int J Syst Bacteriol. 1992, 42: 120-126. 10.1099/00207713-42-1-120.

31. Suitor EC, Weiss E: Isolation of a Rickettsialike Microorganism (Wolbachia persica, n. sp.) from Argas persicus (Oken). J Infect Dis. 1961, 108: 95-106. 10.1093/infdis/108.1.95.

32. Fryer JL, Lannan CN LHG, Larenas JJ, Smith PA: Isolation of a rickettsiales-like organism from diseased coho salmon Oncorhynchus kisutch in Chile. Fish pathology. 1990, 25: 107-114. 10.3147/jsfp.25.107.

33. Whipp MJ, Davis JM, Lum G, de Boer J, Zhou Y, Bearden SW, Petersen JM, Chu MC, Hogg G: Characterization of a novicida-like subspecies of Francisella tularensis isolated in Australia. J Med Microbiol. 2003, 52: 839-842. 10.1099/jmm.0.05245-0.

34. Siddaramappa S, Challacombe JF, Petersen JM, Pillai S, Hogg G, Kuske CR: Common ancestry and novel genetic traits of Francisella novicida-like isolates from North America and Australia as revealed by comparative genomic analyses. Appl Environ Microbiol. 2011, 77: 5110-5122. 10.1128/AEM.00337-11.

35. Darling AE, Mau B, Perna NT: progressiveMauve: multiple genome alignment with gene gain, loss and rearrangement. PLoS One. 2010, 5: e11147-10.1371/journal.pone.0011147.

36. Larsson P, Elfsmark D, Svensson K, Wikström P, Forsman M, Brettin T, Keim P, Johansson A: Molecular evolutionary consequences of niche restriction in Francisella tularensis, a facultative intracellular pathogen. PLoS Pathog. 2009, 5: e1000472-10.1371/journal.ppat.1000472.

37. Marshall SH, Henríquez V, Gómez FA, Cárdenas C: ISPsa2, the first mobile genetic element to be described and characterized in the bacterial facultative intracellular pathogen Piscirickettsia salmonis. FEMS Microbiol Lett. 2011, 314: 18-24. 10.1111/j.1574-6968.2010.02132.x.

38. Champion MD, Zeng Q, Nix EB, Nano FE, Keim P, Kodira CD, Borowsky M, Young S, Koehrsen M, Engels R, Pearson M, Howarth C, Larson L, White J, Alvarado L, Forsman M, Bearden SW, Sjöstedt A, Titball R, Michell SL, Birren B, Galagan J: Comparative genomic characterization of Francisella tularensis strains belonging to low and high virulence subspecies. PLoS Pathog. 2009, 5: e1000459-10.1371/journal.ppat.1000459.

39. Nübel U, Reissbrodt R, Weller A, Grunow R, Porsch-Ozcürümez M, Tomaso H, Hofer E, Splettstoesser W, Finke E-J, Tschäpe H, Witte W: Population structure of Francisella tularensis. J Bacteriol. 2006, 188: 5319-5324. 10.1128/JB.01662-05.

40. Forsman M, Sandström G, Sjöstedt A: Analysis of 16S ribosomal DNA sequences of Francisella strains and utilization for determination of the phylogeny of the genus and for identification of strains by PCR. Int J Syst Bacteriol. 1994, 44: 38-46. 10.1099/00207713-44-1-38.

41. Escudero R, Toledo A, Gil H, Kovácsová K, Rodríguez-Vargas M, Jado I, García-Amil C, Lobo B, Bhide M, Anda P: Molecular method for discrimination between Francisella tularensis and Francisella-like endosymbionts. J Clin Microbiol. 2008, 46: 3139-3143. 10.1128/JCM.00275-08.

42. Berrada ZL, Telford SR: Diversity of Francisella species in environmental samples from Martha's Vineyard, Massachusetts. Microb Ecol. 2010, 59: 277-283. 10.1007/s00248-009-9568-y.

43. Huber B, Escudero R, Busse H-J, Seibold E, Scholz HC, Anda P, Kämpfer P, Splettstoesser WD: Description of Francisella hispaniensis sp. nov., isolated from human blood, reclassification of Francisella novicida (Larson et al. 1955) Olsufiev et al. 1959 as Francisella tularensis subsp. novicida comb. nov. and emended description of the genus Franc. Int J Syst Evol Microbiol. 2010, 60: 1887-1896. 10.1099/ijs.0.015941-0.

44. Alcaraz LDD, Moreno-Hagelsieb G, Eguiarte LE, Souza V, Herrera-Estrella L, Olmedo G: Understanding the evolutionary relationships and major traits of Bacillus through comparative genomics. BMC Genomics. 2010, 11: 332-10.1186/1471-2164-11-332.

45. Rohmer L, Fong C, Abmayr S, Wasnick M, Larson Freeman TJ, Radey M, Guina T, Svensson K, Hayden HS, Jacobs M, Gallagher LA, Manoil C, Ernst RK, Drees B, Buckley D, Haugen E, Bovee D, Zhou Y, Chang J, Levy R, Lim R, Gillett W, Guenthener D, Kang A, Shaffer SA, Taylor G, Chen J, Gallis B, D'Argenio DA, Forsman M, Olson MV, Goodlett DR, Kaul R, Miller SI, Brittnacher MJ: Comparison of Francisella tularensis genomes reveals evolutionary events associated with the emergence of human pathogenic strains. Genome Biol. 2007, 8: R102-10.1186/gb-2007-8-6-r102.

46. Georgiades K, Raoult D: Genomes of the most dangerous epidemic bacteria have a virulence repertoire characterized by fewer genes but more toxin-antitoxin modules. PLoS One. 2011, 6: e17962-10.1371/journal.pone.0017962.

47. Hood AM: Virulence factors of Francisella tularensis. J Hyg. 1977, 79: 47-60. 10.1017/S0022172400052840.

48. McLendon MK, Apicella MA, Allen L-AA: Francisella tularensis: taxonomy, genetics, and Immunopathogenesis of a potential agent of biowarfare. Annu Rev Microbiol. 2006, 60: 167-185. 10.1146/annurev.micro.60.080805.142126.

49. Prior JL, Prior RG, Hitchen PG, Diaper H, Griffin KF, Morris HR, Dell A, Titball RW: Characterization of the O antigen gene cluster and structural analysis of the O antigen of Francisella tularensis subsp. tularensis. J Med Microbiol. 2003, 52: 845-851. 10.1099/jmm.0.05184-0.

50. Didelot X, Maiden MCJ: Impact of recombination on bacterial evolution. Trends Microbiol. 2010, 18: 315-322. 10.1016/j.tim.2010.04.002.

51. Lefébure T, Bitar PDP, Suzuki H, Stanhope MJ: Evolutionary dynamics of complete Campylobacter pan-genomes and the bacterial species concept. Genome Biol Evol. 2010, 2: 646-655. 10.1093/gbe/evq048.

52. Joseph B, Schwarz RF, Linke B, Blom J, Becker A, Claus H, Goesmann A, Frosch M, Müller T, Vogel U, Schoen C: Virulence evolution of the human pathogen Neisseria meningitidis by recombination in the core and accessory genome. PLoS One. 2011, 6: e18441-10.1371/journal.pone.0018441.

53. Achtman M, Morelli G, Zhu P, Wirth T, Diehl I, Kusecek B, Vogler AJ, Wagner DM, Allender CJ, Easterday WR, Chenal-Francisque V, Worsham P, Thomson NR, Parkhill J, Lindler LE, Carniel E, Keim P: Microevolution and history of the plague bacillus, Yersinia pestis. Proc Natl

Acad Sci USA. 2004, 101: 17837-17842. 10.1073/pnas.0408026101.

54. Van Ert MN, Easterday WR, Huynh LY, Okinaka RT, Hugh-Jones ME, Ravel J, Zanecki SR, Pearson T, Simonson TS, U'Ren JM, Kachur SM, Leadem-Dougherty RR, Rhoton SD, Zinser G, Farlow J, Coker PR, Smith KL, Wang B, Kenefic LJ, Fraser-Liggett CM, Wagner DM, Keim P: Global genetic population structure of Bacillus anthracis. PLoS One. 2007, 2: e461-10.1371/journal.pone.0000461.

55. Liu X, Gutacker MM, Musser JM, Fu Y-X: Evidence for recombination in Mycobacterium tuberculosis. J Bacteriol. 2006, 188: 8169-8177. 10.1128/JB.01062-06.

56. Smith JM, Smith NH, O'Rourke M, Spratt BG: How clonal are bacteria?. Proc Natl Acad Sci USA. 1993, 90: 4384-4388. 10.1073/pnas.90.10.4384.

57. Ahmed N: A flood of microbial genomes-do we need more?. PLoS One. 2009, 4: e5831-10.1371/journal.pone.0005831.

58. Enserink M: Anthrax investigation. Full-genome sequencing paved the way from spores to a suspect. Science. 2008, 321: 898-899. 10.1126/science.321.5891.898. New York, N.Y

59. Sandström G, Tärnvik A, Wolf-Watz H, Löfgren S: Antigen from Francisella tularensis: nonidentity between determinants participating in cell-mediated and humoral reactions. Infect Immun. 1984, 45: 101-106.

60. Zerbino DR, Birney E: Velvet: algorithms for de novo short read assembly using de Bruijn graphs. Genome Res. 2008, 18: 821-829. 10.1101/gr.074492.107.

61. Zerbino DR, McEwen GK, Margulies EH, Birney E: Pebble and rock band: heuristic resolution of repeats and scaffolding in the velvet short-read de novo assembler. PLoS One. 2009, 4: e8407-10.1371/journal.pone.0008407.

62. Markowitz VM, Mavromatis K, Ivanova NN, Chen I-MA, Chu K, Kyrpides NC: IMG ER: A system for microbial genome annotation expert re and curation. Bioinformatics Oxford England. 2009, 25: 2271-2278. 10.1093/bioinformatics/btp393.

63. Cole JR, Wang Q, Cardenas E, Fish J, Chai B, Farris RJ, Kulam-Syed-Mohideen AS, McGarrell DM, Marsh T, Garrity GM, Tiedje JM: The Ribosomal Database Project: improved alignments and new tools for rRNA analysis. Nucleic Acids Res. 2009, 37: D141-D145. 10.1093/nar/gkn879.

64. Cole JR, Chai B, Farris RJ, Wang Q, Kulam-Syed-Mohideen AS, McGarrell DM, Bandela AM, Cardenas E, Garrity GM, Tiedje JM: The ribosomal database project (RDP-II): introducing myRDP space and quality controlled public data. Nucleic Acids Res. 2007, 35: D169-D172. 10.1093/nar/gkl889.

65. Stamatakis A: RAxML-VI-HPC: maximum likelihood-based phylogenetic analyses with thousands of taxa and mixed models. Bioinformatics (Oxford, England). 2006, 22: 2688-2690. 10.1093/bioinformatics/btl446.

66. Sjödin A, Svensson K, Ohrman C, Ahlinder J, Lindgren P, Duodu S, Hnath J, Burans JP, Johansson A, Colquhoun DJ, Larsson P, Forsman M: Genome characterisation of the genus Francisella. TreeBASE,http://purl.org/phylo/treebase/phylows/study/TB2:S12723,

67. Anwar N, Hunt E: Improved data retrieval from TreeBASE via taxonomic and linguistic data enrichment. BMC Evol Biol. 2009, 9: 93-10.1186/1471-2148-9-93.

68. Tamura K, Peterson D, Peterson N, Stecher G, Nei M, Kumar S: MEGA5: Molecular Evolutionary Genetics Analysis using Maximum Likelihood, Evolutionary Distance, and Maximum Parsimony Methods. Mol Biol Evol. 2011, 11: 2731-2739.

69. Richter M, Rosselló-Móra R: Shifting the genomic gold standard for the prokaryotic species definition. Proc Natl Acad Sci USA. 2009, 106: 19126-19131. 10.1073/pnas.0906412106.

70. Siguier P, Perochon J, Lestrade L, Mahillon J, Chandler M: ISfinder: the reference centre for bacterial insertion sequences. Nucleic Acids Res. 2006, 34: D32-D36. 10.1093/nar/gkj014.

71. Bruen TC, Philippe H, Bryant D: A simple and robust statistical test for detecting the presence of recombination. Genetics. 2006, 172: 2665-2681.

72. Jakobsen IB, Easteal S: A program for calculating and displaying compatibility matrices as an aid in determining reticulate evolution in molecular sequences. Computer applications in the biosciences: CABIOS. 1996, 12: 291-295.

73. Smith J: Analyzing the mosaic structure of genes. J Mol Evol. 1992, 34: 126-129.

SECTION VIII: MYCOBACTERIUM SPP.– AGENT OF TUBERCULOSIS

CHAPTER 29

DETECTION OF MYCOBACTERIUM AVIUM SUBSPECIES IN THE GUT ASSOCIATED LYMPHOID TISSUE OF SLAUGHTERED RABBITS

Rakel Arrazuria, Iker A Sevilla, Elena Molina, Valentín Pérez, Joseba M Garrido, Ramón A Juste and Natalia Elguezabal

Keywords: Animal pathogens, Epidemiology, *Mycobacterium avium,* subsp, *Mycobacterium avium,* complex, *Thermoactinomyces,* sp, Rabbits, Slaughter

BACKGROUND

Rabbits have been found to be naturally susceptible to *Mycobacterium avium* subsp. *paratuberculosis* (Map) infection in the wild [1, 2, 3, 4], to *Mycobacterium avium* subspecies infection in natural conditions, specifically *Mycobacterium avium* subsp. *avium* (Maa) in pigmy rabbits [5] and moderately susceptible to Map in laboratory conditions [6, 7].

Map and Maa are subspecies of *Mycobacterium avium*, as well as *Mycobacterium avium* subsp. *silvaticum*(Mas) and *Mycobacterium avium* subsp. *hominissuis* (Mah) [8]. From an epidemiologic point of , Maa is typically virulent for birds and small terrestrial mammals causing a range of lesions that go from characteristic tuberculous lesions in parenchymatous organs, to lymphadenitis and disseminated infection [9, 10, 11]. Mah has the human [12] and the pig [13] as its primary hosts and it is frequently found in soil [14]. Map is the causal agent of paratuberculosis in ruminants and it has been controversially associated with human inflammatory bowel disease, more precisely with Crohn's disease [15, 16, 17] and also diabetes mellitus [18]. Its prevalence in slaughtered cattle in Europe has been estimated to be up to 50 % [19]. Mas has been isolated from wood pigeons [20], roe deer [21] and horses causing tuberculous-like lesions in these animals [22]. However, since there is a controversy about the real existence of Mas as a unique subspecies independent of Maa [23], for the present work we will consider Mas as part of Maa, and jointly refer to them as Maa/Mas.

Mycobacterium avium subspecies members are widely spread in the environment and often enter in contact with animals and humans. Transmission from animals to humans can occur either through the consumption of contaminated foods or *via* direct contact with an infected animal. Apparently healthy animals thereby may represent a reservoir for *Mycobacterium avium* subspecies and these pathogens may enter the food chain during slaughter. Most work focused on the detection of *M. avium* subspecies in animal species for human consumption has been performed on meat products. Map has been detected in beef, pork and chicken [24], whereas Mah has been detected in beef, pork and lamb [24]. Detection of non-tuberculous mycobacteria or *Mycobacterium avium* subspecies at slaughter has been described in lymph nodes of pigs [25, 26, 27] and detection of Map has been reported in lymph nodes, muscle and faeces of both dairy and beef cattle [28].

Citation: Rakel Arrazuria, Iker A Sevilla, Elena Molina, Valentín Pérez, Joseba M Garrido, Ramón A Juste and Natalia Elguezabal, Detection of Mycobacterium avium subspecies in the gut associated lymphoid tissue of slaughtered rabbits, DOI: 10.1186/s12917-015-0445-2.

Mycobacterium avium subspecies presence in rabbits in wild conditions led us to hypothesize that these mycobacteria could also be present in commercial rabbits that go to slaughter and thus represent a route of exposure for humans. The aim of the present study was to carry out a small survey on the frequency of mycobacterial microorganisms detected by solid and liquid culture and by a tetraplex real-time PCR for *Mycobacterium* genus, *M. avium* subspecies and *M. tuberculosis* complex in gut associated lymphoid tissue (GALT) and caecal contents of apparently healthy rabbits at slaughter.

METHODS

Ethics statement

Animals used in this study did not undergo any manipulation prior to stunning for standard industrial slaughter according to the pertinent legislation. For this reason, no specific ethical approval was required.

Animals and sampling

We contacted the official veterinarian of the nearest rabbit slaughterhouse to set-up a sampling schedule. This study was based on samplings that took place from May to October of 2013 (decontamination procedure set-up and PCR evaluation) and during January and February of 2014 (proper study) in a rabbit slaughterhouse (Basque Country, Spain) processing 1300000–1400000 rabbits annually. Rabbits are typically slaughtered with an average age of two months and average live weight around 1.8-2.2 kg (http://www.magrama.gob.es/es/ganaderia/temas/produccion-y-mercadosganaderos/INDICADORES_ECONÓMICOS_SECTOR_CUNÍCOLA_2013_tcm7-330314.pdf). Breeding rabbits are slaughtered at about 2–2.5 years of age. Production rabbits are often outbred in order to maximize meat production [29]. This slaughterhouse was operated by an agriculture cooperative company and complied with the pertinent Basque (Basque Government Decree 454/1994), Spanish (Spanish Government Law 32/2007 and Royal decree 731/2007) and European (Council Regulation (EC) No 1099/2009) legislation on animal welfare under the supervision of official veterinarians and the samples obtained were authorized by the slaughterhouse managers.

A total of 12 animals (decontamination procedure set-up and PCR evaluation) and 66 animals (proper rabbit slaughterhouse study) from 21 farms scattered in 6 provinces of North-East Spain were sampled. Samples were drawn from two young animals from each batch of sacrifice and from a third additional breeding animal, if the batch included breeding rabbits. Samples were kept in refrigeration for 6-12h before being processed.

Decontamination procedure

In order to determine the optimum NaOH concentration for decontamination initial set-up experiments were performed. Mucosa from sacculus rotundus and vermiform appendix from 12 rabbits were used to test decontamination with 2 %, 4 %, 6 % and 8 % NaOH. Decontamination procedures were run for 10 and 15 min. Contamination was observed in both solid and MGIT culture at NaOH concentrations lower than 6 % for both 10 and 15 min. 6 % NaOH for 15 min was the lowest concentration that resulted in no contaminated samples. For this reason, the final decontamination procedure was performed with these conditions. Also manufacturer's instructions do not recommend running decontamination for more than 15 min or NaOH concentrations higher than 6 % (BACTEC™ MGIT ™960).

10 ml of sterile water were added to 2 g of sample tissue. Homogenization was then performed on a Stomacher blender for 1 min at medium speed. Afterwards, the homogenized solution was transferred to a tube and 10 ml of 6% NaOH were added. After a vortex mix, the suspension was incubated for 15 min at room temperature before neutralization with 15 ml of phosphate buffer. The suspension was mixed well and centrifuged for 20 min at 2,885 × g and the supernatant was discarded. Pellets were suspended in 2 ml of sterile water.

Culture

Solid culture

Four drops (150 μl)/per tube of the decontaminated suspension were seeded on solid media: Herrold's Egg Yolk Medium (HEYM); Middlebrook 7H10 with penicillin, amphotericin B, and chloramphenicol; Lowenstein-Jensen with penicillin, amphotericin B and supplemented with mycobactin J and Tsukamura minimal media with cycloheximide [30]. All seeded tubes were incubated at 37+/−1 °C and checked for growth at 8, 12, 16 and 20 weeks. After seeding on solid culture, the remaining inoculum was used for liquid culture.

Liquid culture

Pellets destined to liquid culture were seeded on BBL Mycobacteria Growth Indicator Tubes (MGIT) supplemented with BACTEC MGIT growth supplement and BBL MGIT PANTA (Becton, Dickinson and Company). Tubes were incubated for 45 days in a BACTEC MGIT 960 System and time to detection (TTD) values were recorded.

PCR evaluation

PCR performance on spiked mucosa was evaluated since this specimen is known to be tricky because of the presence of PCR inhibitors.

Inocula preparation for tissue spiking

Mah Strain 104 was grown in Middlebrook 7H9 (M7H9) broth supplemented (v/v) with 10 % Middlebrook OADC enrichment (Becton, Dickinson and Company, MD, USA), 0.2 % glycerol and 0.05 % Tween 80 (Sigma-Aldrich, Co. Ltd., Haverhill, UK). Mycobacteria were harvested by centrifugation at 2,800 × g. Pellets were washed twice in phosphate buffered saline (PBS). Mycobacteria were resuspended in PBS containing 0.2 % glycerol and 0.05 % Tween 80 (PBS-GT). Bacterial suspensions were adjusted to 1 McFarland unit after turbidity measurements were performed with a Densicheck densitometer (Bio-Mérieux, Marcy L'Etoile, France). Five ten-fold dilutions of the bacterial suspensions were prepared in PBS-GT and the highest, medium and lowest, with a 2 log difference between each of them were used to inoculate negative tissues. To verify the viable number of CFU, the inocula were plated onto appropriately supplemented agar-solidified M7H9 flasks.

Mucosa spiking

Mucosa was scraped from vermiform appendix tissue from 12 apparently healthy rabbits previously confirmed to be negative for the presence of mycobacteria by PCR, culture and histopathology and it was thoroughly mixed and homogenized. The blended tissues were divided in batches of 1 g of mixture per stomacher bag. The stomacher bags were inoculated with 100 μl of one of each of the previously adjusted bacterial suspensions (high, medium and low). 300 mg of the homogenate spiked tissues were extracted as described in the DNA extraction section and MycMavMtc PCR [31]. In cases where PCR inhibition took place ½ and ¼ dilutions of the extracted DNA were performed previous to PCR reaction and this showed to be enough to prevent inhibition.

Slaughterhouse sample study

A total of 66 animals (48 young and 18 breeding animals) were sampled and different steps that are summarized on Fig. 1 were taken to investigate the specimens.

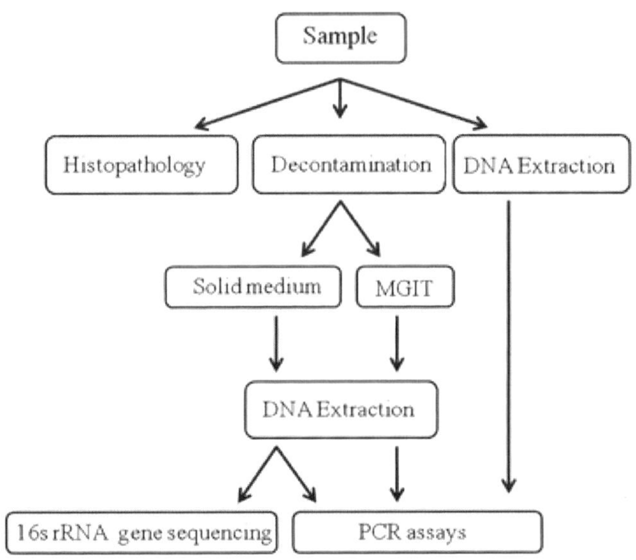

Figure 1: Experimental scheme showing methods followed at each stage.

Briefly, sacculus rotundus and vermiform appendix were scraped for mucosa and caecal contents were collected. Part of each sample was used for direct molecular detection and part for decontamination and subsequent culture. Based on set-up results, the final decontamination procedure was performed with 6 % NaOH as described in the decontamination procedure section because it was the lowest concentration found to inhibit contamination. Both solid and liquid cultures were performed followed by PCR confirmation and sequencing of the 16Sr RNA gene when non-mycobacterial colonies were isolated.

Histopathological analysis was performed on samples of sacculus rotundus and vermiform appendix of a total of 22 rabbits (14 young rabbits and 8 breeding rabbits) including animals with and without macroscopic lesions.

DNA extraction

Spiked tissues and fresh rabbit slaughterhouse samples

DNA extraction was performed on spiked mucosa (PCR evaluation), sacculus rotundus, vermiform appendix and caecal content (slaughterhouse study), using DNA Extract-VK (Vacunek S.L, Bizkaia, Spain) following manufacturer's instructions with modifications. Briefly, 300 mg of tissue or caecal content were weighed in a microtube. 250 μl of sterile distilled water, plus 250 μl of VK-Lysis buffer and 300 mg of VK-extraction beads were added to the tissue and homogenized at 30Hz during 10 min on TissueLyser II (Qiagen). Following homogenization, samples were centrifuged at 7,000 × g for 5 min and 200 μl of the supernatant transferred to a new vial. 25 μl of Proteinase K were added to the previous solution and tubes were incubated at 56 °C for 15 min. Lysis was performed adding 200 μl of Lysis Buffer VL-LB3 to the previous solution and mixing thoroughly. The solution was incubated at 70 °C for 10 min. Then, 210 μl of ethanol (96-100 %) were added and mixed thoroughly. The final mixtures were loaded on VK-DNA binding columns and centrifuged at 11,000 × g for 1 min. Pass-through liquid was discarded. Washing steps were performed with 500 μl of Wash Buffer VK-WB1 and 600 μl of Wash Buffer VK-WB2 with a 11,000 × g 1 min centrifuging step in between. After washes were done, 100 μl of Elution Buffer were added to the column and the column left for 1 min. DNA was recovered by centrifuging at 11,000 × g for 1 min. Extracted DNA was stored at −20 °C until PCRs were performed. Negative DNA extraction controls (for every 23 samples), no template and positive PCR controls (for every PCR) were included in all downstream PCR assays.

Solid medium isolated colonies

A loopful of cells from each colony growing on solid medium was placed in 100 μl of sterile water. Vials were incubated at 95 °C for 10 min and centrifuged at 13,800 × g for 5 min. The supernatant was used as template for further PCR assays.

Positive MGIT liquid medium

One millilitre of vortexed liquid culture from the MGIT tubes was collected and centrifuged at 13,800 × g for 5 min, the supernatant was discarded and after a washing with 1 ml of sterile distilled water, the pellet was suspended in 250 μl of sterile water. Then 300 mg of zirconium beads were added and homogenized at 30Hz for 10 min on TissueLyser II (Qiagen). Following homogenization, samples were centrifuged at 7500 × g for 15 min and the supernatant was collected.

Molecular detection

Detection of mycobacteria by Tetraplex real-time PCR (MycMavMtc)

For initial screening purposes to test the presence of *Mycobacterium* sp., a fourplex real-time PCR described by Sevilla *et al.* [31] was performed. This PCR is able to detect the genus *Mycobacterium* and then distinguish between the *M. tuberculosis* complex and *M. avium* subspecies. The target genes were the internal transcribed spacer (ITS) between 16S and 23SrRNA genes, insertion sequence IS1311 and the devR genr for *Mycobacterium* genus, *M. avium* subspecies and *M. tuberculosis* complex members respectively.

Reactions were carried out in a final volume of 25 μl containing 5 μl of template DNA, and 1X TaqMan Universal PCR MasterMix without AmpErase uracil-DNA glycosylase (Applied Biosystems), 0.3 μM of each primer, 0.2 μM of each probe. An internal amplification control (IAC) was included in the reaction to rule out false negative results due to inhibitors. ROX (6-carboxyl-X-rhodamine) dye was used as passive reference reporter. Amplification was carried out in a 7500 Real-Time PCR instrument (Applied Biosystems) and consisted of one denaturation and polymerase activation cycle of 10 min at 95°C, and 45 cycles of denaturation at 95 °C for 15 s and annealing/extension at 60°C for 1 min. Results were analyzed using the 7500 System SDS software v. 1.4 (Applied Biosystems). Threshold cycle (C_T) and baseline were automatically determined by the software and verified by visual examination of the threshold line in amplification plots.

M. avium subsp. *paratuberculosis* detection by IS*900* & IS*Map02* real-time PCR

To identify Map positive samples, a real time multiplex PCR described by Sevilla *et al.* [32] was performed. This PCR detects IS*900* and IS*Map02* DNA sequences of *M. avium* subsp. *paratuberculosis*.

Briefly, the reaction mixture contained 1× TaqMan Universal PCR Master Mix (Applied Biosystems), 300–400 nM of each primer, 200 nM of each probe, and 5μl of DNA extract in a final volume of 25 μl. An IAC is also included in the PCR reaction.

Amplification and real time measurement were performed in the same system and conditions as described in the previous PCR protocol.

M. avium subsp. *hominisuis* and *M. avium* subsp. *avium/M. avium* subsp. *silvaticum* detection by IS*1245* & IS*901* PCR

In order to identify other *M. avium* subspecies, a previously published real time PCR was carried out, based on the detection of IS*901* and IS*1245* insertion sequences [33]. Maa/Mas organisms are positive for IS*1245* and IS*901*, while Mah is only positive for IS*1245*. The PCR did not include DNA concentration standards for quantification purposes because the objective was just to detect and identify Mah and Maa/Mas.

The final reaction mixture contained the same PCR ingredients at the same concentration indicated above for Map PCR but primers and probes were those previously described by Slana *et al.* [33]. Amplification and real time measurement were performed in the same system and conditions as described in the previous PCR setting.

16S rRNA gene sequencing of colonies on solid medium

The identification of colonies grown on solid media that were not mycobacteria as assessed by previously described PCR methods was performed by 16S rRNA gene sequencing. Amplification of target DNA was performed by PCR using bacterial universal primers pAF (5′- AGA GTT TGA TCC TGG CTC AG-3′) and 530R (5′-CCG CGG CKG CTG GCAC-3′). Amplification was carried out in a 2700 GeneAmp PCR Instrument (Applied Biosystems) and consisted of one denaturation and polymerase activation cycle of 4 min at 94 °C, and 30 cycles of denaturation at 94 °C for 30 s, annealing at 50 °C for 30 s and extension at 72 °C for 40 s. The PCR product was cleaned with Illustra Exoprostar 1-Step (GE Healthcare Life Sciences) following manufacturer's instructions.

The sequencing reaction was carried out with BigDye® Terminator v3.1 cycle sequencing kit (Applied Biosystems) and resolved with a 3130 ABI (Applied Biosystems) capillary sequencer. Sequencing conditions consisted of 30 cycles of denaturation at 96 °C for 10 s, annealing at 50 °C for 5 s and extension at 60 °C for 4 min. Sequence alignment was performed using BLAST (Basic Local Alignment Search Tool) and identification with 100 % of coverage and 99-100 % of identity was made.

Gross pathology

The whole digestive system of the rabbits was inspected for gross anatomical change. Samples from sacculus rotundus and vermiform appendix were collected for solid and/or liquid culture and histopathological analysis. Samples from sacculus rotundus, vermiform appendix and caecal contents were collected for detection of mycobacteria by PCR.

Histopathology

Histopathological analysis was performed on samples of sacculus rotundus and vermiform appendix and on other samples that presented macroscopic lesions. The tissues were fixed in 10 % neutral buffered formalin for a minimum of 24 h, trimmed, dehydrated through graded alcohols, embedded in paraffin wax and sectioned at 5μm. These sections were mounted on glass slides stained with haematoxylin and eosin (HE) or by the Ziehl-Neelsen (ZN) method for acid fast bacteria (AFB) according to standard procedures. Slides were examined under the microscope for granuloma formation and AFB presence.

Statistical analysis

Association of mycobacteria detection and age was tested with the Chi square or Fisher exact probability (FET) tests for the frequencies of PCR results according to age using the PROC FREQ of the SAS statistical package (SAS Institute Inc., Cary, NC, USA). For all analyses, a p value of <0.05 was considered to be statistically significant.

RESULTS

PCR evaluation

MycMavMtc PCR results of the spiked rabbit mucosa are shown in Table 1. Inhibition was observed at all bacterial concentrations when samples were not diluted and only probe IS*1311* was detected in the highest concentration. After dilution steps were performed, inhibitory effects were mitigated. In the medium concentration bacterial suspension a ½ dilution was enough to detect *M. avium* sp. DNA by the IS*1311* probe. However, in the low concentration inoculum after ½ and ¼ dilutions the IS*1311* probe was not positive and only the internal amplification control gave significant C_T values.

Table 1: M. avium subsp hominissuis spiked rabbit mucosa C_Ts of MycMavMtc PCR

		Mah spiked rabbit mucosa		
		high	**medium**	**low**
Dilution	**DNA Probe**	**7.66×10^6 (CFU/g)**	**7.66×10^4 (CFU/g)**	**7.66×10^2 (CFU/g)**
1/1	ITSdenak	UD	UD	UD
	IS*1311*	31.77	UD	UD
	IAC	UD	UD	UD
1/2	ITSdenak	43.56	UD	UD
	IS*1311*	28.5	36.66	UD
	IAC	35.1	41.19	36.00
1/4	ITSdenak	39.7	UD	UD
	IS*1311*	28.85	34.50	UD
	IAC	32.62	33.99	33.63

Mah: *M. avium* subps. *hominissuis*, ITSdenak: detects *Mycobacterium* genus, IS*1311*: detects *Mycobacterium avium*, IAC: internal amplification control, UD: undetermined no threshold-crossing fluorescence, devR detecting Mtb complex members was UD for all assayed conditions

Slaughterhouse sample study

Gross pathology and digestive system parameters

Of the 66 necropsied animals, 6 (9 %) showed visible pathological lesions consistent with mycobacterial infection. They were characterized by the presence of focal thickenings of the intestinal wall in the sacculus rotundus and vermiform appendix together with the presence of pale-whitish spots consistent with lymphoid follicle hyperplasia. Jejunal and ileal wall thickening was observed in one and three animals respectively, affecting some areas of the intestine in these regions. Representative photographs of lesions observed in three different animals are shown in Fig. 2.

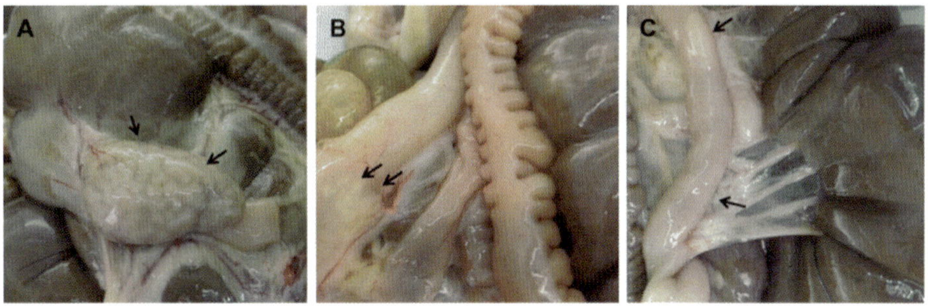

Figure 2: Macroscopic lesions found in slaughtered rabbits. **a** sacculus rotundus with pale white spots and thickened wall (animal D2.B2), **b** vermiform appendix with white spots and thickened wall (animal E1.Y2), **c** ileum with thickened walls and a reactive Peyer's patch (animal C1.Y2).

Molecular detection

Of the 66 analyzed rabbits, 11 were positive for *M. avium* in GALT (16.66 %). Of these, six animals (54.54 %) were positive in vermiform appendix only, 2 (18.18 %) in sacculus rotundus only, and 3 (27.27 %) in both tissue types. C_Ts for IS*1311* probe were 36.48+/−2.32 for undiluted samples and 37.12+/−1.01 for diluted samples. Attending to tissue type, C_Ts were 36.94+/−0.83 for vermiform appendix and 35.83+/−3.88 for sacculus rotundus. Mycobacteria were not detected by PCR in caecal contents.

The 14 *M. avium* positive samples were further analyzed by IS*900* & Is*Map02* PCR for Map detection and IS*1245* & IS*901* PCR for differentiation between Maa/Mas and Mah. All these samples were negative for the first real-time PCR, meaning that Map was not detected in these rabbits. In contrast 13 of the *M. avium*positive samples were identified as Maa/ Mas and 1 was identified as Mah according to the results obtained with IS*1245* & IS*901* PCR (Table 2).

Table 2: Gross pathology and molecular detection of sacculus rotundus and vermiform appendix from analyzed slaughtered rabbits

		Gross pathology	**Molecular detection**	
	Tissues (n)	**Animals (n (%))**	**Animals (n (%))**	**Identity**
Young rabbits	SR (48)	2[a] (11.1)	3 (4.2)	Maa/Mas
			1 (2.0)	Mah
	VA (48)	1 (5.5)	7 (14.6)	Maa/Mas
Breeding rabbits	SR (18)	3[b] (16.6)	2 (11.1)	Maa/Mas
	VA (18)	0 (0)	1 (5.5)	Maa/Mas

n: number of tissues or animals, %: percentage of positive results, SR: sacculus rotundus, VA: vermiform appendix, Maa: *M. avium* subsp. *avium*, Mas: *M. avium* subsp *silvaticum*, Mah: *M. avium* subsp *hominissuis* [a]Lesions spread to the ileum in both animals, [b]Lesions spread to the ileum in one animal

Culture

The culture of samples in BACTEC MGIT recorded contamination of 19.69 % of sacculus rotundus and 7.5 % of vermiform appendix samples. The remaining samples gave TTD readouts compatible with mycobacterial growth patterns on an average of 7.36 days for samples of sacculus rotundus and 6.95 days for samples of vermiform appendix but with a negative result in the MycMavMtc PCR. As a consequence, all MGIT cultures were finally recorded as contaminated.

No contamination on solid media was observed. Four samples cultured on Lowenstein-Jensen solid medium yielded colonies that were negative in the MycMavMTC. Sequencing of 16S rRNA gene identified them as *Thermoactinomycetaceae bacterium W8742* in three cases and *Thermoactinomyces sanguinis* in one case (Table 3).

Table 3: Molecular analysis, gross pathology and histopathology results of animals with at least one positive result in any of the methods

MycMavMtc PCR			**Identity**	**16s rRNA gene sequencing**	**Gross pathology**	**Histopathology**
Animal	**SR**	**VA**				
E1.Y1	-	-	-	*Thermoactinomyceteae* [a]	-	SR (0)/ VA (0)
E1.Y2	-	+	Maa/Mas	NI	VA	SR (0)/ VA (0)
B1.B1	-	-	-	*Thermoactinomyceteae* [b]	-	NA
B1.B2	-	-	-	NI	SR	SR (0)/ VA (0)
E2.Y2	-	-	-	NI	SR/IL[c]/JE[c]	SR (3)/ VA (0)/ IL (1)/ JE (0)
C1.Y2	+	+	Maa/Mas	NI	SR/IL[c]	SR (0)[d]/ VA (1)/ IL (1)
C2.Y1	-	+	Maa/Mas	NI	-	SR (1)/ VA (3)
C2.Y2	-	+	Maa/Mas	NI	-	SR (0)/ VA (0)[d]
B2.Y2	-	-	-	*Thermoactinomyceteae* [a]	-	SR (0)/ VA (0)
A1.Y2	-	+	Maa/Mas	NI	-	NA
E3.Y1	-	+	Mah	NI	-	NA
E3.Y2	-	+	Maa/Mas	NI	-	NA
B7.Y1	-	-	-	*Thermoactinomyces sanguinis* [b]	-	NA
B5.B1	+	+	Maa/Mas	NI	-	NA
D2.Y2	+	+	Maa/Mas	NI	-	NA
D2.B1	-	-	-	NI	SR/IL[c]	SR (2)/ VA (0)/ IL (1)
D2.B2	+	-	Maa/Mas	NI	SR	SR (2)/ VA (0)
D3.Y1	+	-	Maa/Mas	NI	-	NA

SR: sacculus rotundus, VA: vermiform appendix, IL: ileum, JE: jejunum, NI: no isolation. [a]Identified from a colony isolated from sacculus rotundus, [b]Identified from a colony isolated from vermiform appendix. [c]intestinal wall thickening, NA: Not analyzed. (0): Without lesions, (1): Reactive hyperplasia, (2) Unspecific granulomatous lesions (3): Granulomatous lesions,[d]: Ziehl Neelsen positive

Histopathology

Most significant lesions were found in the sacculus rotundus and vermiform appendix lymphoid tissue. In some cases, they were formed by well demarcated granulomas compatible with mycobacterial infection, composed of between 10–50 macrophages with occasional multinucleated Langhan's type giant cells, located in the interfollicular areas of the lymphoid tissue. In other animals, granulomatous lesions were categorized as unspecific and were formed by small granulomas, also seen in the interfollicular areas of lymphoid tissue, with less than 15 macrophages, harbouring variable amounts of a brown pigment in their cytoplasm. Microscopical examination of tissues revealed that wall thickening observed on ileum and jejunum corresponded to reactive lymphoid follicles in the ileal and jejunal Peyer's patches. Remaining samples were classified as reactive hyperplasic or absence of lesion when tissues presented a normal form. AFB were detected on two samples that were classified as absence of lesion and were also PCR positive. Complete results for all animals are shown in Table 3.

Association analysis

Analysis of age and gross pathology results showed that 6 out of 48 (6.25 %) of the young rabbits and 3 out of 18 (16.7 %) breeding rabbits showed some gross changes. However, these frequencies were not statistically significant (FET $p=0.333$).

Microbiological results showed that 9 of 48 (18.7 %) young rabbits and 2 of 18 (11.1%) breeding animals were *M. avium* subspecies positive in the PCR tests, but again, these frequencies were not statistically significant (FET $p=0.713$).

Worth mentioning is that 50 % (2/4) of the samples that presented focal lesions were PCR positive.

The geographical origin of sampled rabbits is shown on Fig. 3a. All geographical areas except for F presented at least one positive farm as shown on Fig. 3b. 8 out of 21 farms were positive (38 %), when positive was considered as having at least one *M. avium* subspecies PCR positive animal. Noticeable, is geographical area E where only 2 animals were sampled and one was positive for Maa and the other for Mah.

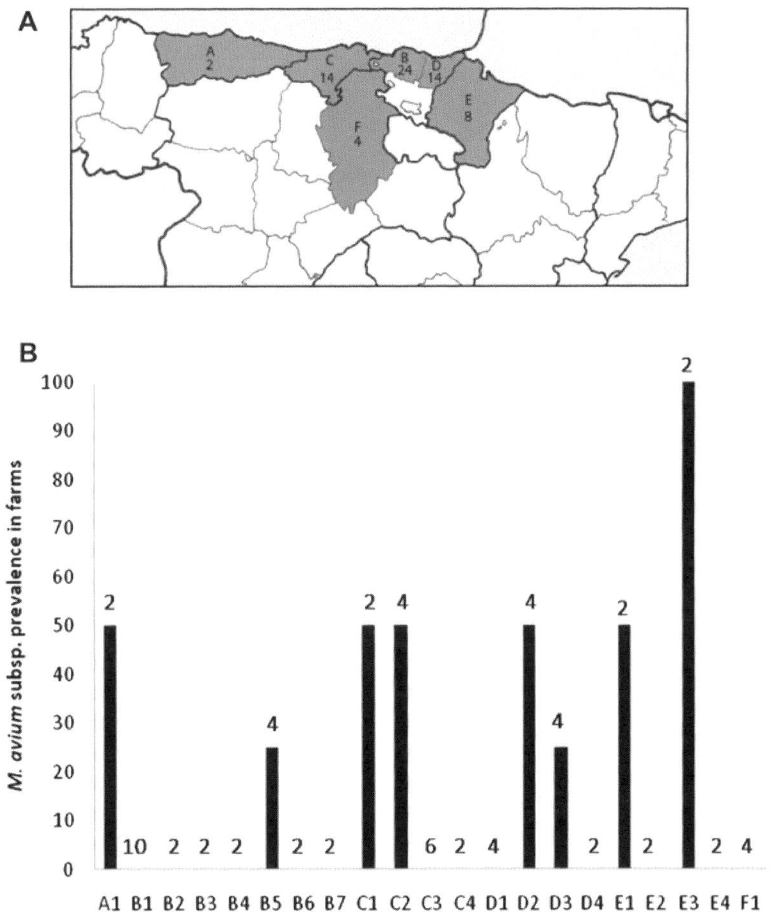

Figure 3: **a** Geographical origin of sampled slaughtered rabbits. A: Asturias, B: Bizkaia, C: Cantabria, D: Gipuzkoa, E: Navarra, F: Burgos and number of analyzed animals per area. **b** *M. avium* subspecies positivity of each farm identified as letters (A-F) representing each geographical area and a number (1–7) identifying the farm. Black bars represent prevalence (%), numbers on bars represent total number of analyzed animals from each farm.

DISCUSSION

There is not much information in the veterinary literature concerning microbiological findings from rabbits at slaughter. A few studies have assessed *Listeria*, *Salmonella*, and *E.coli* among others [34, 35]. It is not surprising then, that data from mycobacteria and more specifically *M. avium* subspecies is scarce and mainly limited to other animal species such as cattle [28] or pigs [26, 27]. Therefore, to the best of our knowledge, this is the first study reporting *M. avium* subspecies detection in slaughtered rabbits.

In rabbits, apart from mesenteric lymph nodes and Peyer's patches, the GALT which accounts for 50 % of the lymphoid tissue includes two specific structures: the sacculus rotundus, and the vermiform appendix. Both tissue types present M cells [36] which actively uptake and present particular antigens and microorganisms to the immune cells of the lymphoid follicle to induce an effective immune response [37]. Map has been reported to enter the domes of the Peyer's patches through M cells [38] so orally ingested mycobacteria should end up in these sites and/or in caecal content and therefore we chose these specimens for our analysis.

Regarding PCR evaluation, the possibility of inhibition was the main concern. MycMavMtc PCR performed well at 10^4-10^6 CFU/g of tissue. According to our results if we had +/−10^2 CFU/g of mycobacteria we would probably not detect them at least in our tissue type because we would necessarily have to perform dilution steps. The detection limit for this PCR for *M. avium hominissuis* in a mixture of bovine tissues has been reported as 1.59×10^2 CFU/g [32] which is in near agreement with our findings. We must add that the DNA extraction methods of both studies are not coincident and that the bovine tissue mixture may present a more favorable chemistry for the DNA extraction and PCR reaction compared to rabbit mucosa. In any case, for the slaughterhouse study we decided to dilute template DNA if inhibition took place, maybe missing positive samples in return.

In the slaughterhouse study, although gross pathology compatible with mycobacterial infection was seen, histological analysis of GALT did not reveal presence of granulomas in all gross pathology positive animals and AFB detected by ZN were only found in two cases. The presence of granulomas in GALT associated to Mah have been reported before in sheep [39]. The unspecific granulomas may not be due to infectious agents and they may be "garbage" granulomas or on the other hand they can be ancient granulomas that accumulate waxy pigments that have been attributed to mycobacteria in previous studies [40].

DNA of *M. avium* was present in 16.6 % of the analyzed GALT samples. If we compare C_T values in sampled tissues with the PCR of artificially spiked tissues we can estimate that the bacterial load is probably below 10^4CFU/g. In an experimental infection in rabbits with Map, isolation was variable, since some sacculus rotundus and vermiform appendix samples that had bacterial loads of 10^2-10^6 genomic equivalents/g estimated by qPCR gave positive solid culture results, whereas the same tissue site samples from other animals with 10^1-10^5 genomic equivalents/g gave negative culture results (unpublished observations). Of course, isolation variability can be affected by the irregular distribution of AFB in the analyzed tissues among other factors. As for, liquid cultures, they were eventually contaminated and other bacteria could have used up the nutrients necessary for mycobacterial growth. MycMavMtc PCR of MGIT cultures was negative meaning that mycobacterial load was possibly under $1{,}59\times10^2$ CFU/g, since this was the reported detection limit for MGIT culture in a bovine tissue mixture using 2 % NaOH [31]. If more than 2 % NaOH were to be used as in the present study (6 % NaOH), it would probably affect mycobacterial viability and interfere with isolation in both solid and liquid media. In solid media, only *Thermoactinomyces*, bacteria were isolated. *Thermoactinomyces*species have been implicated as causal agents of farmer's lung diseases [41] since the disease appears in farmers that are in direct contact with mouldy hay and cereal grains where these bacterial species are known to be abundant. Also they are found in soil, rivers and dairy products [42]. We are not sure about the meaning of this finding but it could be that these bacteria are present in the grains that the rabbits are fed or in the straw litter that maybe used for nesting before kindling. In any case, it is worth mentioning that these bacteria survive decontamination techniques used for mycobacterial culture and that no macro or microscopic signs of pathology in the digestive system were detected in the animals these bacteria were isolated from.

Association analysis revealed that neither gross pathology nor mycobacterial presence was affected by age. Maa has been detected before in rabbits that had been housed with infected pigeons [43] or with doves, ducks and chickens [44] suggesting in both cases that transmission had probably occurred from infected fowl to rabbits. In our case, although not specifically examined, given the standard production housing characteristics in the studied region, it is most probable that rabbits did not have direct contact with fowl. In any case, young rabbits do present Maa implicating an early contact in their life that might point to water or feeding.

The results from this study show that *M. avium* subspecies are widely spread and in contact with farmed rabbits since only 2–3 animals analyzed from each batch of 21 farms has shown 16.6 % positivity among animals and 38 % positivity among farms. Detection of mycobacterial DNA was achieved in 50 % of the tissues with focal lesions, slightly higher than what has been reported for Map in cattle [40, 45]. At this point, we are not sure about the real significance of detecting *M. avium* subspecies in GALT tissue of slaughtered rabbits either from an animal pathological and epidemiological or Public Health perspective. Although detected granulomas suggest the generation of lesions, the focal nature of these granulomas could be compatible with a latent and controlled infection. Rabbit GALT does not enter the food chain, but if it occurred, properly cooked affected parts should not pose a risk to healthy or immunocompromised individuals. Scarcity of previous reports indicates that the problem probably does not compromise rabbit production to a big extent. Lack of other information on the infected animals such as clinical status or weight at slaughter impedes drawing conclusions. It is noteworthy to state that no Map was detected or isolated, therefore indicating that its presence in wild rabbits might be related to environmental factors that do not occur in more controlled farm conditions or that its prevalence is lower and a higher number of animals should be tested.

CONCLUSIONS

This study should be considered as a preliminary survey that might draw attention to a hitherto undetected potential problem. Future studies should consider including other intestinal sites, associated lymph nodes and respiratory tissues as well.

The detection MAC bacteria other than Map indicates that a niche for this group of mycobacteria does exist in farmed rabbits.

DECLARATIONS

Acknowledgements

The authors thank the official veterinarian, Susana Rodríguez and all the employees at the rabbit slaughterhouse for their collaboration in collecting the samples and also Dr. Patricia Vazquez for technical assistance with the histopathological analysis.

Funding

This study was supported by grants (AGL2012-39818-CO2-02) and (INIA, RTA2010-00022) from the Spanish Ministry of Economy and Competitiveness (MINECO) and the Spanish National Institute for Agricultural and Food Research and Technology, respectively. Rakel Arrazuria held a pre doctoral fellowship (BFI-2012-237) from the Basque Government. The funders had no role in study design, data collection and analysis, decision to publish, or preparation of the manuscript.

Authors' contribution

RA collected the samples, participated in all the microbiological and pathological studies and collaborated in the interpretation of the data and writing of the paper, IS participated in the analysis of the data, interpretation of the results and writing of the paper, EM contributed to the sample collection and microbiological studies, VP collaborated in the histopathological interpretation and paper drafting, JG collaborated in the interpretation of the results and the paper drafting, RJ conceived and designed the experiment, performed data analysis and drafting of the paper, NE conceived and designed the experiment, participated in sample collection, pathological studies, interpretation of the results and performed data analysis and writing of the paper. All the authors read and approved the final manuscript.

Authors' information

Rakel Arrazuria, DVMD; Iker A Sevilla, Bsc, PhD; Elena Molina, BSc; Valentín Pérez, DVMD, PhD, Joseba M Garrido, DVMD, PhD; Ramón A Juste, DVMD, PhD; Natalia Elguezabal, BSc, PhD.

REFERENCES

1. Angus KW. Intestinal lesions resembling paratuberculosis in a wild rabbit (*Oryctolagus cuniculus*). J Comp Pathol. 1990;103:101–5.
2. Beard PM, Rhind SM, Buxton D, Daniels MJ, Henderson D, Pirie A, et al. Natural paratuberculosis infection in rabbits in Scotland. J Comp Pathol. 2001;124:290–9.
3. Fuentes O, Cebrian J. El conejo de monte ¿Reservorio de la paratuberculosis ovina y caprina? In: Abstract book. 1988. I Symposium de Patología Ovina y Caprina. Zaragoza, Spain.
4. Maio E, Carta T, Balseiro A, Sevilla IA, Romano A, Ortiz JA, et al. Paratuberculosis in European wild rabbits from the Iberian Peninsula. Res Vet Sci. 2011;91:212–8.
5. Harrenstien LA, Finnegan MV, Woodford NL, Mansfield KG, Waters WR, Bannantine JP, et al. *Mycobacterium avium* in pygmy rabbits (*Brachylagus idahoensis*): 28 cases. J Zoo Wildl Med. 2006;37:498–512.
6. Mokresh AH, Czuprynski CJ, Butler DG. A rabbit model for study of *Mycobacterium paratuberculosis* infection. Infect Immun. 1989;57:3798–807.
7. Vaughan JA, Lenghaus C, Stewart DJ, Tizard ML, Michalski WP. Development of a Johne's disease infection model in laboratory rabbits following oral administration of *Mycobacterium avium* subspecies *paratuberculosis*. Vet Microbiol. 2005;105:207–13.
8. Turenne CY, Wallace Jr R, Behr MA. *Mycobacterium avium* in the postgenomic era. Clin Microbiol Rev. 2007;20:205–29.
9. Biet F, Boschiroli ML, Thorel MF, Guilloteau LA. Zoonotic aspects of *Mycobacterium bovis* and *Mycobacterium avium-intracellulare* complex (MAC). Vet Res. 2005;36:411–36.
10. Pavlik I, Svastova P, Bartl J, Dvorska L, Rychlik I. Relationship between IS901 in the *Mycobacterium avium* complex strains isolated from birds, animals, humans, and the environment and virulence for poultry. Clin Diagn Lab Immunol. 2000;7:212–7.
11. Thorel MF, Huchzermeyer HF, Michel AL. *Mycobacterium avium* and *Mycobacterium intracellulare* infection in mammals. Rev Sci Tech. 2001;20:204–18.
12. Mijs W, de Haas P, Rossau R, Van der Laan T, Rigouts L, Portaels F, et al. Molecular evidence to support a proposal to reserve the designation *Mycobacterium avium* subsp. *avium* for bird-type isolates and *M. avium* subsp. *hominissuis* for the human/porcine type of *M. avium*. Int J Syst Evol Microbiol. 2002;52:1505–18.
13. Alvarez J, Castellanos E, Romero B, Aranaz A, Bezos J, Rodriguez S, et al. Epidemiological investigation of a *Mycobacterium avium* subsp. *hominissuis* outbreak in swine. Epidemiol Infect. 2011;139:143–8.
14. Lahiri A, Kneisel J, Kloster I, Kamal E, Lewin A. Abundance of Mycobacterium avium ssp. hominissuis in soil and dust in Germany - implications for the infection route. Lett Appl Microbiol. 2014;59:65–70.
15. Behr MA, Kapur V. The evidence for *Mycobacterium paratuberculosis* in Crohn's disease. Curr Opin Gastroenterol. 2008;24:17–21.
16. Feller M, Huwiler K, Stephan R, Altpeter E, Shang A, Furrer H, et al. *Mycobacterium avium* subspecies *paratuberculosis*and Crohn's disease: a systematic re and meta-analysis. Lancet Infect Dis. 2007;7:607–13.
17. Juste RA, Elguezabal N, Garrido JM, Pavon A, Geijo MV, Sevilla I, et al. On the prevalence of *M. avium* subspecies *paratuberculosis* DNA in the blood of healthy individuals and patients with inflammatory bowel disease. PLoS ONE. 2008;3:e2537.
18. Masala S, Paccagnini D, Cossu D, Brezar V, Pacifico A, Ahmed N, et al. Antibodies recognizing *Mycobacterium avium paratuberculosis* epitopes cross-react with the beta-cell antigen ZnT8 in Sardinian type 1 diabetic patients. PLoS ONE. 2011;6, e26931.
19. Vazquez P, Garrido JM, Molina E, Geijo MV, Gómez N, Pérez V, et al. Latent infections are the most frequent form of paratuberculosis in slaughtered Friesian cattle.

Span J Agric Res. 2014;12:1049–60.

20. Soltys MA, Wise DR. Atypical mycobacterium in tuberculosis-like lesions in wood pigeons. J Pathol Bacteriol. 1967;93:351–2.

21. Jorgensen JB, Clausen B. Mycobacteriosis in a roe-deer caused by wood-pigeon mycobacteria. Nord Vet Med. 1976;28:539–46.

22. Chiers K, Deschaght P, De BT, Dabrowski S, Kotlowski R, De CD, et al. Isolation and identification of *Mycobacterium avium* subspecies *silvaticum* from a horse. Comp Immunol Microbiol Infect Dis. 2012;35:303–7.

23. Thorel MF, Blom-Potar MC, Rastogi N. Characterization of *Mycobacterium paratuberculosis* and "wood-pigeon" mycobacteria by isoenzyme profile and selective staining of immunoprecipitates. Res Microbiol. 1990;141:551–61.

24. Klanicova B, Slana I, Vondruskova H, Kaevska M, Pavlik I. Real-time quantitative PCR detection of *Mycobacterium avium*subspecies in meat products. J Food Prot. 2011;74:636–40.

25. Agdestein A, Olsen I, Jorgensen A, Djonne B, Johansen TB. Novel insights into transmission routes of *Mycobacterium avium* in pigs and possible implications for human health. Vet Res. 2014;45:46.

26. Muwonge A, Johansen TB, Vigdis E, Godfroid J, Olea-Popelka F, Biffa D, et al. *Mycobacterium bovis* infections in slaughter pigs in Mubende district. Uganda: a public health concern. BMC Vet Res. 2012;8:168.

27. van Ingen J, Wisselink HJ, van Solt-Smits CB, Boeree MJ, van Soolingen D. Isolation of mycobacteria other than *Mycobacterium avium* from porcine lymph nodes. Vet Microbiol. 2010;144:250–3.

28. Alonso-Hearn M, Molina E, Geijo M, Vazquez P, Sevilla I, Garrido JM, et al. Isolation of *Mycobacterium avium* subsp. *paratuberculosis* from muscle tissue of naturally infected cattle. Foodborne Pathog Dis. 2009;6:513–8.

29. Gonzalez P, Caravac FP. Producción de conejos de aptitud cárnica. In: Universidad de Sevilla, editor. *Sistemas ganaderos en el siglo XXI. Volume 30*. 2007. p. 443–61.

30. von Reyn CF, Waddell RD, Eaton T, Arbeit RD, Maslow JN, Barber TW, et al. Isolation of *Mycobacterium avium* complex from water in the United States, Finland, Zaire, and Kenya. J Clin Microbiol. 1993;31:3227–30.

31. Sevilla IA, Molina E, Elguezabal N, Pérez V, Garrido JM, Juste RA. Detection of mycobacteria, *Mycobacterium avium*subspecies and *Mycobacterium tuberculosis* complex by a novel tetraplex real-time PCR. J Clin Microbiol. 2015;53:930–40.

32. Sevilla IA, Garrido JM, Molina E, Geijo MV, Elguezabal N, Vazquez P, et al. Development and Evaluation of a Novel Multicopy-Element-Targeting Triplex PCR for Detection of *Mycobacterium avium* subsp. *paratuberculosis* in Feces. Appl Environ Microbiol. 2014;80:3757–68.

33. Slana I, Kaevska M, Kralik P, Horvathova A, Pavlik I. Distribution of *Mycobacterium avium* subsp. *avium* and *M. a. hominissuis* in artificially infected pigs studied by culture and IS901 and IS1245 quantitative real time PCR. Vet Microbiol. 2010;144:437–43.

34. Kohler R, Krause G, Beutin L, Stephan R, Zweifel C. Shedding of food-borne pathogens and microbiological carcass contamination in rabbits at slaughter. Vet Microbiol. 2008;132:149–57.

35. Rodriguez-Calleja JM, Garcia-Lopez I, Garcia-Lopez ML, Santos JA, Otero A. Rabbit meat as a source of bacterial foodborne pathogens. J Food Prot. 2006;69:1106–12.

36. Beyaz F, Ergun E, Bayraktaroglu AG, Ergun L. The identification of intestinal M cells in the sacculus rotundus and appendix of the Angora rabbit. Vet Res Commun. 2010;34:255–65.

37. Kucharzik T, Lugering N, Rautenberg K, Lugering A, Schmidt MA, Stoll R, et al. Role of M cells in intestinal barrier function. Ann N Y Acad Sci. 2000;915:171–83.

38. Momotani E, Whipple DL, Thiermann AB, Cheville NF. Role of M cells and macrophages in the entrance of *Mycobacterium paratuberculosis* into domes of ileal Peyer's patches in calves. Vet Pathol. 1988;25:131–7.

39. Benavides J, Garcia-Pariente C, Garrido JM, Sevilla IA, Garcia-Marin JF, Perez V, et al. Coexistence of granulomatous enteric inflammation and neoplasia in an adult sheep. Vet Pathol. 2013;50:1158–62.

40. Gonzalez J, Geijo MV, Garcia-Pariente C, Verna A, Corpa JM, Reyes LE, et al. Histopathological classification of lesions associated with natural paratuberculosis infection in cattle. J Comp Pathol. 2005;133:184–96.

41. Pepys J, Jenkins PA, Festenstein GN, Gregory PH, Lacey ME, Skinner FA. Farmer's Lung. Thermophilic actinomycetes as a source of "Farmer's lung hay" antigen. Lancet. 1963;2:607–11.

42. Lacey J&CT. Genus *Thermoactinomyces* Tsiklinsky 1899, 501AL. In: S.T.Williams MES&JGH, editor. Bergey's Manual of Systematic Bacteriology. Baltimore: Williams & Wilkins; 1989. p. 2574–85.

43. Kriz P, Slana I, Kralik P, Babak V, Skoric M, Fictum P, et al. Outbreak of *Mycobacterium avium* subsp. *avium* infection in one flock of domestic pigeons. Avian Dis. 2011;55:503–8.

44. Lehmbecker A, Pfeifer F, Moser I, Wohlsein P. Spontaneous enzootic avian tuberculosis in domestic rabbits (*Oryctolagus cuniculi* f dom). KLEINTIERPRAXIS. 2010;55:21.

45. Vazquez P, Garrido JM, Juste RA. Specific antibody and interferon-gamma responses associated with immunopathological forms of bovine paratuberculosis in slaughtered Friesian cattle. PLoS ONE. 2013;8, e64568.

CHAPTER 30 CURRENT PERSPECTIVES ON MYCOBACTERIUM FARCINOGENES AND MYCOBACTERIUM SENEGALENSE, THE CAUSAL AGENTS OF BOVINE FARCY

Mohamed E. Hamid

INTRODUCTION

Bovine farcy (which is caused by Mycobacterium farcinogenes and M. senegalense) is a chronic granulomatous inflammation of the skin lymphatics and draining lymph nodes of zebu cattle. It has been reported in 19 countries in Africa, Asia, Latin America, and the Caribbean with tropical and subtropical climates. Historically, it existed in a belt that extends east to include south India, Sri Lanka, and Sumatra and west to include north parts of Latin America and the West Indies but mainly dominant in the sub-Saharan African countries [1]. It was in 1888 that Edmond Nocard first isolated and described the causal agent of "bovine farcy" [2]. In his original description, Nocard [2] noted a granulomatous disease of cattle with multiple abscesses, draining sinuses, pulmonary involvement, emaciation, and eventually death. Since then, the classification of theNocardia organisms has undergone several changes.

Literature on the prevalence, transmission patterns, and risk factors of bovine farcy is deficient. The disease is not included within the categories of cattle diseases in List A or List B of the OIE categorization [3] due to its characteristic that it has neither international spread nor significant mortality and morbidity at the level of a country or a zone nor an apparent zoonotic property with severe consequences. Nevertheless, cattlemen and governments in Africa believe that bovine farcy is responsible for certain economic losses as a result of damaged hides. Besides, it is public-health burden since the lymphadenitis due to farcy resembles the lesions of bovine tuberculosis in carcasses and the meat is considered inappropriate for human consumption [1].

Laboratory diagnoses are hardly ever used to make routine diagnosis and to initiate treatment. This is because of logistic and practical difficulties encountered amongst rural communities in Africa. However, laboratory diagnoses can confirm the clinical diagnosis retrospectively on tissues and purulent materials taken during treatment or during meat inspection. Apart from the reasonable use of standard smear-and-culture methods, few diagnostic tests have been developed; the molecular and serological tests have not been evaluated for reproducibility and accuracy.

TAXONOMY

Bovine farcy causing actinomycetes isolated from zebu cattle in eastern Africa were found to belong to the genus Mycobacterium and not to Nocardia [4–10]. The causal agents of bovine farcy contained mycolic acids, the esters of which yielded, on pyrolysis gas chromatography, a single

Citation: Mohamed E. Hamid, "Current Perspectives on Mycobacterium farcinogenes and Mycobacterium senegalense, the Causal Agents of Bovine Farcy," Veterinary Medicine International, vol. 2014, Article ID 247906, 13 pages, 2014. doi:10.1155/2014/247906.

peak that corresponded to the C24 ester characteristic of some mycobacteria. Chamoiseau [7] suggested that these bacteria be allocated in the genusMycobacterium as M. farcinogenes; he distinguished two subspecies, M. farcinogenes subspecies tchadense andM. farcinogenes subspecies senegalense. On the ground of their phenotypic dissimilarity, Chamoiseau [11] raised the two subspecies to species levels as M. farcinogenes and M. senegalense which have first appeared in the 1st edition of Bergey's Manual of Systematic Bacteriology [12].

It is now known that M. farcinogenes and M. senegalense can also be distinguished from one another on the basis of histopathological behavior [11], DNA relatedness [13], mycobactin contents [14], chemotaxonomic and biochemical properties [15–17], pyrolysis mass spectrometry [18], and 16S rRNA sequence data [19–23].

Members of the two species have many properties in common both with one another and with the nonphotochromogenic rapidly growing mycobacteria, namely, M. fortuitum and M. peregrinum, M. septicum (sorbitol negative 3rd M. fortuitum biovar), M. porcinum [24], and, with the recently described species in theM. fortuitum complex, M. boenickei, M. houstonense (sorbitol negative 3rd M. fortuitum biovar), and M. neworleansense (Figure 1; [25, 26]).

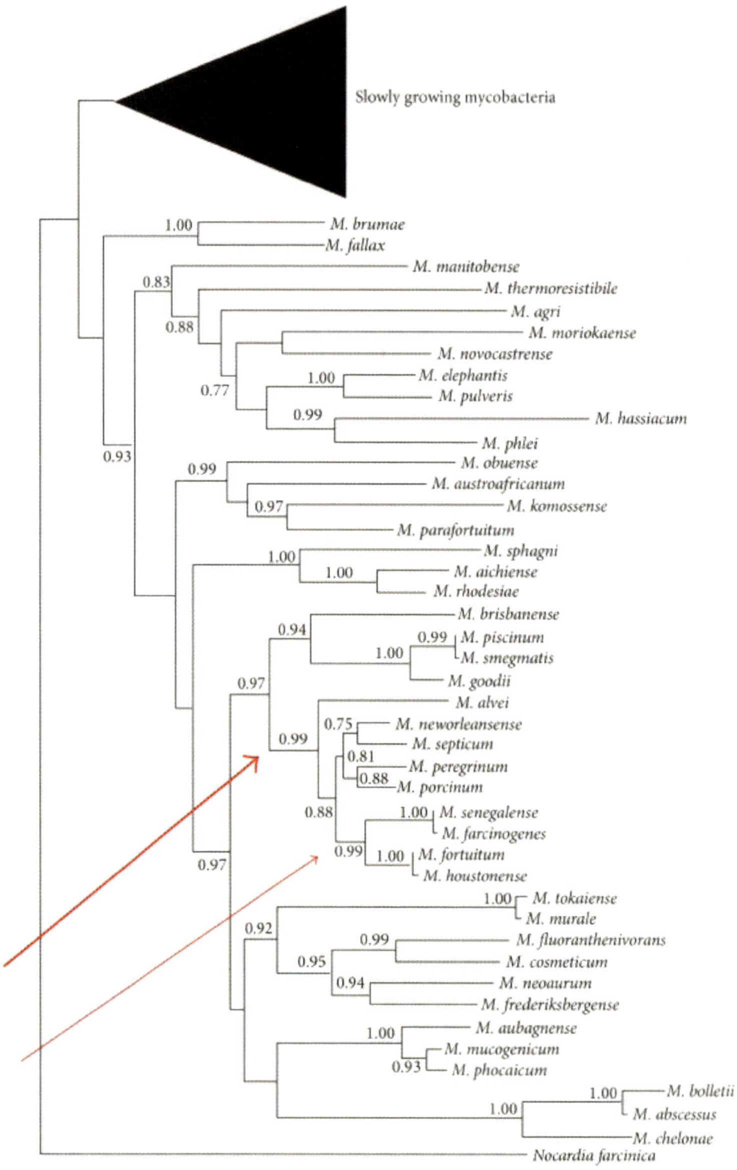

Figure 1: Estimate of mycobacterial phylogeny based on a multilocus seven-gene concatenate (hsp65, rpoB, 16S rRNA, smpB, sodA, tmRNA, and tuf) showing the position of Mycobacterium farcinogenes and M. senegalense within a branch that accommodates the rapidly growing non-photochromogenic mycobacteria (thick arrow) and their close relationship to M. houstonense and M. fortuitum (thin arrow). The percentages of bootstrap values are shown next to the nodes. The tree was modified from Mignard and Flandrois [26].

M. porcinum is a known veterinary pathogen [27]. Phylogenetic tree of the combined rpoB + recA + soda + hsp65 + 16S rRNA gene sequences of 19 rapidly growing mycobacteria using the neighbor-joining method supported the designation of the M. fortuitum grouping into subclades which include M. peregrinum and M. septicum; this is joint by another subclade consisting of M. boenickei, M. neworleansense, and M. porcinum along with subclade in M. fortuitum and M. houstonense, M. farcinogenes and M. senegalense. Both subclades are related to another subclade of M. farcinogenes and M. senegalense. The three are related to the subclade which includes M. fortuitum and M. houstonense [28]. The

99% rpoB gene sequence similarity between M. houstonense and M. fortuitum suggested that these strains may be closely related subspecies, although M. houstonense showed resistance to pipemidic acid, biochemical differences such as mannitol, inositol, sorbitol, and trehalose utilization [22], and three base differences in the 16S rRNA gene sequence [25]. The isolation ofM. fortuitum 3rd variant from cattle specimens [29] may be of epidemiologic and taxonomic implications. TheM. fortuitum 3rd (sorbitol positive) variant is now reclassified as M. houstonense sp. nov. [25]. Recently, Guérin-Faublée et al. [30] described Mycobacterium bourgelatii, a new rapidly growing nonphotochromogenic species which they had isolated from cattle with lymphadenitis. These new isolates need to be compared with other cattle pathogens giving the similarity in both chromogenicity and the rapidly growing property.

N. farcinica is still though not often reported as a causal agent of bovine farcy when diagnosis based on morphological traits, which fail to discriminate Nocardia from other mycolic acid-containing actinomycetes, is used [31–40].

The conclusions from the many taxonomic studies could be summarized as follows:(1)M. farcinogenes and M. senegalense are morphologically similar to each other and to Nocardia farcinica (Figures 2 and 3). But M. farcinogenes is relatively a slow growing Mycobacterium compared to the rapidly growing M. senegalense.(2)On molecular basis, M. farcinogenes and M. senegalense are closely related to M. houstonense. The three species fall ina subclade including M. fortuitum. This subclade is closely linked to the one incorporatingM. peregrinum, M. porcinum, M. septicum, M. neworleansense, and M. alvei (Figure 1).

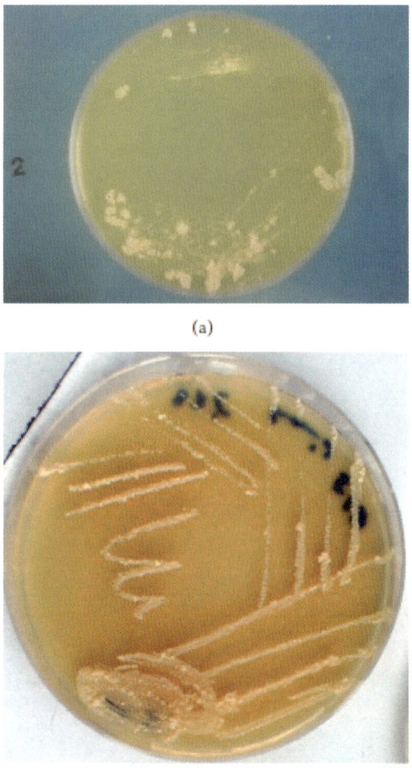

(a)

(b)

Figure 2: Growth of Mycobacterium farcinogenes on glucose yeast extract agar (a) and M. senegalense on glucose yeast extract malt extract agar (b) at 37°C for 7 days, showing nonchromogenic, wheat-colored rough convoluted irregular colonies.

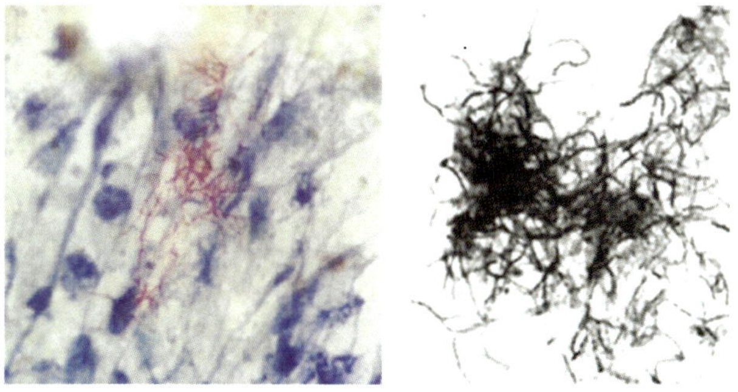

(a) (b)

Figure 3: Smears made from a purulent material of M. farcinogenes-infected cow (a) showing acid fast branching filaments and smear made from a culture of M. senegalense (b). Note short or long filaments, bent and branched, in clumps or tangled lacy network which do not fragment into bacillary forms.

HABITATS

There are no reports on isolating or detecting M. farcinogenes or M. senegalense from environmental samples. Epidemiological data have not reported bovine farcy in wild and other domestic animals. The zoonotic potentials of M. farcinogenes and M. senegalense are unknown; only few reports provided evidence that M. senegalense [41] and M. farcinogenes [42] cause infections in human.

The role of ticks in the transmission of farcy is not understood. Bovine farcy lesions start at the lymph nodes (usually peripheral, femoral, or parotid) and then spread slowly via lymphatic vessel to subcutaneous tissue on the dorsal parts. In contrast, ticks feed mostly on the ventral aspects. Furthermore, tick larvae and nymphs moult before feeding on another animal; therefore, it is not feasible that the bacterium is transferred from one host to another on the outside of ticks. Although transmission of the infection by ticks under field condition has not been established, it has long been believed by locals in the Sudan that the ticks are involved. Some authors associate bovine farcy with tick infestation (notably, the ixodid tick Amblyomma variegatum) [40, 43–45]. Additionally, Al Janabi et al. [46] successfully transmitted N. farcinica (which was believed at that time to be the agent of bovine farcy) from an experimentally infected rabbit to a control one via Amblyomma variegatum.

ISOLATION AND CULTIVATION

Lowenstein-Jensen is the medium commonly used for selective isolation of M. farcinogenes as for many other mycobacteria from infected materials [47]. Glucose yeast extract agar ([48]; GYEA) is used for maintenance and bench work. Modified Sauton's broth [49] is routinely used to cultivate biomass of M. farcinogenes, M. senegalense, and some other mycobacteria for chemotaxonomic studies [16, 50–52]. Mycobacterium medium number 219 is recommended by DSMZ for routine culture [53].

M. farcinogenes and M. senegalense grow on a wide range of common synthetic media. Shigidi et al. [38] used diagnostic sensitivity test (DST) agar for culturing farcy organisms. Out of 13 diverse agar-based media, M. farcinogenes was found to grow particularly well on Mueller Hinton's medium followed by modified Bennett, Tryptic soya, glucose yeast extract, and

DST agars [54]. A broth medium containing (g/L; w/v) yeast extract (4), glucose (15), magnesium sulphate (0.5), trisodium citrate (1.5), potassium sulphate (0.5), and ammonium ferric citrate (trace) and buffered with potassium dihydrogen phosphate (5) was formulated [55] and found to support a luxuriant growth of M. farcinogenes strains than media used before [49].

MORPHOLOGICAL AND CULTURAL CHARACTERISTICS

Colonies appear after 2 to 5 days (M. senegalense) and 5 to 10 days (M. farcinogenes) at 25°C to 37°C on Lowenstein-Jensen medium. Colonies appear rough and convoluted that are firmly attached to the media. The grown colonies are usually nonchromogenic, wheat-colored. Growth on most agar-based media such as GYEA, DST agar, Tryptic Soya agar, and Mueller Hinton agar is seen as nonchromogenic irregular rough colonies (Figure 2) which are not firmly attached to the median (in contrast to their growth Lowenstein-Jensen slants) and are difficult to emulsify [11, 15, 45, 56]. These mycobacteria can be preserved for up to 10 years when cells are suspended in 20% glycerol and kept frozen at −20°C [57].

M. farcinogenes and M. senegalense have short or long filaments, bent and branched, in clumps or tangled lacy network whether seen in smears from culture or from lesions (Figure 3). These filaments do not fragment into bacillary forms and were strongly acid-alcohol fast. Scanning electron microscopy observations have confirmed the true-nonfragmenting filamentous nature of the M. farcinogenes and M. senegalense (Figure 4). It is obvious that these species could be distinguished from other mycobacteria because they form branched substrate mycelia. Moreover, M. senegalense exhibitsa characteristic fungal structure called “synnema” (plural synnemata) which is strand resembling stalks thread together (Figure 4).

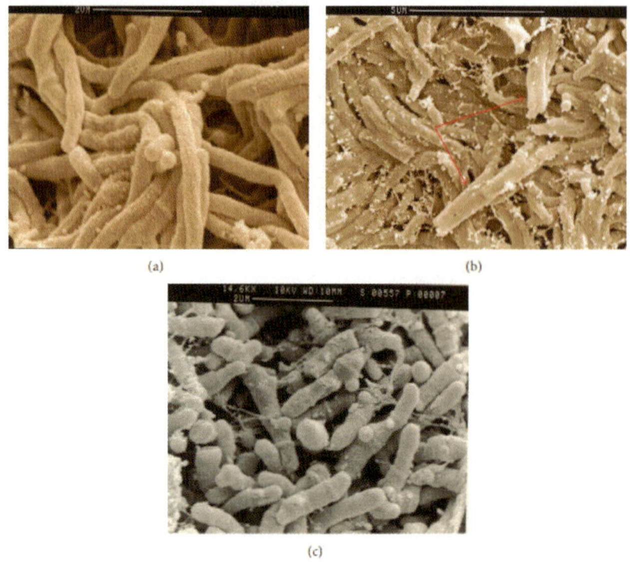

Figure 4: Scanning electron microscopy of M. farcinogenes (a), M. senegalense (b), andNocardia farcinica (c). Note the true-non-fragmenting branched filaments in both species and the presence of “synnemata” in M. senegalense (arrow).

BIOCHEMICAL FEATURES

Members of the M. farcinogenes and M. senegalense produce a positive malonamidase test, an attribute that is rarely shown by other mycobacteria. Routinely, M. senegalense is more active biochemically than M. farcinogenes. Some of the biochemical properties, enzyme profile, tolerance to chemical inhibitors, and resistance pattern to antibiotics as well as morphological and cultural characteristics of the two species are shown in Table 1.

Table 1: Phenotypic characteristics of Mycobacterium farcinogenes and Mycobacterium senegalense

Test	*M. farcinogenes*	*M. senegalense*	References*
Morphology and cultural characteristics			
Growth at 30°C	+	+	[56]
Growth at 35–37°C	+	+	[56]
Growth after 3–5 days	−	+	[11, 15, 56]
Growth after 5–10 days	+	−	[11, 15, 56]
Colony wheat-colored	+	+	[11, 15, 56]
Colony convoluted	+	+	[11, 15, 56]
Colony rough	+	+	[11, 15, 56]
Colony very rough and grainy	+	−	[11, 56]
Colony easily detached from agar	+	−	[15, 56]
Colony relatively emulsifiable	−	+	[11, 56]
Colony nonemulsifiable	+	−	[56]
Aerial hyphae sparse	+	+	[15, 56]
Aerial hyphae abundant	−	−	[15, 56]
Biochemical (enzyme) tests			
Acetamidase	+	+	[11, 15, 82]
Allantoinase	+/−	+	[11]
Arylsulphatase	−	+	[15, 76, 82]
Benzamidase	+/−	+	[11]
Catalase**	+	+	[11, 15, 56, 76, 82]
Iron citrate test	−	−	[11]
Isonicotinamidase	+/−	+	[11]
Beta-lactamase after 60 min	+	+	[15]
Neutral red test	−	−	[11]
Niacin production	−	−	[11]
Nicotinamidase	+/−	+	[11]
Nitrate reductase	+	+	[11, 15, 76]
Nitrophenol oxidase	−	−	[15]
Salicylamidase	+/−	+	[11]

Urease	−/+	+	[11, 15, 82]
Urease	−	ND	[76]
Fluorogenic enzyme tests (cleavage of 4-methylumbelliferone glycosides substrates (4MU))			
4MU-α-L-arabinofuranoside	+	+/−	[56]
4MU-α-L-arabinopyranoside	+	+/−	[56]
4MU-β-D-fucoside	+	+/−	[56]
4MU-β-D-galactoside	+	−	[56]
4MU-β-D-glucoside	−	+	[56]
4MU-β-D-glucoside	+	+	[56]
4MU-p-guanidinobenzoate (HCl)	+	+	[56]
4MU-α-D-mannopyranoside	−	+	[56]
4MU-β-D-ribofuranoside	+	+	[56]
Degradation tests			
Aesculin	+	+	[56]
Arbutin	+	+	[56]
Casein	−	−	[56]
Elastin	−	−	[56]
Guanine	−	−	[56]
Hypoxanthine	−	−	[56]
Keratin	−	−	[56]
Testosterone	+	+	[15]
Tyrosine	−	−	[15, 56]
Tweens	+	+	[56]
Xanthine	−	−	[56]
Growth in the presence of (%)			
Cobalt chloride (0.005)	+	+	[56]
Copper sulphate (0.01)	+	+	[56]
Crystal violet (0.001)	−	−	[15]
Ferrous sulphate (0.01)	+	+	[56]
Hydroxylamine HCl (0.05)	−	−	[56]
Lead acetate (0.01)	+	+	[56]
o-Nitrobenzoic acid (0.05)	−	+	[56]
Oleic acid (0.25, v/v)	+	+	[56]
Phenol (0.01)	+	+	[56]
Phenol (0.1)	−	−	[15, 56, 82]
Phenyl ethanol (0.02%)	−	+	[15, 82]
Potassium tellurite (0.04%)	−	+	[15, 82]
Potassium tellurite (0.5)	−	−	[56]
Pyronin G (0.1)	−	−	[56]
Sodium azide (0.005)	−	+	[56]
Sodium azide (0.01)	−	−	[15, 82]
Sodium chloride (5)	−	−	[56]
Sodium chloride (5%)	−	+	[15, 82]
Sodium deoxycholate (0.01)	−	+	[56]
Sodium nitrate (1)	−	−	[56]
Sodium salicylate (0.1)	−	+	[56]
Sodium selenite (0.001)	−	−	[56]
Thallous acetate (0.05)	−	−	[56]
Tetrazolium chloride (0.01)	−	−	[56]
Toluidine blue (0.03)	−	+	[56]
Teepol HB6 (0.05, v/v)	−	−	[56]
Zinc chloride (0.005)	−	−	[56]
Zinc chloride (0.01)	−	−	[56]
Growth at			
45°C	−	−	[15, 76]
pH4	−	−	[15]
pH5	−	+	[15, 82]
pH10	−	−	[15]
Survival at 60°C for 4 hours	−	−	[15]
Resistance to antibiotics and antibacterial agents (μgmL-1)			
Amikacin (2)	−	−	[55]
p-Aminosalicylic acid, Na salt (64)	−/+	+	[11, 55]
Amoxicillin (64)	+	+	[55]

Ampicillin (64)	+/−	+	[55]
Capreomycin sulphate (10)	−	+	[15]
Capreomycin sulphate (10)	−/+	−	[55]
Cephaloridine (64)	+	+	[55]
Cephapirin Na salt (64)	+	+	[55]
Chlortetracycline HCl (64)	−/+	−/+	[55]
D-Cycloserine (2)	+	+	[55]
Cycloserine	−	−	[11]
Dapsone (16)	+	+	[55]
Dapsone (100)	−	+	[15, 82]
Doxycycline HCl (8)	−	+/−	[55]
Doxycycline HCl (64)	−	−	[55]
Erythromycin (64)	−	+	[55]
Ethambutol HCl (4)	+	+	[15, 55]
Ethambutol HCl (64)	−/+	+	[15, 55, 82]
Ethionamide (5)	+	+	[11, 55]
Gentamycin sulphate (128)	−	−	[55]
Isoniazid (2)	+	+	[15, 55]
Kanamycin sulphate (2)	+	+	[55]
Kanamycin sulphate (16)	−	−	[11]
Lividomycin sulphate (16)	−	−	[55]
Lysozyme (50)	+	+	[15]
Lincomycin HCl (64)	+	+	[55]
Nalidixic acid Na salt (64)	−	+	[55]
Novobiocin (64)	+/−	+	[55]
Neomycin sulphate (128)	−	−	[55]
Oleandomycin phosphate (64)	−	+	[55]
Oxytetracycline HCl (64)	−	−	[55]
Paromomycin sulphate (64)	−	−	[55]
Penicillin (66 IU/mL)	−	+/−	[15]
Polymyxin B sulphate (64)	−	+	[55]
Prothionamide (10)	+	+	[15]
Rifampicin (16)	+	+	[55]
Rifampicin (20)	+	−	[15]
Streptomycin sulphate (1.6)	+	+	[11, 55]
Streptomycin sulphate (64)	−	+	[15]
Sulphamethazine (1.6)	+	+	[55]
Thiacetazone (10)	+	−/+	[55]
Trimethoprim + sulphamethoxazole (8)	+	+	[55]
Vancomycin HCl (64)	−	−	[55]
Viomycin sulphate (64)	−	−	[11, 55]
Growth on sole carbon source (1%)			
Acetamide	+	+	[56]
Acetic acid (Na salt)	+	+	[56]
Butane 1,3 diol	+	−	[15, 82]
Butane 2,3 diol	−	+	[15, 56, 82]
Ethanol	−	−	[15, 82]
Fructose	−	+	[56]
D(+)Galactose	−	−	[56]
D-Gluconic acid	+	+	[56]
D(+)Glucosamine HCl	−	+	[56]
Hippuric acid (Na salt)	−	−	[56]
Lactic acid (Na salt)	−	+	[56]
Malonic acid (Na salt)	−	−	[56]
Maltose	−	−	[56]
Mannitol	−	+	[56]
Oxalic acid (Na salt)	−	−	[56]
1,2-Propanediol	−	+	[56]
Pyruvic acid (Na salt)	−/+	+	[56]
D(+)Raffinose	−	−	[56]
Rhamnose	−	+	[56]
Rhamnose	−	−	[15, 82]
Salicin	−	+	[56]
Sucrose	+	−	[56]
Tartaric acid (Na salt)	−	−	[56]
Trehalose	−	+	[56]
D(+)Turanose	−	−	[56]

* References: Chamoiseau [11]; El Sanousi et al. [76]; Ridell and Goodfellow [15]; Ridell et al. [82]; Hamid [56]; Hamid and Goodfellow, [55]; ** slide catalase test.

CHEMOTAXONOMY

Glycolipids and Phospholipids. M. farcinogenes and M. senegalense have been found to contain trehalose dimycolate (cord factor), phosphatidylethanolamine, and phosphatidylinositol [4, 58]. Glycopeptidolipids (GPL), the so-called C-mycosides, have been found in some M. senegalense strains [16, 58]. Four groups of antigenic glycolipids have been detected in some M. senegalense strains [16]. The M. senegalense strains were considered to belong to two major groups. The first group which includes the majority of the strains as well as the type strain (NCTC 10956) has an alkali-stable glycopeptidolipids class of antigens [16, 59, 60]. The second group belongs to the alkali-labile acyl trehalose lipooligosaccharide class of antigens [16, 60]. The first group was found to share its properties with those described in M. peregrinum [16, 61] and M. porcinum [59], the same unusual distribution of the alaninol end of the molecules. These data reinforce the close taxonomic relationships between the three mycobacterial species and demonstrate the antigenicity of the new variants of mycobacterial glycopeptidolipids, whereas the second group has structures similar to those produced by the antigenic lipooligosaccharides of M. fortuitum [61, 62].

Mycolic acids. M. farcinogenes and M. senegalense strains contain mycolic acids that can be separated into α, α′, and epoxymycolates. Similar mycolic acid patterns are characteristic of M. chitae, M. fortuitum, M. peregrinum, M. smegmatis, and M. porcinum [63, 64]. Mycolic acids are B-hydroxy fatty acids substituted at the a-position with a moderately long aliphatic chain. The distribution of these molecules is restricted to strains in the suborder Corynebacterineae which include the genera Hoyosella, Amycolicicoccus, Corynebacterium, Dietzia, Gordonia, Hoyosella, Millisia, Mycobacterium, Nocardia, Rhodococcus, Segniliparus, Skermania, Smaragdicoccus, Tsukamurella, and Williamsia [65, 66]. These actinomycetes have an arabinogalactan-based cell wall type IV. The causal agents of bovine farcy can easily be discriminated from N. farcinica type strains on the basis of mycolic acid analysis. Nocardia species show a single mycolic acid spot on thin layer chromatography [50, 52, 67].

Members of M. farcinogenes and M. senegalense, like many other mycobacteria, undergo a characteristic cleavage reaction on pyrolysis gas chromatography. In addition to meroaldehyde, they release tetracosanoic acid (C24) as major ester fragment [52, 68]; some other mycobacteria, for example, M. tuberculosis, release hexacosanoic acids (C26).

El Sanousi and Tag El Din [51], using modified precipitation technique of Kanetsuna and Bartoli [69], were able to assign bovine farcy strains to the genus Mycobacterium. Later, Hamid et al. [16] developed a new effective mycolic acid precipitation method for the distinction between mycobacteria and other mycolic acid-containing taxa. The method was based on the precipitation of mycolic acids methyl esters in a mixture of acetonitrile and toluene (3 : 2, v/v). The method was proven to be useful, particularly to accommodate many isolates of bovine farcy to the genus Mycobacterium by giving copious white precipitate when acetonitrile and toluene were used to precipitate mycolic acid methyl esters.

ANTIGENICITY AND IMMUNOGENICITY

Awad and Karib [32] found that bovine farcy animals induced sensitivity to avian and mammalian tuberculins. This finding was later supported by Mostafa [70] who in addition used immunogens prepared from the causal agents of bovine farcy and it was found to give a profound reaction with high specificity and sensitivity than did the preparations from avian and mammalian strains. Magnusson and Mariat [71] have developed an immunological method based on the specificity of delayed-type skin reactions on guinea pigs for comparingNocardia strains including isolates from cases of bovine farcy. The method noticeably differentiated bovine farcy strains, which formed a homogeneous group that was readily separated from reference (type) strains of N. asteroides, N. brasiliensis, and N. farcinica. Comparative immunodiffusion studies by Ridell and Norlin [72], Ridell [73–75], and Ridell et al. [50] indicated that the bovine farcy organisms had stronger affinity to mycobacteria than to Nocardia. From these studies, two serological groups were mainly identified, the first group includes the N. farcinica ATCC 3318, which seemed to belong to the genus Nocardia, whereas members of the other group including farcy strains were more closely related to Mycobacterium strains. The distribution of precipitinogens showed that M. farcinogenes and M. senegalense were closely related and were found to share a large number of precipitinogens. Both species shared visible precipitinogens with some other mycobacterial strains, particularly M. fortuitum, M. peregrinum, and M. smegmatis [75].

Using gel diffusion precipitin test and immunoelectrophoresis, Shigidi et al. [38] found that most of the strains isolated from cases of bovine farcy in Sudan reacted with antiserum from N. farcinica but not with antiserum from M. tuberculosis and M. bovis. In other studies, these strains were proved to be mycobacteria and were classified as M. farcinogenes ([16, 51]). In separate studies, when antigen prepared from whole cells of M. farcinogenes was tested against sera collected from animals infected with bovine farcy, only traces of agglutinin were detected [76] but limited, though sharp, precipitin lines were detected in most of the sera [52]. These two findings imply that circulating antibodies were also involved in the immunity and protection mechanism of infection with M. farcinogenes. Enzyme linked immunosorbent assay (ELISA) was evaluated for the serodiagnosis of bovine farcy among clinically proved cattle. Whole cell homologous suspension of M. farcinogenes was used as antigen and the test revealed a sensitivity of 92.7% and a specificity of 97% [77].

On the basis of antigenic cell surface glycolipids, M. senegalense strains were found to fall into four serological groups [16], whereas the majority of M. farcinogenes did not contain such antigens. The structure of the main group of M. senegalense, which included the type strain, was determined as glycopeptidolipids [59, 60]. These glycolipids were highly reactive to homologous sera prepared from whole cell M. senegalense and to lesser extent with heterologous sera from M. peregrinum [16, 78].

A wild strain of M. farcinogenes (A24) was subjected first to serial passage (20) in modified Sauton's broth then in guinea pigs. The result of the vaccination with the attenuated strain in calves revealed that 75% of calves in the vaccinated group were protected and endured the challenge infection with a virulent freshly isolated M. farcinogenes [79].

MOLECULAR ANALYSIS

DNA-DNA homology studies have indicated that M. farcinogenes and M. senegalense were separate species. According to Baess [13], M. senegalense is moderately related to M. farcinogenes, M. fortuitum, and to M. peregrinum. This fact has been further authenticated by Rogall et al. [19]. Using genus specific oligonucleotide,M. farcinogenes and M. senegalense reacted positively in the mycobacterial system [80].

Earlier sequencing of the 16S rRNA showed a close relationship between M. chelonae, M. farcinogenes, M. fortuitum, and M. senegalense [19, 21]. M. farcinogenes, M. senegalense, M. chelonae, M. fortuitum, and M. peregrinum form a distinct evolutionary branch within the adaptive radiation accommodated by the genusMycobacterium [19–21]. These species form the rapidly growing nonchromogenic mycobacteria.

Consequent studies indicated the close phylogenetic relationship of farcy agents to members of the M. fortuitum complex [81]. With the appearance of new rapidly growing species, Adékambi and Drancourt [28] accommodated these into two subclusters: (i) M. peregrinum, M. septicum, M. neworleansense, and M. porcinum and (ii) M. farcinogenes, M. senegalense, M. houstonense, and M. fortuitum. These clustering and the subclusters agree with that of Schinsky et al. [25].

16S rRNA sequences of M. farcinogenes and M. senegalense are very similar and when using the Kirschner diagnostic helix 10 and helix 18 it is not possible to differentiate between the two species (Table 2). However, when using 16S-23S rDNA spacer, Hamid et al. [23] were able to distinguish between the two species with ample number of base substitution. Two probes designed on the basis of all of the available spacer sequences were evaluated for specificity, namely, biotin–3-TCAGCCAGCATCTGTAG and biotin–3-AGGAGTCTGTGCGCTGT, as probes for the rapid diagnosis of the disease from clinical specimens or for identification of unknown strains of M. farcinogenes or M. senegalense, respectively [23].

Table 2: Comparison of 16S rDNA signature sequences. The alignment comprises the two variable regions found in the 16S rRNA genes of selected members of species closely related to M. farcinogenes and M. senegalense; "-" indicates identity

	16S rRNA position number 177 (*E. coli* position)	16S rRNA position number 254 (*E. coli* position)
M. fortuitum	CGAAT ATGACCAC GCGCTTCAT GGTGT	TTGGTGGGG TAATGGCCT AC
M. houstonense	--G-- -G------ --------- -----	--------- --------- --
M. senegalense	--G-- -G------ --------- -----	--------- --------- --
M. farcinogenes	--G-- -G------ --------- -----	--------- --------- --
M. boenickei	----- -G----G- --T------ --G--	--------- --------- --
M. neworleansense	----- -G----G- --T------ --G--	--------- --------- --
M. porcinum	----- -G----G- --T------ --G--	--------- --------- --
M. septicum	----- ------G- --A----C- -----	--------- --------- --
M. peregrinum	----- ------G- --A----C- -----	--------- --------- --
M. alvei	----- -------T --A----C- -----	--------- --------- --

ANTIMICROBIAL SUSCEPTIBILITY

Most of the M. farcinogenes and M. senegalense strains tested in vitro were found susceptible to cycloserine [11], dapsone [15], or amikacin, doxycycline HCl (64 μg/mL), oxytetracycline HCl (64 μg/mL), and paromomycin sulphate (64 μg/mL) [55]. Susceptibilities to other antimicrobial agents and to various chemical agents are shown in Table 1.

CONCLUSIONS

Basic information about M. farcinogenes and M. senegalense is available in the literature. These actinomycetes are unique in their morphologies and exhibit some distinctive characteristics. These characteristics, notably, cell wall chemical markers and DNA sequence data, separate them from Nocardia farcinica and from closely related nonphotochromogenic rapidly growing mycobacteria. There are hardly any new reports of isolating these bacteria from cattle in recent times. On the contrary, limited numbers of reports have incriminated M. farcinogenes and M. senegalense as causal agents of human diseases.

CONFLICT OF INTERESTS

The author declares that he has no financial or personal relationships which may have inappropriately influenced him in writing this paper.

ACKNOWLEDGMENTS

The author is grateful to Professor M. Goodfellow (University of Newcastle), Professor S.M. El Sanousi, Professor M.T. Abu Samra (University of Khartoum), Professor Galal E. Al Azhari (Sudan University for Science and Technology), Professor D.E. Minnikin (University of Birmingham), Dr. A. Roth (Berlin Frei Universität), and Dr. Moh. Ahmed Hamád (Ministry of Animal Resources, Sudan) for their help and encouragement during previous bovine farcy research projects. These projects received supports from Alexander Humboldt Foundation, The Wellcome Trust (Grant no. 043935/Z/95/A), the International Foundation for Science (IFS; Grant no. B/2903), and the British Council (KHT/991/21/Vet).

REFERENCES

1. M. E. Hamid, "Epidemiology, pathology, immunology and diagnosis of bovine farcy: a review," Preventive Veterinary Medicine, vol. 105, no. 1-2, pp. 1–9, 2012.
2. E. Nocard, "Note sur la maladie de bceufs de la Guadeloupe connue sous le nom de farcin," Annales de l'Institut Pasteur, vol. 2, pp. 293–302, 1888.
3. World Organization for Animal Health (OIE), "Terrestrial Animal Health Code," Chapter 1.2. Criteria for listing diseases, Articles 1.2.1., 1.2.2. and 1.2.3., 2010, http://www.oie.int/fileadmin/Home/eng/Health_standards/tahc/2010/en_chapitre_1.1.2.htm#chapitre_1.1.2.
4. J. Asselineau, M. A. Laneelle, and G. Chamoiseau, "De l'aetiologie du farcin de zebus tchadiens. Nocardiose ou mycobacteriose? II Composition lipidique," Revue d'Elevage et de Medicine Veterinaire des Pays Tropicaux, vol. 22, pp. 205–209, 1969.
5. G. Chamoiseau, "De l'etiologie du farcin de zebus tchadiens Nocardiose ou mycobacteriose? I Etude bacteriologique et biochemique," Revue d'Elevage et de Medicine Veterinaire des Pays Tropicaux, vol. 22, pp. 195–204, 1969.
6. G. Chamoiseau, "De I'etiologie du farcin de zebus tchadiens Nocardiens ou mycobacteriose? I Activite amidasique," Revue d'Elevage et de Medicine Veterinaire des Pays Tropicaux, vol. 25, pp. 191–194, 1972.
7. G. Chamoiseau, "Mycobacterium farcinogenes agent causal du farcin du boeuf en Afrique," Annales de Microbiologie (Institut Pasteur), vol. 124, no. 2, pp. 215–222, 1973.
8. G. Chamoiseau, "Mycobacterium farcinogenes agent causal du farcin du boeuf en Afrique," Revue d›Elevage et de Medicine Veterinaire des Pays Tropicaux, vol. 32, pp. 135–141, 1974.
9. G. Chamoiseau and J. Asselineau, "Examen des lipides d›une souche de N farcinica: presence d›acides mycoloques," Compte Rendu Hebdomadaire des Seances de l›Academie des Sciences D, vol. 270, pp. 2603–2604, 1970.
10. S. M. El Sanousi, M. H. Tag El Din, and S. M. Abdel Wahab, "Classification of the bovine farcy organism," Tropical Animal Health and Production, vol. 9, no. 2, p. 124, 1977.
11. G. Chamoiseau, "Etiology of farcy in African bovines: nomenclature of the causal organisms Mycobacterium farcinogenes (Chamoiseau) and Mycobacterium senegalense (Chamoiseau) comb nov," International Journal of Systematic Bacteriology, vol. 29, no. 4, pp. 407–410, 1979.
12. L. G. Wayne and G. P. Kubica, "Genus Mycobacterium Lehmann and Neumann 1896 363 ALM," in Bergey›s Manual of Systematic Bacteriology, P. H. A. Sneath, N. S. Mair, M. E. Sharpe, and J. G. Holt, Eds., vol. 2, pp. 1436–1457, Williams & Wilkins, Baltimore, Md, USA, 1986.
13. I. Baess, "Deoxyribonucleic acid relatedness among species of rapidly growing mycobacteria," Acta Pathologica et Microbiologica Scandinavica B: Microbiology and Immunology, vol. 90, no. 5, pp. 371–375, 1982.
14. R. M. Hall and C. Ratledge, "Equivalence of mycobactins from Mycobacterium senegalense, Mycobacterium farcinogenes and Mycobacterium fortuitum," Journal of General Microbiology, vol. 131, no. 7, pp. 1691–1696, 1985.
15. M. Ridell and M. Goodfellow, "Numerical classification of Mycobacterium farcinogenes, Mycobacterium senegalense and related taxa," Journal of General Microbiology, vol. 129, no. 3, pp. 599–611, 1983.
16. M. E. Hamid, D. E. Minnikin, and M. Goodfellow, "A simple chemical test to distinguish mycobacteria from other mycolic-acid-containing actinomycetes," Journal of General Microbiology, vol. 139, no. 9, pp. 2203–2213, 1993.
17. M. E. Hamid, J. Chun, J. G. Magee, D. E. Minnikin, and M. Goodfellow, "Rapid characterisation and identification of mycobacteria using fluorogenic enzyme tests," Zentralblatt für Bakteriologie, vol. 280, no. 4, pp. 476–487, 1994.
18. J. G. Magee, M. Goodfellow, P. R. Sisson, R. Freeman, and N. F. Lightfoot, "Differentiation of Mycobacterium senegalense from related non-chromogenic mycobacteria using pyrolysis mass spectrometry," Zentralblatt für Bakteriologie, vol. 285, no. 2, pp. 278–284, 1997. ·
19. T. Rogall, J. Wolters, T. Flohr, and E. C. Bottger, "Towards a phylogeny and definition of species at the molecular level within the genus Mycobacterium," International Journal of Systematic Bacteriology, vol. 40, no. 4, pp. 323–330, 1990.
20. D. A. Stahl and J. W. Urbance, "The division between fast- and slow-growing species corresponds to natural relationships among the mycobacteria," Journal of Bacteriology, vol. 172, no. 1, pp. 116–124, 1990.
21. C. Pitulle, M. Dorsch, J. Kazda, J. Wolters, and E. Stackebrandt, "Phylogeny of rapidly growing members of the genus Mycobacterium," International Journal of Systematic Bacteriology, vol. 42, no. 3, pp. 337–343, 1992.
22. P. Kirschner, M. Kiekenbeck, D. Meissner, J. Wolters, and E. C. Bottger, "Genetic heterogeneity within Mycobacterium fortuitum complex species: genotypic criteria for identification," Journal of Clinical Microbiology, vol. 30, no. 11, pp. 2772–2775, 1992.
23. M. E. Hamid, A. Roth, O. Landt, R. M. Kroppenstedt, M. Goodfellow, and H. Mauch, "Differentiation between Mycobacterium farcinogenes and Mycobacterium senegalense strains based on 16S-23S ribosomal DNA internal transcribed spacer sequences," Journal of Clinical Microbiology, vol. 40, no. 2, pp. 707–711, 2002.
24. B. A. Brown-Elliott and R. J. Wallace Jr., "Clinical and taxonomic status of pathogenic nonpigmented or late-pigmenting rapidly growing mycobacteria," Clinical Microbiology Reviews, vol. 15, no. 4, pp. 716–746, 2002.
25. M. F. Schinsky, R. E. Morey, A. G. Steigerwalt et al., "Taxonomic variation in the Mycobacterium fortuitum third biovariant complex: description of Myobacterium

boenickei sp. nov., Mycobacterium houstonense sp. nov., Mycobacterium neworleansense sp. nov. and Mycobacterium brisbanense sp. nov. and recognition of Mycobacterium porcinum from human clinical isolates," International Journal of Systematic and Evolutionary Microbiology, vol. 54, no. 5, pp. 1653–1667, 2004.

26. S. Mignard and J. Flandrois, "A seven-gene, multilocus, genus-wide approach to the phylogeny of mycobacteria using supertrees," International Journal of Systematic and Evolutionary Microbiology, vol. 58, no. 6, pp. 1432–1441, 2008.

27. M. Tsukamura, H. Menoto, and H. Yugi, "Mycobacterium porcinum sp. nov., a porcine pathogen," International Journal of Systematic Bacteriology, vol. 33, no. 2, pp. 162–165, 1983.

28. T. Adékambi and M. Drancourt, "Dissection of phylogenetic relationships among 19 rapidly growing Mycobacterium species by 16S rRNA, hsp65, sodA, recA and rpoB gene sequencing," International Journal of Systematic and Evolutionary Microbiology, vol. 54, no. 6, pp. 2095–2105, 2004.

29. C. Diguimbaye-Djaibé, V. Vincent, E. Schelling et al., "Species identification of non-tuberculous mycobacteria from humans and cattle of Chad," Schweizer Archiv für Tierheilkunde, vol. 148, no. 5, pp. 251–256, 2006.

30. V. Guérin-Faublée, J. P. Flandrois, C. Pichat, M. L. Boschiroli, and B. Lamy, "Mycobacterium bourgelatiisp. nov., a rapidly growing, non-chromogenic species isolated from the lymph nodes of cattle," International Journal of Systematic and Evolutionary Microbiology, vol. 63, part 12, pp. 4669–4674, 2013.

31. G. Memery, P. Mornet, and A. Camara, "Premiers cas authentiques de farcin du bceuf en Afrique occidentale franaise," Revue d›Elevage et de Medicine Veterinaire des Pays Tropicaux, vol. 11, pp. 11–16, 1958.

32. F. I. Awad and A. A. Karib, "Studies on bovine farcy (nocardiosis) among cattle in the Sudan," Zentralblatt für Veterinärmedizin, vol. 5, no. 3, pp. 265–272, 1958.

33. M. El-Nasri, "Some observation on bovine farcy," The Veterinary Record, vol. 73, pp. 370–372, 1961.

34. I. E. Mostafa, "Studies on cattle nocardiosis (bovine farcy) in the Sudan," Sudan Journal of Veterinary Science and Animal Husbandry, vol. 7, pp. 1–9, 1962.

35. I. E. Mostafa, "Studies of bovine farcy in the Sudan. II. Mycology of the disease," Journal of Comparative Pathology, vol. 77, no. 2, pp. 231–237, 1967.

36. A. Perpezat, P. Destombes, and F. Mariat, "Histopathologic study of nocardiosis in oxen in Chad and biochemical characteristics of Nocardia farcinica," Revue d›Elevage et de Medicine Veterinaire des Pays Tropicaux, vol. 20, no. 3, pp. 429–435, 1967.

37. M. H. A. El-Kareem and A. A. Moustafa, "Bovine nocardiosis, tuberculosis and other caseous infections at Omdurman central abattoir," Sudan Journal of Veterinary Science and Animal Husbandry, vol. 15, pp. 57–60, 1974.

38. M. T. A. Shigidi, T. Mirghani, and M. T. Musa, "Characterisation of Nocardia farcinica isolated from cattle with bovine farcy," Research in Veterinary Science, vol. 28, no. 2, pp. 207–211, 1980.

39. M. A. Oyekunle and M. O. Ojo, "Preliminary observations on bovine cutaneous nocardiosis and dermatophilosis in the subhumid climate of southern Nigeria," Revue d›Elevage et de Medecine Veterinaire des Pays Tropicaux, vol. 41, no. 4, pp. 347–351, 1988.

40. P. H. Marchot, W. Amanfu, and P. L. Leroy, "Bovine farcy in the Accra plains of Ghana," Revue d›Elevage et de Medecine Veterinaire des Pays Tropicaux, vol. 42, no. 2, pp. 173–175, 1989. ·

41. R. J. Wallace Jr., B. A. Brown-Elliott, J. Brown et al., "Polyphasic characterization reveals that the human pathogen Mycobacterium peregrinum type II belongs to the bovine pathogen species Mycobacterium senegalense," Journal of Clinical Microbiology, vol. 43, no. 12, pp. 5925–5935, 2005.·

42. T. C. Wong, W. F. Chan, W. L. Tsang, S. H. Yeung, and F. K. Ip, "Mycobacterium farcinogenes infection after total hip arthroplasty," Journal of Arthroplasty, vol. 20, no. 5, pp. 684–687, 2005.·

43. I. E. Mostafa, "Bovine nocardiosis (cattle farcy): a review," The Veterinary Bulletin, vol. 36, pp. 189–193, 1966.

44. P. A. Olubunmi and A. O. Ayeni, "A description of an outbreak of bovine nocardiosis in Western Nigeria," Journal of Animal Production Research, vol. 3, pp. 127–138, 1983.

45. M. E. Hamid, Identification of bovine farcy by simple lipid analysis and rapid biochemical tests [M.S. thesis], University of Khartoum, Khartoum, Sudan, 1988.

46. B. M. Al Janabi, D. Branagan, and D. Danskin, "The trans stadial transmission of the bovine farcy organism, Nocardia farcinica, by the ixodid Amblyomma variegatum (Fabricius, 1794)," Tropical Animal Health and Production, vol. 7, no. 4, pp. 205–209, 1975.

47. S. T. Cowan and K. J. Steel, Cowan and Steel›s Manual for the Identification of Medical Bacteria, Cambridge University Press, New York, NY, USA, 1974.

48. R. E. Gordon and J. M. Mihm, "Identification of Nocardia caviae (Erikson) nov comb," Annals of the New York Academy of Sciences, vol. 98, pp. 628–636, 1962.

49. H. Mordarska, M. Mordarski, and M. Goodfellow, "Chemotaxonomic characters and classification of some nocardioform bacteria," Journal of General Microbiology, vol. 71, no. 1, pp. 77–86, 1972.

50. M. Ridell, M. Goodfellow, D. E. Minnikin, S. M. Minnikin, and I. G. Hutchinson, "Classification of Mycobacterium farcinogenes and Mycobacterium senegalense by immunodiffusion and thin-layer chromatography of long-chain components," Journal of General Microbiology, vol. 128, no. 6, pp. 1299–1307, 1982.

51. S. M. El Sanousi and M. H. Tag El Din, "On the aetiology of bovine farcy in the Sudan," Journal of General Microbiology, vol. 132, no. 6, pp. 1673–1675, 1986.

52. M. E. Hamid, G. E. Mohamed, M. T. Abu-Samra, S. M.

El-Sanousi, and M. E. Barri, “Bovine farcy: a clinico-pathological study of the disease and its aetiological agent,” Journal of Comparative Pathology, vol. 105, no. 3, pp. 287–301, 1991.

53. Deutsche Sammlung von Mikroorganismen und Zellkulturen (DSMZ), Catalogue Microorganisms, Leibniz-Institut DSMZ-Deutsche Sammlung von Mikroorganismen und Zellkulturen GmbH, 2012, http://www.dsmz.de/catalogues/details/culture/DSM.

54. M. E. Hamid and M. Goodfellow, “Rapid growth and increased biomass yield of Mycobacterium farcinogenes and some related taxa in broth and agar media,” Zentralblatt für Veterinärmedizin B, vol. 42, no. 7, pp. 397–404, 1995.

55. M. E. Hamid and M. Goodfellow, “In vitro antimicrobial susceptibility of bovine farcy organisms,” Revue d›Elevage et de Medicine Veterinaire des Pays Tropicaux, vol. 50, pp. 5–9, 1997.

56. M. E. Hamid, Classification and identification of actinomycetes associated with bovine farcy [Ph.D. thesis], University of Newcastle, Tyne and Wear, UK, 1994.

57. E. M. H. Wellington and S. T. Williams, “Preservation of actinomycete inoculum in frozen glycerol,” Microbios Letters, vol. 6, no. 23-24, pp. 151–157, 1977.

58. G. Laneelle, J. Asselineau, and G. Chamoiseau, “Presence de mycosides C′ (formes simplifiees de mycoside C) dans les bacteries isolees de bovins atteints du farcin,” FEBS Letters, vol. 19, no. 2, pp. 109–111, 1971.

59. L. M. L. Marin, M. Laneelle, D. Prome, and M. Daffe, “Structures of the glycopeptidolipid antigens of two animal pathogens: Mycobacterium senegalense and Mycobacterium porcinum,” European Journal of Biochemistry, vol. 215, no. 3, pp. 859–866, 1993.

60. G. S. Besra, S. S. Gurcha, K.-H. Khoo et al., “Characterization of the specific antigenicity of representatives of M. senegalense and related bacteria,” Zentralblatt für Bakteriologie, vol. 281, no. 4, pp. 415–432, 1994.

61. L. M. Lopez Marin, M. A. Laneelle, D. Prome, M. Daffe, G. Laneelle, and J.-C. Prome, “Glycopeptidolipids from Mycobacterium fortuitum. A variant in the structure of C-mycosides,” Biochemistry, vol. 30, no. 43, pp. 10536–10542, 1991.

62. G. S. Besra, M. R. McNeil, and P. J. Brennan, “Characterization of the specific antigenicity of Mycobacterium fortuitum,” Biochemistry, vol. 31, no. 28, pp. 6504–6509, 1992.

63. D. E. Minnikin, S. M. Minnikin, J. H. Parlett, and M. Goodfellow, “Mycolic acid patterns of some rapidly-growing species of Mycobacterium,” Zentralblatt für Bakteriologie, Mikrobiologie und Hygiene A, vol. 259, no. 4, pp. 446–460, 1985.

64. M. Luquin, V. Ausina, F. Lopez-Calahorra et al., “Evaluation of practical chromatographic procedures for identification of clinical isolates of mycobacteria,” Journal of Clinical Microbiology, vol. 29, no. 1, pp. 120–130, 1991.

65. M. Goodfellow and L. A. Maldonado, “The families Dietziaceae, Gordoniaceae, Nocardiaceae and Tsukamurellaceae,” in The Prokaryotes, M. Dworkin, S. Falkow, E. Rosenberg, K. H. Schleifer, and E. Stackebrandt, Eds., vol. 3 of Archaea and Bacteria: Firmicutes, Actinomycetes, pp. 843–888, Springer, New York, NY, USA, 3rd edition, 2006.

66. M. A. Lanéelle, A. Launay, L. Spina et al., “A novel mycolic acid species defines two novel genera of the Actinobacteria, Hoyosella and Amycolicicoccus,” Microbiology, vol. 158, part 3, pp. 843–855, 2012.

67. D. E. Minnikin, L. Alshamaony, and M. Goodfellow, “Differentiation of Mycobacterium, Nocardia and related taxa by thin layer chromatographic analysis of whole organism methanolysates,” Journal of General Microbiology, vol. 88, no. 1, pp. 200–204, 1975.

68. M. P. Lechevalier, A. C. Horan, and H. A. Lechevalier, “Lipid composition in the classification of nocardiae and mycobacteria,” Journal of Bacteriology, vol. 105, no. 1, pp. 313–318, 1971.

69. F. Kanetsuna and A. Bartoli, “A simple chemical method to differentiate Mycobacterium from Nocardia,” Journal of General Microbiology, vol. 70, no. 2, pp. 209–212, 1972.

70. I. E. Mostafa, “The relationship between bovine farcy and tuberculosis,” The Veterinary Record, vol. 81, no. 3, pp. 74–76, 1967.

71. M. Magnusson and F. Mariat, “Delineation of Nocardia farcinica by delayed type skin reactions on guinea pigs,” Journal of General Microbiology, vol. 51, no. 1, pp. 151–158, 1968.

72. M. Ridell and M. Norlin, “Serological study of Nocardia by using mycobacterial precipitation reference systems,” Journal of Bacteriology, vol. 113, no. 1, pp. 1–7, 1973.

73. M. Ridell, “Taxonomic study of Nocardia farcinica using serological and physiological characters,” International Journal of Systematic Bacteriology, vol. 25, no. 2, pp. 124–132, 1975.

74. M. Ridell, “Immunodiffusion analysis of Mycobacterium farcinogenes, Mycobacterium senegalense and some other mycobacteria,” Zentralblatt für Bakteriologie, Parasitenkunde, Infektionskrankheiten und Hygiene, supplement 2, pp. 235–241, 1981.

75. M. Ridell, “Immunodiffusion analyses of Mycobacterium farcinogenes, Mycobacterium senegalense and some other mycobacteria,” Journal of General Microbiology, vol. 129, no. 3, pp. 613–619, 1983.

76. S. M. El Sanousi, M. A. Salih, M. T. Mousa, M. H. Tag El Din, and S. A. Ali, “Further studies on the properties of the aetiology of bovine farcy isolated from Sudanese cattle,” Revue d›Elevage et de Medecine Veterinaire des Pays Tropicaux, vol. 32, no. 2, pp. 135–141, 1979.

77. H. A. El Hussein and M. E. Hamid, “Evaluation of ELISA in the serodiagnosis of bovine farcy,” Tropical Animal Health and Production, vol. 41, no. 4, pp. 617–622, 2009.

78. M. E. Hamid, M. Ridell, D. E. Minnikin, and M. Goodfellow, “Serotaxonomic analysis of glycolipids

from Mycobacterium chelonae-M. fortuitum complex and bovine farcy strains," Zentralblatt für Bakteriologie, vol. 288, no. 1, pp. 23–34, 1998.

79. E. A. M. Mukhtar, A. A. Alwali, A. M. S. El Eragi, M. E. Hamid, and H. A. El Hussein, "Attenuated Mycobacterium farcinogenes strain A24 as a protective vaccine candidate against bovine farcy," Journal of Animal and Veterinary Advances, vol. 4, pp. 269–273, 2005.

80. B. Boddinghaus, T. Rogall, T. Flohr, H. Blocker, and E. C. Bottger, "Detection and identification of mycobacteria by amplification of rRNA," Journal of Clinical Microbiology, vol. 28, no. 8, pp. 1751–1759, 1990.

81. P. Kirschner, B. Springer, U. Vogel et al., "Genotypic identification of mycobacteria by nucleic acid sequence determination: report of a 2-year experience in a clinical laboratory," Journal of Clinical Microbiology, vol. 31, no. 11, pp. 2882–2889, 1993.

82. M. Ridell, M. Goodfellow, and M. A. Abdulle, "Identification of actinomycetes isolated from cases of bovine farcy in the Sudan," Zentralblatt für Bakteriologie, Mikrobiologie und Hygiene A, vol. 259, no. 1, pp. 43–50, 1985.

CHAPTER 31

ASSOCIATIONS BETWEEN MYCOBACTERIUM AVIUM SUBSP. PARATUBERCULOSIS ANTIBODIES IN BULK TANK MILK, SEASON OF SAMPLING AND PROTOCOLS FOR MANAGING INFECTED COWS

Casey L Cazer, Rebecca M Mitchell, Kellie M Cicconi-Hogan, Michael Gamroth, Roxann M Richert, Pamela L Ruegg and Ynte H Schukken

Keywords: Cattle, *Mycobacteirum avium,* subsp., *paratuberculosis,* Antibodies, Bulk-tank milk, ELISA

BACKGROUND

Johne's disease, a chronic disease caused by infection with *Mycobacterium avium* subsp. *paratuberculosis*(MAP), costs the US dairy industry $200 to $250 million annually due to increased cow replacement costs and reduction in milk production [1] and also decreased fertility in high-shedding animals [2]. The control of Johne's disease requires good herd management practices, such as preventing fecal contamination of feed and water and testing replacement cattle for MAP. Good management procedures focus on reducing transmission and the introduction of MAP into the herd [3]. Because MAP infected cows may not show clinical signs during their productive lifetime [4], it is important to test many cows in a herd to properly assess MAP infection prevalence.

A simple, quick test that provides an estimate of herd-level MAP prevalence would allow herd managers to respond by changing their management strategies, thus improving their probability of eliminating and preventing MAP infection in the long term. MAP surveillance and monitoring has been proposed as an ideal testing strategy to ensure that infection pressures are low while keeping the cost of testing low [5]. Herd-level MAP-prevalence testing often involves pooled fecal samples used for culture or PCR. However pooled sample strategies are still time-consuming because individual cows or environmental areas must be sampled [6].

The magnitude of an ELISA test result for MAP antibodies in the milk of individual cows has been reported to be related to the likelihood of an animal testing positive on a fecal culture for MAP [7]. Collins et al. [7] also reported that the level of MAP shedding, considered a measure of the stage of infection, was directly related to the ability of an individual milk ELISA test to detect an infected animal. The Parachek commercial ELISA tests have been found to have a high specificity and a sensitivity ranging from 21 to 67% on individual milk samples [8]. When used on bulk tank milk, the Pourquier ELISA test had a sensitivity of 57% [9]. Additionally, van Weering et al. [10] demonstrated that certified MAP-negative herds had a low sample/positive (S/P) ratio on bulk milk Pourquier ELISA tests and they showed that the likelihood of a herd having a MAP-infected animal increased with increasing bulk milk ELISA S/P ratio. Finally, bulk milk ELISA tests have been shown to perform similarly to serum ELISA tests at the herd level, with a sensitivity of 56 to 83%, when fecal culture is used as a reference [11]. The sensitivity can be improved by using modified protocols [8, 12]. Together, these published

Citation: Casey L Cazer, Rebecca M Mitchell, Kellie M Cicconi-Hogan, Michael Gamroth, Roxann M Richert, Pamela L Ruegg and Ynte H Schukken, Associations between Mycobacterium avium subsp. paratuberculosis antibodies in bulk tank milk, season of sampling and protocols for managing infected cows, DOI: 10.1186/1746-6148-9-234.

results on bulk milk and individual cow milk provide a logical validation for the use of bulk milk ELISA corrected optical density (OD) as a continuous outcome value to scale the risk of MAP infection in the lactating herd.

Determining associations between management factors and bulk milk ELISA values will provide a simple, efficient method for farms to respond to herd MAP infections by changing their management practices or understanding risks associated with certain management practices. However, few studies have used bulk milk ELISA to identify herd-level risk factors for increased MAP prevalence, while studies relating individual animal fecal or serum test results to management practices are more common (e.g. [13, 14]).

The objective of this study, therefore, is to relate bulk tank milk ELISA optical density with potential risk factors for MAP prevalence in 233 farms. Our aim was to determine if particular management practices and herd characteristics are associated with increased bulk milk ELISA values.

RESULTS

The median herd size was 57 for organic farms and 70 for conventional farms included in the multivariate model. Herd size ranged from 20 to 723 on the organic farms and 26 to 535 on the conventional farms. Organic farms produced an average of 14,900 lbs of milk per cow per year whereas conventional farms in the model produced an average of 20,637 lbs per cow annually. All 170 of the organic farms grazed their cattle whereas 25 conventional herds grazed and 38 conventional farms did not graze. All of the non-grazing farms allowed heifers to graze pasture.

The corrected OD, for all herds, ranged from -0.098 to 0.37 with a mean of -0.023 and a standard deviation of 0.047. The range was -0.098 to 0.17 for herds included in the multivariate model. The mean of the included herds was -0.024 and the standard deviation was 0.037. There were two farms that had a corrected OD greater than 0.17 and these were excluded from the multivariate model due to missing data.

All of the variables initially included in the multivariate model are summarized in Table 1. The stepwise order of removal from the final regression model was as follows: written plan for Johne's disease (P=0.95), parity (P=0.89), calving area (P=0.83), Jersey herd (P=0.82), spreading manure (P=0.75), source of drinking water (P=0.72), open farm (P=0.59), sine seasonality (P=0.48), average yield (P=0.41), heifer and cow contact on pasture (P=0.39), Johne's program (P=0.43), and calf housing (P=0.38). The variables remaining in the final multivariate model are summarized in Table 2.

Table 1: List of variables included in GLMSELECT procedure to produce final multivariate model

Variable	Type	Description
Production	Binary	Organic or Conventional
State	Nominal	NY, OR, or WI
Herd size	Ordinal	< 100, 100 to 200, or > 200
Parity	Continuous	The average lactation of all lactating cows at the time of the survey
Average yield	Continuous	Average annual milk production per cow
Calf housing	Nominal	Always housed in individual pens or areas; sometimes housed in groups or with contact to cows; always housed in groups or with contact to cows
Description of calving area	Nominal	Dedicated calving area; area shared with lactating cows; or area sometimes shared with sick cows
Heifer and cow contact on pasture	Nominal	Heifers grazing a pasture with or after the cows; before the cows; or heifers and cows do not graze the same pasture
Jersey	Binary	Mostly Jersey or not mostly Jersey herd
Johne's procedures	Nominal	Procedures for MAP-positive cows: cull after calving or dry off; cull immediately; keep; never observed clinical Johne's disease
Johne's program	Binary	Participation in Johne's program
Open farm	Binary	Some or no entering animals
Seasonality sine	Continuous	$\mathrm{Sin}(2\pi \frac{\mathrm{Day}}{365})$, where day is a continuous variable from 1 to 365
Seasonality cosine	Continuous	$\mathrm{Cos}(2\pi \frac{\mathrm{Day}}{365})$, where day is a continuous variable from 1 to 365
Source of drinking water	Nominal	Primary source of drinking water for 60 days prior to survey: well; municipal water; or surface water
Spreading manure	Binary	Manure spreading on pasture or fields that will be consumed by animals
Written plan for Johne's disease	Binary	Written herd plan for managing Johne's disease

Table 2: Summary of linear regression model

		Multivariate model		
Variable	**Description**	**β Coefficient**	**Standard error**	**P-value**
Intercept		−0.045	0.008	< .001
Production	Conventional	−0.003	0.004	0.400
	Organic	0	-	-
Herd size	< 100	0.010	0.007	0.175
	100 to 200	0.003	0.008	0.734
	> 200	0	-	-
State	NY	0.003	0.004	0.463
	OR	0.013	0.007	0.069
	WI	0	-	-
Johne's procedures	Cull after calving or dry off	0.020	0.009	0.025
	Cull immediately	0.010	0.005	0.035
	Keep	0.018	0.007	0.019
	Never observed clinical Johne's disease	0	-	-
Seasonality	$Cosine(2\pi \frac{Day}{365})$	−0.030	0.003	< .001

Linear regression model on *Mycobacterium avium* subsp. *paratuberculosis* ELISA optical density from bulk tank milk samples of 233 farms. Multivariate model was built by backwards stepwise elimination and started with all variables listed in Table 1.

The final multivariate model residuals were approximately normal with a slight skew to the right. However, it may be expected that the PROC GLM procedure still produces valid results when the assumption of error normality is mildly violated [15].

None of the included study design variables that were forced into the models were significant in the final multivariate model (Table 2). The cosine seasonality curve was very significant ($P<0.0001$). It demonstrated a peak in OD during the summer months and a trough during the winter months. The regression coefficient of -0.03 indicates the maximum drop in winter of the corrected OD and the maximum increase of +0.03 in summer. The seasonality is most evident in the farms sampled in late 2010 through 2011 (Figure 1). Seasonal calving farms and non-grazing farms were well distributed across the sampling time frame (Figure 1). There were 46 farms in the final multivariate model that indicated they used seasonal calving practices. Of these 46 farms, 42 responded that they tried to calve in the spring, 15 tried to calve in the summer, 21 in the fall and 5 in the winter. Seasonal farms did not necessarily calve over just one season, and all farms with fall or winter calving also had at least one additional calving season. The bulk milk ELISA value of seasonal calving farms differed with season of sampling, with a maximum value in the spring and continually decreasing to a minimum in the winter (Figure 1).

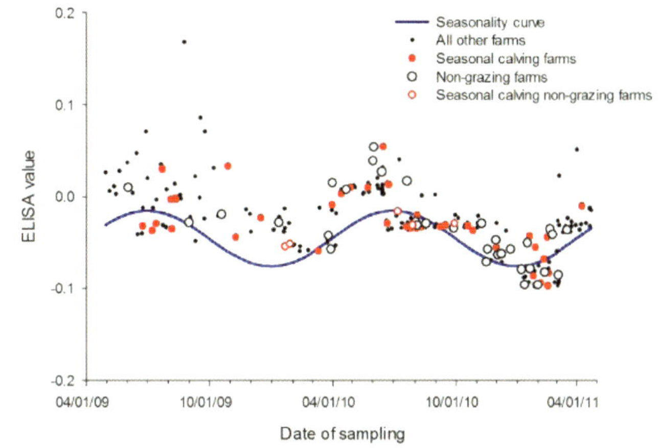

Figure 1: Seasonality in ELISA optical density. Bulk tank milk optical density of *Mycobacterium avium* subsp. *paratuberculosis* ELISA by date of sampling. Solid blue line fitted from cosine seasonality variable with all other variables set to baseline. Herds with seasonal calving practices are red dots. Open circles represent farms that do not graze their cattle. Red open circles are seasonal calving farms that do not graze. Solid dots represent all other farms included in final multivariate model.

The procedure for managing MAP-positive cows was the only other significant variable in the multivariate model. Compared to farms that had never observed clinical Johne's disease, farms that kept MAP-positive cows had a significant increase of 0.018 in their bulk milk OD ($P=0.019$). Farms that culled MAP-positive cows also had significant increases in bulk milk ELISA value when compared to farms without a history of Johne's disease but those that culled the cow immediately had a much smaller increase ($\beta=0.010$, $P=0.035$) than those that culled the cow after a period of delay, such as after her next calving ($\beta=0.020$, $P=0.025$). The final multivariate model explained 40% of the variation in bulk tank ELISA OD.

DISCUSSION

Bulk milk could have a high concentration of MAP antibodies because a dairy herd has a high prevalence of MAP infected cows or because a few infected cows produce large quantities of MAP antibodies. Variation in milk MAP antibody concentration within groups of fecal-positive and groups of fecal-negative cows has been observed due to a small number of cows producing a high level of antibodies and changes in antibody production within individual cows over time [16]. A study by van Weering et al. [10] showed that a 100-fold dilution of a positive individual milk ELISA sample may still result in a positive ELISA result, indicating that a few positive cows may impact the bulk milk ELISA result. Given the relatively small herd sizes in our study, it is clear that a few cows producing high concentrations of antibodies may influence bulk milk ELISA titers. The precise impact of a single ELISA positive cow would depend on the herd size, milk production, and the difference between the individual milk antibody concentration of a particular cow and the average antibody concentration of the rest of the herd. Therefore, some farms may have higher ELISA values than average because they have higher than average MAP infection rates or because they have some cows producing high concentrations of MAP antibodies. Careful comparison of individual cow milk ELISA tests and cow milk production level to a bulk tank test would be required to differentiate between farms that have several infected, average antibody-producing cows, and those that have a limited number of animals with high antibody titers.

In our model, the location of a farm (NY, OR, or WI) was not significantly associated with corrected OD. However, other studies have found that herds in the Midwest are more likely to be positive for Johne's disease [14] and observe clinical signs of Johne's disease in their herd [17]. Herd size, another study design variable, despite not being significantly associated with ELISA results in this study has previously been found to be positively associated with herd infection status, with larger herds having a greater risk [14, 18]. Additionally, Wells and Wagner [14] observed a positive association between group housing for calves and the herd infection status whereas our model did not find a significant association between types of calf housing and ELISA result. Spreading manure on forage fields [13] and open water sources [19] have also been shown to be associated with a higher risk of MAP infection, but were not significantly associated with corrected OD in our model. Finally, other studies have demonstrated an increased risk of Johne's disease with high parity and Jersey breed cows [18], although those variables did not remain in our multivariate model.

The significant seasonal effect, with MAP antibodies highest in the summer and lowest in the winter (Figure 1), represents a change in antibody secretion into bulk milk across the seasons. Seasonal calving could account for this periodic change in antibodies because milk antibodies are, on average, greatest at the beginning and end of lactation [16]. A farm that uses seasonal calving would see a herd-level increase in bulk milk antibodies, including antibodies against MAP, during or shortly after the calving season when most of their cows are just starting to lactate. This could result in high optical densities from the detection of MAP-specific and non-specific antibodies. The bulk milk ELISA value of seasonal calving farms, the majority of which indicated that they attempt to calve their cows in the spring, was greatest during the spring. This supports a days-in-milk dependent change in antibody secretion as a potential explanation for the seasonal trend in MAP antibodies in milk (Figure 1). Thus, seasonal calving could explain some of the seasonal variation but not all since only 46 of the 233 farms in the multivariate model used seasonal calving and non-seasonal calving farms still show a seasonal trend in OD (Figure 1). The seasonal variation also exists in non-grazing conventional farms (Figure 1), suggesting that the seasonal variation in MAP antibodies is not limited to grazing farms, which may have inherent seasonality in their calvings due to seasonal nutritional differences regardless of planned seasonal calving practices. Additionally, the seasonality variable remains significant ($P<0.0001$) after removing all grazing farms from the final multivariate model.

Another possible explanation for the seasonal change in antibodies is a seasonal fluctuation in MAP load. It is unlikely that MAP prevalence changes seasonally on any given farm but the MAP load in the environment or in the cows could potentially change with the seasons. A previous study found a higher prevalence of MAP-positive carcasses, as determined by ileum and lymph node cultures and PCR, in the spring than in other seasons [20]. Additionally, an increase in viable MAP isolated from retail milk in the summer has been shown [21]. Humoral responses are known to occur in subclinical MAP infections, which results in activated B cells producing antibodies [22]. It has previously been suggested that MAP exposure can trigger antibody production in infection-resistant adult cattle, possibly resulting in an increased MAP ELISA titer [7]. Thus it is possible that the increase in MAP load of individual animals during the spring and summer could result in an increased humoral immune response in herdmates and therefore increase antibody levels in milk.

If bulk milk MAP ELISA is used as an indicator of MAP infection, it needs to be corrected for the seasonal changes in MAP milk antibodies. Consistently sampling during only one season may need to be recommended in order to compare ELISA results across time at one farm or among farms. Our results would need to be confirmed by similar studies to make such recommendations with more confidence.

Both culling and keeping cows known to be MAP-infected are associated with an increase in bulk milk ELISA value compared to herds without a history of clinical Johne's disease, which suggests that farms with protocols for MAP-positive cows in place are more likely infected with MAP and possibly have a higher MAP prevalence. The larger increase in bulk milk OD associated with keeping MAP-positive cows or culling them after calving compared to the small increase in OD associated with culling MAP-positive cows immediately was not statistically significant ($P=0.25$). However, it has previously been suggested that culling cows immediately is the best method for controlling MAP antibodies in bulk milk. Lu et al. [23] demonstrated the importance of culling positive animals immediately after detection in order to control MAP transmission. MAP-positive cows that are kept in the herd for any period of time could increase the bulk milk MAP antibody titer by producing MAP antibodies in their milk and by re-exposing other cows, which may then begin secreting MAP antibodies into milk. This would be particularly true for cows with a progressive course of disease, in which antibodies rise rapidly as the cow progresses from moderate to heavy fecal shedding [24].

CONCLUSION

In summary, increased MAP antibody concentrations in bulk milk were associated with season of sampling and the protocols that were used on the farm for managing MAP-positive cows. The association between the season of sampling and MAP antibody concentration could be the result of seasonal variations in MAP in cows and in the environment, and could be related to seasonal calving practices. This seasonal change in MAP antibodies in bulk milk will need to be considered when using bulk milk ELISA as a MAP surveillance tool. The significance of protocols to manage MAP-positive cows pointed towards the importance of culling known MAP-positive cows immediately.

METHODS

Study and survey

Data came from a large cross-sectional study of 292 farms conducted between March 2009 and May 2011 that focused on comparing organic and conventional dairy farms. The study has previously been described in more detail [25]. Briefly, to be included in the study, farms had at least 20 lactating cows and had been shipping milk for 2 full years prior to the study; organic farms must have been shipping certified organic milk for these 2 years. Organic herds in New York, Oregon, and Wisconsin were identified through county extension agents, personal contacts and organic certifying organizations. Conventional herds were identified from lists of licensed dairy farmers, which were obtained from the departments of agriculture in New York, Oregon and Wisconsin, and were located within 50 miles of the identified organic farms. Conventional farms were size-category matched to organic farms based on three herd-size groups: 20 to 99 cows, 100 to 199 cows, and more than 200 cows. Conventional to organic herd ratios were found to be different in each state so farms were matched accordingly: 3 organic to 1 conventional in NY, 1 organic to 1 conventional in OR, and 2 organic to 1 conventional in WI. Conventional herds were designated as non-grazing if less than 30% of the lactating cows' dry matter intake came from pasture during the grazing season. Non-grazing farms could allow heifers to graze pasture.

A questionnaire was used on all farms to identify farm management practice and herd performance. The questionnaire has been described in detail [25] and is available online [26]. All the inters were conducted by a single person within each state. The interers had been trained in administering and scoring the questionnaire in a consistent manner across states. The Institutional Re Board at Oregon State University approved the use of human subjects for the questionnaire, reference number 3995. Herds that indicated that they were seasonal calving herds were further classified by the season in which they tried to calve their cows. Seasonal calving farms were able to designate one or more seasons as a calving season on the questionnaire but the questionnaire did not require specifying a main or primary calving season. Study personnel collected bulk tank samples on the same visit as questionnaire administration. Bulk milk samples were sent to Quality Milk Production Services at Cornell University (Ithaca, NY). Samples were tested for *Salmonella spp.*, *Listeria monocytogenes*, Shiga toxin producing *E. coli*, *Mycoplasma bovis*, Bovine Virus Diarrhea virus, antibodies against *Mycobacterium avium* subsp. *paratuberculosis* (MAP) and mastitis-causing bacteria. Samples were then sent to Dairy One Cooperative in Ithaca, NY for standard milk quality assays.

Enzyme linked immunosorbent assay

Bulk tank samples were analyzed using the commercially available Parachek ELISA (product number 63308) according to the directions provided by the manufacturer (Prionics, Zurich, Switzerland). Briefly, 100 μL of each bulk milk sample was diluted with 100 μL of Green Diluent, containing *Mycobacterium phlei*, and incubated at room temperature for 30-60 minutes. Then 100 μL of each sample and 100 μL of the manufacturer-provided positive and negative controls were added to microtitre plates coated with *M. paratuberculosis*. The plates were shaken and incubated at room temperature for 30 minutes. Plates were washed 6 times with wash buffer at room temperature. Then 100 μL of conjugate reagent (Horseradish peroxidase labeled anti-bovine Ig) was added to each well. The plates were again shaken, incubated at room temperature for 30 minutes, and washed 6 times with wash buffer. Next 100 μL of enzyme substrate solution (DMSO) was added to each well and the plates were incubated and shaken at room temperature until the positive controls reached an optical density of .35 to .40 with a 620-650 nm filter. Finally, 50 μL of enzyme stopping solution (0.5 M H_2SO_4) was mixed into each well and the absorbance of each well was read with a 450 nm filter. The Parachek ELISA optical density result is reported as a numerical value, which is classified as positive or negative in relation to a cut-off value equal to the average negative control plus 0.10. The average optical density of the two negative controls on each plate was subtracted from the sample optical densities of the same plate [11, 27] to account for inter-plate variation. This can result in the corrected optical density being less than 0 [27]. This corrected optical density value (optical density minus average negative control) was used as the continuous outcome variable for statistical analysis.

Statistical analysis

Descriptive analyses were performed on independent and dependent variables included in the multivariate model. The key outcome variable was the corrected bulk milk ELISA optical density. Management factors and other variables of interest were identified in the dataset based on an *a-priori* rationale that they were associated with MAP antibodies in milk (Table 1). These variables of interest included aspects of herd management (production system, written plan for Johne's disease, procedures for MAP-positive cows, participation in a Johne's program), herd descriptors (state, herd size, average parity, average yield, Jerseys), and Johne's disease specific risk factors (spreading manure, contact between heifers and cows on pasture, calf housing, calving area, open farm, source of drinking water). Variables to describe seasonality were developed using sine and cosine functions as previously described: $\text{sine}\left(2\pi\frac{Day}{365}\right)$ and $\text{cosine}\left(2\pi\frac{Day}{365}\right)$ [28]. Stepwise backwards least-squares linear regression (PROC GLMSELECT, SAS 9.3, Inst. Inc., 2011) was used to build a multivariate model with a constant sample size of 233 farms. Fifty-nine farms were excluded from this analysis due to missing data from one or more variables evaluated for inclusion in the multivariate model. The study design variables (state, herdsize size category, production system) were forced into the model (INCLUDE option) because they determined the inclusion of herds in the study. All other variables were selected based on statistical significance at the 0.05 level. The final multivariate model was in the form:

$$
\begin{aligned}
\text{CORRECTED}_{\text{OD}} = {} & \beta 0 + \beta 1(\mathit{HERDSIZE\_} < 100) \\
& + \beta 2(\mathit{HERDSIZE\_}100\text{–}200) \\
& + \beta 3(\mathit{STATE\_NY}) + \beta 4(\mathit{STATE\_OR}) \\
& + \beta 5(\mathit{PRODUCTION\_SYSTEM}) \\
& + \beta 6(\mathit{COSINE\_SEASON}) \\
& + \beta 7(\mathit{SINE\_SEASON}) + \sum_{i=1}^{n} \beta_i X_i + \varepsilon
\end{aligned}
$$

where OD is optical density, β_0 is the intercept, β_1 and β_2 are the coefficients of the herd size variable, β_3 and $\beta_4$are the coefficients of the state variable, β_5 is the coefficient of the production system variable, β_6 and β_7 are the coefficients of the cosine and sine season variables respectively, β_i represents the coefficients of other risk factor variables X_i (i=1 to n), and ϵ is a random error term assumed to be normally distributed with mean 0. This assumption was validated by examining the distribution of residuals.

DECLARATIONS

Competing interests

The authors declare that they have no competing interests.

Authors' contributions

CLC: performed the statistical analysis and drafted the manuscript. RMM: performed the statistical analysis and drafted the manuscript. KMCH: designed and carried out the survey. MG: designed the survey. RMR: designed and carried out the survey. PLR: designed the survey. YHS: assisted with statistical analysis and survey design, and helped draft the manuscript. All authors read and approved the final manuscript.

REFERENCES

1. Ott SL, Wells SJ, Wagner BA: Herd-level economic losses associated with Johne's disease on US dairy operations. Prev Vet Med. 1999, 40: 179-192. 10.1016/S0167-5877(99)00037-9.
2. Smith RL, Strawderman RL, Schukken YH, Wells SJ, Pradhan AK, Espejo LA, Whitlock RH, Van Kessel JS, Smith JM, Wolfgang DR, Gröhn YT: Effect of Johne's disease status on reproduction and culling in dairy cattle. J Dairy Sci. 2010, 93: 3513-3524. 10.3168/jds.2009-2742.
3. Collins MT: Clinical approach to control of bovine paratuberculosis. J Am Vet Med Assoc. 1994, 204: 208-210.
4. Manning EJ, Collins MT: Mycobacterium avium subsp paratuberculosis: Pathogen, pathogenesis and diagnosis. Rev Sci Tech. 2001, 20: 133-150.
5. Collins MT, Gardner IA, Garry FB, Roussel AJ, Wells SJ: Consensus recommendations on diagnostic testing for the detection of paratuberculosis in cattle in the United States. J Am Vet Med Assoc. 2006, 229: 1912-1919. 10.2460/javma.229.12.1912.
6. Collins MT: Diagnosis of paratuberculosis. Vet Clin Food Anim. 2011, 27: 581-591. 10.1016/j.cvfa.2011.07.013.
7. Collins MT, Wells SJ, Petrini KR, Collins JE, Schultz RD, Whitlock RH: Evaluation of five antibody detection tests for diagnosis of bovine paratuberculosis. Clin Diagn Lab Immunol. 2005, 12: 685-692.
8. Slana I, Paolicchi F, Janstova B, Navratilova P, Pavlik I: Detection methods for Mycobacterium avium subsp. paratuberculosis in milk and milk products: a re. Vet Med-Czech. 2008, 53: 283-306.
9. Wilson DJ, Rood K, Biswas P, Byrem TM: Herd-level prevalence of Johne's disease in Utah and adjacent areas of the Intermountain West as detected by a bulk-tank milk surveillance project. J Dairy Sci. 2010, 93: 5792-5797. 10.3168/jds.2010-3481.
10. van Weering H, van Schaik G, van der Meulen A, Waal M, Franken P, van Maanen K: Diagnostic performance of the Pourquier ELISA for detection of antibodies against Mycobacterium avium subspecies paratuberculosis in individual milk and bulk milk samples of dairy herds. Vet Microbiol. 2007, 125: 49-58. 10.1016/j.vetmic.2007.05.010.
11. Lombard JE, Byrem TM, Wagner BA, McCluskey BJ: Comparison of milk and serum enzyme-linked immunosorbent assays for diagnosis of Mycobacterium avium subspecies paratuberculosis infection in dairy cattle. J Vet Diagn Invest. 2006, 18: 448-458. 10.1177/104063870601800504.
12. Nielsen SS, Thamsborg SM, Houe H, Bitsch V: Bulk-tank milk ELISA antibodies for estimating the prevalence of paratuberculosis in Danish dairy herds. Prev Vet Med. 2000, 44: 1-7. 10.1016/S0167-5877(00)00098-2.
13. Obasanjo IO, Gröhn YT, Mohammed OH: Farm factors associated with the presence of Mycobacterium paratuberculosis infection in dairy herds on the New York state paratuberculosis control program. Prev Vet Med. 1997, 32: 243-251. 10.1016/S0167-5877(97)00027-5.
14. Wells SJ, Wagner BA: Herd-level risk factors for infection with Mycobacterium paratuberculosis in US dairies and association between familiarity of the herd manager with the disease or prior diagnosis of the disease in that herd and use of preventive measures. J Am Vet Med Assoc. 2000, 216: 1450-1457. 10.2460/javma.2000.216.1450.
15. SAS/STAT(R) 9.2 User's Guide, Second Edition. [http://support.sas.com/documentation/cdl/en/statug/63033/HTML/default/er.htm#statug_glm_sect026.htm]
16. Nielsen SS, Gröhn YT, Enevoldsen C: Variation of the milk antibody response to paratuberculosis in naturally infected dairy cows. J Dairy Sci. 2002, 85: 795-2802.
17. USDA: APHIS:VS: CEAH: Johne's Disease on U.S. Dairy Operations, 2002. 2005, Fort Collins, CO, http://www.aphis.usda.gov/animal_health/nahms/dairy/#dairy2002,
18. Jakobsen MB, Alban L, Nielsen SS: A cross-sectional study of paratuberculosis in 1155 Danish dairy cows. Prev Vet Med. 2000, 46: 15-27. 10.1016/S0167-5877(00)00138-0.
19. McNab WB, Meek AH, Martin SW, Duncan JR: Associations between dairy production indices and lipoarabinomannan enzyme-immunoassay results for paratuberculosis. Can J Vet Res. 1991, 55: 356-361.
20. McKenna SLB, Keefe GP, Barkema HW, McClure J, VanLeeuwen JA, Hanna P, Sockett DC: Cow-level prevalence of paratuberculosis in culled dairy cows in Atlantic Canada and Maine. J Dairy Sci. 2004, 87: 3770-3777. 10.3168/jds.S0022-0302(04)73515-8.
21. Ellingson JLE, Anderson JL, Koziczkowski JJ, Radcliff RP, Sloan SJ, Allen SE, Sullivan NM: Detection of viable Mycobacterium avium subsp. Paratuberculosis in retail pasteurized whole milk by two culture methods and PCR. J Food Prot. 2005, 68: 966-972.
22. Coussens PM: Mycobacterium paratuberculosis and the bovine immune system. Anim Health Res Rev. 2001, 2: 141-161.
23. Lu Z, Mitchel RM, Smith RL, Van Kessel JS, Chapagain PP, Schukken YH, Gröhn YT: The importance of culling in Johne's disease control. J Theor Biol. 2008, 254: 135-146. 10.1016/j.jtbi.2008.05.008.
24. van Schaik G, Rossiter CR, Stehman SM, Shin SJ, Schukken YH: Longitudinal study to investigate variation in results of repeated ELISA and culture of fecal samples for Mycobacterium avium subsp paratuberculosis in commercial dairy herds. Am J Vet Res. 2003, 64: 479-484. 10.2460/ajvr.2003.64.479.

25. Richert RM, Cicconi KM, Gamroth MJ, Schukken YH, Stiglbauer KE, Ruegg PL: Management factors associated with veterinary usage by organic and conventional dairy farms. J Am Vet Med Assoc. 2012, 2013 (242): 1732-1743.

26. Project C-O-W. [http://milkquality.wisc.edu/organic-dairies/project-c-o-w/]

27. Hendrick SH, Duffield TF, Kelton DF, Leslie KE, Lissemore KD, Archambault M: Evaluation of enzyme-linked immunosorbent assays performed on milk and serum samples for detection of paratuberculosis in lactating dairy cows. J Am Vet Med Assoc. 2005, 226: 424-428. 10.2460/javma.2005.226.424.

28. Schukken YH, Weersink AW, Leslie KE, Martin SW: Dynamics and regulation of bulk milk somatic cell counts. Can J Vet Res. 1993, 57: 131-135.

SECTION IX: CLOSTRIDIUM SPP.– AGENT OF BOTULISM

CHAPTER 32 SYSTEMICALLY ADMINISTERED IGG ANTI-TOXIN ANTIBODIES PROTECT THE COLONIC MUCOSA DURING INFECTION WITH CLOSTRIDIUM DIFFICILE IN THE PIGLET MODEL

Ocean R. Cohen, Jennifer A. Steele, Quanshun Zhang, Diane J. Schmidt, Yuankai Wang, Philip E. S. Hamel, Gillian Beamer, Bingling Xu, Saul Tzipori

INTRODUCTION

Clostridium difficile is an anaerobic, spore-forming, gram-positive bacterium, and the most frequent cause of antibiotic-associated diarrhea in humans. Like other clostridia, *C. difficile* is a toxin-producer, and pathogenic effects are due primarily to the two large clostridial glucosylating toxins, toxin A (TcdA) and toxin B (TcdB). These toxins are enterotoxic and cause increased mucosal permeability by inducing intestinal epithelial cell damage [1]. Both TcdA and TcdB consist of three major domains: the N-terminal catalytic domain, the central translocation domain, and the C-terminal receptor binding domain [2]. By inactivating Rho family GTPases in the gut epithelial cells, the toxins disrupt cell signaling, which leads to disruption of the tight junctions, cytoskeletal degradation, cell rounding, and cell death [1], [2].

The symptoms of *C. difficile* infection (CDI) in humans range from asymptomatic carriage to severe pseudomembranous colitis, toxic megacolon, and death [3]. The historic gold standard treatment for CDI is administration of metronidazole or vancomycin and discontinuation of the previously administered broad-spectrum antibiotics [4]. Treatment failures as well as frequent recurrence in antibiotic-treated patients has led to the search for more effective treatment options, which currently include novel antimicrobials, fecal transplantation, probiotic supplementation, and anti-toxin antibodies [4], [5]. In fact, human monoclonal antibodies (HMab) against TcdA and/or TcdB effectively treat CDI in the hamster model [6] as well as in the piglet model in our laboratory [7], and, in combination with either metronidazole or vancomycin, significantly reduce CDI recurrence rate in humans [5].

These anti-toxin antibodies are administered systemically by intravenous or intraperitoneal injection in the animal models and intravenously in human patients, but little is known as to how these systemically administered IgG antibodies protect the colonic mucosa during CDI. Suggested mechanisms of action for systemically administered HMabs are that they either transfer to the gut lumen via a leaky mucosal barrier [8] or they may be actively transported by an IgG neonatal Fc receptor [9], [10]. Knowing that the *C. difficile* toxins increase intestinal mucosal permeability by disrupting tight junctions, our hypothesis is that the antibodies leak from the mucosal blood capillaries into the lumen through mucosa damaged by CDI. Thus, we expected that intestinal mucosal damage induced by pathogenic *C. difficile* would be associated with greater concentrations of systemically administered HMab in the gut lumen. We investigated this in groups of piglets that were inoculated with either pathogenic (UK6) or non-pathogenic (CD37) strains of *C. difficile* to measure the presence of the HMabs at different sites of the gut mucosa and in the gut lumen of both groups.

METHODS

Monoclonal anti-toxin antibody preparation

The human monoclonal anti-TcdA (CDA1) and anti-TcdB (CDB1) antibodies used in this study were developed by Massachusetts Biologic Laboratories and Medarex, Inc. [6],

Citation: Cohen OR, Steele JA, Zhang Q, Schmidt DJ, Wang Y, Hamel PES, et al. (2014) Systemically Administered IgG Anti-Toxin Antibodies Protect the Colonic Mucosa during Infection with Clostridium difficile in the Piglet Model. PLoS ONE 9(10): e111075. doi:10.1371/journal.pone.0111075.

and were provided for this study and currently licensed by Merck, Inc. These antibodies have already been used in the hamster model [6], the piglet model [7], and in clinical trials in humans [11], [12]. Both CDA1 and CDB1 are IgG1κ antibodies and bind the receptor-binding domain of TcdA and TcdB, respectively [6]. CDA1 and CDB1 were administered to piglets at a dose of 10 mg/kg suspended in sterile PBS via intraperitoneal injection [11], [12]. The dose used in piglets was based on that given to humans in clinical trials, as well as the protective dose in piglets in past experiments in our laboratory [7].

Animals and inoculation

Piglets were derived via Cesarean section from a conventional sow (Parson's Farm) and maintained in sterile isolators for the duration of the experiment, as we have previously described [13]. A total of 23 gnotobiotic piglets were randomly divided into 3 groups: 2 piglets were not infected and treated with CDA1 and CDB1 to determine if these anti-toxin IgGs crossed from the systemic circulation to the gut lumen in the absence of bacterial colonization and to monitor for adverse events associated with CDA1 and CDB1; 9 piglets were orally inoculated with 10^8 vegetative cells of non-pathogenic *C. difficile* strain CD37 and treated with CDA1 and CDB1; and 12 piglets were orally inoculated with 10^8 spores of pathogenic *C. difficile* strain UK6 [14] and treated with CDA1 and CDB1 (Table 1). Randomization was completed immediately after birth by the animal care technicians who were unaware of treatments animals in each group would receive. Additionally, data from 4 UK6-inoculated piglets which received an irrelevant anti-Stx2 HMab from previous experiments in our laboratory [7] were used for antibody controls (Table 1). All animals were cared for according to ethical procedures to reduce pain and suffering by protocol approved by the Institutional Animal Care and Use Committee of Tufts University (protocol #G2013-83).

Table 1: Clinical signs and intestinal lesions in piglets inoculated with *C. difficile*and treated with anti-toxin antibodies

C. difficile strain	clinical signs	mortality	gross intestinal lesions	histopathologic lesions	C. difficile range (cfu/ml)
Pathogenic UK6, treated with CDA1 and CDB1 (n = 12)	mild-moderate diarrhea, transient anorexia	none	mild-moderate mesocolonic edema, rectal dilatation	mild-moderate mesocolonic and submucosal edema	10^5–10^{10}
Pathogenic UK6, treated with irrelevant control[A] (n = 4)	moderate-severe diarrhea, anorexia, lethargy	2/4	moderate-severe mesocolonic edema, pseudomembranous colitis, mucosal congestion	moderate-severe mesocolonic and submucosal edema, marked neutrophilic infiltration, mucosal erosion and ulceration, luminal psueudomembranes	10^6–10^{10}
Nonpathogenic CD37 treated with CDA1 and CDB1 (n = 9)	none	none	none	none or minimal mesocolonic edema	none
Noninfected and treated with CDA1 and CDB1 (n = 2)	none	none	none	none or minimal mesocolonic edema	n/a

Notes: CDA1 = anti-toxin A human monoclonal antibody, CDB1 = anti-toxin B human monoclonal antibody.
[A]control piglets were treated with irrelevant anti-Stx2 human monoclonal antibody [7].
doi:10.1371/journal.pone.0111075.t001

http://dx.doi.org/10.1371/journal.pone.0111075.t001

At 48 hours after inoculation, the piglets receiving the pathogenic strain UK6 developed diarrhea, and at that point a mixture of 10 mg/kg of CDA1 and 10 mg/kg CDB1 was administered by intraperitoneal injection to all piglets in each group. Piglets were observed at least 4 times daily for signs of CDI including diarrhea, perianal inflammation, weakness, lethargy, and anorexia. Piglets were euthanized at a predetermined time between 2 and 4 days post treatment with CDA1 and CDB1 (Table 1). Blood samples were collected immediately prior to euthanasia. Gut luminal contents and tissue samples from the duodenum, jejunum, ileum, cecum, spiral colon, and rectum were harvested after euthanasia.

Human monoclonal antibody quantification

Concentrations of CDA1 and CDB1 in the serum, gastrointestinal contents, and gastrointestinal tissues were measured by ELISA. Prior to use, gastrointestinal contents were diluted at a 1:10 ratio using sterile PBS and centrifuged at 9000 rpm for 3 minutes. The same technique was used for the 6 sections of gastrointestinal tissues prior to homogenization and centrifugation. Serum was not diluted in PBS and was used at body concentrations. High binding capacity 96-well plates were coated with 0.5µg/ml of rTcdA or rTcdB [15] using PBSN coating buffer and left covered overnight at 4°C. Plates were washed using a PBST buffer before being blocked with 0.1% BSA-PBST for 30 minutes at room temperature. Plates were washed, and two-fold serial dilutions of either CDA1 or CDB1 were used as standards beginning at 100 ng/ml and added at 100µl/well followed by the addition of the collected samples and positive and negative controls at 100µl/well and incubated at room temperature for 1 hour. Plates were washed, and donkey anti-human IgG-HRP conjugate was used as the secondary antibody. Plates were developed and the OD_{450} was measured. Mean antibody concentrations were statistically compared using the independent samples t-test for comparisons between the UK6 and CD37-infected groups and using ANOVA for comparisons among the 3 daily time points. Samples from all animals were included in the analysis.

Histopathology

Samples collected for histological examination were fixed in 10% neutral buffered formalin for routine processing, sectioning, and staining with hematoxylin and eosin at TCSVM Histopathology Service Laboratory. We sampled each of the 6 sections of the gastrointestinal tract as well as the heart, lungs, liver, spleen, and kidney. A board certified veterinary pathologist (GB) assessed the tissues for lesions characteristic of CDI including edema, ulceration, erosion, and suppurative (neutrophilic) inflammation.

RESULTS

CDA1 and CDB1 protect against mortality, morbidity, and severity of intestinal lesions

All piglets inoculated with pathogenic UK6 developed typical signs of CDI with diarrhea and anorexia, 2 days post-inoculation, at which point they were treated with CDA1 and CDB1 HMabs. Piglets treated with a mixture of CDA1 and CDB1 two days after inoculation with the UK6 strain of *C. difficile* were protected from development of severe clinical signs of CDI as well as severe injury to the colonic mucosa, systemic intoxication, and mortality, compared with the UK6-infected, irrelevant anti-Stx2 HMab treated controls (Table 1), as well as untreated UK6-infected piglets, which we have previously described [7], [13]. The UK6-infected piglets that received anti-Stx2 HMab instead of CDA1 and CDB1 developed typical CDI disease with moderate to severe pseudomembranous colitis, and half of the piglets developed fatal disease with systemic lesions (Table 1). *C. difficile* cultures for UK6 were performed on large intestinal contents collected during necropsy, but were not significantly different between groups treated with CDA1 and CDB1 vs anti-Stx2 HMabs (Table 1). *C. difficile* cultures for CD37 failed to confirm growth of this strain from the infected group of piglets, likely due to failure of the strain to sporulate and exposure of samples to oxygen during processing (Table 1). Diarrhea improved or resolved in all 12 CDA1 and CDB1 treated piglets following administration (Table 1). On histopathologic examination, lesion severity in UK6-infected, CDA1 and CDB1 treated piglets was reduced to mild-moderate mesocolonic or submucosal edema in the spiral colon and rectum of some of the piglets and there was no evidence of pseudomembranous colitis (Table 1). As expected, the piglets inoculated with the non-pathogenic strain CD37, as well as the uninfected controls treated with CDA1 and CDB1, developed no clinical signs of illness and had either no observed intestinal lesions or minimal mesocolonic edema (Table 1).

CDA1 and CDB1 presence in mucosal tissues and gut contents after systemic administration

CDA1 and CDB1 were measureable in all mucosal tissues evaluated, including the small intestine (Figure 1, B and D). Both HMabs were present in the gut contents in appreciable amounts only in the large intestine of UK6-infected piglets and at significantly higher concentration in the rectum, where most water absorption from the contents has been completed (Figure 1, A and C). Minimal amounts of both HMabs were measured in the small intestinal contents of CD37 or UK6-infected piglets (Figure 1, A and C), which we attribute to the lack of any mucosal lesions in the small intestine in either group. HMab concentrations in the mucosal tissues were ~10 fold greater than in the lumen of the large intestine, with maximal concentrations of nearly 50,000 ng/ml in the large intestinal mucosa (Figure 1, B and D). Figure 1 also reflects the relative distribution of the two HMabs throughout the gut tissues with no trend for significant differences in antibody concentration between CD37 and UK6-infected piglets (Figure 1, B and D). While the focus of analysis was on differences between the two CDI groups, the two uninfected piglets had the same pattern of HMab distribution as the CD37-infected group (data not shown).

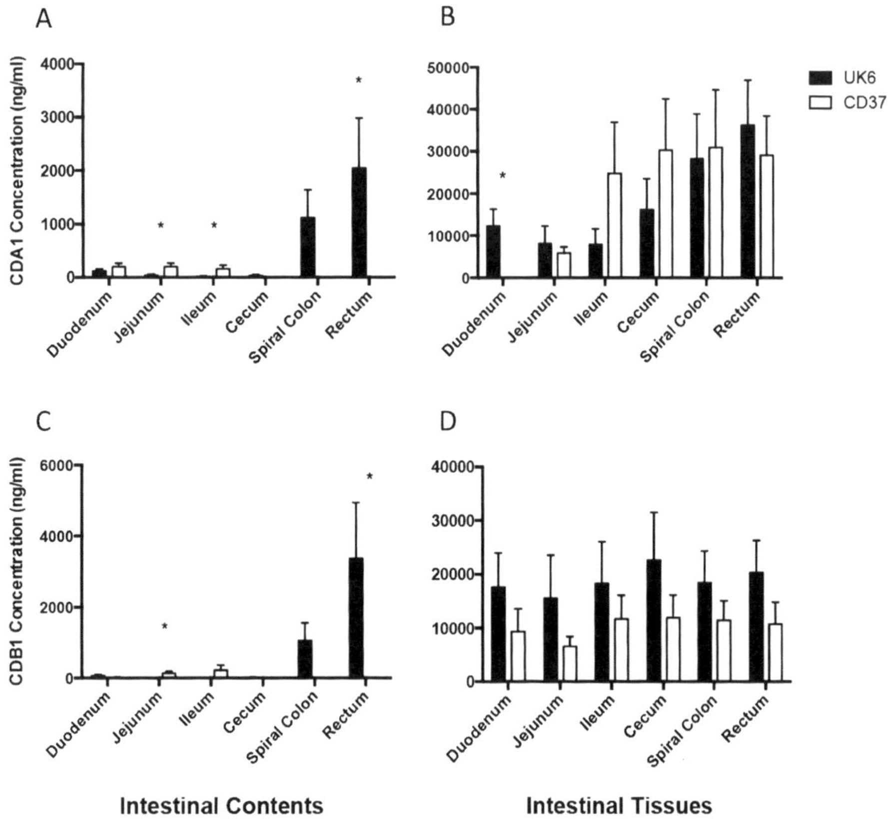

Figure 1: Concentrations of human monoclonal antibodies CDA1 and CDB1 in the intestinal contents and tissues.

Gnotobiotic piglets were inoculated with either pathogenic UK6 or nonpathogenic CD37 and treated systemically with human monoclonal anti-toxin antibodies against TcdA and TcdB (CDA1 and CDB1) 2 days following inoculation. **A.** CDA1 in intestinal contents **B.** CDA1 in intestinal tissues **C.** CDB1 in intestinal contents **D.** CDB1 in intestinal tissues. * $p<0.05$ between groups using the independent samples t-test. Bars represent the mean with standard error.

CDA1 and CDB1 persist in intestinal mucosal tissues and contents

CDA1 and CDB1 were measured in the gut contents and mucosal tissues in groups of piglets infected with UK6 or CD37 and euthanized at 2, 3, and 4 day time points after HMab administration to evaluate the concentration over time. While we found no significant differences in HMab concentrations over this time period in the mucosal tissues or contents (Figure 2), we noticed a trend for increased concentration in the large intestinal contents on days 3 or 4 in the UK6-infected group (Figure 2, A and C). Comparison of CDA1 and CDB1 concentrations in the tissues and contents between the CD37 and UK6-infected groups shows a trend of elevated concentrations in contents of the spiral colon and rectum of the UK6-infected group. The difference was not statistically significant in this analysis, likely due to smaller group sizes when piglets were stratified by day of sampling (Figure 2, A and C).

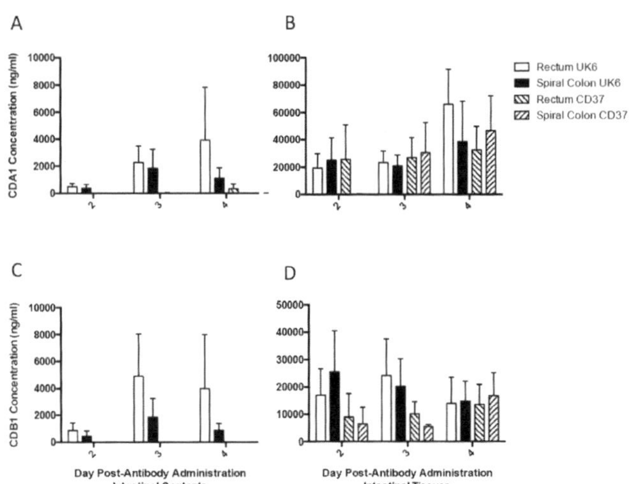

Figure 2: Concentrations of human monoclonal antibodies CDA1 and CDB1 in the large intestinal contents and tissues over time following systemic administration in piglets inoculated with *C. difficile*.

Gnotobiotic piglets were inoculated with pathogenic *C. difficile* strain UK6 and then treated once systemically with human monoclonal anti-toxin antibodies against TcdA and TcdB (CDA1 and CDB1) 2 days following inoculation, at the onset of clinical signs. Piglets were euthanized and tissues collected 2, 3, or 4 days following antibody administration. **A.** CDA1 in large intestinal contents **B.** CDA1 in large intestinal tissues **C.** CDB1 in large intestinal contents **D.** CDB1 in large intestinal tissues. Bars represent the mean with standard error.

DISCUSSION

In this study we show an association between colonic injury due to CDI and the presence of IgG in the gut lumen, as compared with normal intestinal mucosa. The anti-toxin HMabs used in these experiments have been shown to be effective in modifying the clinical outcome of CDI in the hamster and gnotobiotic piglet models, and in clinical trials with human patients [5], [6], [11], [12]. However, it is unclear how systemically administered IgG antibodies are able to provide protection against bacterial toxins liberated in the lumen of the large intestine. We believe that the presence of systemically administered CDA1 and CDB1 HMabs in the gut contents is likely attributed to leakage through the mucosal injury inflicted by the bacteria and/or toxins to the protective mucosal surface, therefore confirming the hypothesis that damage to the gut mucosa facilitates antibody leakage into the gut lumen.

While we cannot entirely rule-out the contribution of active transport of IgG by the neonatal Fc receptor [9], we would not expect the marked difference in HMab concentrations in the gut contents between groups infected with pathogenic and non-pathogenic bacterial strains, as we have shown in these experiments. Antibodies leaking into the gut lumen neutralized the bacterial toxins, thus protecting the mucosa from further damage by the pathogenic strain. Furthermore, the presence of HMab IgG antibody in the mucosal vasculature intercepts and neutralizes toxin uptake from the lumen thus preventing the occurrence of systemic intoxication, which can be observed in patients and consistently in piglets with CDI [16]. Perhaps if HMabs were administered after piglets began to develop more severe clinical signs of CDI after inoculation, a more likely event for human patients, the degree of antibody leakage into the lumen would be even greater. While the contribution of toxin production to *C. difficile*colonization of the large bowel is unknown, Shiga toxin was shown to facilitate the colonic colonization of *E. coli* O157 [17], and it is possible that the same may apply to TcdA and TcdB. It was also difficult to accurately quantify *C. difficile* vegetative cells collected from intestinal contents, as they are quickly destroyed upon contact with oxygen, thus counts likely reflect predominantly spores in the contents samples. As reflected above in the results, we failed to recover CD37 from the intestinal contents of piglets infected with the strain, which may also be due to poor sporulation this strain and exposure of the samples to oxygen. While the degree of colonization of strain CD37 in this group of animals cannot be confirmed, the group still represents a non-pathogenic, non-toxin control with which to compare the clinical and laboratory findings from the group infected with the pathogenic UK6 strain.

We found no significant difference in concentration of either antibody over time between the UK6 and CD37 groups, as seen in Figure 2 depicting the concentration of antibodies in the large intestinal mucosa and contents of the piglets; only in the gut lumen. There was no significant increase in the amount of leakage of antibodies into the lumen over the three days they were quantified, indicating that a single systemic administration of the two HMabs results in greater concentrations in the large intestinal mucosa for at least 4 days, with a trend of increased concentrations in the large intestinal lumen after 2 days in the UK6-infected piglets.

In summary, our investigation has shown that 1) these IgG HMabs were present throughout the gastrointestinal tissues, as shown in the UK6 and the CD37 groups of animals, regardless of pathology; 2) where large intestinal mucosa was damaged by the pathogenic UK6 strain, HMab IgG leaked into the gut lumen in greater concentrations; and 3) the mild mucosal injury observed was presumably because leaked antibodies protected the gut mucosa from further damage and led to rapid recovery.

ACKNOWLEDGMENTS

We would like to give special thanks to the animal care technicians, Patricia Boucher and Rachel Nieminen, who provided care and technical assistance for all of the animals used in these experiments. We would like to thank Merck, Inc. for providing the human monoclonal antibodies used for treatment in these experiments.

AUTHOR CONTRIBUTIONS

Conceived and designed the experiments: ORC JS QZ DJS ST. Performed the experiments: ORC QZ DJS YW PESH GB BX. Analyzed the data: ORC JS GB. Contributed reagents/materials/analysis tools: ST. Wrote the paper: ORC JS ST.

REFERENCES

1. Sun X, Savidge T, Feng H (2010) The enterotoxicity of Clostridium difficile toxins. Toxins (Basel) 2: 1848–1880. doi: 10.3390/toxins2071848
2. Carter GP, Rood JI, Lyras D (2010) The role of toxin A and toxin B in Clostridium difficile-associated disease: Past and present perspectives. Gut microbes 1: 58–64. doi: 10.4161/gmic.1.1.10768
3. McCollum DL, Rodriguez JM (2012) Detection, Treatment, and Prevention of Clostridium difficile Infection. Clinical gastroenterology and hepatology: the official clinical practice journal of the American Gastroenterological Association 10: 581–592. doi: 10.1016/j.cgh.2012.03.008
4. Bakken JS, Polgreen PM, Beekmann SE, Riedo FX, Streit JA (2013) Treatment approaches including fecal microbiota transplantation for recurrent Clostridium difficile infection (RCDI) among infectious disease physicians. Anaerobe 24: 20–24. doi: 10.1016/j.anaerobe.2013.08.007
5. Leav BA, Blair B, Leney M, Knauber M, Reilly C, et al. (2010) Serum anti-toxin B antibody correlates with protection from recurrent Clostridium difficile infection (CDI). Vaccine 28: 965–969. doi: 10.1016/j.vaccine.2009.10.144
6. Babcock GJ, Broering TJ, Hernandez HJ, Mandell RB, Donahue K, et al. (2006) Human monoclonal antibodies directed against toxins A and B prevent Clostridium difficile-induced mortality in hamsters. Infect Immun 74: 6339–6347. doi: 10.1128/iai.00982-06
7. Steele J, Mukherjee J, Parry N, Tzipori S (2013) Antibody against TcdB, but not TcdA, prevents development of gastrointestinal and systemic Clostridium difficile disease. J Infect Dis 207: 323–330. doi: 10.1093/infdis/jis669
8. Hussack G, Tanha J (2010) Toxin-specific antibodies for the treatment of Clostridium difficile: current status and future perspectives. Toxins (Basel) 2: 998–1018. doi: 10.3390/toxins2050998
9. Rath T, Kuo TT, Baker K, Qiao SW, Kobayashi K, et al. (2013) The immunologic functions of the neonatal Fc receptor for IgG. J Clin Immunol 33 Suppl 1S9–17. doi: 10.1007/s10875-012-9768-y
10. Yoshida M, Kobayashi K, Kuo TT, Bry L, Glickman JN, et al. (2006) Neonatal Fc receptor for IgG regulates mucosal immune responses to luminal bacteria. J Clin Invest 116: 2142–2151. doi: 10.1172/jci27821
11. Lowy I, Molrine DC, Leav BA, Blair BM, Baxter R, et al. (2010) Treatment with monoclonal antibodies against Clostridium difficile toxins. The New England journal of medicine 362: 197–205. doi: 10.1056/nejmoa0907635
12. Taylor CP, Tummala S, Molrine D, Davidson L, Farrell RJ, et al. (2008) Open-label, dose escalation phase I study in healthy volunteers to evaluate the safety and pharmacokinetics of a human monoclonal antibody to Clostridium difficile toxin A. Vaccine 26: 3404–3409. doi: 10.1016/j.vaccine.2008.04.042
13. Steele J, Feng H, Parry N, Tzipori S (2010) Piglet models of acute or chronic Clostridium difficile illness. J Infect Dis 201: 428–434. doi: 10.1086/649799
14. Killgore G, Thompson A, Johnson S, Brazier J, Kuijper E, et al. (2008) Comparison of seven techniques for typing international epidemic strains of Clostridium difficile: restriction endonuclease analysis, pulsed-field gel electrophoresis, PCR-ribotyping, multilocus sequence typing, multilocus variable-number tandem-repeat analysis, amplified fragment length polymorphism, and surface layer protein A gene sequence typing. Journal of Clinical Microbiology 46: 431–437. doi: 10.1128/jcm.01484-07
15. Yang G, Zhou B, Wang J, He X, Sun X, et al. (2008) Expression of recombinant Clostridium difficile toxin A and B in Bacillus megaterium. BMC Microbiol 8: 192. doi: 10.1186/1471-2180-8-192
16. Steele J, Chen K, Sun X, Zhang Y, Wang H, et al. (2012) Systemic dissemination of Clostridium difficile toxins A and B is associated with severe, fatal disease in animal models. The Journal of infectious diseases 205: 384–391. doi: 10.1093/infdis/jir748
17. Mohawk KL, Melton-Celsa AR, Robinson CM, O'Brien AD (2010) Neutralizing antibodies to Shiga toxin type 2 (Stx2) reduce colonization of mice by Stx2-expressing Escherichia coli O157:H7. Vaccine 28: 4777–4785. doi: 10.1016/j.vaccine.2010.04.099

CHAPTER 33

INTERNATIONAL CLOSTRIDIUM DIFFICILE ANIMAL STRAIN COLLECTION AND LARGE DIVERSITY OF ANIMAL ASSOCIATED STRAINS

Sandra Janezic, Valerija Zidaric, Bart Pardon, Alexander Indra, Branko Kokotovic, Jose Luis Blanco, Christian Seyboldt, Cristina Rodriguez Diaz, Ian R Poxton, Vincent Perreten, Ilenia Drigo, Alena Jiraskova, Matjaz Ocepek, J Scott Weese, J Glenn Songer, Mark H Wilcox and Maja Rupnik

Keywords: *Clostridium difficile,* Animals, Ribotyping, Geographic distribution, Strain collection

BACKGROUND

Clostridium difficile, an anaerobic sporogenic bacterium, is recognized as the major pathogen in healthcare associated intestinal infections in humans and also as an important animal pathogen. In addition to the potential for serious (including fatal) infections in animals, are companion and food animals considered as an important potential source for human community-acquired infections [1, 2, 3, 4]. This indicates the importance of preventive measures targeting animals and food [5]. Several studies have looked at similarity between strains isolated from humans and animals [1, 6, 7, 8, 9, 10], but typically focusing on limited number of different species and restricted to a narrow geographic region.

PCR ribotyping is currently the method of choice for differentiation of *C. difficile* strains. In humans more than 300 PCR ribotypes are recognized while the number of reported animal associated PCR ribotypes is much lower [1, 8, 11]. It could be expected that variety of animal associated *C. difficile* will increase with the increased number of typed animal isolates. To date piglets and pig farms are hosts and environments where *C. difficile* has been most extensively studied [3, 12, 13, 14, 15, 16, 17, 18]. For this reservoir the modes of transmission and potential association with human infections are also best understood [14, 16].

C. difficile strains can also be differentiated into toxinotypes according to the differences in the toxin A and toxin B encoding region (PaLoc) [19]. Toxinotypes V and XI are particularly often isolated from animals [19], but the reason for this association is not known. Many published studies report *C. difficile* PCR ribotypes, but not many do report the toxinotypes [9, 13].

The aim of this study was to collect *C. difficile* isolates from different countries and different animals and to compare them with classical agarose gel-based and sequencer-based PCR ribotyping and determine the toxinotypes.

RESULTS

Altogether 112 *C. difficile* isolates from 13 animal species were obtained from 14 laboratories from 12 different countries (Austria, Belgium, Canada, Czech Republic, Denmark, Germany, Italy, Scotland, Slovenia, Spain, Switzerland and

---

Citation: Sandra Janezic, Valerija Zidaric, Bart Pardon, Alexander Indra, Branko Kokotovic, Jose Luis Blanco, Christian Seyboldt, Cristina Rodriguez Diaz, Ian R Poxton, Vincent Perreten, Ilenia Drigo, Alena Jiraskova, Matjaz Ocepek, J Scott Weese, J Glenn Songer, Mark H Wilcox and Maja Rupnik, International Clostridium difficile animal strain collection and large diversity of animal associated strains, DOI: 10.1186/1471-2180-14-173.

USA) (Table 1). Inclusion criteria were one strain (PCR ribotype) per animal species per laboratory. Each participating country contributed 1 to 24 isolates. Strains were isolated between 1998 and 2012. Only five isolates were from 1998 to 2002, with the majority of isolates (n=34) from 2011.

Table 1: PCR ribotypes and toxinotypes represented in the international collection of animal *C. difficile* strains

			Number of strains/different countries per animal species						**In total**	
PCR ribotype	**WEBRIBO type**	**Toxinotype***	**Cattle**	**Horse**	**Pig**	**Poultry**	**Cats and dogs**	**Others****	**Nr. of strains (%)**	**Nr. of countries**
078	078, 078/4	V/Btb+	5/4	2/2	8/7			1/1	16 (14,3)	9
014/020	014/0, 014/5, 020, 449,659	0	3/3	1/1	2/1	1/1	4/2	2/2	13 (11,6)	5
002	203, 209	0	2/2		2/2		1/1	1/1	6 (5,4)	5
012	012	0, XIX	2/2		1/1	1/1	1/1	1/1	6 (5,4)	4
010	010	tox-	1/1			1/1	2/2	1/1	5 (4,5)	4
033	033	XIa, XIb/ Btb+	3/3	1/1					4 (3,6)	4
126	126,078ecdc	V/Btb+	2/2	1/1	1/1				4 (3,6)	4
150	AI-12	0			4/4				4 (3,6)	4
045	045, 598, PR4455, 413	V/Btb+	1/1		3/2	1/1		1/1	6 (5,4)	3
001	001, 001ecdc	0				2/2	2/1		4 (3,6)	3
005	005	0	1/1		1/1	1/1			3	3
(CE)013	AI-9-1	0	1/1					2/2	3	3
103	AI-82/1	0	1/1			1/1		1/1	3	3
(CE)288	660	XIb/Btb+	1/1	1/1				1/1	3	3
081	081	0	1/1		2/2				3	2
015	AI-8/0	0	1/1		1/1				2	2
027	027	IIIb/Btb+	1/1	1/1					2	2
029	029	0	1/1			1/1			2	2
(CE)050	050, AI-84	0	1/1		1/1				2	2
056	056	XII			1/1		1/1		2	2
SLO 024	652	V/Btb+					2/1		2	1
003	003	0						1/1	1	1
011/049	049/1	0			1/1				1	1
017	017	VIII						1/1	1	1
018	018	0				1/1			1	1
023	023	IV/Btb+				1/1			1	1
(CE)032	205	tox-						1/1	1	1
(CE)039	039/2	tox-					1/1		1	1
(CE)084	548	tox-						1/1	1	1
(CE)097	AI-60	0					1/1		1	1
127	651	VI/Btb+			1/1				1	1
258	446	XII						1/1	1	1
(CE)342	610	0	1/1						1	1
(CE)365	434	0	1/1						1	1
(CE)448	653	VI/Btb+			1/1				1	1
(CE)602	212	0	1/1						1	1
SLO 133	AI-15	XII			1/1				1	1
SLO 166	661	I						1/1	1	1

All		na	31/7	7/4	31/10	11/2	15/4	17/3	112	12***
Nr. of ribotypes per species			20	6	16	10	9	15		

*Btb + − presence of binary toxin CDT; **including racoons, wild hare, rabbits, goats, partridges, goose, and crow; ***12 countries participated; tox- -nontoxigenic strain (lacking the PaLoc and genes coding for binary toxin CDT); A "CE" prefix, eg. (CE)039, indicates that the PCR ribotype assigment was made in reference laboratory (CDRN Leeds) using the newer capillary electrophoresis-based approach. PCR-ribotypes in the table are ordered according to the number of countries in which the strains were found and then according to the number of strains belonging to that ribotype.

The majority of isolates were from pigs (n=31; 27.7%) and cattle (n=31; 27.7%), followed by poultry (n=11; 9.8%), dogs (n=10; 8.9%), horses, rabbits (7 isolates each; 6.3%), cats (n=5; 4.5%), goats (n=3; 2.7%), partridges and raccoons (2 isolates each; 1.8%), wild hare, crow and goose (1 isolate each; 0.9%).

Only 38 isolates were from animals with clinical signs, 56 were from clinically normal animals and for 18 isolates disease status of the animal was not known.

For 40 animals antibiotic use was unknown and further 52 animals had no history of antibiotic exposure. Prior use of antibiotics was reported for isolates from 20 animals. For 12 of them antibiotic was not specified and for the remaining eight antibiotics given to animals were amoxicillin/clavulanic acid, amoxicillin, colistin, enrofloxacin, cefovecin (6 months before sampling), gentamicin, oxytetracycline, and sulfonamide. Animals treated with antibiotics were cattle (8), cat (1), dog (1), horse (1), pig (2) and rabbit (7). Twenty isolates from animals with reported use of antibiotics belonged to 11 different PCR ribotypes (002, 012, 014/020, 027, 033, 045, 078, 127, (CE)013, (CE)032 and (CE)084). None of those PCR ribotypes was associated with a specific antibiotic.

Molecular characterization of strains with two PCR ribotyping approaches

Results of agarose gel-based and sequencer-based PCR ribotyping for 112 *C. difficile* isolates are presented in Table 1.

Using classical agarose-gel based PCR ribotyping all 112 isolates were distributed into 38 different PCR ribotypes (Table 1). With sequencer-based PCR ribotyping, 50 PCR ribotypes could be identified. This is due to higher discriminatory power of capillary sequencer-based PCR ribotyping for some PCR ribotypes; 001 (001 and 001ecdc), 002 (203 and 209), 014/020 (014/0, 014/5, 020, 449 and 659), (CE)050 (050 and AI-84), 078 (078 and 078/4), 045 (045, 413, 598, PR4455) and 126 (126 and 078ecdc) (Table 1). Comparison of agarose gel PCR ribotypes with the corresponding band profiles generated by capillary electrophoresis-based PCR ribotyping is shown in Figure 1. The discrepancies in the nomenclature between both methods, observed for some of the strains [e.g. PCR ribotype 150 (gel-based) and AI-12 (sequencer-based)], are due to use of a different set of *C. difficile* reference strains and reflects the difficulties in attempts to unify PCR ribotyping nomenclature.

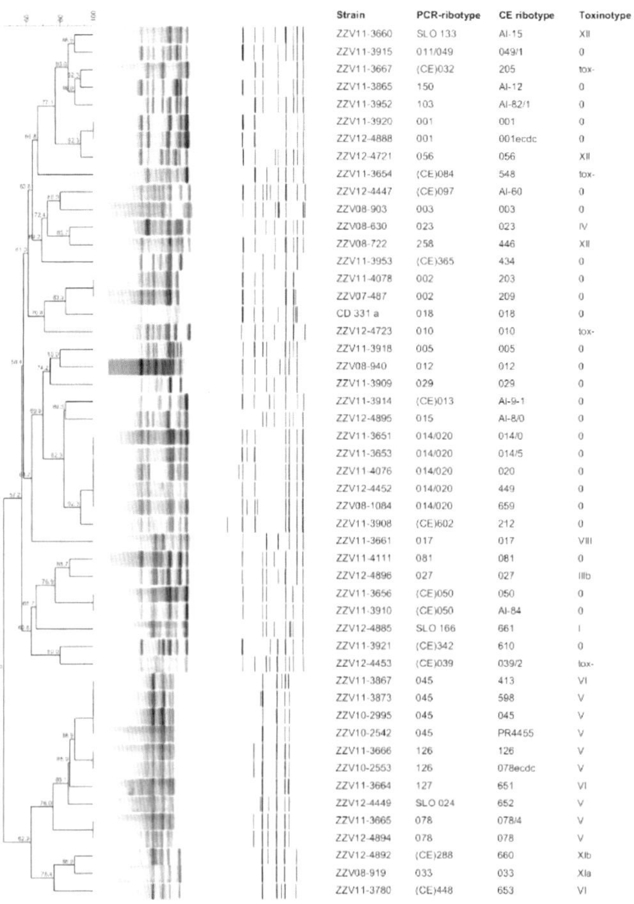

Figure 1: Dendrogram showing similarities of banding patterns generated with classical agarose gel electrophoresis based PCR ribotyping for all 38 different PCR ribotypes included in the collection. For each "gel-based" PCR ribotype all profiles generated with capillary electrophoresis PCR ribotyping are added for comparison. A "CE" prefix, eg. (CE) 039, indicates that the ribotype assigment was made in reference laboratory (CDRN Leeds) using the newer capillary electrophoresis-based approach.

Two most common PCR ribotypes representing 25.9% of all strains were 078 and 014/020. PCR ribotypes with 5 or 6 representatives were 002, 012, 010 (non-toxigenic strain lacking the PaLoc and binary toxin CDT) and 045.

Molecular characterization of strains by toxinotyping

Within toxigenic isolates (n = 104; 92.9%) 11 different toxinotypes were identified (Table 1). More than a half of the isolates belonged to the nonvariant toxinotype 0 (n = 57; 54.9%). The variant toxinotypes were V (n = 27; 26.0%), XII (n = 4; 3.8%), VI (n = 3; 2.9%), XIa (n = 2; 1.9%), XIb (n = 5; 4.7%), III (n = 2; 1.9%), IV, I, VIII and XIX (n = 1; 1%). Eight strains (7.1%) from four different PCR ribotypes (010, (CE)032, (CE)039, (CE)084) were non-toxigenic.

Distribution of PCR ribotypes and toxinotypes in different animal hosts and in different countries

Table 1 shows distribution of *C. difficile* PCR ribotypes and toxinotypes from collected isolates throughout countries and animal species. Isolates from pigs and cattle were the most frequent and were received from 10 and 7 of the 12 participating countries, respectively. The variability of PCR ribotypes was accordingly also the largest in these two hosts; 20 PCR ribotypes came from cattle and 16 from pigs (Table 1). Distribution of the 15 most prevalent PCR ribotypes in countries is presented in Figure 2.PCR ribotype 014/020 was found in the majority of the animal species included in the collection (pig, cattle, horse, poultry, cat, dog, rabbit and a goat) across 5 different countries (Figure 2). PCR ribotypes that were found only in particular animal species, but in several different countries, were PCR ribotype 150, which was found only in pigs but in four different countries, and PCR ribotype 033, which was found in cattle in three different countries and only in a single case in horse.

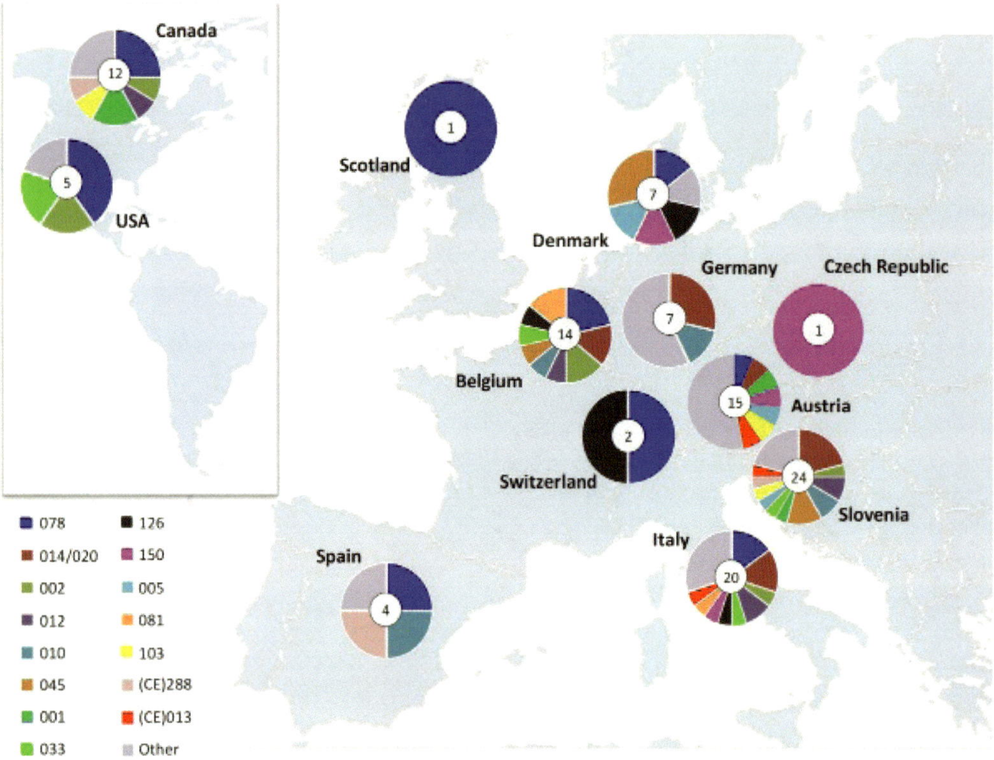

Figure 2: Geographical distribution of animal associated *C. difficile* PCR ribotypes from participating countries. Pie charts show proportion of 15 most prevalent PCR ribotypes in the collection for each participating country. The number in the center of pie chart represents the number of isolates from that country. The diversity of strains per country increases with the total number of strains contributed to the collection but also by strains from certain hosts (poultry in case of Slovenia and rabbits in case of Italy).

Toxinotype V strains of different PCR ribotypes were mainly associated with cattle, horses and pigs and were rarely found in other animals. Also toxinotype XI strains (a and b) were mainly associated with cattle and horses.

DISCUSSION

Several publications are available about isolation and characterization of *C. difficile* from animals, but they are usually limited to a specific geographical region and data of the different studies are sometimes difficult to compare due to nomenclature of PCR ribotypes that is not unified. The advantage of the international animal *C. difficile* strain collection is in performance of strain typing in the single setting, hereby minimizing the ambiguities in PCR ribotype designations. Additionally, two PCR ribotyping approaches have been used; the standard one using 'Cardiff' nomenclature and WEBRIBO based analysis (giving inter-laboratory comparable results independent of Cardiff/Leeds reference strains). This is not a prevalence study with collection of samples from defined number of farms or hosts as was done for hospitals and human isolates in Europe [20]. The isolates in this study were collected from different labs in different countries and the criterion was one PCR ribotype per animal species per lab. Therefore the collected strains are not reflecting the prevalence of PCR ribotypes but are giving a good basis to assess the diversity of animal associated *C. difficile*.

Our results show that variability of PCR ribotypes present in different animal species is large. Isolates from pigs and cattle were most common, perhaps reflecting the importance of *C. difficile* in pigs and concerns about zoonotic transmission from cattle (or more specifically, meat) (Table 1, Table 2). In contrast to cattle and pigs, are cats, dogs, rabbits and poultry clearly understudied and are probably associated with a broader variety of *C. difficile* PCR ribotypes than currently recognized. Only two countries have contributed poultry isolates to the collection, but they represent 10 different PCR ribotypes. Strains from captive rabbits were contributed only by one country, but represent 7 different PCR ribotypes.

Table 2: Comparison of *C. difficile* PCR ribotypes detected in six animal species in different geographical regions

		This study	Netherlands	Germany	Switzerland	Australia	North America
Pigs	Number of ribotypes (reference)	16	3 [10], 1 [7]	20 [15]		1 [18]	7 [21]
	Most prevalent ribotypes	078, 150, 014/020, 045, 002, 081	078	078, 126, 002/2, 126, 413, 049, 598		237	078
Cattle	Number of ribotypes (reference)	20	2 [10]	17 [22]	5 [23]	21 [24]	7 [25] 3 [26]
	Most prevalent ribotypes	078, 014/020, 033, 002, 012, 126	012	033, 078, 045, 126	033, 003, 066, 070, 137	127, 033, 126, 056, 087	078, 017, 027, 014, 033
Cats and dogs	Number of ribotypes (reference)	9	9 [10]	5 [27]			
	Most prevalent ribotypes	014/020, 010, 001	010, 014, 039, 012	010, 014/020, 039, 045			
Goats and sheep	Number of ribotypes (reference)	3			2 [23]	7 [28]	
	Most prevalent ribotypes	010, 014/020, 045			001, 066	101, 137	

Some PCR ribotypes seem to be more often associated with a particular animal host. Many publications report PCR ribotype 078 in pigs [7, 10, 15] and type 033 in cattle [22, 24] (Table 2). Results presented here confirm this observation (Figure 2), but also suggest that the well-known animal-associated PCR ribotype 078 may not be currently present in animals in all countries. In addition to types 078 and 033 some other PCR ribotypes are typically associated with pigs, such as PCR ribotypes 150, 002, 045 and 081 (Table 1). Recent reports from Australia describe a new genotype in terms of PCR ribotype (237) and toxin genes (*tcd* B+, *tcd* A-, *cdt* A+and *cdt* B+) in pigs [18]. PCR ribotype 027 that was prevalent in humans in many countries within the past ten years was in this collection of animal strains found only in USA and Canada.

Toxinotype V and XI and binary toxin positive strains were initially reported to be the prevalent population of strains isolated from animals (70-100%) [19, 29]. However, the results of this study show that nonvariant strains of toxinotype 0 are widespread in animals and that the proportion of binary toxin positive strains can be as low as 35.7%.

All isolates in the collection were distributed into 38 PCR ribotypes, but only a few of those contained five or more isolates, and the majority was represented only by a few or a single isolate (Table 1). This resembles the situation with human strain collections with many different PCR ribotypes, but only a few of them having a large number of isolates [20]. However, as the inclusion criterion for the collection was one PCR ribotype per animal species per laboratory, the number of isolates of a given PCR ribotype does not reflect the actual prevalence of this PCR ribotype in animal host. But the high number of isolates of a given PCR ribotype in the collection does reflect its broader geographic presence and possibly broader spectrum of animal species from which it was isolated.

All animal-associated PCR ribotypes with four or more isolates reported here (Table 1) are among the most prevalent in diverse studies of human isolates [8, 11, 20, 30, 31]. In particular PCR ribotype 014/020 is currently the most prevalent type isolated in Europe and in some USA studies and is the only type that was present here in the majority of animal hosts (Table 1). Although type 014/020 is not recognized as hypervirulent and is not associated with outbreaks or severe disease in humans, its ability to colonize many diverse hosts and its ubiquitous presence indicates considerable endemic potential of this particular PCR ribotype [8].

CONCLUSIONS

PCR ribotype 078 is the most prevalent *C. difficile* type associated with this collection of animal isolates, but only with some hosts and in some countries. The second most prevalent PCR ribotype is 014/020 which, in contrast, has broader range of animal hosts. Variability of animal associated PCR ribotypes is substantial and is likely to increase with the number of typed animal isolates. Large overlap of animal associated *C. difficile*PCR ribotypes with human strains furthers concerns about interspecies, including zoonotic, transmission of this important pathogen. Moreover, strains that are prevalent in humans are also prevalent in different animals from different geographic areas, emphasizing that certain strains have a large potential for global dissemination.

METHODS

Inclusion criteria and requested isolate information

Laboratories from different countries with publications on *C. difficile* in animals were invited to contribute the isolates. Participating laboratories were asked to provide only a single representative PCR ribotype per animal species and laboratory/country. No formal structure was used to guide isolate submission.

Participating laboratories were asked to provide additional information about the individual isolate and the animal host: date and country/city of *C. difficile* isolation or specimen collection, molecular characterization (i.e. PCR ribotype, toxin genes), animal species, age, status (farm, domestic or wild animal), clinical signs and antimicrobial exposure history (when available).

Cultivation and storage of *C. difficile* isolates

Isolates were first inoculated onto selective medium (CLO, bioMerieux) and subcultured on blood agar plates (COH; bioMerieux). Species identification was confirmed by PCR amplification of *C. difficile* specific gene *cdd*using primers Tim 6 (5′-TCCAATATAATAAATTAGCATTCCA) and Struppi 6 (5′-GGCTATTACACGTAATCCAGATA) [32].

All isolates were stored in Microbank cryogenic vials (Pro-lab Diagnostics) at −80°C.

PCR ribotyping and toxinotyping

All isolates were characterized by toxinotyping, agarose gel-based PCR ribotyping and capillary gel electrophoresis-based PCR ribotyping.

Agarose gel-based PCR ribotyping was performed as described elsewhere [33]. PCR ribotypes were determined by comparison of banding patterns with the internal library using the BioNumerics software v7.1 (Applied Maths, Belgium). Banding patterns were compared with a reference library of 48 Cardiff type strains. Strains that were not consistent with those in the library were sent to reference laboratory (CDRN Leeds) for confirmation and are named with prefix (CE), indicating that the assignment was made with the newer capillary electrophoresis-based approach. Three strains generated new ribotyping profiles (not previously recognized in Leeds/Cardiff collection) and are designated with the internal nomenclature (SLO and 3-digit code).

Dendrograms were constructed using the Dice coefficient and the unweighted pair group method with arithmetic means (UPGMA). Position tolerance and optimization were set to 1.1%.

Capillary gel electrophoresis-based PCR ribotyping was performed as described previously [34]. Primers described by Bidet and colleagues [35] were used for amplification of intergenic spacer regions (ISRs), with forward primer labelled with a WellRED dye D4-PA (Sigma-Aldrich, Germany). PCR products were analyzed with CEQ™ 8000 Genetic Analysis System (Beckman Coulter) using a 33 cm capillary and gel LPAI. CEQ 600-bp DNA size standard (Beckman-Coulter) was used to determine fragment lengths. Capillary separation conditions were as follows: samples injection voltage of 2 kV over 60 s, separation voltage of 4.8 kV with a total running time of 75 min and a capillary temperature of 50°C.

PCR ribotypes were determined with WEBRIBO database (https://webribo.ages.at/) [34]. Fragment sizes were also imported into BioNumerics software for comparison of banding patterns generated with classical agarose gel electrophoresis and sequencer-based capillary gel electrophoresis.

Toxinotyping was performed as described previously [36]; http://www.mf.uni-mb.si/mikro/tox). Non-toxigenic strains (without the PaLoc, region encoding toxins A and B) were confirmed by amplification of 115 bp long insert with primer pair Lok1/Lok3 [32]. Presence of binary toxin gene *cdt* B was detected as described previously [37].

DECLARATIONS

Acknowledgements

Part of this research has received funding from European Communities 7th Framework programme (FP7/2007-2011) under grant agreement No. 223585.

Authors' contributions

SJ, VZ and MR have designed the study, SJ and VZ have performed typing, MHW has contributed toward typing, all authors have contributed strains and participated at writing. All authors have read and approved the final manuscript.

REFERENCES

1. Hensgens MP, Keessen EC, Squire MM, Riley TV, Koene MG, de Boer E, Lipman LJ, Kuijper EJ: *Clostridium difficile*infection in the community: a zoonotic disease?. Clin Microbiol Infect. 2012, 18 (7): 635-645. 10.1111/j.1469-0691.2012.03853.x.
2. Rupnik M, Songer JG: *Clostridium difficile* Its Potential as a Source of Foodborne Disease. Adv Food Nutr Res. 2010, 60: 53-66.
3. Squire MM, Riley TV: *Clostridium difficile* Infection in Humans and Piglets: A 'One Health' Opportunity. Curr Top Microbiol Immunol. 2012, 365: 299-314.
4. Weese JS: Clostridium difficile in food–innocent bystander or serious threat?. Clin Microbiol Infect. 2010, 16 (1): 3-10. 10.1111/j.1469-0691.2009.03108.x.
5. Rodriguez-Palacios A, Borgmann S, Kline TR, LeJeune JT: *Clostridium difficile* in foods and animals: history and measures to reduce exposure. Anim Health Res Rev. 2013, 14 (1): 11-29. 10.1017/S1466252312000229.
6. Bakker D, Corver J, Harmanus C, Goorhuis A, Keessen EC, Fawley WN, Wilcox MH, Kuijper EJ: Relatedness

of human and animal *Clostridium difficile* PCR ribotype 078 isolates determined on the basis of multilocus variable-number tandem-repeat analysis and tetracycline resistance. J Clin Microbiol. 2010, 48 (10): 3744-3749. 10.1128/JCM.01171-10.

7. Debast SB, van Leengoed LA, Goorhuis A, Harmanus C, Kuijper EJ, Bergwerff AA: *Clostridium difficile* PCR ribotype 078 toxinotype V found in diarrhoeal pigs identical to isolates from affected humans. Environ Microbiol. 2009, 11 (2): 505-511. 10.1111/j.1462-2920.2008.01790.x.

8. Janezic S, Ocepek M, Zidaric V, Rupnik M: *Clostridium difficile* genotypes other than ribotype 078 that are prevalent among human, animal and environmental isolates. BMC Microbiol. 2012, 12 (1): 48-10.1186/1471-2180-12-48.

9. Jhung MA, Thompson AD, Killgore GE, Zukowski WE, Songer G, Warny M, Johnson S, Gerding DN, McDonald LC, Limbago BM: Toxinotype V *Clostridium difficile* in humans and food animals. Emerg Infect Dis. 2008, 14 (7): 1039-1045. 10.3201/eid1407.071641.

10. Koene MG, Mevius D, Wagenaar JA, Harmanus C, Hensgens MP, Meetsma AM, Putirulan FF, Van Bergen MA, Kuijper EJ: *Clostridium difficile* in Dutch animals: their presence, characteristics and similarities with human isolates. Clin Microbiol Infect. 2011, 18 (8): 778-784.

11. Keel K, Brazier JS, Post KW, Weese S, Songer JG: Prevalence of PCR ribotypes among *Clostridium difficile* isolates from pigs, calves, and other species. J Clin Microbiol. 2007, 45 (6): 1963-1964. 10.1128/JCM.00224-07.

12. Alvarez-Perez S, Blanco JL, Bouza E, Alba P, Gibert X, Maldonado J, Garcia ME: Prevalence of *Clostridium difficile* in diarrhoeic and non-diarrhoeic piglets. Vet Microbiol. 2009, 137 (3–4): 302-305.

13. Avbersek J, Janezic S, Pate M, Rupnik M, Zidaric V, Logar K, Vengust M, Zemljic M, Pirs T, Ocepek M: Diversity of *Clostridium difficile* in pigs and other animals in Slovenia. Anaerobe. 2009, 15 (6): 252-255. 10.1016/j.anaerobe.2009.07.004.

14. Keessen EC, Donswijk CJ, Hol SP, Hermanus C, Kuijper EJ, Lipman LJ: Aerial dissemination of *Clostridium difficile* on a pig farm and its environment. Environ Res. 2011, 111 (8): 1027-1032. 10.1016/j.envres.2011.09.014.

15. Schneeberg A, Neubauer H, Schmoock G, Baier S, Harlizius J, Nienhoff H, Brase K, Zimmermann S, Seyboldt C: *Clostridium difficile* Genotypes in Piglet Populations in Germany. J Clin Microbiol. 2013, 51 (11): 3796-3803. 10.1128/JCM.01440-13.

16. Keessen EC, Harmanus C, Dohmen W, Kuijper EJ, Lipman LJ: *Clostridium difficile* infection associated with pig farms. Emerg Infect Dis. 2013, 19 (6): 1032-1034. 10.3201/eid1906.121645.

17. Noren T, Johansson K, Unemo M: *Clostridium difficile* PCR ribotype 046 is common among neonatal pigs and humans in Sweden. Clin Microbiol Infect. 2014, 20 (1): 2-6. 10.1111/1469-0691.12296.

18. Squire MM, Carter GP, Mackin KE, Chakravorty A, Noren T, Elliott B, Lyras D, Riley TV: Novel molecular type of *Clostridium difficile* in neonatal pigs, Western Australia. Emerg Infect Dis. 2013, 19 (5): 790-792.

19. Rupnik M: Heterogeneity of large clostridial toxins: importance of *Clostridium difficile* toxinotypes. FEMS Microbiol Rev. 2008, 32 (3): 541-555. 10.1111/j.1574-6976.2008.00110.x.

20. Bauer MP, Notermans DW, van Benthem BH, Brazier JS, Wilcox MH, Rupnik M, Monnet DL, van Dissel JT, Kuijper EJ: *Clostridium difficile* infection in Europe: a hospital-based survey. Lancet. 2011, 377 (9759): 63-73. 10.1016/S0140-6736(10)61266-4.

21. Weese JS, Rousseau J, Deckert A, Gow S, Reid-Smith RJ: *Clostridium difficile* and methicillin-resistant Staphylococcus aureus shedding by slaughter-age pigs. BMC Vet Res. 2011, 7: 41-10.1186/1746-6148-7-41.

22. Schneeberg A, Neubauer H, Schmoock G, Grossmann E, Seyboldt C: Presence of *Clostridium difficile* PCR ribotype clusters related to 033, 078 and 045 in diarrhoeic calves in Germany. J Med Microbiol. 2013, 62 (Pt 8): 1190-1198.

23. Romano V, Albanese F, Dumontet S, Krovacek K, Petrini O, Pasquale V: Prevalence and genotypic characterization of *Clostridium difficile* from ruminants in Switzerland. Zoonoses Public Health. 2012, 59 (8): 545-548. 10.1111/j.1863-2378.2012.01540.x.

24. Knight DR, Thean S, Putsathit P, Fenwick S, Riley TV: Cross-sectional study reveals high prevalence of *Clostridium difficile*non-PCR ribotype 078 strains in Australian veal calves at slaughter. Appl Environ Microbiol. 2013, 79 (8): 2630-2635. 10.1128/AEM.03951-12.

25. Rodriguez-Palacios A, Stampfli HR, Duffield T, Peregrine AS, Trotz-Williams LA, Arroyo LG, Brazier JS, Weese JS: *Clostridium difficile* PCR ribotypes in calves, Canada. Emerg Infect Dis. 2006, 12 (11): 1730-1736. 10.3201/eid1211.051581.

26. Hammitt MC, Bueschel DM, Keel MK, Glock RD, Cuneo P, DeYoung DW, Reggiardo C, Trinh HT, Songer JG: A possible role for *Clostridium difficile* in the etiology of calf enteritis. Vet Microbiol. 2008, 127 (3–4): 343-352.

27. Schneeberg A, Rupnik M, Neubauer H, Seyboldt C: Prevalence and distribution of *Clostridium difficile* PCR ribotypes in cats and dogs from animal shelters in Thuringia, Germany. Anaerobe. 2012, 18 (5): 484-488. 10.1016/j.anaerobe.2012.08.002.

28. Knight DR, Riley TV: Prevalence of gastrointestinal *Clostridium difficile* carriage in Australian sheep and lambs. Appl Environ Microbiol. 2013, 79 (18): 5689-5692. 10.1128/AEM.01888-13.

29. Rupnik M: Is *Clostridium difficile*-associated infection a potentially zoonotic and foodborne disease?. Clin Microbiol Infect. 2007, 13 (5): 457-459. 10.1111/j.1469-0691.2007.01687.x.

30. Walk ST, Micic D, Jain R, Lo ES, Trivedi I, Liu EW, Almassalha LM, Ewing SA, Ring C, Galecki AT, Rogers MA, Washer L, Newton DW, Malani PN, Young VB, Aronoff DM: *Clostridium difficile* ribotype does not

predict severe infection. Clin Infect Dis. 2012, 55 (12): 1661-1668. 10.1093/cid/cis786.

31. Waslawski S, Lo ES, Ewing SA, Young VB, Aronoff DM, Sharp SE, Novak-Weekley SM, Crist AE, Dunne WM, Hoppe-Bauer J, Johnson M, Brecher SM, Newton DW, Walk ST: *Clostridium difficile* ribotype diversity at six health care institutions in the United States. J Clin Microbiol. 2013, 51 (6): 1938-1941. 10.1128/JCM.00056-13.

32. Braun V, Hundsberger T, Leukel P, Sauerborn M, von Eichel-Streiber C: Definition of the single integration site of the pathogenicity locus in *Clostridium difficile*. Gene. 1996, 181 (1–2): 29-38.

33. Janezic S, Rupnik M: Molecular typing methods for *Clostridium difficile*: pulsed-field gel electrophoresis and PCR ribotyping. Methods Mol Biol. 2010, 646: 55-65. 10.1007/978-1-60327-365-7_4.

34. Indra A, Huhulescu S, Schneeweis M, Hasenberger P, Kernbichler S, Fiedler A, Wewalka G, Allerberger F, Kuijper EJ: Characterization of *Clostridium difficile* isolates using capillary gel electrophoresis-based PCR ribotyping. J Med Microbiol. 2008, 57 (Pt 11): 1377-1382.

35. Bidet P, Barbut F, Lalande V, Burghoffer B, Petit JC: Development of a new PCR-ribotyping method for *Clostridium difficile* based on ribosomal RNA gene sequencing. FEMS Microbiol Lett. 1999, 175 (2): 261-266. 10.1111/j.1574-6968.1999.tb13629.x.

36. Rupnik M, Avesani V, Janc M, von Eichel-Streiber C, Delmee M: A novel toxinotyping scheme and correlation of toxinotypes with serogroups of *Clostridium difficile* isolates. J Clin Microbiol. 1998, 36 (8): 2240-2247.

37. Stubbs S, Rupnik M, Gibert M, Brazier J, Duerden B, Popoff M: Production of actin-specific ADP-ribosyltransferase (binary toxin) by strains of *Clostridium difficile*. FEMS Microbiol Lett. 2000, 186 (2): 307-312. 10.1111/j.1574-6968.2000.tb09122.x.

CHAPTER 34 THE SYNERGISTIC NECROHEMORRHAGIC ACTION OF CLOSTRIDIUM PERFRINGENS PERFRINGOLYSIN AND ALPHA TOXIN IN THE BOVINE INTESTINE AND AGAINST BOVINE ENDOTHELIAL CELLS

Stefanie Verherstraeten, Evy Goossens, Bonnie Valgaeren, Bart Pardon, Leen Timbermont, Karen Vermeulen, Stijn Schauvliege, Freddy Haesebrouck, Richard Ducatelle, Piet Deprez and Filip Van Immerseel

INTRODUCTION

Since the ban on antimicrobial growth promoters in Europe, necrohemorrhagic enteritis emerged as a major cause of mortality in veal calves in Belgium, causing important economic losses [1, 2, 3]. Bovine necrohemorrhagic enteritis, also known as enterotoxaemia, is most typically characterized by sudden death and macroscopic post-mortem findings are necrotic and hemorrhagic lesions in the small intestine [4, 5]. Microscopically, necrosis of the intestinal mucosa and hemorrhages are observed [1, 5, 6]. *Clostridium perfringens* is considered as the causative agent [1, 7]. This spore-forming, Gram-positive, anaerobic bacterium is often found as a normal inhabitant of the intestine of most animal species and humans [6, 8, 9]. For reasons that are not yet fully understood, *C. perfringens* can, under certain predisposing conditions, proliferate rapidly, concurrently produce toxins and cause disease. Stress, for example, is considered to be such a predisposing factor, and also the feed composition is believed to be of major importance for the development of the disease [7, 10, 11]. The presence of a causative toxin determines the potential of a *C. perfringens* strain to cause lesions in several animal species. Classification of *C. perfringens* strains is based on the production of four major toxins, namely alpha, beta, epsilon and iota toxin. In addition to the major toxins, other toxins can be secreted, such as beta2-toxin and perfringolysin [5, 12].

There has been controversy on the toxins responsible for bovine necrohemorrhagic enteritis. Some studies proposed epsilon toxin as a possible causative toxin [13, 14, 15, 16]. This toxin is produced by type B and D strains and plays a key role in the pathogenesis of sheep and goat enterotoxaemia. Filho et al. could indeed induce clinical signs and lesions, when a type D strain was inoculated intraduodenally in a calf [15]. In an intestinal loop assay comparing alpha and epsilon toxin, only epsilon toxin was able to cause severe oedema and hemorrhages in the lamina propria [9]. These results point to epsilon toxin as causative toxin. More recently, beta2-toxin (CPB2) has been linked to necrohemorrhagic enteritis in calves and cows [2, 6, 17, 18, 19]. Manteca et al. showed that inoculating a beta2-positive type A strain into a bovine ligated intestinal loop caused hemorrhages of the intestinal wall and necrosis [19]. The strain however also produced high levels

Citation: Stefanie Verherstraeten, Evy Goossens, Bonnie Valgaeren, Bart Pardon, Leen Timbermont, Karen Vermeulen, Stijn Schauvliege, Freddy Haesebrouck, Richard Ducatelle, Piet Deprez and Filip Van Immerseel, The synergistic necrohemorrhagic action of Clostridium perfringens perfringolysin and alpha toxin in the bovine intestine and against bovine endothelial cells, DOI: 10.1186/1297-9716-44-45.

of alpha toxin, so a synergistic action between both toxins was proposed. Moreover, allelic variants of the CPB2-gene have been identified and strains from cattle mostly carried the atypical CPB2-gene that is not expressed, in contrast to the "consensus" variant [2, 6, 17]. In addition, a more recent study isolated only beta2-negative type A strains from calves with necrohemorrhagic enteritis and these strains were also able to induce pathological changes in inoculated intestinal loops [10]. We recently developed an experimental intestinal loop model that mimics the typical lesions of calf necrohemorrhagic enteritis both macroscopically and microscopically [20]. In this model, it was demonstrated that type A strains from bovine and non-bovine origin, including both beta2-negative and -positive strains, were able to induce necrohemorrhagic lesions [20]. These results suggest that the causative toxin should be present in all the tested *C. perfringens* strains. This puts forward a potential role for alpha toxin and perfringolysin, since both are produced by nearly all *C. perfringens* strains [21]. The importance of perfringolysin in the pathogenesis of bovine necrohemorrhagic enteritis is not reported before. In gas gangrene or clostridial myonecrosis, perfringolysin is involved in the pathogenesis in synergy with alpha toxin [22, 23, 24]. Additionally, Valgaeren et al. observed that the early pathogenesis of calf necrohemorrhagic enteritis in an experimental loop assay is characterized by congestion of the capillaries resulting in hemorrhages and finally necrosis of the mucosa [20]. This points to the endothelium as a possible target.

Therefore, the objective of the present study was to evaluate the role of perfringolysin in the development of necrohemorrhagic enteritis and its synergism with alpha toxin in calves, by using a calf intestinal loop assay and endothelial cell cytotoxicity assays.

MATERIALS AND METHODS

Bacterial strains and culture conditions

The bacterial strains used were a wild-type gas gangrene strain (JIR325) and its isogenic mutant genetically deficient in the production of perfringolysin and alpha toxin (Δ*pfoA* Δ*plc* double mutant JIR4444) as well as the Δ*pfoA* Δ*plc* double mutant complemented with a plasmid that carried either the perfringolysin gene (*pfoA*-complemented Δ*pfoA* Δ*plc* mutant JIR4460) or the alpha toxin gene (*plc*-complemented Δ*pfoA* Δ*plc* mutant JIR4461) or both toxins (*pfoA plc* double-complemented Δ*pfoA* Δ*plc* mutant JIR4462) (Table 1) [23, 25]. All strains were kindly provided by J.I. Rood (Department of Microbiology, Monash University, Clayton, Victoria, Australia). The strains were grown at 37 °C in Brain Heart Infusion (BHI) broth (Oxoid, Basingstoke, United Kingdom) with 0.375% glucose in an anaerobic (84% N_2, 8% CO_2 and 8% H_2) cabinet (Ruskinn Technology, Bridgend, UK). When required, chloramphenicol (30 µg/mL) was added to the growth media. The supernatants were filter-sterilized over a 0.2 µM filter before use in the experiments (Merck Millipore, Billerica, Massachusetts). When a logarithmic-phase culture was used, a 1/100 dilution from an overnight culture was made 3 h prior to use and was incubated in an anaerobic cabinet.

Table 1: Description of strains and toxin activities in supernatants of an overnight culture

Strain[a]	**Strain number**	**Relevant characteristics**[b]	**Plasmid-encoded toxin gene(s)**[a]	**Plc activity(µg mL^{-1})**[c]	**PFO activity ($\log_2$(titre))**[c]	**Ref.**
Wild-type	JIR325	Strain 13[d]		12.5 ± 2.5	4.8 ± 0.2	[25]
Δ*pfoA* Δ*plc*	JIR4444	JIR325 pfoA::ermB plcΩpJIR1774, suicide plasmid		< 1.0	< 1.0	[23]
pfoA-complemented Δ*pfoA* Δ*plc*	JIR4460	JIR4444(pJIR871), Cm^R	*pfoA* $^+$	< 1.0	4.1 ± 0.3	[23]
plc-complemented Δ*pfoA* Δ*plc*	JIR4461	JIR4444(pJIR1642), Cm^R	*plc* $^+$	6.8 ± 0.7	< 1.0	[23]
double-complemented Δ*pfoA* Δ*plc*	JIR4462	JIR4444(pJIR1720), Cm^R	*pfoA*$^+$*plc*$^+$	8.0 ± 0.5	3.5 ± 0.1	[23]

[a]*pfoA:* perfringolysin gene, *plc* : alpha toxin gene, [b] *Cm*^{r}: chloramphenicol resistant, [c] *Plc* : alpha toxin, PFO: perfringolysin O, [d]JIR325 is a rifampicin and nalidixic acid resistant derivative of strain 13, a gas gangrene strain.

Filter-sterilized supernatant of an overnight culture of each strain was assayed for perfringolysin activity by the doubling dilution hemolytic assay with horse red blood cells as described previously (Table 1) [26]. The perfringolysin activity was expressed as the reciprocal of the last dilution which showed complete hemolysis. The perfringolysin assay was performed in triplicate. For the detection of alpha toxin in the supernatant, the Bio-X Alpha Toxin Elisa Kit (Bio-X Diagnostics, Jemelle, Belgium) was used according to the instructions of the manufacturer (Table 1). The amount of alpha toxin was calculated as described previously in µg mL^{-1}[27]. The alpha toxin ELISA was performed in triplicate.

Assessing the role of perfringolysin by using an intestinal loop model

The animal studies were undertaken with approval (EC2012_056) of the Ethical Committee of the Faculty of Veterinary Medicine (Ghent University). Three 11-week-old Holstein Friesian calves, originating from a commercial veal herd, were used. Intestinal loop assays were conducted as described by Valgaeren et al. [20]. Briefly, the calves were anesthetized and the small intestine was exteriorized. Intestinal loops were ligated and injected with 20 mL logarithmic cultures followed by an injection of 10 mL 25% commercial milk replacer (Vitaspray, Vitamex®, Drongen, Belgium) suspended in sterile 0.9% NaCl solution. Because the gas gangrene strain JIR325 could induce lesions comparable to the bovine strains, this strain was used in combination with its isogenic mutants (Table 1) [20]. Each strain was injected in quintuplicate and as a control BHI was injected in five loops instead. After injection of the loops, the abdomen was closed and the calves were maintained under anesthesia. At 6-h post-inoculation the animals were euthanized and samples were taken. Samples were fixed in 4% phosphate buffered formaldehyde. They were embedded in paraffin wax, sectioned and stained with hematoxylin-eosin by the conventional method for histological examination. The sections were evaluated for presence of necrotic lesions (Leica DM L2 microscope with Leica DFC320 camera and LAS software).

Isolation of bovine umbilical vein endothelial cells

Primary bovine umbilical vein endothelial cells (BUVEC) were isolated from umbilical cord veins by an adaptation of the method of Jaffe et al. [28]. Umbilical cords obtained from calves born by caesarean section, were transported in 0.9% HBSS-HEPES buffer (pH 7.4, Gibco, Grand Island, NY, USA) supplemented with 500 U/mL penicillin (Sigma-Aldrich) and 50 µg/mL streptomycin (Sigma-Aldrich). The umbilical vein was cannulated and flushed with pre-warmed (37 °C) HBSS (Gibco, Grand Island, NY, USA). 0.5% collagenase type IV (Sigma-Aldrich) suspended in HBSS was infused into the lumen of the clamped shut umbilical vein and it was incubated for 30 min at 37 °C. After gently massaging the umbilical vein, the cells were flushed from the vein by perfusion with 10 mL HBSS containing 20% fetal calf serum (FCS, Bockneck Labs Inc., Toronto, Canada). After rinsing (250 × g, 5 min), a single cell suspension was obtained by filtration through a 70 µm cell strainer (BD Labware, San Jose, CA, USA). The pelleted (250 × g, 10 min) cells were resuspended in endothelial cell growth medium containing 20% FCS (EGM-2; Lonza, Basel, Switzerland) and seeded in 25 cm^2 plastic tissue culture flasks. After 24 h incubation at 37 °C in the presence of 5% CO_2, the cell medium was changed. Bovine umbilical vein endothelial cells were grown to confluence. The endothelial origin and purity was verified by immunocytochemistry using anti-mouse CD31 antibody (Dako, Heverlee, Belgium).

Assessing the cytotoxic effects of perfringolysin on bovine endothelial cells

In order to visually assess cytotoxicity, BUVEC were seeded on 13-mm-circular glass slides (VWR International BVBA, Leuven, Belgium) in a 24-well plate at a concentration of 1×10^5 cells/mL and were incubated at 37 °C in the presence of 5% CO_2. After 36 h, the cells were exposed to 3% filter-sterilized supernatant of an overnight culture diluted in serum-free endothelial cell growth medium (SFM). The strains used for producing the supernatants were the wild-type strain JIR325 and its isogenic mutants (Table 1). SFM was used as a control. After 1.5 h incubation, the cells were rinsed three times with HBSS containing Ca^{2+} and Mg^{2+}. They were fixed with 100% methanol and stained with Haemacolor-stain (Merck, Darmstadt, Germany). The glass slides were mounted on a microscope slide and observed microscopically.

To quantify the cytotoxicity, BUVEC were seeded in a 96-well plate at a concentration of 1×10^5 cells/mL and incubated for 36 h as described above. 1% or 6% of the above mentioned supernatants in SFM was added to the cells. SFM was used to determine reference values. After 1.5 h incubation, a Neutral Red Uptake Assay was performed [29]. Briefly, Neutral Red Medium (EGM-2 medium containing neutral red (Merck N.V./S.A., Overijse, Belgium)) was added to the cells and the plates were incubated at 37 °C. After 3 h of incubation, the cells were rinsed with HBSS containing Ca^{2+} and Mg^{2+} and treated with extracting solution (50% absolute ethanol, 49% distilled water and 1% glacial acetic acid) for 15 min at room temperature on a shaker to extract the neutral red from the cells. The absorbance was determined at 550 nm and cell viability was expressed as the percentage of viable cells compared to untreated cells (negative control) and cells treated with the supernatant of the wild-type (positive control). Each culture supernatant was tested in duplicate in three independent assays.

Statistical analysis

Significant differences in the number of loops with necrosis between the wild-type and the mutants were determined using a two-tailed Fisher Exact test ($P < 0.05$). Significant differences between the relative viability of the mutants and 0%, which corresponds with the relative viability of the wild-type strain, were investigated using a two-tailed Wilcoxon signed rank test ($P < 0.05$). A one-way analysis of variance (ANOVA) with the post hoc Tukey-Kramer multiple-comparison test was used to identify significant differences in the relative viability of cells after contact with the supernatants of the mutants ($P < 0.001$). All statistical analyses were performed using GraphPad Prism Software 5.0 (GraphPad Software, Inc., USA).

RESULTS

Assessing the role of perfringolysin by using an intestinal loop model

Histological examination of loops inoculated with the wild-type strain showed necrosis of the tips of the villi and congestion of the capillaries and hemorrhages in the underlying viable tissue (Figure 1). Rod-shaped bacteria were found attached to cellular debris in the lumen and to the mucosa. To elucidate the relative contribution of perfringolysin and alpha toxin in the induction of necrohemorrhagic enteritis a wild-type strain and its Δ*pfoA* Δ*plc* mutant was used in combination with the Δ*pfoA* Δ*plc* mutant complemented with either the *pfoA* or the *plc* gene or both (Figure 2). Using the same intestinal loop model, Valgaeren et al. observed mucosal hemorrhages, not only in the challenge strain inoculated loops, but also in some control loops. Necrosis only occured after inoculation of a *C. perfringens* strain [20]. Therefore, in the present study we focussed on the presence of necrosis to compare the mutants with the wild-type strain. Significantly fewer loops injected with the Δ*pfoA* Δ*plc* mutant or the *pfoA*-complemented Δ*pfoA* Δ*plc* mutant (or *plc*-deficient strain) showed necrosis in comparison to the wild-type strain ($P<0.01$). The *plc*-complemented Δ*pfoA* Δ*plc*mutant (or *pfoA*-deficient strain) could induce necrotic lesions in fewer loops as compared to the wild-type strain, but the difference in number of necrotic loops did not reach statistical significance. The double-complemented Δ*pfoA* Δ*plc* mutant showed necrosis in as many loops as the wild-type. Apparently, only the complementation of both toxins could restore the activity to that of the wild-type. In the control loops no necrotic lesions were detected.

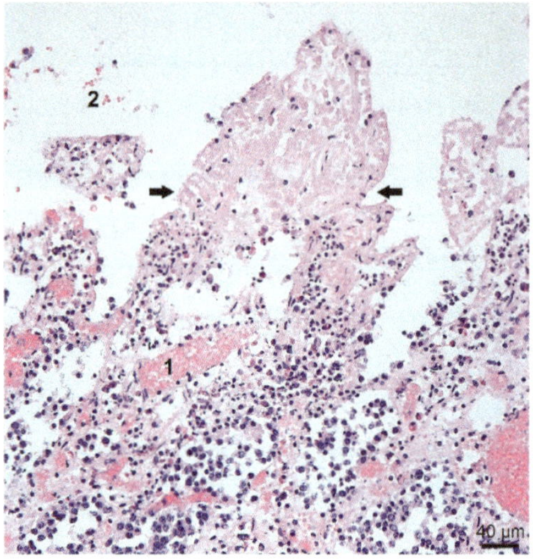

Figure 1: Histological section from an intestinal loop inoculated with wild- type. Hematoxylin and eosin stained histological section from an intestinal loop inoculated with a logarithmic culture of the wild-type strain and milk replacer, sampled after 6 h incubation. Arrows indicate the demarcation of the necrosis of the villus tip with loss of epithelial cells. Also capillary congestion (1) and hemorrhage (2) are present.

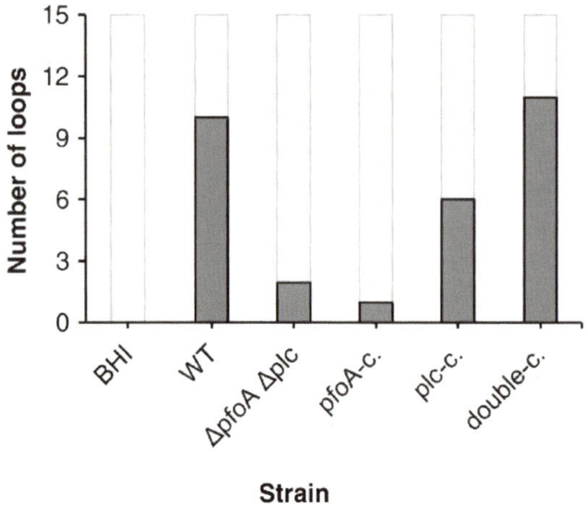

Figure 2: Number of loops with necrosis for wild- type and isogenic mutants. The graph shows the total number of loops in which necrosis was present, evaluated 6 h after inoculation with a logarithmic-phase culture of the wild-type strain (WT), Δ*pfoA* Δ*plc* mutant (Δ*pfoA* Δ*plc*), *pfoA*-complemented Δ*pfoA* Δ*plc* mutant (*pfoA*-c.), *plc*-complemented Δ*pfoA*Δ*plc* mutant (*plc*-c.), double-complemented Δ*pfoA* Δ*plc* mutant (double-c.) and BHI as a control in three calf intestinal loop assays. Each strain was inoculated in quintuplicate. A significant difference was found between the wild-type and the Δ*pfoA* Δ*plc* double mutant ($P<0.01$) and the *pfoA*-complemented Δ*pfoA* Δ*plc* mutant ($P<0.01$).

Assessing the cytotoxic effects of perfringolysin on bovine endothelial cells

To determine whether perfringolysin and alpha toxin have cytotoxic effects on endothelial cells, bovine umbilical cord endothelial cells were exposed to supernatant of a wild-type strain and its isogenic mutants. Almost all cells detached after exposure to supernatant of the wild-type strain (Figure 3). No cytotoxicity could be observed visually when using the supernatant of the Δ*pfoA* Δ*plc* mutant as compared to the control. The supernatants of the *pfoA*-complemented Δ*pfo* Δ*plc* mutant and the *plc*-complemented Δ*plc* Δ*pfo* mutant were less cytotoxic in comparison with supernatant of the wild-type strain, but more cytotoxic as compared to supernatant of the Δ*plc* Δ*pfo* mutant. Complementation of the Δ*plc* Δ*pfo* mutant with both the *plc* and *pfo*gene restored cytotoxic effects to the wild-type levels. These data indicate that perfringolysin and alpha toxin are important factors for cytotoxicity on bovine endothelial cells and have a synergistic effect.

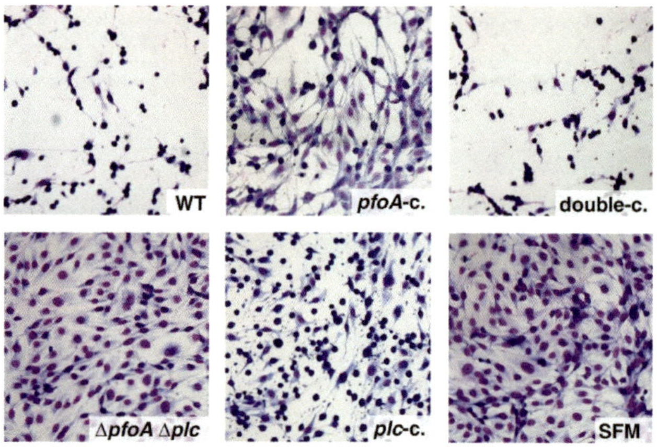

Figure 3: Cytotoxic effect of the supernatant of wild-type and isogenic mutants on bovine umbilical vein endothelial cells(BUVEC.) Photomicrograph of Haemacolor-stained cells after 1.5 h exposure to 3% supernatant of the wild-type strain (WT), Δ*pfoA* Δ*plc* double mutant (Δ*pfoA* Δ*plc*), *pfoA*-complemented Δ*pfoA* Δ*plc* mutant (*pfoA*-c.), *plc*-complemented Δ*pfoA* Δ*plc* mutant (*plc*-c.), double-complemented Δ*pfoA* Δ*plc* mutant (double-c.) and SFM as a negative control. Magnification, ×400.

To quantify the relative contribution of alpha toxin and perfringolysin on endothelial cell cytotoxicity, the viability was assessed by a Neutral Red Uptake Assay. The percentage viability after 1.5 h incubation with 1 and 6% supernatant of the isogenic mutants relative to viable untreated cells (negative control) and cells treated with supernatant of the wild-type strain (positive control) are shown in Figure 4. The cytotoxic effect of 6% supernatant of the Δ*pfoA* Δ*plc* mutant was significantly lower than the wild-type ($P<0.05$) and all other tested strains ($P<0.001$). The cytotoxicity of 1% supernatant of Δ*pfoA* Δ*plc* mutant, *pfoA*-complemented Δ*pfoA*Δ*plc* mutant and the *plc*-complemented Δ*pfoA* Δ*plc* mutant was significantly lower as compared to that of the wild-type ($P<0.05$) and that of the double-complemented Δ*pfoA* Δ*plc* mutant ($P<0.001$). These results confirm that perfringolysin as well as alpha toxin contribute to the cytotoxic effect of a *C. perfringens* culture, and show a synergistic effect of perfringolysin and alpha toxin.

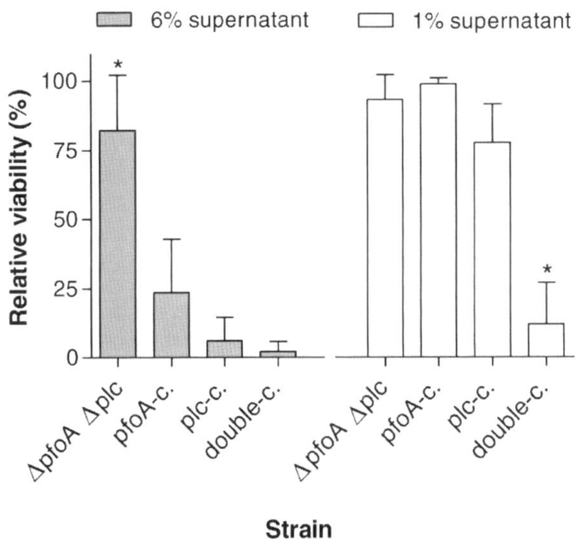

Figure 4: Effect of the supernatant of wild-type and isogenic mutants on the viability of bovine umbilical vein endothelial cells. The graph shows the percentage of viable cells relative to viable untreated cells (negative control) and cells treated with supernatant of the wild-type strain (positive control) after 1.5 h incubation with 6 and 1% supernatant of Δ*pfoA* Δ*plc* double mutant (Δ*pfoA* Δ*plc*), *pfoA*-complemented Δ*pfoA* Δ*plc* mutant (*pfoA*-c.), *plc*-complemented Δ*pfoA* Δ*plc* mutant (*plc*-c.) and double-complemented Δ*pfoA* Δ*plc* mutant (double-c.). The values are the average of three independent experiments conducted in duplicate with error bars representing the standard deviations (SD). Asterisks indicate significant difference between that strain and all other strains for each concentration ($p<0.001$).

DISCUSSION

The presence of a causative toxin in a *C. perfringens* strain determines its potential to cause lesions and subsequently diseases in several animal species. However, there is still controversy on the toxin responsible for bovine necrohemorrhagic enteritis. In a previous study, it was demonstrated that type A strains from bovine and non-bovine origin can induce necrohemorrhagic lesions in a calf intestinal loop assay [20]. These results suggest that the causative toxin is one of the toxins produced by all *C. perfringens* type A strains. In the present study, it was shown that perfringolysin and alpha toxin are involved in the induction of necrohemorrhagic lesions. Indeed, a *plc*-complemented Δ*pfoA* Δ*plc* mutant (or *pfoA*-deficient strain) and a *pfoA*-complemented Δ*pfoA* Δ*plc* mutant (or *plc*-deficient strain) of a gas gangrene strain had a decreased ability to induce necrohemorrhagic lesions in a calf intestinal loop assay. The gas gangrene strain JIR325 was used, because perfringolysin- and alpha toxin-deficient mutants of this strain were already available and because this strain was able to induce mucosal hemorrhages and necrosis of the villus tips comparable to the lesions induced by bovine strains in a calf intestinal loop model [20]. In previous studies, it was suggested that epsilon toxin and beta2-toxin are essential in the development of necrosis. Filho *et al.* induced lesions in a calf intraduodenally inoculated with a type D strain [15]. The authors proposed epsilon toxin as causative toxin. However, based on our results, alpha toxin and perfringolysin may also have been involved in lesion development, since both toxins are produced by type D strains as well. In an intestinal loop assay, comparing alpha and epsilon toxin, only epsilon toxin was able to cause severe oedema and hemorrhages in the lamina propria [9], but these authors did not observe necrosis, in contrast to our results which showed necrohemorrhagic lesions comparable to field cases. Manteca et al. stated that beta2-toxin was an essential toxin, because inoculation of a beta2-positive type A strain into a bovine ligated intestinal loop caused necrohemorrhages of the intestinal wall [19]. However, the strain also produced a high level of alpha toxin and the authors proposed a synergistic effect of alpha toxin and beta2-toxin. Since nearly all type A strains produce perfringolysin as well, this toxin may also have been important in the development of the lesions. In addition, our results agree with a recent study in which only beta2-negative type A strains were isolated from calves with necrotic enteritis and these strains were able to induce pathologic changes when inoculated in intestinal loops [10]. It is still possible that beta2-toxin or other toxins can have supplementary effects.

Valgaeren et al. also found indications that endothelial damage may be involved in the early stages of intestinal lesion development [20]. Our results suggest perfringolysin-induced cytotoxic effects on endothelial cells may play a potential role in the development of necrohemorrhagic enteritis. We showed that the *plc*-complemented Δ*pfoA* Δ*plc* mutant (or *pfoA*-deficient strain) was significantly less cytotoxic for bovine umbilical cord endothelial cells (BUVEC). Endothelial cells form a vital barrier that controls the exchange of cells, macromolecules and fluids between the vascular lumen and the surrounding tissue. They also maintain the normal blood flow due to their antiplatelet, anticoagulant and fibrinolytic properties. Disruption of the endothelial barrier leads to increased vascular permeability along with tissue edema and hemorrhage. Furthermore, it augments local coagulation and vascular thrombosis, and subsequent hypoxic tissue necrosis [30]. In order to confirm that the endothelium is the target cell of perfringolysin or alpha toxin in bovine necrohemorrhagic enteritis, it would be interesting to localize the toxin in lesions, as already been done for beta toxin in necrotic enteritis in piglets and in a human case [31, 32]. Beta toxin has been shown to induce porcine endothelial cell damage in vitro and to bind to endothelial cells, and not to epithelial cells, in the gut of diseased animals, suggesting that disruption of endothelial cells plays a role in type C enteritis [30, 31, 33].

Additionally, our results show that perfringolysin and alpha toxin act synergistically in inducing BUVEC cytotoxicity and necrohemorrhagic lesions in a calf intestinal loop model. In gas gangrene, perfringolysin and alpha toxin also act synergistically [22, 23, 24, 34]. Alpha toxin is a phospholipase C that hydrolyzes phosphatidylcholine and sphingomyelin, both of which are important constituents of eukaryotic cell membranes. Perfringolysin is a cholesterol-dependent cytolysin and oligomerizes upon contact with cholesterol-containing membranes to form large transmembrane pores by inserting a beta-barrel into the membrane [24]. It has been stated that the ability of perfringolysin to perforate the membrane of target cells, is determined by the amount of free cholesterol molecules present [35, 36]. Moe and Heuck found that alpha toxin cleaves the phosphocholine headgroup of phosphatidylcholine, increasing the number of free cholesterol molecules in the membrane and by doing so, facilitating the interaction of perfringolysin and cholesterol [36]. This concerted action of alpha toxin and perfringolysin may contribute to the synergistic effect between both toxins in gas gangrene and in bovine necrohemorrhagic enteritis.

In gas gangrene, perfringolysin modulates the host inflammatory response by upregulating leukocyte and endothelial adhesion molecules. This causes leukocyte accumulation within the blood vessels and inhibits the normal influx of phagocytic cells into infected host tissue, reducing inflammation [22, 23, 37]. Additionally, alpha toxin enhances the expression of platelet adhesion molecules, contributing to the formation of freely moving intravascular aggregates of platelets, fibrin and neutrophils. This leads to the obstruction of the vessels and contributes to a decreased blood flow [34]. Gas gangrene is characterized by tissue necrosis, thrombosis and a lack of leukocyte infiltration at the site of infection. On the contrary, bovine necrohemorrhagic enteritis is associated with congestion of the capillaries, hemorrhages and inflammation [7, 10, 20]. So perfringolysin and alpha toxin appear to be involved in both diseases, but may act in a different way. The use of mutants deficient in the production of alpha toxin or perfringolysin in a mouse myonecrosis model showed that alpha toxin is essential for thrombosis formation [22, 23]. Furthermore, when rabbits were treated intravenously with recombinant perfringolysin a vasodilatory effect and a reduced systemic vascular resistance was observed. On the other hand, in rabbits treated with recombinant alpha toxin the vascular resistance was maintained and the arterial pressure was reduced [23, 38, 39]. Altered vascular integrity, but not vascular occlusion, seems to be in accordance with the role of perfringolysin in bovine necrohemorrhagic enteritis. This may also explain partly the inflammation present in necrohemorrhagic enteritis as opposed to the lack of leukocyte infiltration in gas gangrene.

Next to the toxic effect of perfringolysin on endothelial cells, other effects on the gastro-intestinal mucosa are most likely of importance in the development of necrohemorrhagic enteritis. Indeed, before perfringolysin can target the endothelial cells, it has to cross the epithelial barrier. While cytotoxic effects of perfringolysin and alpha toxin on intestinal epithelial cells cannot be excluded, also other *C. perfringens* toxins, enzymes or other molecules could affect the intestinal integrity. Intestinal integrity disturbances can also be caused by *C. perfringens* independent factors in the field, such as viral and parasitological pathogens. The most well-known example of a predisposing pathogen for necrotic enteritis is coccidiosis in broilers [40, 41], but also in calves several infectious agents, such as coccidia, enteropathogenic bacteria, corona- and rotaviruses can affect the intestinal barrier integrity [40, 41, 42, 43, 44]. In addition, certain feed components can act as predisposing factors for the induction of gut lesions. These include high non-starch polysaccharide containing diets and high protein diets, the latter most likely feeding the auxotrophy *C. perfringens* has for many amino acids [45, 46]. The diet can have a direct effect on the virulence of *C. perfringens*, but it can as well affect the intestinal tract. In calves fed with milk replacing proteins an increase in permeability of the intestinal mucosa was observed, which caused leakage of macromolecules from the gut into the tissues [41, 47, 48, 49]. This might also facilitate the uptake of toxins through the epithelial barrier.

In conclusion, our study indicates that perfringolysin is involved in the pathogenesis of bovine necrohemorrhagic enteritis and acts synergistically with alpha toxin. We hypothesize that both toxins may induce intestinal lesions by targeting the endothelial cells.

DECLARATIONS

Acknowledgements

The authors thank J.I. Rood for providing the bacterial strains used in this study. The authors acknowledge support from all veterinary surgeons from the division of anesthesia for their assistance in the intestinal loop assays, the PhD students from the pathology-department who assisted in the sampling and the department of obstetrics, reproduction and herd health for the supply of bovine umbilical cords. The authors would like to thank Christian Puttevils, Delphine Ameye and Astra Dhanijns for the technical assistance. This project was supported by the Institute for Science and Technology, Flanders under contract number 090910.

Authors' contributions

SV, EG, BV, BP, LT, RD, PD and FVI participated in the design of the study. SV, EG, BV, BP, KV, SS and RD performed the calf intestinal loop assays. SV carried out the cell cytotoxicity assays and analyzed the data. SV, FH, RD, PD and FVI wrote the manuscript. All authors revised the manuscript and read and approved the final manuscript.

REFERENCES

1. Manteca C, Daube G, Pirson V, Limbourg B, Kaeckenbeeck A, Mainil JG: Bacterial intestinal flora associated with enterotoxaemia in Belgian Blue calves. Vet Microbiol. 2001, 81: 21-32. 10.1016/S0378-1135(01)00329-7.
2. Muylaert A, Lebrun M, Duprez JN, Labrozzo S, Theys H, Taminiau B, Mainil J: Enterotoxaemia-like syndrome and *Clostridium perfringens* in veal calves. Vet Rec. 2010, 167: 64-65. 10.1136/vr.b4869.
3. Pardon B, De Bleecker K, Hostens M, Callens J, Dewulf J, Deprez P: Longitudinal study on morbidity and mortality in white veal calves in Belgium. BMC Vet Res. 2012, 8: 26-10.1186/1746-6148-8-26.
4. Valgaeren BR, Pardon B, Verherstraeten S, Goossens E, Timbermont L, Haesebrouck F, Ducatelle R, Deprez PR, Van Immerseel F: Intestinal clostridial counts have no diagnostic value in the diagnosis of enterotoxaemia in veal calves. Vet Rec. 2013, 172: 237-10.1136/vr.101236.
5. Songer JG: Clostridial enteric diseases of domestic animals. Clin Microbiol Rev. 1996, 9: 216-234.
6. Lebrun M, Filee P, Mousset B, Desmecht D, Galleni M, Mainil JG, Linden A: The expression of *Clostridium perfringens*consensus beta2 toxin is associated with bovine enterotoxaemia syndrome. Vet Microbiol. 2007, 120: 151-157. 10.1016/j.vetmic.2006.10.020.
7. Lebrun M, Mainil JG, Linden A:Cattle enterotoxaemia and*Clostridium perfringens*: description, diagnosis and prophylaxis.Vet Rec. 2010, 167: 13-22. 10.1136/vr.167.1.12.

8. Rood JI: Virulence genes of *Clostridium perfringens*. Annu Rev Microbiol. 1998, 52: 333-360. 10.1146/annurev.micro.52.1.333.

9. Morris WE, Dunleavy MV, Diodati J, Berra G, Fernandez-Miyakawa ME: Effects of *Clostridium perfringens* alpha and epsilon toxins in the bovine gut. Anaerobe. 2012, 18: 143-147. 10.1016/j.anaerobe.2011.12.003.

10. Morris WE, Venzano AJ, Elizondo A, Vilte DA, Mercado EC, Fernandez-Miyakawa ME: Necrotic enteritis in young calves. J Vet Diagn Invest. 2011, 23: 254-259. 10.1177/104063871102300209.

11. Nowell VJK, Kropinsky AM, Songer JG, Macinnes JI, Parreira VR, Prescott JF: Genome sequencing and analysis of a type A *Clostridium perfringens* isolate from a case of bovine clostridial abomasitis. PLoS One. 2012, 7: e32271-10.1371/journal.pone.0032271.

12. Songer JG, Miskimmins DW: *Clostridium perfringens* type E enteritis in calves: two cases and a brief re of the literature. Anaerobe. 2004, 10: 239-242. 10.1016/j.anaerobe.2004.05.001.

13. Niilo L, Avery RJ: Bovine "enterotoxemia" I. *Clostridium Perfringens* types isolated from animal sources in Alberta and Saskatchewan. Can Vet J. 1963, 4: 31-36.

14. Uzal FA, Kelly WR, Morris WE, Assis RA: Effects of intravenous injection of *Clostridium perfringens* type D epsilon toxin in calves. J Comp Pathol. 2002, 126: 71-75. 10.1053/jcpa.2001.0514.

15. Filho EJ, Carvalho AU, Assis RA, Lobato FF, Rachid MA, Carvalho AA, Ferreira PM, Nascimento RA, Fernandes AA, Vidal JE, Uzal FA: Clinicopathologic features of experimental *Clostridium perfringens* type D enterotoxemia in cattle. Vet Pathol. 2009, 46: 1213-1220. 10.1354/vp.08-VP-0304-U-FL.

16. Uzal FA, Rolfe BE, Smith NJ, Thomas AC, Kelly WR: Resistance of ovine, caprine and bovine endothelial cells to *Clostridium perfringens* type D epsilon toxin in vitro. Vet Res Commun. 1999, 23: 275-284. 10.1023/A:1006362819202.

17. Gibert M, Jolivet-Reynaud C, Popoff MR: Beta2 toxin, a novel toxin produced by *Clostridium perfringens*. Gene. 1997, 203: 65-73. 10.1016/S0378-1119(97)00493-9.

18. Bueschel DM, Jost BH, Billington SJ, Trinh HT, Songer JG: Prevalence of cpb2, encoding beta2 toxin, in *Clostridium perfringens* field isolates: correlation of genotype with phenotype. Vet Microbiol. 2003, 94: 121-129. 10.1016/S0378-1135(03)00081-6.

19. Manteca C, Daube G, Jauniaux T, Linden A, Pirson V, Detilleux J, Ginter A, Coppe P, Kaeckenbeeck A, Mainil JG: A role for the *Clostridium perfringens* beta2 toxin in bovine enterotoxaemia?. Vet Microbiol. 2002, 86: 191-202. 10.1016/S0378-1135(02)00008-1.

20. Valgaeren B, Pardon B, Goossens E, Verherstraeten S, Schauvliege S, Timbermont L, Ducatelle R, Deprez P, Van Immerseel F: Lesion development in a new intestinal loop model indicates the involvement of a shared *Clostridium perfringens* virulence factor in haemorrhagic enteritis in calves. J Comp Pathol. 2013, 149: 103-112. 10.1016/j.jcpa.2012.11.237.

21. Rood JI, Cole ST: Molecular genetics and pathogenesis of Clostridium perfringens. Microbiol Rev. 1991, 55: 621-648.

22. Ellemor DM, Baird RN, Awad MM, Boyd RL, Rood JI, Emmins JJ: Use of genetically manipulated strains of *Clostridium perfringens* reveals that both alpha-toxin and theta-toxin are required for vascular leukostasis to occur in experimental gas gangrene. Infect Immun. 1999, 67: 4902-4907.

23. Awad MM, Ellemor DM, Boyd RL, Emmins JJ, Rood JI: Synergistic effects of alpha-toxin and perfringolysin O in *Clostridium perfringens*-mediated gas gangrene. Infect Immun. 2001, 69: 7904-7910. 10.1128/IAI.69.12.7904-7910.2001.

24. O'Brien DK, Melville SB: Effects of *Clostridium perfringens* alpha-toxin (PLC) and perfringolysin O (PFO) on cytotoxicity to macrophages, on escape from the phagosomes of macrophages, and on persistence of C. perfringens in host tissues. Infect Immun. 2004, 72: 5204-5215. 10.1128/IAI.72.9.5204-5215.2004.

25. Lyristis M, Bryant AE, Sloan J, Awad MM, Nisbet IT, Stevens DL, Rood JI: Identification and molecular analysis of a locus that regulates extracellular toxin production in *Clostridium perfringens*. Mol Microbiol. 1994, 12: 761-777. 10.1111/j.1365-2958.1994.tb01063.x.

26. Awad MM, Bryant AE, Stevens DL, Rood JI: Virulence studies on chromosomal alpha-toxin and theta-toxin mutants constructed by allelic exchange provide genetic evidence for the essential role of alpha-toxin in *Clostridium perfringens*-mediated gas gangrene. Mol Microbiol. 1995, 15: 191-202. 10.1111/j.1365-2958.1995.tb02234.x.

27. Zhang G, Darius S, Smith SR, Ritchie SJ: In vitro inhibitory effect of hen egg white lysozyme on *Clostridium perfringens*type A associated with broiler necrotic enteritis and its alpha-toxin production. Lett Appl Microbiol. 2006, 42: 138-143. 10.1111/j.1472-765X.2005.01812.x.

28. Jaffe EA, Nachman RL, Becker CG, Minick CR: Culture of human endothelial cells derived from umbilical veins. Identification by morphologic and immunologic criteria. J Clin Invest. 1973, 52: 2745-2756. 10.1172/JCI107470.

29. Van Parys A, Boyen F, Verbrugghe E, Leyman B, Bram F, Haesebrouck F, Pasmans F: *Salmonella* Typhimurium induces SPI-1 and SPI-2 regulated and strain dependent downregulation of MHC II expression on porcine alveolar macrophages. Vet Res. 2012, 43: 52-10.1186/1297-9716-43-52.

30. Gurtner C, Popescu F, Wyder M, Sutter E, Zeeh F, Frey J, Von Schubert C, Posthaus H: Rapid cytopathic effects of *Clostridium perfringens* beta-toxin on porcine endothelial cells. Infect Immun. 2010, 78: 2966-2973. 10.1128/IAI.01284-09.

31. Miclard J, Jäggi M, Sutter E, Wyder M, Grabscheid B, Posthaus H: *Clostridium perfringens* beta-toxin targets endothelial cells in necrotizing enteritis in piglets. Vet Microbiol. 2009, 137: 320-325. 10.1016/j.vetmic.2009.01.025.

32. Miclard J, Van Baarlen J, Wyder M, Grabscheid B, Posthaus H: *Clostridium perfringens* -toxin binding to vascular endothelial cells in a human case of enteritis necroticans. J Med Microbiol. 2009, 58: 826-828. 10.1099/jmm.0.008060-0.

33. Schumacher VL, Martel A, Pasmans F, Van Immerseel F, Posthaus H:Endothelial binding of beta toxin to small intestinal mucosal endothelial cells in early stages of experimentally induced*Clostridium perfringens*type C enteritis in pigs. Vet Pathol. in press,

34. Hickey MJ, Kwan RY, Awad MM, Kennedy CL, Young LF, Hall P, Cordner LM, Lyras D, Emmins JJ, Rood JI: Molecular and cellular basis of microvascular perfusion deficits induced by *Clostridium perfringens* and *Clostridium septicum*. PLoS Pathog. 2008, 4: e1000045- 10.1371/journal.ppat.1000045.

35. Flanagan JJ, Tweten RK, Johnson AE, Heuck AP: Cholesterol exposure at the membrane surface is necessary and sufficient to trigger perfringolysin O binding. Biochemistry. 2009, 48: 3977-3987. 10.1021/bi9002309.

36. Moe PC, Heuck AP: Phospholipid hydrolysis caused by *Clostridium perfringens* alpha-toxin facilitates the targeting of perfringolysin O to membrane bilayers. Biochemistry. 2010, 49: 9498-9507. 10.1021/bi1013886.

37. Stevens DL, Tweten RK, Awad MM, Rood JI, Bryant AE: Clostridial gas gangrene: evidence that alpha and theta toxins differentially modulate the immune response and induce acute tissue necrosis. J Infect Dis. 1997, 176: 189-195. 10.1086/514022.

38. Asmuth DM, Olson RD, Hackett SP, Bryant AE, Tweten RK, Tso JY, Zollman T, Stevens DL: Effects of *Clostridium perfringens* recombinant and crude phospholipase C and theta-toxin on rabbit hemodynamic parameters. J Infect Dis. 1995, 172: 1317-1323. 10.1093/infdis/172.5.1317.

39. Stevens DL, Bryant AE: The role of clostridial toxins in the pathogenesis of gas gangrene. Clin Infect Dis. 2002, 35: S93-S100. 10.1086/341928.

40. Drew MD, Syed NA, Goldade BG, Laarveld B, Van Kessel AG: Effects of dietary protein source and level on intestinal populations of *Clostridium perfringens* in broiler chickens. Poult Sci. 2004, 83: 414-420.

41. Van Immerseel F, De Buck J, Pasmans F, Huyghebaert G, Haesebrouck F, Ducatelle R: *Clostridium perfringens* in poultry: an emerging threat for animal and public health. Avian Pathol. 2004, 33: 537-549. 10.1080/03079450400013162.

42. Lindsay DS, Dubey JP, Fayer R: Extraintestinal stages of *Eimeria bovis* in calves and attempts to induce relapse of clinical disease. Vet Parasitol. 1990, 36: 1-9. 10.1016/0304-4017(90)90088-S.

43. Chase CC, Hurley DJ, Reber AJ: Neonatal immune development in the calf and its impact on vaccine response. Vet Clin North Am Food Anim Pract. 2008, 24: 87-104. 10.1016/j.cvfa.2007.11.001.

44. Wei S, Gong Z, Che T, Guli A, Tian F: Genotyping of calves rotavirus in China by reverse transcription polymerase chain reaction. J Virol Methods. 2013, 189: 36-40. 10.1016/j.jviromet.2013.01.002.

45. Boyd MJ, Logan MA, Tytell AA: The growth requirements of *Clostridium perfringens* (*welchii*) BP6K. J Biol Chem. 1948, 174: 1013-1025.

46. Fuchs AR, Bonde GJ: The nutritional requirements of *Clostridium perfringens*. J Gen Microbiol. 1957, 16: 317-329. 10.1099/00221287-16-2-317.

47. Barratt ME, Strachan PJ, Porter P: Antibody mechanisms implicated in digestive disturbances following ingestion of soya protein in calves and piglets. Clin Exp Immunol. 1978, 31: 305-312.

48. Kilshaw PJ, Slade H: Passage of ingested protein into the blood during gastrointestinal hypersensitivity reactions: experiments in the preruminant calf. Clin Exp Immunol. 1980, 41: 575-582.

49. Silva AG, Huber JT, Herdt TH, Holland R, Degregorio RM, Mullaney TP: Morphological alterations of small intestinal epithelium of calves caused by feeding soybean protein. J Dairy Sci. 1986, 69: 1387-1393. 10.3168/jds.S0022-0302(86)80545-8.

CHAPTER 35

THE EPIDEMIOLOGY OF CLOSTRIDIUM PERFRINGENS TYPE A ON ONTARIO SWINE FARMS, WITH SPECIAL REFERENCE TO CPB2-POSITIVE ISOLATES

Gloria Chan, Abdolvahab Farzan, Glenn Soltes, Vivian M Nicholson, Yanlong Pei, Robert Friendship and John F Prescott

Keywords: *Clostridium perfringens,* type A, *cpb2,* Pig, Epidemiology

BACKGROUND

Clostridium perfringens type A is considered by some to be one of the most common causes of diarrhea in neonatal pigs [1, 2]. However, the pathogenic basis of *C. perfringens* type A diarrhea is unclear, and the current diagnostic methods for this disease are not specific.

Clostridium perfringens are ubiquitous Gram-positive anaerobes that can be isolated from many environments, and their spore-forming ability allows them to persist in the swine ecosystem [2]. Currently, *C. perfringens* are divided into five toxinotypes (A to E) depending on their production of four major toxins. Isolates of any toxinotype may also produce enterotoxin (CPE) and beta2 toxin (CPB2) [3].

In the past decade, diagnosis of neonatal piglet diarrhea due to *C. perfringens* type A has increased, and has been associated with increased pre-weaning mortality [1]. Disease can develop in suckling pigs in the first week of life, and typical clinical signs include non-hemorrhagic, mucoid diarrhea seen within 48 h of birth, and lasting for 5 d [2]. The current method of diagnosis is based on isolation of large numbers of *C. perfringens*type A possessing the consensus CPB2 gene (*cpb2*) detected by polymerase chain reaction (PCR) from the feces or intestinal contents, and the exclusion of other known causes of neonatal diarrhea [3]. There is currently no commercial test available for detecting CPB2 in isolates [1, 3]. Most porcine isolates carry and express *cpb2* [4].

There is poor understanding of most aspects of *C. perfringens* type A as a possible cause of neonatal diarrhea in piglets, and the prevalence and types of *C. perfringens* present on Ontario swine farms is unknown. The objectives of this study were to compare the prevalence of *C. perfringens* and selected toxin genes among pigs at different stages of production, and to identify farm factors affecting this prevalence.

METHODS

Farm selection

Forty-eight farms in Ontario were conveniently selected and visited once or twice between two periods of sample collection from August to December 2010, and from January 2011 and May 2011. For the first period of sample collections, 28 farms were visited. One farm was visited twice in the first period, and visited again in the second period. In the second period, a total of 11 farms from the first period were visited again, and 20 farms were visited for the first time. Some farms that were visited from the first period were not re-visited because they did not have suckling pigs or they were no longer in business.

Citation: Gloria Chan, Abdolvahab Farzan, Glenn Soltes, Vivian M Nicholson, Yanlong Pei, Robert Friendship and John F Prescott, The epidemiology of Clostridium perfringens type A on Ontario swine farms, with special reference to cpb2-positive isolates, DOI: 10.1186/1746-6148-8-156.

Sample collection

In both periods of sample collection, for farrowing operations, pooled-fecal samples were collected from gestating sows, weanling pigs, and grower-finisher pigs. In addition, a pooled sample was taken from the manure pit. In the second period of sample collection, fecal samples were also collected from lactating sows and their litters. A lactating sow fecal sample was collected by randomly selecting a sow, and manually obtaining a rectal sample with a gloved hand. A pooled-fecal sample of the lactating sow's litter was also obtained by selecting three suckling pigs in the litter and collecting the feces from the piglet's rectum. If suckling pigs did not defecate sufficient material during the sampling process, fresh piglet feces were obtained from the farrowing area of the litter. Three fecal samples were collected from lactating sows, and three pooled fecal samples were collected from their respective litters from each farrowing operation.

A pooled-fecal sample of gestating sows was obtained by selecting 6 sows from different areas of the barn, and obtaining a rectal sample. A pooled-fecal sample of weanling pigs or grower-finisher pigs was obtained from randomly selecting 6 pens, observing the pigs defecating, and then immediately collecting the fresh feces from the floor of the pens. On farrow-to-feeder farms sampling was similar to farrow-to-finish farms except two pooled samples were collected from weaning pigs. On grower-finisher farms, 3 pooled-fecal samples were taken from the pigs present, as well as a pooled manure pit sample. All farms on the study used a liquid manure system and a sample from the holding tank or manure pit was obtained by filling a plastic bottle from the manure pit. Liquid manure from 3 locations in the pit and at 3 different depths was combined to create the pooled sample.

Questionnaire

A survey was administered to collect information on each farm for different management factors including the following: type of operation (farrowing-to-finish, farrowing-to-feeder, or grower-finisher operation), total number of barns, herd size (number of sows, gilts, weanling pigs, and grower-finisher pigs), sow flow, weanling flow, grower-finisher flow (all-in/all-out or continuous), number of farrowing rooms and crates, the presence of other agricultural species (other species), drug usage and vaccination, history of diarrhea outbreak in suckling pigs or post-weaning pigs in the past year, and treatment of the diarrhea problem. A total of 46 farms were surveyed; two farms were not surveyed because they were no longer in business.

Bacterial isolation

For bacterial culture, samples were weighed and 4–5 serial 10-fold dilutions were performed in phosphate buffered saline, pH 7.2. Fecal dilutions were plated onto selective SFP (Shahadi Ferguson Perfringens) medium (Difco, Detroit, MI, USA). The SFP media contains 5% egg yolk emulsion (Oxoid, Nepean, ON), 12 μg/ml kanamycin sulphate, and 30 IU/ml polymyxin B sulphate (SFP Selective Supplement, Oxoid). The plates were transferred to an anaerobic jar, with anaerobic atmosphere provided by GasPak (BD, Sparks, MD, USA) and incubated at 37°C overnight. Colonies with characteristic *C. perfringens* colonial and microscopic morphologies, as well as lecithinase activity on the egg yolk agar, were counted and counts converted to colony-forming units (CFU) per gram.

Genotyping of isolates

Clostridium perfringens colony lysates were examined by multiplex polymerase chain reaction (PCR) for toxin genes using the method described by Albini and colleagues [5]. Five isolates per sample were genotyped for *cpa*, consensus *cpb2* (*cpb2*) and atypical *cpb2* (*atyp-cbp2)*. The isolates recovered during the first period of the study were also genotyped for the major toxin genes beta toxin (*cpb*), enterotoxin (*cpe*), epsilon toxin (*etx*), and iota toxin (*itx*), NetB toxin (*netB*) and large clostridial cytotoxin (*tpeL*). Since these were all found to be absent they were not examined in the second period. The primer sets for the major toxin genes and *cpb2*used were designed using the reported nucleotide sequences [5]. The primer sets for *netB*, *tpeL*, and *atyp-cpb2* were designed for this study using standard approaches and appropriate bacterial control strains. The Roche LightCycler® 480 SW 1.5 software package was used to analyze the data. Relevant positive control strains were included in all batched PCR tests.

Data analysis

The data were entered in a spreadsheet (Microsoft Excel 2007; Microsoft Corp., Redmond, WA) and imported to Stata 10 Intercooled for Windows XP (StataCorp LP, College Station, TX) for statistical analysis.

Three outcomes were measured, which included *C. perfringens* type A (*Cp*A) count in fecal samples, the presence of *cpb2*-carrying *C. perfringens* type A (*cpb2-Cp*A) isolates in fecal samples, and the presence of *atyp-cpb2*-carrying *C. perfringens* type A (atyp-cpb2-*Cp*A) isolates in fecal samples. The independent variables included in multivariable analysis were stage of production (main effect), type of operation, total number of barns, herd size (small or <1000, medium or ≥ 1000–3000, and large or >3000), and the presence of other species.

A mixed linear regression modeling method with farm as a random effect was used to analyze the association between *CpA* count in fecal samples and independent variables. Intra-class correlation coefficient was calculated as $ICC = \sigma^2_{farm}/(\sigma^2_{farm} + \sigma^2_{sample})$. In addition, two separate logistic regression models were fitted to investigate the association between the presence of *cpb2-Cp*A and *atyp-cpb2-Cp*A in fecal samples and independent variables. Intra-cluster coefficient was calculated as $ICC = \sigma^2_{farm}/(\sigma^2_{farm} + \pi^2/3)$ by assuming that sample level variance on the logit scale was $\pi^2/3$, $\pi=3.1416$.

Univariable analysis of independent variables and their association with *Cp*A count, and presence of *cpb2-Cp*A and *atyp-cpb2-Cp*A isolates in fecal samples was performed using a single linear or logistic regression. Variables with $P < 0.20$ were selected for inclusion in multivariable analyses which was modeled at the sample level with farm as random variable.

A manual stepwise procedure was used to build the multivariable models. Pair-wise correlation coefficients were calculated between independent variables, and coefficients with an absolute value greater than 0.8 were considered colinear. If two independent variables were significantly correlated, the more informative variable was used in the final model. A variable was identified as a confounder if it changed the coefficient of the main effects by 20% or more when the potential confounder variable was removed. If a variable was determined to be a confounder, it was included in the final model regardless of its statistical significance. Interaction was evaluated between all independent variables and the main effects model. Each interaction term was assessed for statistical significance with the main effects, and the interaction terms with $P < 0.05$ were included in the final model. Interaction terms that were not significant in the final model were removed if removal of the interaction term did not result in a significant change in the likelihood ratio test (logistic regression) and partial F-test (linear regression).

For linear multivariable analysis, a $\log_{10}$ transformation was used on the *C. perfringens* count (CFU/g) in order to meet the normal distribution and homoscedasticity assumptions for the outcome of interest. The Cook-Weisberg test was performed for the linear multivariable model with farm as a fixed effect, and the assumption of homoscedasticity was met if $P > 0.05$. The Shapiro-Wilk normality test was used to test the normal distribution of $\log_{10}$ CFU/g with farm as a fixed effect, and the assumption of normality was met if $P > 0.05$. The standardized residuals were graphically assessed for outliers, and the leverage values were graphically assessed.

The logistic regression multivariable model with farm as a fixed effect for the presence of *cpb2* in *C. perfringens* type A isolates was assessed for goodness-of-fit, which was indicated by $P > 0.05$ in the Hosmer-Lemeshow test. Pearson residuals were graphically assessed for outliers, and the leverage values were graphically assessed.

The Spearman's rank correlation test was used to analyze the association between the toxin genes in lactating sows and their litters.

RESULTS

A total of 354 fecal samples were collected, distributed between the sources shown in Table 1. Overall, *Clostridium perfringens* was isolated from 225 (64%) of 354 fecal samples (98% of suckling piglets, 34% of weanling pigs, 18% of grower-finisher pigs, 89% of gestating sows, 96% of lactating sows, and 75% of manure pit samples) (Table 1). A farm was considered positive for *C. perfringens* if *cpa* was detected in the isolate of at least one fecal sample, and a farm was considered positive for consensus *cpb2* if it was detected in the *C. perfringens* isolate of at least one fecal sample. A total of 42 farms (87.5%) were positive for *C. perfringens*, and 25 farms (52%) were positive for *cpb2*. *C. perfringens* was not recovered from samples collected on 6 (12.5%) of 48 farms, all of which were grower-finisher operations. Within-herd prevalence of *C. perfringens* type A ranged between 0 and 100% with a mean of 53.5±32%.

Table 1: Log $_{10}$CFU/g of *C. perfringens* in fecal samples and the positive proportion of toxin genes

	Log_{10}(CFU/g)	**Percentage of positive samples**		**Total No. of Samples**
	Mean±SD	***Cpb2***	***Atyp-cpb2***	
Suckling pigs	5.0±1.70	77	44	57
Lactating Sows	4.0±1.86	26	16	57
Gestating Sows	4.3±1.85	5	0	37
Weanling pigs	1.3±1.87	18	7	44
Grower-finisher pigs	0.6±1.24	2	5	99
Manure Pit	2.7±1.82	27	17	60
Total	2.7±2.38	25	15	354

Clostridium perfringens count ($\log_{10}$CFU/g)

The mean of $\log_{10}$ CFU/g of *Clostridium perfringens* in fecal samples is shown in Table 1. The total mean count was 2.7±2.4 $\log_{10}$ CFU/g. The distribution of independent variables on 46 surveyed farms is shown in Table 2. Independent variables with $P < 0.20$ that were initially included in the multivariable linear regression analysis were the stage of production, type of operation, total herd size, presence of other species, and sampling period. The type of operation and total herd size did not significantly affect the *C. perfringens* count of fecal samples in the final model ($P > 0.05$). The $\log_{10}$*C. perfringens* count for fecal samples collected from the first and second sampling period was not significantly different ($P > 0.05$); the sampling period was included in the final model because *C. perfringens* count in the samples collected from different stage of production was confounded by sampling period. In multivariable analysis, the $\log_{10}$*C. perfringens* count was higher in suckling pig fecal samples compared to that of weanling pigs, grower-finisher pigs, and the manure pit ($P < 0.05$) (Table 3). The $\log_{10}$*C. perfringens* count was higher in gestating sow samples, lactating sow samples, or the manure pits, respectively, compared to that of weanling pigs and grower-finisher pigs ($P < 0.05$). In the final model, *C. perfringens* count in fecal samples collected from sows (both gestating and lactating) was interacted by the presence of other species on farms ($P < 0.05$) (Table 3). Overall, the $\log_{10}$*C. perfringens* count was higher in the fecal samples collected from sows on farms where other species were absent. The $\log_{10}$*C. perfringens* in gestating sows versus piglets was $4.1 = [(-1.35) + (-0.93) + 1.5 + 4.9 \text{ (constant)}]$ and $5.0 = [(-1.35) + 1.5 + 4.9 \text{ (constant)}]$ in the presence and absence of other species, respectively. Similarly, the $\log_{10}$*C. perfringens* in lactating sows versus piglets was $3.88 = [(-1.93) + (-0.93) + 1.84 + 4.9 \text{ (constant)}]$ and $4.81 = [(-1.93) + 1.84 + 4.9 \text{(constant)}]$ in the presence and absence of other species, respectively.

Table 2: The distribution of independent variables among 46 surveyed farms

Independent Variable		**Percentage of *Cpb2*-positive farms**	**Univariable analysis *P*-value (sample level)**
Type of operation (sample n=220)	Farrowing (farm n=30)	73	0.012
	Grower-finisher (farm n=16)	25	
Other species (sample n=212)	Not present (farm n=23)	57	0.004
	Present (farm n=23)	57	
Herd Size (sample n=217)	Small (<1000) (farm n=9)	33	Referent
	Medium (≥1000-3000) (farm n=28)	61	0.272
	Large (>3000) (farm n=9)	67	0.018
Sow Flow (sample n=84)	All-in/all-out (farm n=16)	75	0.417
	Continuous (farm n=14)	71	
Weanling Flow (sample n=15)	All-in/all-out (farm n=23)	70	0.326
	Continuous (farm n=8)	87.5	
Grower-Finisher Flow (sample n=20)	All-in/all-out (farm n=27)	48	0.327
	Continuous (farm n=13)	54	
Antibiotic usage (sample n=66)	Yes (farm n=7)	100	0.304*
	No (farm n=23)	65	
Diarrhea (sample n=58)	Yes (farm n=11)	82	0.792*
	No (farm n=19)	68	

*Exact logistic regression.

Table 3: Multivariable linear regression model of factors associated with fecal *C. perfringens* count ($\log_{10}$ CFU/g)

Variables		**Coefficient**	**Standard Error**	**95% Confidence Interval**	***P*-value**
Stage	Suckling pig	Referent			
	Lactating sow	−1.9	0.367	(−2.7)-(−1.2)	<0.001
	Gestating sow	−1.4	0.438	(−2.2)-(−0.50)	0.002
	Weanling	−3.8	0.398	(−4.6)-(−3.1)	<0.001
	Grower-finisher	−4.4	0.413	(−5.2)-(−3.6)	<0.001
	Manure pit	−1.7	0.403	(−2.5)-(−0.93)	<0.001
Other species	Absent	Referent			
	Present	−0.93	0.484	(−1.9)-(−0.019)	0.055
	Present x Gestating sow	1.5	0.626	0.30-2.75	0.015
	Present x Lactating sow	1.8	0.533	0.79-2.9	0.001
Sampling Period	First	Referent			
	Second	0.34	0.234	(−0.12)-(−0.80)	0.144

The Intraclass Correlation Coefficient (ICC) was 0.24, indicating a low level of clustering in which the within-farm variation of the *C. perfringens* count accounted for almost a quarter of the total variation of the count.

Potential outliers were identified for two farms, of which the weanling fecal samples had a *C. perfringens*count of 6.0 and 6.7 $\log_{10}$ CFU/g, respectively. Potential extreme observations were identified for two farms, of which *C. perfringens* was not isolated from weanling fecal samples.

Clostridium perfringens-associated toxin genes

The distribution of *cpb2* and *atyp-cbp2* genes among *Clostridium perfringens* isolates cultured from fecal samples is presented in Table 1.

The independent variables initially included in the multivariable logistic analysis were the stage of production, presence of *atyp-cpb2*, type of operation, presence of other species, total herd size, and sampling period. The type of operation, presence of other species, and total herd size did not significantly affect the likelihood of detecting *cpb2*-positive *C. perfringens* isolates in the final model ($P > 0.05$). The variable of vaccination was not included in the statistical analysis because none of the farms surveyed vaccinated sows or pigs for *C. perfringens*.

Cpb2 was more likely found in the isolates of suckling pigs compared to those of lactating sows, gestating sows, and grower-finisher pigs, and manure pits ($P < 0.05$) (Table 4). The likelihood of finding *cpb2* in *C. perfringens* isolates recovered from weanling pigs was higher compared to that of gestating sows (OR=0.077, P=0.011) and grower-finisher pigs (OR=0.065, P=0.027).

Table 4: Multivariable logistic regression model of factors associated with *cpb2* -positive *C. perfringens* isolates

Variables		Odds Ratio	Standard Error	95% Confidence Interval	*P*-value
Stage	Suckling pig	Referent			
	Lactating sow	0.069	0.0437	0.020-0.24	<0.001
	Gestating sow	0.020	0.0189	3.2×10^{-3}-0.13	<0.001
	Weanling	0.26	0.216	0.052-1.3	0.103
	Grower-finisher	0.017	0.0185	2.0×10^{-3}-0.14	<0.001
	Manure pit	0.11	0.0677	3.2×10^{-2}-0.37	<0.001
Atyp-cpb2	Negative	Referent			
	Positive	19	12.0	5.7-65	<0.001

The Intraclass Correlation Coefficient (ICC) that compared the within-farm and between-farm variance was 0.24 and 0.25, respectively for linear regression and logistic regression, indicating a low level of clustering in which the within-farm variation of *C. perfringens* count and the presence of *cpb2* accounted for almost a quarter of the total variation.

The likelihood of detecting *atyp-cpb2* was higher in *cpb2*-positive isolates compared to *cpb2*-negative isolates ($P < 0.001$) (Table 4). The percentages of samples that had *atyp-cpb2* were 51% in *cpb2*-positive samples, and 6% in *cpb2*-negative samples.

Clostridium perfringens isolates recovered from lactating sows (OR=0.20, P=0.001), weanlings (OR=0.20, P=0.039), and the manure pits (OR=0.32, P=0.022) were less likely to be positive for *atyp-cpb2* than isolates recovered from suckling pigs. The correlation of *cpb2* or *atyp-cpb2* in isolates of lactating sows and in isolates from their litters was not statistically significant.

Potential outliers were identified for two farms. On one farm, *cpb2* nor *atyp-cpb2* were detected in the *C. perfringens* isolates of a suckling pig fecal sample. On the other farm, *cpb2* was not detected in the *atyp-cpb2*positive *C. perfringens* isolates of the manure pit fecal sample. Potential extreme observations were identified for one farm, of which the *cpb2*-positive *C. perfringens* isolates were only recovered from two of three suckling pig fecal samples.

The isolates recovered during the first period of the study were all negative for *cpb*, *cpe*, *etx*, *itx*, *netB* and *tpeL*. For this reason, they were not examined in the second period.

DISCUSSION

The current study of enteric *Clostridium perfringens* in pigs identified novel findings that may increase the understanding of the epidemiology of infection and possible diagnosis of the suckling pig diarrhea thought to be caused by this organism. *Clostridium perfringens* type A is speculated to be an emerging pathogen associated with neonatal piglet diarrhea [6, 7, 8, 9], although not all prevalence studies conducted on infectious causes of piglet diarrhea have included *C. perfringens* type A in the analysis [6, 10, 11]. Isolates recovered from diarrheic piglets could not be differentiated genetically from isolates recovered from non-diarrheic piglets in the United States [12] or on genotype in Canada [13].

This study is the first to examine systematically the quantitative prevalence of *C. perfringens,* as well as an expanded range of toxin genes, in pigs of different ages on multiple farms. Our results showed that the number of *C. perfringens* type A isolates was higher in suckling pigs compared to pigs in other stages of production. High numbers of *C. perfringens* were also isolated from gestating and lactating sows. The pattern of decline in colonization by *C. perfringens* with age has been noted previously in the intestine of individual pigs but not at the farm level [14]. The decrease in *C. perfringens* count for fecal samples in weanling and grower-finisher pigs was generally expected, since the population of *C. perfringens* decreases in the pig intestine as other bacterial species establish their populations [2]. Host-related factors that affect the decline in colonization may include diet, changes in large intestinal microflora with time, age-related changes in host physiology, or the development of intestinal immunity. The decline in numbers of *C. perfringens* in pigs in the grower-finisher stage may also be partly due to changes in management factors including the use of antimicrobials during the nursery and grower-finisher stages. The effect of other species on the farm in increasing *C. perfringens* counts in sows (Table 3) was an unexpected observation that factors other than "host" can affect colonization by this organism.

Many *C. perfringen*s isolated from pigs are relatively unusual among isolates from different animal sources in that they belong to a clonal population [15]. Unusually, these isolates are characterized both by being consensus *cpb2* positive and by expressing CPB2 [4]. There thus appears to be an adaptation of this lineage to swine. Although we did not however examine the isolates made here for their phylogenetic relationships, on the basis of the present study, the adaptation of this lineage appears to be to the young pig, and notably to the suckling piglet. This relationship of *cpb2*-positive *C. perfringens* to the young piglet (Tables 2, 4) has not previously been demonstrated at the farm level. Most of the suckling pig isolates in this study were positive for consensus *cpb2* as noted in other studies [4, 7, 8, 9]. The gestating sow isolates were usually not positive for *cpb2* and lacked the *atyp-cpb2* gene that was found in lactating sow and suckling pig isolates, which appear to be specifically colonized by *cpb2*-positive strains [3]. It is possible that the sows in the lactating stage acquired *cpb2*-positive *C. perfringens* strains from suckling pigs in the litter, but that strains were not always maintained when the suckling pigs were weaned and sows returned to the gestating stage. However, there was no significant correlation of the presence of *cpb2* and *atyp-cpb2* in *C. perfringens* type A isolates from sows and their litters, suggesting that the source of the strains in suckling pigs may be different from sows, or that *cpb2* and/or *atyp-cpb2* positive isolates are more likely to proliferate in suckling pigs. Interestingly, there was a dominance of *atyp-cpb2* isolates in *C. perfringens* isolated from grower-finisher pigs. It is possible that other factors contributed to the decline in consensus *cpb2*-positive *C. perfringens* isolates seen in grower-finisher pigs, such as antimicrobial usage; a negative association between *cpb2*-positive *C. perfringens* isolates and resistance to erythromycin and clindamycin was documented in an Ontario study [16]. The isolates from the manure pit were unexpectedly similar to isolates from suckling pigs, reasons for which are unclear.

This study identified genes in the most abundant isolate of *C. perfringens*, so that the less abundant genotypes may not have been detected. *C. perfringens* isolates positive for *cpb2* were more likely to be positive for *atyp-cpb2*, suggesting a linkage between these genes. Further research on the genetic diversity of *C. perfringens* type A isolates in clinically healthy and diarrheic suckling pigs, and the conditions of which *cpb2*and *atyp-cpb2* toxin genes are expressed, may help clarify the role of this agent in neonatal piglet diarrhea.

Since the farms in our study were conveniently selected, the results may not apply to the general population of Ontario swine farms. The difference in bacterial count of *C. perfringens* in fecal samples from pigs at different stages of production might have been affected by the sampling procedure, since samples for weanling pigs and grower-finisher pigs were collected from feces on the pen floor whereas the samples for sows and suckling pigs were collected from the rectum. The fecal samples collected from gestating sows, weanling pigs, grower-finisher pigs, and the manure pits were pooled, so it is conceivable that some samples were misclassified. Fecal samples collected from farrowing operations in the first period of the study did not include those of suckling pigs or lactating sows, which could affect the farm-level sensitivity for the detection of *cpb2*-positive *C. perfringens* isolates from these farms.

This is the first time that *C. perfringens* type A from swine has been examined for *netB* and *tpeL*, genes that are common in isolates from chickens with necrotic enteritis [17]. Their absence further supports the idea of host adaptation of strains of *C. perfringens*, as apparent here in the association of *cpb*2-positive strains with piglets. The absence of *cpb* is consistent with the absence of *C. perfringens* type C in enteric disease in swine and other animals in Ontario. The lack of *cpe* in *C. perfringens* isolates confirms earlier studies [18, 19].

CONCLUSIONS

To our best knowledge, this is the first study on the epidemiology of *C. perfringens* in the swine population. This study provides baseline data from healthy pigs at different stages of production as well as in the manure pits for future studies to investigate the role of *C. perfringens* in swine enteric diseases. The study suggests that if C. *perfringens* type A are involved in neonatal enteritis, there may be strains with specific characteristics that cannot be identified by the existing genotyping system. Further work is required to determine whether this is the case.

DECLARATIONS

Acknowledgments

The research was funded by the Ontario Ministry of Agriculture Food and Rural Affairs. We also thank the Natural Sciences and Engineering Research Council for support. We thank Bryan Bloomfield for technical assistance and the swine producers for participating in the research.

Authors' contributions

JP, RF, and AF designed the study. GC and AF performed the data collection, and statistical analysis. GS, VN, and YP performed the bacterial isolation. GS and VN performed the multiplex polymerase chain reaction. All authors contributed to drafting and revising of the manuscript. All authors read and approved the final manuscript.

REFERENCES

1. Lehe K: Successful control of clostridial enteritis: A report from the back forty. Proceedings of American Association of Swine Veterinarians. Perry, IA, USA: American Association of Swine Veterinarians, Dallas; 2009.

2. Schwartz KJ: *Clostridium*-associated diseases in swine. Proceedings of American Association of Swine Veterinarians. Perry, IA, USA: American Association of Swine Veterinarians, Dallas; 2009.
3. Songer JG, Uzal FA: Clostridial enteric infections in pigs. J Vet Diag Invest. 2005, 17: 528-536. 10.1177/104063870501700602.
4. Jost BH, Billington SJ, Trinh HT, Bueschel DM, Songer JG: Atypical *cpb2* genes, encoding beta2-toxin in *Clostridium perfringens* isolates of nonporcine origin. Infect Immun. 2005, 73: 652-656. 10.1128/IAI.73.1.652-656.2005.
5. Albini S, Brodard I, Jaussi A, Wollschlaeger N, Frey J, Miserez R, Abril C: Real-time multiplex PCR assays for reliable detection of *Clostridium perfringens* toxin genes in animal isolates. Vet Microbiol. 2008, 127: 179-185. 10.1016/j.vetmic.2007.07.024.
6. Yaeger M, Funk N, Hoffman L: A survey of agents associated with neonatal diarrhea in Iowa swine including *Clostridium difficile* and porcine reproductive and respiratory syndrome virus. J Vet Diagn Invest. 2002, 14: 281-287. 10.1177/104063870201400402.
7. Garmory HS, Chanter N, French NP, Bueschel D, Songer JG, Titball RW: Occurrence of *Clostridium perfringens* beta2-toxin amongst animals, determined using genotyping and subtyping PCR assays. Epidemiol Infect. 2000, 124: 61-67. 10.1017/S0950268899003295.
8. Bueschel DM, Jost BH, Billington SJ, Trinh HT, Songer JG: Prevalence of cbp2, encoding beta2 toxin, in Clostridium perfringens field isolates: correlation of genotype with phenotype. Vet Microbiol. 2002, 94: 121-129.
9. Waters M, Savoie A, Garmory HS, Bueschel D, Popoff MR, Songer GJ, Titball RW, McClane BA, Sarker MR: Genotyping and phenotyping of beta2-toxigenic *Clostridium perfringens* fecal isolates associated with gastrointestinal diseases in piglets. J Clin Microbiol. 2003, 41: 3584-3591. 10.1128/JCM.41.8.3584-3591.2003.
10. Wieler LH, Ilieff A, Herbst W, Bauer C, Vieler E, Bauerfeind R, Failing K, Klos H, Wengert D, Baljer G, Zahner H: Prevalence of enteropathogens in suckling and weanling suckling pigs with diarrhea in southern Germany. J Vet Med B. 2001, 48: 151-159. 10.1046/j.1439-0450.2001.00431.x.
11. Katsuda K, Kohmoto M, Kawashima K, Tsunemitsu H: Frequency of enteropathogen detection in suckling and weanling pigs with diarrhea in Japan. J Vet Diagn Invest. 2006, 18: 350-354. 10.1177/104063870601800405.
12. Baker AA, Davis E, Rehberger T, Rosener D: Prevalence and diversity of toxigenic *Clostridium perfringens* and *Clostridium difficile* among swine herds in the midwest. Appl Environ Microbiol. 2010, 76: 2961-2967. 10.1128/AEM.02459-09.
13. Farzan A, Kircanki J, DeLay J, Soltes G, Songer GJ, Friendship R, Prescott JF: An investigation into the association between *cpb2*-encoding *Clostridium perfringens* type A and diarrhea in neonatal piglets. Can J Vet Res. in press
14. Smith WH, Jones JET: Observations on the alimentary tract and its bacterial flora in healthy and diseased pigs. J Path Bact. 1963, 84: 387-412.
15. Jost HB, Trinh TH, Songer GJ: Clonal relationships among *Clostridium perfringens* of porcine origin as determined by multilocus sequence typing. Vet Microbiol. 2006, 116: 158-165. 10.1016/j.vetmic.2006.03.025.
16. Slavic D, Boerlin P, Fabri M, Klotins KC, Zoethout JK, Weir PE, Bateman D: Antimicrobial susceptibility of *Clostridium perfringens* isolates of bovine, chicken, porcine, and turkey origin from Ontario. Can J Vet Res. 2011, 75: 89-97.
17. Chalmers G, Bruce HL, Hunter DB, Parreira VR, Kulkarni RR, Jiang YF, Prescott JF, Boerlin P: Multilocus sequence typing analysis of *Clostridium perfringens* isolates from necrotic enteritis outbreaks in broiler chicken populations. J Clin Microbiol. 2008, 46: 3957-3964. 10.1128/JCM.01548-08.
18. Kanakaraj R, Harris DL, Songer GJ, Bosworth B: Multiplex PCR assay for detection of *Clostridium perfringens* in feces and intestinal contents of pigs and in swine feed. Vet Microbiol. 1998, 63: 29-38. 10.1016/S0378-1135(98)00229-6.
19. Klaasen HL, Molkenboer MJ, Bakker J, Miserez R, Häni H, Frey J, Popoff MR, van den Bosch JF: Detection of the beta2 toxin gene of Clostridium perfringens in diarrhoeic piglets in The Netherlands and Switzerland. FEMS Immunol Med Microbiol. 1999, 24 (3): 325-332.

CHAPTER 36

PREVALENCE AND MOLECULAR CHARACTERIZATION OF CLOSTRIDIUM DIFFICILE ISOLATED FROM FEEDLOT BEEF CATTLE UPON ARRIVAL AND MID-FEEDING PERIOD

Marcio C Costa, Richard Reid-Smith, Sheryl Gow, Sherry J Hannon, Calvin Booker, Joyce Rousseau, Katharine M Benedict, Paul S Morley and J Scott Weese

Keywords: Public health, Foodborne, Oxytetracycline, Antimicrobials

BACKGROUND

Clostridium difficile is a Gram-positive, spore-forming bacterium responsible for *C. difficile* infection (CDI) in humans [1], a serious and increasingly problematic disease. A remarkable change in the epidemiology of CDI has been encountered over the past 10 years, with increasing incidence, mortality and relapse rates in humans [2, 3]. Additionally, while classically a hospital-associated pathogen predominantly affecting elderly individuals, there are increasing reports of community-associated CDI, including disease in younger individuals and people with few or no traditional risk factors [1, 4, 5].

The source of infection for community-associated cases of CDI remains uncertain, however foodborne infection has been suggested [4]. Indeed, several studies have recovered spores of *C. difficile* from food products including retail meat [6, 7, 8, 9], yet the source of contamination for food products has not been identified. Contamination of carcasses during slaughter and processing is most likely [10, 11], but the presence of dormant spores of the bacterium in the muscle tissues of food animals should also be considered [12].

While currently unproven, concerns about zoonotic and foodborne transmission of CDI are reasonable considering reports of isolation of *C. difficile* from animals. Concern has been heightened by the apparent increase in CDI in humans caused by the *C. difficile* ribotype 078 [4, 13, 14], a strain that has been associated with community-associated infection [15, 16] since this is the dominant *C. difficile* strain among food animals [15, 17, 18, 19] and has also been recovered from meat products [8, 9].

High prevalences of *C. difficile* shedding have been reported in food animals, yet most studies have involved young animals well before the time of slaughter. Studies of animals performed nearer to the time of slaughter are likely more relevant for assessment of the potential for foodborne exposure, yet limited epidemiological investigations have been performed in feedlot cattle [11, 20].

The objectives of this study were to evaluate the shedding of *C. difficile* by adult feedlot cattle upon arrival and after acclimation to the feedlot diet and environment, and to characterize the recovered isolates. In addition, the potential association between the use of antimicrobial drugs and shedding of the bacterium was also investigated.

RESULTS

A total of 539 cattle were sampled from 4 feedlots, ranging from 121 to 179 cattle per feedlot (mean 135). Adjusting for lack of independence in pens, *C. difficile* was isolated overall from 3.7% of 539 (CI = 2.3-6.1) animals at the time of feedlot

---

Citation: Marcio C Costa, Richard Reid-Smith, Sheryl Gow, Sherry J Hannon, Calvin Booker, Joyce Rousseau, Katharine M Benedict, Paul S Morley and J Scott Weese, Prevalence and molecular characterization of Clostridium difficile isolated from feedlot beef cattle upon arrival and mid-feeding period, DOI: 10.1186/1746-6148-8-38.

arrival in 34 unique pens and from 6.2% of 335 (CI = 2.9-13.1) cattle at mid-feeding period in 22 unique pens. No individuals were positive at both sampling times.

Results of the regression analysis using generalized estimating equation (GEE), accounting for the date of sampling during the feeding period (< 62 days on feed (DOF), 62-71 DOF, or > 71DOF) and for the effects of repeated sampling are presented in Table 1. There was no statistically detectable difference in the likelihood of recovery of *C. difficile* based on DOF ($P = 0.47$).

Table 1: Univariable associations of use of antimicrobials with prevalence of *C.difficile* and prevalence at different periods*

Class of antimicrobial	Odds ratio	95% CI	*P*-value
IN FEED			0.33
Tetracycline	0.77	0.55-1.08	
DAYS ON FEED			0.47
< 62	4.25	0.73-24.63	
62-71	1.07	0.21-5.38	
> 71	Referent	Referent	

* controlling for lack of independence sampling

Sixty-four individuals were treated with parenteral antimicrobials during the study period including beta-lactams (2), macrolides (32), phenicols (1), quinolones (1), sulfonamides (1) and tetracyclines (27). The sum of the Animal Defined Daily Dose (ADD), which quantifies the total amount of antimicrobials administered for each period and for the total risk period were 11, 96, 3, 3, 3 and 54 for each of the drug classes, respectively. Tetracycline was the only in-feed antimicrobial used and was given to all individuals, with a summed ADD of 1278.4. As shown in Table 1, there was no significant association between the use of tetracycline and the prevalence of *C. difficile* in these animals ($P = 0.33$). Results for models regarding the remaining antimicrobials are not shown, as the univariable logistic regression models did not converge.

One isolate could not be recovered after storage and therefore, molecular analysis was performed on the remaining 35 isolates. All the isolates recovered were classified as ribotype 078 and were positive for the toxin producing genes *tcd*A, *tcd*B and *cdt*A. All isolates were indistinguishable on PFGE and classified as North American pulsotype 7 (NAP 7) (Figure 1). As expected, sequencing of the *tcd*C gene identified a 39 bp deletion and C184T upstream truncating mutation, consistent with the *tcd*C-A genotype according to Curry et al. [21].

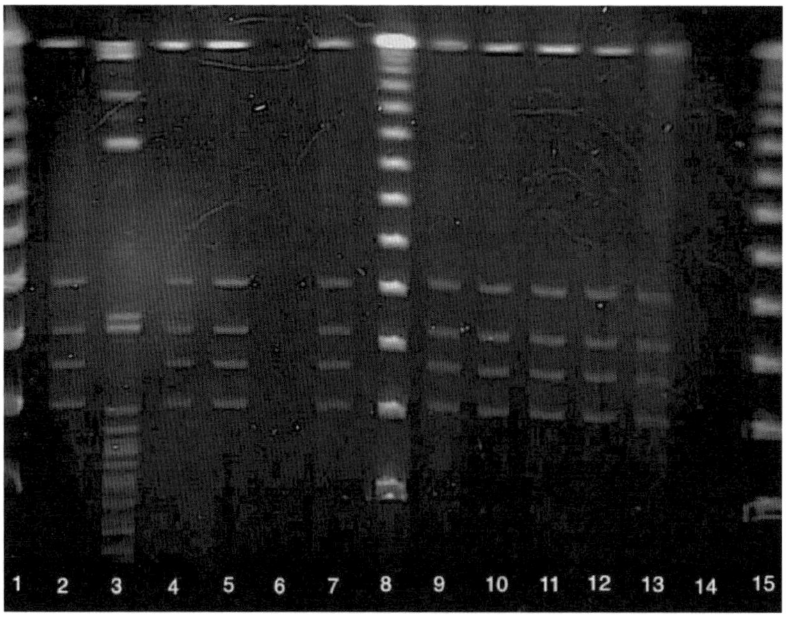

Figure 1: Pulsed-field gel electrophoresis of *Clostridium difficile* isolates recovered from beef cattle entering feedlots. Pulsed-field gel electrophoresis of *Clostridium difficile* isolates recovered from beef cattle entering feedlots. Figure 1 legend: Lanes 1, 8 and 15 contain a PFGE ladder (50-1000 kb). Lane 3 has an unrelated sample and lanes 6 and 14 are empty. The remaining lanes show NAP7 *C. difficile*.

DISCUSSION

The prevalence of feedlot cattle shedding *C. difficile* was low at both sampling times. There is a limited number of studies concerning the epidemiology of *C. difficile* in the bovine species and the data available in the literature are largely restricted to calves [17, 18, 22, 23, 24]. The low shedding prevalence of *C. difficile* in cattle arriving at feedlots reported here is in agreement with the prevalence reported by Indra et al. [2] in cows (4.5%) and slightly higher than the one reported by Rodriguez-Palacios et al. [20] in feedlot cattle at harvest age (1.8%). However, our results indicate a lower shedding prevalence than the one found by Rodriguez-Palacios et al. [11] whom isolated the bacterium from 12.9% of animals arriving to feedlot. The reasons for this difference cannot be explained, however stressing from shipping and different management conditions prior to arrival such as hygiene, population, stocking density, animal mixing and antimicrobial administration should be considered, along with potential geographic variation and differences in methodology.

A high prevalence of *C. difficile* shedding has been reported in young calves. The bacterium was recovered from 14.9% of healthy calves in one study [24] and from 12.7% in another [18], but it can be as high as 51% in veal calves [17]. In addition, *C. difficile* has been detected by PCR in feces of 33.8% of calves submitted for post-mortem examination [23]. The lower prevalence in this and the above-cited studies of older animals is perhaps not surprising given increasing evidence of a strong effect of age on *C. difficile* shedding prevalence, something that has been noted in swine [25, 26, 27] and horses, [28], as well as humans [29]. Costa et al. [17] also observed a significant decrease in shedding prevalence (from 32% to 2%) as veal calves became older, which is in agreement with Hoffer et al. [22], who isolated *C. difficile* from only one out of 204 veal calves sampled at slaughter. The reasons for a higher shedding prevalence in young individuals are uncertain but competition from a more adapted intestinal microflora in older animals may make colonization more difficult. In addition, stress from birth adaptation, a naïve immune response, the type of feeding and the different management systems could also explain the increased prevalence in younger animals.

The potential for antimicrobial drugs to disrupt the normal intestinal microflora leading to *C. difficile*overgrowth has been shown in other species, including humans [30] and horses [28]. Therefore, in order to further investigate the effect of *C. difficile* shedding by animals from feedlot, antimicrobial exposure of cattle was investigated. Antimicrobial exposure, particularly tetracyclines, was common however no influence on *C. difficile* shedding was identified. The lack of an identifiable association between the use of antimicrobials and shedding of *C. difficile* reported here agrees with the findings of Rodriguez-Palacios et al. [11].

Ribotype 078, the only strain found here, can cause CDI in humans [4, 14] and has been increasingly associated with community-associated CDI [13, 15]. A study of human and animal ribotype 078 isolates using highly discriminatory multilocus variable number tandem repeat analyses indicated they were closely related, suggesting that the bacterium may be transmitted between humans and animals [31]. The predominance of this strain was not particularly surprising since it is typically associated with food animals, has been found in various studies of pigs and cattle and it is the most commonly reported strain in pigs in Canada [2, 17, 18, 19, 22, 31, 32]. In addition, the strain has been prevalent (between 73% and 86%) among isolates recovered from some retail beef samples [8, 9]. Another interesting aspect was the finding that no cattle were positive at both sampling times. This suggests that persistent carriers are not common, and that *C. difficile* may be transiently shed and circulated throughout animal populations. Inconsistent or transient shedding has also been reported in dogs [33] and horses [34]. Further studies involving more frequent sampling would help elucidate the on-farm cycling of *C. difficile*.

The predominance of clones classified as ribotype 078/NAP7 recovered from beef cattle reported here (100%) reinforces the results of other studies in the bovine species [17, 18, 19, 22]. However, other researchers found that only 2 out of 24 [11] and 1 out of 17 [20] isolates recovered from cattle were ribotype 078. In addition, it was interesting that other strains, including 027/NAP III, found in retail beef [6, 8, 9] were not isolated in the present study.

The prevalence of shedding of *C. difficile* ribotype 078 by feedlot cattle reported here is an important information for a better understanding of *C. difficile* epidemiology in adult beef cattle. The low prevalence upon feedlot arrival and later in the feeding period must be considered when interpreting food contamination and foodborne risks. The lack of an effect of antimicrobials exposure was interesting and while a study such as this cannot completely discount a role of antimicrobials in the epidemiology of *C. difficile* in cattle, it is clearly not a major determinant, at least on these farms.

CONCLUSIONS

We conclude that the prevalence of *C. difficile* in adult cattle was low at arrival and at mid-feeding period from feedlots. No association was found between exposure to antimicrobial drugs or between days on feed and the prevalence of *C. difficile* in this collection of samples. Ribotype 078/NAP7 was the only strain present among all isolates recovered. It is apparent that *C difficile* is carried in the intestinal tracts of a small percentage of beef cattle going to slaughter, but its public health significance requires further study.

METHODS

Animal selection

Cattle enrolled in this study were managed at four western Canadian feedlots in south Alberta, under production conditions that are typical of those used at large commercial cattle feedlots throughout western Canada and the United States. Feedlots had one-time capacities between 15,000 and 20,000 animals, with pens capable of housing 50 to 350 animals. Animals are housed in open-air, dirt-floor pens arranged side by side with feed alleys and 20% porosity wood-fence windbreaks. All feedlots have modern cattle handling facilities. Each animal handling facility has a hydraulic chute equipped with an individual animal scale, a chute-side computer with software for individual animal data collection and management (*iFHMS*, Feedlot Health Management Services Ltd., Okotoks, Alberta) and separation alleys to facilitate the return of animals to designated pens. All animal handling and sampling procedures were approved prior to the initiation of the study by the University of Guelph Animal Care Committee, the Animal Care Committee of Feedlot Health Management Services (FHMS) and the Institutional Animal Care and Use Committee of Colorado State University.

Candidate animals utilized in the study were procured through the auction market system across western Canada. Various cattle types were fed at these feedlots including cattle of various entry weights, age classes (calves and yearlings), frame sizes, sources (e.g., ranch-direct cattle and back-grounded cattle), and genders (bulls, steers and heifers). A 2-stage random sampling plan was used to determine which pens and animals within those pens were selected for enrolment. Animals were allocated to the study from January 17, 2009 to September 11, 2009. During the enrolment period, 30% of all new pens of cattle were randomly selected for inclusion in the study using a pen randomization table as the cattle arrived at the feedlot. Within each selected pen, 10% of all animals in that pen were then randomly enrolled in the study at initial processing using an individual animal randomization table. Cattle enrolled in the study weighed a mean of 375 kg (152 to 513 kg).

All animals enrolled in the study were subject to standardized animal health management and feedlot production procedures as per the protocols developed by the feedlot animal health/production consultants (FHMS). In brief, each animal received a unique individual animal identification ear tag, a trial-specific ear tag to help identify individuals for future sample collection, a subcutaneous hormonal growth implant in the middle third of the ear, vaccine(s) to immunize against selected bacteria and viruses that cause disease in feedlot cattle, and application of topical avermectin for internal and external parasite control. In animals at higher risk of developing disease, a parental antimicrobial was administered as part the prevention and control strategies for bovine respiratory disease. Water and standard mixed complete feedlot diets, formulated to meet or exceed the National Research Council nutritional requirements for beef cattle feedlot cattle, were offered *ad libitum* throughout the feeding period.

Individual animals enrolled in the trial were sampled twice over the course of the study: at the time of arrival and initial processing, and then again at various times in the middle of the feeding period when cattle were processed again to perform standard feedlot management procedures. Feces were collected from individual animals per rectum using a new palpation sleeve (#33, Almedic, Montreal, Canada) for collection and transfer (minimum 4 g) into a new sterile plastic fecal cup (# 109117, Globe Scientific, Paramus, New Jersey). Fecal samples were labelled, refrigerated (4°C) and transported to FHMS within 7 days of collection. At FHMS, samples were placed into ZipLoc bags and shipped (once a week in a chilled cooler, by air courier (Purolator Corporation) from Calgary, Alberta to the microbiology laboratory (University of Guelph, Guelph, Ontario) for further processing.

Each fecal sample collected over the course of the trial was assigned a unique identification number to ensure blinding of the laboratory staff and uniform labelling of samples. All treatments of cattle housed in the pens of cattle that were enrolled and sampled for the Individual antimicrobial use data were recorded at each feedlot over the course of the study using a chute-side computer system (*i*FHM*S*, FHMS). These data were available for each animal and included the product, the dose, the route and the number of days administered. Data on both individual animal and in-feed antimicrobial exposure were collected, with the in-feed data compiled from the pen-based feeding records. All study data were subsequently compiled, collated in a computer spreadsheet program (Microsoft Office Excel 2003), and verified.

Clostridium difficile culture

Approximately 2 g of feces were inoculated into 9 mL of *C. difficile* moxalactam norfloxacin (CDMN) enrichment broth (Oxoid Ltd; Nepean, ON Canada) containing 0.1% sodium taurocholate and incubated anaerobically at 37°C for 7 days. Two millilitres of broth were then added to 2 mL of anhydrous alcohol and incubated at room temperature for 60 min. After centrifugation (3,980 rcf for 10 min), the pellet was inoculated onto CDMN (Oxoid Ltd; Nepean, ON Canada) agar and incubated in an anaerobic chamber at 37°C for 48 h and, if negative, re-checked 3 days later. Isolation and identification of *C. difficile* was based on the characteristic morphology and odour of the colonies, Gram stain and the presence of the L-proline aminopeptidase activity (Remel Inc, Lenexa, KS, USA). One single colony for each isolate was subcultured and stored at -80°C and re-cultured prior to molecular analysis.

Molecular analysis

Clostridium difficile was grown on blood agar for 24 h and approximately 10 colonies were suspended in 1 mL of distilled water and centrifuged at 12,100 rcf for 1 min. The supernatant was discarded and 200 μL of a commercial DNA extraction kit (InstaGene Matrix; Bio-Rad, Richmond, CA, USA) were added and incubated at 56°C for 30 min and at 100°C for 8 min. The mixture was centrifuged and 200 μL of the supernatant were frozen at -20°C until processing.

Ribotyping was performed as described by Bidet et al. [35]. Ribotype patterns were evaluated visually and compared to an internal library of ribotypes. The international numerical designation (e.g., ribotype 078) was used for bacterial strains recognized as a known international ribotype based on comparison with reference strains. A multiplex PCR was used for detection of genes encoding toxin A (*tcdA*) and toxin B (*tcdB*) as described by Lemee et al. [36]. A second PCR was performed for detection of toxin A gene constitutive difference between A-/B+ strains and A+/B+ strains, and thus, identification of toxin A negative strains was performed according to Kato et al. [37]. Detection of *cdt*A, the gene encoding for the enzymatic component of CDT, was performed according to Stubbs et al. [38]. Sequence analysis of the *tcd*C gene was performed [39] and the result was classified according to Curry et al. [21].

Pulsed-field gel electrophoresis was performed following the protocol used by Miller et al. [40] with modifications. Briefly, *C. difficile* was cultured for 48 h and inoculated into 3 mL of pre-reduced brain and heart infusion (BHI) solution and grown anaerobically for 6 h. The solution was then adjusted to have an optical density $(OD)_{600}$ between 0.3 and 0.7. Four hundred microlitres of the solution were centrifuged at 12,000 rcf for 1 min and the pellet suspended in 150 μL of cell lysis buffer and added 150 μL of melted 1% SeaKem Gold PFGE agarose (Cambrex BioScience Rockland Inc., ME, USA) plus 1% SDS for pipetting into plug molds. After solidified, plugs were transferred into 500 μL of lysis buffer added by 25 μL of lysozyme (final concentration 20 mg/mL) and 25 μL of mutanolysin (final concentration 12.5 U/mL) and incubated at 37°C overnight. The solution was then replaced by 500 μL of proteinase K (PK) buffer added by 25 μL of PK (final concentration 20 mg/mL) and incubated overnight at 56°C for 4 h. Plugs were rinsed three times with 1 × TE buffer and placed on a shaker for 5 min. The last step was repeated once and three more washes were performed with intervals of 10, 15 and 20 min. The solution was replaced by 150 μL of buffer A (New England Biolabs, ON, Canada) and after 10 min replaced by buffer A plus 60 U of restriction enzyme *Sma*I and incubated at 25°C overnight. Half of the plug was cut off and transferred to wells of a 1.3% pulsed-field certified agarose gel (BioRad, CA, USA). DNA separation was performed in a CHEF-DR II chamber (BioRad, CA, USA) added of 2.2 L of 0.5× TBE buffer plus 500 μL of 0.2 M thiourea, set to run for 22 h at 6 V/cm with initial switch time of 1 sec and final switch time of 40 sec. The gel was stained in ethidium bromide and images were obtained using a computerized system (SynGene, Synoptics, MD, USA).

Antimicrobial use data

Individual animal exposure data regarding antimicrobial drugs were recorded at each feedlot over the course of the study using a chute-side computer system (iFHMS, Okotoks, Alberta). These data included the product used, the dose, and the date and route of administration. All study data were subsequently compiled, collated in a computer spreadsheet and verified. Ionophores, and coccidiostats were not included in this analysis.

Dosage information for exposures to antimicrobial drugs was converted into an Animal Defined Daily Dose (ADD). The ADD metric represents the number of days of treatment for an animal based on an assumed average maintenance dosage needed for clinical therapy. Dosage conversion to ADD was based on the expected length of drug effect as indicated by approved dosages.

Statistical analysis

The least square means estimates and 95% confidence intervals for the prevalence of *C. difficile* at arrival and the second (post-arrival) time point were modelled using logistic regression. Regression analysis using generalized estimating equation (GEE) methods, was used to correct prevalence estimates for lack of independence related to sampling of multiple individuals from the same pens using a compound symmetry (exchangeable) correlation structure. Logistic regression was performed using commercially available software (SAS version 9.2, SAS Institute Inc, Cary, NC).

Date of sampling during the feeding period (< 62 days on feed (DOF), 62-71 DOF, or > 71DOF) and exposure of cattle to antimicrobial drugs. Antimicrobial exposure data were summarized as ADDs administered parenterally or in feed between arrival and second sampling, by class of antimicrobial drug, and by route of administration (beta lactams, macrolides, phenicols, quinolones, tetracyclines, and sulfonamides for parenteral exposures and tetracyclines for in-feed exposures).

The outcome for the logistic models was the presence or absence of *C. difficile*. Variables were screened in univariable models to determine those to be included in multivariable model building using a critical alpha for inclusion of 0.25. Multivariable models were not assessed since none of the antimicrobial exposure variables met the inclusion criteria. Odds ratios, 95% confidence intervals (95%CI), and the associated P-values were reported from logistic regression models.

DECLARATIONS

Acknowledgements

This study was supported by Alberta Beef Producers, the Agriculture and Food Council of Alberta's Advancing Canadian Agriculture and Agri-Food (ACAAF) program, and the Public Health Agency of Canada.

Authors' contributions

MC: Molecular analysis of isolates. Analysis and interpretation of data. Writing manuscript. CB and SH: Participated in study design, coordinated sample collection and antimicrobial use data collection, and assisted with interpretation of data analysis. RR-S and SG: Participated in study design, project coordination, and project oversight, and assisted with interpretation of data analysis. JSW: Principal investigator in charge of study design and laboratory procedures. Analysis and interpretation of data. Critical re. JR: Isolation of *C. difficile*. PM and KB: Participated in study design, project coordination and oversight, conducted and interpreted statistical analyses. All authors read and approved the final manuscript.

REFERENCES

1. Warny M, Pepin J, Fang A, Killgore G, Thompson A, Brazier J, et al: Toxin production by an emerging strain of *Clostridium difficile* associated with outbreaks of severe disease in North America and Europe. Lancet. 2005, 366: 1079-1084. 10.1016/S0140-6736(05)67420-X.
2. Indra A, Lassnig H, Baliko N, Much P, Fiedler A, Huhulescu S, Allerberger F: *Clostridium difficile*: a new zoonotic agent?. Wien Klin Wochenschr. 2009, 121: 91-95. 10.1007/s00508-008-1127-x.
3. Zilberberg MD, Shorr AF, Kollef MH: Increase in adult *Clostridium difficile*-related hospitalizations and case-fatality rate, United States, 2000-2005. Emerg Infec Dis. 2008, 14: 829-831.
4. Jhung MA, Thompson AD, Killgore GE, Zukowski WE, Songer G, Warny M, Johnson S, Gerding DN, McDonald LC, Limbago BM: Toxinotype V *Clostridium difficile* in humans and food animals. Emerg Infect Dis. 2008, 14: 1039-1045. 10.3201/eid1407.071641.
5. Kuntz JL, Chrischilles EA, Pendergast JF, Herwaldt LA, Polgreen PM: Incidence of and risk factors for community-associated *Clostridium difficile* infection: a nested case-control study. BMC Infect Dis. 2011, 11: 194-10.1186/1471-2334-11-194.
6. Rodriguez-Palacios A, Staempfli HR, Duffield T, Weese JS: *Clostridium difficile* in retail ground meat,

Canada. Emerg Infect Dis. 2007, 13: 485-487. 10.3201/eid1303.060988.

7. Simango C, Mwakurudza S: Clostridium difficile in broiler chickens sold at market places in Zimbabwe and their antimicrobial susceptibility. Int J Food Microbiol. 2008, 124: 268-270. 10.1016/j.ijfoodmicro.2008.03.020.

8. Songer JG, Trinh HT, Killgore GE, Thompson AD, McDonald LC, Limbago BM: *Clostridium difficile* in retail meat products, USA, 2007. Emerg Infect Dis. 2009, 15: 819-821. 10.3201/eid1505.081071.

9. Weese JS, Avery BP, Rousseau J, Reid-Smith RJ: Detection and enumeration of *Clostridium difficile* spores in retail beef and pork. Appl Environ Microbiol. 2009, 75: 5009-5011. 10.1128/AEM.00480-09.

10. Jöbstl M, Heuberger S, Indra A, Nepf R, Köfer J, Wagner M: *Clostridium difficile* in raw products of animal origin. Int J Food Microbiol. 2010, 138: 172-175. 10.1016/j.ijfoodmicro.2009.12.022.

11. Rodriguez-Palacios A, Pickworth C, Loerch S, LeJeune JT: Transient fecal shedding and limited animal-to-animal transmission of *Clostridium difficile* by naturally infected finishing feedlot cattle. Appl Environ Microbiol. 2011, 77: 3391-3397. 10.1128/AEM.02736-10.

12. Rupnik M: Is *Clostridium difficile*-associated infection a potentially zoonotic and foodborne disease?. Clin Microbiol Infect. 2007, 13: 457-459. 10.1111/j.1469-0691.2007.01687.x.

13. Bauer MP, Notermans DW, van Benthem BH, Brazier JS, Wilcox MH, Rupnik M, Monnet DL, van Dissel JT, Kuijper EJ: ECDIS Study Group. *Clostridium difficile* infection in Europe: a hospital-based survey. Lancet. 2011, 377: 63-73. 10.1016/S0140-6736(10)61266-4.

14. Rupnik M, Widmer A, Zimmermann O, Eckert C: *Clostridium difficile* Toxinotype V, Ribotype 078, in animals and humans. J Clin Microbiol. 2008, 46: 2146-10.1128/JCM.00598-08.

15. Goorhuis A, Bakker D, Corver J, Debast SB, Harmanus C, Notermans DW, et al: Emergence of *Clostridium difficile*infection due to a new hypervirulent strain, polymerase chain reaction ribotype 078. Clin Infect Dis. 2008, 47: 1162-1170. 10.1086/592257.

16. Mulvey MR, Boyd DA, Gravel D, Hutchinson J, Kelly S, McGeer A, Moore D, Simor A, Suh KN, Taylor G, Weese JS, Miller M, the Canadian Nosocomial Infection Surveillance Program: Hypervirulent *Clostridium difficile* strains in hospitalized patients, Canada. Emerg Infect Dis. 2010, 16: 678-681.

17. Costa MC, Stämpfli HR, Arroyo LG, Pearl DL, Weese JS: Epidemiology of *Clostridium difficile* on a veal farm: prevalence, molecular characterization and tetracycline resistance. Vet Microbiol. 2011, 152: 379-384. 10.1016/j.vetmic.2011.05.014.

18. Hammitt MC, Bueschel DM, Keel MK, Glock RD, Cuneo P, Deyoung DW, Reggiardo C, Trinh HT, Songer JG: A possible role for *Clostridium difficile* in the etiology of calf enteritis. Vet Microbiol. 2008, 127: 343-352. 10.1016/j.vetmic.2007.09.002.

19. Keel MK, Brazier JS, Post KW, Weese S, Songer JG: Prevalence of PCR ribotypes among *Clostridium difficile* isolates from pigs, calves, and other species. J Clin Microbiol. 2007, 45: 1963-1964. 10.1128/JCM.00224-07.

20. Rodriguez-Palacios A, Koohmaraie M, Lejeune JT: Prevalence, enumeration, and antimicrobial agent resistance of *Clostridium difficile* in cattle at harvest in the United States. J Food Prot. 2011, 74: 1618-1624. 10.4315/0362-028X.JFP-11-141.

21. Curry SR, Marsh JW, Muto CA, O'Leary MM, Pasculle AW, Harrison LH: *tcd*C genotypes associated with severe TcdC truncation in an epidemic clone and other strains of *Clostridium difficile*. J Clin Microbiol. 2007, 45: 215-221. 10.1128/JCM.01599-06.

22. Hoffer E, Haechler H, Frei R, Stephan R: Low occurrence of *Clostridium difficile* in fecal samples of healthy calves and pigs at slaughter and in minced meat in Switzerland. J Food Prot. 2010, 73: 973-975.

23. Houser BA, Hattel AL, Jayarao BM: Real-time multiplex polymerase chain reaction assay for rapid detection of *Clostridium difficile* toxin-encoding strains. Foodborne Pathog Dis. 2010, 7: 719-726. 10.1089/fpd.2009.0483.

24. Rodriguez-Palacios A, Staempfli HR, Duffield T, Peregrine AS, Trotz-Williams L, Arroyo L, Brazier JS, Weese JS: *Clostridium difficile* PCR ribotypes in calves, Canada. Emerg Infect Dis. 2006, 12: 1730-1736. 10.3201/eid1211.051581.

25. Alvarez-Perez S, Blanco JL, Bouza E, Alba P, Gibert X, Maldonado J, Garcia ME: Prevalence of *Clostridium difficile* in diarrhoeic and non-diarrhoeic piglets. Vet Microbiol. 2009, 137: 302-305. 10.1016/j.vetmic.2009.01.015.

26. Norman KN, Harvey RB, Scott HM, Hume ME, Andrews K, Brawley AD: Varied prevalence of *Clostridium difficile* in an integrated swine operation. Anaerobe. 2009, 15: 256-260. 10.1016/j.anaerobe.2009.09.006.

27. Songer JG, Post KW, Larson DJ, Jost BH, Glock RD: Enteric infection of neonatal swine with *Clostridium difficile*. Swine Health Prod. 2000, 8: 185-189.

28. Baverud V, Gustafsson A, Franklin A, Aspán A, Gunnarsson A: *Clostridium difficile*: prevalence in horses and environment, and antimicrobial susceptibility. Equine Vet J. 2003, 35: 465-71.

29. Alfa MJ, Du T, Beda G: Survey of incidence of *Clostridium difficile* infection in Canadian hospitals and diagnostic approaches. J Clin Microbiol. 1998, 36: 2076-2080.

30. Pépin J, Saheb N, Coulombe MA, Alary ME, Corriveau MP, Authier S, Leblanc M, Rivard G, Bettez M, Primeau V, Nguyen M, Jacob CE, Lanthier L: Emergence of fluoroquinolones as the predominant risk factor for *Clostridium difficile*-associated diarrhea: a cohort study during an epidemic in Quebec. Clin Infect Dis. 2005, 41: 1254-1260. 10.1086/496986.

31. Debast SB, van Leengoed LA, Goorhuis A, Harmanus C, Kuijper EJ, Bergwerff AA: *Clostridium difficile* PCR ribotype 078 toxinotype V found in diarrhoeal pigs identical to isolates from affected humans.

Environ Microbiol. 2009, 11: 505-511. 10.1111/j.1462-2920.2008.01790.x.

32. Weese JS, Rousseau J, Deckert A, Gow S, Reid-Smith RJ: *Clostridium difficile* and methicillin-resistant *Staphylococcus aureus* shedding by slaughter-age pigs. BMC Vet Res. 2011, 7: 41-10.1186/1746-6148-7-41.

33. Weese JS, Finley R, Reid-Smith RR, Janecko N, Rousseau J: Evaluation of *Clostridium difficile* in dogs and the household environment. Epidemiol Infect. 2010, 138: 1100-1114. 10.1017/S0950268809991312.

34. Schoster A, Arroyo LG, Stämpfli HR, Shewen P, Sigismondo LM, Reid-Smith RJ, Janecko N, Weese JS: Longitudinal study of *Clostridium difficile*, *Clostridium perfringens*, *Salmonella* and *Escherichia coli* in healthy horses. Proceedings of the. 2011, ACVIM Forum: 15-18 June 2011; Denver

35. Bidet P, Barbut F, Lalande V, Burghoffer B, Petit J: Development of a new PCR ribotyping method for *Clostridium difficile*based on ribosomal RNA gene sequencing. FEMS Microbiol Lett. 1999, 175: 261-266. 10.1111/j.1574-6968.1999.tb13629.x.

36. Lemee L, Dhalliun A, Testelin S, Mattrat M, Maillard K, Lemeland J, Pons J: Multiplex PCR targeting tpi (triose phosphate isomerase), tcdA (Toxin A), and tcdB (Toxin B) genes for toxigenic culture of *Clostridium difficile*. J Clin Microbiol. 2004, 42: 5710-5714. 10.1128/JCM.42.12.5710-5714.2004.

37. Kato H, Kato N, Watanabe K, Iwai N, Nakamura H, Yamamoto T, Suzuki K, Kim SM, Chong Y, Wasito EB: Identification of toxin A-negative, toxin B-positive *Clostridium difficile* by PCR. J Clin Microbiol. 1998, 36: 2178-2182.

38. Stubbs S, Rupnik M, Gibert M, Brazier J, Duerden B, Popoff M: Production of actin-specific ADP-ribosyltransferase (binary toxin) by strains of *Clostridium difficile*. FEMS Microbiol Lett. 2000, 186: 307-312. 10.1111/j.1574-6968.2000.tb09122.x.

39. Spigaglia P, Mastrantonio P: Molecular analysis of the pathogenicity locus and polymorphism in the putative negative regulator of toxin production (TcdC) among *Clostridium difficile* clinical isolates. J Clin Microbiol. 2002, 40: 3470-3475. 10.1128/JCM.40.9.3470-3475.2002.

40. Miller M, Gravel D, Mulvey M, Taylor G, Boyd D, Simor A, Gardam M, McGeer A, Hutchinson J, Moore D, Kelly S: Health-care associated *Clostridium difficile* infection in Canada: patient age and infecting strain type are highly predictive of severe outcome and mortality. Clin Infect Dis. 2010, 50: 194-201. 10.1086/649213.

SECTION X: BRUCELLA ABORTUS - ABORTION

CHAPTER 37

BAYESIAN ESTIMATION OF SENSITIVITY AND SPECIFICITY OF ROSE BENGAL, COMPLEMENT FIXATION, AND INDIRECT ELISA TESTS FOR THE DIAGNOSIS OF BOVINE BRUCELLOSIS IN ETHIOPIA

T. Getachew, G. Getachew, G. Sintayehu, M. Getenet, and A. Fasil

INTRODUCTION

Brucellae are Gram-negative, facultative intracellular bacteria that can infect many species of animals and man. Ten species are recognized within the genus Brucella. There are 6 "classical" species: B. abortus, B. melitensis, B. suis, B. ovis, B. canis, and B. neotomae [1, 2] and, more recently, other four species have been recognized [3]. The principal manifestations of brucellosis are reproductive failure such as abortion or birth of unthrifty newborn and infertility [4, 5]. Brucellosis in animals and humans is still common in the Middle East, Asia, Africa, South and Central America, the Mediterranean Basin, and the Caribbean. Brucella melitensis is particularly common in the Mediterranean basin and it has also been reported in Africa, India, and Mexico [6].

Previous studies carried out in Ethiopia on bovine brucellosis using Rose Bengal and complement fixation tests described higher prevalence in intensive and semi-intensive dairy farms than extensive farms [1, 7, 8]. In 1987, the World Organization for Animal Health reported 20% prevalence of brucellosis, being higher around large towns than in rural areas [9]. In central highlands of Ethiopia, 4.2% prevalence of brucellosis was reported in zebu cattle [7]. Eshetu et al. [10] reported a prevalence of 10% in smallholder farms of central Ethiopia (Wuchale-Jida district) near Addis Ababa in 2005. Kebede et al. [11] reported a prevalence of 11% in cattle under extensive management systems. Studies conducted in different regions in 2003 and 2005 have reported animal level prevalence of 0.8% and 3.2% and herd prevalence of 2.9% and 42.3% [8, 12]. Another study in Ethiopia from 2003 to 2004 has reported a prevalence of 1.6% and a herd level prevalence of 13.7% [1]. A more recent study from 2011 to 2012 on exotic and crossbred dairy cattle and breeding farms has reported animal level prevalence of 1.9% and herd level prevalence of 10.6% in Ethiopia [13].

Serological tests are widely used to conduct several epidemiological studies and diagnostic purposes, but there is no perfect serological test [14, 15]. However, the diagnostic performance and discriminative ability of a test could be evaluated by comparing the sensitivity and specificity of several tests analytically [14, 16]. The diagnostic performance of a test could be evaluated by comparison with standard reference test and analyzed using latent models [17–19]. The objective of this studywas to evaluate diagnostic performance and discriminative ability of Rose Bengal Plate Test (RBPT), complement fixation test (CFT), and indirect enzyme linked immunosorbent assay (I-ELISA) tests used for screening and confirmatory diagnosis of bovine brucellosis in Ethiopia using Bayesian method. This study is one of a kind in the context of field diagnostic test evaluation for bovine brucellosis in Ethiopia which has significant importance for disease surveillance and future control endeavors.

MATERIALS AND METHODS

Study Area and Population

The study was conducted in five dairy farms, namely, Sululta, Awash, Wonji, Adami Tulu, and Alage located at 35, 100,

Citation: T. Getachew, G. Getachew, G. Sintayehu, M. Getenet, and A. Fasil, "Bayesian Estimation of Sensitivity and Specificity of Rose Bengal, Complement Fixation, and Indirect ELISA Tests for the Diagnosis of Bovine Brucellosis in Ethiopia," Veterinary Medicine International, vol. 2016, Article ID 8032753, 5 pages, 2016. doi:10.1155/2016/8032753.

90, 170, and 200 km from Addis Ababa, respectively. The management system and breed of the farms were similar and the disease status was unknown. Thus, the farms were assumed as one population. All animals aged above six months in the farm were included in the sampling and the total number of the study animals was 278 pure and crossbreed Holstein Frisian dairy cows.

The farm history during sampling showed that there was no vaccination against brucellosis in all farms. Blood samples of 5–7 mL were collected in plain vacutainer tube from the jugular vein. The samples were allowed to clot for 2-3 h at room temperature. Then the serum was extracted by spinning at 2500 rpm for five minutes and kept in refrigerator at −20°C until the test is conducted. All farms except Sululta are located in the Great Rift Valley area of Ethiopia.

Diagnostic Tests

All serological tests conducted for test evaluation were performed at NAHDIC, Sebeta, Ethiopia (Bacterial Serology Laboratory).

Rose Bengal Test

Rose Bengal Test was conducted following the procedure described by OIE 2009. Antigen for the Rose Bengal Test was prepared from B. abortus strain 99 stained with Rose Bengal dye and suspended in acid buffer pH 3.65. Equal volume (30 μL) of antigen and test serum is brought together using a micropipette channel; then after thorough mixing it was rocked for four minutes; finally the result was read using magnifying glass and recorded as positive or negative based on the absence or presence of agglutination due to antigen-antibody reaction in the serum. Rose Bengal antigen was purchased from Lillidale Diagnostics, UK.

Complement Fixation Test

Complement fixation test was conducted using Alton et al. [20] Method. As a principle, if a specific antibody against bovine Brucella is present in the serum, then antigen-antibody complex is formed and the complement will bind. The positive result of the test was when no hemolysis of the sheep RBC occurs. If there is no specific antibody against Brucella, the free complement exists which will cause sensitization of sheep RBC and lead to hemolysis. The validation of the result was done using positive and negative controls. Result interpretation based on the titration scale considered strong reaction when more than 75% fixation of the complement (3+) occurred at a dilution of 1 : 5 and the reaction was classified as weak positive with 50% fixation of complement (2+) that occurred at a dilution of 1 : 10 and above. Brucella antigen for the complement fixation test was prepared from B. abortus S99 and standardized against the OIEISS to give 50% fixation at a dilution of 1/200.Brucella antigen and positive control for complement fixation test were obtained from AH-VLA (Animal Health Veterinary Laboratory Agency), UK. Hemolytic serum and guinea pig complement was obtained from ID VET (Innovative Veterinary Diagnostic) Company.

Indirect ELISA Test

Test was performed according to the manufacturer's instructions and procedures. Indirect ELISA kit obtained from VLA Lillidale Animal Health Limited, Badbury View, Bothenwood, Wimborne, Dorset BH214HU, UK (https://www.gov.uk/government/organisations/animal-health-and-veterinary-laboratories-agency).

Reagent Preparation. The dilution buffer was prepared by adding 5 tablets PBS 0.5 mL phenol red indicator and 250 μL of Tween 20 to 500 mL distilled water; the pH was adjusted to 7.2. Then solution was prepared by adding the contents of the ampoule of Na_2HPO_4 and 1 mL of Tween 20 to 10 liters of distilled water. The substrate buffer prepared was by dissolving 1 tablet in 120 mL distilled water. The chromogen was prepared by dissolving 2 tablets in 1 mL of sterile distilled water. The stopping solution was prepared by diluting the ampoule of sodium azide with 500 mL of distilled water. Antigen was prepared from approved smooth lipopolysaccharides B. abortus strain 99 1 μg/m/L coated in 0.05 M carbonate/bicarbonate buffer, pH 9.6 onto flat bottom microplate wells. Positive and negative controls were reconstituted with 1 mL sterile distilled water and allowed until an even suspension is obtained before use. The test procedure, first a 1/40 predilution of all tests and control sera was made; then the plate was prepared by adding 80 μL of diluting buffer to wells followed by transferring of 20 μL of prediluted samples into a 96-well microplate coated with Brucellalipopolysaccharides (LPS). The optical density (OD0) was set at 405 nanometers blanked on well H12 and the presence or absence of antibodies against LPS of Brucella was determined by comparing the mean OD of positive controls. Color development within a well indicates that the sample has antibodies to Brucella. The validation criteria are as follows the cut-off value for positive/negative was calculated as 10% of the mean OD of positive control wells. Any test sample giving an OD equal to or above this value should be considered positive.

Test Evaluation Using Bayesian Model

Estimation of diagnostic test sensitivity and specificity through Bayesian modeling has an advantage to provide more stable point and interval estimates without the necessity of large sample sizes [21, 22]. One of the reasons why Bayesian approach was employed was that it can give good estimates of sensitivity and specificity in the absence of gold standard method like culture and isolation. The Bayesian approach is a well-established methodology for robust diagnostic test evaluation. We could not culture samples for bacterial isolation ofBrucella in our laboratory because of biorisk and biosecurity concern. Finally, we consider that this does not affect the results of our study.

The sensitivity and specificity of the three tests were evaluated using a total of 278 sera samples collected from five dairy farms. Each serum sample was subjected to the three tests and the results were entered into the computer. The observed data of the three tests' results was summarized in cross tabulation. Bayesian model without gold standard was applied to estimate the sensitivity and specificity estimates. Prior information for the unknown data in the model was used from published data on bovine brucellosis [15, 23].

Gall and Nielsen [15] reviewed over 50 publications in which sensitivity and specificity values of assays used for the detection of exposure to Brucella abortus where the sum of sensitivity and specificity values for each test was averaged to give a performance index. Similarly, comparison was made of sensitivity and specificity of I-ELISA RBT that thus we used as prior information for our data analysis.

The uncertainty of an average sensitivity and specificity obtained from the published data was transformed to the beta distribution using Betabuster free software (http://www.epi.ucdavis.edu/diagnostictests [22]). The prior information for sensitivity of RBP, I-ELISA, and CFT was of modes 0.91, 0.97, and 0.94, respectively, and the transformed beta (a, b) was beta (49.4, 6.0); (103.2, 3.73); and (89.27, 6.14), respectively. Prior mode for specificity of RBP, I-ELISA, and CFT was 0.86, 0.97, and 0.89, respectively, and the transformed beta distribution (a, b) was (22.76, 4.43); (102.1, 4.23); and (83.05, 11.14), respectively (Table 1).

Table 1: Prior information used for sensitivity and specificity of RBT, I-ELISA, and CFT

	RBT	I-ELISA	CFT	
Se	81.2 (66.4–96)	96 (90.2–99.8)	89 (81.3–96.7)	Gall and Nielsen (2004) [15]
Sp	86.3 (71.64–99)	93.8 (88–99.6)	83.5 (75.8–91.2)	
Se	100 (96.7–100)	98.9 (96.2–99.8)	100 (96.7–100)	Mainar-Jaime et al. (2005) [23]
Sp	86.4 (79.1–91.9)	100 (97.1–100)	94.4 (88.8–97.7)	
Âse	90.6 (81.6–98)	97.4 (93.2–99.9)	94.5 (89–98.3)	Mean Se and Sp
ÂSp	86.4 (71–99)	96.9 (92.5–99.8)	89 (82.3–94.4)	

The Bayesian model for one population-three tests was modified and applied for the data using WinBUGS free software. The median value of the posterior distributions was built after 50,000 iterations and the burnout of the initial 5,000 iterations. The model sensitivity was checked using kernel density and autocorrelation graphs that showed the posterior distribution fit fairly to the data. Conditional dependence of the tests was also checked because the tests are based on similar biological basis which might lead to correlated errors leading to incorrect estimation of sensitivity and specificity [22]. Then, conditional independent Bayesian model was applied which allowed us to estimate the conditional correlations (rhoD and rhoDc) for Se and Sp, respectively, for the three tests.

RESULTS

All sera samples were tested blindly by all the three tests (RBT, I-ELISA, and CF) independently. The tests result showed 5/278; 8/278 and 2/278 positive for RBT, I-ELISA, and CF, respectively; this indicated that I-ELISA is superior in sensitivity and specificity, followed by CF. Kappa test of the three tests showed moderate agreement (kappa = 0.70); the rhoD and rhoDc values were small and clustered around zero which indicates that the tests are conditionally independent (Table 2).

Table 2: Cross tabulation of the three tests' results

	CFT pos.		CFT neg. I-ELISA		Total
	I-ELISA pos.	I-ELISA neg.	Pos.	neg.	
RBT pos.	2	0	2	1	5
RBT neg.	0	0	4	269	273
Total	2	0	6	270	278

The posterior inference for the true sensitivity of RBT, I-ELISA, and CFT was 89.6 (95% PI: 79.9–95.8), 96.8 (95% PI: 92.3–99.1), and 94 (95% PI: 87.8–97.5) and true specificity was 84.5 (95% PI: 68–94.98), 96.3 (95% PI: 91.7–98.8), and 88.5 (81–93.8), respectively. In this study, the true sensitivity and specificity of I-ELISA (96.8 95% PI (92.3–99.1) and 96.3 95% PI (91.7–98.8), resp.) were found higher than RBPT and CFT. The seroprevalence of brucellosis in these farms was estimated to be 4 (95% PI: 0.8–11.45).

The conditional correlation to evaluate conditional dependence of the three tests showed that the value estimate for both rhoD (for sensitivity) and rhoDc (for specificity) was small with the probability interval clustering around zero which showed the tests were conditionally independent. The sensitivity analysis based on the posterior distribution kernel density and autocorrelation graphs showed that the observed data fairly fit the model and prior information has not significantly influenced the median estimate (Table 3).

Table 3: Observed estimate of sensitivities and specificities

Test	Parameter	Posterior estimation
RBT	Se	89.6 (95% PI: 79.9–95.8)
	Sp	84.5 (95% PI: 68–94.8)
I-ELISA	Se	96.8 (95% PI: 92.3–99.1)
	Sp	96.3 (95% PI: 91.7–98.8)
CFT	Se	94 (95% PI: 87.8–97.5)
	Sp	88.5 (95% PI: 81–93.8)
Prevalence		4 (95% PI: 0.8–11.45)
rhoD		0.22 (95% PI: −0.05–0.71)
rhoDc		0.176 (95% PI: −0.082–0.64)

95% PI = 95% probability interval.

DISCUSSION

Screening and confirmatory diagnostic tests are the primary tools for successful epidemiological study. In Ethiopia, although many papers were published to determine the prevalence of bovine brucellosis in different farm settings, we could not find any published data on sensitivity and specificity of the serological tests. The knowledge on the diagnostic sensitivity and specificity of a test would help to limit diagnostic errors in classifying infected and noninfected animals correctly and to prevent excessive economical losses when the animals are wrongly classified by the tests [24].

No single serological test is appropriate in all epidemiological situations and all animal species; all tests have limitations especially when screening individual animals. Consideration should be given to all factors that impact on the relevance of the test method and test results to a specific diagnostic interpretation or application. Antigen for the Rose Bengal Test was prepared by depositing killed B. abortus strain 99 (Weybridge) cells stained with Rose Bengal dye and suspended in acid buffer pH 3.65. Antigen for complement fixation test was prepared from B. abortus strain 99 (Weybridge) and standardized against the OIEISS to give 50% fixation at a dilution of 1/200. The same B. abortus strain 99 (Weybridge) was also used as a source of soluble antigen extracts (smooth lipopolysaccharide (S-LPS) for the indirect ELISA). Therefore, antigen for indirect ELISA was prepared from approved smooth lipopolysaccharides B. abortus strain 99 1 μg/m/L coated in 0.05 M carbonate/bicarbonate buffer, pH 9.6, onto flat bottom microplate wells. All the three antigens are used to detect infections due to smooth Brucella species as per information obtained from the manufacturer. All diagnostic kit components (i.e., antigen, reference sera, and complements) used for the test evaluation purpose were of highest quality obtained from VLA, UK, internationally recognized diagnostic kit supplier with good manufacturing practice.

Estimation of diagnostic sensitivity and specificity of a test requires knowledge of the true disease status of the animals on which the test is to be applied using the gold standard test; however, in the absence of such a gold standard test a Bayesian approach is a useful tool to evaluate the characteristics of the tests [18, 19, 25].

Bayesian method has an advantage as it provides a stable point and interval estimates without the necessity of large sample size [21, 26]. It is widely accepted that screening tests should have a higher sensitivity but could have a lower specificity. The sensitivity of RBT in the current study was fairly high (89.6 (95% PI: 79.9–95.8)) which was higher than the previous finding by Sanogo et al. (2013) [27] (54.9% (cr 23.5–95.1)).

Previous studies suggested that CFT is an appropriate confirmatory test with high specificity [16] but this was not consistent with the current finding that the specificity of CFT was moderate (88.5 (95% PI: 81–93.8)) which might be due to small population size in our study. However, Gall and Nielsen (2004) [15] reported the sensitivity and specificity of CFT as Se 81.2 and Sp 83.5, respectively, which is in agreement with our current finding. The I-ELISA was found to be the best sensitive and specific test (95% PI: 92.3–99.1 and 95% PI: 91.7–98.8, resp.) for bovine brucellosis compared to both CFT and RBPT. The possible reason for this high accuracy might be due to the fact that I-ELISA detects all isotopes of immunoglobulin IgG while CFT cannot detect them [14]. The mean sensitivity and specificity for indirect ELISA were reported as Se 96.0 and Sp 93.8 by Gall and Nielsen (2004) which was in agreement with our estimates.

The conditional dependence of the tests is that the conditional correlation rhoD and rhoDc values for sensitivity and specificity, respectively, were small and clustered around zero which indicates that the tests are conditionally independent and could be an advantage while using in test combinations [28]. The sensitivity analysis using different prior information showed that the posterior distribution kernel density and autocorrelation graphs showed that the observed data fairly fit the model and prior information has not significantly influenced the median estimates.

CONCLUSION AND RECOMMENDATION

Based on this observation I-ELISA had the best performance followed by CFT and RBPT in descending order of accuracy. However, the decision for the choice of diagnostic test for different purposes not only does rely on the accuracy, but also should take into consideration the capacity for the test throughput, technical complexity, and cost effectiveness. Regardless of its lower sensitivity, RBT remains the most widely used screening test because of its rapid result and cost effectiveness. Therefore, conducting test verification is very essential to know the test characteristics and to determine the type of test we require to use for the study purpose, epidemiological surveillance, or international trade. We recommend further studies should be conducted on the performance of these tests in the field setting for the diagnosis of sheep and goat brucellosis to generate sufficient information.

ACKNOWLEDGMENTS

The research team acknowledges the National Animal Health Diagnostic and Investigation Center for facilitating field programs and Mr. Belachew Dura, Mr. Mengistu Nemera, and Mr. Tafesse Koran for collecting serum samples from different dairy farms for the study.

REFERENCES

1. K. Asmare, Y. Asfaw, E. Gelaye, and G. Ayelet, "Brucellosis in extensive management system of Zebu cattle in Sidama Zone, Southern Ethiopia," African Journal of Agricultural Research, vol. 5, no. 3, pp. 257–263, 2010.
2. M. J. Corbel, M. Banai, and I. Genus, "Brucella Meyer and Shaw 1920, 173AL," in Bergey's Manual of Systematic Bacteriology, D. J. Brenner, N. R. Krieg, and J. T. Staley, Eds., pp. 370–386, Springer, New York, NY, USA, 2005.
3. V. L. Atluri, M. N. Xavier, M. F. de Jong, A. B. den Hartigh, and R. M. Tsolis, "Interactions of the human pathogenic Brucella species with their hosts," Annual Review of Microbiology, vol. 65, pp. 523–541, 2011. ·
4. O. M. Radostits, C. C. Gay, D. C. Blood, and K. W. Hinchcliff, Veterinary Medicine: A Textbook of the Diseases of Cattle, Sheep, Pigs, Goats and Horses, WB Saunders, London, UK, 9th edition, 2000.
5. World Organization for Animal Health (OIE), "Ovine and Caprine Brucellosis," 2009, http://web.oie.int/eng/normes/MMANUAL/2008/pdf/2.07.02_CAPRINE_OVINE_BRUC.pdf.
6. Center for Food Security and Public Health (CFSPH), 2009, http://www.cfsph.iastate.edu/Factsheets/pdfs/brucellosis.pdf.
7. B. Tekleye, O. B. Kassali, M. Mugurewa, R. G. Sholtens, and Y. Tamirat, "The prevalence of brucellosis in indigenous cattle in central Ethiopia," Bulletin of Animal Health and Production in Africa, vol. 37, pp. 97–98, 1989.
8. T. Tolosa, F. Regassa, K. Belihu, and Inter-African Bureau for Animal Resources, "Sero-prevalence study of bovine brucellosis in extensive management system

in selected sites of Jimma zone, Western Ethiopia," Bulletin of Animal Health and Production in Africa, vol. 56, pp. 25–37, 2008.

9. World Organization for Animal Health (OIE), "Bovine brucellosis and brucellosis of small ruminants," Technical Series Office International des Epizooties, vol. 6, pp. 48–49, 1987.
10. Y. Eshetu, J. Kassahun, P. Abebe, M. Beyene, B. Zewdie, and A. Bekele, "Seroprevalence study of Brucellosis on dairy cattle in Addis Ababa, Ethiopia," Bulletin of Animal Health and Production in Africa, vol. 53, pp. 211–214, 2005.
11. T. Kebede, G. Ejeta, G. Ameni, and École Nationale Vétérinaire de Toulouse, "Seroprevalence of bovine brucellosis in smallholder farms in central Ethiopia (Wuchale-Jida district)," Revue de Médecine Vétérinaire, vol. 159, pp. 3–9, 2008.
12. G. Berhe, K. Belihu, and Y. Asfaw, "Seroepidemiological investigation of bovine brucellosis in the extensive cattle production system of Tigray region of Ethiopia," International Journal of Applied Research in Veterinary Medicine, vol. 5, pp. 65–71, 2007.
13. K. Asmare, B. Sibhat, W. Molla et al., "The status of bovine brucellosis in Ethiopia with special emphasis on exotic and cross bred cattle in dairy and breeding farms," Acta Tropica, vol. 126, no. 3, pp. 186–192, 2013.
14. F. P. Poester, K. Nielsen, L. E. Samartino, and W. L. Yu, "Diagnosis of Brucellosis," The Open Veterinary Science Journal, vol. 4, pp. 46–60, 2010.
15. D. Gall and K. Nielsen, "Serological diagnosis of Bovine brucellosis: a review of test performance and cost comparison," Revue Scientifique et Technique, vol. 23, no. 3, pp. 989–1002, 2004.
16. I. R. Dohoo, P. F. Wright, G. M. Ruckerbauer, B. S. Samagh, F. J. Robertson, and L. B. Forbes, "A comparison of five serological tests for bovine brucellosis," Canadian Journal of Veterinary Research, vol. 50, no. 4, pp. 485–493, 1986.
17. R. Poulloit and R. Gerbier, "A Bayesian method for the evaluation of the sensitivity and specificity of correlated diagnostic tests in the absence of gold standard," in Proceeding of the 9th International Symposium on Veterinary Epidemiology and Economics, 2000, http://www.sciquest.org.nz/.
18. R. Pouillot, G. Gerbier, and I. A. Gardner, "'TAGS', a program for the evaluation of test accuracy in the absence of a gold standard," Preventive Veterinary Medicine, vol. 53, pp. 67–81, 2002.
19. C. Enøe, S. Andersen, V. Sørensen, and P. Willeberg, "Estimation of sensitivity, specificity and predictive values of two serologic tests for the detection of antibodies against Actinobacillus pleuropneumoniaeserotype 2 in the absence of a reference test (gold standard)," Preventive Veterinary Medicine, vol. 51, no. 3-4, pp. 227–243, 2001.
20. G. G. Alton, L. M. Jones, R. D. Angus, and J. M. Verger, Techniques for the Brucellosis Laboratory, Institut National de la Recherche Agronomique, Paris, France, 1988.
21. C. Enøe, M. P. Georgiadis, and W. O. Johnson, "Estimation of sensitivity and specificity of diagnostic tests and disease prevalence when the true disease state is unknown," Preventive Veterinary Medicine, vol. 45, no. 1-2, pp. 61–81, 2000.
22. A. J. Branscum, I. A. Gardner, and W. O. Johnson, "Estimation of diagnostic-test sensitivity and specificity through Bayesian modeling," Preventive Veterinary Medicine, vol. 68, no. 2–4, pp. 145–163, 2005.
23. R. C. Mainar-Jaime, P. M. Muñoz, M. J. de Miguel et al., "Specificity dependence between serological tests for diagnosing bovine brucellosis in Brucella-free farms showing false positive serological reactions due to Yersinia enterocolitica O:9," Canadian Veterinary Journal, vol. 46, no. 10, pp. 913–916, 2005.
24. B. W. Stemshorn, L. B. Forbes, M. D. Eaglesome, K. H. Nielsen, F. J. Robertson, and B. S. Samagh, "A comparison of standard serological tests for the diagnosis of bovine brucellosis in Canada," Canadian Journal of Comparative Medicine, vol. 49, no. 4, pp. 391–394, 1985.
25. N. Toft, E. Jørgensen, and S. Højsgaard, "Diagnosing diagnostic tests: evaluating the assumptions underlying the estimation of sensitivity and specificity in the absence of a gold standard," Preventive Veterinary Medicine, vol. 68, no. 1, pp. 19–33, 2005.
26. G. Gari, F. Biteau-Croller, C. Le Goff, P. Caufour, and F. Roger, "Evaluation of the indirect fluorescent antibody test for the diagnosis and screening of lumpy skin disease," Veterinary Microbiology, vol. 129, no. 3-4, pp. 269–280, 2008.
27. M. Sanogo, E. Thys, Y. L. Achi et al., "Bayesian estimation of the true prevalence, sensitivity and specificity of the Rose Bengal and indirect ELISA tests in the diagnosis of bovine brucellosis," Veterinary Journal, vol. 195, no. 1, pp. 114–120, 2013.
28. N. Dendukuri and L. Joseph, "Bayesian approaches to modeling the conditional dependence between multiple diagnostic tests," Biometrics, vol. 57, no. 1, pp. 158–167, 2001.

CHAPTER 38

RECENT ADVANCES IN BRUCELLA ABORTUS VACCINES

Elaine MS Dorneles, Nammalwar Sriranganathan and Andrey P. Lag

INTRODUCTION

B. abortus is the main causative agent of brucellosis in cattle, causing abortion and infertility in adult animals [1]. Bovine brucellosis is a worldwide zoonotic disease, endemic in some regions of the world such as Latin America, Middle East, Africa and Asia [1] and responsible for large economic losses due to animal and human health problems.

Due to public health importance of brucellosis and the damage that it causes to the livestock industry, much effort has been expended to control and eradicate the disease in cattle. The development of an efficacious vaccine for brucellosis control/ eradication has been a challenge for scientists for many years. Despite enormous advances and the development of *B. abortus* S19 and RB51 vaccines, the search for improved vaccines has never ends. Although the available vaccines are effective in controlling brucellosis, they have numerous drawbacks, such as interference with diagnostic tests, pathogenicity for humans, potential to cause abortion in pregnant animals, among others. In this paper, we present a re of the main aspects of the vaccines that have been used in the bovine brucellosis control and eradication over the years and some of the current advances in the research for a new *B. abortus* vaccine.

VACCINES, VACCINATION AND THEIR USE IN BRUCELLOSIS CONTROL AND ERADICATION PROGRAMS

According to Schurig et al. [2] and Ko and Splitter [3], an ideal vaccine against brucellosis should possess the following characteristics: (i) be live and able to provide a strong type 1 T helper immune response (Th1); (ii) do not induce antibodies that interfere with the serological tests employed in the diagnosis of infected cattle, regardless of route, dose of administration, age or sex of the animals; (iii) be attenuated and do not cause disease or persistent infection in immunized animals nor be pathogenic for humans; (iv) be able to induce a strong and long-lasting protection against systemic and uterine infection, besides preventing abortion, even in pregnant animals inoculated with a single dose; (v) do not lead to seroconversion on revaccination; (vi) be stable and do not revert virulence in vivo nor in vitro; and (vii) be inexpensive, easy to produce and to administer.

Even though we still do not have an ideal vaccine, vaccination with available vaccine strains remains the most successful method for the prevention and control of brucellosis in cattle, being a critical component of most brucellosis control and eradication programs throughout the world [4]. Numerous countries have adopted control measures against bovine brucellosis in order to reduce the prevalence or eradicate the disease from domestic livestock, in an effort to prevent transmission to humans and mitigate economic losses. Vaccination of female calves is the point of any brucellosis control program, since it has performed well in the reduction of disease prevalence, therefore useful at the disease control stage. Considering that vaccination alone is not enough to control and eradicate the disease, it should be associated with continuous elimination of infected animals, as they are the source of new infections. Thus, besides vaccination, most bovine brucellosis eradicate programs also include test–and–slaughter policies, surveillance and hygiene measures [4].

The aim of vaccination is the reduction of susceptibly individuals in the population and the success of any vaccination program depends mainly on the effectiveness of the vaccine used and its coverage in the target population. Vaccines against

Citation: Elaine MS Dorneles, Nammalwar Sriranganathan and Andrey P. Lage, Recent advances in Brucella abortus vaccines, DOI: 10.1186/s13567-015-0199-7.

brucellosis have been evaluated with respect to their potency by three different approaches: (i) testing in laboratory animals or (ii) testing in natural hosts experimentally challenged and (iii) testing under natural conditions [5]. Of these, test in natural hosts shows more significant response and is the only one able to measure the efficacy of *B. abortus* vaccines [6,7]. In experimental studies of vaccine efficacy, vaccinated and non-vaccinated controls will receive a known infectious dose of a virulent *B. abortus* strain at the most susceptible period (mid-gestation), and the protection is measure by the ability of the vaccine in preventing abortion [4]. However, it is important to emphasize that the experimentally obtained effectiveness may differ from field efficacy that can be influenced by other factors, such as nutrition, environmental stress, age at vaccination, vaccination management or immunological status [4]. Besides, the above three classical methodologies, *B. abortus* vaccines could also be assessed by measuring the immune responses and determination of correlates of protection by mathematical modeling. The identification of protection markers can be an useful approach to screen vaccine candidates whether validated by vaccine potency tests [8]. Since experiments involving challenge of pregnant cattle are very expensive, time-consuming and requires large animal biosafety level 3 facilities, the rational way for the future of *B. abortus* vaccines testing and development could be the characterization and identification of the correlates of protection.

Another important aspect related to the success of brucellosis control programs is the quality of the vaccine used. Despite the cost of the vaccine being just one fraction of the total cost of a control program, its quality will affect directly and dramatically the outcome of the program. Assessing the quality of live *Brucella* vaccines is usually based on in vitro criteria, including physico-chemical and microbiological in vitro tests as to purity, dissociation, and determination of pH, humidity and count of viable bacteria [9]. Recently, genetic stability has also been proposed as an additional criterion in assessing of the quality of *Brucella* spp. vaccines [10, 11, 12]. Although less frequently, immunogenicity in mouse can also be included in *Brucella* vaccines tests, however not having cutoff points (protection zone) defined for RB51 vaccine [9, 10, 11] and as mouse immune system does not accurately represent bovine immune system, it is very difficult to use such data.

Attenuated *B. abortus* strains have demonstrated the best results in the prevention of bovine brucellosis. *B. abortus* live modified vaccines are highly effective in decreasing transmission and production losses caused by brucellosis, but are less effective at preventing infection by field strains [4]. Since, abortion is the key for the brucellosis transmission in cattle, a vaccine that can effectively prevent abortion is able to reduce disease transmission and largely reduce economic losses caused by the disease. Immunization with live modified *B. abortus* vaccines is generally performed in young female calves in a single dose by intramuscular or subcutaneous injection [5]. However, in zones of high prevalence of brucellosis, massive vaccination, including adult cows, is performed.

It is also important to take into account that although cattle are the main target of the vaccination against *B. abortus* within bovine brucellosis control and eradication programs, they are not the unique species infected by this agent. Goats, feral swine, elks, bison and other hosts can also be infected by *B. abortus* and some of them are even able to sustain the disease, being considered an important source of the re-emergency of the disease in cattle [1].

Only a few vaccines have been used massively in cattle immunization against *B. abortus,* S19, RB51, 45/20 and SR82, being S19 and RB51 the most widely used vaccines [4]. However, many *B. abortus* vaccine candidates have been developed, including DNA, subunit, recombinant *B. abortus* and recombinant vector vaccines. All of them are evaluated principally in mouse model [13, 14, 15, 16, 17, 18, 19, 20, 21, 22, 23, 24, 25, 26, 27, 28, 29, 30, 31, 32, 33, 34, 35, 36, 37, 38, 39, 40, 41, 42, 43, 44, 45, 46], and with a few exceptions, the majority of these new vaccines, have not been tested in cattle or were not protective in cattle, the target species.

S19 VACCINE

Strain 19 is a live attenuated vaccine and the first *B. abortus* vaccine to be used extensively for bovine brucellosis control [47]. In USA, this vaccine was used for more than five decades from 1941 and is still being used in several other countries [4].

Brucella abortus S19 was isolated in 1923 from milk of a Jersey cow by Dr John Buck [48]. This virulent culture was accidentally left out at room temperature for one year and when tested in guinea pigs showed lower virulence compared with previous tests [49]. Subsequently, S19 showed to be highly successful in immunization of calves [48,50]. The efficacy of *B. abortus* S19 was proved by experimental tests in cattle [47,51] and under field conditions [5,52]. Its main characteristics are stable low pathogenicity, relatively high immunogenicity, and moderate antigenicity [53]. Strain 19 is a smooth attenuated *B. abortus* biovar 1 that induces antibody response that cannot be distinguished from the antibody response induced by infection with field strains [4,50]. The lipopolysaccharide (LPS) O-side chain is an immunodominant antigen to which the majority of antibodies resulting from S19 immunization or natural infection are directed [54]. Antibody titers resulting from vaccination may persist for a prolonged period in a small proportion of vaccinated calves: approximately two animals per 100 000 calfhood vaccinated ones [54]. Residual antibody titers increase with the age at which the animal was vaccinated [5], and to address this issue, vaccination is usually performed on young female calves between three and eight months of age [47]. However, vaccination of this age group does not appear to significantly differ in immunity induced [47]. Restriction on age of vaccination, due to the interference in the brucellosis diagnosis, is the main disadvantage of vaccination with S19. This has contributed greatly to their replacement by RB51 vaccine strain, which does not have this problem.

In calves, S19 vaccination can be performed with full dose [$2.5 - 12 \times 10^{10}$ colony forming units (CFU)], original dosage used in S19 classical experiments, or with reduced dosage ($3–10 \times 10^9$ CFU) to minimize residual antibody titers and to prevent occasional persistent vaccinal infection [4]. After calfhood-vaccination, S19 is usually cleared from superficial cervical lymph node within 10 to 12 weeks. Vaccination of adult cattle with S19, low dosage ($0.3-3 \times 10^9$ CFU), was also successfully employed in infected herds [5,55,56]. S19-adult vaccination was tested as a strategy to be used in infected herds in order to reduce abortions and subsequently brucellosis transmission; however, it was discontinued because vaccination of pregnant animals can cause abortion and mainly because of the persistence of vaccinal antibodies [56,57].

In general, after calfhood vaccination, S19 does not persist in the reproductive tracts of mature heifers and does not cause abortion in these animals [54]. Nonetheless, even with markedly infrequent occurrence, some cattle remain chronically infected and may abort and excrete the vaccine strain in the milk. Another disadvantage of S19 vaccination includes the fact that in some circumstances S19 can cause abortion in pregnant animals [57]. After vaccination of cattle with one, two or three doses prior to breeding age, McDiarmid [51] recovered S19 from 10% of milk samples and 1.5% of samples from cases of abortion. In males, calfhood S19 vaccination usually results in persistent antibody titers, testicular infection, and hence infertility [58]. Furthermore, the vaccination of infected animals with S19 does not cure nor alter the normal course of the disease [47,50].

On the other hand, duration of immunity induced by S19 in cattle vaccinated as calves has proven to be quite long, reaching almost the entire productive lifespan of the animal [47,51]. The immunity in cattle vaccinated between 6 and 8 months of age does not decrease from the first through the fifth pregnancy [47,51]. Moreover, revaccination experiments with S19 and killed *B. abortus* vaccines demonstrated no apparent benefit in cattle-challenge experiments compared with just S19-calfhood immunization [47], despite McDiarmid [51] having observed a small gain from S19 revaccination. Under field conditions 82 to 95% of vaccinated cattle have been shown to have complete protection against infection with virulent strains [50]. However, it has also been demonstrated that the effectiveness of the vaccine decreases proportionally with an increasing dose of bacterial exposure [47,50].

Regarding the immune response triggered by S19 vaccination, most of our knowledge comes from mice studies, which have been shown a strong Th1 immune response with production of IFN-γ and high levels of antigen-specific $CD4^+$ and granzyme B-secreting $CD8^+$ T-cell responses [32].

Being pathogenic to man, the utilization of S19 requires safety training of the personal involved and the use of personal protection equipment as gloves, long sleeve coats, protection glasses, and N95 masks.

RB51 VACCINE STRAIN

B. abortus strain RB51 is a rough rifampicin-resistant strain, which exhibited a lack of expression of the LPS O-side chains (OPS) [59]. RB51 vaccine strain was developed in 1982 by Prof. Gerhardt Schurig's group and is derived from a virulent smooth *B. abortus* biovar 1 strain 2308 [59]. This is a natural mutant derived by a serial passages on media containing subinibitory concentrations of rifampicin or penicillin and by selecting single colonies with rough morphology [59]. The rough characteristic is stable during in vitro and in vivo passages and does not revert to virulent phenotype [59].

The protection against abortion and infection induced by RB51 vaccination in cattle has been sufficiently demonstrated under experimental conditions [6,7,60,61,64]. Also, the use of RB51 is highly effective under field conditions, in herds with high and low brucellosis prevalence [62,63].

The literature shows that calves vaccinated with RB51 at three, five and seven months of age are protected against infection and abortion [64], as well as heifers vaccinated at age of 10 or 24 months, after challenge with the virulent *B. abortus* 2308 [6,60]. Nevertheless, it has been suggested that under experimental circumstances the vaccination with S19 is slightly (not significant) more efficacious than RB51 [4,64]. After vaccination, RB51 is usually cleared from calf superficial cervical lymph node within 6 to 10 weeks [64]. RB51 is considered more attenuated than S19, based on results of clearance and histologic examination of infected tissues of vaccinated animals.

In general, the recommended dosage for RB51 calfhood vaccination is $1.0 - 3.4 \times 10^{10}$ CFU [4]. Protection against *B. abortus* infection is similar through the suggested dosage, although higher antibody titers and longer persistence of bacteria had been associated with the full dose (3.4×10^{10} CFU) [8]. Reduced dosage (1×10^9 CFU), generally recommended for adult animals, also protects against infection and abortion caused by virulent 2308 [61]. Despite RB51 having highly reduced abortifacient characteristics [59,65], it is not completely safe for pregnant cow, mainly when full dose is administrated [66]. However, some results indicate that non-vaccinated cattle and cattle vaccinated with S19 as calves can be safely vaccinated with RB51 (full dose) during the pregnancy [6,67,68]. Furthermore, data indicates that RB51 vaccination is a safe procedure also for males [69].

In addition, as S19 vaccine, RB51 can cause infection in humans especially immunosuppressed individuals [70]. RB51 is resistant to rifampicin, one of the antibiotics of choice in the treatment of human brucellosis, and failure to be detected by routine serological tests are the two most important points one has to be aware during diagnosis and treatment of humans. Therefore, the same protective measures recommended for S19 also applies to RB51 use.

Because of the rough phenotype, RB51 does not induce the production of anti-OPS antibodies in immunized animals, overcoming the serologic problems observed after S19 vaccination [7,59,61]. Consequently, RB51 vaccinated cattle can be easily and accurately differentiated from naturally infected animals, allowing the effective use of the test-and-slaughter and vaccination policies simultaneously. Vaccination with RB51 does not induce antibodies detectable by routine serologic brucellosis diagnostic tests, even after S19 calfhood vaccination and multiple RB51 boosters or use of full dose of RB51 (3.4×10^{10} CFU) [7,61,68]. However, RB51-specific antibodies can be detected by dot enzyme-linked immunosorbent assay or ELISA using killed RB51 antigens [71,72], until approximately 12 weeks after vaccination, with the peak occurring four weeks after vaccination or revaccination with decreasing titers after ten weeks [61,73]. Interestingly, S19-vaccinated cattle exhibit higher titers against RB51 antigens in ELISA than animals vaccinated with RB51, probably due to persistence of S19, which may result in high levels of cross-reacting antibodies against RB51 antigens [73].

So far, there are no experiments that evaluated the duration of immunity, but Olsen and Stoffregen [4] suggest that a booster vaccination is required between 4 and 5 years of age to maintain high levels of protection after RB51 calfhood vaccination. Also, RB51 revaccination has been recommended six months and one year after calfhood vaccination in northern Mexico [74]. Nonetheless, findings from blastogenic response of $CD4^+$ and $CD8^+$ T-cells and the production of IFN- and IL-4 by the lymphocyte subsets six months after RB51 revaccination indicate that there was no increase or improvement in the immunological response resulting from RB51-revaccination of adult cattle [75]. Even though, RB51 revaccination may still be considered as a tool for increasing herd immunity, since not all animals are completely protected after primary immunization [50]. Furthermore, it has been demonstrated that RB51 induces a strong Th1 cellular immune response with production of IFN-γ and $CD8^+$ specific cytotoxic cells, but not IL-4 after vaccination of mice [76].

45/20 VACCINE

This vaccine is prepared with heat-killed *B. abortus* biovar 1 strain 45/20 combined with oil adjuvant [77]. The 45/20 is a rough *B. abortus,* derived of smooth strain 45/0 after 20 passages through guinea pigs [78]. This bacterin was used in some European Union countries for *B. abortus* control replacing S19, in order to eliminate the problems related to the induction of antibodies interfering in the routine diagnosis of infection [5]. However, data of experimental efficacy and immunologic response are contradictory and mostly show the superiority of vaccination with S19 [79,80]. Furthermore, its use has some drawbacks such as the use of oil adjuvant, needing of repeat vaccination and reversion to smooth strain when used as a live vaccine [5,78]. Furthermore, some studies have also indicated that 45/20 is not completely free of the O-side chain [81], hence this vaccine can induce antibodies detectable by routine serologic tests employed in the diagnosis of bovine brucellosis. The variability in reported protection, along with unpredictable serological effects and the occurrence of reactions at the site of vaccine injection in some animals led to the interruption of the use of 45/20 vaccine.

SR82 VACCINE STRAIN

The SR82 strain is a *B. abortus* biovar 6 live attenuated vaccine used since 1974 by the former Union of Soviet Socialist Republics (USSR) for bovine brucellosis control [82]. This vaccine agglutinates in both rough and smooth anti-sera, but does not induce positive response in brucellosis agglutination tests [82,83]. Moreover, SR82 induced protection level similar to S19, after challenge with virulent *B. abortus*, and it has been shown to be effective under field conditions [82,83]. Currently the SR82 strain is still massively used in the Russian Federation, Azerbaijan, Tejikistan and other countries in the region [82].

VACCINATION WITH RECOMBINANT GENES, PROTEINS, VECTORS AND *B. ABORTUS* RECOMBINANT MUTANTS

Classically and historically the vaccines used in the bovine brucellosis control are live attenuated vaccines produced from spontaneously attenuated or randomly selected strains. Nonetheless, the numerous advances in genomics, proteomics, recombinant DNA technology and even in vaccinology, allowed the exploration of other tools for the development of safer vaccines, without drawbacks observed in classical vaccines. In this context, several studies aimed to develop, test the efficacy or assess the immulogical responses of the *B. abortus* genetically engineered vaccines (recombinant genes, proteins, vectors and modified *B. abortus*strains) have been performed essentially in mice. However, with a few exceptions the majority of these recombinant vaccines, have not been tested or did not protect cattle, their target species. Moreover, it is important to take into account that recombinant vaccines, especially non-living ones, have limitations regarding economic viability, need for multiple doses and the need for combination of antigens.

DNA vaccines

DNA vaccines offer the possibility of inducing both cellular and humoral responses, expression of antigens is prolonged, they have better stability and do not require refrigeration under storage. Therefore, several antigens have been explored for their value as DNA vaccines against *B. abortus* challenge, providing various levels of protection. DNA vaccines encoding ribosomal *L7/L12,* lumazine synthase (*BLS*), *P39* (a putative periplasmic binding protein), *Omp16* (outer membrane protein) and *BAB1_0278* genes have demonstrated to confer protection against *B. abortus* challenge in mice [22,23,27,42]. Moreover, Cu/Zn superoxide dismutase (Cu-Zn SOD) DNA vaccine induced a protection level similar to the one induced by RB51 [25]. All these genes also proved capable of eliciting a desirable cellular immune response in mice [22,23,32,33,42]. In contrast, plasmid DNA carrying the *BAB1_0263* and bacterioferritin (*BFR*) genes did not induce significant level of protection against challenge with virulent *B. abortus* in mice.

Combined DNA vaccines have also demonstrated their ability to protect better against challenge. DNA vaccines of genes coding for an immundominant *Brucella*-antigen (BCSP31) and promising *Brucella*-antigens (SOD and L7/L12) provided significantly better protection than S19 in mice [32]. This combined DNA vaccine also elicited significantly higher cytotoxic response (granzyme B–producing $CD8^+$ T cells) compared to S19-vaccinated mice [32]. Likewise, divalent fusion DNA vaccine encoding *L7/L12* and *Omp16* genes also proved to be effective and able to elicit a strong T-cell proliferative response and induce a large amount of IFN-γ producing T cells [27]. Additionally, data showed that combination of these *B. abortus* genes (*BCSP31, SOD*and *L7/L12*) with *Mycobacterium tuberculosis* (*Ag85B, MPT64*, and *MPT83*) or *Mycobacterium bovis* (*Ag85B, MPT64,* and *MPT83*) genes are very promising for both agents [33,34]. DNA vaccine containing six genes encoding immunodominant antigens from *M. bovis* and *B. abortus* induced protection comparable to S19 and better than Bacillus Calmette-Guerin (BCG) vaccine in cattle, suggesting that this is a highly promising vaccine for both diseases [34]. Combined DNA vaccine containing *M. tuberculosis* and *B. abortus* genes with added IL-12 adjuvant system showed that besides the high level of protection, IL-12 acts as an adjuvant to enhance protective immunity against *M. tuberculosis* and *B. abortus* in challenge mice [33]. Conversely, results suggest that a SOD DNA vaccine fused to IL-2 did not improve protection efficacy [29].

However, despite some of *B. abortus* DNA vaccine candidates have shown very promising results in mice, the need of at least four booster vaccinations to be effective as well as the high cost for use in large animals, make this type of vaccine impractical for cattle, the main target of brucellosis vaccination. Moreover, excluding mouse studies practically no DNA vaccine has been explored in natural hosts.

Subunit vaccines

Many of the same antigens tested as DNA vaccines have also been evaluated as potential antigens for subunit vaccines (L7/L12 ribosomal protein; P39; BLS; Omp16; Cu/Zn SOD) [14,21,24,37,40]. The outer membrane proteins (OMPs) of *B. abortus*, potential immunogenic antigens, have been widely explored as subunit vaccines [37,39,43,45]. Unlipidated recombinant Omp16 and Omp19, and recombinant Omp25 liposome encapsulated gave protection comparable to S19 in vaccinated mice following challenge [37,39,45]. Also, Omp28 subunit vaccine increased resistance against challenge with virulent *B. abortus* but at lower level than live attenuated vaccines [43].

Similarly, flagellar proteins have been screened in search for a subunit vaccine antigen candidate. Five flagellar genes, although *Brucella* spp. are non-motile, (*BAB1_0260* (FlgJ); *BAB2_0122* (FliN); *BAB2_0150*; *BAB2_1086*; *BAB2_1093*) were evaluated for their ability to induce humoral and cell-mediated responses and protect mice against *B. abortus* challenge [84]. Of these, FlgJ and FliN were found to be protective antigens that produced humoral and cell-mediated responses in mice.

Moreover, recombinant proteins of other proven or putative pathogenesis-associated genes such as L7/12, BLS, rSurA and rDnaK induced different levels of protective immunity and cellular immune response in mice against brucellosis [14,24,31]. Whereas, dihydrolipoamide succinyltransferase (rE2o) and cysteine synthase A (rCysK) provided partial protection against *B. abortus* challenge and induced primarily Th2 type of immune response [41,46]. Furthermore, CobB, AsnC and P39 elicit protective immunity similarly to Cu/Zn SOD and S19, which is marked by both humoral and cellular immune responses [21,85]. Also, Cu/Zn SOD recombinant protein (liposomes encapsulated) confers resistance in mice, further increased upon co-immunization with recombinant IL-18 [40]. In contrast, BAB1_0560, BAB1_1108, BAB2_0059 (VirB10), BAB2_0191, BAB2_0423 (GntR) and BRF protein vaccines did not induce protective immune response [21,85].

The potential use of *B. abortus* subunit vaccines under field conditions is very limited, although some encouraging results showed. The requirement of multiple boosters, adjuvants and combination of several antigens makes it economically unsuitable for cattle. Moreover, it is important to consider that the response observed in mice may not reflect the protection achieved in natural hosts after vaccination. Furthermore, to generate a strong and protective immune response that can mimic the natural infection from a combination of few proteins of the pathogen is a hard and complex challenge.

Vector vaccines

Alternatively, genes encoding immunodominant *B. abortus* antigens can be introduced into attenuated viruses or bacteria that serve as vector vaccines. *B. abortus* genes have been successfully expressed in viruses (Semliki Forest virus and Vaccinia virus) and bacteria (*Escherichia coli, Ochrobactrum anthropi, Lactococcus lactis*, *Salmonella enterica* subsp *enterica* serovar Typhimurium and *B. abortus*) [16,20,26,28,35,38,44,86]. *Escherichia coli, O. anthropi* (plus unmethylated CpG motifs) and *L. lactis* expressing Cu/Zn SOD antigen of *B. abortus* were able to elicit a Th1 immune response and to protect mice following challenge with virulent *B. abortus* [20,28,44,86]. Likewise, Semliki Forest virus-based vector carrying RNA encoding *Brucella* translation initiation factor 3 (IF3) showed a significant level of protection against a challenge with *B. abortus* 2308 in mice [35]. L7/L12 protein carried by *S. enterica* serovar typhimurium but not by Vaccinia virus conferred protective efficacy and immunogenicity [26,38]. Also, vaccinia virus carrying 18-kDa OMP of *B. abortus* were not able to protect mice against a challenge with the virulent strain *B. abortus* 2308 [87].

The expression of *B. abortus* antigens on viral or bacterial vectors is a superior alternative to DNA and subunit vaccines, as it closely mimics the natural infection, allowing the modulation of the host immune response and the multiplication of the initial number of antigen copies within the host. However, despite not having some of the inconveniences observed in non-living vaccines, as multiple doses, need for adjuvant and high cost, other organisms expressing *B. abortus* proteins still need the perfect grouping of antigens, expressed in high amount to be effective. The amount of foreign protein expressed by the carrier organism needs to be able to promote a specific protection. Moreover, the use of viral platform implies in small chance that the vector DNA is integrated into the genome of the host cell. In addition, although promising most of these above vaccines have failed or have not been tested in cattle, the target species, so no conclusion could be drawn at this time.

B. abortus recombinant mutants

Another focus of research for new vaccines to protect against *B. abortus* infection has been the construction of RB51 recombinant mutants, which retain the rough phenotype and attenuation but have improved characteristics such as immunogenicity and protection against a challenge [17, 18, 19]. Hence, some studies have shown that the complementation of RB51 with a functional *wbo*A gene (RB51*Wbo*A), which lead to the expression of O-side chain in its cytoplasm, or the overexpression of Cu/Zn SOD protein (RB51SOD) results in significant enhancement of the vaccine efficacy against challenge with virulent *B. abortus* in mice [17,18]. Furthermore, the combination of these two genes in a single RB51 strain (RB51SOD/*wbo*A) also significantly increased the protective ability of this RB51 recombinant vaccine in mice and did not alter its desirable characteristics [19]. Nonetheless, this RB51-recombinant strain was not as effective as the parental RB51 strain in calfhood vaccination of bison after challenge with 2308 [36].

Besides RB51, *B. abortus* strain 2308 has also been tested as recombinant mutant vaccine; the deletion of the gene *znuA,* important protein for survival and normal growth under low Zn^{2+} concentrations, generated a mutant capable of conferring protection similar to S19 or RB51 against challenge with parental 2308 in mice [30]. Experiments in natural hosts, cattle, showed that the double gene deletion (*htrA cycL*) PHE1 was attenuated in the bovine host when compared to the virulent parental 2308 [88]. However, due the absence of a standard challenge study using this potential vaccine, the meaning of such data is unclear. Recombinant mutants based on deletion of ABC transporter ATPase (*BAB1_0542*) or phosphoglycerate kinase (*pgk*) gene of *B. abortus* 2308 also showed protection against challenge with virulent strain in mice and the critical role of these genes for full bacterial virulence [89,90]. In addition to the virulence attenuation, it is desired that these *B. abortus* mutants also show no interference with the diagnostics tests, hence genes associated to the smooth phenotype have been explored in the generation of deleted vaccines. Rough mutant generated by *wboA* gene deletion of S19 protected mice against challenge with 2308 and did not induce abortion in pregnant sheep, showing promising results to be explored in the future development of rough vaccines [91].

The improvement of the existing *B. abortus* vaccines or the creation of new attenuated vaccines by deletion or complementation of some genes seems to be the most promising direction to find a safer and more efficient substitute for the known *B. abortus* vaccines. Modified live vaccines are highly effective in comparison to killed vaccines. This is most likely due to strong and protective cellular immune response induced by live vaccines [2,3]. The use of this platform avoids the main disadvantages related to the non-living vaccines, as multiple delivery, low immunogenicity, need for adjuvants and high cost. Furthermore, *B. abortus* strains, even if genetically modified, can colonize, be immunogenic, and therefore perfectly simulate the natural infection. They are able to multiply within animals for a short period expressing in vivo protective antigens. The major advantage of this approach over the use of vectors is that recombinant mutants share most of proteins with *B. abortus* field strains, whereas carrier organisms are able of expressing only few *Brucella* antigens. However, a real concern on *B. abortus* mutant strains is the presence of antibiotic selection marker. The antibiotic marker is used in the screening of transformed clones, but it is not desirable in the final vaccine due to the potential of spreading antibiotic resistance genes. Options, as an RB51 leucine auxotroph, have been explored to avoid this issue [92]. Additionally, so far, there is no data available to exclude the possibility that these live mutants will not have similar safety and diagnostic issues as live strains, especially if made from smooth strains. Also, to move forwards in the control of bovine brucellosis, these recombinant mutants must be evaluated in cattle and other target animal species. There is still a worldwide need for a vaccine that is safe and highly efficacious in natural hosts, since the transmission of disease occurs from cattle to people. The results obtained in mice, although favorable for some vaccines, have to be interpreted according to their limitations, as they cannot be directly extrapolated to cattle.

On another point of about the usefulness of *B. abortus* mutant as vaccines, S19 and RB51, the widely used *B. abortus* vaccines, has been investigated as potential vectors for heterologous protein expression, mainly using protective antigens important for other diseases of veterinary interest [93, 94, 95, 96]. In this context, multivalent recombinant RB51 vaccines expressing *Neospora caninum* or *M. bovis* proteins have been shown to induce antigen specific immune response to heterologous antigens and, in the case of *N. caninum,* was also achieved significant level of protection in mice [93,94]. Likewise, S19 carrying the genes encoding for the heterologous antigens of *Babebia bovis* or *M. bovis* demonstrated successful specific cellular immune response to recombinant proteins in mouse model [95,96]. These above bivalent live modified *B. abortus* candidate vaccines need further evaluation as to their ability to induce protective immune response as well lack of interference in the diagnostic tests.

OTHER *B. ABORTUS* POTENTIAL VACCINES

Besides *B. abortus* recombinants vaccines, also vaccines based on outer membrane vesicles (OMVs) has been exploited as an acellular alternative to live vaccines [97]. OMVs are bilayer membrane vesicles release by Gram-negative and Gram-positive bacteria, which have been associated to many processes such as release of virulent factors, DNA transfer, regulation of host immune response and survival in the host cell [98]. *B. abortus* OMVs are mainly composed for outer membrane proteins (Omps) and have been associated with modulation of host immune response by inhibition of TNF-α and IL-8 response, inhibition of IFN-γ induced expression of MHC class II molecules on human monocytes and increase in expression of adhesion molecules [97, 98, 99]. A *Brucella melitensis* vaccine based on OMVs has been tested and showed promising results in BALB/c mice [100]. Furthermore, it is already available a vaccine based on OMVs, against meningococcus serogroup B (*Neisseria meningitides*) in some countries as Cuba, Norway and New Zealand [97]. Therefore, it is possible to speculate that an OMV vaccine against *B. abortus* has a great potential to be considered as part of the continuous efforts to reach safer and more effective *B. abortus* vaccine. Nonetheless, due to its high cost and laborious production, OMV is a more suitable approach for human vaccines, being impracticable for cattle bearing in mind the technologies currently available.

CONCLUSIONS

Vaccination is a determinant strategy for brucellosis control and eradication programs, therefore it has been the target of innumerous studies over decades. Nowadays, some effective vaccines are available to control the disease in cattle. S19 and RB51 are the officially approved *B. abortus* vaccine strains more widely and successfully used to prevent bovine brucellosis worldwide. However, due to some side effects shown by these current vaccines, plus the advances in recombinant DNA technology and the lack of a vaccine for humans, there is an on going extensive efforts focused on the development of new and better vaccines. Engineered vaccines have the potential to be the future of the bovine and human brucellosis control, but many studies are still needed to develop a better vaccine than the current vaccines in terms of safety, efficacy and other desirable characteristics. Moreover, it is important to consider that, mainly non-living recombinant vaccines, also present important issues, as the requirement of multiple boosters, adjuvants, and optimal combination of antigens, besides usually inducing poor cellular immune response. In addition, although the excellent results observed for some recombinant vaccines in mice, very few of these candidate vaccines have been evaluated in cattle. The recent studies indicate that the future of a new *B. abortus* vaccine will be the construction of directed mutants, which exclude the drawbacks and simultaneously increase immunogenic characteristics presented by S19 and RB51. Furthermore, concerning the immune response induced after S19 and RB51 vaccination in cattle, as well as after RB51 revaccination, very little is understood. Efforts to find out the principal characteristics of the immune response triggered in cattle by the two most used and successful *B. abortus* vaccine strains are essential to try to establish an ideal vaccine. The definition of immune markers correlated with protection, by mathematical modeling or evaluation of the immune response in vaccine - challenge studies - would be very helpful in the screening of *B. abortus* candidate vaccines.

DECLARATIONS

Acknowledgements

A.P. Lage were indebted to Conselho Nacional de Desenvolvimento Científico e Tecnológico – CNPq for his fellowship. EMSD thanks CNPq and Capes (Ciência Sem Fronteiras 8808–13) for her fellowship as well. APL lab was supported by CNPq, Fundação de Amparo à Pesquisa do Estado de Minas Gerais - Fapemig and FEP – MVZ Coordenação Preventiva.

Authors' contributions

EMSD wrote the paper. APL and NS critically reed the manuscript. All authors read and approved the final manuscript.

REFERENCES

1. Corbel MJ, Elberg SS, Cosivi O (2006) Brucellosis in humans and animals. World Health Organization, Geneva
2. Schurig G, Boyle S, Sriranganathan N (1995) Brucella abortus vaccine strain RB51: a brief re. Arch Med Vet 27:19–22
3. Ko J, Splitter GA (2003) Molecular host-pathogen interaction in brucellosis: current understanding and future approaches to vaccine development for mice and humans. Clin Microbiol Rev 16:65–78
4. Olsen SC, Stoffregen WS (2005) Essential role of vaccines in brucellosis control and eradication programs for livestock. Expert Rev Vaccines 4:915–928
5. Nicoletti P (1990) Vaccination. In: Nielsen K, Duncan JR (eds) Animal Brucellosis. CRC Press, Boca Raton
6. Poester FP, Goncalves VS, Paixao TA, Santos RL, Olsen SC, Schurig GG, Lage AP (2006) Efficacy of strain RB51 vaccine in heifers against experimental brucellosis. Vaccine 24:5327–5334
7. Olsen SC, Bricker B, Palmer MV, Jensen AE, Cheville NF (1999) Responses of cattle to two dosages of Brucella abortus strain RB51: serology, clearance and efficacy. Res Vet Sci 66:101–105
8. Thakur A, Pedersen LE, Jungersen G (2012) Immune markers and correlates of protection for vaccine induced immune responses. Vaccine 30:4907–4920
9. Miranda KL, Dorneles EM, Pauletti RB, Poester FP, Lage AP (2015) *Brucella abortus* S19 and RB51 vaccine immunogenicity test: evaluation of three mice (BALB/c, Swiss and CD-1®) and two challenge strains (544 and 2308). Vaccine 33:507–511
10. Garcia-Yoldi D, Le Fleche P, Marin CM, De Miguel MJ, Munoz PM, Vergnaud G, Lopez-Goni I (2007) Assessment of genetic stability of Brucella melitensis Rev 1 vaccine strain by multiple-locus variable-number tandem repeat analysis. Vaccine 25:2858–2862
11. Miranda KL, Poester FP, Minharro S, Dorneles EM, Stynen AP, Lage AP (2013) Evaluation of Brucella abortus S19 vaccines commercialized in Brazil: immunogenicity, residual virulence and MLVA15 genotyping. Vaccine 31:3014–3018
12. Dorneles EM, de Faria AP, Pauletti RB, Santana JA, Caldeira GA, Heinemann MB, Titze-de-Almeida R, Lage AP (2013) Genetic stability of Brucella abortus S19 and RB51 vaccine strains by multiple locus variable number tandem repeat analysis (MLVA16). Vaccine 31:4856–4859
13. Oliveira SC, Harms JS, Banai M, Splitter GA (1996) Recombinant Brucella abortus proteins that induce proliferation and gamma-interferon secretion by CD4+ T cells from Brucella-vaccinated mice and delayed-type hypersensitivity in sensitized guinea pigs. Cell Immunol 172:262–268
14. Oliveira SC, Splitter GA (1996) Immunization of mice with recombinant L7/L12 ribosomal protein confers protection against Brucella abortus infection. Vaccine 14:959–962
15. Vemulapalli R, Duncan AJ, Boyle SM, Sriranganathan N, Toth TE, Schurig GG (1998) Cloning and sequencing of yajC and secD homologs of Brucella abortus and demonstration of immune responses to YajC in mice vaccinated with B. abortus RB51. Infect Immun 66:5684–5691
16. Vemulapalli R, Cravero S, Calvert CL, Toth TE, Sriranganathan N, Boyle SM, Rossetti OL, Schurig GG (2000) Characterization of specific immune responses of mice inoculated with recombinant vaccinia virus expressing an 18-kilodalton outer membrane protein of Brucella abortus. Clin Diagn Lab Immunol 7:114–118
17. Vemulapalli R, He Y, Buccolo LS, Boyle SM, Sriranganathan N, Schurig GG (2000) Complementation of Brucella abortus RB51 with a functional wboA gene results in O-antigen synthesis and enhanced vaccine efficacy but no change in rough phenotype and attenuation. Infect Immun 68:3927–3932
18. Vemulapalli R, He Y, Cravero S, Sriranganathan N, Boyle SM, Schurig GG (2000) Overexpression of protective antigen as a novel approach to enhance vaccine efficacy of Brucella abortus strain RB51. Infect Immun 68:3286–3289
19. Vemulapalli R, Contreras A, Sanakkayala N, Sriranganathan N, Boyle SM, Schurig GG (2004) Enhanced efficacy of recombinant Brucella abortus RB51 vaccines against B. melitensis infection in mice. Vet Microbiol 102:237–245
20. He Y, Vemulapalli R, Schurig GG (2002) Recombinant Ochrobactrum anthropi expressing Brucella abortus Cu,

Zn superoxide dismutase protects mice against B. abortus infection only after switching of immune responses to Th1 type. Infect Immun 70:2535–2543

21. Al-Mariri A, Tibor A, Mertens P, De Bolle X, Michel P, Godefroid J, Walravens K, Letesson JJ (2001) Protection of BALB/c mice against Brucella abortus 544 challenge by vaccination with bacterioferritin or P39 recombinant proteins with CpG oligodeoxynucleotides as adjuvant. Infect Immun 69:4816–4822
22. Al-Mariri A, Tibor A, Mertens P, De Bolle X, Michel P, Godfroid J, Walravens K, Letesson JJ (2001) Induction of immune response in BALB/c mice with a DNA vaccine encoding bacterioferritin or P39 of Brucella spp. Infect Immun 69:6264–70
23. Velikovsky CA, Cassataro J, Giambartolomei GH, Goldbaum FA, Estein S, Bowden RA, Bruno L, Fossati CA, Spitz M (2002) A DNA vaccine encoding lumazine synthase from Brucella abortus induces protective immunity in BALB/c mice. Infect Immun 70:2507–2511
24. Velikovsky CA, Goldbaum FA, Cassataro J, Estein S, Bowden RA, Bruno L, Fossati CA, Giambartolomei GH (2003) Brucella lumazine synthase elicits a mixed Th1-Th2 immune response and reduces infection in mice challenged with Brucella abortus 544 independently of the adjuvant formulation used. Infect Immun 71:5750–5755
25. Onate AA, Cespedes S, Cabrera A, Rivers R, Gonzalez A, Munoz C, Folch H, Andrews E (2003) A DNA vaccine encoding Cu, Zn superoxide dismutase of Brucella abortus induces protective immunity in BALB/c mice. Infect Immun 71:4857–4861
26. Baloglu S, Boyle SM, Vemulapalli R, Sriranganathan N, Schurig GG, Toth TE (2005) Immune responses of mice to vaccinia virus recombinants expressing either Listeria monocytogenes partial listeriolysin or Brucella abortus ribosomal L7/L12 protein. Vet Microbiol 109:11–17
27. Luo D, Ni B, Li P, Shi W, Zhang S, Han Y, Mao L, He Y, Wu Y, Wang X (2006) Protective immunity elicited by a divalent DNA vaccine encoding both the L7/L12 and Omp16 genes of Brucella abortus in BALB/c mice. Infect Immun 74:2734–2741
28. Andrews E, Salgado P, Folch H, Onate A (2006) Vaccination with live Escherichia coli expressing Brucella abortus Cu/Zn superoxide-dismutase: II. Induction of specific CD8+ cytotoxic lymphocytes and sensitized CD4+ IFN-gamma-producing cell. Microbiol Immunol 50:389–393
29. Gonzalez-Smith A, Vemulapalli R, Andrews E, Onate A (2006) Evaluation of Brucella abortus DNA vaccine by expression of Cu-Zn superoxide dismutase antigen fused to IL-2. Immunobiology 211:65–74
30. Yang X, Becker T, Walters N, Pascual DW (2006) Deletion of znuA virulence factor attenuates Brucella abortus and confers protection against wild-type challenge. Infect Immun 74:3874–3879
31. Delpino MV, Estein SM, Fossati CA, Baldi PC, Cassataro J (2007) Vaccination with Brucella recombinant DnaK and SurA proteins induces protection against Brucella abortus infection in BALB/c mice. Vaccine 25:6721–6729
32. Yu DH, Hu XD, Cai H (2007) A combined DNA vaccine encoding BCSP31, SOD, and L7/L12 confers high protection against Brucella abortus 2308 by inducing specific CTL responses. DNA Cell Biol 26:435–443
33. Yu DH, Li M, Hu XD, Cai H (2007) A combined DNA vaccine enhances protective immunity against Mycobacterium tuberculosis and Brucella abortus in the presence of an IL-12 expression vector. Vaccine 25:6744–6754
34. Hu XD, Yu DH, Chen ST, Li SX, Cai H (2009) A combined DNA vaccine provides protective immunity against Mycobacterium bovis and Brucella abortus in cattle. DNA Cell Biol 28:191–199
35. Cabrera A, Saez D, Cespedes S, Andrews E, Onate A (2009) Vaccination with recombinant Semliki Forest virus ps expressing translation initiation factor 3 of Brucella abortus induces protective immunity in BALB/c mice. Immunobiology 214:467–474
36. Olsen SC, Boyle SM, Schurig GG, Sriranganathan NN (2009) Immune responses and protection against experimental challenge after vaccination of bison with Brucella abortus strain RB51 or RB51 overexpressing superoxide dismutase and glycosyltransferase genes. Clin Vaccine Immunol 16:535–540
37. Pasquevich KA, Estein SM, Garcia Samartino C, Zwerdling A, Coria LM, Barrionuevo P, Fossati CA, Giambartolomei GH, Cassataro J (2009) Immunization with recombinant Brucella species outer membrane protein Omp16 or Omp19 in adjuvant induces specific CD4+ and CD8+ T cells as well as systemic and oral protection against Brucella abortus infection. Infect Immun 77:436–445
38. Zhao Z, Li M, Luo D, Xing L, Wu S, Duan Y, Yang P, Wang X (2009) Protection of mice from Brucella infection by immunization with attenuated Salmonella enterica serovar typhimurium expressing A L7/L12 and BLS fusion antigen of Brucella. Vaccine 27:5214–5219
39. Pasquevich KA, Ibanez AE, Coria LM, Garcia Samartino C, Estein SM, Zwerdling A, Barrionuevo P, Oliveira FS, Seither C, Warzecha H, Oliveira SC, Giambartolomei GH, Cassataro J (2011) An oral vaccine based on U-Omp19 induces protection against B. abortus mucosal challenge by inducing an adaptive IL-17 immune response in mice. PLoS One 6:e16203
40. Singha H, Mallick AI, Jana C, Fatima N, Owais M, Chaudhuri P (2011) Co-immunization with interlukin-18 enhances the protective efficacy of liposomes encapsulated recombinant Cu-Zn superoxide dismutase protein against Brucella abortus. Vaccine 29:4720–4727
41. Verma SK, Jain S, Kumar S (2012) Immunogenicity and protective potential of a bacterially expressed recombinant dihydrolipoamide succinyltransferase (rE2o) of Brucella abortus in BALB/c mice. World J Microbiol Biotechnol 28:2487–2495
42. Sislema-Egas F, Cespedes S, Fernandez P, Retamal-Diaz A, Saez D, Onate A (2012) Evaluation of protective effect of DNA vaccines encoding the BAB1_0263 and BAB1_0278 open reading frames of Brucella abortus in

BALB/c mice. Vaccine 30:7286–7291

43. Lim JJ, Kim DH, Lee JJ, Kim DG, Min W, Lee HJ, Rhee MH, Kim S (2012) Protective effects of recombinantBrucella abortusOmp28 against infection with a virulent strain of Brucella abortus544 in mice. J Vet Sci 13:287–292
44. Saez D, Fernandez P, Rivera A, Andrews E, Onate A (2012) Oral immunization of mice with recombinant Lactococcus lactis expressing Cu, Zn superoxide dismutase of Brucella abortus triggers protective immunity. Vaccine 30:1283–1290
45. Goel D, Rajendran V, Ghosh PC, Bhatnagar R (2013) Cell mediated immune response after challenge in Omp25 liposome immunized mice contributes to protection against virulent Brucella abortus 544. Vaccine 31:1231–1237
46. Jain S, Afley P, Kumar S (2013) Immunological responses to recombinant cysteine synthase A of Brucella abortus in BALB/c mice. World J Microbiol Biotechnol 29:907–913
47. Manthei CA (1959) Summary of controlled research with strain 19, Proceedings 63rd Ann Meet US Livestock Sanitary Association.
48. Buck JM (1930) Studies on vaccination during calfhood to prevent bovine infectious abortion. J Agri Res 41:667–689
49. Graves RR (1943) The story of John M. Buck's and Matilda's contribution to the cattle industry J Am Vet Med Assoc 102:193–195
50. Jones FM, Hooper JA (1976) Brucella abortus strain 19 calfhood vaccination – a re. Southwest Vet 29:219–225
51. McDiarmid A (1957) The degree and duration of immunity in cattle resulting from vaccination with S. 19 Br. abortus vaccine and its implication in the future control and eventual eradication of Brucellosis. Vet Rec 69:877–879
52. Koh SH, Morley FH (1981) The effect of calfhood vaccination with strain 19 on the serological diagnosis and eradication of bovine brucellosis. Aust Vet J 57:551–553
53. Mingle CK, Manthei CA, Jasmin AM (1941) The stability of reduced virulence exhibited by Brucella abortus strain 19. J Am Vet Med Assoc 99:203–205
54. Meyer ME, Nelson CJ (1969) Persistence of Brucella abortus, strain 19 infection in immunized cattle. Proc Annu Meet U S Anim Health Assoc 73:159–165
55. Breitmeyer RE, Hird DW, Carpenter TE (1992) Serologic and bacteriologic test results after adult vaccination with strain 19 in three dairy herds infected with brucellosis. J Am Vet Med Assoc 200:806–811
56. Nicoletti P (1981) Prevalence and persistence of Brucella abortus strain 19 infections and prevalence of other biotypes in vaccinated adult dairy cattle. J Am Vet Med Assoc 178:143–145
57. Corner LA, Alton GG (1981) Persistence of Brucella abortus strain 19 infection in adult cattle vaccinated with reduced doses. Res Vet Sci 31:342–344
58. Lambert G, Manthei CA, Deyoe BL (1963) Studies on Brucella abortus infection in bulls. Am J Vet Res 24:1152–1157
59. Schurig GG, Roop RM 2nd, Bagchi T, Boyle S, Buhrman D, Sriranganathan N (1991) Biological properties of RB51; a stable rough strain of Brucella abortus. Vet Microbiol 28:171–188
60. Cheville NF, Stevens MG, Jensen AE, Tatum FM, Halling SM (1993) Immune responses and protection against infection and abortion in cattle experimentally vaccinated with mutant strains of Brucella abortus. Am J Vet Res 54:1591–1597
61. Olsen SC (2000) Immune responses and efficacy after administration of a commercial Brucella abortus strain RB51 vaccine to cattle. Vet Ther 1:183–191
62. Lord VR, Schurig GG, Cherwonogrodzky JW, Marcano MJ, Melendez GE (1998) Field study of vaccination of cattle with Brucella abortus strains RB51 and 19 under high and low disease prevalence. Am J Vet Res 59:1016–1020
63. Dorneles EM, Santana JA, Alves TM, Pauletti RB, Mol JP, Heinemann MB, Lage AP (2014) Genetic stability of Brucella abortus isolates from an outbreak by multiple-locus variable-number tandem repeat analysis (MLVA16). BMC Microbiol 14:186
64. Cheville NF, Olsen SC, Jensen AE, Stevens MG, Palmer MV, Florance AM (1996) Effects of age at vaccination on efficacy of Brucella abortus strain RB51 to protect cattle against brucellosis. Am J Vet Res 57:1153–1156
65. Palmer MV, Cheville NF, Jensen AE (1996) Experimental infection of pregnant cattle with the vaccine candidate Brucella abortus strain RB51: pathologic, bacteriologic, and serologic findings. Vet Pathol 33:682–691
66. Palmer MV, Olsen SC, Cheville NF (1997) Safety and immunogenicity of Brucella abortus strain RB51 vaccine in pregnant cattle. Am J Vet Res 58:472–477
67. Martins H, Garin-Bastuji B, Lima F, Flor L, Pina Fonseca A, Boinas F (2009) Eradication of bovine brucellosis in the Azores, Portugal-Outcome of a 5-year programme (2002–2007) based on test-and-slaughter and RB51 vaccination. Prev Vet Med 90:80–89
68. Samartino LE, Fort M, Gregoret R, Schurig GG (2000) Use of Brucella abortus vaccine strain RB51 in pregnant cows after calfhood vaccination with strain 19 in Argentina. Prev Vet Med 45:193–199
69. Edmonds MD, Schurig GG, Samartino LE, Hoyt PG, Walker JV, Hagius SD, Elzer PH (1999) Biosafety of Brucella abortus strain RB51 for vaccination of mature bulls and pregnant heifers. Am J Vet Res 60:722–725
70. Ashford DA, di Pietra J, Lingappa J, Woods C, Noll H, Neville B, Weyant R, Bragg SL, Spiegel RA, Tappero J, Perkins BA (2004) Adverse events in humans associated with accidental exposure to the livestock brucellosis vaccine RB51. Vaccine 22:3435–3439
71. Olsen SC, Stevens MG, Cheville NF, Schurig G (1997) Experimental use of a dot-blot assay to measure serologic responses of cattle vaccinated with Brucella abortus strain RB51. J Vet Diagn Invest 9:363–367
72. Nielsen K, Smith P, Yu W, Nicoletti P, Elzer P, Vigliocco

A, Silva P, Bermudez R, Renteria T, Moreno F, Ruiz A, Massengill C, Muenks Q, Kenny K, Tollersrud T, Samartino L, Conde S, Draghi De Benitez G, Gall D, Perez B, Rojas X (2004) Enzyme immunoassay for the diagnosis of brucellosis: chimeric Protein A-Protein G as a common enzyme labeled detection reagent for sera for different animal species. Vet Microbiol 101:123–129

73. Stevens MG, Olsen SC, Cheville NF (1995) Comparative analysis of immune responses in cattle vaccinated with Brucella abortus strain 19 or strain RB51. Vet Immunol Immunopathol 44:223–235

74. Luna-Martinez JE, Mejia-Teran C (2002) Brucellosis in Mexico: current status and trends. Vet Microbiol 90:19–30

75. Dorneles EM, Teixeira-Carvalho A, Araujo MS, Lima GK, Martins-Filho OA, Sriranganathan N, Lage AP (2014) T lymphocytes subsets and cytokine pattern induced by vaccination against bovine brucellosis employing S19 calfhood vaccination and adult RB51 revaccination. Vaccine 32:6034–6038

76. He Y, Vemulapalli R, Zeytun A, Schurig GG (2001) Induction of specific cytotoxic lymphocytes in mice vaccinated with Brucella abortus RB51. Infect Immun 69:5502–5508

77. McEwen AD, Samuel JMD (1955) Brucella abortus: heat stable protective antigen revealed by adjuvant and present in a rough variant strain 45/20: immunization experiments on guinea pigs. Vet Rec 67:546–548

78. McEwen AD (1940) Experiments on contagious abortion. The immunity of cattle inoculated with vaccines of graded virulence. Vet Rec 52:815

79. Cunningham B (1977) The effect of immaturity of the calf on immunological responses to strain 19 and killed 45/20 adjuvant vaccines. Vet Rec 101:283–285

80. Woodard LF, Jasman RL (1983) Comparative efficacy of an experimental S45/20 bacterin and a reduced dose of strain 19 vaccine against bovine brucellosis. Am J Vet Res 44:907–910

81. Schurig GG, Hammerberg C, Finkler BR (1984) Monoclonal antibodies to Brucella surface antigens associated with the smooth lipopolysaccharide complex. Am J Vet Res 45:967–971

82. Ivanov AV, Salmakov KM, Olsen SC, Plumb GE (2011) A live vaccine from Brucella abortus strain 82 for control of cattle brucellosis in the Russian Federation. Anim Health Res Rev 12:113–121

83. Salmakov KM, Fomin AM, Plotnikova EM, Safina GM, Galimova GM, Salmakova AV, Ivanov AV, Panin AN, Sklyarov OD, Shumilov KV, Klimanov AI (2010) Comparative study of the immunobiological properties of live brucellosis vaccines. Vaccine 28(Suppl 5):F35–40

84. Li X, Xu J, Xie Y, Qiu Y, Fu S, Yuan X, Ke Y, Yu S, Du X, Cui M, Chen Y, Wang T, Wang Z, Yu Y, Huang K, Huang L, Peng G, Chen Z, Wang Y (2012) Vaccination with recombinant flagellar proteins FlgJ and FliN induce protection against Brucella abortus 544 infection in BALB/c mice. Vet Microbiol 161:137–144

85. Fu S, Xu J, Li X, Xie Y, Qiu Y, Du X, Yu S, Bai Y, Chen Y, Wang T, Wang Z, Yu Y, Peng G, Huang K, Huang L, Wang Y, Chen Z (2012) Immunization of mice with recombinant protein CobB or AsnC confers protection against Brucella abortus infection. PLoS One 7:e29552

86. Onate AA, Vemulapalli R, Andrews E, Schurig GG, Boyle S, Folch H (1999) Vaccination with live Escherichia coli expressing Brucella abortus Cu/Zn superoxide dismutase protects mice against virulent B. abortus. Infect Immun 67:986–988

87. Vemulapalli R, Cravero S, Calvert CL, Toth TE, Sriranganathan N, Boyle SM, Rossetti OL, Schurig GG (2000) Characterization of specific immune responses of mice inoculated with recombinant vaccinia virus expressing an 18-kilodalton outer membrane protein of Brucella abortus. Clin Vaccine Immunol 7:114–118

88. Edmonds M, Booth N, Hagius S, Walker J, Enright F, Roop RM 2nd, Elzer P (2000) Attenuation and immunogenicity of a Brucella abortus htrA cycL double mutant in cattle. Vet Microbiol 76:81–90

89. Zhang M, Han X, Liu H, Tian M, Ding C, Song J, Sun X, Liu Z, Yu S (2013) Inactivation of the ABC transporter ATPase gene in Brucella abortus strain 2308 attenuated the virulence of the bacteria. Vet Microbiol 164:322–329

90. Trant CG, Lacerda TL, Carvalho NB, Azevedo V, Rosinha GM, Salcedo SP, Gorvel JP, Oliveira SC (2010) The Brucella abortus phosphoglycerate kinase mutant is highly attenuated and induces protection superior to that of vaccine strain 19 in immunocompromised and immunocompetent mice. Infect Immun 78:2283–2291

91. Wang Z, Niu J, Wang S, Lv Y, Wu Q (2013) In vivo differences in the virulence, pathogenicity, and induced protective immunity of wboA mutants from genetically different parent Brucella spp. Clin Vaccine Immunol 20:174–180

92. Rajasekaran P, Seleem MN, Contreras A, Purwantini E, Schurig GG, Sriranganathan N, Boyle SM (2008) Brucella abortus strain RB51 leucine auxotroph as an environmentally safe vaccine for plasmid maintenance and antigen overexpression. Applied Environ Microbiol 74:7051–7055

93. Vemulapalli R, He Y, Boyle SM, Sriranganathan N, Schurig GG (2000) Brucella abortus strain RB51 as a vector for heterologous protein expression and induction of specific Th1 type immune responses. Infect Immun 68:3290–3296

94. Ramamoorthy S, Sanakkayala N, Vemulapalli R, Jain N, Lindsay DS, Schurig GS, Boyle SM, Sriranganathan N (2007) Prevention of vertical transmission of Neospora caninum in C57BL/6 mice vaccinated with Brucella abortus strain RB51 expressing N. caninum protective antigens. Int J Parasitol 37:1531–1538

95. Sabio y García JV, Bigi F, Rossetti O, Campos E (2010) Expression of MPB83 from Mycobacterium bovis in Brucella abortus S19 induces specific cellular immune response against the recombinant antigen in BALB/c mice. Microbes Infect 12:1236–1243

96. Sabio y García JV, Farber M, Carrica M, Cravero S, Macedo GC, Bigi F, Oliveira SC, Rossetti O, Campos E (2008) Expression of Babesia bovis rhoptry-associated

protein 1 (RAP1) in Brucella abortus S19. Microbes Infect 10:635–641

97. Avila-Calderón E, Araiza-Villanueva M, Cancino-Diaz J, López-Villegas E, Sriranganathan N, Boyle S, Contreras-Rodríguez A (2015) Roles of bacterial membrane vesicles. Arch Microbiol 197:1–10

98. Pollak CN, Delpino MV, Fossati CA, Baldi PC (2012) Outer membrane vesicles from Brucella abortus promote bacterial internalization by human monocytes and modulate their innate immune response. PLoS One 7:e50214

99. Lamontagne J, Butler H, Chaves-Olarte E, Hunter J, Schirm M, Paquet C, Tian M, Kearney P, Hamaidi L, Chelsky D, Moriyon I, Moreno E, Paramithiotis E (2007) Extensive cell envelope modulation is associated with virulence in Brucella abortus. J Proteome Res 6:1519–1529

100. Jain-Gupta N, Contreras-Rodriguez A, Vemulapalli R, Witonsky SG, Boyle SM, Sriranganathan N (2012) Pluronic P85 enhances the efficacy of outer membrane vesicles as a subunit vaccine against Brucella melitensis challenge in mice. FEMS Immunol Med Microbiol 66:436–444

CHAPTER 39 WITHIN-HOST EVOLUTION OF BRUCELLA CANIS DURING A CANINE BRUCELLOSIS OUTBREAK IN A KENNEL

Miklós Gyuranecz, Brandy D Rannals, Christina A Allen, Szilárd Jánosi, Paul S Keim and Jeffrey T Foster

Keywords: *Brucella canis,* Brucellosis, Evolution, MLVA, VNTR

BACKGROUND

Brucella canis, the etiologic agent of canine brucellosis, can lead to severe economic loss in infected kennels. Canine brucellosis is a contagious disease transmitted via contaminated reproductive, oronasal, or conjunctival fluids [1]. The bacteria are particularly associated with reproductive tissue, causing abortion in females and epididymitis and prostatitis in males [2]. *Brucella canis* affects human beings, but few cases are reported in humans [1, 3] or other animals, suggesting either host-preference for dogs or limited opportunities for transmission to other species.

Several multi-locus, variable-number tandem repeat (VNTR) analysis (MLVA) systems have been developed and described for *Brucella* species [4, 5, 6, 7]. MLVA is a rapid, reproducible molecular typing system providing high discriminatory power among closely related strains [8, 9]. These characteristics make MLVA a potentially powerful tool for epidemiological (e.g. to follow local epidemics) and forensic investigations of events involving *Brucella* species [10, 11, 12, 13, 14] and many other bacterial agents. This molecular approach specifically allows for fine-scale detail on likely source populations of new brucellosis cases in human cases [14, 15, 16] and tracking outbreaks in wildlife and livestock [7, 17].

The first known outbreak of *B. canis* infection in Hungary was described in 2009 [18]. The affected kennel population consisted of 31 dogs of various ages. The disease was most likely introduced to the kennel by a pregnant female whose abortion was the first obvious reproductive disorder in October 2008 [18]. Sporadic reproductive clinical symptoms were detected by the breeder during the eight months preceding the first laboratory examination.

The aim of this study was to genetically characterize the eight strains of *B. canis* isolated from three dogs in a kennel during three months of the outbreak. Our goal was to use MLVA to assess the level of within-host genetic variation at different dates and sampling sites on the dogs for a better understanding of rapid *Brucella*evolution and its use for epidemiology.

METHODS

Samples of blood, vagina and throat swabs and lymph nodes (mesenteric and sublingual lymph nodes) were obtained from every resident dog at 1-month intervals in June, July and August 2009. All experiments were performed in accordance with all applicable institutional and national guidelines and regulations and with the consent of the dog owner. The samples were collected from tissues typical for clinical brucellosis investigations and submitted for bacteriological examination as described previously [18]. Eight *B. canis*isolates (Bc 1-8) were recovered from three animals on selective *Brucella* agar plates (Oxoid Ltd., Cambridge, United Kingdom) (Table 1). Primary isolates were subcultered on trypticase soy agar plates (Difco, BD Diagnostic Systems, Sparks, MD) three times to reveal pure culture before DNA extraction (QIAamp DNA Mini Kit, Qiagen Inc., Valencia, CA).

Citation: Miklós Gyuranecz , Brandy D Rannals , Christina A Allen, Szilárd Jánosi, Paul S Keim and Jeffrey T Foster, Within-host evolution of Brucella canis during a canine brucellosis outbreak in a kennel, DOI: 10.1186/1746-6148-9-76.

Table 1: Summary of host, isolation date, source and primary and alternate VNTR alleles of the studied strains

				Polymorphic VNTR							Monomorphic VNTR										
Isolate ID	**Host**	**Isolation date**	**Isolation source**	**1**	**1 alt**	**2**	**2 alt**	**30**	**33**	**33 alt**	**3**	**7**	**14**	**16**	**20**	**21**	**25**	**27**	**28**	**29**	**31**
Bc 1	female, abortion in June	June	foetus	234		214		568	295	303	417	306	121	233	439	100	490	413	198	260	507
Bc 2		July	blood	234	242	206	214	568	303		-	306	121	233	439	100	490	413	198	260	507
Bc 3		July	vagina	234		206		568	263		417	306	121	233	439	100	490	413	198	260	507
Bc 4	stud dog, without clinical symptoms	July	blood	234		214		568	303	311	417	306	122	233	439	100	490	413	198	260	507
Bc 5		August	lymph node	234		231		568	295		417	306	121	233	439	100	490	413	198	260	507
Bc 6	female puppy, born with infection in March	July	blood	242	250	150	214	574	255	263	417	306	121	233	439	100	490	413	198	260	507
Bc 7		August	blood	234		214		568	255	263	417	306	121	233	439	100	490	413	198	260	507
Bc 8		August	lymph node	234	242	214		568	255	263	417	306	121	233	439	100	490	413	198	260	507

Species identity for all isolates was confirmed by real-time PCR by a *B. canis*-specific assay [19]. The eight isolates were screened with a 15-marker MLVA system as previously described [5], with modifications. We redesigned the three largest VNTR primer sets (VNTRs 2, 29, 33) to create smaller amplicons to reduce this potential source of allelic variation (Table 2). Larger amplicons generally exhibit greater variation in sizing due to loss of linearity for ladder fragment standards above ~500 bp. We ran these new primers in 10 μl reactions in singleplex under the following conditions: 1× PCR buffer, 2 mM $MgCl_2$, 0.2 mM dNTPs, 0.04 U platinum Taq DNA polymerase (Invitrogen, Carlsbad, CA), 0.10 μM forward primer and 0.08 μM reverse primer. Thermocycling parameters were an initial denaturation at 94°C for 5 min, followed by 94°C for 45 s, 65°C for 45 s and 72°C for 45 s for 35 cycles, and a final annealing step at 72°C for 5 min.

Table 2: Newly designed primers for three largest amplicons from Huynh et al. 2008

Locus	**Amplicon size**	**F primer (5′-3′)**	**R primer (5′-3′)**
VNTR 2	178 bp	cgctctcctcgcccgcttcttctt	tgtttttggttgcgcatggccg
VNTR 29	150 bp	gtttgtcgtcgcgggagagattagggg	cggcaggcgcttgaggatgagg
VNTR 33	213 bp	cggataggcgcggcgtgagtaagg	acaacatggcgcgtgaaaggccc

VNTR PCR amplicons were discriminated through electrophoretic analysis with an ABI PRISM 3130xl automated fluorescent capillary DNA sequencer (Applied Biosystems Inc., Foster City, CA). All samples were run in triplicate with three different PCR steps each as well as on different fragment analysis runs to examine the reproducibility of the analyses. Each run contained validated *B. melitensis* and *B. suis* DNA standards as positive controls. Fragment analysis was performed with GeneMapper software (Applied Biosystems). Fragment sizing was accomplished by comparison to a 1200 base LIZ-labelled size standard (Applied Biosystems). Customized bins for allele calls in GeneMapper allowed automated scoring of the VNTR alleles. When isolates had more than one amplification peak (i.e. multiple alleles at a locus), we chose the highest peak as the main allele but also recorded alternate alleles. Phylogenetic relationships derived from complete MLVA genotypes were determined using maximum parsimony algorithm in PAUP 4.0 Beta 10 (Sinauer Associates Inc., Sunderland, MA).

RESULTS

Ten of the 15 MLVA loci did not mutate in any of the strains (Table 1). VNTR 3 had the same allele for 7 isolates and had a null allele for 1 isolate so was considered monomorphic in our analyses. For polymorphic loci, VNTRs 1 and 30 had single repeat insertions in isolate Bc 6. Both VNTR 2 and 33 were highly variable among the eight isolates and demonstrated multiple repeat changes. Alternate alleles occurred in three of these loci, VNTRs 1, 2, and 33. In 8 of 10 instances the alternate allele was present as the primary allele in at least one other isolate. Phylogenetic analysis of the eight samples placed the isolates onto three branches with genetic differences among the strains within each branch (Figure 1a). Six of the eight isolates had unique genotypes. Strains from the same dog but taken at different dates or collection sources occurred on different branches. For instance, strain Bc 1 appears more closely related to strains Bc 4, 5, 6, 7 and 8 than it does to Bc 2 and 3, although Bc 1, 2, and 3 all came from the same female dog. Isolates Bc 4 and 5 came from the same stud dog a month apart but were more closely related to other isolates on the tree from different dogs. Isolate Bc 6 from the puppy (from another female than the one described here) was genetically quite distinct from any other isolates and had different alleles at VNTRs 1 and 30. Interestingly, Bc 6 was collected a month earlier than two additional isolates from this dog (Bc 7 & 8).

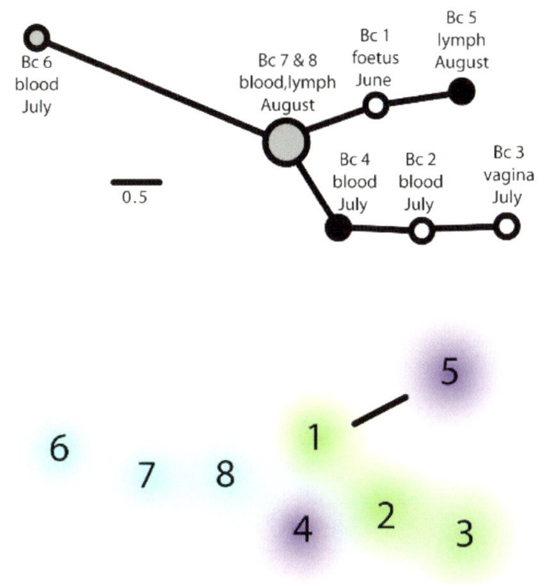

Figure 1: MLVA-15-based phylogeny. a) MLVA-15-based phylogram of *Brucella canis* isolates from the affected kennel. Scale bar indicates number of substitutions per position. Circle colour indicates isolates from same individual. **b**) Cloud phylogeny indicating the overlap among primary and alternate alleles. All isolates except Bc 5 share primary and alternate alleles. Cloud colour indicates isolates from same individual.

Including alternate alleles in the analysis by using clouds instead of circles and lines allows illustration of the high degree of overlap among primary and alternate alleles (Figure 1b). For VNTR 1, the primary allele for Bc 6 was shared with Bc 2 & 8. VNTR 2 had the primary allele for Bc 1, 4, 7, & 8 shared with Bc 2 & 6. Finally, VNTR 33 had Bc 2 & 4 share an allele with Bc 1 and the primary allele in Bc 3 was shared with Bc 6, 7 & 8. Thus, there was considerable overlap among genotypes when primary and alternate alleles were evaluated.

DISCUSSION

MLVA provided discrimination among the otherwise indistinguishable isolates from different animals and from within each host, with VNTR mutations being detected at multiple dates and tissue sites. It is strongly suspected that the strains isolated from the dogs originated from the same recent introduction to the kennel, with subsequent rapid *in vivo* mutations. Strain Bc 1 was isolated from the foetus of the female in June. This isolate is distantly related in the tree to Bc 2 & 3 originating from the blood and vagina, respectively, from that female in July. Since these genotypes are closely related to the rest of the isolates and these isolates came from a foetus, the female parent was almost certainly infected as well. Additional *in vivo* evolution route also occurred in the stud dog with VNTR mutations between the collections of the July (Bc 4) and August (Bc 5) isolates. Similar *in vivo* evolution was observed in the case of the isolates (Bc 6-8) of the female puppy as well. These results are consistent with rapid within-host evolution of *Burkholderia pseudomallei* in acute infections in humans [9], demonstrating that VNTR changes can happen within weeks, as well as data from *Yersinia pestis* in fleas their prairie dog hosts that are consistent with within host evolution [20]. High mutation rates are inferred for several of the loci we used in our MLVA. Although Huynh et al. [5] found that average allelic diversity for *B. suis* (of which *B. canis* is a distinct lineage within it) was a moderate 0.49, allelic diversity in VNTRs 2, 3, 1, 33, 30 was quite high at 0.77-0.88, with the number of alleles per locus ranging from 6-13, indicating that these loci account for much of the diversity seen over short time periods. We must note that although minimal generations occurred during culturing during the short incubation period, we cannot rule out some mutations occurring *in vitro*. Direct MLVA testing on samples prior to culturing is recommended in future studies to rule out this possibility, although the number of generations within the dogs would be expected to be much higher than what is typical under standard culturing. We also note that the variation we are detecting is for neutral genetic markers, those presumably not under selection, and thus do not know what changes may be occurring in loci potentially under selection such as those involved in pathogenicity.

The emergence of alternate alleles that become primary alleles shows the fluidity of genetic variation when assessed by MLVA and are a particularly important aspect of this study. Alternate alleles are traditionally ignored as noise in phylogenetic analyses. Rather than making the determination of relationships among isolates more confusing, however, alternate alleles reveal the potential mutations that connect isolates. Nonetheless, a simple depiction of the relatedness of the isolates was not possible in this study. Several of the loci were so variable that determining the direct relationship of isolates was challenging since isolates from the same animal were not always adjacent to each other on the tree. High amounts of mutations at the most variable loci and the subsequent occurrence of homoplasy reduces the utility of VNTRs for some investigations, as seen in *B. melitensis*[21] and leading to lowered weights of these types of loci in analyses [22]. If the most variable markers are excluded from analyses however, then few or no isolates are distinguishable since variation is exclusively within the most polymorphic loci. There is a fine line between adding more polymorphic loci and having that addition variation being less reliable. The application of the study is that rapid within-host evolution is occurring in *Brucella* infections and that we can detect it. However, this evolution is so rapid for some genetic markers that complete knowledge of the relationships of various isolates is not clear, especially for isolates collected from outbreak cases, so that fine-scale epidemiological studies are not possible in all instances.

CONCLUSIONS

The current study is the first to employ fine-scale genotyping on a comprehensive *in vivo* isolate collection derived from a *B. canis* outbreak. This investigation highlights the rapid genetic changes of several VNTRs of *B. canis* and the emergence of alternate alleles at some loci but also shows that MLVA was not an ideal method to analyse the epidemiological relationship of strains in the same outbreak. Nonetheless, the ability for *B. canis* to diversify over a short time frame has substantial implications for our understanding of infection caused by *B. canis*.

DECLARATIONS

Acknowledgements

MG was supported by the Lendület program (grant number: LP2012-22) of the Hungarian Academy of Sciences.

Funding from the U.S. Department of Homeland Security (DHS) supported this work. Use of product or trade names does not constitute endorsement by the U.S. Government.

Authors' contributions

MG conceived of the study and with JTF wrote the manuscript and analysed the data. BDR and CAA performed the genotyping. SJ performed the bacteriological examination. PSK helped write the manuscript. All authors have read and approved the final manuscript.

REFERENCES

1. Hollett RB: Canine brucellosis: Outbreaks and compliance. Theriogenology. 2006, 66 (3): 575-587. 10.1016/j.theriogenology.2006.04.011.
2. Wanke MM: Canine brucellosis. Anim Reprod Sci. 2004, 82–3: 195-207.
3. Lucero NE, Corazza R, Almuzara MN, Reynes E, Escobar GI, Boeri E, Ayala SM: Human Brucella canis outbreak linked to infection in dogs. Epidemiol Infect. 2010, 138 (2): 280-285. 10.1017/S0950268809990525.
4. Bricker BJ, Ewalt DR, Halling SM: *Brucella* 'HOOF-Prints': strain typing by multi-locus analysis of variable number tandem repeats (VNTRs). BMC Microbiol. 2003, 3: 15-10.1186/1471-2180-3-15.
5. Huynh LY, Van Ert MN, Hadfield T, Probert WS, Bellaire BH, Dobson M, Burgess RJ, Weyant RS, Popovic T, Zanecki S: Multiple locus variable number tandem repeat (VNTR) analysis (MLVA) of *Brucella* spp. identifies species-specific markers and provides insights into phylogenetic relationships. National Institute of Allergy and Infectious Disease, NIH: Frontiers in Research. Edited by: St. Georgiev V. 2008, Totowa, New Jersey: Humana Press, 47-54.
6. Le Fleche P, Jacques I, Grayon M, Al Dahouk S, Bouchon P, Denoeud F, Nockler K, Neubauer H, Guilloteau LA, Vergnaud G: Evaluation and selection of tandem repeat loci for a *Brucella* MLVA typing assay. BMC Microbiol. 2006, 6: 9-10.1186/1471-2180-6-9.
7. Whatmore AM, Shankster SJ, Perrett LL, Murphy TJ, Brew SD, Thirlwall RE, Cutler SJ, MacMillan AP: Identification and characterization of variable-number tandem-repeat markers for typing of *Brucella* spp. J Clin Microbiol. 2006, 44 (6): 1982-1993. 10.1128/JCM.02039-05.
8. Pearson T, Okinaka RT, Foster JT, Keim P: Phylogenetic understanding of clonal populations in an era of whole genome sequencing. Infect Genet Evol. 2009, 9 (5): 1010-1019. 10.1016/j.meegid.2009.05.014.
9. Price EP, Hornstra HM, Limmathurotsakul D, Max TL, Sarovich DS, Vogler AJ, Dale JL, Ginther JL, Leadem B, Colman RE: Within-host evolution of *Burkholderia pseudomallei* in four cases of acute melioidosis. PLoS Pathog. 2010, 6 (1): e1000725-10.1371/journal.ppat.1000725.
10. Abril C, Thomann A, Brodard I, Wu N, Ryser-Degiorgis MP, Frey J, Overesch G: A novel isolation method of *Brucella*species and molecular tracking of *Brucella suis* biovar 2 in domestic and wild animals. Vet Microbiol. 2011, 150 (3–4): 405-410.
11. Bricker BJ, Ewalt DR: Evaluation of the HOOF-Print assay for typing *Brucella abortus* strains isolated from cattle in the United States: results with four performance criteria. BMC Microbiol. 2005, 5: 37-10.1186/1471-2180-5-37.
12. Garcia-Yoldi D, Le Fleche P, De Miguel MJ, Munoz PM, Blasco JM, Cvetnic Z, Marin CM, Vergnaud G, Lopez-Goni I: Comparison of multiple-locus variable-number tandem-repeat analysis with other PCR-based methods for typing *Brucella suis* isolates. J Clin Microbiol. 2007, 45 (12): 4070-4072. 10.1128/JCM.01096-07.
13. Kang SI, Heo EJ, Cho D, Kim JW, Kim JY, Jung SC, Her M: Genetic comparison of *Brucella canis* isolates by the MLVA assay in South Korea. J Vet Med Sci. 2011, 73 (6): 779-786. 10.1292/jvms.10-0334.
14. Al Dahouk S, Fleche PL, Nockler K, Jacques I, Grayon M, Scholz HC, Tomaso H, Vergnaud G, Neubauer H: Evaluation of *Brucella* MLVA typing for human brucellosis. J Microbiol Meth. 2007, 69 (1): 137-145. 10.1016/j.mimet.2006.12.015.
15. Kilic S, Ivanov IN, Durmaz R, Bayraktar MR, Ayaslioglu E, Uyanik MH, Aliskan H, Yasar E, Bayramoglu G, Arslanturk A: Multiple-vocus variable-number tandem-repeat analysis genotyping of human *Brucella* isolates from Turkey. J Clin Microbiol. 2011, 49 (9): 3276-3283. 10.1128/JCM.02538-10.
16. Valdezate S, Navarro A, Villalon P, Carrasco G, Saez-Nieto JA: Epidemiological and phylogenetic analysis of Spanish human *Brucella melitensis* strains by multiple-locus variable-number tandem-repeat typing, hypervariable octameric oligonucleotide fingerprinting, and rpoB typing. J Clin Microbiol. 2010, 48 (8): 2734-2740. 10.1128/JCM.00533-10.
17. Higgins J, Stuber T, Quance C, Edwards WH, Tiller RV, Linfield T, Rhyan J, Berte A, Harris B: Molecular epidemiology of *Brucella abortus* isolates from cattle, elk, and bison in the United States, 1998 to 2011. Appl Environ Microbiol. 2012, 78 (10): 3674-3684. 10.1128/AEM.00045-12.
18. Gyuranecz M, Szeredi L, Ronai Z, Denes B, Dencso L, Dan A, Palmai N, Hauser Z, Lami E, Makrai L: Detection of *Brucella canis*-induced reproductive diseases in a kennel. J Vet Diagn Invest. 2011, 23 (1): 143-147. 10.1177/104063871102300127.
19. Foster JT, Okinaka RT, Svensson R, Shaw K, De BK, Robison RA, Probert WS, Kenefic LJ, Brown WD, Keim P: Real-time PCR assays of single-nucleotide polymorphisms defining the major *Brucella* clades. J Clin Microbiol. 2008, 46: 296-301. 10.1128/JCM.01496-07.
20. Girard JM, Wagner DM, Vogler AJ, Keys C, Allender CJ, Drickamer LC, Keim P: Differential plague-transmission dynamics determine *Yersinia pestis* population genetic structure on local, regional, and global scales. Proc Natl Acad Sci USA. 2004, 101 (22): 8408-10.1073/pnas.0401561101.
21. Jiang H, Fan M, Chen J, Mi J, Yu R, Zhao H, Piao D, Ke C, Deng X, Tian G: MLVA genotyping of Chinese

human *Brucella melitensis* biovar 1, 2 and 3 isolates. BMC Microbiol. 2011, 11: 256-10.1186/1471-2180-11-256.

22. Kattar MM, Jaafar RF, Araj GF, Le Fleche P, Matar MG, Rached RA, Khalife S, Gilles Vergnaud G: Evaluation of a multilocus variable-number tandem-repeat analysis scheme for typing human *Brucella* isolates in a region of brucellosis endemicity. J Clin Microbiol. 2008, 45: 3935-3940.

CHAPTER 40 RISK FACTORS FOR CONTACTS BETWEEN WILD BOAR AND OUTDOOR PIGS IN SWITZERLAND AND INVESTIGATIONS ON POTENTIAL BRUCELLA SUIS SPILL-OVER

Natacha Wu, Carlos Abril, Andreas Thomann, Eleonore Grosclaude, Marcus G Doherr, Patrick Boujon and Marie-Pierre Ryser-Degiorgis

Keywords: *Brucella suis,* Brucellosis, Interactions, Outdoor pigs, Risk factors, Spill-over, Wild boar

BACKGROUND

The wild boar (*Sus scrofa*) population is expanding in Europe [1, 2, 3]. Rearing domestic pigs outdoor also shows an increasing trend [4]. Although this type of animal husbandry provides a better quality of life for pigs [5, 6], it exposes them to a higher risk of contact with wild boar, which can carry pathogens with various routes of transmission [7].

Important air-born pig diseases include porcine reproductive and respiratory syndrome (PRRS) and enzootic pneumonia (EP; [8]). In contrast to the PRRS virus, *Mycoplasma hyopneumoniae* (causing EP) seems to be widespread in Swiss wild boar, which are considered a potential reservoir for this pathogen [9]. Classical swine fever (CSF) virus and *Mycobacterium bovis* (causing tuberculosis) are transmitted by indirect or direct close contact [2, 10]. These pathogens are currently not an issue in Switzerland [11, 12] but they could be introduced by wild boar emigrating from neighbouring countries [13, 14, 15]. *Sarcoptes scabiei* (causing sarcoptic mange) is transmitted by close contact [16]. While efforts are done to eradicate the mite from Swiss piggeries [17], infestations have been recently diagnosed in wild boar (FIWI, unpublished observations). In wild boar, Aujeszky›s disease (AD) virus and *Brucella suis* (causing brucellosis) are transmitted mainly by the venereal route [18, 19]. While AD virus infection is rare in Swiss wild boar [11], nearly 30% of them are carrier of *B. suis*, including adults with genital organ infection [1].

The objectives of this study were (a) to document the occurrence of contacts between wild boar and outdoor pigs in Switzerland, (b) to identify risk factors for such contacts in order to propose risk-adapted protection measures for piggeries, and (c) to test exposed pigs for a possible pathogen spill-over, taking *B. suis* as an example. This pathogen was selected because infections have been well documented in Swiss wild boar [1, 11, 20], while domestic pigs are officially free of brucellosis [21]. A re-emergence of brucellosis in outdoor pigs has been observed in France following intrusions of and/or mating with wild boar [22], indicating a substantial risk of losing the "free from disease" status in Switzerland if close contacts between wild boar and pigs occur. Furthermore, since transmission of *B. suis* mostly requires the closest type of contact (mating), *B. suis* spill-over would suggest that transmission of all other pathogens is possible.

Here we report different types of interactions between wild boar and outdoor pigs and show that risk factors are not only related to wild boar presence, piggery location and fence characteristics but also include pig breed. We additionally report field investigations performed in the frame of a brucellosis outbreak in domestic pigs with a history of contacts with wild boar.

Citation: Natacha Wu, Carlos Abril, Andreas Thomann, Eleonore Grosclaude, Marcus G Doherr, Patrick Boujon and Marie-Pierre Ryser-Degiorgis, Risk factors for contacts between wild boar and outdoor pigs in Switzerland and investigations on potential Brucella suis spill-over, DOI: 10.1186/1746-6148-8-116.

RESULTS

Contacts between wild boar and pigs

Questionnaire surveys among game-wardens and pig farmers

Thirty-one percent (26/82) of the game-wardens who participated to the study observed contacts at least once between 1995 and 2008, and additionally before 1995 for four of them. Overall, contacts of any category (categories 1–4, see definitions in Methods) were reported in 13 Swiss cantons. Observations included tracks but also intrusions (N=10) and domestic sows with cross-bred piglets (N=9). Births of cross-bred animals were reported from 7/13 cantons.

Of the 322 pig farmers who replied the questionnaire, 175 had fattening/finishing pigs, 77 had breeding pigs, 59 kept both types of animals, one held pigs as a hobby, and no information was available for 10 piggeries. Two hundred twenty-two piggeries had concrete run-out, 62 had pure pasture run-out, 21 had mixed run-out (concrete and pasture), five had another type of ground (e.g. chipped wood or gravel), and 12 did not answer the question. Herd size ranged from 2 to more than 1500 pigs, with an average of 303 animals per farm. The most represented breeds were Landrace and Large White pigs (L/LW; N=275) followed by Duroc (N=31) and Mangalitza (also called curly-hair hogs; N=25). Concrete run-outs were fenced with concrete walls, metallic bars, wooden boards, wire mesh, or various combinations of those. In the case of pasture run-outs, fences consisted in electric wires (ranging from 20 cm to 60 cm height), wire mesh, wooden boards, metallic bars, or combinations. None of these pasture fences were fixed deep in the ground.

Eighty farmers (24.8%) reported contacts of any category. They mentioned at least one contact since they acquired the piggery, which could go back to the 1970's. The frequency of contacts ranged from one in 39 years to 50 per year. From these 80 piggeries, the majority had a pure pasture run-out. Contacts were significantly more reported from piggeries with pasture and mixed run-out than with concrete run-out ($P<0.001$ and $P=0.011$, respectively). Overall, there was an average of 178 contacts of any type per year for a total of 322 outdoor farms, or 0.55 contact/farm/year (95% CI 0.50–0.61). Contacts were reported in all calendar seasons and in all 17 cantons with wild boar presence.

Cases of cross-breeding (or intra-specific hybridization) of wild boar with different pig breeds were reported in 17/322 piggeries (5.3%; seven of them had already been announced by game-wardens). Most of them were cross-bred with L/LW (N=6) and Mangalitza sows (N=6). Cross-breeding additionally occurred twice with a pure Duroc, once with a cross-bred Duroc x L/LW, once with a Pot-bellied pig, and once with a Minipig. In one of these piggeries holding Mangalitza, single and multiple births of cross-bred piglets following intrusions of wild boar or excursions of domestic sows have been observed (at least once a year for the past 3–4 years). In one instance, eight sows gave simultaneously birth to cross-bred piglets (P9, Table 1). Cross-breeding occurred more often with Mangalitza than L/LW ($P=0.0003$). Overall, there was an average of five mating events per year for a total of 85 farms with pure pasture or mixed run-out, which corresponded to an estimated rate of 0.06 mating/farm/year (95% CI 0.02–0.13). Cross-bred piglets were reported in 10 cantons, and in one case no information was obtained on piggery location.

Table 1: Outdoor pigs from regions with wild boar presence sampled for serological and microbiological testing for *Brucella suis*

Farm Nr	N pigs	Run-out	Farm type	Pig breed	Contact category	Particularities	N tested	Alive vs slaughtered
P1	1000	Pasture	F[1]+B[1]	L/LW[2]	3	Close contact with wild boar shedding *Brucella suis*	51/27 19	A[3] / S[3] A+S
P2	5	Concrete	F	L/LW	2		7	S
P3	9	Mixed	F	M[2]	1		4	S
P4	70	Pasture	F	L/LW	3		30	S
P5	45[4]	Pasture	F+B	M	4	Reproduction problems	5/6 16	A / S[5] A+SO[3]
P6	12	Pasture	F+B	L/LW+hybrids[6]	1		3	S
P7	30	Pasture	F	M	None	Reproduction problems	14	A
P8	24	Pasture	F+B	M	4		2	A
P9	29	Pasture	F+B	M+hybrids	4		5	A
P10	14	Pasture	B	M+hybrids[7]	2		5/6	A / S
P11	23	Pasture+mixed	F+B	M	None[8]		3	A
P12	4	Concrete	B	M+Duroc	1	Boar borrowed from and sow lent to P5	4	A+S

P13	11	Pasture	F+B	M	None	Fattening pigs bought from *B. suis*infected piggery (P5)	6 5	A A+S

[1] F: Fattening, B: Breeding.

[2] L/LW: Large white or Landrace, M: Mangalitza.

[3] A: Alive, S: Slaughtered, SO: Stamped-out.

[4] Including 17 newborn piglets.

[5] Pigs slaughtered before the discovery of the outbreak.

[6] Hybrids were bought from another outdoor piggery for breeding purposes. In this other piggery, however, hybridization had been accidental (wild boar intrusion).

[7] A breeding domestic sow, which had mated with a wild boar (accidental intrusion), was bought pregnant of hybrid piglets from another outdoor piggery

[8] Sampling on request of the pig owner.

Sampled domestic pigs from Swiss outdoor piggeries (P) in 2008–2010 in a study on risk factors for contacts between wild boar and outdoor pigs. Categories of contacts: (1) presence of wild boar around the enclosure (> 2 m); (2) presence of wild boar just outside the fence (< 2 m); (3) wild boar intrusions without mating; and (4) mating (hybrid births).

Surveillance of piggeries with camera traps

During one year of surveillance in two piggeries at risk (P1 and P4, Table 1), wild boar were detected only in piggery P1. There were four detections in nearly 16 months, always just outside the enclosure (< 2 m) on the pedestrian way between the forest and the fence, at night (between 6 p.m. and 2 a.m.), from December to March: (1) single juvenile; (2) wild sow with offspring; (3) single adult (sex not identifiable); (4) two animals (undetermined age and sex).

Assessment of risk factors for contacts

Information on potential risk factors for contacts between wild boar and domestic pigs (Table 2) were obtained from 322 pig farmers. The final multivariable models, one for each outcome (Table 3, 4, 5, 6), showed that (1) pigs in enclosures separated from the piggery building (> 5 m) or/and located away from other houses (> 500 m) or/and close to a forest (< 500 m) were most at risk for indirect contacts with wild boar roaming around the piggery (2–500 m); (2) pigs in enclosures separated from the piggery building (> 5 m) or/and protected with an electric fence were most at risk for closer indirect contacts with wild boar (< 2 m from the fence), (3) pigs in enclosures located far from the piggery building (> 500 m) or/and protected by an electric fence or/and any fence ≤ 60 cm, were most at risk for an intrusion; and (4) piggeries holding Mangalitza or/and protected by an electric fence were most at risk for the occurrence of cross-breeding (i.e., for mating with wild boar). When comparing the most represented breeds with each other, cross-breeding was more frequent among Mangalitza than L/LW (odds ratio: 11.55, 95% CI_{OR} = 3.41–39.13).

Table 2: Explicative variables and hypotheses

Variables	Hypotheses: situations increasing the risk of contacts between pigs and wild boars
Run-out type: concrete vs mixed vs pure pasture	Pure pasture as run-out (is less protected than concrete or mixed run-out)
Fattenig vs mixed vs breeding farm	Breeding farm (presence of several sexually mature sows attractive for boars)
Corn culture	Corn culture next to the enclosure (food source)
Grass cutlure	Grass culture next to enclosure (food source)
Distance enclosure-farm < 5 m	The larger the distance between the pig enclosure and the farm buildings, the higher the risk (lower disturbance by human presence)
Distance enclosure-farm < 50 m	
Distance enclosure-farm < 100 m	
Distance enclosure-farm < 500 m	
Distance enclosure-houses < 5 m	The larger the distance between the pig enclosure and the houses, the higher the risk (lower disturbance by human presence)
Distance enclosure-houses < 50 m	
Distance enclosure-houses < 100 m	
Distance enclosure-houses < 500 m	

Distance enclosure-forest < 5 m	The shorter the distance between the pig enclosure and the forest, the higher the risk (proximity to wild boar habitat)
Distance enclosure-forest < 50 m	
Distance enclosure-forest < 100 m	
Distance enclosure-forest < 500 m	
Herd size: < 50 pigs vs > 50 pigs	Small herd size (less intimidating and thus more attracting to wild boar).
Breeding sow: absence vs presence	Presence of breeding sow in the enclosure (attractive to wild boar males)
Breeding hog: absence vs presence	Absence of breeding hog in the enclosure (presence is considered a protective factor)
Landrace/Large White vs other breeds vs Mangalitza	A specific pig breed may be more attractive to wild boars
Other animal species near the enclosure: absence vs presence	Absence of other animals near the enclosure (less disturbance)
Access to run-out whole year vs part year	Access of domestic pigs to run-out the whole year (higher exposure, in particular potential higher contact risk for sows during the wild boar rut)
Presence of farmer around the farm	Absence of farmer near the enclosure (lower disturbance by human presence)
Presence of walkers around the farm	Absence of walkers near the enclosure (lower disturbance by human presence)
Fence type: solid vs flexible	Flexible fence (solid walls provide better protection against wild boar intrusions)
Fence height: < 60 cm vs > 60 cm	Low fences (<60 cm; easily passed by wild boars)

Single variables and hypotheses regarding their influence on the occurrence of contacts between outdoor pigs and wild boar.

Table 3: Final multivariable model 1 for risk factors for contacts between outdoor pigs and wild boar in Switzerland

Model 1 (N=253, Pseudo-R^2=0.78)				
Risk factors significantly associated with presence of wild boar around a farm (2–500 m)				
		p	**OR**	**95% CI_{OR}**
distance enclosure-farm	< 5 m	baseline		
	> 5 m	0.001	2.80	1.52–5.14
distance enclosure-houses	< 500 m	baseline		
	> 500 m	0.005	5.06	1.44–18.12
distance enclosure-forest	> 500 m	baseline		
	< 500 m	0.012	5.10	1.65–15.52

Multivariable logistic regression models of risk factors in a study performed in 2008–2010. Significant associations with wild boar contacts are expressed by odds ratios (OR) and respective 95% confidence intervals (95% CI). The number of records considered in each model is indicated in parentheses (N).

Table 4: Final multivariable model 2 for risk factors for contacts between outdoor pigs and wild boar in Switzerland

Model 2 (N=254, Pseudo-R^2=0.98)				
Risk factors significantly associated with wild boar at the fence (0–2 m)				
		p	**OR**	**95% CI_{OR}**
distance enclosure-farm	< 5 m	baseline		
	> 5 m	0.026	2.68	1.12–6.38
fence type	solid fence	baseline		
	flexible fence	0.003	3.75	1.58–8.89

Table 5: Final multivariable model 3 for risk factors for contacts between outdoor pigs and wild boar in Switzerland

Model 3 (N=207, Pseudo-R^2=0.76)				
Risk factors significantly associated with intrusion of wild boar				
		p	**OR**	**95% CI$_{OR}$**
distance enclosure-farm	< 500 m	baseline		
	> 500 m	0.036	8.28	1.15–59.73
fence type	solid fence	baseline		
	flexible fence	0.040	4.71	1.08–20.61
fence height	> 60 cm	baseline		
	< 60 cm	0.038	4.81	1.09–21.24

Table 6: Final multivariable model 4 for risk factors for contacts between outdoor pigs and wild boar in Switzerland

Model 4 (N=236, Pseudo-R^2=0.97)				
Risk factors significantly associated with cross-breeding with wild boar				
		p	**OR**	**95% CI$_{OR}$**
breed	Large white/Landrace	baseline		
	Mangalitza	0.003	11.19	2.30–54.50
fence type	solid fence	baseline		
	flexible fence	0.003	10.49	2.18–50.48

Testing for *B. suis* infection of exposed pigs

Tested animals of 10/11 initially selected piggeries (P1-11, Table 1) were negative both by serology and qPCR, including the pigs from P1, which had been in close contact with an infected wild boar (for piggery history, see Methods). In parallel to these investigations, a recently acquired breeding boar (B2) from P5 died of a peritonitis thought to be due to a foreign body, and bacteriological culture performed post-mortem revealed a concurrent infection with *B. suis* Biovar 2 in the epididymidis [23]. All pigs older than six months subsequently tested seropositive to *B. suis* (both in the RBT and CFT) in this piggery were stamped out (Figure 1, P5). Six of 16 were positive by qPCR and five of them in culture [23]. Five qPCR-positive adult sows (of which four were also culture-positive) presented severe macroscopic lesions: metritis with miliary abscesses (N=3), mastitis, and pyometra.

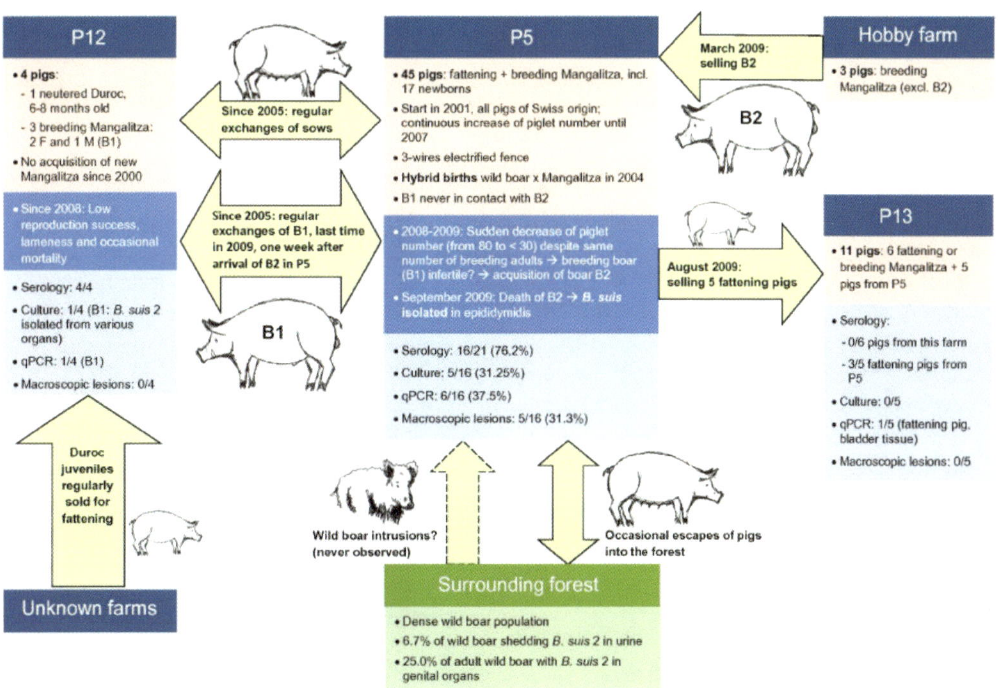

Figure 1: Summary of information collected on the brucellosis outbreak in domestic pigs in Switzerland in 2009. Piggeries where microbiological investigations could be carried out (P5, P12, P13) are numbered according to Table 1. Pink text boxes: piggery characteristics. Pig numbers are given for the time period of the outbreak. Dark blue text boxes: summary of unusual events noticed in the piggeries in 2008–2009. Light blue text boxes: results of bacteriological tests for *Brucella* sp. performed in the context of the outbreak. Yellow arrows show animal movements among piggeries.

Epidemiological investigations on the brucellosis outbreak in Mangalitza pigs

Animal movements from and to P5 and results of bacteriological investigations in the concerned piggeries are presented in Figure 1. Two potential sources of infection were considered for P5: (1) Spill-over from wild boar: births of cross-bred piglets in 2004 indicated successful mating between domestic sows and wild boar. A prevalence of 22.4% has been documented for *B. suis* in wild boar from this area, including adults shedding bacteria [1]. Animals had regularly been exchanged between P5 and another piggery (P12) since 2005, and health problems had been observed since 2008 in both P5 and P12. Therefore, P5 could have been infected by wild boar, and P12 by P5. P5 also infected P13 in selling fattening pigs. However, comparison of strains from selected wild boar, brown hares (*Lepus europaeus*) and affected pigs revealed distinct clusters, and wild boar were considered an unlikely source of infection [23]. (2) Introduction of infected pigs: While B2 was introduced after the decrease of reproduction and therefore considered an unlikely source of infection, P12 could have been contaminated by young piglets bought from other farms and have been the origin of the outbreak in P5.

DISCUSSION

A considerable geographical overlap between the wild boar population and outdoor piggeries in Switzerland was previously documented, pointing at a risk of contacts between wild boar and pigs [1]. Here, the occurrence of contacts was assessed, risk factors for these interactions were identified, and pigs from farms at risk were tested for *B. suis* as an example of pathogen transmissible from wild boar to pigs.

Occurrence of contacts between wild boar and pigs

To obtain a data set as complete as possible on the occurrence of contacts between wild boar and domestic pigs, we combined several methodical approaches. First, we carried out two parallel questionnaire surveys among different target groups, namely pig farmers (who are mostly present in proximity of pig enclosures but may not want to announce observed contacts by fear of sanctions by the local authorities) and game-wardens (who are usually called in case of wild boar intrusions and do not mind reporting such information). This proved to be efficient as obtained information was largely complementary. Because questionnaire surveys can be easily performed at a large scale, they give access to a large amount of data within a limited time period and increase the chance to record rare events. In a second step, we completed the questionnaire surveys by telephone inters and visits of selected piggeries with the aim to validate information received in written form. Past and present occurrence of cross-bred animals was mostly recorded during such visits, revealing that cross-breeding was under-reported in mailed questionnaires filled by farmers. This is probably due to the fact that farmers are worried about the consequences it may have for their piggery if close contacts with wild boar are known to occur, such as the request of expensive fence transformations by the veterinary authorities or the loss of the official "piggery health status" attributed by the Swiss Pig Health Service. Personal contacts allow to gain the trust of the farmers and thus to obtain more truthful data. The final data set indicated that the observed yearly contact rate between wild boar and pigs per farm is low but that the number of observed contacts varies greatly among farms. Overall, contacts are not rare and sometimes even lead to cross-breeding.

Additionally, we surveyed two selected piggeries at risk with camera traps. Because this method is work-intensive and requests expensive material, it is not applicable on a large number of farms. Also, as contacts with wild boar on a single farm may not be frequent, the expected number of detections is disproportionally low compared to the invested effort. However, results of camera surveillance confirmed our assumption that many contacts are not observed by the farm personal since they occur at night, which is to be expected given that wild boar are mainly nocturnal [1]. Consequently, the derived contact rates are conservative since they underestimate reality.

Intrusions of wild boar and mating with domestic sows have been documented in France and Germany [22, 24] but to our knowledge this study is the first to quantify contacts between pigs and wild boar including cross-breeding in piggeries. Established populations of hybrids are numerous in the United States [25], Sardinia [2], and also exist in southern Switzerland (canton of Ticino) [26]. However, these cross-bred animals are free-ranging and related to feral pigs and are relevant rather for conservation issues than for pig farming.

Risk factors for contacts

This study is also the first one investigating risk factors for contacts between wild boar and domestic pigs. Because of the limited number of participants and the fact that some farmers had omitted to announce observed close contacts in the mail questionnaire, bias cannot be excluded. However, most identified factors corresponded to our expectations (pig enclosure location away from buildings and close to a forest, protection by low and flexible fences). The fact that risk factors for distant contacts were not necessarily identified for closer contact categories may have two explanations. Firstly, the backward selection procedure targeted the most significant factors for each category, some factors may have been eliminated even if playing a certain role once a strong factor was already part of the respective model. Secondly, data sets to a certain extent varied among contact categories, thus potentially influencing the weight of each considered factor. Nevertheless, a large distance to buildings of any kind and poor fence protection were repeatedly identified as risk factors in the final models. Overall, piggeries with concrete run-out (i.e., with solid fences such as metallic bars and concrete walls, and usually adjacent to buildings) are less at risk for any kind of contact with wild boar than piggeries with pasture run-out (which are mostly protected by electric fences and often located on pastures distant from the farm).

Interestingly, our analysis revealed that the pig breed is also important, Mangalitza being more at risk for mating with wild boar than other breeds. There is a higher proportion of Mangalitza pigs kept on pasture run-out than L/LW pigs, but these are generally closer to forested areas. Nevertheless, the final model showed that the enclosure location and the breed are independent risk factors and not confounders. In Switzerland, Mangalitza is the breed looking most similar and genetically most closely related to wild boar [27], and it could be more attracting to wild boar than other breeds.

Infection status of exposed pigs

Pig owner compliance for visits and pig testing was moderate. This was partly due to the fact that positive results have to be announced to the veterinary authorities with severe consequences for the piggery. Only few piggeries and sometimes only a small proportion of the stock could be sampled but an outbreak of brucellosis was documented. The piggery first found to be infected (P5) gathered all identified risk factors and had experienced a hybrid birth, suggesting an infection through contacts with wild boar, as documented in other countries [22, 24]. However, phylogenetic analysis of *B. suis* isolated from pigs and wild boar from the surrounding areas revealed distinct clusters and it was considered unlikely that wild boar were the direct origin of the outbreak, although possibly not all wildlife strains were included in the analysis [23]. To our knowledge, spill-over from wild boar to pigs has so far always been concluded from field evidence but not proven by strain analysis. Due to the regular pig exchanges between P5 and P12, it was not possible to determine which piggery had infected the other, and to date the source of infection remains unidentified.

Risk of pathogen spill-over from wild boar to outdoor pigs

Wild boar can carry many pathogens and contacts between wild boar and pigs bear a considerable risk of spill-over [28, 29]. Although the risk of transmission is expected to increase from category 1 to 4, it is largely dependent on the transmission route of the pathogens [4, 30]. Thus, the risk of spill-over is highest for infectious agents transmitted by aerosols, to which all outdoor piggeries in areas with wild boar presence may be exposed (contact categories 1–4), whereas a spill-over is least likely for agents transmitted mainly via the venereal route.

Here, investigations focussed on *B. suis*, which is one of the wild boar pathogen of major concern for domestic pigs in Switzerland [1, 20]. Although *B. suis* infection is widespread in Swiss wild boar and mating of wild boar with pig sows regularly occurs, a spill-over from wild boar to pigs could not be documented, suggesting that the risk of transmission of *B. suis* from wild boar to pigs is negligible. However, a spill-over cannot be completely ruled out because the number of sampled piggeries was low, mating had been documented in only few of them, and the origin of the brucellosis outbreak could not be definitely elucidated. Furthermore, while the risk of *B. suis* spill-over to pigs may have been very low up to now, the situation could change due to the significant increase of both wild boar abundance and prevalence of *B. suis* in wild boar [1].

Prevention strategies

The outbreak was discovered in the frame of a research project. Brucellosis may be unapparent among living animals since infected sows can still give birth, though after few oestrous cycles of sexual rest [31], and infected boars can remain fertile [28]. Furthermore, metritis can easily be overlooked at slaughter, and infections are not always associated to pathological changes. Despite decreased reproduction success in two affected piggeries (P5, P12), veterinary investigations were not carried out and pigs were further exchanged. This indicates a need to increase the awareness of farmers for infectious diseases.

In Switzerland, targeted surveillance of porcine brucellosis is carried out only for breeding boars of conventional breeds. Mangalitza pigs are not represented in semen collection centres but boars are exchanged for mating, and they are not tested for brucellosis because Switzerland is considered free of this disease. It is therefore difficult to completely exclude *B. suis* infection in the pig population. Based on the present results, serological testing should be carried out before exchanging animals.

Our data indicate that outdoor piggeries with low electric fence (i.e., pasture run-out), located up to 500 m to a forest within the wild boar range and distanced from buildings, in particular those holding Mangalitza, are exposed to a serious risk of interactions with wild boar and need better protection. Significant seasonal differences regarding the spatial movements of wild boar were not observed [1] and contacts with domestic pigs were reported in all calendar season. Thus, this protection should be present the whole year round. Because wild boar seem to be generally more attracted by sows than by food [32, 33], it seems appropriate to have the most reliable protection where mature sows are held. Most fences are not wild boar-proof, but wire-mesh fencing added to an electrified wire are most effective [34]. To avoid intrusions and escapes, the Swiss Pig Health Service recommends building two 1.50 m wire-mesh fences in parallel, fixed 30 cm deep in the ground to avoid the fence to be sapped, or reinforced by an additional electric fence around the pasture. However, the implementation of this type of fencing is challenging because it is perceived as not feasible by large piggeries regularly performing pasture rotations, both on a financial and practical point of .

CONCLUSIONS

This study shows that interactions between wild boar and outdoor pigs are not uncommon, pointing at the risk of pathogen spill-over even if a wild boar origin could not be documented in the case of the outbreak described here. It also provides data on risk factors that could help the risk-based implementation of protection measures for piggeries. Since a further augmentation of the wild boar population is expected [1] and modern animal welfare requirements are in favour of outdoor facilities for domestic livestock, interactions between wild boar and pigs will likely increase in the future. Our study underlines the importance of improving surveillance strategies for pathogens shared between wildlife and domestic animals and the need to increase disease awareness of farmers and veterinary practitioners.

METHODS

Study area

The study was conducted in Switzerland (4284.57 km^2) from March 2008 to March 2010. No reliable data are available on wild boar numbers but the hunting bag has shown an exponential increase in the past decade [1], reaching 6’878 hunted wild boar in 2010 [4]. Official statistics reported

1'588'998 domestic pigs in 2010 for 8'848 farmers [35], including 4'426 outdoor farms in 2008–2009 [1]. Wild boars are most widespread in the mountain range along the western and northern Swiss borders, while the majority of outdoor piggeries are located in lowlands [1].

Contacts between wild boar and domestic pigs

Definition of contact

Four categories of contacts were defined according to the risk of pathogen transmission: (1) presence of wild boar around the pig enclosure (2 m to 500 m; indicators: tracks, direct observations); (2) presence of wild boar just outside the fence (up to 2 m; indicators: tracks, direct observations); (3) wild boar intrusions into the pig enclosure without documented mating (indicators: direct observations); (4) mating following intrusions or escapes (indicators: births of cross-bred piglets).

Questionnaire survey among game-wardens

In spring 2008, a questionnaire was sent to the wildlife services of all Swiss cantons, which are usually informed about wild boar intrusions into domestic pig enclosures. Game-wardens (or hunters, depending on the hunting system of the canton, but referred to as game-wardens here for simplification) with wild boar in their areas of surveillance were asked to report contacts observed within the past 15 years. Questions concerned the presence of outdoor pigs, and the occurrence, categories and frequency of contacts with wild boar. Responses were sent by 302 game-wardens from 15 cantons, while 11 cantons did not participate. Reasons for not participating were: absence of wild boar hordes in these regions, no wild boar hunt, or impossibility to provide data at the time of the study. Eighty-two questionnaires reporting presence of both wild boar and outdoor pigs were considered for this study, and 236 responses were excluded for the following reasons: no outdoor piggeries (N = 205), no wild boar in the region (N = 29) or incomplete questionnaires (N = 2).

Questionnaire to owners of outdoors pigs

Subsequently, based on hypotheses regarding factors which could influence the occurrence of contacts between outdoor pigs and wild boar (Table 2), a more detailed questionnaire was designed for owners of outdoor pigs, asking about the location and characteristics of piggeries, and the occurrence and categories of contacts between pigs and wild boar (full questionnaire available from the corresponding author). The questionnaire was improved after inters with two selected farmers and sent between January and July 2009 to all 1279 piggeries with concrete and pasture run-out located in Swiss communes with reported wild boar presence [1] (Figure 2), excepting the canton of Zurich, for which data were not available at the time of the survey. Thanks to telephone inters and visits of selected farmers (see below), we additionally obtained information on known piggeries where contacts with wild boar had occurred but that were either not included in the official databases or had originally not been selected due to their location just outside regions at risk or which had initially not answered our questionnaire. These farms were then contacted for a telephone inter or personal visit. Participation was voluntary and data were treated anonymously.

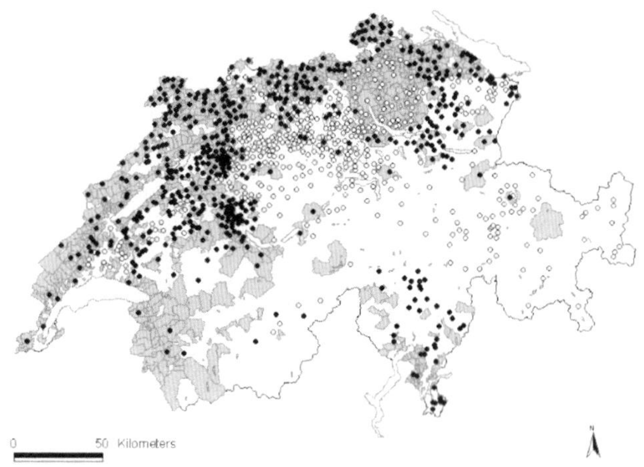

Figure 2: Occurrence of wild boar and outdoor pigs, and location of selected pig farms. Map of Switzerland showing communes with wild boar occurrence (grey areas) and outdoor piggeries (dots). Black dots: farms selected to study risk factors for contacts between wild boar and outdoor pigs in 2009–2010; white dots: not selected farms.

Three hundred and seventy-one pig owners (29% response rate) participated to the survey; 322 responses were included in the study (including partially filled questionnaires) and 49 excluded (no pigs anymore, or no wild boar in the region). Missing information from 32 piggeries with reported contacts was gathered by telephone inters.

To validate answers from completed questionnaires, selected piggeries were personally visited between April 2009 and March 2010. Following piggeries were contacted: all which announced contacts (N = 80), and a selection with pasture or mixed run-out but without observed contacts (N = 33); 48 owners gave their agreement (33 pure pasture run-out, 13 mixed pasture/concrete run-out, and two pure concrete run-out).

Finally, data obtained through both questionnaire surveys (farmers and game-wardens/hunters) were confronted to remove unnecessary data on contacts announced in both surveys, and data sets were merged. In the questionnaire, farmers could report observed contacts either as mean number of contacts per year or as total number of contact since they own the farm. An estimated contact rate per farm and year was obtained by first calculating the average number of recorded contacts per year for each farm (if not already indicated by the farmer), and subsequently summing these averages to obtain the average number (over all farms) of contacts per year.

Surveillance of outdoor piggeries with camera traps

Two piggeries with L/LW on pure pasture run-out (piggeries P1 and P4, Table 1) which had participated in the questionnaire survey, were monitored with infrared camera traps (Reconyx 55, http://www.reconyx.com) to attempt to directly document contacts between wild boar and outdoor pigs at any time of the day and night over four seasons. In both piggeries, wild boar had been previously observed around and inside the enclosures situated between agricultural fields and a forest. The cameras, which detect movement up to 15.2 m away and record date and time of the pictures, were placed along the forest, in opposite direction to the enclosure. They shot five pictures per trigger with one second of delay between two triggers, and remained constantly active.

In P1, two to three cameras (depending on the location) were installed from December 2008 to March 2010, in three different locations due to pasture rotations, and for a duration of six, seven, and three months, respectively. This piggery was protected by a three-wires electrified fence (60 cm high). In P4, two cameras were installed from September to November 2009. The pasture was surrounded by a single-wire electrified fence additionally to a wire-mesh fence fixed above the ground. Animal number, date and age (defined according to Wu and others [1]) were recorded for each photographed wild boar.

Statistical analyses for risk factors

For risk factor analyses, piggeries were considered “positive” for the closest reported contact category and all other more distant categories, e.g., piggeries with evidence of mating were also considered “positive” for the presence of wild boar around the enclosure and for wild boar intrusions, even if these contacts were not directly observed.

Analysis of risk factors for contacts between wild boar and domestic pigs was carried-out in a two-stage analysis with the NCSS 2007 software (Hintze J., 2006; NCSS, Kaysville, Utah, http://www.ncss.com). First, significant potential risk factors were separately identified for the four outcomes (different categories of contacts based on intensity) in a univariable approach, using Chi-square or Fisher’s exact test and logistic regression.

Subsequently, for each of the four outcomes (models) risk factors with statistical significance ($P<0.05$) at the univariable level were tested in a Spearman rank correlation matrix to identify and remove strongly correlated factors and therefore reduce the potential for multicollinearity in the final multivariable models [36]. For this procedure, contact categories were numerically coded according to the expected direction of effect (contact risk increase). Variables with a large proportion of missing values (e.g., pigs kept outside 24 h a day versus only part of the day, composition of wild boar group, wild boar sex and age category) or with imprecise records (e.g., seasonal occurrence and day time of different contact categories) were also excluded from the models.

The remaining variables were submitted to the second modeling step. Here final multivariable models (Table 3, 4, 5, 6) were obtained with a manual stepwise backward elimination procedure with a cut-off level at $P<0.05$. A manual inclusion procedure was applied to test whether factors previously eliminated but considered important from a biological point of would be significant in the final risk factor models. However, because none of these factors became significant, the final models arose from the stepwise backward elimination procedure only. Statistical significance of the risk factors in the models was determined by the Wald test.

Survey for *B. suis* infection in selected outdoor piggeries

Following the questionnaire surveys and visits of piggeries, 11 farmers (piggeries P1-11, Table 1) gave their oral consent to let us sample their animals alive (breeding pigs) or at slaughter (fattening and finishing pigs). Sampling procedures were performed in accordance with the Swiss legislation. They were approved by the committee for animal experiments of the canton of Bern (authorization no. 102/09) and the concerned cantonal veterinary offices. Two piggeries that acquired pigs from a piggery infected with *B. suis* were additionally included in the study (P12-13, Table 1). Sampling related to the brucellosis outbreak was mandatory according to the Swiss legislation and performed under the supervision of the cantonal veterinary authorities. Altogether, 218 pigs were sampled: EDTA blood, serum and urine (whenever possible) were collected from all animals, and tissues (spleen, urinary bladder, uterus) were additionally taken from slaughtered pigs.

The majority of the tested pigs were from 10 piggeries with reported contacts with wild boar (Table 1). In P1, which reported regular wild boar presence around the pig enclosure and recurrent intrusions on the pasture, a wild boar shedding *B. suis* Biovar 2 in urine [1] had entered an enclosure of breeding sows and piglets for several hours in 2008. Blood samples ($N=46$) and urine ($N=3$) were subsequently collected from nine sows and 37 fattening pigs, which had been on the same pasture as the infected wild boar. All sows and 9/37 fattening pigs could be sampled alive twice at 90 days interval, as required in the Swiss federal ordinance on epizootics; 4/9 sows and 11/37 fattening pigs were sampled at slaughter. More pigs from P1 were sampled alive, at slaughter, or both (Table 1).

In living pigs, blood samples were taken on or close to the outdoor pasture by puncturing the jugular vein after manual contention of the animal by a pig farmer. Adults were immobilized with a snout rope placed behind the canine teeth, juveniles < 30 kg were placed in dorsal recumbency with their front limbs and head pulled cranially in order to better expose the jugular vein. Urine was collected with a plastic cup in case of spontaneous urination. Blood from slaughtered pigs was collected at the slaughterhouse with a plastic cup when carcasses were bled by the butcher. Urine was punctured from the urinary bladder immediately after extraction of the organs from the carcass. Tissue samples were also collected on site. After collection, urine samples were transferred into uncoated tubes, and blood samples into EDTA-coated and serum tubes. All samples were transported to the laboratory in a cool box. Serum tubes were centrifuged upon arrival and sera were immediately analyzed. All other samples were stored at −20°C until further analysis.

Sera were directly analysed with the rose bengal test (RBT) and with a complement fixation test (CFT), as recommended by the OIE [37]. Bacterial DNA was extracted with QIAamp® DNA Mini Kit (QIAGEN, Basel, Switzerland) from collected tissue samples and EDTA blood after thawing, and analysed by a qPCR targeting the *Brucella* spp. specific IS*711* insertion element [38].

DECLARATIONS

Acknowledgements

Stephanie Speiser, Linus Eichhorn, Werner Zimmermann (Swine Clinic of Bern), Stefanie Rossteuscher, Patricia Scheer (Swiss Pig Health Service), Naomi Goy (Institute of Veterinary Bacteriology, University of Bern) and Christian Hebeisen (Institute of Zoology, University of Neuchâtel) provided addresses of outdoor piggeries, support for pig sampling, and/or advices about the questionnaire design. We thank all cantonal wildlife services, game-wardens, hunters, butchers and pig farmers who participated to our study. Manuela Weber, Helena Greter, Fabien Mavrot, Simon Röösli (Centre for Fish and Wildlife Health FIWI) and Antonella Reber (Veterinary Public Health Institute VPHI) helped in the field, in the laboratory and/or with data management. The laboratory staff of the Centre for Zoonoses, Bacterial Animal Diseases and Antimicrobial Resistance (ZOBA) provided technical support. We are thankful to the wildlife and veterinary services of the canton of Geneva for their support to collect wild boar and pig samples, in particular to Grégoire Seitert, Gottlieb Dändliker, Alain Rauss, David Badstuber, and Jean-Pierre Perruchoud. Vladimira Hiníc (ZOBA), Mainity Batista Linhares (FIWI) and Anna Fahrion (VPHI) assisted us when stamping-out infected domestic pigs. We acknowledge Helmut Segner (FIWI) and Andreas Waldvogel (Institute Galli-Valerio) for critical reading of the manuscript. Financial support was provided by the Swiss Federal Veterinary Office and the Swiss Federal Office of Environment.

Authors' contributions

NW carried out the questionnaire survey, farm visits, inters and camera trapping, collected the blood and tissue samples, performed qPCR and part of the serological tests, contributed to field investigation of the brucellosis outbreak, analysed the data, and drafted the manuscript. CA and AT supervised the sampling of the pigs stamped out in the frame of the outbreak and the follow up of all laboratory work. PB performed the necropsy of the first pig affected by brucellosis and contributed to the isolation and analysis of this *Brucella* strain. EG contributed to sample collection and carried out most field investigations in the frame of the brucellosis outbreak. MD contributed to statistical analysis of risk factors. MPR designed the study, coordinated the project, contributed to sample collection, field investigations and data analysis, and drafted the manuscript. MPR and CA contributed to the acquisition of the funds. All authors have critically revised and approved the final version of the manuscript.

REFERENCES

1. Wu N, Abril C, Vladimira H, Brodard I, Thür B, Fattebert J, Hüssy D, Ryser-Degiorgis M-P: Free-ranging wild boar: a disease threat to domestic pigs in Switzerland?. Journal of Wildlife Diseases. 2011, 47 (4): 868-879.
2. Artois M, Depner KR, Guberti V, Hars J, Rossi S: Classical swine fever (hog cholera) in wild boar in Europe. Revue Scientifique et Technique de l'Office International des Epizooties. 2002, 21 (2): 287-303.
3. Sáez-Royuela C, Tellería JL: The increased population of the Wild Boar (*Sus scrofa* L.) in Europe. Mammal Re. 1986, 16 (2): 97-101. 10.1111/j.1365-2907.1986.tb00027.x.
4. Hars J, Albina E, Artois M, Boireau P, Crucière C, Garin B, Gauthier D, Hathier C, Lamarque F, Mesplède A, et al: Epidémiosurveillance des maladies du sanglier transmissibles aux animaux domestiques et à l'Homme. Épidémiologie et Santé Animale. 2000, 37: 31-43.
5. Presto MH, Andersson HK, Folestam S, Lindberg JE: Activity behaviour and social interactions of pigs raised outdoors and indoors. Archives Animal Breeding. 2008, 51: 338-350.
6. Bremermann N: Vergleichende Untersuchungen zur Gesundheit. Freien Universität Berlin: Mastleistung und Fleischqualität von Schweinen in derStall- bzw. Freilandhaltung. Doctoral thesis; 2001.
7. Meng XJ: Wild boars as sources for infectious diseases in livestock and humans. Philosophical Transactions: Biological Sciences. 2009, 364 (1530): 2697-2707. 10.1098/rstb.2009.0086.
8. Otake S, Dee S, Corzo C, Oliveira S, Deen J: Long-distance airborne transport of infectious PRRSV and *Mycoplasma hyopneumoniae* from a swine population infected with multiple viral variants. Veterinary Microbiology. 2010, 145 (3–4): 198-208.
9. Kuhnert P, Overesch G, Belloy L: Genotyping of *Mycoplasma hyopneumoniae* in wild boar lung samples. Veterinary Microbiology. 2011, 152 (1–2): 191-195.
10. Cousins DV: *Mycobacterium bovis* infection and control in domestic livestock. Revue scientifique et technique de l'Office International des Epizooties. 2001, 20 (1): 71-85.
11. Köppel C, Knopf L, Ryser M-P, Miserez R, Thur B, Stark K: Serosurveillance for selected infectious disease agents in wild boars (*Sus scrofa*) and outdoor pigs in Switzerland. European Journal of Wildlife Research. 2007, 53: 212-220. 10.1007/s10344-006-0080-0.
12. Leuenberger R: Surveillance of wild boar in Switzerland: prevalence of infections relevant to domestic pigs. Basel: University of Basel; 2004.PhD Thesis.
13. Hofmann MA, Thür B, Vanzetti T, Schleiss W, Schmidt J, Griot C: Klassische Schweinepest beim Wildschwein in der Schweiz. Schweizer Archiv für Tierheilkunde. 1999, 141: 185-190.
14. Dondo A, Zoppi S, Rossi F, Chiavacci L, Barbaro A, Garrone A, Benedetto A, Goria M: Mycobacteriosis in wild boar : Results of 2000–2006 activity in North-Western Italy. Épidémiologie et Santé Animale. 2007, 51: 35-42.
15. Gortázar C, Ferroglio E, Höfle U, Frölich K, Vicente J: Diseases shared between wildlife and livestock: a European perspective. European Journal of Wildlife Research. 2007, 53 (4): 241-256. 10.1007/s10344-007-0098-y.
16. Cargill C, Davis PR: External Parasites. In Diseases of Swine. 8th edition.Edited by Straw BE, D'Allaire S, Mengling WL, Taylor DJ. Iowa: Iowa StatePress; 1999:669–683.
17. Zimmermann W, Neff F, Birrer S: Serologische Bestandsuntersuchung der Sarcoptes scabiei var. suis Infektion mit Kolostralmilchproben: vorläufige Resultate. Schweizer Archiv für Tierheilkunde. 2001, 143 (2): 70-76.
18. Cvetnic Z, Spicic S, Curic S, Jukic B, Lojkic M, Albert D, Thiebaud M, Garin-Bastuji B: Isolation of *Brucella suis* biovar 3 from horses in Croatia. Veterinary Record. 2005, 156 (18): 584-585.

19. Romero C, Meade P, Shultz J, Chung H, Gibbs E, Hahn E, Lollis G: Venereal transmission of pseudorabies viruses indigenous to feral swine. Journal of Wildlife Diseases. 2001, 37 (2): 289-296.

20. Leuenberger R, Boujon P, Thur B, Miserez R, Garin-Bastuji B, Rufenacht J, Stark KD: Prevalence of classical swine fever, Aujeszky's disease and brucellosis in a population of wild boar in Switzerland. Veterinary Record. 2007, 160 (11): 362-368. 10.1136/vr.160.11.362.

21. Brucellose porcine. http://www.bvet.admin.ch/gesundheit_tiere/01065/01083/01105/index.html?lang=fr.

22. Garin-Bastuji B, Hars J, Calvez C, Thiébaud M, Artois M: Brucellose du porc domestique et du sanglier sauvage due à *Brucella suis* biovar 2 en France. Epidemiologie et santé animale. 2000, 38: 1-5.

23. Abril C, Thomann A, Brodard I, Wu N, Ryser-Degiorgis M-P, Frey J, Overesch G: A novel isolation method of *Brucella*species and molecular tracking of *Brucella suis* biovar 2 in domestic and wild animals. Veterinary Microbiology. 2011, 150 (3–4): 405-410.

24. Kautzsch S, Seyfarth D, Schöne R, Stehmann R: Ein Fall von Brucellose der Schweine und daraus abgeleitete Überlegungen zur Epidemiologie dieser Tierseuche. Berliner und Münchener Tierärtzliche Wochenschrift. 1995, 108: 201-205.

25. Gipson PS, Lee CD: Wild hogs in the United States: A New Management Challenge. In Proceedings of the first national Feral Swine Conference: June 2nd to 3rd: Texas. United States. 1999, 1999: 5-10.

26. Moretti M: Biometric data growth rates of mountain population of wild boar (Sus scrofa L.), Ticino, Switzerland. IBEX Journal of Mountain Ecology. 1995, 3: 56-59.

27. Manea MA, Georgescu SE, Kevorkian S, Costache M: Genetic diversity analyses of seven Romanian pig populations based on 10 microsatellites. Romanian Biotechnological Letters. 2009, 14 (6): 4827-4834.

28. EFSA: Scientific Opinion of the panel on Animal Health and Welfare (AHAW) on a request from the Commission on porcine brucellosis (*Brucella suis*). The EFSA Journal. 2009, 1144: 1-112.

29. Hartley M: Qualitative risk assessment of the role of the feral wild boar (*Sus scrofa*) in the likelihood of incursion and the impacts on effective disease control of selected exotic diseases in England. European Journal of Wildlife Research. 2010, 56 (3): 401-410. 10.1007/s10344-009-0334-8.

30. Corn JL, Cumbee JC, Chandler BA, Stallknecht DE, Fischer JR: Implication of feral swine expansion: expansion of feral swine in the United States and potential implication for domestic swine. In Feral Swine Subcommittee on Brucellosis and Pseudorabies: November 6th to 9th: St- Joseph. Missouri, United States: United State Animal Health Association. 2005, 2005: 295-297.

31. MacMillan AP: Brucellosis. In Diseases of swine. 8th edition. Edited by StrawBE, D'Allaire S, Mengling WL, Taylor DJ. Iowa, USA: Iowa State Press;1999:385–393.

32. Garin-Bastuji B, Hars J: La brucellose du porc et du sanglier en France, état des connaissances au 1er juillet 2001. 2001, 1-16. In *2001*: Agence française de sécurité sanitaire des aliments (AFSSA Alfort).

33. Wyckoff AC, Henke SE, Campbell TA, Hewitt DG, Vercauteren KC: Feral swine contact with domestic swine: a serologic survey and assessment of potential for disease transmission. Journal of Wildlife Diseases. 2009, 45 (2): 422-429.

34. Hone J, Atkinson B: Evaluation of fencing to control feral pig-movement. Australian Wildlife Research. 1983, 10 (3): 499-505. 10.1071/WR9830499.

35. Landwirtschaft – Detaillierte Daten, Nutztiere, Interaktive Karten.

36. Dohoo I, Martin W, Stryhn H: Model building strategies. In Veterinary Epidemiologic Research. 2nd edition. Charlottetown, Prince Edward Island,Canada: VER Inc; 2009:365–369.

37. Chapter 2.8.5 Porcine brucellosis. 8http://www.oie.int/fileadmin/Home/eng/Health_standards/tahm/2.08.05_PORCINE_BRUC.pdf.

38. Hiníc V, Brodard I, Thomann A, Holub M, Miserez R, Abril C: IS711-based real-time PCR assay as a tool for detection of *Brucella* spp. in wild boars and comparison with bacterial isolation and serology. BMC Veterinary Research. 2009, 5 (1): 22-10.1186/1746-6148-5-22.

CHAPTER 41

EVALUATION OF THE HOOF-PRINT ASSAY FOR TYPING BRUCELLA ABORTUS STRAINS ISOLATED FROM CATTLE IN THE UNITED STATES: RESULTS WITH FOUR PERFORMANCE CRITERIA

Betsy J Bricker and Darla R Ewalt

BACKGROUND

During the epidemiological inquiry into a disease outbreak, investigators try to trace the outbreak strain back to the original source of infection. If a potential index strain is identified, the strains are compared to establish a genetic connection between them. To help in this endeavor, a variety of approaches to characterize and classify disease strains have been developed that exploit genotypic and/or phenotypic markers. However, it can be difficult to determine which approaches are practical and informative for routine investigation of the disease agent of choice. Furthermore, direct comparisons of published methods may not be possible because different types of data are generated. At the request of the European Society of Clinical Microbiology and Infectious Diseases, these questions and others were discussed by a panel of international experts, resulting in the formation of the European Study Group on Epidemiological Markers (ESGEM) in 1994. The result of the meeting was a published set of guidelines for the evaluation of epidemiological typing systems [1]. The guidelines describe the performance criteria that should be considered when evaluating a typing system for widespread use. These criteria include: typeability, reproducibility, stability, discriminatory power, epidemiologic concordance, and typing system concordance.

Recently, a new approach has been developed for genetic typing that exploits the greater than normal amount of polymorphism observed within genomic regions containing short (2 to a few tens of base-pairs), tandemly repeated DNA sequences [2, 3, 4]. The accelerated mutation rates associated with the repeated sequences are thought to be due to slip-strand mispairing (SSM) [5] and recombination (most likely in the form of gene conversion arising from double-strand break repair [6]), resulting in rapid micro-evolution within the locus. SSM occurs when DNA polymerase misreads the number of repeats on the template strand, typically causing step-wise mutations (the addition or loss of single repeat units). Recombination mechanisms can cause more dramatic expansions or contractions of repeat strings, especially within the very large repeat strings found in eukaryotes [6]. Each variable number tandem repeat (VNTR) locus mutates independently and at an individual rate determined by a number of factors including: the repeat sequence, the size and number of repeat units, the flanking sequence, DNA secondary structure and sequence function [7]. Characterization of these continuously evolving targets has facilitated differentiation of bacterial strains [8, 9]. Examination of multiple tandem repeat loci enhances subtype characterization in two ways: firstly, the capacity for genetic discrimination increases when multiple VNTR loci are examined; secondly, the effects of homoplasy (identical alleles arising independently through convergence, reversal or parallelism) may be diminished. Multilocus VNTR analysis (MLVA) has become an effective technique that can discriminate many difficult-to-type bacteria, including many human pathogens such as *Haemophilus influenzae*

Citation: Betsy J Bricker and Darla R Ewalt, Evaluation of the HOOF-Print assay for typing Brucella abortus strains isolated from cattle in the United States: results with four performance criteria, DOI: 10.1186/1471-2180-5-37.

[10]; *Bacillus anthracis* [11]; *Yersinia pestis*[12]; *Francisella tularensis* [13] and *Mycobacterium tuberculosis* [14].

Brucellosis is an economically important zoonotic disease found throughout many regions of the world, and until recently, throughout the U.S. One causative agent, *Brucella abortus*, is predominantly pathogenic for its natural hosts, cattle and bison (Bovidae family); but it is also pathogenic for humans and several incidental animal species including elk. The disease causes reproductive failure in the host species and chronic health problems in humans.

B. abortus is a member of a highly homogenous genus, exhibiting ~98.5% nucleotide sequence homology among species [15]. Conventional subtyping of *Brucella* strains into biovars, for epidemiological trace-back, relies on a large array of tests including phage susceptibility, metabolic, biochemical, and serological characterization [16]. Often the differences are subtle. Few biovars are recognized within most *Brucella*species and some species cannot be subtyped at all. Worldwide, *B. abortus* has seven biovars; only biovars 1, 2 and 4 occur in the U.S. Differences among these three biovars are minor; discrimination is based on serology and the ability to grow in culture media with certain dyes [16]. Historically, about 85% of U.S. strains were typed as biovar-1.

Previously, we reported the discovery of a reiterated 8-bp sequence, arrayed in tandemly ordered strings [17], that is present in at least eight loci within the sequenced genomes of three *Brucella* species [15, 18, 19]. A protocol was developed for assessing the number of repeats at each of the eight loci by PCR amplification. The resulting amplicons, containing the entire array of tandem repeats and a small amount of flanking sequence, are sized and the number of repeats is deduced from the length. Since all eight loci have the same 8-bp repeat sequence, the technique was named «HOOF-Prints», an acronym for h ypervariable o ctameric oligonucleotide f ingerprints[17].

This paper evaluates the HOOF-Prints technique as it is applied to a diverse collection of *B. abortus* field strains representing all three biovar subtypes isolated from throughout the U.S. Our primary goal was to assess how well HOOF-Print genotyping can discriminate among unrelated field strains. Genotyping performance is compared to conventional subtyping into biovars. Individual fingerprint patterns and allelic diversity are presented. The HOOF-Prints technique is also assessed by four of the performance criteria recommended by the ESGEM: typeability, reproducibility, power of discrimination, and concordance with other typing methods. Recommendations for test population criteria are also addressed.

RESULTS AND DISCUSSION

Selection of the test group

An important consideration for evaluating an epidemiological typing system is the selection of a suitable test population. The test population should be large ($N > 100$), consisting of a diverse collection of unrelated strains that is representative of the natural population in which the test is intended to be used [1]. Information about biovar type, herd location and year of isolation is also included.

All of the strains tested, except for the reference strains, were randomly chosen from diagnostic specimens that had been cultured, positively identified as *B. abortus*, biovar typed, and archived by the diagnostic laboratory at the National Veterinary Services Laboratories (APHIS, USDA). As suggested by the ESGEM, the test population was diverse based on the location and date of collection. The field strains originated from 97 different cattle herds, including both dairy and market cattle. Most of the isolates (n = 95) were from the US, but one isolate from Mexico and one isolate from El Salvador were also included. Over half of the isolates (n = 54) were collected in 1991 when brucellosis was still widely disseminated over the country, but on the decline due to the success of the national brucellosis eradication program. In subsequent years, there was a dramatic decrease in outbreaks, so fewer isolates were available. Currently, reports of new outbreaks in the U.S. are uncommon. The primary source of new outbreaks has shifted from domestic cattle to wildlife reservoirs.

To measure the assay's power of discrimination, only one isolate from each herd was included in the test group to prevent statistical over-representation of genotypes. When possible, the infected herds originated from different cities, and in all cases the herds had different owners. However, information regarding possible epidemiological links among the herds was unavailable. A disproportionate number of *B. abortus* biovar-2 and biovar-4 isolates were selected to assess the level of natural genotypic diversity within these subtypes. These two biovars are relatively more common in wildlife reservoirs and have recently been on the increase in cattle, due to more cattle outbreaks originating from wildlife. Six common laboratory strains of *B. abortus* including the reference strains of *B. abortus* biovars 1, 2, and 4, and the two major vaccine strains were also included in this study. Only *B. abortus* biovars 1, 2 and 4 were included in the test group, since these are the biovars that occur naturally in the United States.

HOOF-Print analysis

Eight loci containing octameric tandem repeats were characterized for each of the 103 isolates in the test population. Tandem repeat loci were amplified by PCR with primers directed to the conserved sequences flanking the repeat regions and the total number of repeat units at each locus was deduced from the size of the corresponding amplicon [17]. The HOOF-Print profiles of some of the strains used in this study have been previously reported in earlier studies [17, 20].

At each locus, the alleles are named for the calculated number of repeat units at that locus, such that Allele-4 contains 4 repeat units and Allele-8 contains 8 repeat units. The HOOF-Print (genotypic fingerprint) for an isolate was generated from the allelic profile at all eight loci of that isolate.

Typeability

An important feature of any typing method is the ability of that method to conclusively classify every sample to a specific type defined by the test parameters. The ESGEM recommends that "*T*" be as close to 1.0 as possible [1]. In the case of the HOOF-Print assay, all isolates produced an amplified product at each of the eight loci. *Taq* DNA Polymerase adds a non-template nucleotide resulting in 2 products differing by 1-bp. With this protocol, the majority of amplicon products contain the extra nucleotide, but a significant portion of amplicons without the non-template nucleotide are also produced, resulting in the resolution of 2 peaks, 1-bp apart, by capillary electrophoresis. Nevertheless, since the repeat units increased in increments of 8-bp, allele assignment was clear-cut and an allele was assigned for all eight loci, giving the method a typeability index of 1.0. It should be noted that some strains were assigned an allele called M for Locus-6 and also for Locus-1. These isolates repeatedly produced single amplicons that were outside the predicted size range. For Locus-6, all M amplicons were the same size. Sequence analysis of the amplicons from several of these isolates showed a specific deletion in the flanking sequence region. All of the sequenced mutants produced the same aberrant sequence. Sequence analysis of the M allele at Locus-1 also showed a deletion in the flanking region of the DNA. Although these isolates did not fall in the normal expected range of alleles, they gave consistent results and could be assigned to a new allele that was called M for mutant.

Reproducibility

Like typeability, it is critical that a typing method reliably produce the same result for a given sample. The ESGEM recommends a reproducibility index of $R \geq 0.95$. This feature was continuously tested during the study since every isolate was independently tested twice. However, in a more structured evaluation, 20 isolates were analyzed in triplicate in a randomized sequence. In a blinded fashion, one individual was responsible for preparing the assay, performing the assay, and interpreting the results. The HOOF-Print Assay had an $R = 0.998$ at the locus level and an $R = 0.983$ at the composite fingerprint level. The reason that R was less than 1.0 was because in one test, Locus-6 was incorrectly recorded as containing Allele-2 instead of Allele-5. This was an obvious clerical error, not an experimental failure, since the raw data clearly showed Allele-5 as the only form present in the sample. Nevertheless, the assay easily met the suggested limit for reproducibility.

Allelic diversity among the HOOF-Print loci

The *B. abortus* strains exhibited extensive variability in the number and range of alleles at each locus (Table 1). Similar levels of locus diversity were observed among each of the three biovars individually and within the test population as a whole. For example, Loci 5 and 8 had very little diversity, regardless of the biovar designation. By contrast, Locus-7 is highly diverse in all three biovars, with the same alleles occurring in multiple biovars.

Table 1: Allelic diversity among B. abortus VNTR loci

	No. of Alleles	Range of Repeats	Discrimination Index[a]
Biovar 1 strains			
Locus-1	14	2 – 14, M[c]	0.90
Locus-2	4	3 – 6	0.66
Locus-3	9	3 – 16	0.78
Locus-4	7	2 – 10	0.77
Locus-5	2	2 – 3	0.07
Locus-6	3	2 – 3, M	0.17
Locus-7	12	3 – 14	0.87
Locus-8	1	2	0.00
Biovar 2 strains			
Locus-1	8	2 – 10	0.80
Locus-2	5	3 – 7	0.71
Locus-3	8	2 – 13	0.86
Locus-4	6	2 – 7	0.78
Locus-5	2	2 – 5	0.14
Locus-6	4	2 – 4, M	0.39
Locus-7	12	3 – 15	0.93
Locus-8	1	2	0.00
Biovar 4 strains			
Locus-1	10	2 – 12	0.92
Locus-2	2	4 – 5	0.53
Locus-3	5	1 – 6	0.74
Locus-4	5	2 – 6	0.77
Locus-5	1	2	0.00
Locus-6	2	2, M	0.43
Locus-7	9	3 – 12	0.90

Locus-8	1	2	0.00
All strains [b]			
Locus-1	14	2 – 14, M	0.87
Locus-2	5	3 – 7	0.67
Locus-3	11	1 – 16	0.82
Locus-4	7	2 – 13	0.78
Locus-5	3	2 – 5	0.04
Locus-6	5	2 – 5, M	0.40
Locus-7	13	3 – 15	0.89
Locus-8	1	2	0.00

a-The Discrimination Index was calculated for each locus by the method of Hunter and Gaston as described in the Materials and methods section; *b* -These numbers were calculated from the entire 103-sample test population. *c* – "M" indicates an atypical (mutant) allele.

Among the loci with multiple alleles, the distribution of alleles by size resembled an asymmetrical bell shaped curve skewed towards smaller repeat numbers (data not shown). This pattern of distribution is consistent with step-wise mutations resulting from SSM. The overall trend in allele frequency is toward short strings of repeats ranging from 2 to 5 repeat units per locus.

Power of discrimination

A fundamental question addressed in epidemiological investigations is whether the outbreak strain is derived from or genetically related to the proposed index strain. The answer requires a method for differentiation of genetically related and unrelated strains. The more genetic markers that are available to define isolates, the easier it becomes to discriminate among related and unrelated strains. Therefore, the discriminatory power of a test indicates how successful the test will be in identifying genetic relationships among strains. The ESGEM recommends evaluating a large group ($\geq$ 100 samples) of genetically diverse samples by the Hunter-Gaston Discrimination Index (HGDI) [21], and proposes as a limit that HGDI is $\geq$ 0.95. In other words, for any two randomly-chosen, unrelated isolates, there is a 95% or greater probability that they will be placed in separate groups. Since the HGDI is heavily influenced by the level of genetic diversity within the test population, our test population consisted of only one isolate per herd to avoid over-representation of related fingerprint profiles. To assess the demonstrable diversity within the less common biovars, a disproportionate number of randomly selected *B. abortus* biovar-2 and biovar-4 isolates was included. Despite all attempts to use genetically unrelated isolates, the level of genetic relatedness among outbreaks from the different herds is not known, and some isolates may be epidemiologically linked.

The discriminatory power of the conventional typing method for *Brucella*, biovar typing, was examined. The calculated HGDI for the total test population based solely on biovar typing was 0.60. It should be noted that this value is artificially high due to disproportionate representation of biovar-2 and biovar-4 isolates in the test population. Historically, about 85% of *B. abortus* infections in the U.S. were caused by biovar 1, which would result in an HGDI $\approx$ 0.2. Even with the disproportionate biovar representation, the discrimination index is well below the recommended power of discrimination, $\geq$ 0.95, but for many years it has been the only subtyping method available.

The discriminatory power of HOOF-Print genotyping was determined for each of the three biovar subpopulations and for the entire test population (n = 103). When the HGDI was calculated on a locus-by-locus basis within the biovar specific subgroups and within the total test population, the results were variable, ranging from 0 (no discrimination; Locus-8, all populations) to 0.93 (Locus-7; biovar-2 subgroup) as seen in Table 1. Although the locus-specific HGDI values varied slightly among the biovar subgroups, the trends were similar, indicating that HOOF-Print genotyping is equally discriminating for each biovar subgroup. On a single locus basis, none of the loci met the minimal discrimination level of $\geq$ 0.95.

When the alleles from all eight loci were combined into a composite HOOF-Print genotype, the test group of 103 samples exhibited 98 different fingerprint patterns (HGDI = 0.99). This is well above the recommended limit set by ESGEM. In only four cases did two isolates have the same fingerprint: isolates #16 and #17 [strains 1–2361 and 1–2385]; isolates #46 and #47 [strains 1–2421 and 1–2040]; isolates #79 and #96 [strains 98-0689 and 4-0213]; and isolates #102 and #103 [strains 6-0242 and 4-1303]. One field isolate, #25 [strain1-2052] matched the fingerprint pattern for the vaccine strain S19. Independent analysis of phenotypic and biochemical characteristics also identified this isolate as vaccine strain S19. Another field isolate, #31 [strain 1-2050], was previously characterized by biovar typing as vaccine strain S19. While the fingerprint pattern for this isolate was not an exact match for the fingerprint patterns for the other S19 samples, it differed by only 1 repeat unit at Locus-1. This type of difference is consistent with micro-evolution from a step-wise mutation event.

Cluster analysis of HOOF-Print genotypes from the test populations

The HOOF-Print assay was designed to complement epidemiological investigations. Genotypic similarities are assumed to demonstrate genetic linkage among related lineages, and conversely, related lineages would be expected to have genotypic similarities. However, since the mutation rates for the selected loci among *Brucella* strains have yet to be determined, the evolutionary distance defined by HOOF-Print genotyping is unclear. We used cluster analysis to see if the HOOF-Print genotypes could be used to infer long and short term evolutionary history. Pairwise genetic distances within the total 103 strain test population were calculated from the absolute difference in repeat units at each of the eight loci, consistent with the stepwise model of mutation. A dendrogram was created by the neighbor-joining method (Figure 1). The clusters appear to be independent of the time or location of strain isolation (e.g. isolates #18 and #19 that were isolated in 1999 and 1994, respectively). This is not surprising since the test population is presumably composed of unrelated strains. As expected, the few strains known to be genetically related did cluster appropriately (e.g. field isolates of the vaccine strain S19; RB51 and its parental strain 2308). Unfortunately, epidemiological information and comprehensive histories are not routinely submitted with diagnostic samples and so specific information about the selected test isolates was not available, making it impossible to assess the validity of the cluster results for these data. If VNTR polymorphism in *Brucella* is generated by a mechanism other than the stepwise mutation model, then the genetic relationships proposed in Figure 1 could be invalid.

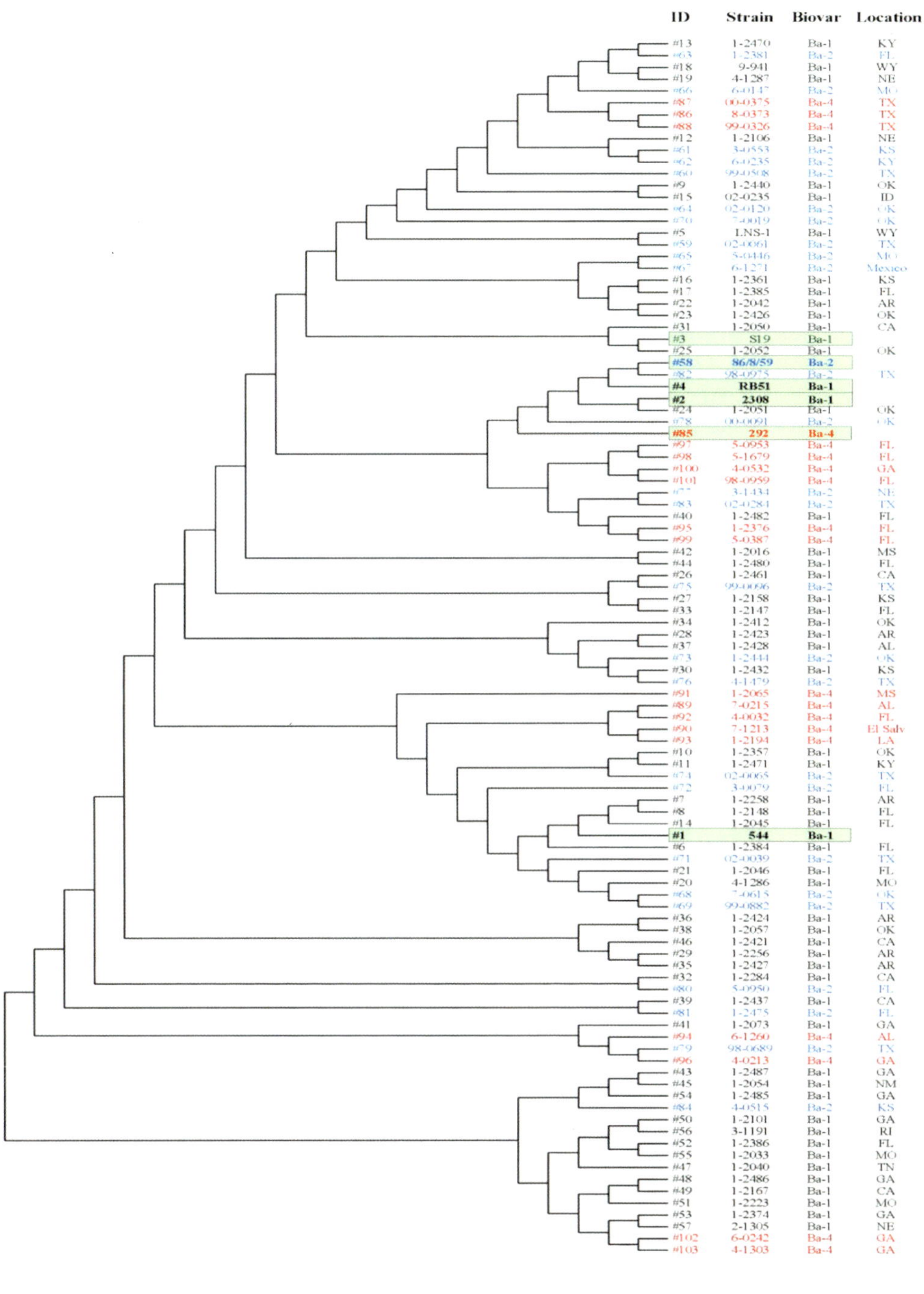

Figure 1: Neighbor-joining dendrogram of clustered HOOF-Print genotypes. Genotyped were clustered into groups based on the differences in the numbers of repeat units at the eight VNTR loci. Biovars are differentiated by colored text: black = biovar-1; green = biovar-2 and red = biovar-4.

Distribution of HOOF-Print genotypes and alleles by geographic region

We wanted to see if there was a connection between geographic region and the HOOF-Print genotypes or alleles. The multilocus genotype clusters shown in the dendrogram in (Figure 1) do not correspond to specific states or regions. However, because multilocus genotyping is so highly discriminating, nearly every HOOF-Print genotype that was identified is unique. It is possible that the rapid evolution of the most variable loci could potentially mask regional influences in genotype composition. To detect regional relationships at the locus level, the alleles for each locus were examined for asymmetrical geographic distribution. To simplify the data and assure that sufficient data was available for statistical analysis, the US was divided into 2 regions: the east and the west, separated by the Mississippi River. For loci that contain a large number of alleles, the alleles were grouped so that no more that 4 or 5 groups were compared. Only data from *B. abortus* field strains from the US were included (n = 95). The data for each locus was cross tabulated and analyzed by the chi-square test statistic to see if a statistically significant association between alleles and geographic region could be demonstrated. Note that for Locus-6, Fisher›s exact test was used instead of the chi-square test, because of the small number of strains carrying alleles with more than 2 repeat units. The data indicate that within most loci there are no significant associations between alleles and geographic region (p values ranging from 0.1739 to 0.8563). For Locus 1, there may be a slight imbalance in distribution, with smaller alleles (7 or less repeat units) appearing more often in the west and larger alleles (8 or more repeat units) appearing more often in the east ($p = 0.0400$).

Table 2: Statistical analysis of the allelic distributions within each VNTR locus by geographic region [a]

VNTR Locus	*P* value
Locus-1	0.0400
Locus-2	0.1739
Locus-3	0.8365
Locus-4	0.4147
Locus-6	0.2824
Locus-7	0.8563

While it is reasonable to expect a relationship between genotypes/alleles and geographic region, several factors can affect geographic distributions. In the case of brucellosis, the government sponsored eradication program is drawing to a close. As a result, the incidence of *Brucella* has decreased dramatically to nearly complete eradication. Many states have been disease free for decades. Therefore, the initial source of a new infection is often found outside of the local area and involves the importation of diseased cattle from elsewhere. In a few areas, transmission from wildlife to cattle has become the leading source of disease outbreaks. Only a very small number of residual endemic bovine infections continue to be identified and eradicated. As the number of infected herds decrease, each outbreak is more isolated and can be quickly contained so that subsequent regional spread of the associated genotype is less likely. Therefore, it is likely that with so the few infected herds, the remaining *B. abortus* genotypes in the US are no longer representative of the natural distribution of genotypes that were present prior to the eradication program.

Finally, the selection criteria for the test population used in this study were designed to maximize the number of unrelated strains. Strains were selected from a large number of different states, and when possible, only one isolate from each city was included. Thus, possible links between alleles and geographic region may not be represented in the test population.

Comparison of biovar typing and HOOF-Print genotyping

The fourth performance criterion recommended by the ESGEM is concordance of the typing results with the results of other typing methods. When HOOF-Print genotyping was compared with conventional biovar typing, the most obvious difference was the high discriminatory power of the genotyping method and low discriminatory power of the biovar typing method. This complicates the direct comparison of typing results because the numbers of subtypes generated vary greatly between the two methods. In the dendrogram shown in Figure 1, all 103 strains were clustered by genotypic similarity. However, the hierarchical groups assembled by genotype were not homogeneous for biovar type. Most genotype clusters contain an assortment of biovars (shown by color coding in Figure 1), although some small clusters of biovars were found (e.g. biovar-4 isolates #89, 90, 91, 92 and 93). It is important to keep in mind that the dendrogram in Figure 1is only one of many possible arrangements of the data. Furthermore, the method used for clustering the data was based on the step-wise model of mutation. If a different mechanism or a combination of mechanisms is involved, then the clustering parameters used in this study do not apply and the clusters are invalid.

In the most extreme case, two isolates with identical fingerprints were identified as belonging to different biovars. This result was somewhat surprising, considering the clonal nature of *Brucella*, but there are at least two possible explanations for this observation. One possible cause is homoplasy, resulting from convergent evolution among unrelated strains. The hypermutability of VNTR loci results in continuous micro-evolution, and HOOF-Print genotyping reveals the most recent mutation events in a strain's genetic history. Even among the most variable loci in this study, a limited repertoire of alleles was found. Although the total number of allelic combinations is large, random convergence of genotype patterns between genetically unrelated strains is likely to occur occasionally. Incorporation of additional polymorphic loci into the assay may help resolve inconsistencies caused by homoplasy.

Alternatively, the strain could have typed as a different biovar type due to mutation(s) in genes that affect biovar phenotype. Only two differences distinguish *B. abortus* biovar 2 and biovar 4: biovar 2 strains are A-antigen dominant/fuchsin dye sensitive while biovar 4 strains are M-antigen dominant/ fuchsin dye insensitive [16]. Both traits are associated with the bacterial surface and may require common genes. Although spontaneous mutations are much less common than VNTR polymorphisms, atypical biovar profiles are occasionally found among field isolates. Thus, this argument cannot be ruled out without further study.

CONCLUSION

The HOOF-Print Assay is a rapid, easy to perform technique for subtyping *B. abortus* strains. When the assay was evaluated with a test population consisting of a large number of unrelated, naturally occurring field isolates, the selected tandem repeat loci displayed considerable polymorphism as evidenced by the large number of alleles found at many of the loci. The study demonstrates that the HOOF-Print assay meets or exceeds the minimum limits recommended by the ESGEM for epidemiological typing, based on the performance criteria: typeability, reproducibility, and power of discrimination. When compared to conventional biovar typing, HOOF-Print genotyping is considerably more discriminating. However, some inconsistencies with conventional biovar typing were observed. Caution will be needed in interpreting the data, to prevent drawing incorrect conclusions from artificial genotypic similarity caused by homoplasy. Incorporation of additional polymorphic loci may help identify convergent evolution among unrelated strains. In practice, HOOF-Print genotyping should be utilized as a complement to conventional epidemiological investigations into the short-term history of localized brucellosis outbreaks. In the future, we plan to look at genotypic variability among related isolates to better understand how HOOF-Print genotypes evolve and to experimentally measure the VNTR mutation rates among the polymorphic *B. abortus* loci.

METHODS

Disclaimer: Mention of trade names or commercial products in this article is solely for the purpose of providing specific information and does not imply recommendation or endorsement by the U.S. Department of Agriculture.

Isolation and characterization of the bacterial strains used in this study

The bacterial field strains used in this study were originally isolated in the Bacterial Diagnostic Laboratory at the USDA National Veterinary Services Laboratories, Ames, IA, as part of the USDA Brucellosis Eradication Program. The suspect bacteria were subcultured, identified by conventional microbiological tests and biotyped by additional biochemical and phenotypic characteristics [16] prior to archiving at -70°C. The type strains were originally obtained from the American Type Culture Collection bank and stored at -70°C until propagated.

The selected strains were thawed, grown, harvested and preserved in 66% methanol. Many of the isolates were retrieved and prepared specifically for this study while other strains had been preserved in methanol for a number of years with no apparent DNA degradation.

HOOF-Print analysis

The HOOF-Print technique was performed as previously described [17] with minor modifications as follows: PCR amplification was performed with 1 unit of FastStart Taq polymerase (cat no. 2-032-902; Roche Biochemicals, Indianapolis, IN) in 50-mM Tris, 10-mM KCl, 1.5-mM $MgCl_2$, and 5-mM $(NH_4)_2SO_4$, pH 8.3, with the addition of dGTP, dATP, dCTP and dTTP at 250-µM each, primers at 250-nM each, and GC-Rich Resolution Solution (included with the polymerase) at 1X concentration, per manufacturer's instructions. Primer pairs [17] consisted of one primer fluorescently labeled with HEX, FAM or NED and one unlabeled primer. Both primers were designed to anneal to the conserved sequences flanking the repeat region. Amplification was done one locus at a time (8 assays per sample) or multiplexed with up to three primer sets per reaction (with a different dye for each primer set). Cycling parameters were as follows: 95°C for 5 min to activate the modified polymerase, followed by 37 cycles of 95°C for 30 sec, 53°C for 30 sec and 75°C for 45 sec; and ending with a 60-min incubation at 75°C to promote maximal addition of the non-templated nucleotide to the amplicons. The higher extension temperature increased amplicon yield, possibly by denaturing short hairpin formations in the target sequence. The amplified samples were maintained at 4°C prior to analysis.

The degree of amplification success was monitored by gel electrophoresis through 4% agarose. Before size analysis, the fluorescent amplicons were diluted in water, usually in a 1:100 or 1:200 ratio, then separated by capillary electrophoresis on an ABI Prism 3100 Genetic Analyzer with GeneScan-500 [ROX] size markers (cat. no. 401734; Applied BioSystems, Foster City, CA). Data were collected and the amplicon sizes were determined with GeneScan Data Analysis Software, ver 3.7 (Applied BioSystems). The number of repeat copies was deduced from the amplicon size.

For some isolates, more than one product was reproducibly synthesized for a given locus, typically differing by a single repeat unit. This phenomenon, which was especially common in reference strains, is thought to be the result of micro-evolution. Minor heterogeneity at some loci was not unexpected since many of these samples were primary isolates that had not been propagated clonally. In these cases the dominant allele was used for analysis.

Reproducibility analysis

A reproducibility evaluation was integrated into the protocol by analyzing every sample twice in independent assays. To formally evaluate the reproducibility of the HOOF-Print technique an additional blinded survey was performed. Twenty isolates were prepared in triplicate and randomized in order. A different individual prepared the reaction mixes, performed the assay and analyzed the data, unaware of the identities of the samples.

Statistical analyses

The following statistical analyses were performed as suggested by the ESGEM [1].

Typeability is the success in determining an unambiguous type for each isolate, calculated by the formula $T = \frac{N_t}{N}$ where T is the typeability, N_t is the number of strains characterized by a complete array of alleles, and N is the size of the test population. If a complete 8-allele fingerprint can be determined for all strains in the test population, then $T = 1$.

Reproducibility is the ability to assign the same type to an isolate in independently repeated tests. It is calculated from the equation $R = \frac{Nr}{N}$ where R is the reproducibility index, N_r is the number of strains that are repeatedly assigned a single type and N is the total number in the test sample.

Allele frequency is the relative proportion of each allele, given as a percentage by the formula $p_j = \frac{n_j}{N}(100)$ where n_j is the number of strains with the allele «*j*"; and N is the size of the test population.

The *Hunter-Gaston Discrimination Index* [21] measures the power of discrimination for a typing method by calculating the probability that two unrelated strains will be correctly assigned to different types. The equation used is

$$DI = 1 - \frac{1}{N(N-1)} \sum_{j=1}^{S} n_j(n_j - 1)$$

where DI is the index of discrimination; N is the size of the test population; s is the total number of alleles per locus or fingerprint patterns in the population, and n_j is the number of isolates with the allele «*j*".

Cluster and molecular evolutionary analyses were conducted using MEGA version 2.1 [22]. A distance matrix was created using pairwise comparison of HOOF-Print genotypes from all of the 103 isolates in the test population. The genetic distance was calculated from the absolute difference in repeat units at each locus, assuming that each incremental change in repeat number represents an equal and independent mutation event. The distance matrix was used to make an unrooted tree using the neighbor-joining method [23].

Statistical analysis of the distribution of alleles by geographic region was done by creating a cross tabulation of each locus into two regions, defined as east or west of the Mississippi River. For the loci that contain a large number of alleles, the alleles were grouped so that no more than four or five groups were compared to make sure that enough data for each locus would be compared. Differences among the data were analyzed using the chi-square test statistic or, in the case of Locus-6, the Fisher's exact test (Table 2). Statistical analyses were performed with the SAS system version 8 (SAS Institute, Cary, N.C.) using the FREQ Procedure based on a sample size of 95. A P value < 0.05 was considered to be significant.

DECLARATIONS

Acknowledgements

We would like to thank Dr. Bruce Wagner of the Centers for Epidemiology and Animal Health, Veterinary Services, Animal and Plant Health Inspection Service, USDA, for his statistical assistance; and Nancy Koster for her technical assistance in this project.

Authors' contributions

DRE isolated, cultivated, harvested and processed most of the bacterial strains used in this study; typed each strain by conventional biotyping methods and compiled the available background information for each isolate. BJB performed the HOOF-Print assay on all strains, determined the genotypes, performed most of the statistical analyses of the data, and wrote the manuscript. Both authors contributed to discussions about the data, read and approved the final manuscript.

REFERENCES

1. Struelens MJ: Consensus guidelines for appropriate use and evaluation of microbial epidemiologic typing systems. Clin Microbiol Infect. 1996, 2: 2-11.
2. Field D, Wills C: Abundant microsatellite polymorphism in *Saccharomyces cerevisiae*, and the different distributions of microsatellites in eight prokaryotes and S. *cerevisiae*, result from strong mutation pressures and a variety of selective forces. Proc Natl Acad Sci USA. 1998, 95: 1647-1652. 10.1073/pnas.95.4.1647.
3. van Belkum A, Scherer S, van Alphen L, Verbrugh H: Short-sequence DNA repeats in prokaryotic genomes. Microbiol Mol Biol Rev. 1998, 62: 275-293.
4. Le Fleche P, Hauck Y, Onteniente L, Prieur A, Denoeud F, Ramisse V, Sylvestre P, Benson G, Ramisse F, Vergnaud G: A tandem repeats database for bacterial genomes: application to the genotyping of *Yersinia pestis* and *Bacillus anthracis*. BMC Microbiol. 2001, 1: 2-10.1186/1471-2180-1-2. Epub 2001 Mar 30
5. Levinson G, Gutman GA: Slipped-strand mispairing: A major mechanism for DNA sequence evolution. Mol Biol Evol. 1987, 4: 203-221.
6. Paques F, Leung W-Y, Haber JE: Expansions and contractions in a tandem repeat induced by double-strand break repair. Mol Cell Biol . 1998, 18: 2045-2054.
7. Brinkmann B, Klintschar M, Neuhuber F, Huhne J, Rolf B: Mutation rate in human microsatellites: influence of the structure and length of the tandem repeat. Am J Hum Genet. 1998, 62: 1408-1415. 10.1086/301869.
8. van Belkum A: The role of short sequence repeats in epidemiologic typing. Curr Opin Microbiol. 1999, 2: 306-311. 10.1016/S1369-5274(99)80053-8.
9. Keim P, Klevytska AM, Price LB, Schupp JM, Zinser G, Smith KL, Hugh-Jones ME, Okinaka R, Hill KK, Jackson PJ: Molecular diversity in *Bacillus anthracis*. J Appl Microbiol. 1999, 87: 215-217. 10.1046/j.1365-2672.1999.00873.x.
10. van Belkum A, Scherer S, van Leeuwen W, Willemse D, van Alphen L, Verbrugh H: Variable number of tandem repeats in clinical strains of *Haemophilus influenzae*. Infect Immun. 1997, 65: 5017-5027.
11. Keim P, Price LB, Klevytska AM, Smith KL, Schupp JM, Okinaka R, Jackson PJ, Hugh-Jones ME: Multiple-locus variable-number tandem repeat analysis reveals genetic relationships within *Bacillus anthracis*. J Bacteriol. 2000, 182: 2928-2936. 10.1128/JB.182.10.2928-2936.2000.
12. Klevytska AM, Price LB, Schupp JM, Worsham PL, Wong J, Keim P: Identification and characterization of variable-number tandem repeats in the *Yersinia pestis* genome. J Clin Microbiol. 2001, 39: 3179-3185. 10.1128/JCM.39.9.3179-3185.2001.
13. Johansson A, Goransson I, Larsson P, Sjostedt A: Extensive allelic variation among *Francisella tularensis* strains in a short-sequence tandem repeat region. J Clin Microbiol. 2001, 39: 3140-3146. 10.1128/JCM.39.9.3140-3146.2001.
14. Le Fleche P, Fabre M, Denoeud F, Koeck JL, Vergnaud G: High resolution, on-line identification of strains

from the *Mycobacterium tuberculosis* complex based on tandem repeat typing. BMC Microbiol. 2002, 2: 37-10.1186/1471-2180-2-37.

15. Paulsen IT, Seshadri R, Nelson KE, Eisen JA, Heidelberg JF, Read TD, Dodson RJ, Umayam L, Brinkac LM, Beanan MJ, Daugherty SC, Deboy RT, Durkin AS, Kolonay JF, Madupu R, Nelson WC, Ayodeji B, Kraul M, Shetty J, Malek J, Van Aken SE, Riedmuller S, Tettelin H, Gill SR, White O, Salzberg SL, Hoover DL, Lindler LE, Halling SM, Boyle SM, Fraser CM: The *Brucella suis* genome reveals fundamental similarities between animal and plant pathogens and symbionts. Proc Natl Acad Sci USA. 2002, 99: 13148-13153. 10.1073/pnas.192319099.
16. Alton GG, Jones LM, Pietz DE: Laboratory Techniques in Brucellosis. Monograph Series No 55. 1975, Geneva, Switzerland: World Health Organization, 34-59. 2
17. Bricker BJ, Ewalt DR, Halling SM: *Brucella* 'HOOF-Prints': strain typing by multi-locus analysis of variable number tandem repeats (VNTRs). BMC Microbiol. 2003, 3: 15-10.1186/1471-2180-3-15.
18. DelVecchio VG, Kapatral V, Redkar RJ, Patra G, Mujer C, Los T, Ivanova N, Anderson I, Bhattacharyya A, Lykidis A, Reznik G, Jablonski L, Larsen N, D'Souza M, Bernal A, Mazur M, Goltsman E, Selkov E, Elzer PH, Hagius S, O'Callaghan D, Letesson JJ, Haselkorn R, Kyrpides N, Overbeek R: The genome sequence of the facultative intracellular pathogen *Brucella melitensis*. Proc Natl Acad Sci USA. 2002, 99: 443-448. 10.1073/pnas.221575398.
19. Halling SM, Peterson-Burch BD, Bricker BJ, Zuerner RL, Qing Z, Li L-L, Kapur V, Alt DP, Olsen SC: Completion of the genome sequence of *Brucella abortus* and comparison to the highly similar genomes of *B. melitensis* and *B. suis*. J Bacteriol. 2005, 187: 2715-2726. 10.1128/JB.187.8.2715-2726.2005.
20. Bricker BJ: Molecular diagnostics of animal brucellosis: A re of PCR-based assays and approaches. Brucella molecular and cellular biology. Edited by: Lopez-Goni I, Moriyon, I. 2004, Wymondham, UK: Horizon Bioscience, 25-51.
21. Hunter PR, Gaston MA: Numerical index of the discriminatory ability of typing systems: an application of Simpson's index of diversity. J Clin Microbiol. 1988, 26: 2465-2466.
22. Kumar S, Tamura K, Jakobsen IB, Nei M: MEGA2: molecular evolutionary genetics analysis software. Bioinformatics. 2001, 17: 1244-1245. 10.1093/bioinformatics/17.12.1244.
23. Saitou N, Nei M: The neighbor-joining method: A new method for reconstructing phylogenetic trees. Molec Biol Evol. 1987, 4: 406-425.

SECTION XI: COXIELLA BURNETTI– AGENT OF Q FEVER

CHAPTER 42

SEROLOGICAL AND MOLECULAR EVIDENCE OF Q FEVER IN DOMESTIC RUMINANTS IN BANGLADESH

Md. Arifur Rahman Md. Mahbub Alam Md. Aminul Islam A. K. Fazlul Haque Bhuiyan and A. K. M. Anisur Rahman

INTRODUCTION

Q (for Query) fever is a ubiquitous zoonosis caused by an obligate intracellular bacterium Coxiella (C.) burnetii. It has been reported from all over the world except Antarctica and possibly New Zealand [1, 2]. The primary reservoirs of C. burnetii are cattle, sheep, and goats. However, the infection has been reported in other mammals (humans, cats, dogs, rodents, rabbits, horses, swine, camels, water buffalo, and marine mammals), ticks and other arthropods, birds, fish, and reptiles [3, 4]. The common manifestations of Q fever in ruminants are abortion, stillbirth, premature delivery, and delivery of weak offspring [2]. Indeed these clinical manifestations are usually observed in sheep and goats and Q fever is mostly asymptomatic in cattle. Clinically infected cows may develop infertility, metritis, and mastitis [5].

In humans, Q fever is mostly asymptomatic but may be responsible for acute or chronic disease conditions such as influenza-like illness, pneumonia, hepatitis, meningoencephalitis, myocarditis, endocarditis, and chronic fatigue syndrome in persistently infected patients and may contribute to abortion and stillbirth in pregnant women [2, 6].

Diagnosis of Q fever in animals is based on detection of bacteria, bacterial DNA, or antibodies [7]. Although these bacteria can grow in axenic (host cell-free) media, isolation is time consuming and hazardous for the laboratory workers [8]. In addition, Q fever isolation techniques require a Biosafety Level 3 Laboratory (BSL-3). Mostly, C. burnetii exposure in animals can be screened indirectly by serological tests. The CFT (OIE recommended test) and ELISA (EU recommended test) are the two most commonly used serological tests in this purpose. However, CFT protocol is complex and fails to detect antibodies in sheep or goats [9]. The ELISA is reported to be highly sensitive and specific for the diagnosis of Q fever [10]. Moreover, ELISA can be used to detect antibodies in bulk milk and individual animal serum. The bacterial DNA can be detected by using PCR [11]. Although Q fever is present worldwide, its status in animals, humans, arthropods, birds, wild animals, and other reservoirs in Bangladesh is not known except one report on serological evidence in cattle and goats [12]. Nevertheless, the reproductive diseases in dairy cattle [13–15] are endemic in Bangladesh. So the objectives of this paper are to determine the herd level prevalence of Q fever in dairy cattle and goats, to estimate the animal level prevalence of Q fever in cattle, sheep, and goats originated from herds having previous history of abortion, and to detect C. burnetii DNA from aborted fetal membranes of cattle, goat, and sheep.

MATERIALS AND METHODS

Milk Samples

This study used milk samples from two previous studies, which were undertaken in the Department of Medicine, BAU, Mymensingh 2202. In one study, 399 randomly collected bulk milk samples were examined for somatic cell count from where 94 samples were used in this study. The history of reproductive failure in the selected dairy herds was not known. In another study, 17 milk ring test positive samples were sent to Belgium for isolation of Brucella spp., which were also used for this study. The districts of Bangladesh included in this study are shown in Figure 1.

Citation: Md. Arifur Rahman, Md. Mahbub Alam, Md. Aminul Islam, A. K. Fazlul Haque Bhuiyan, and A. K. M. Anisur Rahman, "Serological and Molecular Evidence of Q Fever in Domestic Ruminants in Bangladesh," Veterinary Medicine International, vol. 2016, Article ID 9098416, 7 pages, 2016. doi:10.1155/2016/9098416.

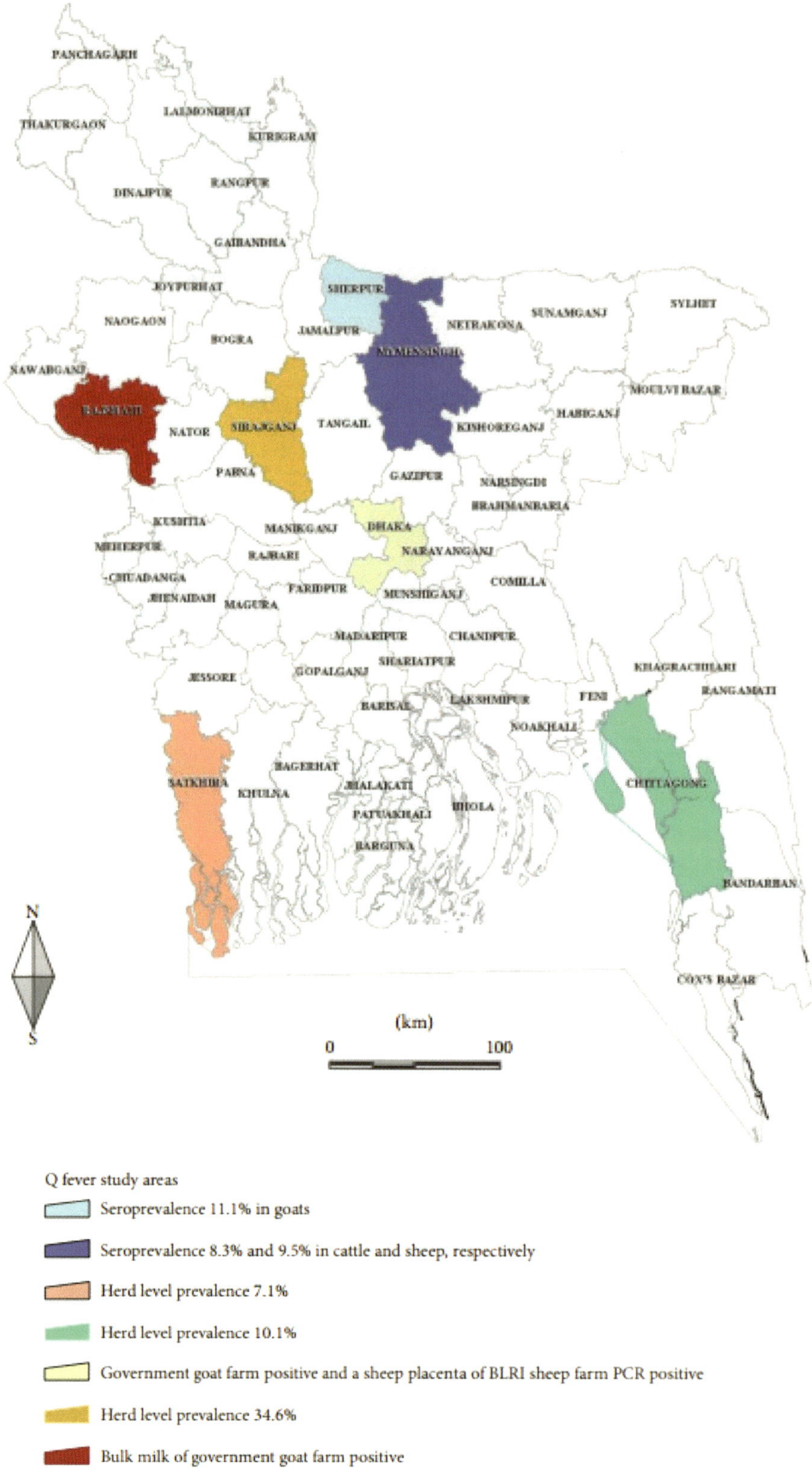

Figure 1

Serum Sample Collection

Serum samples were collected from a serum bank in the Department of Medicine, BAU, Mymensingh. Those samples were randomly collected to study brucellosis in cattle, sheep, and goats in different districts of Bangladesh in 2007 and 2008 [16]. Ninety-four (94) serum samples were collected from 40 herds of the Mymensingh and Sherpur Districts out of 58 having some abortion (known from the owners) in the last year.

DNA Samples of Placentas

Twenty-three DNA samples (5 from cattle, 10 from goats, and 8 from sheep) extracted from aborted fetal membranes for the detection of Brucella spp. were also used in this study. DNA was extracted using the DNeasy spin column kit (QIAGEN) according to the manufacturer's protocol.

Herd and Animal Level Data Collection

Animal level data on age, breed, sex, and pregnancy status and herd level data on herd size, herd composition, and location of the herd were collected from available database of serum samples.

For milk samples, the location of the farm and number of lactating cows in herd were collected from the bovine mastitis database.

Indirect ELISA Test

Preparation of Milk and Sera Samples

The milk and sera samples were prepared according to the instructions of commercial kit. In brief, 10 milliliters of milk from each selected herd was collected for testing antibody against C. burnetii exposure. The samples were centrifuged and the nonfat fraction was stored at −20°C until tested for antibodies against C. burnetii. Before testing, herd milk samples were prepared at 1 : 5 dilution using diluted (1 : 10) wash solution. Sera of the selected animals were removed from the serum bank and prepared at 1 : 400 dilution by using diluted wash solution.

Test Procedure

All reagents were taken into 18–26°C before use. The reagents were mixed by shaking gently. All samples were tested in duplicate and the optical densities (OD) of the samples were averaged and corrected by subtracting the OD of the negative control. Both milk and serum based tests were performed using the commercial CHEKIT Q Fever Antibody ELISA Test Kit (IDEXX, Liebefeld-Bern, Switzerland) based on C. burnetii inactivated phase 1 and phase 2 antigens [10]. The positive cut-off value (S/P ratio) of iELISA in bulk milk and individual animal sera was ≥30% and ≥40%, respectively.

Real Time PCR

The real time (rt) PCR assay was performed using a 7500 rt PCR System (Applied Biosystems). Samples were considered positive with a cycle threshold (Ct) < 40 [17]. It was performed in Veterinary Agrochemical Research Centre (CODA-CERVA) in Brussels, Belgium.

Statistical Analysis

The association of herd and animal level factors with Q fever prevalence was analyzed by χ^2 test using R 3.1.0 (The R Foundation for Statistical Computing 2014).

RESULTS

Descriptive Statistics

The serum samples were collected from 40 herds where there was history of abortion in any of the three domestic ruminant species in the last year. The herd size varied from 1 to 20 with a median of 3 animals. Thirteen herds consisted of only cattle, 13 of only goats, 8 of both cattle and goats, and 6 of only sheep. In 55.0% (22/40) herd's aborted materials were disposed by burial but in the rest of the herds the materials were thrown away in the field or in nearby water bodies. About 35% (14/40) farmers were found to keep sheep (7.5%) or goats (27.5%) inside their house at night.

The age of cattle varied from 4 months to 12 years with a median of 6 years. The range and median age of goats and sheep, respectively, were 2.5 months to 4 years and 2 years, 1 month to 4 years and 8 months. Among cattle 82.0% were female and indigenous and all of the sheep were indigenous and 74.2% of them were female but 80.0% and 94.0% goats were female and Black Bengal breed type, respectively. The range of positive S/P value in cattle herds was 41.4 to 123.0.

Herd Level Prevalence of Q Fever in Dairy Cattle

A summary of ELISA test results on the presence of C. burnetii antibodies in herd milk is presented in Table 1. An overall herd level prevalence of Q fever in dairy cattle was 15.6% (95% Confidence Interval (CI): 9.4–23.8) (Table 1). The distribution of Q fever in dairy herds is shown in Table 2. The prevalence of Q fever was significantly higher in Sirajganj (34.6%) in comparison to Satkhira District (P<0.01). Although statistically insignificant, the prevalence of Q fever was relatively higher in herds having only Friesian cross (13.7%) and both Sahiwal and Friesian breed together (27.8%) in comparison to Sahiwal cross.

Table 1: Summary of iELISA tests results on the presence of Coxiella burnetii antibodies (S/P values) in milk samples

Test result	Number of herds/flocks	Apparent prevalence	95% CI	Range of S/P values (%)	Mean S/P values (%)
Positive (S/P ≥ 30%)	17 (cattle)	15.6%	9.4–23.8	41.4–123.0	81.3
Negative (S/P < 30%)	92	84.4%	76.2–90.6	0–25.9	5.6
Positive (S/P ≥ 30%)	2 (goats)*			421.6 and 424.2	

*Both goat flocks were positive; CI: Confidence Interval.

Table 2: Distribution of herd level prevalence of Q fever based on iELISA using bulk milk

Variable	Tested	Positive (>40%)	Prevalence	95% CI	χ^2 test P value
District					<0.01
Satkhira	28	2	7.1	0.9–23.5	
Chittagong	55	6	10.9	4.1–22.2	
Sirajganj	26	9	34.6	17.2–55.6	
Number of lactating cows					1
>5	22	3	13.6	2.9–34.9	
1 to 5	87	14	16.1	9.1–15.5	
Breed composition					0.29
Sahiwal cross	18	2	11.1	1.4–34.7	
Friesian cross	73	10	13.7	6.8–23.8	
Both	18	5	27.8	9.7–53.5	

The other two bulk milk samples were collected from two government goat farms in Savar, Dhaka, and Rajshahi Districts; CI: Confidence Interval

Seroprevalence of Q Fever in Cattle, Goats, and Sheep

The summary of ELISA test results on the presence of C. burnetii antibodies in serum samples is provided in Table 3. Out of 94 sera samples tested, the ages of 15 (10 sheep and 5 goats) animals were below six months (two seropositive sheep), which were excluded from the result in estimating seroprevalence (maternal immunity). The overall seroprevalence of Q fever in domestic ruminants was 5.06% (95% CI: 1.63–13.14). Three point seven nine percent (3.79%) sera samples were Q fever suspect and 91.13% were Q fever negative. The range of positive S/P value was 42.70 to 49.80%. The distribution of Q fever seroprevalence in domestic ruminants is shown in Table 4. The seroprevalence of Q fever was found to be higher in sheep (9.52%, 95% CI: 1.67–31.83) in comparison to goat (3.33%, 95% CI: 0.17–19.05) and cattle (3.57%, 95% CI: 0.18–20.24) but it was statistically insignificant. The seroprevalence of Q fever varied according to sex, pregnancy status, and study areas but none was significant statistically.

Table 3: Summary of iELISA tests results on the presence of Coxiella burnetii antibodies (S/P values) in serum samples

Test result	Number	Prevalence (%)	95% Confidence Interval	Range of S/P values (%)	Mean S/P values (%)
Positive (S/P ≥ 40%)	4	5.06	1.63–13.14	42.70–49.80	45.35
Suspect (30% ≤ S/P < 40%)	3	3.79	0.98–11.45	30.10–34.50	32.40
Negative (S/P < 30%)	72	91.13	82.04–96.06	0–29.80	5.13

Table 4: The distribution of seroprevalence of Q fever in domestic ruminants

Variable	Tested	Positive	Prevalence (95% CI)	χ^2 test P value
Species				0.55
Cattle	28	1	3.57 (0.18–20.24)	
Sheep	21	2	9.52 (1.67–31.83)	
Goats	30	1	3.33 (0.17–19.05)	
Sex				1.00
Male	15	1	6.67 (0.34–33.96)	
Female	64	3	4.69 (1.22–13.96)	
Pregnancy				0.63
No	38	1	2.63 (0.14–15.43)	
Yes	26	2	7.69 (1.34–26.59)	
Male	15	1	6.67 (0.34–33.96)	
District				1.00
Sherpur	25	1	4.0 (0.21–22.32)	
Cattle	16	0	0 (0–24.07*)	
Sheep	0	0		
Goats	9	1	11.11 (0.58–49.33)	
Mymensingh	54	3	5.56 (1.44–16.34)	
Cattle	12	1	8.33 (0.44–40.25)	
Sheep	21	2	9.52 (1.67–31.83)	
Goats	21	0	0 (0–19.24*)	

CI: Confidence Interval; *97.5% Confidence Interval.

The demographic characteristics of the four Q fever seropositive domestic ruminants are shown in Table 5. Both seropositive sheep were from the same location (Unions/Sub-Upazila of Mymensingh Sadar Upazila/subdistrict).

Table 5: Characteristics of the four Q fever seropositive domestic ruminants

Farmer ID	Area	Species	Age	Breed	Sex	Body weight	S/P value (%)
Fa 50	Sirta, Mymensingh Sadar	Cattle	6 years	Indigenous	Female	200	42.7
Fa 268	Noyabil, Sherpur	Goat	1 year	Black Bengal	Female	6	49.8
Fa 543	Buror Chor, Mymensingh Sadar	Sheep	10 months	Indigenous	Male entire	12	43.4
Fa 548	Buror Chor, Mymensingh Sadar	Sheep	1.5 years	Indigenous	Female	18	45.5

Real Time PCR Result

Coxiella burnetii DNA was detected from only one sheep placenta. The remaining 22 samples were negative.

DISCUSSION

In this study the herd level prevalence of Q fever in cattle based on bulk milk and animal level seroprevalence of Q fever in cattle, goats, and sheep were estimated by using indirect ELISA test. The overall prevalence of Q fever in bulk cow milk was 15.6% indicating that Q fever is an existing disease in dairy cattle population in Bangladesh. The herds under study were originated from major milk pockets of Bangladesh like Sirajganj, Chittagong, and Satkhira Districts (Figure 1). The sample size was very small and the sample does not represent the dairy herds of Bangladesh. It was also a limitation of this study. Due to the lack of fund it was not possible to include more samples in this study. So the herd level prevalence of Q fever we obtained may not represent the true status of this disease in dairy herds of the study areas. A widely variable and much higher herd level prevalence of Q fever (57.8 to 78.6%) was reported from different corners of the world [18–21]. Dairy cattle are usually chronically infected with Q fever and shed C. burnetii in the milk [22]. It is also stated that chronically infected dairy cattle are the most important source of human infection [1]. Another important source of human infection is the manipulation of fetus and its fluids and placentas from aborted small ruminants without safety protection measures. As Q fever is a zoonosis and it exists in animals of Bangladesh it is also supposed to be present in humans. Due to lack of reporting, awareness, and nonspecific influenza-like symptoms of this disease in humans, it may be overlooked and remained undiagnosed in human diagnostic laboratories. Due to lack of reporting from animals, the physicians are also unaware about this disease in humans. As a result, physicians usually do not refer flu-like cases for Q fever diagnosis. Both in humans and in animals, inhalation of bacteria present in the environment is the main route of infection. So dairy workers, animal caretakers, and pyrexia of unknown origin cases should be regularly tested for Q fever. Moreover, consumption of contaminated raw milk may produce infection in humans [1]. Indeed, the Bangladeshi population seldom ingests the raw milk.

We have tested only bulk milk, which does not allow identification of individual cows infected with Q fever. However, it is very useful for screening herds under disease surveillance system. A large epidemiologic study including representative dairy herds of Bangladesh will help to reveal the herd level status of this disease in Bangladesh. Out of three study areas, significantly higher prevalence of Q fever was found in dairy herds of Sirajganj than Satkhira District. The cattle management system in Sirajganj area slightly varies from that of other parts of Bangladesh. In the dry season, the cattle graze freely and remain in the pasture ("Bathan") for almost six months (December to May). As a result, a lot of intermingling among cattle of different owners occurs during that period. Intermixing of cattle from different owners may facilitate the transmission of infection in dairy cattle herds of this area. In some herd, presence of sheep is also noticed in that period. Environment conditions in dry season could play a role in the survival of the bacteria and facilitate the transmission between animals as well. Similarly, higher prevalence of Q fever in loose housing system was also reported by Paul et al. [10]. Capuano et al. [23] also reported relatively higher seroprevalence of Q fever in herds housed in winter but turned out in spring than those housed permanently. Like other infectious diseases, Q fever was reported to be significantly associated with increased herd size [23, 24]. In this study, the prevalence of Q fever in contrast was a bit higher in smaller herds. However, the difference was not significant statistically. The prevalence of Q fever was relatively higher in herds having Friesian cross and in herd containing both Sahiwal and Friesian breed together although the difference was not significant statistically. Other authors had also reported significantly higher level of Q fever prevalence in Holstein breed [10, 23].

We have observed relatively higher seroprevalence of Q fever in sheep than cattle and goats. Similar observations were also reported by other authors [25, 26]. The prevalence of Q fever was reported to be significantly higher with the age of the animals [27–29]. We have also observed that the age of the seropositive animals is ≥10 months.

In our study, serum samples of the animals were originated from herds where there was history of abortion in previous year. Out of four seropositive cases two were in sheep indicating that Q fever might have some role in sheep abortion. Our rt PCR result also supports this hypothesis. An rt PCR Q fever positive result in the placenta means a contact with the bacteria. To confirm an abortion caused by Coxiella burnetii is necessary to detect histopathology lesions in the aborted fetus and placenta. Significantly higher seroprevalence of Q fever in sheep had also been reported by Berri et al. [30]. The immunosuppressive effects of pregnancy may be responsible for the increased multiplication of the organism in the placenta and thereby the higher seroprevalence [31].

It is revealed from this study that Q fever is present in all of the three important domestic ruminant species in Bangladesh. It may have some role in sheep abortion as the seroprevalence is relatively higher and one sheep placenta is rt PCR positive.

ACKNOWLEDGMENTS

This research work was funded by the Seed Bull Production Project (SPGR fund) in the Department of Animal Breeding and Genetics, BAU, and the NST Authority. The authors are grateful to Professor Dr. Md. Taohidul Islam, Department of Medicine, BAU, Mymensingh, for providing bulk milk samples and to Dr. David Fretin of Veterinary Agrochemical Research Centre, Brussels, Belgium, for the support on real time PCR.

REFERENCES

1. M. Maurin and D. Raoult, "Q fever," Clinical Microbiology Reviews, vol. 12, no. 4, pp. 518–553, 1999.
2. E. Angelakis and D. Raoult, "Q fever," Veterinary Microbiology, vol. 140, no. 3-4, pp. 297–309, 2010.
3. B. Babudieri, "Q fever: a zoonosis," Advances in Veterinary Science, vol. 5, pp. 81–182, 1959.
4. S. R. Porter, G. Czaplicki, J. Mainil, R. Guattéo, and C. Saegerman, "Q fever: current state of knowledge and perspectives of research of a neglected zoonosis,"

International Journal of Microbiology, vol. 2011, Article ID 248418, 22 pages, 2011.

5. H. To, K. K. Htwe, N. Kako et al., "Prevalence of Coxiella burnetii infection in dairy cattle with reproductive disorders," Journal of Veterinary Medical Science, vol. 60, no. 7, pp. 859–861, 1998.
6. M. J. Wildman, E. G. Smith, J. Groves, J. M. Beattie, E. O. Caul, and J. G. Ayres, "Chronic fatigue following infection by Coxiella burnetii (Q fever): ten-year follow-up of the 1989 UK outbreak cohort," Quarterly Journal of Medicine, vol. 95, no. 8, pp. 527–538, 2002.
7. A. Rodolakis, "Q fever, state of art: epidemiology, diagnosis and prophylaxis," Small Ruminant Research, vol. 62, no. 1-2, pp. 121–124, 2006.
8. A. Omsland, T. Hackstadt, and R. A. Heinzen, "Bringing culture to the uncultured: Coxiella burnetii and lessons for obligate intracellular bacterial pathogens," PLoS Pathogens, vol. 9, no. 9, Article ID e1003540, 2013.
9. E. Kováčová, J. Kazár, and A. Šimková, "Clinical and serological analysis of a Q fever outbreak in western Slovakia with four-year follow-up," European Journal of Clinical Microbiology and Infectious Diseases, vol. 17, no. 12, pp. 867–869, 1998.
10. S. Paul, J. F. Agger, B. Markussen, A.-B. Christoffersen, and J. S. Agerholm, "Factors associated with Coxiella burnetii antibody positivity in Danish dairy cows," Preventive Veterinary Medicine, vol. 107, no. 1-2, pp. 57–64, 2012.
11. E. Rousset, V. Duquesne, P. Russo, and M. F. Aubert, "Q fever," in Manual of Diagnostic Tests and Vaccines for Terrestrial Animals, World Organisation for Animal Health (OIE), Paris, France, 2010.
12. N. Haider, M. S. Rahman, S. U. Khan et al., "Serological evidence of Coxiella burnetii infection in cattle and goats in Bangladesh," EcoHealth, vol. 12, no. 2, pp. 354–358, 2015.
13. M. A. S. Talukder, M. A. M. Y. Khandoker, M. G. M. Rahman, M. R. Islam, and M. A. A. Khan, "Reproductive problems of cow at Bangladesh Agricultural University Dairy Farm and possible remedies," Pakistan Journal of Biological Sciences, vol. 8, pp. 1561–1567, 2005.
14. A. Khair, M. M. Alam, A. K. M. A. Rahman, M. T. Islam, A. Azim, and E. H. Chowdhury, "Incidence of reproductive and production diseases of cross-bred dairy cattle in Bangladesh," Bangladesh Journal of Veterinary Medicine, vol. 11, no. 1, pp. 31–36, 2014.
15. M. A. S. Sarker, M. Aktaruzzaman, A. K. M. A. Rahman, and M. S. Rahman, "Retrospective study of clinical diseases and disorders of cattle in Sirajganj district in Bangladesh," Bangladesh Journal of Veterinary Medicine, vol. 11, no. 2, pp. 137–144, 2014.
16. A. K. M. A. Rahman, C. Saegerman, D. Berkvens et al., "Bayesian estimation of true prevalence, sensitivity and specificity of indirect ELISA, Rose Bengal Test and Slow Agglutination Test for the diagnosis of brucellosis in sheep and goats in Bangladesh," Preventive Veterinary Medicine, vol. 110, no. 2, pp. 242–252, 2013.
17. S. Boarbi, M. Mori, E. Rousset, K. Sidi-Boumedine, M. Van Esbroeck, and D. Fretin, "Prevalence and molecular typing of Coxiella burnetii in bulk tank milk in Belgian dairy goats, 2009–2013," Veterinary Microbiology, vol. 170, no. 1-2, pp. 117–124, 2014.
18. J. F. Agger, A.-B. Christoffersen, E. Rattenborg, J. Nielsen, and J. S. Agerholm, "Prevalence of Coxiella burnetii antibodies in Danish dairy herds," Acta Veterinaria Scandinavica, vol. 52, article 5, 2010.
19. J. Muskens, E. Van Engelen, C. Van Maanen, C. Bartels, and T. J. G. M. Lam, "Prevalence of Coxiella burnetii infection in Dutch dairy herds based on testing bulk tank milk and individual samples by PCR and ELISA," Veterinary Record, vol. 168, no. 3, p. 79, 2011. ·
20. G. Czaplicki, J.-Y. Houtain, C. Mullender et al., "Apparent prevalence of antibodies to Coxiella burnetii (Q fever) in bulk tank milk from dairy herds in southern Belgium," The Veterinary Journal, vol. 192, no. 3, pp. 529–531, 2012.
21. I. Astobiza, F. Ruiz-Fons, A. Piñero, J. F. Barandika, A. Hurtado, and A. L. García-Pérez, "Estimation of Coxiella burnetii prevalence in dairy cattle in intensive systems by serological and molecular analyses of bulk-tank milk samples," Journal of Dairy Science, vol. 95, no. 4, pp. 1632–1638, 2012. ·
22. G. H. Lang, "Q fever: an emerging public health concern in Canada," Canadian Journal of Veterinary Research, vol. 53, no. 1, pp. 1–6, 1989.
23. F. Capuano, M. C. Landolfi, and D. M. Monetti, "Influence of three types of farm management on the seroprevalence of Q fever as assessed by an indirect immunofluorescence assay," Veterinary Record, vol. 149, no. 22, pp. 669–671, 2001.
24. E. D. Ryan, M. Kirby, D. M. Collins, R. Sayers, J. F. Mee, and T. Clegg, "Prevalence of Coxiella burnetii (Q fever) antibodies in bovine serum and bulk-milk samples," Epidemiology and Infection, vol. 139, no. 9, pp. 1413–1417, 2011.
25. M. Khalili and E. Sakhaee, "An update on a serologic survey of Q fever in domestic animals in Iran," The American Journal of Tropical Medicine and Hygiene, vol. 80, no. 6, pp. 1031–1032, 2009.
26. F. Ruiz-Fons, I. Astobiza, J. F. Barandika et al., "Seroepidemiological study of Q fever in domestic ruminants in semi-extensive grazing systems," BMC Veterinary Research, vol. 6, article 3, 2010.
27. A. L. García-Pérez, I. Astobiza, J. F. Barandika, R. Atxaerandio, A. Hurtado, and R. A. Juste, "Short communication: investigation of Coxiella burnetii occurrence in dairy sheep flocks by bulk-tank milk analysis and antibody level determination," Journal of Dairy Science, vol. 92, no. 4, pp. 1581–1584, 2009.
28. E. Kennerman, E. Rousset, E. Gölcü, and P. Dufour, "Seroprevalence of Q fever (coxiellosis) in sheep from the Southern Marmara region, Turkey," Comparative Immunology, Microbiology and Infectious Diseases, vol. 33, no. 1, pp. 37–45, 2010.
29. S. Esmaeili, F. B. Amiri, and E. Mostafavi, "Seroprevalence survey of Q fever among sheep in northwestern Iran," Vector-Borne and Zoonotic Diseases, vol. 14, no. 3, pp. 189–192, 2014.

30. M. Berri, A. Souriau, M. Crosby, and A. Rodolakis, "Shedding of Coxiella burnetii in ewes in two pregnancies following an episode of Coxiella abortion in a sheep flock," Veterinary Microbiology, vol. 85, no. 1, pp. 55–60, 2002.

31. K. Polydorou, "Q fever in Cyprus: a short review," The British Veterinary Journal, vol. 137, no. 5, pp. 470–477, 1981.

CHAPTER 43

PREVALENCE OF COXIELLA BURNETII IN CLINICALLY HEALTHY GERMAN SHEEP FLOCKS

Angela Hilbert, Gernot Schmoock, Hannah Lenzko, Udo Moog, Roland Diller, Andreas Fröhlich, Lothar Hoffmann, Steffen Horner, Michael Elschner, Herbert Tomaso, Klaus Henning, Heinrich Neubauer and Lisa D Sprague

Keywords: *Coxiella (C.) burnetii,* Zoonosis, Sheep, Prevalence

BACKGROUND

C. burnetii is an obligate intracellular bacterial pathogen and the causative agent of Q- fever, a worldwide occurring zoonosis, and notifiable disease in many countries including Germany. The organism is very resistant and can persist in the environment in a spore-like state for weeks; once airborne it can be transported long distances by the wind [1, 2, 3]. Numerous species including dogs, cats, birds, arthropods, and wildlife can harbour the agent, however, cattle, sheep, and goats are considered to be the main reservoir [4]. Infection in animals is mostly subclinical or inapparent but can occasionally lead to abortions or birth of weak offspring. During parturition, large numbers of the organism are shed into the birth fluids, but smaller amounts can also be found in milk, faeces, and urine [5]. Transmission to humans occurs mainly via inhalation of fomites, seldom through ingestion of contaminated raw milk, and very rarely via person-to-person contact [4]. In humans, disease ranges from asymptomatic to severe and can be fatal. The clinical picture presents itself with fever or influenza-like illness. Pneumonia, hepatitis, meningoencephalitis, myocarditis, and pericarditis can occur as life-threatening complications. Infection in early pregnancy can lead to abortion and in later stages of pregnancy to premature labour [6].

According to the Federal Statistical Office, there are approx. 2.35 million sheep in Germany. Despite the gradual decline in the German sheep population and falls in the price of wool over the past years, foodstuffs obtained from sheep (i.e. meat and milk) are enjoying an increase in popularity. In the state of Thuringia, the stock of sheep amounts to nearly 190.000 and serves not only as a source of meat and milk, but also plays an important role in landscape management and nature conservation. The sheep are distributed among approx. 6300 flocks of which 252 contain more than 100 ewes. Although several German studies describing the seroprevalence of *C. burnetii* in sheep during outbreaks of Q-fever exist [7, 8, 9], no current prevalence data are available. Moreover, seroprevalence studies in asymptomatic, i.e. clinically healthy flocks, and in flocks with prevailing infections are missing, making risk assessment and the implementation of counteractive measures and regulations difficult.

Accordingly, the aim of this study was to estimate the sero- and antigen prevalence of *C. burnetii* at flock level among clinically healthy non-vaccinated sheep flocks using the state of Thuringia as a model example.

RESULTS

Serology

Based on the sensitivity and specificity of the used test of 100% a flock was considered sero-positive if at least one animal tested positive in the ELISA. Of the 39 evaluated flocks with more than 100 ewes, 11 were serologically positive (28%; Table 1). The exact 95% confidence interval for the flock-level prevalence was estimated as 15-45%.

Citation: Angela Hilbert, Gernot Schmoock, Hannah Lenzko, Udo Moog, Roland Diller, Andreas Fröhlich, Lothar Hoffmann, Steffen Horner, Michael Elschner, Herbert Tomaso, Klaus Henning, Heinrich Neubauer and Lisa D Sprague, Prevalence of Coxiella burnetii in clinically healthy German sheep flocks, DOI: 10.1186/1756-0500-5-152.

Table 1: Summary of flocks, collected -, positive serum-, and DNA (PCR positive) samples

			# positive samples vs. # of samples taken					
flock #	**flock size (ewes)**	**abortion rate (%)[§]**	**serum**		**vaginal swab**	**rectal swab**	**afterbirth**	**foetus/foetal swab**
1	500	0	**1/28**	0/11	0/11	0/11	-	-
2	1000	0	0/29	0/11	0/11	0/11	0/9	-
3	1800	< 1	**4/29**	**2/11**	0/11	0/11	0/11	-
4	1300	0	0/29	0/11	0/11	0/11	-	-
5	1200	3	**4/29**	**3/11**	0/11	0/11	0/3	0/4
6	500	0	0/29	0/11	0/11	0/11	-	-
7	450	0	0/29	0/11	0/11	0/11	0/9	-
8	1100	< 1	**3/30**	**1/11**	0/11	0/11	-	-
9	1800	0	**1/29**	0/11	0/11	0/11	-	-
10	550	0	**4/29**	**2/11**	0/11	0/11	0/3	-
11	700	< 1	**2/29**	**2/11**	0/11	0/11	-	-
12	330	0	0/30	0/11	0/11	0/11	0/2	-
13*	2500	2	**6/30**	**1/11**	**11/11**	**11/11**	**7/11****	-
14	400	< 1	0/29	0/11	0/11	0/11	-	-
15	700	< 1	0/29	0/11	0/11	0/11	-	-
16	750	< 1	0/29	0/11	0/11	0/11	-	-
17	900	< 1	0/29	0/11	0/11	0/11	0/3	0/2
18	250	< 1	0/29	0/11	0/11	0/11	-	-
19	450	< 1	0/29	0/11	0/11	0/11	0/1	-
20	1000	< 1	0/29	0/11	0/11	0/11	-	-
21	500	< 1	0/29	0/11	0/11	0/11	-	-
22	406	< 1	0/29	0/11	0/11	0/11	-	-
23	700	< 1	**3/29**	**2/11**	0/11	0/11	-	-
24	700	0	0/29	0/11	0/11	0/11	-	-
25	550	< 1	**5/29**	**1/11**	0/11	0/11	-	-
26	1000	1	0/29	0/11	0/11	0/11	-	-
27	317	< 1	0/29	0/11	0/11	0/11	-	-
28	350	6	0/29	0/11	0/11	0/11	0/1	-
29	420	0	0/29	0/11	0/11	0/11	-	-
30	1178	< 1	0/29	0/11	0/11	0/11	-	-
31	500	< 1	0/29	0/11	0/11	0/11	-	-
32	120	0	0/29	0/11	0/11	0/11	0/4	-
33	115	< 1	**17/29**	**6/11**	**1/11**	**1/11**	-	-
34	400	< 1	0/29	0/11	0/11	0/11	0/1	-
35	650	< 1	0/29	0/11	0/11	0/11	-	-
36	133	0	0/29	0/11	0/11	0/11	-	-
37	377	< 1	0/29	0/11	0/11	0/11	0/2	-
38	409	< 1	0/29	0/11	0/11	0/11	-	-
39[&]	25	0	25		11	11	-	-
40	460	< 1	0/29	0/11	0/11	0/11	-	-
total			**1158**		**440**	**440**	**71**	**6**

[§]according to farmers and Thuringian sheep health authority; *history of *C. burnetii* infection; **7/11 DNA positive, from 3/7 isolation of *C. burnetii;* - no samples; [&]excluded from study

Isolation of *C. burnetii*

C. burnetii was isolated and propagated from nine afterbirths acquired from flock 13. Three of these isolates were obtained from samples collected during the prevalence study in May 2009 (Table 1), one isolate was obtained from a sample collected before initiation of the study, and the remaining five isolates originated from additional samples collected in June 2009 (Table 2).

Table 2: Additional samples collected in flocks 3, 13 and 33 (analysed by ELISA or PCR)

			# positive samples vs. # of samples taken				
flock # date	**flock size (ewes)**	**abortion rate (%)**	**serum**	**vaginal swab**	**rectal swab**	**afterbirth**	**foetus/foetal swab**
3 (01/2010)	1800	< 1	1/34	0/11	0/11	0/5	0/8
13							
(07/2005)		-	-	1/51	-	-	-
(12/2005)		-	-	-	-	-	1/14
(01/2008)	2500	-	-	-	-	0/18	-
(04/2008)		2	-	-	-	2/34*	-
(05/2009)		-	1/6	-	-	8/19*	0/1
(06/2009)		-	-	-	-	18/24*	-
(07/2010)		-	-	-	-	0/58	-
(03/2011)		-	-	0/107	-	-	-
33							
(02/2010)	115	< 1	42/89	5/26	-	-	-
(07/2010)		-	-	-	-	0/11	-

- no samples; *1/34 *C. burnetii* isolate; *1/19 *C. burnetii* isolate; *4/24 *C. burnetii* isolates

Detection of *C. burnetii* by means of PCR

Based on the specificity and sensitivity of the PCR assay of 100% a flock was considered antigen-positive if at least one animal tested positive in the PCR. *C. burnetii* DNA was detected in two flocks (5%; Table 1). The exact 95% confidence interval for the flock-level prevalence was estimated as 0.6-17%.

Genotyping of *C. burnetii* by means of MLVA and plasmid type determination

In order to investigate the genetic relationship among the isolates obtained from afterbirths collected in flock 13, MLVA were done. These revealed identical VNTR profiles all clustering into the same group (Figure 1). All tested isolates were shown to contain the plasmid QpH1.

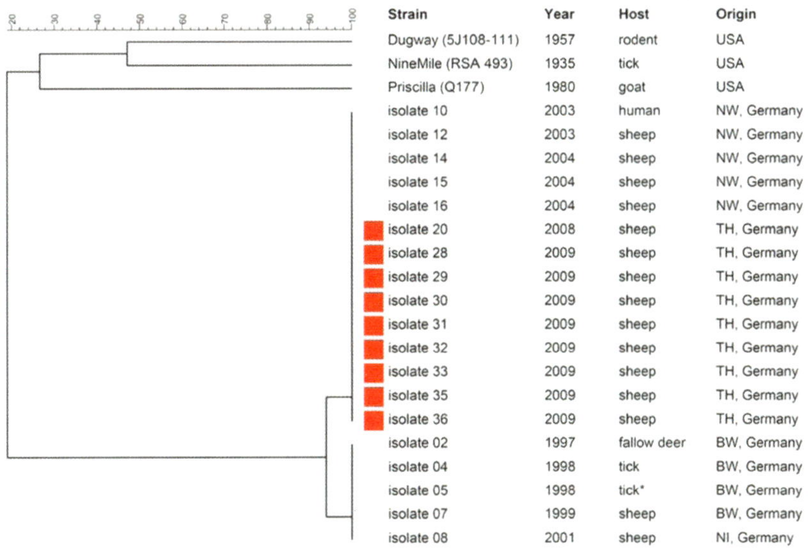

Figure 1:

Phylogenetic tree of German *C. burnetii* isolates on the basis of 17 multilocus variable number of tandem repeat analyses (MLVA).

DISCUSSION

Epidemiological data regarding the distribution of *C. burnetii* in sheep in Germany are scarce and based on data obtained during Q-fever outbreaks [7, 8] and on materials submitted for routine laboratory examination [9]. Data describing the epidemiological situation in clinically inconspicuous flocks and between outbreaks are missing. The present study, therefore, aimed at estimating the sero- and antigen prevalence of *C. burnetii* in randomly chosen non-vaccinated sheep flocks throughout the state of Thuringia with unknown abortion status.

Our study revealed that 28% of the tested flocks were serologically positive. Other studies assessing the seroprevalence of *C. burnetii* in sheep found rates ranging between 1% to 47% in Germany [8, 9, 10], 3% to 22% in Turkey [11, 12], 12% in northern Spain and 31.7% in Gran Canaria [13, 14], 11.8% in southern Italy [15], and up to 73% in Bulgaria [16]. However, the direct comparison of our results with the prevalences found in the above listed studies is problematic, due to considerable differences in study design and evaluation methods (prevalence in single animals vs. flock prevalence), flock size, flock management, abortion rate, number of samples tested and the detection methods applied (CFT, IFAT, competitive ELISA).

We next compared our data with the results obtained from the ovine samples (> 1500) submitted to the German National Reference Laboratory (NRL) for Q-fever. Evaluation of the samples sent to the NRL between August 2007 and July 2010 determined a seroprevalence of 10.8%, which is in agreement with our estimated prevalence value; yet one has to bear in mind that the evaluation of these samples is biased. We also compared our results with those acquired from the contemporaneous Thuringian *Brucella* screening in which the ovine samples were additionally tested for the presence of *C. burnetii* antibodies with the CHEKIT™ Q-fever Test Kit. The screening revealed a seroprevalence of 31% (4/13 flocks) when evaluating the results from the flocks with > 100 ewes which is also in agreement with our results (data not shown). We can not rule out a possible lower sensitivity of the used ELISA due to the fact that it does not use ruminant antigen. However, this particular ELISA is the only one on the "List of certified products pursuant to section 17c Animal Diseases Act" in Germany. Moreover, even if we had found more positive animals within a flock, it would not have had an influence on the flock prevalence. Further positive flocks on the other hand, would have altered the flock prevalence.

Despite the fact that serological screening to test for antibodies against *C. burnetii* is carried out on a regular basis, results should be interpreted with caution. Recent evaluation studies on serum samples obtained from cattle, sheep and goats showed that shedding animals are not always reliably detected; single animals may seroconvert but not shed the agent, whereas others shed the agent without or with delayed production of antibodies [17, 18, 19]. One also has to bear in mind that antibodies may continue to circulate long after the agent has been cleared from the organism [20].

Our PCR analyses detected *C. burnetii* DNA in 5% of the flocks assessed in the study. Recent PCR-based studies identified *C. burnetii* in 9% of tested sheep flocks in northern Spain [21] and in 18.6% of farms with small ruminants in southern Italy [22]. Two further studies on samples obtained from either ovine abortions in Sardinia [23] or ovine foetal organ samples and placentae in Portugal [24] discovered *C. burnetii* in 10.9% and in 36% of the cases, respectively. A Turkish study assessing milk samples collected from 22 flocks determined 6.5% *C. burnetii* positive animals in 12 flocks with a history of abortion and no positives in flocks without a history of abortion [25]. But again, comparison of the data is difficult due to the differences in study design, sampling, and methods applied. However, the evaluation of the *C. burnetii*-tested samples of the contemporaneous Thuringian *Brucella* screening using different sampling criteria, e.g. health status, flock size, etc. revealed an antigen prevalence of 25%, which is in agreement with our estimated prevalence.

Although we found eleven seropositive flocks, only two of the flocks (13, 33) were DNA-positive. Nonetheless, we were able to obtain nine isolates from flock 13 in afterbirths collected between April 2008 and June 2009. All isolates were genetically identical as shown by MLVA and determination of the plasmid type. The QpH1 plasmid, first isolated from a tick [26], has been regularly found in isolates obtained from cattle, sheep, and goats [27]. We were intrigued to find that our nine isolates clustered into the same group as the isolates obtained from sheep and a human isolate linked to a Q-fever outbreak back in 2003 in North Rhine Westphalia [28]. Our findings argue for the circulation of a particular *C. burnetii* strain infecting both man and animal in central Germany, however, more isolates must be tested to corroborate this hypothesis. We did not observe any genetic variations as described in the exceptional Dutch outbreak (2007-2010) [29, 30] in our comparatively small panel, although we used more loci and purified DNA from isolates. It is worthwhile mentioning that *C. burnetii* was already detected back in 2005 in flock 13, indicating the persistence of infection in this flock. However, since no isolates were obtained in 2005 we can not confirm the circulation of one particular strain or exclude re-introduction.

Identification of shedders is central to any eradication or surveillance programme. We believe that monitoring of clinically inconspicuous sheep flocks for the presence of *C. burnetii* infection can be reliably done by analysing the afterbirths. As shown in Table 2, in January 2008, none of the examined afterbirths reacted positive in the PCR assays but by June 2009, 75% of the tested afterbirths were positive. Samples obtained from afterbirths and vaginal swabs taken between July 2010 and March 2011 were again negative. Our observations are in agreement with the findings of others, describing that shedding is not a continuous process [31, 32]. However, it is also possible that the amounts of shed or circulating bacteria might not suffice to maintain an infection cycle. The threshold level of bacteria required to produce a clinically apparent infection in an animal and to what extent virulence of the circulating strain affects infection and clinical presentation are still unknown. Studies assessing possible individual or breed related immunity are also missing.

CONCLUSIONS

Based on the assumed prevalence at flock level, we were able to demonstrate that *C. burnetii* is present in clinically inconspicuous sheep flocks. Although *C. burnetii* infections are not a primary veterinary concern, due to the lack of significant impact on animal health, the zoonotic risk for humans should not be underestimated. Therefore, strategies combining the interests of public and veterinary public health should include the identification and culling of shedders as well as the implementation of protective vaccines.

MATERIALS AND METHODS

Sheep flocks and sampling procedures

The present study was designed as a cross sectional study. Forty unvaccinated flocks (Table 1) distributed throughout the state of Thuringia with more than 100 ewes and an unknown abortion rate, were chosen at random from the given population of 252 flocks. Flocks were kept on pasture, lambing took place in-doors. Based on the reported cases to the German animal disease reporting system, the sample size was calculated as such that with an assumed minimum seroprevalence of 10% and an antigen prevalence of 25% within the flock, at least one infected animal would be detected with 95% confidence under the assumption of 100% sensitivity and specificity of the diagnostic test used [33].

Sera and swabs were collected at random during the lambing seasons by and under the supervision of a veterinarian (UM) from the Thuringian sheep health service during his regular flock management visits between February 2009 to June 2009 (flocks 1-13) and December 2009 to April 2010 (flocks 14-40). In practice, the sampling was carried out as follows: Serum samples were collected from 29 ewes per flock on day 1 or day 2 post partum. For cultivation and PCR assays, one vaginal and one rectal swab were obtained from 11/29 ewes. Afterbirths and foetuses were collected when available. Of the 1281 serum samples, 477 vaginal swabs, 451 rectal swabs, 188 afterbirths and 15 foetuses/foetal/pharyngeal swabs collected, a total of 1158 serum samples, 440 vaginal swabs, 440 rectal swabs, 71 afterbirths and 6 foetuses/foetal swabs from 39 flocks were evaluated (Table 1). Since *Coxiella* and *Chlamydia* spp screening is part of the Thuringian flock management system no ethics approval and consent was necessary [34].

Additional samples (not included in the study) were obtained from flocks 3 (January 2010), 13 (January and April 2008, May and June 2009, and July 2010) and 33 (July 2010) (Table 2).

Sample preparation and conservation

Blood was drawn from the jugular vein with a 14 gauge needle into 7.5 mL serum Monovettes (Kabe GmbH, Nümbrecht-Elsenroth, Germany) and stored upright at RT for 12 h. The Monovettes were then centrifuged at 1500 ×*g* for 10 min, the supernatant serum removed and stored at -20°C until further use. Swabs collected for nucleic acid extraction were transferred to 200 µL lysis buffer [(6 M guanidiumisothiocyanate, 10 mM urea, 20% (v/v) Triton X-100 and 10 mM Tris HCl (pH 4.4))] (Roche Diagnostics, Mannheim, Germany) and stored at 4°C. Afterbirths and organ samples from aborted foetuses were stored at -80°C until further use.

ELISA

Serum samples were tested for the presence of antibodies to *C. burnetii* using the CHECKIT™ Q-fever Test Kit (Idexx GmbH, Liebefeld-Bern, Switzerland) according to the manufacturer's instructions. All measurements were performed in duplicate. Results were normalised using the positive and negative control sera provided in the kit and expressed as percentage of the positive control according to the following formula: [(OD sample - OD negative control)/(OD positive control - OD negative control)] × 100. Sera with values below 30% were considered negative, sera with values between 30 and 40% were considered inconclusive, and sera with values greater 40% were considered as positive.

Cell culture

Propagation and isolation of *C. burnetii* was performed using Buffalo Green Monkey (BGM) cells in UltraCulture medium (Bio Whittaker, Walkersville, USA) supplemented with 1% non essential amino acids (100×), 1% vitamins, and 2 mmol L-glutamine (all Biochrom, Berlin, Germany). Cells were seeded into 25 cm^{2}tissue culture flasks (Greiner Bio-One GmbH, Frickenhausen, Germany) and maintained in a humidified atmosphere with 5% CO_2 at 37°C. The cell monolayers were assessed for confluent growth on the day of inoculation.

Vaginal swabs were rehydrated in 2000 µL of Hank›s medium, centrifuged at 15 000 ×*g* for 10 min at RT, and the resulting pellet resuspended in 1000 µL Hank's medium (Biochrom). Organ samples (approx. 10 g) were mechanically disrupted, homogenised and resuspended in 40 mL Hank's medium. This solution was subsequently filtered through 0.45 - 0.2 µm syringe filters (Minisart, Sartorius, Hannover, Germany). Between 100 µL - 500 µL of the resuspended pellet or the final filtrate was used for inoculation. After 12-24 h, the medium was replaced by fresh UltraCulture medium, also used for further propagation. Cell cultures were monitored weekly by phase contrast microscopy and propagated for up to six months. Specimens that showed intracellular growth of microorganisms were stained according to the method of Giménez [35]. Cultures were regarded as positive when small red inclusions containing coccoid rods were observed.

DNA extraction from samples

DNA from vaginal, rectal, and foetal swabs as well as from foetal organs was isolated using the High Pure PCR Template Preparation Kit™ (Roche Diagnostics) according to the manufacturer's instructions. Organ samples were cut into 50 mg sections, mechanically disrupted and digested over night in 200 µL lysis buffer with 40 µL proteinase K (20 mg/mL) (Roche Diagnostics) at 37°C.

Polymerase chain reaction (PCR)

Conventional PCR

In order to avoid abortive cell cultivation, samples for cultivation were tested beforehand at the National Reference Laboratory for Q-fever in Wusterhausen with a nested PCR method targeting the *com 1* gene encoding a 27 kDa outer membrane protein of *C. burnetii*[36]. Conventional PCR was carried out in a TC-412 Thermocycler (Techne AG, Burkhardtsdorf, Germany). From each PCR reaction, 15 µL were analysed by agarose gel electrophoresis (1.5% w/v in Tris Borate EDTA buffer).

Real-time PCR

Detection of *C. burnetii* was performed with a TaqMan based real-time PCR assay targeting the transposase element IS1111 as described by Klee et al. [37] using a Stratagene Mx3000P Thermocycler (Agilent Technologies, Santa Clara, CA, USA). Tenfold serial dilution of cloned IS1111 gene fragments ranging from 1×10^0 to 1×10^5 plasmid copy numbers were added for *Coxiella* DNA quantification and sensitivity control of the assay. The cycle threshold value (Ct) was calculated by the instrument's software MxPro3000P v 4.01. A negative result was assigned when no amplification occurred or when the cycle threshold value was ≥ 40.

Identification of the plasmid type in the C. burnetii isolates

Identification of the plasmid type of the isolates was done according to a modified procedure described by Zhang et al. [36]. PCR assays were conducted on a MasterCycler ep Thermocycler (Eppendorf, Germany). From each PCR reaction, 5 µL were analysed by agarose gel electrophoresis (1.5% w/v in Tris Borate EDTA buffer).

Genotyping of *C. burnetii* isolates by means of multiple-loci variable number of tandem repeats analysis (MLVA)

Genotyping of the 9 *C. burnetii* isolates obtained from flock 13 was done according to the VNTR method described by Arricau-Bouvery et al. [32] using 17 markers. PCR assays were conducted on a MasterCycler ep Thermocycler (Eppendorf, Germany). Compatible primer pairs were subsequently multiplexed and the forward primer for each pair labelled at the 5'-end with a fluorescent dye (dye set G5, Applied Biosystems). The PCR products were pooled according to their group and diluted 1:100 in LiChrosol water (VWR International, Germany). One µL of this solution was mixed with 13.7 µL Hi-Di formamide and 0.3 µL GeneScan™ 1200 LIZ Size Standard (both Applied Biosystems) for the reproducible sizing of the fragments, denatured for 3 min at 93°C, and cooled on ice. The PCR products were separated in an ABI 3130 Genetic Analyzer (Applied Biosystems) using a 36 cm array and POP7 polymer. Data obtained from the PeakScanner Ver.1.0 (Applied Biosystems) were analysed with the Bionumerics 6.0 software package (Applied Maths). The clustering analysis was based on the categorical coefficient and unweighted pair group method using arithmetic averages (UGPMA).

DECLARATIONS

Acknowledgements

We are greatly indebted to all the sheep farmers who joined the study. We thank Dr. R. Teuscher for his support. We are especially grateful to Prof. M. D. Salman and Prof. M. Greiner for their very helpful comments and suggestions. We appreciate the help of Dr. M. J. Sprague and Dr. C. Bartling for their critical reading of the manuscript. N. Lemser, K. Nitsche, S. Schwarz and R. Wehr, are thanked for their excellent technical assistance.

This study was supported by the German Ministry for Education and Research (BMBF), "Epizootiology of Q-fever in ruminants and wild mammals and differentiating molecular pathogenesis of *Coxiella burnetii* in humans and animals." Grant # 01 KI ts.

Authors' contributions

AH: processed the samples for ELISA and cultivation and evaluated the data. GS: processed the DNA samples for PCR and MLVA and evaluated the data. HL: collected the samples. UM: collected the samples and helped with the contacting of the sheep farmers. RD: designed the study. AF: carried out additional statistics. LH and SH: evaluated the samples from the Thuringian Brucellosis screening for the presence of *C. burnetii*. ME: contributed to the study design. HT: helped with editing the manuscript. KH: helped with the ELISA and cultivation of the *C. burnetii* isolates. HN: contributed to the study design, obtained the funding, contributed to the interpretation of the data, and helped with editing and revision of the manuscript; LDS: contributed to the study design, evaluated the data, drafted, and wrote the manuscript. All authors read and approved the final manuscript.

REFERENCES

1. Tissot-Dupont H, Amadei MA, Nezri M, Raoult D: Wind in November, Q-fever in December. Emerg Infect Dis. 2004, 10: 1264-uloolar
2. Gilsdorf A, Kroh C, Grimm S, Jensen E, Wagner-Wiening C, Alpers K: Large Q-fever outbreak due to sheep farming near residential areas, Germany, 2005. Epidemiol Infect. 2008, 136: 1084-uoolar
3. Wallensten A, Moore P, Webster H, Johnson C, van der Burgt G, Pritchard G, Ellis-Iversen J, Oliver I: Q-fever outbreak in Cheltenham, United Kingdom, in 2007 and the use of dispersion modelling to investigate the possibility of airborne spread. Euro Surveill. 2010, 15 (12): 1oolar
4. Maurin M, Raoult D: Q fever. Clin Microbiol Rev. 1999, 12: 518uoolar
5. Rodolakis A: Q-fever in dairy animals. Ann N Y Acad Sci. 2009, 1166: 90-93. 10.1111/j.1749-6632.2009.045doolar

6. Carcopino X, Raoult D, Bretelle F, Boubli L, Stein A: Q-fever during pregnancy: a cause of poor fetal and maternal outcome. Ann N Y Acad Sci. 2009, 1166: 79-89. 10.1111/j.1749-6632.2009.045doolar

7. Lange S, Klaus G: Seroepidemiological studies on the detection of Q fever in sheep in middle Thuringia. Berl Munch Tierarztl Wochenschr. 1992, 105: 333oolar

8. Lange S, Söllner H, Dittmar H, Hofmann J, Lange A: Q fever antibody titre-follow-up study in cattle with special reference to pregnancy. Berl Munch Tierarztl Wochenschr. 1992, 105: 260oolar

9. Sting R, Breitling N, Oehme R, Kimmig P: The occurrence of *Coxiella burneti* in sheep and ticks of the genus Dermacentor in Baden-Württemberg. Dtsch Tierarztl Wochenschr. 2004, 111: 390oolar

10. Hellenbrand W, Breuer T, Petersen L: Changing epidemiology of Q fever in Germany, 1947-1999. Emerg Infect Dis. 2001, 7: 789-796. 10.3201/eid0705.01uloolar

11. Kilic S, Pasa S, Babur C, Özlem MB: Investigation of Coxiella burnetii antibodies in sheep in Aydin region, Turkey. Rev Med Vet. 2005, 156: 336oolar

12. Kennerman E, Rousset E, Gölcü E, Dufour P: Seroprevalence of Q fever (coxiellosis) in sheep from the Southern Marmara Region, Turkey. Comp Immunol Microbiol Infect Dis. 2010, 33: 37-45. 10.1016/j.cimid.2008.07doolar

13. Ruiz-Fons F, Astobiza I, Barandika JF, Hurtado A, Atxaerandio R, Juste RA, García-Pérez AL: Seroepidemiological study of Q fever in domestic ruminants in semi-extensive grazing systems. BMC Vet Res. 2010, 6: 3-10.1186/1746-6148uloolar

14. Rodríguez NF, Carranza C, Bolaños M, Pérez-Arellano JL, Gutierrez C: Seroprevalence of *Coxiella burneti* in domestic ruminants in Gran Canaria Island, Spain. Transbound Emerg Dis. 2010, 57: 66-67. 10.1111/j.1865-1682.2010.011doolar

15. Capuano F, Parisi A, Cafiero MA, Pitaro L, Fenizia D: *Coxiella burneti*: what is the reality?. Parassitologia. 2004, 46: 131oolar

16. Serbezov VS, Kazár J, Novkirishki V, Gatcheva N, Kovácová E, Voynova V: Q fever in Bulgaria and Slovakia. Emerg Infect Dis. 1999, 5: 388-394. 10.3201/eid0503.99uloolar

17. Guatteo R, Beaudeau F, Berri M, Rodolakis A, Joly A, Seegers H: Shedding routes of *Coxiella burneti* in dairy cows: implications for detection and control. Vet Res. 2006, 37: 827-833. 10.1051/vetres:200doolar

18. Rousset E, Durand B, Berri M, Dufour P, Prigent M, Russo P, Delcroix T, Touratier A, Rodolakis A, Aubert M: Comparative diagnostic potential of three serological tests for abortive Q fever in goat herds. Vet Microbiol. 2007, 124: 286-297. 10.1016/j.vetmic.2007.04doolar

19. Rodolakis A, Berri M, Héchard C, Caudron C, Souriau A, Bodier CC, Blanchard B, Camuset P, Devillechaise P, Natorp JC, Vadet JP, Arricau-Bouvery N: Comparison of *Coxiella burneti* shedding in milk of dairy bovine, caprine, and ovine herds. J Dairy Sci. 2007, 90: 5352-5360. 10.3168/jds.2006doolar

20. Berri M, Souriau A, Crosby M, Rodolakis A: Shedding of *Coxiella burneti* in ewes in two pregnancies following an episode of Coxiella abortion in a sheep flock. Vet Microbiol. 2002, 85: 55-60. 10.1016/S0378-1135(01)004doolar

21. Oporto B, Barandika JF, Hurtado A, Aduriz G, Moreno B, Garcia-Perez AL: Incidence of ovine abortion by *Coxiella burneti*in northern Spain. Ann N Y Acad Sci. 2006, 1078: 498-501. 10.1196/annals.1374doolar

22. Parisi A, Fraccalvieri R, Cafiero M, Miccolupo A, Padalino I, Montagna C, Capuano F, Sottili R: Diagnosis of *Coxiella burneti*-related abortion in Italian domestic ruminants using single-tube nested PCR. Vet Microbiol. 2006, 118: 101-106. 10.1016/j.vetmic.2006.06doolar

23. Masala G, Porcu R, Sanna G, Tanda A, Tola S: Role of *Chlamydophila abortu* in ovine and caprine abortion in Sardinia, Italy. Vet Res Commun. 2005, 29: 117doolar

24. Clemente L, Barahona MJ, Andrade MF, Botelho A: Diagnosis by PCR of *Coxiella burneti* in aborted fetuses of domestic ruminants in Portugal. Vet Rec. 2009, 164: 373-374. 10.1136/vr.164.12doolar

25. Öngör H, Cetinkaya B, Karahan M, Açik MN, Bulut H, Muz A: Detection of *Coxiella burneti* by immunomagnetic separation-PCR in the milk of sheep in Turkey. Vet Rec. 2004, 154: 570-572. 10.1136/vr.154.18doolar

26. Samuel JE, Frazier ME, Kahn ML, Thomashow LS, Mallavia LP: Isolation and characterization of a plasmid from phase I *Coxiella burneti*. Infect Immun. 1983, 41: 488uoolar

27. Willems H, Thiele D, Krauss H: Plasmid based differentiation and detection of *Coxiella burneti* in clinical samples. Eur J Epidemiol. 1993, 9: 411-418. 10.1007/BF0015doolar

28. Porten K, Rissland J, Tigges A, Broll S, Hopp W, Lunemann M, van Treeck U, Kimmig P, Brockmann SO, Wagner-Wiening C, Hellenbrand W, Buchholz U: A super-spreading ewe infects hundreds with Q fever at a farmers' market in Germany. BMC Infect Dis. 2006, 6: 147-10.1186/1471-2334-6uloolar

29. Klaassen CH, Nabuurs-Franssen MH, Tilburg JJ, Hamans MA, Horrevorts AM: Multigenotype Q fever outbreak, the Netherlands. Emerg Infect Dis. 2009, 15: 613-614. 10.3201/eid1504.08uloolar

30. Roest HI, Ruuls RC, Tilburg JJ, Nabuurs-Franssen MH, Klaassen CH, Vellema P, van den Brom R, Dercksen D, Wouda W, Spierenburg MA, van der Spek AN, Buijs R, de Boer AG, Willemsen PT, van Zijderveld FG: Molecular epidemiology of Coxiella burnetii from ruminants in Q fever outbreak, the Netherlands. Emerg Infect Dis. 2011, 17: 668uloolar

31. Enright JB, Franti CE, Longhurst WM, Behymer DE, Wright ME, Dutson VJ: *Coxiella burneti* in a wildlife-livestock environment. Antibody response of ewes and lambs in an endemic Q fever area. Am J Epidemiol. 1971, 94: 6oolar

32. Arricau-Bouvery N, Hauck Y, Bejaoui A, Frangoulidis D, Bodier CC, Souriau A, Meyer H, Neubauer H, Rodolakis A, Vergnaud G: Molecular characterization of *Coxiella burneti* isolates by infrequent restriction

site-PCR and MLVA typing. BMC Microbiol. 2006, 6: 38-10.1186/1471-2180-uloolar

33. Cannon RM, Roe TM: Livestock disease surveys: a field manual for veterinarians. 1982, Canberra: Australian Government Publishing Seoolar

34. Programm zur Förderung der Tiergesundheit in den Schaf- und Ziegenbeständen in Thüringen. Thüringer Staatsanzeiger. 2008, 16: 564-565.

35. Giménez DF: Staining *Rickettsia* in yolk-sac cultures. Stain Technol. 1964, 39: 135oolar

36. Zhang GQ, Hotta A, Mizutani M, Ho T, Yamaguchi T, Fukushi H, Hirai K: Direct identification of *Coxiella burneti* plasmids in human sera by nested PCR. J Clin Microbiol. 1998, 36: 2210-uoolar

37. Klee SR, Tyczka J, Ellerbrok H, Franz T, Linke S, Baljer G, Appel B: Highly sensitive real-time PCR for specific detection and quantification of *Coxiella burneti*. BMC Microbiol. 2006, 6: 2-10.1186/1471-2180-6-2.

CHAPTER 44

SEROEPIDEMIOLOGICAL STUDY OF Q FEVER IN DOMESTIC RUMINANTS IN SEMI-EXTENSIVE GRAZING SYSTEMS

Francisco Ruiz-Fons, Ianire Astobiza, Jesús F Barandika, Ana Hurtado, Raquel Atxaerandio, Ramón A Juste, Ana L García-Pérez

BACKGROUND

Q fever is a worldwide distributed zoonosis caused by *Coxiella burnetii*, a ubiquitous Gram-negative bacterium that is able to infect humans and a wide range of animals, both aquatic and terrestrial [1, 2, 3]. Q fever is a polymorphic disease in humans with subclinic, acute and chronic forms [1, 3]. Several groups in Spain have studied the clinical aspects and the distribution of the disease in different regions [5, 6, 7]. The disease seems to be more prevalent in northern Spain than in the and southern regions of the country, and it is especially high in the Basque Country (northern Spain) where large series of human pneumonia cases due to *C. burnetii* have been reported [1, 8]. It is proposed that *C. burnetii* is maintained in nature following two different cycles, the wild cycle in which ticks and wild animals are involved, and the domestic cycle, where ruminant and other animal species such as dogs and cats are the main reservoirs [1, 3]. Nonetheless, the link between both proposed cycles is currently weakly known, especially because the domestic cycle has been considered the main source for human infection [9] and has therefore been the focus of most studies.

Clinical outcome of *C. burnetii* infection in domestic ruminants consists of abortion and stillbirths in sheep and goats while it causes infertility and mastitis in cattle [10]. No clinical signs are evidenced in non-pregnant animals. When abortion occurs, or even when ewes lamb normally, animals shed a high number of *C. burnetii*through placenta, vaginal fluids, faeces and milk [1, 11, 12]. Infectious abortion in domestic ruminants is a multi-etiologic process that causes important losses in the livestock industry. Furthermore, the zoonotic nature of most of the abortifacient pathogens is a cause for concern from the perspective of Public Health. While attention has been paid to most of these pathogens, such as *Brucella*, *Chlamydophila* or *Toxoplasma* in sheep, others like *C. burnetii* have not been routinely investigated in cases of abortion. The recent application of molecular techniques to study fetal tissues and placenta indicates that *C. burnetii* could be more prevalent than previously thought [13, 14].

Serological surveys have been carried out in many countries to evaluate the distribution of *C. burnetii* in domestic ruminants. In some areas bovine seems to be the main reservoir [15, 16, 17] whereas in others, goats [18, 19] or sheep [20, 21, 22] are the main domestic reservoir. However in other studies, serological surveys indicate that the different domestic ruminant species can play together a relevant role in the domestic cycle of *C. burnetii* [3, 23, 24, 25]. In addition, different management systems showed different degree of exposure to infection [26]. Regarding Spain, few serological evidences have been reported both in domestic and wild ruminants [5, 27].

Under the current panorama of Q fever re-emergence and the lack of information on the current status of *C. burnetii* infection in domestic ruminants in one of the most traditional livestock producing regions in Spain, we aimed to determine the epidemiological situation of this pathogen in the framework of a larger project on coxiellosis in livestock and wildlife. This study updates the status of this zoonotic pathogen in the ruminants population of the Basque Country and highlights the main risks for human infection in a hyperendemic Q fever region. We also evaluated if the age of the animals might account for differences in exposure to *C. burnetii*. Moreover, relationships between *C. burnetii* contact rate and abortion history at the herd level were also investigated.

Citation: Francisco Ruiz-Fons, Ianire Astobiza, Jesús F Barandika, Ana Hurtado, Raquel Atxaerandio, Ramón A Juste and Ana L García-Pérez, Seroepidemiological study of Q fever in domestic ruminants in semi-extensive grazing systems, DOI: 10.1186/1746-6148-6-3.

METHODS

Study area

The Basque Country (7,234 km^2) is a region located in northern Spain (Figure 1). Livestock production is one of the pillars of the rural economy of the region, with a total amount of 344,288 sheep, 160,000 cattle (dairy and beef) and 28,500 goats [28]. Livestock production is widely scattered throughout the region and the number of herds is high, with approximately 5,300 sheep, 6,915 cattle (dairy and beef) and 2,000 goat herds. Semi-extensive production is predominant for sheep, beef cattle and goats, and it is characterized by housing in winter months until early spring, when parturition occurs, and extensive grazing the rest of the year.

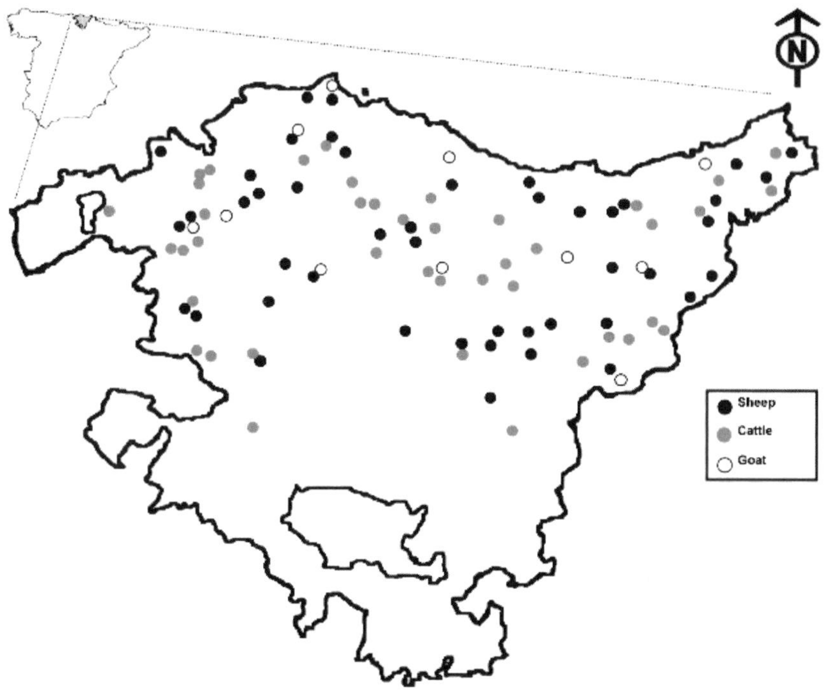

Figure 1: Geographic distribution of the sampled herds in the study area.

Sampling approach

The survey was carried out from October 2007 to April 2008. Overall regional census was compiled for each ruminant species (data from the Basque Statistics Institute) and sample size was proportionally calculated according to the number of herds per county with a maximum number of 2,000 animals from 100 herds. Individuals (females) older than one year were randomly selected within herds to a maximum of 30 sheep, 15 beef cattle and 10 goats per herd. Finally, 1,379 sheep, 626 beef cattle and 115 goats from 46, 42 and 11 herds, respectively, were surveyed (Figure 1). Whole blood extractions were carried out by the veterinary practitioner groups in charge of the Official Sanitary Campaigns in the Basque Country, directed and supervised by the local Animal Health and Welfare Authorities (Diputaciones Forales).

After individual collection of blood into tubes without anticoagulant, sera were obtained by centrifugation and stored at -20°C until serological analyses were performed. History of recent abortion (*i.e.*, occurrence of abortions during the two previous breeding seasons) was obtained from a number of the surveyed herds by intering the farmers during sample collection.

Serological analyses

Sera were tested for the presence of anti-*C. burnetii* antibodies by means of an ELISA test (ELISA Cox kit, LSI-Laboratoire Service International, Lyon, France) according to manufacturer›s instructions. Sensitivity of this ELISA test reaches 100% whereas specificity was determined to be of 95% (manufacturer›s data). ELISA positive sera were retested for anti-*C. burnetii* antibodies by means of the Complement Fixation test (CFT) following standard procedures [29]. *C. burnetii* antigen was provided by Dade Behring (Marburg, Germany) using Nine Mile and Henzerling strains produced on embryonated eggs. According to the standards of the OIE, samples with CFT titres ≤ 1/5 were considered negative. Titres between 1/10 and 1/40 were representative for latent infection while titres ≥ 1/80 revealed an evolutive phase of the infection [29].

Statistical analyses

For statistical analysis purposes, two age categories were established for each animal species (Table 1) in relation to the age at first parturition. Sheep and goats were classified in two groups, yearlings (1-2 years old) and adults (>2 years old), while beef cattle was classified as heifer (1-3 years old) or adult (>3 years old). Several animals younger than 1 year-old (73 sheep, 8 cattle and 6 goats) were sampled but were not considered for age-associated seroprevalence pattern analyses because of the smaller sample size.

Table 1: Mean anti-*C. burnetii* antibody prevalence (Serop.) and its associated standard error (SE) throughout ruminant species-by-age class

	Age class	N	Pos	Serop. (%)	SE
Sheep	1-2 yr.	225	21	9.3	0.02
	Adult	1073	139	13.0	0.01
Subtotal sheep		*1298*	*160*	*12.3*	*0.01*
Beef cattle	Heifer	97	6	6.2	0.02
	Adult	521	35	6.7	0.01
Subtotal cattle		*618*	*41*	*6.6*	*0.01*
Goats	1-2 yr.	40	1	2.5	0.03
	Adult	69	8	11.6	0.04
Subtotal goats		*109*	*9*	*8.3*	*0.03*

N: Number of animals analyzed; Pos: Number of seropositive animals.

ELISA anti-*C. burnetii* antibody prevalence was calculated at individual and at herd level for each ruminant species. Rogan-Gladen correction (RGC) according to the sensitivity and specificity of the ELISA test was used for population seroprevalence calculation [30]. A herd was considered positive when at least one animal showed antibodies by ELISA. Thus, differences on antibody prevalence (continuous) between ruminant species, age classes (categorical) and abortion history (categorical, reported/non-reported) were statistically assessed by means of Chi-square tests. Statistical uncertainty was assessed by calculating the 95% confidence interval for each of the proportions according to the expression $S.E._{95\%C.I.} = 1.96\,[p(1 - p)/n]^{1/2}$ [31].

RESULTS

ELISA test showed an average *C. burnetii* seroprevalence of 11.8 ± 2.0% (RGC: 7.1 ± 1.4%) in sheep, 8.7 ± 5.9% (RGC: 3.9 ± 3.5%) in goats and 6.7 ± 2.0% (RGC: 1.8 ± 1.0%) in beef cattle. Statistically significant differences were found between cattle and sheep seroprevalences ($\chi^2 = 11.7$, $p < 0.001$). The percentage of seropositive herds was 74% (34/46) for sheep, 43% (18/42) for cattle and 45% (5/11) for goats. Within-herd seroprevalence values ranged 0-80% for sheep, 0-53% for cattle and 0-30% for goats, with 21%, 14% and 27% of the herds, respectively, showing a *C. burnetii* seroprevalence ≥ 20%.

Eight out of 162 (4.9 ± 3.3%), 6 out of 42 (14.3 ± 10.6%) and 1 out of 10 (10.0 ± 18.6%) ELISA-positive sheep, cattle and goats, respectively, also reacted positive in the CFT giving titres ≥ 1/10. CFT positive ewes belonged to 5 herds (5/46, 8.7%) and antibody titres did not exceed 1/20. In cattle, CFT positive animals belonged to 3 herds (3/42, 7.1%) and antibody titres did not exceed 1/40. Finally, only one goat reacting positive in ELISA also reacted in the CFT showing a titre of 1/10.

ELISA seroprevalence-age associated patterns differed between ruminant species (Table 1). While *C. burnetii*seroprevalence tended to increase from yearlings to adults in sheep and goats, seroprevalence values remained similar for heifer and adult cattle. Nonetheless, no statistically significant differences between age class seroprevalence values were found. In addition, anti-*C. burnetii* antibody prevalence did not differ statistically in relation to herd abortion history, neither in sheep (9.1 ± 3.9% for flocks reporting abortion and 9.0 ± 2.0% for non-reporting flocks) nor in cattle (10.7 ± 7.8% and 9.4 ± 3.9%, respectively). Seven of the 23 intered sheep flock owners reported recent problems of abortion. Five of these flocks were positive for ELISA anti-*C. burnetii* antibodies, with seroprevalences ranging between 3.3% and 36.7%. Interestingly, CFT titres ≥ 1/10 were detected in only one of those flocks. Meanwhile, 5 of 18 cattle herds reported abortion problems and showed seroprevalences between 0% and 20%, but none of the ELISA positive animals from those herds reporting abortion had significant CFT titres. Conversely, 6 of 13 cattle herds reporting no reproductive problems showed seroprevalences between 6.6% and 53.3% by ELISA, and in 2 of these herds several animals showed titres ≥ 1/10 against *Coxiella* by CFT. Recent abortion history could only be obtained from a small number of goat herds (n = 4) and consequently we did not considered them in the analysis.

DISCUSSION

Q fever is considered a strongly endemic disease in humans in the Basque Country [32, 33]. Contact with domestic ruminants was considered one of the most relevant risk factors for *C. burnetii* infection. Moreover, *C. burnetti* was found to be widespread in sheep flocks [34] and is known to be a relevant agent for ovine abortion [13] that causes important economic losses to livestock producers. Nevertheless, very scarce information on the current status of this pathogen in other ruminant species, such as cattle or goats, was available for this region. As a first approach to improve knowledge on the current status of *C. burnetii* among livestock in the Basque Country, we studied the seroprevalence in beef cattle, sheep and goats, which are reared in semi-extensive conditions, while intensively managed species (dairy cattle) will be the subject of a future study.

Comparison of herein reported ELISA results with other epidemiological surveys has to be carefully considered due to the different serological techniques employed. While recent studies tend to use the indirect fluorescence assay (IFA) or ELISA, those carried out some decades ago used mainly CFT. Whereas IFA and ELISA tests on ruminant sera showed similar results, low agreement was observed between ELISA and CFT [35, 36], which agrees with our observations in sheep (unpublished data). CFT has a good specificity but a low sensitivity [29]; in fact, only 15 out of 214 ELISA positive animals gave CFT titres ≥ 1/10. The highest sensitivity associated to the ELISA test together with the high duration of detectable levels of circulating anti-*C. burnetii*antibodies were the reasons for using this technique for epidemiological purposes in the current study. Although ELISA test can fail to detect *C. burnetii* contact at an individual level [36], it becomes very useful for studies at the population level like the one presented herein. On the other hand, molecular methods are highly sensitive tools for detecting *C. burnetii* infected animals. Nonetheless, the high variability of *C. burnetii*excretion by animals throughout the year limits the reliability of molecular methods for epidemiological purposes, especially if sampling takes place outside of the reproductive season.

The seroprevalence found in sheep was comparable to that reported in other Spanish regions where seroprevalence ranged between 1.7% and 18.8% [5] or in some Mediterranean regions, with values between 9% and 25% [19, 22, 24, 37, 38]. These data highlight the risk of *C. burnetii* zoonosis associated to sheep in all the Mediterranean countries. Nevertheless, seroprevalence of cattle and goats in some of these countries suggest that these species would also represent a potential risk. In fact, cattle seropositivity ranged between 5.8% and 25% [24, 37], and in goats between 13% and 51% [19, 24, 38]. In Spain, the highest prevalences found in these species were 66.9% for cattle and 32.7% for goats in different production systems from and southern Spain, respectively [5], and more recently, 35% of southern Spanish cattle in extensive production have been found to have contact with *C. burnetii* [27].

The lower seroprevalence observed in the present study in cattle and goats could be explained by the semi-extensive management conditions in which animals are moving during part of the year in large land surfaces thus reducing the contact between animals. Therefore, the different prevalences of *C. burnetii* in livestock suggest that local productive system and management factors might influence the life cycle of *C. burnetii*. Moreover, wildlife could play a relevant role as reservoir for livestock [27], especially where extensive productive systems are predominant, which increases the risk of wildlife/livestock contact. The significantly higher seroprevalence observed in sheep with regard to beef cattle could not be explained by differences in the sampling dates in relation to the lambing/calving season. Both beef cattle and sheep were surveyed coinciding with the end of the gestation period, when the excretion of *C. burnetii* by infected animals is higher because of parturition [10]. Interestingly, when CFT was analysed in ELISA positive animals, beef cattle had a higher percentage of reactors (14.3%) compared to sheep (4.9%) indicating a higher number of latent infections in cattle than in sheep. Nevertheless, the small size of the sample and the concentration of CFT-positive animals in a reduced number of herds make it difficult to reach a definitive explanation. Other management factors, like closer contact among ewes during milking, which implies overnight housing, could be the reason for a higher overall ELISA seroprevalence in sheep than in cattle.

Age-related *C. burnetii* serological patterns have been seldom reported in the scientific literature in regard to domestic ruminants [24, 34]. Pathogen contact rate tends to increase with age simply as a consequence of a higher probability of contact with life span, a feature that herein was observed for sheep and goats.

Long-time contact with *C. burnetii* in the surveyed herds together with the random selection of sampled animals could explain the lack of association found between herd seroprevalence and abortion reports. Different results have been reported in this regard, with significant associations between seroprevalence and abortion reported for cattle and sheep in several studies [16, 37], whereas in other reports infection with *C. burnetii* in cattle did not result in abortion, suggesting that infection sometimes can pass unnoticed [39]. In the current study, in 6 cattle herds without reproductive problems within-herd seroprevalence by ELISA ranged between 6.6 and 53% and in 2 of these herds several animals had CFT titers ≥ 1/10 indicating a recent contact with *C. burnetii*. Although several farmers did not report abortion or reproductive problems, high seroprevalences can be associated with the presence of *C. burnetii* in the herd. Similarly, Astobiza et al. [12] found a high within-flock seroprevalence (54%) and a high percentage of *C. burnetii* shedders at lambing (55-79%) in a sheep flock with a low rate of abortion (3.4%). These observations indicate that there are several epidemiological and clinical aspects of *C. burnetii* infection that need to be elucidated and require further investigation.

CONCLUSIONS

The results reported herein showed that sheep had the highest contact rate with *C. burnetii* in the region, but also that cattle and goats should not be neglected as part of the domestic cycle of *C. burnetii*. Based on our observations, we can conclude that measures are to be implemented for the control of *C. burnetii* and Q fever in the study region along the line of those currently in operation in other European countries. Moreover, further epidemiological research on herd, local and regional factors influencing *C. burnetii* life cycle is needed in order to establish more efficient control measures that prevent spread of the infection and its associated effects on livestock and humans. At present, a control programme based on vaccination using a Phase I vaccine is in progress and its efficacy will be assessed in the near future.

DECLARATIONS

Acknowledgements

We acknowledge the collaboration of farmers from the different Breed Farmers Associations. This work was supported by funding from INIA (FAU2006-00002-C04-01), FEDER, and the Department of Agriculture, Fisheries and Food of the Basque Government. F. Ruiz-Fons is supported by a research contract from the 'Instituto de Salud Carlos III' of the Spanish Ministry for Health.

Authors' contributions

FR was responsible for data collection and statistical analysis, and wrote the manuscript; JFB, JA and RA helped in the samplings and performed the serological tests; AH assisted with the interpretation and discussion of results and correcting the manuscript; RAJ advised on statistical analysis and critically revised the manuscript. ALG is head of the project and had primary responsibility for the investigations reported here. All authors revised the manuscript and approved it in its final version.

REFERENCES

1. Maurin M, Raoult D: Q fever. Clin Microbiol Rev. 1999, 12: 518-553.
2. Lapointe JM, Gulland FM, Haines DM, Barr BC, Duignan PJ: Placentitis due to *Coxiella burnetii* in a Pacific harbour seal (*Phoca vitulina richardsi*). J Vet Diagn Invest. 1999, 11: 541-543.
3. Arricau-Bouvery N, Rodolakis A: Is Q Fever an emerging or re-emerging zoonosis?. Vet Res. 2005, 36: 327-349. 10.1051/vetres:2005010.
4. Kovácová E, Kazar J: Q fever--still a query and underestimated infectious disease. Acta Virol. 2002, 46: 193-210.
5. Pascual-Velasco F: [Fiebre Q]. Zamora: Junta de Castilla y León Press 1996.
6. Bolaños M, Santana OE, Pérez-Arellano JL, Ángel-Moreno A, Moreno G, Burgazzoli JL, Martín-Sánchez AM: Q fever in Gran Canaria: 40 new cases. Enferm Infecc Microbiol Clin. 2003, 21: 20-23. 10.1157/13042133.
7. Cardenosa N, Sanfeliu I, Font B, Muñoz T, Nogueras MM, Segura F: Short report: seroprevalence of human infection by *Coxiella burnetii* in Barcelona (northeast of Spain). Am J Trop Med Hyg. 2006, 75: 33-35.
8. Sobradillo V, Ansola P, Baranda F, Corral C: Q fever pneumonia: a re of 164 community-acquired cases in the Basque country. Eur Respir J. 1989, 2: 263-266.
9. Lang GH: Coxiellosis (Q fever) in animals. Q fever: The disease. Edited by: Marrie TJ. Boca Raton: CRC Press, 1990, 1: 24-42.
10. Woldehiwet Z: Q fever (coxiellosis): epidemiology and pathogenesis. Res Vet Sci. 2004, 77: 93-100. 10.1016/j.rvsc.2003.09.001.
11. Rodolakis A, Berri M, Hechard C, Caudron C, Souriau A, Bodier CC, Blanchard B, Camuset P, Devillechaise P, Natorp JC, Vadet JP, Arricau-Bouvery N: Comparison of *Coxiella burnetii* shedding in milk of dairy bovine, caprine, and ovine herds. J Dairy Sci. 2007, 90: 5352-5360. 10.3168/jds.2006-815.
12. Astobiza I, Barandika JF, Hurtado A, Juste RA, García-Pérez AL: Kinetics of *Coxiella burnetii*excretion in a commercial dairy sheep flock after treatment with oxytetracycline. Vet J.
13. Oporto B, Barandika JF, Hurtado A, Adúriz G, Moreno B, García-Pérez AL: Incidence of ovine abortion by *Coxiella burnetii*in northern Spain. Ann N Y Acad Sci. 2006, 1078: 498-501. 10.1196/annals.1374.095.
14. Perugini AG, Capuano F, Esposito A, Marianelli C, Martucciello A, Iovane G, Galiero G: Detection of *Coxiella burnetii* in buffaloes aborted fetuses by IS111 DNA amplification: A preliminary report. Res Vet Sci. 2009, 87: 189-191. 10.1016/j.rvsc.2009.01.005.
15. To H, Htwe KK, Kako N, Kim HJ, Yamaguchi T, Fukushi H, Hirai K: Prevalence of *Coxiella burnetii* infection in dairy cattle with reproductive disorders. J Vet Med Sci. 1998, 60: 859-861. 10.1292/jvms.60.859.
16. Cabassi CS, Taddei S, Donofrio G, Ghidini F, Piancastelli C, Flammini CF, Cavirani S: Association between *Coxiella burnetii*seropositivity and abortion in dairy cattle of Northern Italy. New Microbiol. 2006, 29: 211-214.
17. Kim WJ, Hahn TW, Kim DY, Lee MG, Jung KS, Ogawa M, Kishimoto T, Lee ME, Lee SJ: Seroprevalence of *Coxiella burnetii*infection in dairy cattle and non-symptomatic people for routine health screening in Korea. J Korean Med Sci. 2006, 21: 823-826. 10.3346/jkms.2006.21.5.823.
18. Hatchette TF, Hudson RC, Schlech WF, Campbell NA, Hatchette JE, Ratnam S, Raoult D, Donovan C, Marrie TJ: Goat-associated Q fever: a new disease in Newfoundland. Emerg Infect Dis. 2001, 7: 413-419.
19. Loukaides F, Hadjichristodoulou C, Soteriades ES, Kolonia V, Ioannidou MC, Psaroulaki A, Tselentis Y: Active surveillance of Q fever in human and animal population of Cyprus. BMC Infect Dis. 2006, 6: 48-10.1186/1471-2334-6-48.
20. Hellenbrand W, Breuer T, Petersen L: Changing epidemiology of Q fever in Germany, 1947-1999. Emerg Infect Dis. 2001, 7: 789-796. 10.3201/eid0705.010504.
21. Tissot-Dupont H, Amadei MA, Nezri M, Raoult D: Wind in November, Q fever in December. Emerg Infect Dis. 2004, 10: 1264-1269.
22. Kennerman E, Rousset E, Gölcü E, Dufour P: Seroprevalence of Q fever (coxiellosis) in sheep from the southern Marmara Region, Turkey. Comp Immunol Microbiol Infect Dis. 2010, 33: 37-45. 10.1016/j.cimid.2008.07.007.
23. Hatchette T, Campbell N, Whitney H, Hudson R, Marrie TJ: Seroprevalence of *Coxiella burnetii* in selected populations of domestic ruminants in Newfoundland. Can Vet J. 2002, 43: 363-364.
24. Psaroulaki A, Hadjichristodoulou C, Loukaides F, Soteriades E, Konstantinidis A, Papastergiou P, Ioannidou MC, Tselentis Y: Epidemiological study of Q fever in humans, ruminant animals, and ticks in Cyprus using a geographical information system. Eur J Clin Microbiol Infect Dis. 2006, 25: 576-586. 10.1007/s10096-006-0170-7.
25. Çekani M, Papa A, Kota M, Velo E, Berxholi K: Report of a serological study of *Coxiella burnetii* in domestic animals in Albania. Vet J. 2008, 175: 276-278. 10.1016/j.tvjl.2007.01.005.
26. Capuano F, Landolfi MC, Monetti DM: Influence of three types of farm management on the seroprevalence of Q fever as assessed by an indirect immunofluorescence assay. Vet Rec. 2001, 149: 669-671.
27. Ruiz-Fons F, Rodriguez O, Torina A, Naranjo V, Gortázar C, de la Fuente J: Prevalence of *Coxiella burnetti* infection in wild and farmed ungulates. Vet Microbiol. 2008, 126: 282-286. 10.1016/j.vetmic.2007.06.020.
28. Eustat: Basque Statistics Institute. [http://www.eustat.es/bancopx/spanish/Economía/Sector%20primario/Censo%20agrario/Ganadería/Ganadería.html]
29. World Organization for Animal Health. [http://www.oie.int/eng/normes/mmanual/2008/pdf/2.01.12_Q-FEVER.pdf]

30. Rogan WJ, Gladen B: Estimating prevalence from the results of a screening test. Am J Epidemiol. 1978, 107: 71-76.

31. Martin SW, Meek AH, Willeberg P: Veterinary Epidemiology. Measures of disease frequency. Ames: Iowa State University Press 1987.

32. Sanzo JM, García MA, Sáez MP, Sarobe V, Audikana A, Dehesa V: [Fiebre Q]. Vitoria-Gasteiz: Servicio de Publicaciones del Gobierno Vasco Press 1991.

33. Montes M, Cilla G, Vicente D, Nieto D, Ercibengoa M, Pérez-Trallero E: Gipuzkoa, Basque Country, Spain (1984-2004): A hyperendemic area of Q fever. Hospital Donostia. Ann N Y Acad Sci. 2006, 1078: 129-132. 10.1196/annals.1374.020.

34. García-Pérez AL, Astobiza I, Barandika JF, Atxaerandio R, Hurtado A, Juste RA: Investigation of *Coxiella burnetii*occurrence in dairy sheep flocks by bulk-tank milk analysis and antibody levels determination. J Dairy Sci. 2009, 92: 1581-1584. 10.3168/jds.2008-1672.

35. Kovácová E, Kazar J, Spanelova D: Suitability of various *Coxiella burnetii* antigen preparations for detection of serum antibodies by various tests. Acta Virol. 1998, 42: 365-368.

36. Rousset E, Durand B, Berri M, Dufour P, Prigent M, Russo P, Delcroix T, Touratier A, Rodolakis A, Aubert M: Comparative diagnostic potential of three serological tests for abortive Q fever in goat herds. Vet Microbiol. 2007, 124: 286-297. 10.1016/j.vetmic.2007.04.033.

37. Cetinkaya B, Kalender H, Ertas HB, Muz A, Arslan N, Ongor H, Gurcay M: Seroprevalence of coxiellosis in cattle, sheep and people in the east of Turkey. Vet Rec. 2000, 146: 131-136.

38. Masala G, Porcu R, Sanna G, Chessa G, Cillara G, Chisu V, Tola S: Occurrence, distribution, and role in abortion of *Coxiella burnetii* in sheep and goats in Sardinia, Italy. Vet Microbiol. 2004, 99: 301-305. 10.1016/j.vetmic.2004.01.006.

39. Paiba GA, Lloyd G, Bewley K, Webster GJ, Green LE, Morgan KL: An investigaton of *Coxiella burnetii* infection at calving within a herd of dairy cows in England using PCR. Rickettsiae and rickettsial diseases at the turn of the third millennium. Edited by: Brouqui P, Raoult D. Amsterdam: Elsevier, 1999:387-392.

SECTION XII BORRELIA BURGDORFERI – TICK-BORN DISEASE, AGENT OF LYME DISEASE

CHAPTER 45

SURVEY OF BORRELIAE IN TICKS, CANINES, AND WHITE-TAILED DEER FROM ARKANSAS, U.S.A.

Rebecca T Trout Fryxell, C Dayton Steelman, Allen L Szalanski, Ken L Kvamme, Peggy M Billingsley and Philip C Williamson

Keywords: *Borrelia,* Ticks, Vector borne, Surveillance, Deer

BACKGROUND

In the Eastern and Upper Midwestern regions of North America, *Ixodes scapularis* (L.) is the most abundant tick species encountered by humans and the primary vector of *Borrelia burgdorferi* (causative agent of Lyme disease), whereas in the southeastern region *Amblyomma americanum* (Say) is the most abundant tick species encountered by humans but it cannot transmit *B. burgdorferi*[1, 2]. Since its first description in the 1970s, Lyme disease is the most frequently reported vector-borne disease in the northern hemisphere [3]. However, in some areas of the world Lyme borreliosis may be caused by *Borrelia* genotypes other than *B. burgdorferi* and includes a range of symptoms and pathologies [3, 4]. In the southern United States *B. lonestari* is associated with Southern Tick Associated Rash Illness (STARI) or Masters disease [5, 6]. This bacteria is common throughout the southeast and has been identified primarily in *A. americanum;* however, the etiology of *B. lonestari* remains undetermined [7, 8, 9, 10, 11, 12, 13, 14, 15] and recent reports indicate *B. lonestari* may not be pathogenic [16].

Health professionals often question cases of Lyme disease from the southeastern United States because symptoms may be confused with other tick-borne illnesses and not all patients produce the erythema migrans or bull's eye rash used for diagnosis [15, 17]. Additionally, these cases are rarely fatal, but can cause cardiac, neurological and joint problems [17]. However, the potential vectors (*I. scapularis*), pathogens (*B. burgdorferi*) and hosts (*Peromyscus* species) are all present in the south [17]. In Georgia, *B. burgdorferi* was isolated and characterized from field collected *I. scapularis* and cotton mice (*Peromyscus gossypinus*); and these field isolates were transmitted via *I. scapularis* to hamsters (Cricetidae) and mice (Muridae) [1]. Field collected *I. scapularis* from Alabama could acquire, maintain, and transmit *B. burgdorferi*[18] and field collected ticks and rodents from the southern U.S. were positive for *B. burgdorferi*[1, 19, 20, 21, 22]. Previously in Arkansas, ticks and reservoir species were screened for *Borrelia* in nine northeast Arkansas counties using indirect fluorescence antibody (IFA), both *I. scapularis* and *A. americanum* were identified as potential vectors, and deer mice (*Peromyscus* spp.) and marsh rice rats (*Oryzomys palustris* Harlan) as potential reservoir hosts [23]. Although the environment is suitable for *Borrelia* transmission [17], many researchers and physicians do not believe the southern U.S. is at risk for *Borrelia* related diseases [2, 4, 15]. The exact cause for the reduced incidence for Lyme disease in the southern United States is unknown, but hypotheses include the abundance of other tick species in the area, the habitat, host dynamics, and tick genetics [2, 24].

Previous research indicates that *B. burgdorferi* IFA positive canines geographically associated with *I. scapularis*infested deer, increase the likelihood of *B. burgdorferi* transmission to humans because the nymphs that feed on the deer may also feed on canines and their owners [25, 26]. Recent Arkansas tick studies identified five tick species infesting canines and white-tailed deer with *A. americanum* infesting canines and *I. scapularis*primarily infesting white-tailed deer [27]. A population genetic study of *I. scapularis* based on the 16S mtDNA identified both the American and Southern lineages (formerly known as *I. scapularis* and *I. dammini*) on canines and white-tailed deer [28], which is a concern because the American *I. scapularis* lineage is more likely than the Southern *I. scapularis* lineage to transmit Lyme disease [29]. The

Citation: Rebecca T Trout Fryxell, C Dayton Steelman, Allen L Szalanski, Ken L Kvamme, Peggy M Billingsley and Philip C Williamson, Survey of Borreliae in ticks, canines, and white-tailed deer from Arkansas, U.S.A., DOI: 10.1186/1756-3305-5-139.

objective of this study was to identify *Borrelia* species within Arkansas ticks, canines, and white-tailed deer to determine the identity and locations of Borreliae endemic to Arkansas using PCR amplification of the flagellin (*flaB)* gene. The CDC defines an endemic county as "endemic for Lyme disease if there are at least two confirmed human cases that were acquired in that county or there are established populations of *I. scapularis* infected with *B. burgdorferi"*[30].

METHODS

Tick, canine, and white-tailed deer collections

This project used the collections reported in Trout and Steelman [27]. Briefly, ticks were collected from canines (March 2006 to November 2007) and white-tailed deer (Oct. 2007 – Jan. 2008) and stored in 80% ethanol until visual identification of species and life stage [31, 32, 33]. Additionally, a small volume of canine or white-tailed deer blood (0.5-1 cc) was obtained from each host and stored on a FTA card (FTA ® Indicating Micro Card, Whatman International Ltd, Maidstone, England) in an envelope labeled with collection information. FTA cards were stored at room temperature until DNA extraction. All FTA cards, all ticks from canines, and at least one specimen of each tick species from each white-tailed deer were subjected to further analyses.

Tick DNA extraction and detection for *Borrelia* species

To minimize DNA contamination, DNA extractions and PCR were conducted in different laboratories and reagents and equipment were dedicated to each procedure. Tick identification and extractions were conducted in the Veterinary Entomology Laboratory (VELUA) and PCR reactions were conducted in the Insect Genetics Laboratory (IGLUA) at the University of Arkansas. During each PCR, at least one blank reagent to detect contamination (negative control) and an appropriate positive control ensured PCR reagents and conditions were used. PCR and reaction product analyses were performed on the ticks according to the protocols of Trout *et al.*[28]. After tick identification to species, each specimen was dried on a paper towel to allow the residual ethanol to evaporate and was then cut longitudinally and half of the tick was subjected to the Qiagen Dneasy Insect Protocol (Qiagen Inc., Valencia, CA). Extracted DNA from half of the tick was stored at −20°C until further analyses. The remaining tick half was stored at −20°C for additional analysis or morphological confirmation as required. To evaluate the tick DNA, each sample was first assessed by PCR with Ixodidae specific mitochondrial primers (16 S + 2/16 S-1) using previously described cycling parameters [34]. If the mitochondrial marker amplified, then the tick was subjected to a genus specific *flaB* PCR to identify the presence of *Borrelia* DNA [6, 35].

Host DNA extraction and detection for *Borrelia* species

Each canine and white-tailed deer FTA card was screened in duplicate to determine the presence of *Borrelia*DNA. The FTA card was cut into halves, where half of the card remained at VELUA for an initial screening and the other half was sent to the University of North Texas Health Science Center in Ft. Worth (UNTHSC) for verification screening. Each FTA card half was removed from its envelope and a 1.2 mm disc was punched from the card using a sterilized Harris Micro Punch and the paper disc was washed for DNA extraction according to the Whatman protocol (Harris MicroPunch®, Whatman International Ltd, Maidstone, England). After the punch had dried at room temperature, it was subjected to PCR analyses. To ensure DNA detection from FTA punches were not inhibited in any manner, FTA punches were assessed for PCR amplification of host cytochrome b genes [36]. As with the ticks, canines and white-tailed deer specimens were screened for *Borrelia* species by PCR in a genus specific manner [6, 35].

Statistical analyses

Summary statistics and relative abundance of each tick species were calculated to determine overall trends within the population using JMP ($\alpha=0.05$) [37]. Fisher's exact tests and two-tailed T-tests were performed in Excel 2007 to determine if the species of tick or tick host had any effect on the probability that the tick would be PCR positive for *Borrelia*[38]. Since spatial and temporal sampling of ticks and hosts were different (e.g., ticks from white-tailed deer were collected only in the fall) and this sampling structure may affect findings, comparisons across and among cohorts were not conducted.

Sequence identification of *Borrelia* species

PCR products, from *flaB* positive samples, were sent to UNTHSC for DNA sequence analysis. The PCR reaction products were hydrolyzed with ExoSAP-IT (USB Corporation, Cleveland, OH) and sequence determination was performed using a BigDYE Terminator v.3.1 Cycle Sequencing kit (Applied Biosystems, Inc., Foster City, CA) followed by capillary electrophoresis on a ABI PRISM 310 Genetic Analyzer (Applied Biosystems Inc., Foster City, CA) using the method of Williamson *et al.* [39]. Sequences were edited, aligned, and analyzed with Sequencher 4.7 (Gene Codes, Corporation, Ann Arbor MI) and compared with sequences in GenBank (National Center for Biotechnology Information, Bethesda, MD).

Spatial identification of *Borrelia* species

Canine and deer collection data along with their corresponding tick collections and *Borrelia* DNA presence/absence data were georeferenced into ArcMap 9.0 (ESRI Redlands, CA USA) and projected to the NAD 1983 UTM Zone 15 N of the GCS North American 1983 Geographic coordinate system. Boolean operations and symbology were used to identify locations with PCR positive ticks and hosts. The resulting Boolean map was overlaid on an existing county map of Arkansas [40].

RESULTS

Identification of *Borrelia* DNA in the tick population

A total of 2123 ticks were included in this study and represented five tick species; *I. scapularis* (33%), *A. americanum* (31%), *R. sanguineus* (16%), *D. variabilis* (9%), and *A. maculatum* (8%). An additional 3% were *Amblyomma* ticks that could not be identified to species because the tick specimens were damaged. The tick population was comprised of each life stage, but most were adults (83%) and more were collected from domesticated canines (67%) than from hunter-killed white-tailed deer (33%). Overall, 583 of the 2123 (27.5%) ticks tested by PCR produced an amplicon for the *Borrelia flaB* gene (Table 1). The prevalence of *flaB*amplicons for each tick species were 36.4% (252/692) *I. scapularis*, 27.9% (50/179) *A. maculatum*, 25.8% (88/341) *R. sanguineus*, 24.5% (161/657) *A. americanum*, and 10.3% (19/184) *D. variabilis*. Fifty percent of the 583 *flaB* amplicons from PCR positive ticks were sequenced, representing approximately one fourth of the specimens from each tick species (Table 2). DNA sequences produced from the tick *flaB* amplicons represented multiple genotypes of *Borrelia*. These sequences align with *B. burgdorferi* strain B31 (AB035617), OK-strain HS-2 (FJ871032), *Borrelia lonestari* Clone Scc26 (DQ100451), isolate MO2002-V1 (AY850063), isolate TX076 (EF689742), strain NC/MD (AF273670), and clone AA115 (AY654945) (Figure 1). The majority (136/296) of *flaB* sequences matched *B. lonestari* strain NC/MD (AF273670) which was amplified from all five tick species. Locations of all *Borrelia* isolated from ixodid ticks collected from Arkansas canines and white-tailed deer during 2007 were mapped because *B. burgdorferi* ticks were few (Figure 2).

Table 1: Almost a third of each Ixodid ticks [a] species collected from Arkansas canines and white-tailed deer generated amplicons by PCR for the *Borrelia flaB* gene indicating Borreliae are endemic to Arkansas

Tick species	**No. PCR positive ticks / No. Screened for *flaB*(%)**					
	Larvae	**Nymphs**	**Males**	**Females**	**Adults[a]**	**Total**
Ticks Collected from Canines						
Amblyomma spp.	0 / 18 (0%)	4 / 15 (26.7%)	2 / 11 (18.2%)	0 / 7 (0%)	2 / 11 (18.2%)	8 / 62 (12.9%)
Amblyomma americanum	0 / 0 (0%)	37 / 162 (22.8%)	58 / 237 (24.5%)	56 / 233 (24%)	0 / 2(0%)	151 / 634 (23.8%)
Amblyomma maculatum	0 / 2 (0%)	2 / 9 (22.2%)	22 / 95 (23.2%)	2 / 9 (22.2%)	0 / 0 (0%)	26 / 115 (22.6%)
Dermacentor variabilis	0 / 1 (0%)	0 / 41 (0%)	7 / 52 (13.5%)	11 / 84 (13.1%)	0 / 0 (0%)	18 / 178 (10.1%)
Ixodes scapularis	0 / 0 (0%)	3 / 7 (42.9%)	21 / 42 (50%)	18 / 69 (26.1%)	1 / 3 (33.3%)	43 / 121 (35.5%)
Rhipicephalus sanguineus	0 / 0 (0%)	28 / 97 (28.9%)	19 / 94 (20.2%)	22 / 105 (21%)	9 / 21 (42.9%)	78 / 317 (24.6%)
Total	0 / 21 (0%)	74 / 331 (22.4%)	129 / 531 (24.3%)	109 / 507 (21.5%)	12 / 37 (32.4%)	324 / 1427 (22.7%)
Ticks Collected from White-tailed Deer						
Amblyomma spp.	0 / 0 (0%)	4 / 7 (57.1%)	0 / 0 (0%)	1 / 1 (100%)	0 / 0 (0%)	5 / 8 (62.5%)
Amblyomma americanum	0 / 0 (0%)	0 / 2 (0%)	2 / 7 (28.6%)	8 / 14 (57.1%)	0 / 0 (0%)	10 / 23 (43.5%)
Amblyomma maculatum	0 / 0 (0%)	0 / 1 (0%)	9 / 35 (25.7%)	15 / 28 (53.6%)	0 / 0 (0%)	24 / 64 (37.5%)
Dermacentor variabilis	0 / 0 (0%)	0 / 2 (0%)	0 / 2 (0%)	1 / 2 (50%)	0 / 0 (0%)	1 / 6 (16.7%)
Ixodes scapularis	0 / 1 (0%)	4 / 6 (66.7%)	86 / 231 (37.2%)	119 / 333 (35.7%)	0 / 0 (0%)	209 / 571 (36.6%)
Rhipicephalus sanguineus	0 / 0 (0%)	0 / 0 (0%)	5 / 10 (50%)	5 / 14 (35.7%)	0 / 0 (0%)	10 / 24 (41.7%)
Total	0 / 1 (0%)	8 / 18 (44.4%)	102 / 285 (35.8%)	149 / 392 (38%)	0 / 0 (0%)	259 / 696 (37.2%)
Total Ticks Collected from Canines and White-tailed Deer						
Amblyomma spp.	0 / 18 (0%)	8 / 22 (36.4%)	2 / 11 (18.2%)	1 / 8 (12.5%)	2 / 11 (18.2%)	13 / 70 (18.6%)
Amblyomma americanum	0 / 0 (0%)	37 / 164 (22.6%)	60 / 244 (24.6%)	64 / 247 (25.9%)	0 / 2 (0%)	161 / 657 (24.5%)
Amblyomma maculatum	0 / 2 (0%)	2 / 10 (20%)	31 / 130 (23.8%)	17 / 37 (45.9%)	0 / 0 (0%)	50 / 179 (27.9%)
Dermacentor variabilis	0 / 1 (0%)	0 / 43 (0%)	7 / 54 (13%)	12 / 86 (14%)	0 / 0 (0%)	19 / 184 (10.3%)

Ixodes scapularis	0 / 1 (0%)	7 / 13 (53.8%)	107 / 273 (39.2%)	137 / 402 (34.1%)	1 / 3 (33.3%)	252 / 692 (36.4%)
Rhipicephalus sanguineus	0 / 0 (0%)	28 / 97 (28.9%)	24 / 104 (23.1%)	27 / 119 (22.7%)	9 / 21 (42.9%)	88 / 341 (25.8%)
Total	0 / 22 (0%)	82 / 349 (23.5%)	231 / 816 (28.3%)	258 / 899 (28.7%)	12 / 37 (32.4%)	583 / 2123 (27.5%)

[a] Damaged adult specimens could not be properly sexed.

Table 2: Multiple Borreliae genotypes [a] were identified in Arkansas ticks [b], canines and white-tailed deer including *B. burgdorferi*and *B. lonestari;* however, *B. lonestari* was significantly more prevalent than *B. burgdorferi* in the tick population

Host pecies	**Seq. / PCR Pos. / screened**	**No. hosts-*flaB* positive with amplicons homologous to*B. burgdorferi* sequences**		**No. Hosts*flaB* positive with amplicons homologous to*B. lonestari* sequences**					
		B31	**OK HS-2**	**IP2**	**Scc26**	**MO2002-V1**	**TX076**	**NC/MD**	**AA115**
Tick Collections from Canines									
*Amblyomma*species	6/8/62	0	0	0	0	0	1N, 1M	1N, 1M, 2A	0
Amblyomma americanum	105/151/634	0	0	0	2N, 4M, 10F	3N, 3M, 9F	3N, 2M, 5F	15N, 31M, 13F	1N
Amblyomma maculatum	24/26/115	0	0	0	1N, 1M	0	8M, 1F	12M, 1F	0
Dermacentor variabilis	17/18/178	0	0	0	2M, 2F	1M, 3F	3M, 1F	3F	0
Ixodes scapularis	28/43/121	0	0	0	1F	1M, 1F	1M, 4F	2N, 11M, 6F, 1A	0
Rhipicephalus sanguineus	54/78/317	0	0	0	6N, 8M, 6F, 2A	3N, 2F	1M	8N, 5M, 3F, 5A	2N, 1F
Total Ticks From Canines	234/324/1427	0	0	0	9N, 15M, 19F, 2A	6N, 5M, 15F	4N, 16M, 11F	26N, 60M, 26F, 8A	3N, 1F
Tick Collections from White-tailed Deer									
*Amblyomma*species	1/5/8	1N	0	0	0	0	0	0	0
Amblyomma americanum	2/10/23	0	0	0	0	1F	0	1F	0
Amblyomma maculatum	15/24/64	1M	1F	0	0	2M, 5F	1F	3M, 2F	0
Dermacentor variabilis	1/1/6	0	0	0	0	1F	0	0	0
Ixodes scapularis	39/209/571	1M	4M, 7F	0	0	6M, 10F	2M, 1F	4M, 4F	0
Rhipicephalus sanguineus	4/10/24	0	0	0	0	1F	1F	1M, 1F	0
Total Ticks From Deer	62/259/696	1N, 2M	4M, 8F	0	0	8M, 18F	2M, 3F	8M, 8F	0
Ticks, Canines, and White-tailed Deer									
Canine	10/10/173	0	1	6	0	1	0	2	0

Deer	49/49/250	0	21	1	0	3	0	24	0
Total Ticks	296/583/2123	1 N, 2 M	4 M, 8 F	0	9 N, 15 M, 19 F, 2A	6 N, 13 M, 33 F	4 N, 20 M, 14 F	26 N, 68 M, 34 F, 8A	3 N, 1 F
Total	355/642/2546	3	33	7	45	56	38	162	4

[a] Genbank identities for *Borrelia* strains include strain B31 (AB035617), strain OK HS-2 (FJ871032), strain *IP2* (AY345236), clone Scc26 (DW100451), isolate MO2001-V1 (AY850063), isolate TX076 (EF689742), strain NC/MD (AF273670), and clone AA115 (AY654945).

[b] Number of larva (L), nymph (N), adult male (M), adult female (F), and damage adult specimens could not be properly sexed (A).

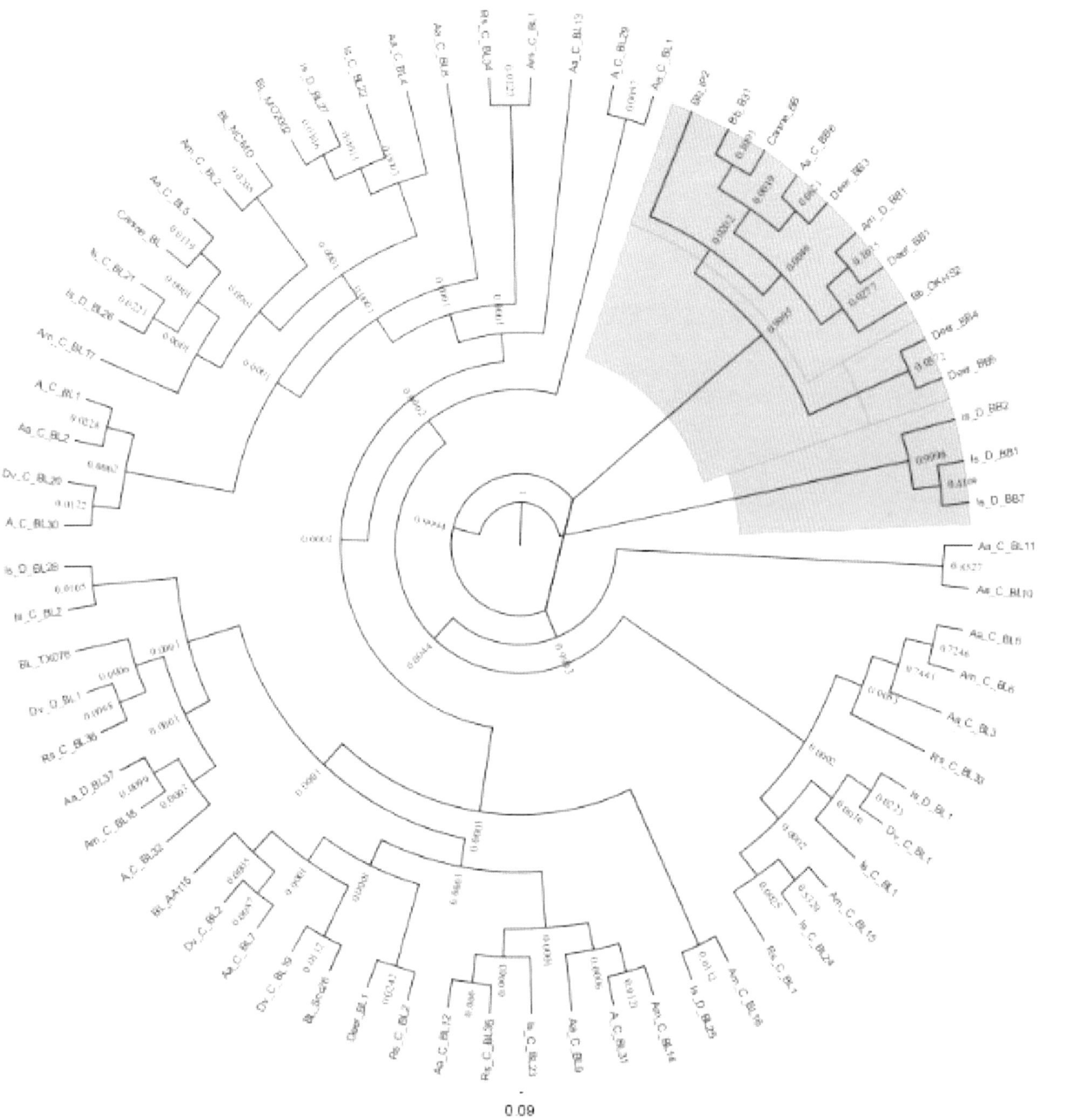

Figure 1: Polar tree layout of the phylogenetic relationship of the *Borrelia* flagellin B (*flaB*) gene fragment (330 bp) amplified from ticks collected from Arkansas canines and white-tailed deer, and host blood samples[a]. Those specimens aligning with *B. burgdorferi* are highlighted in gray[b]. [a] The different tick species are abbreviated *A. americanum* (Aa), *A. maculatum* (Am), *D. variabilis* (Dv), *I. scapularis* (Is), and *R. sangineus* (Rs). Ticks from canines (c), ticks from deer (d), and blood samples (Canine or Deer) are also represented. [b]The different *Borrelia* species are abbreviated as BL for *B. lonestari* and BB for *B. burgdorferi.*

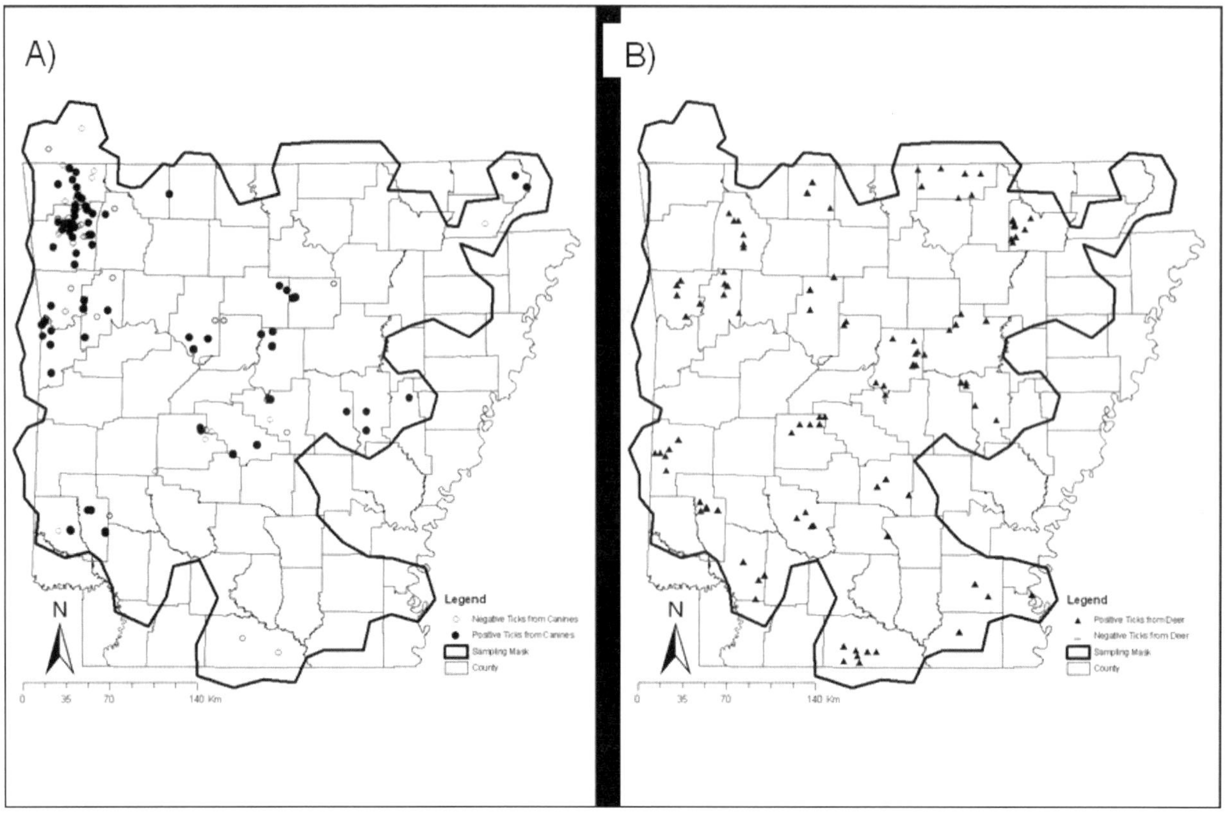

Figure 2: Locations of *Borrelia flaB* amplicons isolated from ixodid ticks collected from Arkansas canines (A) and white-tailed deer (B) during 2007.

Identification of *Borrelia* DNA in canines and their ticks

Of the 173 canines and their 1427 ticks subjected to the *flaB* PCR, 5.8% (n=10) and 22.7% (n=324) were positive respectively. All ten positive canine *flaB* amplicons were sequenced and six samples were homologous to *B. burgdorferi IP2* (AY345236), two were homolgous to *B. lonestari* NC/MD (AF273670), one was homologous to *B. lonestari* fragments MO2002-V1 (AY850063), and one was homologous to strain *B. burgdorferi* OK HS-2 (FJ871032) (Table 2). Contingency tests revealed that the number of *flaB* positive and negative ticks were significantly different based on tick species ($\times^2$=31.9; df=5; P<0.0001) such that *I. scapularis* (35.5%) had the highest *flaB* positive rate. The most frequently encountered tick on canines was *A. americanum* and 23.8% (151/634) were *flaB* PCR positive. Of the 173 canines, 87 canines did not have a positive tick, 27 canines had one positive tick, and 59 canines had more than one positive tick. Of the 59 canines with more than one positive tick, 18 canines had multiple specimens of the same species that were positive, 13 canines had specimens of two separate tick species positive, and two canines had specimens of three separate tick species PCR positive.

In canine collected ticks, the *B. lonestari* strain NC/MD (AF273670) was also the most common amplicon and amplified in nymphs, males, and females. Positive ticks were identified primarily in northwest Arkansas where many of the canines were collected (Figure 2A). Ticks from *B. burgdorferi* positive canines did not generate *B. burgdorferi* sequences. Instead these ticks were either negative for *flaB* or produced *flaB* positive amplicons that were homologous with *B. lonestari*.

Identification of *Borrelia* DNA in white-tailed deer and their ticks

Of the 250 white-tailed deer and the 696 ticks subjected to the *flaB* PCR, 19.6% (n=49) and 37.2% (n=259) were positive for *flaB*. Of the 49 white-tailed deer *flaB* amplicons, 24 amplicons were homologous to *B. lonestari* NC/MD (AF273670), 21 amplicons were homologous to *B. burgdorferi* OK HS-2 (FJ871032), 3 amplicons were homolgous to *B. lonestari* MO2002-V1 (AY850063), and one amplicon was homolgous to *B. burgdorferi* IP2 (AY345236) (Table 2). Contingency tests revealed that the number of *flaB* positive and negative ticks were not significantly different based on tick species (X^2=3.96; df=5; P=0.556). *flaB* prevalence rates in ticks from white-tailed deer was 62.5% (5/8) in unknown *Amblyomma*, 41.7% (10/24) in *R. sanguineus*, 43.5% (10/23) in *A. americanum*, 37.5% (24/64) in *A. maculatum*, 36.6% (209/571) in *I. scapularis*, and 16.7% (1/6) in *D. variabilis*. A majority of white-tailed deer did not have a positive tick (n=91), but 70 white-tailed deer had more than one PCR positive tick of which 24 deer had more than one *flaB* positive tick species and one deer had three different tick species *flaB* positive. Fragments amplified from all five deer-collected tick species were most similar to the *B. lonestari* sequence AY850063. Positive ticks were identified throughout Arkansas (Figure 2B).

DISCUSSION

Borreliae were identified in field collected ticks, canines, and white-tailed deer throughout the state suggesting the bacteria (as a family) are endemic in Arkansas. Of interest was the diversity of *Borrelia*genotypes identified from the variety of different field collections (Figure 1, Table 2). Five different

*B. lonestari*genotypes and three different *B. burgdorferi* genotypes were identified in Arkansas. None of the genotypes appeared to be more common in one tick species or host; however, *B. burgdorferi* genotypes were only identified in ticks collected from deer - the significance of this finding remains to be determined. Specifically, *B. burgdorferi* genotypes were amplified only from twelve *I. scapularis,* two *A. maculatum*, and an *Amblyomma* tick that was too damaged for the species to be determined. Only one *I. scapularis* nymph was homologous with *B. burgdorferi,* consequently there is insufficient data to consider the area endemic for Lyme disease. This damaged *Amblyomma* nymph was collected in Washington County of northwest Arkansas. *B. burgdorferi* transmission by *A. maculatum* needs additional attention and previous studies with *A. americanum* have indicated that *A. americanum* cannot transmit *B. burgdorferi*[1, 2]. Due to the low prevalence of *B. burgdorferi* in nymphal ticks, Arkansas should not be considered a Lyme disease endemic area [30]. *B. lonestari* NC/MD was the most common sequence amplified (45.6%) and it is homologous to the sequence previously isolated from a patient's skin with Lyme-like symptoms [41] suggesting this genotype is the most common *Borrelia* in Arkansas. In 2007, four Arkansas counties reported human cases of Lyme disease (Benton, Carroll, Washington, Crawford, and Saline Co.). Ticks collected from these counties in this study primarily produced amplicons homologous to *B. lonestari*, and a few ticks produced amplicons homologous to *B. burgdorferi.* If these human cases of Lyme disease are 'real' then they are most likely either rare, acquired from a different location, or are false positives. Collections of field collected ticks near the site of transmission (e.g., where the tick attached to the human) would answer these questions. Data presented here corroborate with Texas collected ticks identified with *B. lonestari* DNA in *A. americanum A. cajennense, A. maculatum, D. variabilis, I. scapularis*, and *R. sanguineus* and relatively few samples of *B. burgdorferi* DNA (AE000783) [39] and with *B. lonestari* in Arkansas white-tailed deer serum [26].

We documented *Borrelia* in five tick species infesting domesticated canines and white-tailed deer; consequently, Borreliae are likely endemic in Arkansas and in the southeastern U.S. by a more diverse tick repertoire than previously thought. Identifying *Borrelia* in ticks indicates that field collected ticks have fed on infected animals at some point in their life cycle and identifying *Borrelia* in canines and white-tailed deer indicates that infected ticks have transmitted *Borrelia* to these hosts. We observed a trend for ticks collected from canines to be positive with *B. lonestari* whereas ticks from deer could be positive with either *B. lonestari*or *B. burgdorferi.* This may be related to the species of tick collected on each host and the sampling periods, as canines were primarily infested with *A. americanum* and collected year round whereas white-tailed deer were primarily infested with *I. scapularis* and collected in the fall. Also, ticks feeding on white-tailed deer may actually be feeding on hosts that are incompetent reservoirs of Lyme disease [42]. Additional evidence is required to assert the potential for each role in transmission. Past research has indicated that several tick species are not active vectors of *B. burgdorferi* (e.g., transmission through salivary glands) [18, 20], but additional research should isolate Borrelias from the study area and confirm these tick species are not passive vectors (e.g., transmission studies in a suitable animal model). Additionally, often ticks are misidentified and physicians do not think "beyond Lyme disease" to diagnose the patient properly [2]. Other tick-borne diseases transmitted in Arkansas include rickettsia spotted fevers [32, 43] and Ehrlichiosis [13, 39], perhaps the cases of Lyme disease reported in 2007 were actually misdiagnosed.

Monitoring tick populations on canines could provide reliable early detection of tick-borne disease outbreaks [44]. Monitoring field populations of ticks for *B. burgdorferi* and other tick-borne diseases is essential to minimize transmission and maximize management. Recent landscape changes in Arkansas are expanding urban environments into deer habitats [45, 46]. Previously, this pattern of urban development into previous deer habitats in Lyme Connecticut led to the increased diagnoses of Lyme disease in the northeastern United States [47]; similar reports have indicated *B. burgdorferi* emerged independently in the Midwest and eastern United States [48, 49, 50].

Additional research into the involvement of *Borrelia* spp. in the southeastern zoonotic cycle (e.g., abundance of tick/host infection, reservoir maintenance, vector competency) should be conducted in order to determine the life cycle and etiology of the various Borreliae detected in this survey and what roles, if any, they may play relative to subsequent borreliosis observed in humans. Future work should also evaluate the interaction of *A. americanum* carrying *B. lonestari, A. maculatum* carrying *B. burgdorferi*, and *I. scapularis* carrying *B. burgdorferi* and what effect, if any, this might have on the pathogenicity of the Borreliae, as both tick species have been identified simultaneously infesting the same host [27, 51]. It is possible that there are multiple interactions occurring between tick species (e.g., species competition for host), the variety of hosts (e.g., Ixodid ticks feed on three different hosts), and the different Borreliae (infesting both the tick and the host), which warrants additional research.

CONCLUSIONS

Data from this study indicate multiple *Borrelia* genotypes are endemic to Arkansas because *flaB* was amplified from ticks, canines, and white-tailed deer, but the exact role each genotype plays in transmission and epidemiology remains undetermined. There were significantly more amplicons of *B. lonestari* than *B. burgdorferi* present suggesting that the majority of tick-borne diseases in Arkansas are not *B. burgdorferi*.

DECLARATIONS

Acknowledgments

We thank veterinarians with the Arkansas Veterinarian Society, Cory Gray with the Arkansas Game and Fish Commission, and the personnel involved with each association for collecting the tick samples from the various hosts. Special thanks to the Department of Forensic and Investigative Genetics at the University of North Texas Health Science Center in Ft. Worth Texas for conducting the sequence analyses and screening the FTA cards for *Borrelia.* We would also like to acknowledge the Department of Entomology at the University of Arkansas for additional support with this project. This research was supported in part by the University of Arkansas, Arkansas Agricultural Experiment Station.

Authors' contributions

RTF, CDS, and ALS conceived the study and designed the experiments. PMB and PCW conducted the work in Texas, and RTF conducted the work in Arkansas. RTF, KLK, PMB, and PCW analyzed the results. RTF and PCW wrote and edited the manuscript. All authors read and approved the final version of the manuscript.

REFERENCES

1. Oliver JH, Owsley MR, Hutcheson HJ, James AM, Chen C, Irby WS, Dotson EM, McLain DK: Conspecificity of the ticks Ixodes scapularis and I. dammini (Acari: Ixodidae). J Med Entomol. 1993, 30: 54-63.
2. Stromodahl EY, Hickling GJ: Beyond Lyme: etiology of tick-borne human diseases with emphasis on the southeastern United States. Zoonoses and Public Health. 2012, in press
3. Dennis DT, Piesman JF: Over of tick-borne infections of humans. Tick-borne Diseases of Humans. Edited by: Goodman JL, Dennis DT, Sonenshine DE. 2005, ASM Press, Washington, D.C, 3-11.
4. Bacon RM, Kiersten MS, Kugeler J, Mead PS: Surveillance for Lyme Disease—United States, 1992–2006. MMWR. 2008, 57 (Suppl 10): 1-9.
5. Armstrong PM, Rich SM, Smith RD, Hart DL, Spielman A, Telford SR: A new Borrelia infecting lone star ticks. Lancet. 1996, 347: 67-68.
6. Barbour AG, Maupin GO, Teltow GJ, Carter CJ, Piesman J: Identification of an uncultivatable Borrelia species in the hard tick Amblyomma americanum: possible agent of a Lyme disease-like illness. J Infect Dis. 1996, 173: 403-9. 10.1093/infdis/173.2.403.
7. Burkot TR, Mullen GR, Anderson R, Schneider BS, Happ CM, Zeidner NS: Borrelia lonestari DNA in Adult Amblyomma americanum Ticks, Alabama. Emerg Infect Dis. 2001, 7: 471-473.
8. Stegall-Faulk T, Clark DC, Wright SM: Detection of Borrelia lonestari in Amblyomma americanum (Acari: Ixodidae) from Tennessee. J Med Entomol. 2003, 40: 100-102. 10.1603/0022-2585-40.1.100.
9. Stromdahl EY, Williamson PC, Kollars TM, Evans SR, Barry RK, Vince MA, Dobbs NA: Evidence of Borrelia lonestari DNA in Amblyomma americanum (Acari: Ixodidae) removed from humans. J Clin Microbiol. 2003, 41: 5557-62. 10.1128/JCM.41.12.5557-5562.2003.
10. Clark K: Borrelia species in host-seeking ticks and small mammals in northern Florida. J Clin Microbiol. 2004, 42: 5076-5086. 10.1128/JCM.42.11.5076-5086.2004.
11. Varela-Stokes AS: Transmission of bacterial agents from lone star ticks to white-tailed deer. J Medical Entomol. 2007, 44: 478-483. 10.1603/0022-2585(2007)44[478:TOBAFL]2.0.CO;2.
12. Taft SC, Miller MK, Wright SM: Distribution of Borreliae among ticks collected from eastern states. Vector Borne Zoonot Dis. 2005, 5: 383-389. 10.1089/vbz.2005.5.383.
13. Mixson TR, Campbell SR, Gill JS, Ginsberg HS, Reichard MV, Schulze TL, Dasch GA: Prevalence of Ehrlichia, Borrelia, and Rickettsial Agents in Amblyomma americanum (Acari: Ixodidae) Collected from nine states. J Med Entomol. 2006, 43: 1261-1268. 10.1603/0022-2585(2006)43[1261:POEBAR]2.0.CO;2.
14. Schulze TL, Jordan RA, Healy SP, Roegner VE, Meddis M, Jahn MB, Guthrie DL: Relative abundance and prevalence of selected Borrelia infections in Ixodes scapularis and Amblyomma americanum (Acari: Ixodidae) from publicly owned lands in Monmouth County, New Jersey. J Med Entomol. 2006, 43: 1269-1275. 10.1603/0022-2585(2006)43[1269:RAAPOS]2.0.CO;2.
15. (CDC) Centers for Disease Control: Lyme Disease. Division of Vector Borne Infectious Diseases, National Center for Zoonotic, Vector-Borne, and Enteric Diseases. 2007,http://www.cdc.gov/ncidod/dvbid/lyme/ld_transmission.htm,
16. Vaughn MF, Sloane PD, Knierim K, Varkey D, Pilgad MA, Johnson BJB: Practice based research network partnership with CDC to acquire clinical specimens to study the etiology of Southern Tick-Associated rash illness (STARI). JABFM. 2010, 23: 720-727. 10.3122/jabfm.2010.06.100098.
17. Goddard J: What's going on with Lyme disease in the South?. Inf Med. 2001, 18: 132-133.
18. Piesman J, Sinsky RJ: Ability of Ixodes scapularis, Dermacentor variabilis, and Amblyomma americanum (Acari: Ixodidae) to acquire, maintain, and transmit Lyme disease spirochetes (Borrelia burgdorferi). J Med Entomol. 1998, 25: 336-339.
19. Magnarelli LA, Oliver JH, Hutcheson HJ, Boone JL, Anderson JF: Antibodies to Borrelia burgdorferi in rodents in the eastern and southern United States. J Clin Microbiol. 1992, 30: 1449-1452.
20. Sanders FH, Oliver JH: Evaluation of Ixodes scapularis, Amblyomma americanum, and Dermacentor variabilis (Acari: Ixodidae) from Georgia as Vectors of a Florida Strain of the Lyme Disease Spirochete, Borrelia burgdorferi. J Med Entomol. 1995, 32: 402-406.
21. Durden LA, McLean RG, Oliver JH, Ubico SR, James AM: Ticks, Lyme disease spriochetes, trypanosomes, and antibody to encephalitis viruses in wild birds from coastal Georgia and South Carolina. J Parasitol. 1997, 83: 1178-1182. 10.2307/3284382.
22. Weller SJ, Baldridge GD, Munderloh UG, Noda H, Simser J, Kurtti TJ: Phylogenetic placement of rickettsiae from the ticks Amblyomma americanum and Ixodes scapularis. J Clin Microbiol. 1998, 36: 1305-1317.
23. Simpson KK, Hinck LW: The prevalence of Borrelia burgdorferi, the Lyme disease spirochete, in ticks and rodents in northeast Arkansas. Proc Arkansas Academy of Sci. 1993, 47: 110-115.
24. Diuk-Wasser MS, Hoen AG, Cislo P, Brinkerhoff R, Hamer SA, Rowland M, Cortinas R, Vourc'h G, Melton F, Hickling GJ, Tsao JI, Bunikis J, Barbour AG, Kitron U, Piesman J, Fish D: Human risk of infection with Borrelia burgdorferi, the Lyme disease agent, in eastern United States. Am Soc Trop Med Hyg. 2012, 86: 320-327. 10.4269/ajtmh.2012.11-0395.
25. Daniels TJ, Fish D, Levine JF, Greco MA, Eaton AT,

Padgett PJ, LaPointe DA: Canine exposure to Borrelia burgdorferi and prevalence of Ixodes dammini (Acari: Ixodidae) on deer as a measure of Lyme disease risk in the northeastern United States. J Med Entomol. 1993, 30: 171-178.

26. Murdock JH, Yabsley MJ, Little SE, Chandrashekar R, O'Connor TP, Caudell JN, Huffman JE, Langenberg JA, Hollamby S: Distribution of antibodies reactive to Borrelia lonestari and Borrelia burgdorferi in white-tailed deer (Odocoileus virginianus) populations in the eastern United States. Vector borne and Zoonotic Dis. 2009, 9: 729-736. 10.1089/vbz.2008.0144.

27. Trout RT, Steelman CD: Ticks parasitizing canines and deer in Arkansas. J Entomol Sci. 2010, 45: 140-148.

28. Trout RT, Steelman CD, Szalanski AL: Population Genetics and Phylogeography of Ixodes scapularis from Canines and Deer in Arkansas. Southwestern Entomol. 2009, 34: 273-287. 10.3958/059.034.0308.

29. Qiu WG: Geographic uniformity of the Lyme disease spirochete (Borrelia burgdorferi) and its shared history with tick vector (Ixodes scapularis) in the northeastern United States. Genetics. 2002, 160: 833-849.

30. (CDC) Centers for Disease Control: Lyme Disease Division of Vector Borne Infectious Diseases, National Center for Zoonotic, Vector-Borne, and Enteric Diseases. 2012,http://www.cdc.gov/lyme/faq/index.html#endemic,

31. Arthur DR: Ticks and Disease. 1961, Row, Peterson and Company, Evanston, IL

32. Lancaster JL, Patrick JK: Rocky mountain spotted fever in northwest Arkansas. J Arkansas Med Soc. 1977, 74: 156-158.

33. Goddard J, Norment BR: A guide to the ticks of Mississippi. 1985, Mississippi Agric For Expnt Stat Bull, Mississippi, 935-

34. Black WC, Piesman J: Phylogeny of hard- and soft- tick taxa (Acari: Ixodida) based on mitochondrial 16 S rDNA sequences. Proc Natl Acad Sci. 1994, 91: 10034-10038. 10.1073/pnas.91.21.10034.

35. Bacon RM, Gilmore RD, Quintana M, Piesman J, Johnson BJB: DNA evidence of Borrelia lonestari in Amblyomma americanum (Acari: Ixodidae) in Southeast Missouri. J Med Entomol. 2003, 40: 590-592. 10.1603/0022-2585-40.4.590.

36. Gilbert C, Ropiquet A, Hassanin A: Mitochondrial and nuclear phylogenies of Cervidae (Mammalia, Ruminantia): Systematics, morphology, and biogeography. Mol Phylogenet Evol. 2006, 40: 101-117. 10.1016/j.ympev.2006.02.017.

37. Sall J, Creighton L, Lehman A: JMP Start Statistics: A guide to statistics an data analysis using JMP and JMP IN Software. 2005, SAS Institute Inc., Cary, NC, 3

38. Dodge M, Stinson C: What's new in Microsoft Office Excel 2007. Microsoft Office Excel 2007 inside out. 2007, Microsoft Press, Indianapolis, IN

39. Williamson PC, Billingsley PM, Teltow GJ, Seals JP, Turnbough MA, Atkinson SF: Borrelia, Ehrlichia, and Rickettsia spp. in ticks removed from persons, Texas, USA. Emerg Infect Dis. 2010, 16: 441-446.

40. Arkansas State Land Information Board: Natural color Select 1-Foot county Mosaic. Digital Orthrophoto Quadrangles, Color Infrared and Natural Color. 2006, AR Counties, Little Rock, Arkansas,http://www.geostor.arkansas.gov/G6/Home.html?id=bbf7f1801f53d2c3a3fcf719bef46f84,

41. James AM, Liveris D, Wormser GP, Schwartz I, Montecalvo MA, Johnson MJB: Borrelia lonestari infection after a bite by an Amblyomma americanum tick. J Infect Dis. 2001, 183: 1810-1814. 10.1086/320721.

42. Telford SR, Mather TN, Moore SI, Wilson ML, Spielman A: Incompetence of deer as reservoirs of the Lyme disease spirochete. Am J Trop Med Hyg. 1988, 39: 105-109.

43. Kardatzke JT, Neidhardt K, Dzuban DP, Sanchez JL, Azad AF: Cluster of tick-borne infections at Fort Chaffee, AR: Rickettsiae and Borrelia burgdorferi in Ixodid ticks. J Med Entomol. 1992, 29: 669-672.

44. Rhea SK, Glickman SW, Waller A, Ising A, Maillard JM, Lund EM, Glickman LT: Evaluation of routinely collected veterinary and human health data for surveillance of human tick-borne diseases in North Carolina. Vector-Borne and Zoonotic Diseases. 2011, 11: 9-14. 10.1089/vbz.2009.0255.

45. DeFries RS, Foley JA, Asner GP: Land-use choices: balancing human needs and ecosystem function. Front Ecol Environ. 2004, 2: 249-257. 10.1890/1540-9295(2004)002[0249:LCBHNA]2.0.CO;2.

46. Lepczyk CA, Hammer RB, Stewart SI, Radeloff VC: Spatiotemporal dynamics of housing growth hotspots in the North U.S. from 1940 to 2000. Landscape Ecol. 2007, 22: 939-952. 10.1007/s10980-006-9066-2.

47. Spielman A: The emergence of Lyme disease and human babesiosis in a changing environment. Ann New York Acad of Sci. 2006, 740: 146-156.

48. Pinger RR, Timmons L, Karris K: Spread of Ixodes scapularis (Acari: Ixodidae) in Indiana: collections of adults in 1991–1994 and description of a Borrelia burgdorferi infected populations. J Med Entomol. 1996, 33: 852-855.

49. Diuk-Wasser MA, Gatewood AG, Cortinas MR, Yaremych-Hamer S, Tsao J, Kitron U, Hickling G, Brownstein JS, Walker E, Piesman J, Fish D: Spatiotemporal patterns of host-seeking Ixodes scapularis nymphs (Acari: Ixodidae) in the United States. J Med Entomol. 2006, 43: 166-176. 10.1603/0022-2585(2006)043[0166:SPOHIS]2.0.CO;2.

50. Hoen AG, Margos G, Bent SJ, Diuk-Wasser MA, Barbour A, Kurtenbach K, Fish D: Phylogeography of Borrelia burgdorferi in the eastern United States reflects multiple independent Lyme disease emergence events. Proc Natl Acad Sci. 2009, 106: 15013-15018. 10.1073/pnas.0903810106.

51. Koch HG: Seasonal incidence and attachment sites of ticks (Acari: Ixodidae) on domestic dogs in southeastern Oklahoma and northwestern Arkansas. J Med Entomol. 1982, 19: 293-298.

SECTION XIII: RICKETTSIA SPP.- TICK-BORNE DISEASES

CHAPTER 46 ACUTE FEBRILE ILLNESS IS ASSOCIATED WITH RICKETTSIA SPP INFECTION IN DOGS

Laia Solano-Gallego, Alessandra Caprì, Maria Grazia Pennisi, Marco Caldin, Tommaso Furlanello and Michele Trotta

Keywords: Dog, Febrile illness, *Rickettsia conorii, Ehrlichia, Anaplasma, Babesia, Hepatozoon, Leishmania,* Serology, PCR

BACKGROUND

Rickettsia conorii is a Spotted Fever Group (SFG) *Rickettsia* that causes Mediterranean Spotted Fever (MSF) in humans in Mediterranean countries and Sub-Saharan Africa. The onset of MSF is abrupt and typical human cases present with high fever, flu-like symptoms, a black eschar at the tick bite site and a maculo-papular rash. Severe forms of the disease may present with major neurological manifestations and multi-organ involvement may occur. The mortality rate is estimated at around 2.5% and classical risk factors for severe forms include elderly age, cirrhosis, chronic alcoholism and glucose-6-phosphate dehydrogenase deficiency [1,2]. In Italy, more than 1000 human cases of MSF are reported annually mainly in Sicily, Sardinia, Lazio and Liguria [2,3]. Moreover, a more pathogenic subspecies of *R. conorii*, *R. conorii israelensis*, has been described in human cases in Sicily [4]. In addition, *R. conorii* Indian tick typhus strain has also been diagnosed in human patients in Sicily [5].

The organism is transmitted in the Mediterranean basin by the brown dog tick *Rhipicephalus sanguineus*. Mediterranean spotted fever is a human seasonal disease that is frequently diagnosed between April and October with a maximum peak in June-August [2] and it is well correlated with the presence of *Rh. sanguineus*. Ticks are possibly the main reservoir of *R. conorii* infection due to the existence of both transtadial and transovarial transmission and cofeeding in this tick sp. [1,2,6]. The role of dogs in maintaining zoonotic foci remains unclear [1]. Although dogs are the natural host of the vector, there is limited information on their susceptibility to Rickettsiae infection and on the development of long duration rickettsiemia able to allow transmission to a feeding vector tick [7]. However, experimental infections suggest that dogs can be competent reservoirs for *R. conorii* [6,7]. Due to high levels of *Rh. sanguineus* exposure, dogs have been used in epidemiological studies as sentinels for human MSF [8] and proximity to seroreactive dogs has been found as a risk factor for MSF in humans [9]. Several studies have reported anti-*R. conorii* antibodies by the indirect fluorescent antibody test (IFA) in dogs in *R. conorii* endemic countries such as Italy with seroprevalence rates ranging from 15.5% to 74% [10]. The very high seroprevalences detected in Italian dogs would suggest frequent exposure to *Rickettsia* spp. or persistent low-grade infection with a rickettsial organism or organisms that cross react with *R. conorii* antigens by IFA testing.

Studies reported the detection of *Rickettsia* DNA in the blood of Spanish and Italian dogs [11-14]. However, evidence that natural *R. conorii* infection causes illness in dogs remains limited. Illness has been associated with *R. conorii* natural infection in only a few dogs since human MSF was described in 1910 [15]. The possibility that *R. conorii* may cause a clinical disease in dogs is supported by the evidence of seroconversion in three sick dogs from Israel [16] and the association between anemia and seroreactivity to *R. conorii*antigens [17]. In addition, a study reported the association between male dogs and seroreactivity to *R. conorii*antigens as found in humans where males have higher rates of infection [2,17]. Moreover, febrile illness has been associated with *R. conorii* infection in three dogs from Sicily by means of seroconversion and PCR [13] and in seven dogs from Portugal by PCR [18]. For this reason, the clinical significance of infection with *R. conorii*, or other SFG rickettsiae in dogs, remains unclear and requires further characterization.

Citation: Laia Solano-Gallego, Alessandra Caprì, Maria Grazia Pennisi, Marco Caldin, Tommaso Furlanello and Michele Trotta, Acute febrile illness is associated with Rickettsia spp infection in dogs, DOI: 10.1186/s13071-015-0824-3.

The aims of this prospective case–control study were: 1) to investigate the presence of *Rickettsia* spp. infection in dogs from southern Italy (Sicily and Reggio Calabria) with fever by means of serological and molecular tests when compared with case control dogs with normal body temperatures; 2) to evaluate whether *Rickettsia* spp. infection causes clinical disease and clinicopathological abnormalities by clinical history, physical examination and baseline laboratory tests; and 3) to evaluate co-infections with other microorganisms that cause canine vector borne diseases such as *Leishmania infantum*, *Ehrlichia* spp., *Anaplasma* spp., *Babesia* spp. and *Hepatozoon canis* and their clinical importance in sick dogs.

METHODS

Dogs

The study was carried out between August-November 2009 and between April-November 2010 in Sicily, Italy. Dogs were enrolled in the study from 20 Veterinary clinics throughout Sicily (Catania, Caltanissetta, Enna, Messina, Palermo, Siracusa and Trapani) and from the south of Calabria (Reggio Calabria).

Physical and laboratory examinations were performed during the study at the time of onset of clinical signs and after one month or later. MSF is most commonly described in humans with a maximum peak in June and August [2]. Clinical questionnaires were distributed and filled by veterinarians to obtain detailed clinical data at the time of onset of clinical signs and after one month or later. Information collected from the questionnaires included the date of sample collection, age, sex, breed, type of housing (indoor *versus*outdoor), flea and tick exposure, presence of vectors on clinical examination, vaccination status, presenting complaint, clinical signs observed, previous medical history, clinical response to specific therapy and clinical status of the dog's owner.

Blood serum samples were taken two times (first and second visit) when possible with an interval between samplings of one month in the majority of dogs or two months in few dogs, in order to evaluate acute (first visit) and convalescent (second visit) antibodies and seroconversion. Blood was taken in EDTA tubes at the time of diagnosis prior to doxycycline treatment and after one month or more. One hundred and seventy-one dogs were included in the study and they were divided into two groups: febrile dogs and afebrile dogs.

Febrile dogs

Ninety-nine dogs with febrile illness were enrolled in the study. The inclusion criteria were: 1) Dogs with an acute onset (less than 10 days of duration) of fever (≥39.5°C) were included. 2) Only dogs with informed consent signed by the owner were enrolled. The exclusion criteria were: 1) Dogs with an acute onset of fever and evidence of another disease involved such as heat-stroke, neoplasia, bacterial abscesses and pyometra; 2) Dogs with a recent history of doxycycline administration during the past two months; 3) Dogs without signed informed consent by the owner.

Matched case afebrile dogs

A case control set of dogs (n=72) with no apparent disease or other diseases unrelated to febrile illness was randomly selected from dogs seen at the same veterinary clinics during the same month as the febrile dogs. The inclusion criteria were: 1) Healthy dogs evaluated for routine procedures such as vaccinations, elective surgery (neutering/spaying); 2) Sick dogs that did not present with acute fever (≥39.5°C) or suspicion of tick-transmitted disease; 3) Only dogs with informed consent signed by the owner were enrolled in the study. The exclusion criteria were: 1) Dogs recently treated with doxycycline during the last two months; 2) Dogs without signed informed consent by the owner.

Only privately owned dogs were included in the study and examined by routine non-invasive diagnostic procedures. Owners were accurately informed and an informed consent was signed by both owner and veterinarian. Eight dogs presented clinical signs but not fever.

Blood samples from dogs were taken for diagnostic purposes as part of clinical management and, therefore, no ethical approval was needed.

Unfortunately, only 92 out of 171 dogs enrolled in the study came back for a second visit a month or more after the first visit.

Laboratory procedures

Routine laboratory tests

Complete blood count (CBC) with blood smear examination and platelet concentration, complete biochemical profile including C-reactive protein and serum electrophoresis were performed in all dogs at the time of diagnosis and second visit as previously described [19]. The samples were submitted in less than 24 hours from blood withdrawal to *Laboratorio Privato di Analisi Veterinarie San Marco* (Padua, Italy). Whole EDTA blood and serum samples for PCR and serology were stored at −20°C until used for molecular and serological testing.

Serological techniques (IFA or ELISA)

Indirect immunofluorescence assays (IFA) kits from Fuller Laboratories (Fullerton, CA, USA) were used for IgG antibodies detection against *R. conorii, E. canis* and *A. phagocytophilum* antigens following manufacturer's instructions.

IFA does not distinguish between canine antibodies against *A. phagocytophilum* and *Anaplasma platys* [20]. In addition, the IFA test used for *Rickettsia conorii* is known to cross-react with other species of spotted fever group *Rickettsia* such as *R. rickettsii*, *R. helvetica*, *R. slovaca* and *R. massiliae* as stated in manufacturer's instructions.

An antibody titer of 1:64 or greater was considered positive for *R. conorii* antigen. An antibody titer of 1:80 or greater was considered positive for *E. canis* and *A. phagocytophilum* antigens.

Seroconversion was defined as≥2–4 fold increase convalescent antibody titers (second visit) when acute (first initial visit) titers were positive or as any positive antibody titers when acute (first initial visit) titers were negative. High antibody titers were defined as equal or greater of 1:512 (*R.*

conorii) or 1:640 (*E. canis* and *A. phagocytophilum*). Paired samples were run the same day.

ELISA was performed to detect antibodies against *L. infantum* as previously described [21].

DNA extraction, real-time PCR for Rickettsia spp. and other infectious agents and DNA sequencing

DNA extraction was performed from EDTA-anticoagulated whole blood sample by the High Pure PCR Template Preparation Kit (Roche Applied Science, GmbH, Mannheim, Germany) in accordance with the manufacturer's protocol with some modifications. Two hundred μL of blood were incubated with 40 μL of Proteinase K and with 200 μL of Binding Buffer at 72°C for 1 h. Subsequent steps were carried out according to the manufacturer's instructions (Roche Applied Science, GmbH, Mannheim, Germany). DNA was eluted in 50 μL of elution buffer at 72°C [13].

A quantitative PCR (qPCR) for the detection of *Rickettsia* spp., *A. phagocytophilum/A. platys*, *E. canis* and *L. infantum* in DNA samples was performed. PCR amplifications were carried out for *Rickettsia* spp. [13,14], *E. canis*, *A. phagocytophilum/A. platys* (fragment of 16S rRNA gene) [22], and *L. infantum* (fragment of kinetoplast minicircle) [23] using LCSet primers and probes following manufacturer's instructions (TIB MOLBIOL). Real-time PCR amplifications were carried out in Roche LightCycler, version 3.5.17, (Roche Diagnostic, GmbH, Mannheim, Germany), with a final volume of 10 μL, including 2.5 μL of the DNA template, 2 μL of Light Cycler Fast start reaction mix (FastStart DNA Master^{PLUS}, Roche Diagnostic, GmbH, Mannheim, Germany), and 0.5 μL of LCSet primers and probes according to the manufacturer's instructions (TIB Molbiol, Berlin, Germany). Amplifications were conducted in sealed 20 μL Light Cycler glass capillaries (Roche Diagnostic, GmbH, Mannheim, Germany). Thermal cycling for *Rickettsia* spp qPCR comprised an initial denaturation step at 95°C for 8 min, followed by 55 cycles of a denaturation at 95°C for 5 s, annealing at 59°C for 7 s, and extension at 72°C for 7 s, with quantification of fluorescence signal [13,14]. Thermal cycling for *A. phagocytophilum/A. platys* qPCR comprised an initial denaturation step at 95°C for 8 min, followed by 45 cycles of a denaturation at 95°C for 5 s, annealing at 61°C for 10 s, and extension at 72°C for 11 s, with quantification of fluorescence signal [22]. Thermal cycling for *E. canis* qPCR comprised an initial denaturation step at 95°C for 8 min, followed by 60 cycles of a denaturation at 95°C for 5 s, annealing at 61°C for 10 s, and extension at 72°C for 11 s, with quantification of fluorescence signal [22]. Thermal cycling for *Leishmania infantum* qPCR comprised an initial denaturation step at 37°C for 10 min, 95°C for 8 min, followed by 45 cycles of a denaturation at 95°C for 5 s, annealing at 60°C for 5 s, and extension at 72°C for 4 s, with quantification of fluorescence signal [23]. A real-time PCR reaction was considered positive when the normalized fluorescence signal [ratio of the signal from detection channel F2 (640 nm) to the signal from detection channel F1 (495 nm) at the end of the annealing step] showed an exponential increase in fluorescence. The melting temperature of probe–template hybrids was automatically determined by the analysis of the software, and was useful for species identification of *Rickettsia rickettsii versus* other *Rickettsia* species and *A. phagocytophilum versus A. platys. Rickettsia rickettsii* had a melting temperature of approximately 65°C, while *R. conorii* had a melting temperature of approximately 58.2°C. *Anaplasma phagocytophilum* had a melting temperature of approximately 66°C, while *A. platys* had a melting temperature of approximately 57°C. Each real-time PCR run include a blank, a negative control, and a DNA cloned amplicon as a positive control (LCSet positive control; TIB Molbiol, Berlin, Germany).

Conventional PCRs for the detection of fragment of 18S rRNA gene of *Babesia* spp. [24] and of 18S rRNA gene of *Hepatozoon* spp. [25] were also carried out, as previously described. The partial 18S rRNA gene for *Babesia*spp. was amplified by using conventional PCR analysis in a final volume of 50 μL, containing 2.5 μL of DNA template from each sample, 1 μL (10 pmol/ μl) of each of the primers, PIRO-A and PIRO-B, 1 μL (10 pmol/μl) of deoxyribonucleotide triphosphates (dNTPs) (Roche Diagnostics, GmbH, Mannheim, Germany), 5 μL of PCR buffer 10X (5 PRIME GmbH, Hamburg, Germany), and 1U of recombinant Taq DNA polymerase (5 PRIME GmbH, Hamburg, Germany). DNA amplification was performed with the Thermal Cycler 2720 (Applied Biosystems, Europe) at the following temperature profiles: initial denaturation at 95°C for 5 minutes, denaturation at 95°C for 30 seconds, annealing at 58°C for 30 seconds, extension at 72°C for 30 seconds, and repeated for 35 cycles, with a final extension for 7 minutes at 72°C. The partial 18S rRNA gene (666 bp) for *Hepatozoon canis* was amplified by using conventional PCR analysis in a final volume of 50 μL, containing 5 μL of DNA template from each sample, 1 μL (10 pmol/μl) of each of the primers, HEP-F and HEP-R, 1 μL (10 pmol/μl) of dNTPs (Roche Diagnostics, GmbH, Mannheim, Germany), 5 μL of PCR buffer 10X (5 PRIME GmbH, Hamburg, Germany), and 1 U of recombinant Taq DNA polymerase (5 PRIME GmbH, Hamburg, Germany). DNA amplification was performed with the Thermal Cycler 2720 (Applied Biosystems, Europe) at the following temperature profiles: initial denaturation at 95°C for 5 minutes, denaturation at 95°C for 30 seconds, annealing at 53°C for 30 seconds, extension at 72°C for 30 seconds, and repeated for 35 cycles, with a final extension for 7 minutes at 72°C.

DNA electrophoresis for amplicons detection was carried out in 2.2% FlashGel System (Lonza, Rockland, ME USA), and DNA fragments were visualized. For subsequent sequencing of *Babesia* spp. and *Hepatozoon* spp. positive samples, amplification product from PCR was submitted for direct sequencing.

Rickettsia positive samples by qPCR for 16S gene were also amplified for the OmpA gene by a conventional PCR for further molecular characterization [13,14]. The partial OmpA gene for *Rickettsia* spp was amplified by PCR in a final volume of 50 μL, containing 5 μL of DNA template from each sample, 1 μL (10 pmol/μl) of each of the primers, 107F and 299R 1 μL (10 pmol/μl) of dNTPs (Roche Diagnostics, GmbH, Mannheim, Germany), 5 μL of PCR buffer 10X (5 PRIME GmbH, Hamburg, Germany), and 1U of recombinant Taq DNA polymerase (5 PRIME GmbH, Hamburg, Germany). DNA amplification was performed with the Thermal Cycler 2720 (Applied Biosystems, Europe) at the following temperature profiles: initial denaturation at 95°C for 5 minutes, denaturation at 95°C for 30 seconds, annealing at 54°C for 30 seconds, extension at 72°C for 30 seconds, and repeated for 35 cycles, with a final extension for 7 minutes at 72°C.

The samples were sequenced and compared to known sequences deposited in GenBank®. The sequencing reaction was performed with the Applied Biosystem 3730xl DNA Analyzer on both strands by BMR Genomics srl (Padua, Italy) by using the dideoxychain-termination method [26]. Consensus sequences were aligned [(BIOEDIT version 7.0 (ClustalW)] with known sequences in GenBank® using the basic local alignment search tool (BLAST) available from (http://blast.ncbi.nlm.nih.gov/Blast.cgi?PROGRAM=blastn&PAGE_TYPE=BlastSearch&LINK_LOC=blasthome). Sequences were deposited in GenBank®.

Current *Rickettsia* infection was considered when dogs were positive to *Rickettsia* PCR and/or demonstrated seroconversion to *R. conorii* antigen.

Statistical analysis

For univariate analysis, Chi-square and Fisher's exact tests were used to test for associations between proportions and putative explanatory factors and univariate Odds ratios (OR) were calculated. The differences were considered significant if the *P*-value was<0.05. SPSS (IBM, USA) statistical software (version 19) was used for statistical analyses.

RESULTS

Dogs

The dog population characteristics including breed, gender, age and presence or absence of ticks per each group are described in Table 1. Statistical associations were found between breed and presence or absence of ticks and febrile *versus* afebrile group (Table 1).

Table 1: Description of dog population characteristics

DOGS	BREED		GENDER		AGE*		TICKS	
	N=159		N=171		n=161		N=121	
	Mixed	Pure	Male	Female	Young	Adult	Presence	Absence
Total	58/159 (37.1%)	101/159 (63.5%)	94/171 (54.9%)	77/171 (45%)	16/161 (9.9%)	145/161 (90%)	31/121 (25.6%)	90/121 (74.3)
Febrile	40/58** (68.9%)	53/101 (52.4%)	40/94 (42.5%)	45/77 (58.4%)	13/16 (81.2%)	85/145 (58.6%)	29/31*** (93.5%)	46/90 (51.1%)
Afebrile	18/58 (31%)	48/101 (47.5%)	54/94 (57.4%)	32/77 (42.8%)	3/16 (18.7%)	60/145 (41.3%)	2/31 (6.4%)	44/90 (48.8%)

*For age classification, young was considered as less than 12 months of age and adult was considered as above 12 months of age
**Chi-square=4.126, *P*=0.042 ***Chi-square=17.622, *P*<0.0001.

Serological and PCR results for all pathogens

The serological results in febrile and afebrile dogs at the time of the first and second visits are shown in Table 2. The total first visit seropositivity rates for *R. conorii*, *E. canis*, *A. phagocytophilum* and *L. infantum*were 44.8%, 48.5%, 37.8% and 17.6%, respectively. The seroconversion results for *R. conorii*, *E. canis* and *A. phagocytophilum* antigens in both groups of dogs are displayed in Table 3. The total seroconversion rates for *R. conorii*, *E. canis* and *A. phagocytophilum* were 20.7%, 14.3% and 8.8%, respectively. Seroconversion rates for *R. conorii* were significantly higher in febrile dogs when compared with afebrile dogs (Chi-square=4.070, *P*=0.0436). The seroconversion rates for *E. canis* and *A. phagocytophilum* were not different among the groups studied (Table 3).

Table 2: Seroreactivity to several tick-borne pathogens antigens in febrile and afebrile dogs at the time of first and second visit

Pathogens	Initial serology (first visit)			Convalescent serology (second visit)		
	Febrile	Afebrile	Total	Febrile	Afebrile	Total
	N=95	N=70	N=165	N=44	N=48	N=92
R. conorii	53 (55.8%)*	21 (30.0%)	74 (44.8%)	29 (65.9%)**	15 (31.2%)	44 (47.8%)
E. canis	47 (50.0%)	32 (46.4%)	79 (48.5%)	15 (34.1%)	11 (22.9%)	26 (28.2%)
A. phagocytophilum	38 (40.4%)	24 (34.3%)	62 (37.8%)	9 (20.4%)	7 (14.6%)	16 (17.4%)
L. infantum* **	20 (20.2%)	10 (14.1%)	30 (17.6%)	Not determined		

*Chi-square=10.837, *P*=0.001;**Chi-square=11.052, *P*=0.002; *** Number of febrile dogs was 99; Number of afebrile dogs was 71; total number of dogs was 170.

Table 3: Seroconversion results for *R. conorii* , *E. canis* , *A. phagocytophilum* in febrile and afebrile dogs

Pathogens	**Seroconversion**		
	Number of positive dogs (%, CI 95%)		
	Febrile	**Afebrile**	**Total**
	N=44	**N=48**	**N=92**
R. conorii	13 (29.5%, 18-44%)*	6 (12.5%, 5-25%)	19 (20.7%, 13-30%)
E. canis**	7 (16.3%, 7-29%)	6 (12.5%, 5-25%)	13 (14.3%, 8-22%)
A. phagocytophilum**	3 (7.0%, 1-18%)	5 (10.4%, 4-22%)	8 (8.8%, 4-16%)

*Chi-square=4.070, P=0.0436;**Number of febrile dogs was 43; number of total dogs was 91.

The total first visit molecular positive rates for *Rickettsia* spp., *E. canis*, *A. phagocytophilum*, *A. platys*, *L. infantum*, *Babesia* spp. and *Hepatozoon* spp. were 1.8%, 4.1%, 0%, 2.3%, 11.1%, 2.3% and 0.6%, respectively. Positive PCR for *E. canis* (7.1%), *Rickettsia* spp. (3%), *Babesia* spp. (4%) and *Hepatozoon* spp. (1%) were only found in febrile dogs (Table 4).

Table 4: Molecular prevalence of all pathogens in febrile and afebrile dogs at the first visit

Pathogens	**PCR**		
	Febrile	**Afebrile**	**Total**
	n=99	**n=71**	**n=170**
R. conorii	3 (3.0%)*	0 (0%)	3 (1.8%)
E. canis	7 (7.1%)**	0 (0%)	7 (4.1%)
A. platys	3 (3.0%)	1 (1.4%)	4 (2.3%)
B. vogeli	4 (4.0%)	0 (0%)	4 (2.3%)
H. canis	1 (1.0%)	0 (0%)	1 (0.6%)
L. infantum	14 (14.1%)	5 (6.9%)	19 (11.1%)

*All dogs were positive to 16SrRNA and OmpA PCRs; ** Fisher's exact test, P=0.042

Fourteen febrile dogs (31.8%) were diagnosed with *Rickettsia* spp. infection based on seroconversion and/or PCR while only six afebrile dogs (12.5%) seroconverted (Chi-square=5.036; P=0.0248; Fisher's exact test; P=0.0414).

Febrile illness was statistically significant associated with: acute *R conorii* positive antibody reaction (Chi-square=10.837; univariate Odds ratio=2.944; P=0.001); convalescent *R. conorii* positive antibody reaction (Chi-square=7.312; univariate Odds ratio=4.253; P=0.001); seroconversion to *R. conorii* (Chi- square=4.070; univariate Odds ratio=2.935; P=0.044); *E. canis* positive PCR (Chi-square=5.236; univariate Odds ratio=1.247; P calculated with Fisher's exact test=0.042); *E. canis* or *Rickettsia* or *Anaplasma* PCRs positive (Chi-square=6.835; univariate Odds ratio=9.793; P=0.009); positivity to any tick pathogen PCRs (Chi-square=10.161; univariate odds ratio=13.687; P=0.001).

Twelve febrile dogs (12.6%) displayed initial high *R. conorii* antibody titers while only five afebrile dogs (7.1%) presented initial high *R. conorii* antibody titers (Chi-square=1.314; P=0.252). Eleven febrile dogs (25%) displayed convalescent high *R. conorii* antibody titers while only 4 afebrile dogs (8.3%) presented convalescent high *R. conorii* antibody titers (Chi-square=2.860; P=0.091).

Five febrile dogs (35.7%) displayed initial high *E. canis* antibody titers while none the afebrile dogs (0.0%) presented initial high *E. canis* antibody titers (Chi-square=3.840; P=0.050). Five out of seven febrile dogs (71.4%) diagnosed with *E. canis* infection by means of PCR were seronegative (n=2) or presented a low positive antibody titer (1:80; n=3) at the time of illness and seroconverted suggesting acute infection. Only two febrile dogs diagnosed by positive *E. canis* PCR presented an initial high antibody titer (1:1280).

Three out of three febrile dogs (100%) diagnosed with *A. platys* infection by means of PCR were seronegative or presented a low positive antibody titer (1:80) by *A. phagocytophilum* IFA at the time of illness and only one seroconverted suggesting acute infection. Only one febrile dog diagnosed by positive *A. platys* PCR presented high antibody titer (1:1280).

Initial *E. canis* IFA was statistically associated with *A. phagocytophilum* IFA (Chi-square=93.490; P<0.0001).

Co-infections

Seven febrile dogs diagnosed with *Rickettsia* spp. infection based on seroconversion and/or PCR presented coinfections with *A. platys* diagnosed by PCR (n=2), or with *E. canis* diagnosed by seroconversion (n=1) or with both *E. canis* and *A. phagocytophilum* diagnosed by seroconversion (n=2) or with *Babesia* diagnosed by PCR (n=2). Two afebrile dogs diagnosed with *Rickettsia* spp infection based on seroconversion presented coinfections with *E. canis* diagnosed by seroconversion (n=1) and with both *E. canis* and *A. phagocytophilum*diagnosed by seroconversion (n=1).

Only febrile dogs presented coinfections with more than one pathogen demonstrated by molecular analysis: one coinfected with *R. conorii* and *A. platys*, one with *E. canis* and *H. canis*; one with *L. infantum* and *E. canis*, one with *L. infantum* and *A. platys* and two coinfected with *L. infantum* and *B. vogeli*.

Clinical manifestations and clinicopathological abnormalities

The most common clinical signs and laboratory abnormalities of febrile dogs diagnosed with *Rickettsia*infection based on seroconversion and/or PCR were fever, lethargy, myalgia, lameness, elevation of C-reactive protein, hypoalbuminemia, thrombocytopenia and mild non-regenerative anemia. However, other less common clinical signs and clinicopathological abnormalities included orchitis, lymphadenomegaly, splenomegaly, abdominal pain/hunched posture, vomiting and diarrhea, hyperglobulinemia, elevation liver enzymes (ALP, AST) and mature neutrophilic leukocytosis.

Anemia was statistically associated with the presence of an initial high *R. conorii* antibody titer (Chi-square=3.877; $P=0.049$), positive serology for *L. infantum* (Chi-square=4.229; $P=0.040$), positive *E. canis* PCR (Fisher's exact test; $P=0.048$), with positivity for *E. canis* or *Rickettsia* or *Anaplasma* PCR (Chi-square=4.229; $P=0.040$) and with positivity for any of the pathogens studied by PCR (Chi-square=4.561; $P=0.033$). Thrombocytopenia was statistically associated with the presence of positive convalescent *R. conorii* antibody titer (Chi-square=4.227; $P=0.040$), with acute high *E. canis* antibody titer (Chi-square=10.809; $P=0.001$), with positive convalescent *E. canis* antibody titer (Chi-square=4.463; $P=0.035$). It was also significantly associated with positive acute *A. phagocytophilum* antibody titer (Fisher's exact test; $P=0.005$), with high convalescent *A. phagocytophilum* antibody titers (Fisher's exact test; $P=0.037$), with *E. canis* positive PCR (Fisher's exact test; $P=0.002$), with positivity for *E. canis* or *Rickettsia* or *Anaplasma* PCR (Chi-square=9.888; $P=0.002$) and with positivity for any of the pathogens studied by PCR (Chi-square=14.457; $P<0.0001$). Hemoparasites were not found by blood smear examination in any of the dogs included in the study.

DNA sequences

The OmpA gene DNA sequences (170 bp) obtained from three *Rickettsia* positive PCR samples (GenBank® accession numbers KP896303, KP896304 and KP896305) were 100% identical to several *R. conorii* sequences present in GenBank® (e.g.: GenBank® accession number KJ433804 and KF245453). The above OmpA gene DNA sequences were only 95% identical to the *R. parkeri* sequences present in GenBank® (GenBank® accession number: KJ158741, KJ174528, JQ906784) which were the second BLAST match.

The 18SrRNA gene DNA sequence (412 bp) obtained from four *Babesia* spp. positive PCR samples (GenBank® accession numbers KP896299, KP896300, KP896301 and KP896302) were 100% identical to the *B. vogeli*sequences present in GenBank® (GenBank® accession number: HQ148663). The positive amplicon for *Hepatozoon* spp. PCR was not sequenced due to the low amount of DNA in the sample.

DISCUSSION

This study demonstrates acute febrile illness associated with natural *Rickettsia* infection in dogs living in endemic areas of human MSF by means of seroconversion alone and the combination of seroconversion and/or PCR in comparison to an afebrile control group. Since human MSF was first described in 1910 by Conor and Bunch, canine illness associated with naturally occurring *R. conorii* infection has been described in only a few dogs. *Rickettsia conorii* infection associated with febrile illness was described in three dogs from Sicily by means of seroconversion and PCR [13] and seven dogs from Portugal by serology and PCR [18]. In addition, this study found significantly higher acute and convalescent *R. conorii* antibody titers in febrile dogs when compared with afebrile-control dogs.

Spotted fever group *Rickettsia* infection have so far only been recognized as causing acute infections in humans and dogs [1,27]. Therefore, acute and convalescent antibodies and PCR at the time of diagnosis were employed as diagnostic tools in this study to allow the detection of canine *Rickettsia* spp. infection. Interestingly, the majority of febrile dogs were diagnosed based on seroconversion to *Rickettsia* antigen and only three febrile dogs were diagnosed by molecular analysis in agreement with human MSF diagnostic findings [1,28,29]. Molecular detection of *Rickettsia* spp. such as *R. conorii* in blood appears to be of low to moderate sensitivity in humans [1,29,30] and in dogs [14] as found also in this study. The discrepancy between serological and molecular testing is likely due to the fact that *Rickettsia* spp. circulate in blood in low numbers during the acute phase of infection [2,31] and are probably rapidly cleared from blood. Accordingly, experimental infections of dogs with *R. conorii* resulted in a short rickettsiemia of 2–10 days post-infection [6,7] which did not recur following immunosuppression [15].

Clinical signs and clinicopathological abnormalities detected in febrile dogs diagnosed with *Rickettsia* spp. infection based on seroconversion or positive PCR at initial examination were similar to abnormalities associated with SFG rickettsiosis in humans [2,3,32,33] and Rocky Mountain Spotted Fever rickettsiosis in dogs [34,35] and in experimental infections of dogs with *R. conorii* [6,7]. The majority of experimentally *R. conorii*infected dogs presented acute fever, anorexia and lethargy [6,7]. In addition, similar clinical signs and clinicopathological abnormalities were detected in three client-owned Yorkshire terriers living in Sicily [13] and in seven client-owned Portuguese dogs [18].

Due to the fact that the majority of febrile dogs with *Rickettsia* spp. infection were diagnosed by seroconversion and the detection of rickettsiemia was not successful by molecular techniques in the majority of dogs, the *Rickettsia* species infecting the majority of these dogs remains unclear. It is well known that serological cross-reaction exists between different species of *Rickettsia* [28] and, therefore, *R. conorii* might not be the only pathogen infecting these dogs. However, based on current knowledge, the most likely species infecting dogs is *R. conorii* due to the fact that, so far, only *R. conorii* has been diagnosed by molecular techniques in the Mediterranean region [13,18] in dogs. In addition, the most common *Rickettsia* pathogen recognized in Sicily in humans and ticks is *R. conorii* [36] including different strains [4,5]. Other *Rickettsia*species such as *R. slovaca* [5], *R. africae*, *R. aeschlimannii* [37] and a new spotted fever group *Rickettsia* [38] have been occasionally found in Sicily in ticks and *R. massiliae* has been isolated from one human patient [39]. Additionally, three febrile dogs from the present study were diagnosed by DNA amplification and sequencing of *R. conorii* as the most likely infecting pathogen. Moreover, the three previous canine rickettsiosis cases reported in Sicily were diagnosed as *R. conorii* infection as well [13]. However, the pathogenic role of *R. massiliae* might be more important than previously thought and this rickettsia might cause MSF in humans [39-41] and subclinical [6] or febrile illness in dogs [42]. This is due to the facts that a moderate proportion of *Rh. sanguineus* ticks are infected with this microorganism [42-46], human cases of this infection have occasionally been reported [39-41] and *R. massiliae* antibodies are present in dogs [42,47] and humans [48,49]. Further studies should try to improve diagnostic techniques to better characterize the species of *Rickettsia* infecting dogs in Sicily and in the Mediterranean basin.

The findings of *Rickettsia* seroconversion in afebrile control dogs including healthy dogs suggest that, in some dogs, *Rickettsia* infection is subclinical. This finding is in agreement with experimental infections [6,7] and previous literature where dogs have been considered only sentinels of this infection [50,51]. Clinical manifestations of *R. conorii* or *Rickettsia* spp. infections can vary from subclinical to commonly mild disease in humans and other mammals including dogs, as demonstrated in the present study [2].

Serological and molecular positive rates obtained for *E. canis*, *A. phagocytophilum*, *A. platys*, *B. vogeli* and *L. infantum* are similar to previous studies performed in southern Italy [52,53] and other Mediterranean areas [54]. In contrast, there is insufficient information on seroconversion of tick-transmitted pathogens in sick and healthy dogs in endemic areas. Interestingly, higher seroconversions were found with *R. conorii* than with *E. canis* and *A. phagocytophilum* and *R. conorii* seroconversion was the only infection significantly associated with febrile illness in this study.

In the present study, febrile illness was associated with several tick pathogens and detection of DNA of pathogens was mainly observed in febrile dogs. In addition, coinfections were only detected by molecular techniques in dogs with febrile illness. The pathogenic role of coinfections remains unclear and is scarcely investigated [55,56]. However, the findings of this study suggest that coinfections diagnosed by PCR demonstrating active infection might aggravate clinical manifestations as previously reported [55,57].

In this study, the majority of febrile cases were diagnosed as associated with acute *E. canis* infection based on PCR-positive and acute negative or low positive antibody titers and evidence of seroconversion. Interestingly, it is thought that the majority of clinical cases of *E. canis* infection correspond to the chronic phase of this disease [58-60] while, in our study, clinical signs and laboratory abnormalities were mainly found during acute infections. The association of antibody reactivity found between *E. canis* and *A. phagocytophilum* is not surprising due to the well-known cross-reaction that occurs between *Ehrlichia* and *Anaplasma* species [60]. In the present study, we consider that the *A. phagocytophilum* positive serological results are most likely due to *A. platys* infection in dogs rather than a true infection with *A. phagocytophilum* due to the fact that only *A. platys* was diagnosed by molecular techniques and the location of tested dogs in Sicily where only *A. platys* is prevalent in dogs [61].

There is limited clinical knowledge about *B. vogeli* infection in dogs in endemic areas. *Babesia vogeli* infection is considered to cause subclinical infection or a mild to moderate diseases in some dogs [24,62,63]. Surprisingly, in the present study, *B. vogeli* infection was only detected in febrile dogs while subclinical infection was not evident based on molecular analysis in this study. Unfortunately, *Babesia* serology and seroconversion were not performed as this could have decreased the number of truly infected dogs diagnosed in this study. Although blood molecular analysis is probably the most sensitive and accurate diagnostic technique for active *Babesia* infection in dogs [62], it is important to highlight that *Babesia*parasites were not observed on blood smear examination. Based on the present findings, *B. vogeli* should be included in the differential diagnosis of dogs with febrile illness and blood PCR appears to be the best diagnostic technique to use for its detection.

Hepatozoon canis infections in dogs are frequently subclinical in endemic areas and clinical cases are sporadically reported [64]. Interestingly, in the present study, only one young febrile dog was diagnosed with *H. canis* infection. These findings are unusual due to the fact that higher rates of *H. canis* infection are reported in Mediterranean endemic areas [54,64,65] and that subclinical infections were not found. In addition, the dog with hepatozoonosis was coinfected with an acute *E. canis* infection diagnosed by PCR. Unfortunately, the dog was lost during follow-up and clinical data about response to treatment was lacking. Whether the clinical signs and clinicopathological abnormalities observed were attributed only to *E. canis*infection or to both infections remains unclear and further studies would need to elucidate the role of coinfections and *H. canis* in febrile illness in endemic areas.

CONCLUSIONS

In conclusion, this study demonstrates acute febrile illness associated with natural *Rickettsia* infection in dogs living in MSF endemic areas based on acute and convalescent antibody titers, seroconversion alone and the combination of seroconversion and PCR. The most common clinical signs and clinicopathological abnormalities were similar to those described in human and canine spotted fever rickettsiosis. Additional febrile illness was associated with *E. canis* infection demonstrated by PCR, and with detection of tick pathogens and co-infection demonstrated by molecular techniques.

DECLARATIONS

Acknowledgments

The authors thank all veterinarians and dog owners that contributed to this study. The authors thank also Martina Nicetto for her help on molecular analysis and the staff of *Laboratorio Privato di Analisi Veterinarie San Marco* (Padua, Italy) for their support to this study. We are grateful to Dr Ruby Chang (Royal Veterinary College) for assistance with statistical analyses. The authors are also grateful to Bayer Animal Health

(Germany) and Bayer Italia S.p.A. and *Laboratorio Privato di Analisi Veterinarie San Marco* (Padua, Italy) for funding this study. Publication fees of this manuscript have been sponsored by Bayer HealthCare - Animal Health division.

Dr. Laia Solano-Gallego hold a Ramón y Cajal senior researcher contract awarded by the *Ministerio de Ciencia e Innovación* (Spain) and the European Social Fund.

Authors' contributions

LSG and MGP designed the research study. LSG set up ELISA and IFAs, contributed with data analysis and interpretation and wrote the manuscript. AC coordinated the veterinary clinics enrolled, set up and performed ELISAs and IFAs, contributed with data analysis and interpretation and revised the manuscript. MGP contributed with data analysis and interpretation and revised the manuscript. MC and TF contributed with routine laboratory testing and revised the manuscript. MT performed DNA extraction, real-time PCR and conventional PCR and revised the manuscript. All authors read and approved the final version of the manuscript.

REFERENCES

1. Brouqui P, Parola P, Fournier PE, Raoult D. Spotted fever rickettsioses in southern and eastern Europe. FEMS Immunol Med Microbiol. 2007;49(1):2–12.
2. Parola P, Paddock CD, Raoult D. Tick-borne rickettsioses around the world: emerging diseases challenging old concepts. Clin Microbiol Rev. 2005;18(4):719–56.
3. Cascio A, Iaria C. Epidemiology and clinical features of Mediterranean spotted fever in Italy. Parassitol. 2006;48(1–2):131–3.
4. Giammanco GM, Vitale G, Mansueto S, Capra G, Caleca MP, Ammatuna P. Presence of *Rickettsia conorii* subsp. *israelensis*, the causative agent of Israeli spotted fever, in Sicily, Italy, ascertained in a retrospective study. J Clin Microbiol. 2005;43(12):6027–31.
5. Torina A, de Mera IG F, Alongi A, Mangold AJ, Blanda V, Scarlata F, et al. *Rickettsia conorii* Indian tick typhus strain and *R. slovaca* in humans, Sicily. Emerg Infect Dis. 2012;18(6):1008–10.
6. Levin ML, Zemtsova GE, Montgomery M, Killmaster LF. Effects of homologous and heterologous immunization on the reservoir competence of domestic dogs for *Rickettsia conorii* (*israelensis*). Ticks Tick-borne Dis. 2014;5(1):33–40.
7. Levin ML, Killmaster LF, Zemtsova GE. Domestic dogs (*Canis familiaris*) as reservoir hosts for *Rickettsia conorii*. Vector Borne Zoonotic Dis. 2012;12(1):28–33.
8. Delgado S, Carmenes P. Canine seroprevalence of *Rickettsia conorii* infection (Mediterranean spotted fever) in Castilla y Leon (northwest Spain). Eur J Epidemiol. 1995;11(5):597–600.
9. Mannelli A, Mandola ML, Pedri P, Tripoli M, Nebbia P. Associations between dogs that were serologically positive for *Rickettsia conorii* relative to the residences of two human cases of Mediterranean spotted fever in Piemonte (Italy). Prev Vet Med. 2003;60(1):13–26.
10. Torina A, Caracappa S. Dog tick-borne diseases in Sicily. Parassitol. 2006;48(1–2):145–7.
11. Estrada-Pena A, Venzal Bianchi JM. Efficacy of several anti-tick treatments to prevent the transmission of *Rickettsia conorii* under natural conditions. Ann New York Acad Sci. 2006;1078:506–8.
12. Torina A, Vicente J, Alongi A, Scimeca S, Turla R, Nicosia S, et al. Observed prevalence of tick-borne pathogens in domestic animals in Sicily, Italy during 2003–2005. Zoonoses Public Health. 2007;54(1):8–15.
13. Solano-Gallego L, Kidd L, Trotta M, Di Marco M, Caldin M, Furlanello T, et al. Febrile illness associated with *Rickettsia conorii* infection in dogs from Sicily. Emerg Infect Dis. 2006;12(12):1985–8.
14. Solano-Gallego L, Trotta M, Caldin M, Furlanello T. Molecular survey of *Rickettsia* spp. in sick dogs in Italy. Zoonoses Public Health. 2008;55(8–10):521–5.
15. Kelly PJ, Matthewman LA, Mason PR, Courtney S, Katsande C, Rukwava J. Experimental infection of dogs with a Zimbabwean strain of *Rickettsia conorii*. J Trop Med Hyg. 1992;95(5):322–6.
16. Baneth G, Breitschwerdt EB, Hegarty BC, Pappalardo B, Ryan J. A survey of tick-borne bacteria and protozoa in naturally exposed dogs from Israel. Vet Parasitol. 1998;74(2–4):133–42.
17. Solano-Gallego L, Llull J, Osso M, Hegarty B, Breitschwerdt E. A serological study of exposure to arthropod-borne pathogens in dogs from northeastern Spain. Vet Res. 2006;37(2):231–44.
18. Alexandre N, Santos AS, Bacellar F, Boinas FJ, Nuncio MS, de Sousa R. Detection of *Rickettsia conorii* strains in Portuguese dogs (*Canis familiaris*). Ticks Tick-borne dis. 2011;2(2):119–22.
19. Furlanello T, Fiorio F, Caldin M, Lubas G, Solano-Gallego L. Clinicopathological findings in naturally occurring cases of babesiosis caused by large form *Babesia* from dogs of northeastern Italy. Vet Parasitol. 2005;134(1–2):77–85.
20. Stillman BA, Monn M, Liu J, Thatcher B, Foster P, Andrews B, et al. Performance of a commercially available in-clinic ELISA for detection of antibodies against *Anaplasma phagocytophilum*, *Anaplasma platys*, *Borrelia burgdorferi*, *Ehrlichia canis*, and *Ehrlichia ewingii* and *Dirofilaria immitis* antigen in dogs. J Am Vet Med Assoc. 2014;245(1):80–6.
21. Riera C, Valladares JE, Gallego M, Aisa MJ, Castillejo S, Fisa R, et al. Serological and parasitological follow-up in dogs experimentally infected with *Leishmania infantum* and treated with meglumine antimoniate. Vet Parasitol. 1999;84(1–2):33–47.
22. Solano-Gallego L, Trotta M, Razia L, Furlanello T, Caldin M. Molecular survey of *Ehrlichia canis* and *Anaplasma phagocytophilum* from blood of dogs in Italy. Ann N Y Acad Sci. 2006;1078:515–8.
23. Solano-Gallego L, Rodriguez-Cortes A, Trotta M, Zampieron C, Razia L, Furlanello T, et al. Detection of *Leishmania infantum* DNA by fret-based real-time PCR in urine from dogs with natural clinical leishmaniosis. Vet Parasitol. 2007;147(3–4):315–9.

24. Solano-Gallego L, Trotta M, Carli E, Carcy B, Caldin M, Furlanello T. *Babesia canis canis* and *Babesia canis vogeli*clinicopathological findings and DNA detection by means of PCR-RFLP in blood from Italian dogs suspected of tick-borne disease. Vet Parasitol. 2008;157(3–4):211–21.
25. Inokuma H, Okuda M, Ohno K, Shimoda K, Onishi T. Analysis of the 18S rRNA gene sequence of a *Hepatozoon* detected in two Japanese dogs. Vet Parasitol. 2002;106(3):265–71.
26. Sanger E, Nicklen S, Coulson AR. DANN sequencing with chain terminating inhibitors. Proc Natl Acad Sci U S A. 1977;74:5463–7.
27. Nicholson WL, Allen KE, McQuiston JH, Breitschwerdt EB, Little SE. The increasing recognition of rickettsial pathogens in dogs and people. Trends Parasitol. 2010;26(4):205–12.
28. Brouqui P, Bacellar F, Baranton G, Birtles RJ, Bjoersdorff A, Blanco JR, et al. Guidelines for the diagnosis of tick-borne bacterial diseases in Europe. Clin Microbiol Infect. 2004;10(12):1108–32.
29. Santibanez S, Portillo A, Santibanez P, Palomar AM, Oteo JA. Usefulness of rickettsial PCR assays for the molecular diagnosis of human rickettsioses. Enferm Infecc Microbiol Clin. 2013;31(5):283–8.
30. Znazen A, Sellami H, Elleuch E, Hattab Z, Ben Sassi L, Khrouf F, et al. Comparison of two quantitative real time PCR assays for *Rickettsia* detection in patients from Tunisia. PLoS Negl Trop Dis. 2015;9(2):e0003487.
31. Breitschwerdt EB, Levy MG, Davidson MG, Walker DH, Burgdorfer W, Curtis BC, et al. Kinetics of IgM and IgG responses to experimental and naturally acquired *Rickettsia rickettsii* infection in dogs. Am J Vet Res. 1990;51(8):1312–6.
32. Rovery C, Brouqui P, Raoult D. Questions on Mediterranean spotted fever a century after its discovery. Emerg Infect Dis. 2008;14(9):1360–7.
33. Colomba C, Saporito L, Polara VF, Rubino R, Titone L. Mediterranean spotted fever: clinical and laboratory characteristics of 415 Sicilian children. BMC Infect Dis. 2006;6:60.
34. Ober CP, Spaulding K, Breitschwerdt EB, Malarkey DE, Hegarty BC. Orchitis in two dogs with Rocky Mountain spotted fever. Vet Radiol Ultrasound. 2004;45(5):458–65.
35. Gasser AM, Birkenheuer AJ, Breitschwerdt EB. Canine rocky mountain spotted fever: a retrospective study of 30 cases. J Am Anim Hosp Assoc. 2001;37(1):41–8.
36. Giammanco GM, Di Rosa S, Ammatuna P, Mansueto P, Micalizzi A, Vitale G. Continous alert for rickettsiosis in Sicily: molecular characterization of *Rickettsia* sp. obtained from ticks and human beings (1986–2001). New Microbiol. 2005;28(4):377–9.
37. Beninati T, Genchi C, Torina A, Caracappa S, Bandi C, Lo N. Rickettsiae in ixodid ticks, Sicily. Emerg Infect Dis. 2005;11(3):509–11.
38. Eremeeva ME, Stromdahl EY. Short report: New spotted fever group *rickettsia* in a *Rhipicephalus turanicus* tick removed from a child in eastern Sicily, Italy. Am J Trop Med Hyg. 2011;84(1):99–101.
39. Vitale G, Mansuelo S, Rolain JM, Raoult D. *Rickettsia massiliae* human isolation. Emerg Infect Dis. 2006;12(1):174–5.
40. Parola P, Socolovschi C, Jeanjean L, Bitam I, Fournier PE, Sotto A, et al. Warmer weather linked to tick attack and emergence of severe rickettsioses. PLoS Negl Trop Dis. 2008;2(11):e338.
41. Garcia-Garcia JC, Portillo A, Nunez MJ, Santibanez S, Castro B, Oteo JA. A patient from Argentina infected with *Rickettsia massiliae*. Am J Trop Med Hyg. 2010;82(4):691–2.
42. Beeler E, Abramowicz KF, Zambrano ML, Sturgeon MM, Khalaf N, Hu R, et al. A focus of dogs and *Rickettsia massiliae*-infected *Rhipicephalus sanguineus* in California. Am J Trop Med Hyg. 2011;84(2):244–9.
43. Marquez FJ, Rodriguez-Liebana JJ, Soriguer RC, Muniain MA, Bernabeu-Wittel M, Caruz A, et al. Spotted fever group *Rickettsia* in brown dog ticks *Rhipicephalus sanguineus* in southwestern Spain. Parasitol Res. 2008;103(1):119–22.
44. Mura A, Masala G, Tola S, Satta G, Fois F, Piras P, et al. First direct detection of rickettsial pathogens and a new rickettsia, 'Candidatus Rickettsia barbariae', in ticks from Sardinia. Italy Clin Microbiol Infect. 2008;14(11):1028–33.
45. Harrus S, Perlman-Avrahami A, Mumcuoglu KY, Morick D, Baneth G. Molecular detection of *Rickettsia massiliae*, *Rickettsia sibirica mongolitimonae* and *Rickettsia conorii israelensis* in ticks from Israel. Clin Microbiol Infect. 2011;17(2):176–80.
46. Sarih M, Socolovschi C, Boudebouch N, Hassar M, Raoult D, Parola P. Spotted fever group rickettsiae in ticks, Morocco. Emerg Infect Dis. 2008;14(7):1067–73.
47. Pons I, Nogueras MM, Sanfeliu I, Ortuno A, Segura F. Serological evidence of infection with Bar29 in dog population of Catalonia, in the northeast of Spain. 5th International Meeting on Rickettsiae and Rickettsial Diseases, Marseille, France. Abstract book. 2008.
48. Cardenosa N, Segura F, Raoult D. Serosurvey among Mediterranean spotted fever patients of a new spotted fever group rickettsial strain (Bar29). Eur J Epidemiol. 2003;18(4):351–6.
49. Bernabeu-Wittel M, del Toro MD, Nogueras MM, Muniain MA, Cardenosa N, Segura F, et al. Presence of human past infections due to the Bar29 rickettsial strain in Southern Spain. J Infect. 2006;52(4):e117–9.
50. Ortuno A, Pons I, Nogueras MM, Castella J, Segura F. The dog as an epidemiological marker of *Rickettsia conorii*infection. Clin Microbiol Infect. 2009;15 Suppl 2:241–2.
51. Segura-Porta F, Diestre-Ortin G, Ortuno-Romero A, Sanfeliu-Sala I, Font-Creus B, Munoz-Espin T, et al. Prevalence of antibodies to spotted fever group rickettsiae in human beings and dogs from and endemic area of Mediterranean spotted fever in Catalonia, Spain. Eur J Epidemiol. 1998;14(4):395–8.

52. Otranto D, Dantas-Torres F. Canine and feline vector-borne diseases in Italy: current situation and perspectives. Parasit Vectors. 2010;3:2.

53. Otranto D, Testini G, Dantas-Torres F, Latrofa MS, Diniz PP, de Caprariis D, et al. Diagnosis of canine vector-borne diseases in young dogs: a longitudinal study. J Clin Microbiol. 2010;48(9):3316–24.

54. Rene-Martellet M, Lebert I, Chene J, Massot R, Leon M, Leal A, et al. Diagnosis and incidence risk of clinical canine monocytic ehrlichiosis under field conditions in Southern Europe. Parasit Vectors. 2015;8(1):3.

55. Rojas A, Rojas D, Montenegro V, Gutierrez R, Yasur-Landau D, Baneth G. Vector-borne pathogens in dogs from Costa Rica: first molecular description of *Babesia vogeli* and *Hepatozoon canis* infections with a high prevalence of monocytic ehrlichiosis and the manifestations of co-infection. Vet Parasitol. 2014;199(3–4):121–8.

56. Baneth G, Harrus S, Gal A, Aroch I. Canine vector-borne co-infections: *Ehrlichia canis* and *Hepatozoon canis* in the same host monocytes. Vet Parasitol. 2015;208:30–4.

57. Andrade GB, Barreto WT, Santos LL, Ribeiro LR, Macedo GC, Sousa KC, et al. Pathology of dogs in Campo Grande, MS, Brazil naturally co-infected with *Leishmania infantum* and *Ehrlichia canis*. Rev Bras Parasitol Vet. 2014;23(4):509–15.

58. Harrus S, Kass PH, Klement E, Waner T. Canine monocytic ehrlichiosis: a retrospective study of 100 cases, and an epidemiological investigation of prognostic indicators for the disease. Vet Rec. 1997;141(14):360–3.

59. Mylonakis ME, Koutinas AF, Breitschwerdt EB, Hegarty BC, Billinis CD, Leontides LS, et al. Chronic canine ehrlichiosis (*Ehrlichia canis*): a retrospective study of 19 natural cases. J Am Anim Hosp Assoc. 2004;40(3):174–84.

60. Little SE. Ehrlichiosis and anaplasmosis in dogs and cats. Vet Clin North Am Small Anim Pract. 2010;40(6):1121–40.

61. de la Fuente J, Torina A, Naranjo V, Nicosia S, Alongi A, La Mantia F, et al. Molecular characterization of *Anaplasma platys*strains from dogs in Sicily,Italy. BMC Vet Res. 2006;2:24.

62. Solano-Gallego L, Baneth G. Babesiosis in dogs and cats-Expanding parasitological and clinical spectra. Vet Parasitol. 2011;181(1):48–60.

63. Salem NY, Farag HS. Clinical, Hematologic, and Molecular Findings in Naturally Occurring *Babesia canis vogeli* in Egyptian Dogs. Vet Med Internat. 2014;2014:270345.

64. Baneth G. Perspectives on canine and feline hepatozoonosis. Vet Parasitol. 2011;181(1):3–11.

65. Otranto D, Dantas-Torres F, Weigl S, Latrofa MS, Stanneck D, Decaprariis D, et al. Diagnosis of *Hepatozoon canis* in young dogs by cytology and PCR. Parasit Vectors. 2011;4:55.

CHAPTER 47 SEROLOGICAL DIFFERENTIATION OF ANTIBODIES AGAINST RICKETTSIA HELVETICA, R. RAOULTII, R. SLOVACA, R. MONACENSIS AND R. FELIS IN DOGS FROM GERMANY BY A MICRO-IMMUNOFLUORESCENT ANTIBODY TEST

Miriam Wächter, Silke Wölfel, Martin Pfeffer, Gerhard Dobler, Barbara Kohn, Andreas Moritz, Stefan Pachnicke and Cornelia Silaghi

Keywords: *Rickettsia Helvetica, R. raoultii, R. slovaca, R. monacensis, R. felis,* Seroprevalence, Differentiation, DogsTicks

BACKGROUND

Rickettsiae are short rod-shaped gram-negative, obligate intracellular bacteria [1]. They are, regarding the clinical and serological perspective, divided into two major groups: the Typhus Group (TG) and the Spotted Fever Group (SFG). The TG includes two members: *R. typhi* and *R. prowazekii*, the causative agents of murine typhus and epidemic typhus, respectively. The heterogeneous SFG contains >20 Rickettsiae, mainly transmitted by ticks, except for *R. felis* which is transmitted by fleas and *R. akari* which is transmitted by mites [2-4]. Recent genomic analyses indicate the divison into four groups: the TG, the SFG, the ancestral group (AG) and the transitional group (TRG), which includes *R. felis* [5]. Rickettsiae of the SFG are able to cause mild to severe rickettsioses in humans [6]. Rickettsioses are considered emerging infectious diseases worldwide [1,7]. To evaluate the epidemiological situation in different countries it is necessary to examine vectors and reservoir hosts for the occurrence of different rickettsial species. Various molecular and serological methods have been described for the detection and differentiation of *Rickettsia* species. Real-time polymerase chain reaction (PCR) is frequently applied to detect *Rickettsia* in biopsies, blood and arthropods [7]. Several conventional PCRs targeting different genomic regions for subsequent sequencing and phylogenetic analysis of rickettsiae have been published in the last decades [4,8,9]. Species-specific real-time PCRs are only available for some rickettsial species (e.g. *R. conorii*, *R. rickettsii*) [10,11]. Due to the strong serological cross-reactions among SFG Rickettsiae, the availability of serological tools for differentiation is limited, so far. Commercially available IFA and ELISA tests are only suitable for the discrimination between SFG- and TG-Rickettsiae [1]. Brouqui et al. [12] described a micro-immunofluorescence method which allows the investigation of up to nine different rickettsial antigens in one spot as a suitable method to differentiate the causative *Rickettsia*species by determination of endpoint titres. Absorption western blotting can also be used to identify rickettsial species [13]. The rickettsial IFA adapted to the micro-method format (micro-IFA) is the test of choice for the serodiagnosis of rickettsial disease in human medicine [1]. In Germany, six species of the SFG Rickettsiae have been detected in ticks by molecular methods (Table 1). All of them have been described to cause diseases in humans. *R. helvetica* is generally associated with uneruptive fever, but cases with more severe clinical signs such as endocarditis or meningitis have been reported [14-16]. *R. monacensis*, *R. massiliae* and *R. felis* can cause classical spotted fevers and

Citation: Miriam Wächter, Silke Wölfel, Martin Pfeffer, Gerhard Dobler, Barbara Kohn, Andreas Moritz, Stefan Pachnicke and Cornelia Silaghi, Serological differentiation of antibodies against Rickettsia helvetica, R. raoultii, R. slovaca, R. monacensis and R. felis in dogs from Germany by a micro-immunofluorescent antibody test, DOI: 10.1186/s13071-015-0745-1.

additional constitutional symptoms like fatigue, headache and myalgia [7,17-23]. Nevertheless the pathogenicity of *R. felis* is still discussed controversially [24]. *R. raoultii* and *R. slovaca* cause TIBOLA (tick-borne lymphadenopathy) or DEBONEL (*Dermacentor*-borne necrosis erythema lymphadenopathy) with a typical clinical syndrome including an eschar at the site of the tick bite and lymphadenopathy [25-27]. Data concerning clinical human cases in Germany are rare. In the recent years only a few cases have been published, among them cases of *R. slovaca* infection in 2009 and one in 2010 [27,28] and a case of *R. felis* infection in 2000 [29]. So far no clinical cases caused by *R. monacensis*, *R. helvetica*, *R. massiliae* or *R. raoultii* were described in Germany. In 2008, 9.1% of 256 examined hunters in Germany had antibodies against the SFG Rickettsiae in an IFA [30]. In 2012, an average of 27.7% of forestry workers had antibodies against the SFG Rickettsiae in the IFA with seroprevalences up to 55% in particular geographical regions (Wölfel et al., Seroprevalence of IgG against Rickettsiae of the Spotted Fever Group in Forestry Workers in State Brandenburg, Eastern Germany, unpublished). In 2014, we detected antibodies against the SFG Rickettsiae in 77.9% of 605 dogs examined with ELISA (Wächter et al., Seroprevalence of Spotted Fever Group Rickettsiae in dogs in Germany, in press). Until now no clinical cases in dogs involving the rickettsial species *R. helvetica*, *R. raoultii*, *R. slovaca*, *R. massiliae*, *R. felis* or *R. monacensis* have been reported. However, *R. rickettsii* in the USA and *R. conorii* in southern Europe can cause symptomatic diseases of variable severity in dogs [31,32]. *Rickettsia rickettsii* causes a severe vasculitis leading to symptoms like lethargy, anemia and neurologic symptoms [31]. *Rickettsia conorii*, causing the Mediterranean Spotted Fever in humans, can lead to symptoms like fever, diarrhea, vomiting and petechial rash in dogs [32]. In our previous study statistically significant correlations between age, tick infestation and seropositivity of the dogs were found, but no differentiation of rickettsial species was possible by ELISA (Wächter et al., Seroprevalence of Spotted Fever Group Rickettsiae in dogs in Germany, in press). Therefore, the aims of the study were (i) to establish the micro-IFA as a tool to distinguish antibodies against different rickettsial species in dogs (ii) to differentiate the antibody responses in dogs previously found positive by ELISA and (iii) to compare the micro-IFA to a commercial ELISA with regard to sensitivity and specificity.

Table 1: Prevalence rates of Spotted Fever Group Rickettsiae in ticks in Germany, according to the geographic region

***Rickettsia* species**	**Tick species**	**% pos**	**Number of ticks tested**	**Region**	**Reference**
R. helvetica	*Ixodes ricinus*	5.6-13.3%	1187	BW	[33]
		12.0%	2141	BY	[34]
		4.8%	2861	BY	[35]
		6.0%	4459	BY	[36]
		14.2%	127	BE	[37]
		3.5-6.2%	3591	south of Germany	[7]
		32.9%	1089	NI	[38]
		13.4-17.4%	1702	BY/ SL/ SN	[39]
		8.5%	2186	BY	[40]
		52.5%	1400	Hamburg	[41]
		26.2%	2100	Hannover	[42]
R. raoultii	*Dermacentor*	30.0%	666	BW	[43]
	spp.	56.7%	1359	BY/ SL/ SN	[39]
R. slovaca	*Dermacentor*	0.8%	666	BY	[43]
	spp.	13.3%	15	BY/ SL/ SN	[39]
R. monacensis	*I. ricinus*	0.5%	2861	BY	[35]
		0.6%	3591	BY	[7]
		0.4%	4459	BY	[36]
		0.4%	1089	NI	[38]
		0.2%	2186	BY	[40]
R. felis	*I. ricinus*	0.4%	1450	BY/NRW	[7]
R. massiliae	*I. ricinus*	1.7%	57	eastern BY	[7]

BE: Berlin; BY: Bavaria; BW: Baden-Wurttemberg; NI: Lower Saxony; NRW: North Rhine-Westphalia; SL: Saarland; SN: Saxony.

METHODS

Samples

Altogether 605 serum samples of dogs from a previous study (Wächter et al., Seroprevalence of Spotted Fever Group Rickettsiae in dogs in Germany, in press) were tested for antibodies against five SFG Rickettsiae by micro-IFA. These samples had previously been tested for antibodies against SFG Rickettsiae by a commercial ELISA (Canine Spotted Fever Rickettsia EIA IgG Antibody Kit, Fuller Laboratories, Fullerton, California, USA) (Wächter et al., Seroprevalence of Spotted Fever Group Rickettsiae in dogs in Germany, in press). Dogs included in this study were (i) born in Germany, (ii) had never left Germany and (iii) data on sex, age, breed, location, clinical status (healthy or sick), tick infestation and date of blood collection were available.

Production of micro-IFA-slides

Rickettsia helvetica strain AS 819, *R. raoultii* strain *Khabarovsk* (kindly provided by Lee Fuller, Fuller Laboratories), *R. slovaca* strain RU 828, *R. monacensis* strain AS 787 and *R. felis* strain ELB (kindly provided by Lee Fuller, Fuller Laboratories) were cultivated in 75 cm^2 tissue culture flasks containing either Vero cells or Drosophila melanogaster cells (only *R. felis*). Readily infected cell cultures were harvested after 8 to 19 days, depending on the growth characteristics of the respective *Rickettsia* species. Identity and purity of the strains was confirmed by sequencing a part of the ompB gene following a protocol of Roux and Raoult [2]. After inactivation by adding formalin in a final concentration of 1% the Rickettsiae were released from their host cells by needle disruption. The suspension was centrifuged twice at 1,000 g, 4°C for 5 minutes to remove cell debris. The supernatant was collected. Centrifugation at 17,000 g, 4°C for 5 minutes followed twice. Every time the supernatant was discarded and the pellet was resuspended in 1.8 ml phosphate buffered saline (PBS). The final pellet was resuspended in 100 µl PBS. Serial dilutions in PBS (1:2, 1:5, 1:10) of the antigens were applied with a 10 µl piston-operated pipette to empty slides to estimate the density of rickettsial antigen by IFA and Diff-Quick ® (Polysciences, Warrington, USA) staining to equalize the density of all five rickettsial species. *R. felis*, *R. monacensis* and *R. slovaca* were diluted with PBS 1:10, *R. helvetica* and *R. raoultii* were used as undiluted solutions. The different rickettsial antigens were applied to a 10-well microscope slide with a pen-point as shown in Figure 1. The slides were air dried and fixed in methanol-acetone (1:1) for 30 min, air-dried again and stored at 4°C until use.

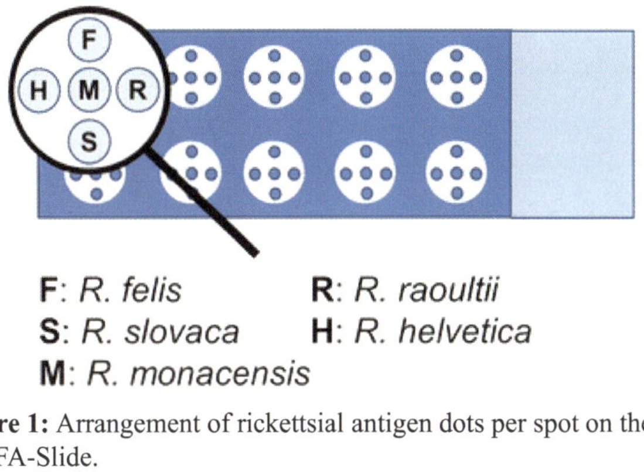

Figure 1: Arrangement of rickettsial antigen dots per spot on the Micro IFA-Slide.

Micro-IFA

A twofold serial dilution of the serum samples with PBS was made and the screening dilution of 1:128 was applied to the slide wells and incubated at 37°C for 45 min in a humid chamber. The slide was washed with 0.2% PBS-Tween (Euroimmun, Lübeck, Germany) three times for 5 min. Fluorescein isothiocyanate (FITC)-labelled rabbit anti-dog immunoglobulin G (Sigma-Aldrich, St. Louis, USA) was applied in a 1:20 dilution and incubated at 37°C for 30 min in a humid chamber, washed with 0.2% PBS-Tween three times for 5 min and mounted with fluorescence mounting medium (Dako, Carpinteria, California, USA). Reactions were read with a fluorescence microscope (Leica 5000, Wetzlar, Germany) by two independent investigators. Suitable positive and negative control dog sera that had been identified in a previous study (Wächter et al., Seroprevalence of Spotted Fever Group Rickettsiae in dogs in Germany, in press) were included in each assay. Samples were considered positive for antibodies of the SFG Rickettsiae when any of the five antigens showed distinct fluorescence patterns at the 1:128 dilution (Figure 2). Fifty positive samples of each of the five regions (Figure 1) were chosen with a random generator (source: http://rechneronline.de/zufallszahlen/, 20-05-2014) and subjected to end-point titration. If one rickettsial species showed at least twofold higher antibody titres than the others, it was considered the species responsible for the antibody induction. If more than one species showed fluorescence at the same end point titre the results were considered not distinguishable.

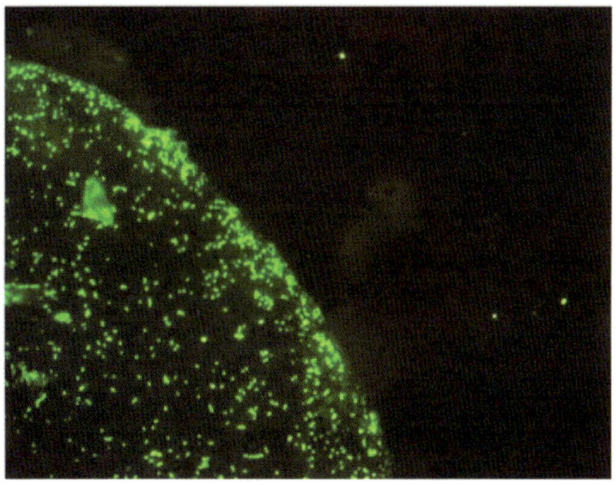

Figure 2: Positive reaction for antibodies against *Rickettsia raoultii* antigen on the Micro IFA-Slide (dilution 1:128).

Comparison ELISA-micro-IFA

The results of the screening dilution (1:128, n=605) of this study obtained with micro-IFA were compared to results obtained with ELISA from a previous study (Wächter et al., Seroprevalence of Spotted Fever Group Rickettsiae in dogs in Germany, in press).

Statistical analysis

Statistical analysis was performed with SPSS® version 21.0.1., SPSS Inc., Chicago, IL, USA. Correlations between location and seropositivity were compared by χ^2-test, for small sample sizes the Fishers exact test was used. Statistical significance was considered at a p-value <0.05. Multiple comparisons were corrected with the Bonferroni adjustment to p<0.01.

Confidence intervals (95% CI) were calculated individually for each proportion with the Clopper and Pearson method. Sensitivity and specificity of the ELISA was calculated as follows: Sensitivity (true positive rate=TPR)=TP (true positive)/ P (positive) and specificity (SPC, true negative rate)=TN (true negative)/ N (negative). The TP and the TN were the sera seropositive and seronegative for antibodies for the SFG tested with the micro-IFA, P and N were the sera tested seropositive and seronegative with the ELISA, respectively.

RESULTS

At the screening serum dilution of 1:128, 568 out of 605 (93.9%; CI: 91.7%-95.7%) of the dogs showed antibodies against at least one of the SFG Rickettsiae. Out of the 93.9% anti-*Rickettsia* positive dog specimens 70.4% showed at least twofold higher antibody titres against one *Rickettsia* species and were therefore considered as clearly differentiable. In 23.6% of the dogs equal antibody titers against two and in 5.6% against three rickettsial antigens were observed. Only one specimen (0.4%) was reactive against four of the five *Rickettsia* species (Table 2). All of those were considered as non-differentiable with regard to the antibody-inducing *Rickettsia* species. Considering only the 70.4% clearly differentiable serum samples the total seroprevalence rates were 66.0% (CI: 59.8%-71.9%) for *R. helvetica,* 2.8% (CI: 1.1%-5.7%) for *R. raoultii*, 1.6% (CI: 0.4%-4.1%) for *R. slovaca*, 0.0% (CI: 0.0%-0.1%) for *R. monacensis* and 0.0% (CI: 0.0%-0.1%) for *R. felis*. If all positive serological reactions against the tested rickettsial species, including cross-reactive antibodies, in the randomly selected 250 positive sera (50 from each of the five regions in Germany) were considered, 94.0% (CI: 90.3%-96.6%) for *R. helvetica,* 22.8% (CI: 17.8%-28.5%) for *R. raoultii*, 5.2% (CI: 2.8%-8.7%) for *R. slovaca*, 2.0% (CI: 0.7%-4.6%) for *R. monacensis* and 0.4% (CI: 0.0%-0.2%) for *R. felis* could be observed. Titres varied for *R. helvetica* from 1:128 to 1:4096, for *R. raoultii* from 1:128 to 1:4096, for *R. slovaca* from 1:256 to 1:2048, for *R. monacensis* from 1:256 to 1:2048 and for *R. felis* from 1:128 to 1:512 (Table 3). No statistically significant different infection rates for *R. helvetica* (p=0.038), *R. slovaca* (p=0.105) and *R. raoultii* (p=0.131) were observed comparing the five different regions of Germany (Figure 3). Statistically significant differences for *R. helvetica* were seen comparing north and south (p=0.042), south and middle (p=0.042) and south and west (p=0.007). Comparison of ELISA (Wächter et al., Seroprevalence of Spotted Fever Group Rickettsiae in dogs in Germany, in press) and micro-IFA yielded the following results. All serum samples (n=605) were tested at a cut-off titre of 1:128. With the ELISA 77.6% (CI: 74.1%-80.9%) of the samples were positive, whereas with the micro-IFA 93.9% (CI: 91.7%-95.7%). Altogether 102 samples were tested positive in the micro-IFA and negative in the ELISA and 6 samples were tested positive in the ELISA and negative in the micro-IFA. Considering this data at a cut-off titre of 1:128 the ELISA shows a sensitivity of 82.0% and a specificity of 83.8%.

Table 2: Seropositivity for SFG Rickettsiae of the dogs with regard to number and association of the different rickettsial species

Number of rickettsial species with seropositivity in dogs	Rickettsial species					No. of positive animals (%)
	RH	**RR**	**RS**	**RM**	**RF**	
One	x					165
		x				7
			x			4
				x		0
					x	0
Total						**176 (70.4%)**
Two	x	x				32
	x		x			2
	x			x		1
	x				x	20
		x			x	2
		x		x		1
		x	x			1
Total						**59 (23.6%)**
Three	x	x	x			4
	x	x		x		2
	x	x			x	7
	x		x		x	1
Total						**14 (5.6%)**
Four	x	x	x	x		1

Total						1 (0.4%)
					Total	250 (100.0%)

RH: *Rickettsia helvetica.*

RR: *Rickettsia raoultii.*

RS: *Rickettsia slovaca.*

RM: *Rickettsia monacensis.*

RF: *Rickettsia felis.*

SFG: Spotted fever group.

Table 3: Seropositivity for 50 sera/region for *R. helvetica* , *R. raoultii* , *R. slovaca* , *R. monacensis and R. felis* in serum samples of dogs tested at serial dilutions

Rickettsial species	RH		RR		RS		RM		RF	
	No seropositive (%)		No seropositive (%)		No seropositive (%)		No seropositive (%)		No seropositive (%)	
Titre	Differentiable	Not differentiable	Differentiable	Not differentiable	Differentiable	Not differentiable	Differentiable	Not differentiable	Differentiable	Not differentiable
1:128	1 (0.6%)	2 (2.9%)	5 (71.4%)	2 (4.0%)	0 (0.0%)	0 (0.0%)	0 (0.0%)	0 (0.0%)	0 (0.0%)	1 (100.0%)
1:256	10 (6.1%)	5 (7.1%)	1 (14.3%)	3 (6.0%)	0 (0.0%)	1 (11.1%)	0 (0.0%)	1 (20.0%)	0 (0.0%)	0 (0.0%)
1:512	36 (21.8%)	12 (17.1%)	0 (0.0%)	9 (18.0%)	2 (50.0%)	2 (22.2%)	0 (0.0%)	1 (20.0%)	0 (0.0%)	0 (0.0%)
1:1024	86 (52.1%)	29 (41.4%)	0 (0.0%)	23 (46.0%)	1 (25.0%)	5 (55.5%)	0 (0.0%)	1 (20.0%)	0 (0.0%)	0 (0.0%)
1:2048	12 (7.3%)	9 (12.9%)	1 (14.3%)	6 (12.0%)	1 (25.0%)	1 (11.1%)	0 (0.0%)	2 (40.0%)	0 (0.0%)	0 (0.0%)
1:4096	20 (12.1%)	13 (18.6%)	0 (0.0%)	7 (14.0%)	0 (0.0%)	0 (0.0%)	0 (0.0%)	0 (0.0%)	0 (0.0%)	0 (0.0%)
No total	**165**	**70**	**7**	**50**	**4**	**9**	**0**	**5**	**0**	**1**

RH: *Rickettsia helvetica.*
RR: *Rickettsia raoultii.*
RS: *Rickettsia slovaca.*
RM: *Rickettsia monacensis.*
RF: *Rickettsia felis.*

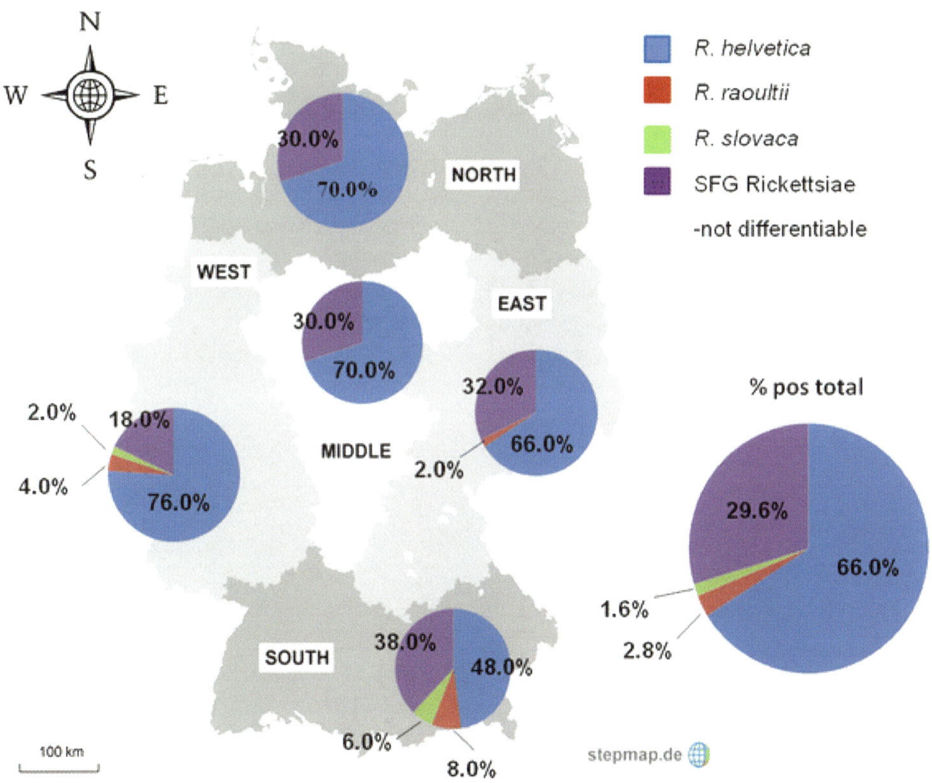

Figure 3: Division of Germany for sample assessment in five regions and seroprevalence rates of the tested *Rickettsia*spp. based on the 50 positive samples tested in the five different regions.

DISCUSSION

Our study presents the first findings about serological differentiation of rickettsial species in dogs in Germany. The serological differentiation of antibodies against SFG Rickettsiae is difficult due to their strong cross reactivity [12]. The micro-IFA method has already been used by several authors to differentiate between antibodies against SFG-Rickettsiae. Breitschwerdt et al. [44] used micro-IFA for a seroepidemiological study in dogs testing for *R. rickettsii*, *R. rhipicephali, R. montana* and *R. bellii*. In Germany, nine different rickettsial antigens were investigated in hunters to differentiate antibodies against indigenous German SFG Rickettsiae as well as species endemic in regions were the hunters had travelled before [30]. The use of a micro-IFA method enables to a certain extent the differentiation of the antibodies leading to the most dominant serological response. However, a prerequisite is the knowledge of which Rickettsiae occur in the investigated region [45]. We included antigens of SFG Rickettsiae that have been repeatedly detected in Germany and have been described to cause clinical manifestations. *R. massiliae* was not used because a single detection exclusively by molecular tools in Germany was described so far (Table 1) [7]. In this study we examined dogs as potential hosts for the *Rickettsia* species previously described in Germany and showed that, to a certain extent, it is serologically possible to distinguish between them. In 29.6% of the cases the detected antibodies were not differentiable and thus did not allow a clear species allocation. Some authors state that if two or more rickettsial species show distinct fluorescence at the end-titre they may be co-infectious rickettsial species [44,46]. As dogs are more frequently exposed and infested with ticks and the pathogens they harbor than humans, dogs might likely be infected with more than one *Rickettsia* species sequentially during their lifetime, thus explaining the high percentage of not distinguishable seropositive animals (Wächter et al., Seroprevalence of Spotted Fever Group Rickettsiae in dogs in Germany, in press). For the major part (66%) of the samples at least twofold higher antibody titres against *R. helvetica* could be observed. These findings are consistent with the fact that the vector for *R. helvetica* is *Ixodes ricinus*, the most abundant tick species in Germany. Prevalence rates of *R. helvetica* in *I. ricinus* ticks were found in Bavaria, Baden-Wurttemberg, Berlin, Saarland, Lower Saxony and Saxony ranging from 3.5% up to 52.5% (Table 1). The lowest prevalence rates in ticks were found in southern Germany. Accordingly, the lowest seroprevalence rate was found in dogs originating from there. The highest prevalence rates were found in Lower Saxony, which is partly identical with the middle and northern region of Germany where high seroprevalence rates in dogs were found [7,38], (Table 3). Regarding the distribution of dogs with antibodies against *R. raoultii* and *R. slovaca* the distribution areas of the vectors have to be considered. So far, in Germany *R. raoultii* has only been detected in *Dermacentor reticulatus*, *R. slovaca* only in *D. marginatus* [28,39]. Spitalska et al. [47] described in the Slovak Republic that *D. marginatus* and *D. reticulatus* could also be host for *R. raoultii* and *R. slovaca*, respectively. However, comparing the geographic distribution in Germany for *D. reticulatus* and *D. marginatus* [48] with the distribution of seropositive dogs there is a partial concordance. The reason why the seroprevalence comparing the different regions is not statistically significant may be due to the fact that the number of cases were very small (Table 3). *R. monacensis* was detected in low prevalences in ticks (0.2%-0.6%) nearly exclusively in Bavaria, only one study reported *R. monacensis* in ticks in Lower Saxony (Table 1). Regarding the dogs with cross-reactive antibodies against *R. monacensis*, these five dogs were nearly all located in the south of Germany. When comparing the vectors and their infection rates of *I. ricinus* for *R. helvetica* (3.5%-52.5%) and of the cat flea *Ctenocephalides felis* for *R. felis* (25.0%-56.0%) it may be surprising that the seroprevalence rate in dogs for *R. helvetica* is 66.0% and for *R. felis* is 0.0%. However, looking at the infestation of dogs with their vectors, a study about population dynamics of fleas in Germany showed that just 5.1% of the dogs are infested with fleas [49,50]. We showed in our previous study that 91.1% of the examined dogs were infested with ticks up to five ticks/month, and 17.5% even up to 20 ticks/month (Wächter et al., Seroprevalence of Spotted Fever Group Rickettsiae in dogs in Germany, in press). Therefore infestation rates with ticks seem higher than with fleas which may lead to higher seroprevalence rates of *R. helvetica* compared to *R. felis*although the infection rates in the vector population are approximately even (Table 1), [50]. There were no dogs with antibodies exclusively against *R. felis*. The cross-reaction of *R. felis* with other members of the SFG is discussed controversially in the literature. The antibodies have been reported to show stronger reactivity to *R. typhi* from the Typhus Group than to members of the Spotted Fever Group [22,51-53]. Fang and Raoult [54] described that mouse polyclonal antisera against *R. felis* only cross-reacted to members of the SFG Rickettsiae but not to the TG. However, in contrast to the study of Fang and Raoult [54], serum of a classical human case of murine typhus showed exclusive reactivity with TG-Rickettsiae and *R. felis* antigen but none with SFG-Rickettsiae. The same results were obtained when testing a commercially available positive anti-TG Rickettsia positive control (Fuller Laboratories, Fullerton, California, USA) (Wölfel et al., personal communication). In summary this indicates that *R. felis* might be the only SFG Rickettsia to show antigenic relation to the TG Rickettsiae, but can show reactivity to other SFG Rickettsia as well [55]. *R. felis* was the only antigen for which titres above 1:512 were not observed. However, it remains unclear, if the reactivity against several rickettsial antigens including *R. felis* was caused by multiple infections or by cross reaction. The serologic test systems micro-IFA and ELISA are used for seroepidemiologic surveys as well as diagnosing acute cases. The micro-IFA is the gold standard in human medicine, its sensitivity is indicated with over 97%, its specificity with over 99% if a dilution of 1:64 or higher is used [7]. Clements et al. [56] compared the two test systems for diagnosing Rocky Mountain Spotted Fever in humans and in this study the ELISA was as sensitive and as specific as the IFA. Compared to the adapted micro-IFA test in this study the ELISA of the previous study had a moderate sensitivity (82.0%) and specificity (83.8%). These results are in line with non-published results of a comparable study with human sera. In that study, titres lower than 1:128 in an IFA could not be detected by ELISA (Dobler et al., personal communication). One reason for this reduced sensitivity might be that ELISA systems usually are designed for the clinical diagnosis of acute infections with high antibody titres instead of epidemiological studies (Dobler et al., personal communication). Lower antibody titres as expected after a longer post infection interval therefore might remain undetected by ELISA. The sensitivity of a serological assay also depends on the used antigen. In this case the ELISA used in the previous study was produced with *R. rickettsii*antigen, the causative agent of RMSF. Lower sensitivity and specificity rates for antibodies against other rickettsial species might be explained by that, as this *Rickettsia* species is not endemic in Germany. If no differentiation between rickettsial species is needed, ELISA assays might be reliable diagnostic tools for diagnosing acute cases where high antibody titres in sera can be expected and no differentiation between rickettsial species is needed. It is also a good screening tool for high numbers of samples, when the reduction of sensitivity is acceptable. The resulting seroprevalence rate then adds up all the rickettsial species occurring in the tested area. The micro-IFA on the other hand can be used to differentiate several rickettsial species and to determine the different antibody-titres, needed for example to monitor clinical cases.

CONCLUSION

This study reports the first results of a reliable serological test differentiating antibodies against rickettsial SFG species in dogs in Germany. The micro-IFA is a suitable tool for dogs to differentiate antibodies of the SFG Rickettsiae. Dogs are able to produce antibodies against SFG-Rickettsiae. The results reflect the natural exposure of dogs in Germany and could be related to the known infection rates in ticks. When compared to the micro-IFA the ELISA of the previous study showed acceptable sensitivity and specificity making both tests suitable for diagnostic purposes. For epidemiological studies the IFA should be preferred due to its higher sensitivity and specificity.

DECLARATIONS

Acknowledgements

We thank the following persons for providing the blood samples: Prof. Dr. Ingo Nolte and Jan-Peter Bach, Small Animal Clinic, Foundation University of Veterinary Medicine, Hannover; Nicole Schulz, Department of Veterinary Clinical Sciences, Clinical Pathology and Clinical Pathophysiology, Justus-Liebig-University, Gießen; Anneliese Balling, Institute of Animal Hygiene and Veterinary Public Health, University of Leipzig, Leipzig; Aleksandra Chirek, Small Animal Clinic, Faculty of Veterinary Medicine, Freie Universität Berlin, Berlin; Dr. Sabine Schall, Schifferstadt; Elisabeth Stemmler, Hohenwestedt, Veterinary clinic Dr. Stefan Reindl, Ingolstadt, veterinary practice Dr. Ebenboeck and colleagues, Traunstein, Dr. Uwe Urban, Amerang, Anuschka Winkelmann, St. Wolfgang, Johanna Gude, Eckental, Dr. Martin Steffl, University of Hohenheim, Stuttgart, Dr. Armin Reinle, Weil am Rhein, Veterinary clinic Neckarwiesen, Esslingen, Femke Mortier, Clinic of small animal medicine, Munich. Michael Leschnik, University of Veterinary Medicine, Vienna, Austria is acknowledged for providing the positive controls. The work of Martin Pfeffer and Cornelia Silaghi was done under the frame of EurNegVec COST Action TD1303. Finally we want to thank Bayer Vital GmbH for supporting Miriam Wächter with a grant. The paper has been sponsored by Bayer HealthCare – Animal Health Division in the framework of the 10th CVBD World Forum Symposium.

Authors' contributions

MW, SW and GD performed the laboratory analyses. CS and MP had the idea for the concept of the study. CS developed the experimental design. MW and CS analysed the data and wrote the manuscript. MP, SP and SW reed and critically corrected the manuscript. GD, BK, MP and AM provided study material. All authors read and approved the final manuscript.

REFERENCES

1. Parola P, Paddock CD, Raoult D. Tick-borne rickettsioses around the world: emerging diseases challenging old concepts. Clin Microbiol Rev. 2005;18:719–56.
2. Roux V, Raoult D. Phylogenetic analysis of members of the genus *Rickettsia* using the gene encoding the outer-membrane protein rOmpB (ompB). Int J Syst Evol Microbiol. 2000;50(Pt 4):1449–55.
3. Dumler JS, Barbet AF, Bekker CP, Dasch GA, Palmer GH, Ray SC, et al. Reorganization of genera in the families *Rickettsiaceae* and *Anaplasmataceae* in the order *Rickettsiales*: unification of some species of *Ehrlichia* with *Anaplasma*, *Cowdria* with *Ehrlichia* and *Ehrlichia* with *Neorickettsia*, descriptions of six new species combinations and designation of *Ehrlichia equi* and 'HGE agent' as subjective synonyms of *Ehrlichia phagocytophila*. Int J Syst Evol Microbiol. 2001;51:2145–65.
4. Roux V, Rydkina E, Eremeeva M, Raoult D. Citrate synthase gene comparison, a new tool for phylogenetic analysis, and its application for the *rickettsiae*. Int J Syst Bacteriol. 1997;47:252–61.
5. Gillespie JJ, Beier MS, Rahman MS, Ammerman NC, Shallom JM, Purkayastha A, et al. Plasmids and rickettsial evolution: insight from *Rickettsia felis*. PLoS One. 2007;2:e266.
6. Parola P, Paddock CD, Socolovschi C, Labruna MB, Mediannikov O, Kernif T, et al. Update on tick-borne rickettsioses around the world: a geographic approach. Clin Microbiol Rev. 2013;26:657–702.
7. Dobler G, Wölfel R. Typhus and other rickettsioses: emerging infections in Germany. Dtsch Arztebl Int. 2009;106:348–54.
8. Raoult D, Roux V. Rickettsioses as paradigms of new or emerging infectious diseases. Clin Microbiol Rev. 1997;10:694–719.
9. Raoult D, Fournier PE, Fenollar F, Jensenius M, Prioe T, de Pina JJ, et al. *Rickettsia africae*, a tick-borne pathogen in travelers to sub-Saharan Africa. N Engl J Med. 2001;344:1504–10.
10. Fournier PE, Raoult D. Suicide PCR on skin biopsy specimens for diagnosis of rickettsioses. J Clin Microbiol. 2004;42:3428–34.
11. Jiang J, You BJ, Liu E, Apte A, Yarina TR, Myers TE, et al. Development of three quantitative real-time PCR assays for the detection of *Rickettsia raoultii*, *Rickettsia slovaca*, and *Rickettsia aeschlimannii* and their validation with ticks from the country of Georgia and the Republic of Azerbaijan. Ticks Tick Borne Dis. 2012;3:327–31.
12. Brouqui P, Bacellar F, Baranton G, Birtles RJ, Bjoersdorff A, Blanco JR, et al. Guidelines for the diagnosis of tick-borne bacterial diseases in Europe. Clin Microbiol Infect. 2004;10:1108–32.
13. Teysseire N, Raoult D. Comparison of Western immunoblotting and microimmunofluorescence for diagnosis of Mediterranean spotted fever. J Clin Microbiol. 1992;30:455–60.
14. Nilsson K, Elfving K, Pahlson C. *Rickettsia helvetica* in patient with meningitis, Sweden, 2006. Emerg Infect Dis. 2010;16:490–2.
15. Nilsson K, Lindquist O, Pahlson C. Association of *Rickettsia helvetica* with chronic perimyocarditis in sudden cardiac death. Lancet. 1999;354:1169–73.

16. Fournier PE, Grunnenberger F, Jaulhac B, Gastinger G, Raoult D. Evidence of *Rickettsia helvetica* infection in humans, eastern France. Emerg Infect Dis. 2000;6:389–92.

17. Jado I, Oteo JA, Aldamiz M, Gil H, Escudero R, Ibarra V, et al. *Rickettsia monacensis* and human disease, Spain. Emerg Infect Dis. 2007;13:1405–7.

18. Madeddu G, Mancini F, Caddeo A, Ciervo A, Babudieri S, Maida I, et al. *Rickettsia monacensis* as cause of Mediterranean spotted fever-like illness, Italy. Emerg Infect Dis. 2012;18:702–4.

19. Vitale G, Mansuelo S, Rolain JM, Raoult D. *Rickettsia massiliae* human isolation. Emerg Infect Dis. 2006;12:174–5.

20. Parola P, Socolovschi C, Jeanjean L, Bitam I, Fournier PE, Sotto A, et al. Warmer weather linked to tick attack and emergence of severe rickettsioses. PLoS Negl Trop Dis. 2008;2:e338.

21. Garcia-Garcia JC, Portillo A, Nunez MJ, Santibanez S, Castro B, Oteo JA. A patient from Argentina infected with *Rickettsia massiliae*. Am J Trop Med Hyg. 2010;82:691–2.

22. Schriefer ME, Sacci Jr JB, Dumler JS, Bullen MG, Azad AF. Identification of a novel rickettsial infection in a patient diagnosed with murine typhus. J Clin Microbiol. 1994;32:949–54.

23. Zavala-Velazquez JE, Ruiz-Sosa JA, Sanchez-Elias RA, Becerra-Carmona G, Walker DH. *Rickettsia felis* rickettsiosis in Yucatan. Lancet. 2000;356:1079–80.

24. Labruna MB, Walker DH. *Rickettsia felis* and changing paradigms about pathogenic rickettsiae. Emerg Infect Dis. 2014;20:1768–9.

25. Ibarra V, Oteo JA, Portillo A, Santibanez S, Blanco JR, Metola L, et al. *Rickettsia slovaca* infection: DEBONEL/TIBOLA. Ann N Y Acad Sci. 2006;1078:206–14.

26. Oteo JA, Ibarra V, Blanco JR, Martinez de Artola V, Marquez FJ, Portillo A, et al. Dermacentor-borne necrosis erythema and lymphadenopathy: clinical and epidemiological features of a new tick-borne disease. Clin Microbiol Infect. 2004;10:327–31.

27. Rieg S, Schmoldt S, Theilacker C, de With K, Wolfel S, Kern WV, et al. Tick-borne lymphadenopathy (TIBOLA) acquired in Southwestern Germany. BMC Infect Dis. 2011;11:167.

28. Pluta S, Tewald F, Hartelt K, Oehme R, Kimmig P, Mackenstedt U. *Rickettsia slovaca* in *Dermacentor marginatus* ticks, Germany. Emerg Infect Dis. 2009;15:2077–8.

29. Richter J, Fournier PE, Petridou J, Haussinger D, Raoult D. *Rickettsia felis* infection acquired in Europe and documented by polymerase chain reaction. Emerg Infect Dis. 2002;8:207–8.

30. Jansen A, La Scola B, Raoult D, Lierz M, Wichmann O, Stark K, et al. Antibodies against *Rickettsia* spp. in hunters, Germany. Emerg Infect Dis. 2008;14:1961–3.

31. Piranda EM, Faccini JL, Pinter A, Saito TB, Pacheco RC, Hagiwara MK, et al. Experimental infection of dogs with a Brazilian strain of *Rickettsia rickettsii*: clinical and laboratory findings. Mem Inst Oswaldo Cruz. 2008;103:696–701.

32. Solano-Gallego L, Kidd L, Trotta M, Di Marco M, Caldin M, Furlanello T, et al. Febrile illness associated with *Rickettsia conorii* infection in dogs from Sicily. Emerg Infect Dis. 2006;12:1985–8.

33. Hartelt K, Oehme R, Frank H, Brockmann SO, Hassler D, Kimmig P. Pathogens and symbionts in ticks: prevalence of *Anaplasma phagocytophilum* (*Ehrlichia* sp.), *Wolbachia* sp., *Rickettsia* sp., and *Babesia* sp. in Southern Germany. Int J Med Microbiol. 2004;293 Suppl 37:86–92.

34. Wölfel R, Terzioglu R, Kiessling J, Wilhelm S, Essbauer S, Pfeffer M, et al. *Rickettsia* spp. in *Ixodes ricinus* ticks in Bavaria, Germany. Ann N Y Acad Sci. 2006;1078:509–11.

35. Silaghi C, Gilles J, Höhle M, Pradel I, Just FT, Fingerle V, et al. Prevalence of spotted fever group rickettsiae in *Ixodes ricinus* (Acari: Ixodidae) in southern Germany. J Med Entomol. 2008;45:948–55.

36. Schorn S, Pfister K, Reulen H, Mahling M, Silaghi C. Occurrence of *Babesia* spp., *Rickettsia* spp. and *Bartonella* spp. in *Ixodes ricinus* in Bavarian public parks, Germany. Parasit Vectors. 2011;4:135.

37. Pichon B, Kahl O, Hammer B, Gray JS. Pathogens and host DNA in *Ixodes ricinus* nymphal ticks from a German forest. Vector Borne Zoonotic Dis. 2006;6:382–7.

38. Schicht S, Schnieder T, Strube C. *Rickettsia* spp. and coinfections with other pathogenic microorganisms in hard ticks from northern Germany. J Med Entomol. 2012;49:766–71.

39. Silaghi C, Hamel D, Thiel C, Pfister K, Pfeffer M. Spotted fever group rickettsiae in ticks, Germany. Emerg Infect Dis. 2011;17:890–2.

40. Overzier E, Pfister K, Thiel C, Herb I, Mahling M, Silaghi C. Diversity of *Babesia* and *Rickettsia* Species in Questing *Ixodes ricinus*: A Longitudinal Study in Urban, Pasture, and Natural Habitats. Vector Borne Zoonotic Dis. 2013;13:559–64.

41. May K, Strube C. Prevalence of *Rickettsiales* (*Anaplasma phagocytophilum* and *Rickettsia* spp.) in hard ticks (*Ixodes ricinus*) in the city of Hamburg, Germany. Parasitol Res. 2014;113:2169–75.

42. Tappe J, Strube C. *Anaplasma phagocytophilum* and *Rickettsia* spp. infections in hard ticks (*Ixodes ricinus*) in the city of Hanover (Germany): revisited. Ticks Tick Borne Dis. 2013;4:432–8.

43. Pluta S, Hartelt K, Oehme R, Mackenstedt U, Kimmig P. Prevalence of *Coxiella burnetii* and *Rickettsia* spp. in ticks and rodents in southern Germany. Ticks Tick Borne Dis. 2010;1:145–7.

44. Breitschwerdt EB, Moncol DJ, Corbett WT, MacCormack JN, Burgdorfer W, Ford RB, et al. Antibodies to spotted fever-group rickettsiae in dogs in North Carolina. Am J Vet Res. 1987;48:1436–40.

45. La Scola B, Raoult D. Laboratory diagnosis of rickettsioses: current approaches to diagnosis of old and new rickettsial diseases. J Clin Microbiol. 1997;35:2715–

27.

46. Segura F, Pons I, Miret J, Pla J, Ortuno A, Nogueras MM. The role of cats in the eco-epidemiology of spotted fever group diseases. Parasit Vectors. 2014;7:353.

47. Spitalska E, Stefanidesova K, Kocianova E, Boldis V. *Rickettsia slovaca* and *Rickettsia raoultii* in *Dermacentor marginatus*and *Dermacentor reticulatus* ticks from Slovak Republic. Exp Appl Acarol. 2012;57:189–97.

48. Rubel F, Brugger K, Monazahian M, Habedank B, Dautel H, Leverenz S, et al. The first German map of georeferenced ixodid tick locations. Parasit Vectors. 2014;7:477.

49. Mackensen H. Study about the population dynamics of fleas at dogs and cats in the area of Karlsruhe, Germany, Ludwig-Maximilians-University, Comparative Tropical Medicine and Parasitology. 2006.

50. Gilles J, Just FT, Silaghi C, Pradel I, Passos LM, Lengauer H, et al. *Rickettsia felis* in fleas, Germany. Emerg Infect Dis. 2008;14:1294–6.

51. Williams M, Izzard L, Graves SR, Stenos J, Kelly JJ. First probable Australian cases of human infection with *Rickettsia felis*(cat-flea typhus). Med J Aust. 2011;194:41–3.

52. Abdad MY, Stenos J, Graves S. *Rickettsia felis*, an emerging flea-transmitted human pathogen. Emerg Health Threats J. 2011;4:7168.

53. Adams JR, Schmidtmann ET, Azad AF. Infection of colonized cat fleas, *Ctenocephalides felis* (Bouche), with a rickettsia-like microorganism. Am J Trop Med Hyg. 1990;43:400–9.

54. Fang R, Raoult D. Antigenic classification of *Rickettsia felis* by using monoclonal and polyclonal antibodies. Clin Diagn Lab Immunol. 2003;10:221–8.

55. Znazen A, Rolain JM, Hammami A, Jemaa MB, Raoult D. *Rickettsia felis* infection, Tunisia. Emerg Infect Dis. 2006;12:138–40.

56. Clements ML, Dumler JS, Fiset P, Wisseman Jr CL, Snyder MJ, Levine MM. Serodiagnosis of Rocky Mountain spotted fever: comparison of IgM and IgG enzyme-linked immunosorbent assays and indirect fluorescent antibody test. J Infect Dis. 1983;148:876–80.

CHAPTER 48 THE ROLE OF CATS IN THE ECO-EPIDEMIOLOGY OF SPOTTED FEVER GROUP DISEASES

Ferran Segura, Immaculada Pons, Jaime Miret, Júlia Pla, Anna Ortuño and María-Mercedes Nogueras

Keywords: Spotted fever group Rickettsiae, *Rickettsia conorii, Rickettsia massiliae-,* Bar29, *Rickettsia felis,* Cats, Molecular detection, Epidemiology

BACKGROUND

Spotted fever group (SFG) rickettsiae are Gram negative bacteria, obligate intracellular microorganisms, and widely distributed throughout the world. They are associated with arthropods, mainly with ticks, but also with fleas and mites. Some SFG rickettsiae can cause human disease. Clinical cases have been described in nearly every continent.

Mediterranean Spotted Fever (MSF) is one of the oldest described vector-borne infectious diseases. Many clinical cases have been reported since its etiological agent, *Rickettsia conorii,* was isolated in 1932. The usual vector is *Rhipicephalus sanguineus,* the brown dog tick [1]. This disease is endemic in the Mediterranean area [2] where *R. conorii* has also been isolated in different studies [3]. However, clinical cases have also been reported in other regions, such as Northern and Europe, Northern Africa, Middle East, the Indian subcontinent and Asia [1, 4]. Moreover, *R. conorii* has also been detected in ticks from outside Europe. The main symptoms of MSF are fever and rash. A *tache noire*, arthralgia, myalgia, and headache are usually present [5]. Even though MSF is a benign disease in most cases, severe manifestations and cases of death have also been reported.

Initially, MSF had been considered the only tick-borne rickettsial disease in the Mediterranean area. However, new species have been described as a consequence of the improvement of molecular techniques. Some clinical cases of MSF showed different severity in manifestations and a different pattern of antibiotic sensitivity than those described classically [6]. As a consequence, it had been strongly suspected that other SFG rickettsiae could be involved in some MSF cases [1, 7]. In 1992, *Rickettsia massiliae* was isolated from ticks [1]. In 1996, the strain *R. massiliae-* Bar29 was isolated from ticks collected in our area [8]. A study conducted using sera from MSF patients suggested that *R. massiliae-* Bar29 could have been involved in cases of MSF [7]. In addition, sero-epidemiological studies showed *R. massiliae–* Bar29 past infection in humans [9, 10]. *R. massiliae* was confirmed as a human pathogen in 2006, when an isolate from an Italian patient, obtained 20 years before, was identified [11]. Up to now, two more human cases of *R. massiliae* infection have been described [12, 13]. *R. massiliae* strains are one of the most widely distributed *Rickettsia.* It has been described in all five continents. Nowadays, it is considered prevalent in America [1, 6, 8, 9, 10, 11, 12, 13, 14, 15, 16, 17, 18, 19, 20, 21, 22, 23, 24, 25].

In 1990, *Rickettsia felis* was isolated from the flea *Ctenocephalides felis,* its main vector. *R. felis* is the etiological agent of Flea-borne spotted fever. Its main clinical

Citation: Ferran Segura, Immaculada Pons, Jaime Miret, Júlia Pla, Anna Ortuño and María-Mercedes Nogueras, The role of cats in the eco-epidemiology of spotted fever group diseases, DOI: 10.1186/1756-3305-7-353.

manifestations are fever, headache, myalgia, and macular rash. In addition, severe manifestations have been described. Human clinical cases have been reported worldwide [1].

Prevention of zoonoses depends on detection of reservoirs, vectors, routes of transmission, and risk factors for infection. Although cats can be reservoirs of some microorganisms, they are very popular as pets around the world. Flea exposure is very frequent in cats [26]. Experimental cats exposed to *R. felis* infected fleas became seropositive and *R. felis* was detected in blood by PCR [27]. Naturally exposed cats were also seroreactive [27]. However, the role of cats in the *R. felis* transmission cycle has not been elucidated.

Nowadays, the dog is considered the sentinel of *R. conorii* infection [2, 28]. However, since cats can be exposed to ticks [26], antibodies against *R. conorii* have also been detected in cats [29, 30, 31]. Likewise, since *R. massiliae* strains have been found in *Rhipicephalus* spp. [6, 8, 12, 14, 15, 16, 17, 18, 19, 20, 21, 24, 25], cats may also be seroreactive to this microorganism. To our knowledge, this fact has not been studied up to now.

In this study, we attempted to examine the antibodies against these three SFG rickettsiae in cats living in an area where these microorganisms are present [2, 3, 5, 8, 28, 32, 33]. In addition, we will analyze the possible infection of cats using molecular detection and culture.

METHODS

Ethics statement

This study was approved by the Ethical Committee of Corporació Sanitària i Universitària Parc Taulí. This study was adherent to the Animal Protection Law (5/1995) of the Government of Catalonia, and RD1201/2005 of the Government of Spain, based on European Union directives 86/609/CEE and 2003/65/CE.

Sample collection

The study was undertaken in Northeastern Spain. Twenty municipalities of seven regions participated in the study. Blood samples of 212 cats were collected from January 2001 to March 2009. Thirty-nine cats were stray cats that were kept as a strategy of control of rodent populations by municipalities. Their samples were provided by the municipal veterinarians when they carried out routine health care and reproductive controls. One hundred and seventy-one samples were collected at different veterinary clinics. One hundred and forty-seven of these cats were pets. One veterinary clinic worked together with Progat. Progat is a non-profit organization dedicated to the protection of stray cats, the sterilization of urban cat colonies, and the promotion of sterilization. This organization takes care of the health of stray cats. These cats undergo a veterinary examination when they are sterilized. In this study, 24 cats surveyed in veterinary clinics had been collected by Progat and, therefore, they were stray cats.

The following variables were registered: date of sample collection, age, sex, municipality, source (veterinary clinics, control of stray cats), living place (apartment, house, street), outdoor activities, health status, type of disease, contact with other animals, and ectoparasite infestation.

Blood samples were aseptically collected from the external jugular vein of each cat. One millilitre of blood was introduced in a serum-separating tube for serologic analyses, and the remainder was placed into a paediatric isolator 1.5 tube (Isolator™ 1.5; Oxoid, Ogdensburg, NY). Sera were obtained by centrifugation of blood at 1,500 rpm for 10 minutes. When it was possible, whole-blood samples were collected in sterile EDTA and heparin vacutainers. Samples were frozen at -80°C until used.

Serological technique

Antibody titres against *Rickettsia conorii, Rickettsia felis*, and *Rickettsia massiliae*-Bar29 were evaluated by IFA using an anti-cat IgG (Sigma-Aldrich Química,S.A., Madrid). A commercial antigen (*R. conorii* spot, BioMérieux, Marcy l'Étoile, France) was used to determine antibodies to *R. conorii*. *R. felis* antigen was kindly provided by the Unité de Rickettsies, Marseille, France. *R.massiliae*-Bar29 antigen was obtained from that strain previously isolated from *Rhipicephalus sanguineus* in our region [8].

Briefly, 25 µL of twofold dilutions of cat sera in phosphate-buffered saline (PBS) – 3% non-fat dry milk were applied to the antigens. The slides were incubated in a humidified chamber at 37°C for 30 min. Two washes in PBS and one wash in water were performed to remove unbound immunoglobulins. Binding sera were detected using a fluorescein isothiocyanate-labelled anti-cat IgG (Sigma-Aldrich Química, S.A., Madrid) diluted 1/128 in PBS – 0.01% Evans Blue (Biomerieux, S.A., Madrid). The slides were incubated and washed as described above. The slides were examined with a fluorescence microscope at 400x. The highest dilution, at which distinct and specific fluorescence was seen, was scored as the end-point titre for the serum sample. The intensity of each specific fluorescence was evaluated and independently graded by two of the authors.

Molecular detection

DNA from those samples collected in an EDTA vacutainer was obtained using the Masterpure DNA purification kit (Epicentre, Madison, Wisconsin) according to the manufacturer's instructions. This kit was also used to obtain DNA from cultures of *R. conorii* and *R. massiliae*- Bar29 (obtained previously by our group, [3, 8]), and *R. felis*, kindly provided by the Unité de Rickettsies. These samples were used as positive controls. The DNA samples were stored at -20°C until used. Measures to avoid contamination were carried out using separate and dedicated rooms for DNA extraction and molecular detection.

The presence of a rickettsial agent was assessed by following real-time PCR assays: *R. felis*-specific PCR targeting the rickettsial gene for outer membrane protein B (*ompB*) [34], *Rickettsia*-specific PCR assays targeting 17 kDa antigen gene [35], *rickA* gene [36], and *ompA* gene. The *omp* A PCR assay, which was designed by our laboratory previously, amplified a fragment of 316 nucleotides within *omp* A gene (314-FOR: 5'-GGGCATTTACTTACGGTGGTGAT-3'; 630-REV: 5'-CTTTGACGGAGCTGCAGATTGTAT). The PCR targeting *rick* A and *omp* A genes used SYBGreen as an intercalant. The *Rickettsia*-specific PCR targeting 17 kDa gene and the *R. felis*-specific PCR targeting *omp* B gene used a probe. Sensimix dU kit (Quantance) was used. This kit included a Uracil DNA Glycosylase (UNG) and deoxyuracil triphosphates (dUTP) as well as a Hot start DNA polymerase. Concentrations used were as follows, 5 mM of $MgCl_2$, 0.4 µM of probe and 0.5 µM of each primer for *omp* B PCR assay; and 5 mM of $MgCl_2$, 0.4 µM of probe and 0.3 µM of each primer for 17 kDa PCR assay. Concentrations used in *omp* A PCR assay were 4.5 mM of $MgCl_2$, and 0.2 µM of each primer. Concentrations used in *rick* A PCR assay were 5 mM of $MgCl_2$, and 0.2 µM of each primer. Real-time PCR assays were carried out and analyzed using 7500 thermocycler (Applied Biosystems). PCRs were set up in a UV-sterilized workstation. Negative control consisted of PCR reagents and DNA-free water as template. Two negative controls and one positive control were included in all assays. Each sample was assayed twice.

Amplification products were purified by Exosap-it (GE Healthcare, Buckinghamshire, UK). DNA obtained was directly sequenced using forward and reverse primers. A new reverse primer was designed into the sequence amplified by the PCR targeting 17 kDa gene. For this purpose, FASTA sequences of 17 kDa genes of *Rickettsia*strains shown in Table 1 were obtained and aligned by CLUSTAL.W and Nucleotide Basic Local Alignment Search Tool - BLAST programs. Primers were designed using Primer BLAST program (NCBI). The primer selected was that located in a region where all sequences are identical (primer N8: 5'-TCCAACAAGCT GTCCTTTGCCCTT-3'). DNA sequencing was performed twice with each forward and reverse primers. When there was a sufficient amount of PCR product, this was also sequenced with primer N8. DNA was sequenced on a 3130 Genetic Analyser (Applied Biosystems) using a BigDye Terminator v3.1 Cycle Sequencing Kit (Applied Biosystems, Foster City, CA). Sequences obtained were compared with those in the GenBank nucleotide database by Nucleotide BLAST program. Sequences of cats were aligned with each other and with the rest of the *Rickettsia* strains (Table 1) using CLUSTAL.W and BLAST programs.

Table 1: *Rickettsia* sequences used in this study

Rickettsia	Sequence in GenBank (accession number)	Group[a]
R. massiliae	*R. massiliae* MTU5 (CP000683.1), strain Alowo_68 (JN871729.1), strain AZT80 (CP003319.1), *Rickettsia* sp. TwKM01 (AY445821.1), Uncultured *Rickettsia* sp. clone 57 (GU353185.1)	Group-M
R. africae	*R. africae* ESF-5 (CP001612.1)	
R. amblyommii	*R. amblyommii* (AY375162.1), isolate AL-1 (EU828788.1), isolate TX051(EF689730.1), Candidatus *R. amblyommii* str. GAT-30 V (CP003334.1)	
R. conorii	strain Malish 7 (AE006914.1), RIRANT17KA *R.conorii* (M28480.1)	
R. honei	*R. honei* str. thai tick typhus (AF060706.1), *R. honei* (AF027124.1), strain RB (AF060704.1)	
R. parkeri	strain Portsmouth (CP003341.1), *R. parkeri* (U17008.1), isolate TX116 (EF689732.1), strain At24 (EF102237.1)	
R. peacockii	strain Rustic (CP001227.1), *R. peacockii* (AF260571.1)	
R. philipii	*R. philipii* str. 364D (CP003308.1)	
R. rickettsii	from Mexico (DQ176856.1), strain Hauke (CP003318.1), strain Hlp#2 (CP003311.1), strain Hino (CP003309.1), strain Iowa (CP000766.2), strain 'Sheila Smith' (CP000848.1), *R. rickettsii* (AY281069.1), strain Arizona (CP003307.1), strain Colombia (CP003306.1), strain Brazil (CP003305.1), strain ai103.1 (GU723477.1), strain ai101.1 (GU723476.1)	
R. sibirica	*R. sibirica* (AF445384.1)	Group-C
R. slovaca	clone 50 (JN182788.1), strain D-CWPP (CP003375.1), strain D-CWPP (CP003375.1), 13-B (CP002428.1)	
Candidatus *R. andeanae*	isolate T163 (GU395295.1)	
Candidatus R. gravesii	Candidatus *R. gravesii* (DQ269436.1)	
Rickettsia sp.	ARANHA (AY360215.1), 'Argentina' clone htrA_RArg_Apsd (EU826507.1), , COOPERI (AY362705.1), GRA-1 (AB444097.1), Hf332 (AB114804.1), , HpunctITA10 (AJ781417.1), HymargITA12 (AJ781419.1), RhturITA11 (AJ781418.1), R300 (AY472039.1), RpA4 (EF392727.1), scc31 (DQ105801.1), Is-1 (DQ344620.1), Tselentii (GU353184.1), TwKM03 (AY445822.1), DmargITA9 (AJ781416.1), HJ126 (ABAA4810.1), Ibadan (JN871831), Elepo (JN871731.1)	
Rickettsia endosymbiont of	*A. maculatum* isolate TX012 (EF689728.1), *Carios kelleyi* (AY763102.1)	
Uncultured *Rickettsia sp.* clone	UnfedWild17.32 (GQ302897.1), UnfedWild17.10 (GQ302898.1), UnfedWild17.2 (GQ302894.1), FedWild17.57 (GQ302890.1), UnfedWild17.18 (GQ302896.1)	
R. australis	strain Cutlack (CP003338.1), RIRTRAPRO *R.australis* (M74042.1)	
R. felis	*R. felis* (GU447234.1), scc50 (DQ102709.1), URRWXCal2 (CP000053.1), 17 (AF195118.1), California (AF210693.1)	
R. heilongjiangensis	*R. heilongjiangensis* 054 (CP002912.1)	
R. japonica	*R. japonica* YH (AP011533.1)	
R. marmionii	strain KB (AY737683.1)	
R. montana	*R. montana* (U11017.1)	
R. montanensis	strain. OSU 85–930 (CP003340.1)	
R. prowazekii	*R. prowazekii* Rp22 (CP001584.1), strain GvF12 (DQ926851.1)	
R. rhipicephali	*R. rhipicephali* (U11020.1), strain HJ5 (DQ865207.1), *R. rhipicephali* (CP003342.1)	
R. typhi	strain Wilmington (AE017197.1), RIRANT17KB *R.typhi* (M28481.1 strain TH1527 (CP003397.1)	
Candidatus *R. antechini*	Candidatus *R. antechini* (DQ372953.1)	
Candidatus *R. hoogstraalii*	Candidatus *R. hoogstraalii* (FJ767736.1), (EF629538.1)	
Rickettsia sp.	HymargITA13 (AJ781420.1), HOT2 (AF483199.1), cf1and5 (AY953286.1)	
Uncultured Rickettsia sp.	clone FedWild17.12 (GQ302888.1), Clone Shimane 042 (AB699875)	

[a]Considering the region amplified by 17 kDa PCR, those sequences identical have been grouped.

Culture

Cultures were carried out using the blood samples collected in the heparin vacutainers. For each animal, 150 microlitres of whole-blood was added to six shell vials (SVs) seeded with Vero cells (African green monkey epithelial cells). The SVs were centrifuged at 700 × g for 1 h at 22°C. The inoculum was discarded, and 1 mL of minimal essential medium (MEM) (Lonza, Basel, Switzerland), supplemented with 10% of fetal bovine serum (Lonza, Basel, Switzerland) and 1 mM of glutamine (Lonza, Basel, Switzerland), was added to each one. Three SVs were incubated at 32°C, and three at 28°C. Every week, the medium was replaced with a new medium.

After 5 weeks, a cell monolayer from each SV was scraped with glass beads and transferred to a confluent monolayer of Vero cells in a 25 cm^2 cultured flask. Each flask was incubated at the same temperature used for SV incubation. Every week, a slide with medium and monolayer scraped from each flask was prepared for Gimenez staining.

After three weeks, cell monolayers were scraped with glass beads and cultures were collected. Cultures corresponding to the same cat incubated at the same temperature were joined. For each one, three slides were prepared for Gimenez staining and two IFA assays. One of the IFA assays was performed using a serum sample with antibodies against *R. conorii* (1/1024) and *R. felis* (1/1024). The other IFA assay was performed using a serum sample with antibodies against *R. massiliae*- Bar29 (1/256). Moreover, 0.8 mL of each cell monolayer scraped was used to obtain DNA. The presence of rickettsial DNA was analyzed using the PCRs described above.

Statistical analysis

To achieve an accuracy of 5.0% in the estimation of a confidence interval using a normal asymptotic finite population correction for the bilateral 95%, assuming that the expected proportion was the highest prevalence found in the literature (worst cases) and that the total size of the populations were 1000, sample size was calculated.

The following variables were built: adult/kitten, demography, street, activities, and season of collection. The age was classified into categories [adult (≥1 year) and kitten (<1 year)]. The demographic area was determined considering the number of inhabitants of the municipality where the sample was collected. Municipalities with<5,000 inhabitants were included in the rural area group, municipalities with 5,000 to 50,000 inhabitants were considered suburban areas, and municipalities with>50,000 inhabitants were regarded as urban areas. The variable "Street" included stray cats and pets with outdoor activities. The variable "Activities" classified cats into three categories: indoor (pets without outdoor activities), outdoor (cats living at the street), indoor-outdoor (pets with outdoor activities).

Data analysis was carried out using the software application SPSS Statistics 18.0. A univariate analysis was performed to determine risk factors. Univariate group comparisons were performed using Chi-square and Fisher exact tests. Quantitative variables were compared by Mann–Whitney U test. A $p<0.05$ was considered statistically significant.

RESULTS

Study population

Samples were collected in twenty municipalities of seven regions. They are both urban and rural regions, as well as coastal and mountainous regions. The clinical and epidemiological characteristics of the study population are shown in Table 2. Of the 212 cats, 147 (69.3%) cats were pets and 65 (30.7%) stray cats. Outdoor activities were reported in 46 pets. Age ranged from 5 months to 17 years. The mean age was 3.7±4.1 years. Sixty (29.1%) cats were kittens and 146 (70.9%) were adults. In six cats, age was not surveyed.

Table 2: Demographic information from cats tested for antibodies to SFG rickettsiae

Variable	Total population	Seropositive population[a]
Age		
Kitten	60 (29.1)	16 (27.1)
Adult	146 (70.9)	43 (72.9)
Sex		
Male	99 (47.4)	23 (39.7)
Female	110 (52.6)	35 (60.3)
Demographical area		
Urban	172 (81.1)	46 (78)
Suburban	29 (13.7)	7 (11.8)
Rural	11 (5.2)	6 (10.2)
Habitat		
Apartment	53 (25)	14 (23.7)
House	94 (44.3)	24 (40.7)
Stray (PROGAT Foundation)	24 (11.3)	8 (13.6)
Stray cats controlled by municipalities	41 (19.4)	13 (22)
Activities		
Indoor	101 (47.6)	26 (44.1)

Outdoor	65 (30.7)	21 (35.6)
Indoor & Outdoor	46 (21.7)	12 (20.3)
Ectoparasites	65 (30.6)	20 (33.9)
Fleas	54 (25.5)	14 (23.7)
Ticks	12 (5.6)[b]	6 (10.2)[c]
Health status		
Healthy	156 (82.5)	40 (75.5)
Sick	33 (17.5)[d]	13 (24.5)[e]
Contact with animals	166 (78.3)	46 (77.9)
Contact with cats	129 (60.8)	38 (64.4)
Contact with dogs	48 (22.6)	15 (25.4)
Contact with other animals	5 (2.3)	0 (0)
Season of collection		
Winter	46 (21.7)	13 (22)
Spring	105 (49.5)	30 (50.9)
Summer	31 (14.6)	10 (16.9)
Autumn	30 (14.2)	6 (10.2)

[a]Cats with antibodies against one or more SFG rickettsiae (*R. conorii, R. felis, R. massiliae*-Bar29).

[b]*Rhipicephalus pusillus* on 1 cat, *Rhipicephalus sanguineus* on 6 cats, *Rhipicephalus sanguineus* and *R. turanicus* on 1 cat, *R. sanguineus*, *R. turanicus* and *R. pusillus* on 1 cat. In two cats, tick specie was not determined.

[c]($p=0.051$) *Rhipicephalus pusillus* on 1 cat, *Rhipicephalus sanguineus* on 2 cats, *Rhipicephalus sanguineus* and *R. turanicus* on 1 cat, two ticks not identified.

[d]Dehydration, anaemia, cough, apathy, diabetes mellitus, hepatic diseases, respiratory diseases, Feline immunodeficiency, Feline leukaemia, breast lump, nasal lump, bacteraemia, cystitis, diarrhoea, fever, gingivitis, mouth infection, urinary tract infection, and uterus infection.

[e]Uterus infection, bacteraemia, fever, cough, listlessness, anaemia, respiratory disease, gingivitis, anaemia, dehydration, Feline immunodeficiency, and Diabetes mellitus.

Most samples were collected between March and July (65%). Samples of cats attended at veterinary clinics were collected throughout the year. All samples of stray cats controlled by municipalities and 82.6% of samples of stray cats from Progat foundation were collected between March and July.

Sixty-five (30.6%) cats were infested. Most of them were collected in April (12.7%), May (42.9%), and June (15.9%), ($p<0.001$). There was higher proportion of infested cats among stray cats. In fact, 65.1% of stray cats have ectoparasites, whereas 12.4% of indoor pets and 23.9% of pets with outdoor activities had ectoparasites ($p<0.001$). There was higher percentage of infested cats among those living in rural areas (63.6%) and suburban areas (50%) than among those living in urban environment (27.3%) ($p=0.006$). Of infested cats, 98.4% had contact with animals ($p<0.001$), 95% had contact with cats ($p<0.001$), and 45.9% had contact with dogs ($p=0.016$).

Fleas were found on 54 (25.5%) cats. Although most fleas (73.2%) were collected between February and July, no statistical association was found between infestation by fleas and month of collection. Ticks were collected on 12 (5.6%) cats. Ticks were identified as *Rhipicephalus pusillus, R. sanguineus,* and *R. turanicus.* Eleven ticks were collected in May and one in June ($p<0.001$). All cats infested by ticks were stray cats controlled by municipalities in urban areas.

The health status was surveyed in 189 cats. Thirty-three (17.5%) cats showed some type of disease. These were: dehydration, anaemia, cough, apathy, Diabetes mellitus, hepatic diseases, respiratory diseases, Feline immunodeficiency, Feline leukaemia, breast lump, nasal lump, bacteraemia, cystitis, diarrhoea, fever, gingivitis, mouth infection, urinary tract infection, and uterus infection. Fifty percent of sick cats were stray cats ($p=0.030$). A higher proportion of sick cats were found among infested cats (31%, $p=0.01$) and cats with ticks (72.7%, $p<0.001$).

Sero-epidemiological study

Considering titres ≥ 1/64 as positive, there were 59 (27.8%) cats with antibodies against one or more of the antigens analyzed. Table 2 shows demographic information of these seropositive cats. A weak association was observed between SFG seropositivity and tick infestation ($p=0.051$). Seropositive cats had a tick infestation rate twice as much as the overall study population (10.2% *vs.* 5.6%). Ticks found on seropositive cats were *Rhipicephalus pusillus, R. sanguineus* and *R. turanicus.*

Seropositive cats had a higher percentage of sick cats than the study population (24.5% *vs.* 17.5%). However, it was not statistically significant ($p=0.085$). The diseases observed in seropositive cats were: Uterus infection, bacteraemia, fever, cough, listlessness, anaemia, respiratory disease, gingivitis, dehydration, Feline immunodeficiency, and Diabetes mellitus.

Thirteen (6.1%) cats had antibodies against *Rickettsia conorii* (1/64: 12 [5.6%], 1/128: 1 [0.5%]). Forty-one (19.3%) cats were seroreactive to *Rickettsia massiliae*- Bar29 (1/64:23 cats [10.8%], 1/128: 13 [6.1%], 1/256: 3 [1.4%], ≥ 1/512: 2 [1%]). In 16 cats (7.5%) antibodies against *Rickettsia felis* were detected (1/64: 14 [6.6%], 1/128: 1 [0.5%], 1/256: 1 [0.5%]).

There were 11 (5.2%) cats with cross-reactions. It means that 19% of seropositive cats had antibodies against two or three species. Thirty-three (15.6%) cats were seropositive against *R. massiliae*- Bar29 exclusively, 4 (1.9%) cats against *R. conorii,* and 11 (5.2%) cats against *R. felis*. Cross-reaction between *R. massiliae*- Bar29 and *R. conorii* were observed in five cats, between *R. massiliae*-Bar29 and *R. felis* in 2 cats, and 3 cats presented cross-reactions between *R. conorii* and *R. felis*. One cat was seroreactive against the three species. Considering as a minimum value the percentage of cats seroreactive exclusively against each antigen, and the maximum value the percentage of all cats seroreactive against each antigen, seroprevalence of *R. massiliae*-Bar29 would range from 15.6% to 19.5%, seroprevalence of *R. conorii*from 1.9% to 6.2%, and that of *R. felis* from 5.2% to 7.5%. The titres as well as the clinico-epidemiological features of each seroreactive cat are shown in Table 3.

Table 3: Information of seropositive cats

Cat's number	17 kDa PCR[a]	Titres RC	RF	B29	Habitat	Outdoor activity	Month of collection	Age[b]	Sex[c]	Demography[d]	Ectoparasites[e]	Sick[f]	Contact with animals
100	+ (GM)	-	-	≥512	Apartment	Yes	January	17 y.	F	U	No	Bact	Cats, dogs
102	-	128	-	≥512	Apartment	No	February	4 y.	F	U	No	No	-
50	+ (GM,GC)	-	-	256	Apartment	Yes	May	6 y.	F	U	No	No	Cats
89	ND [g]	-	-	256	Street	Yes	October	<1 y.	F	U	No	No	Cats
104	+ (GM,GC)	-	-	256	House	No	March	12 y.	F	U	No	No	Cats
51	+ (GM,GC)	64	-	128	Apartment	No	May	<1 y.	F	U	No	No	No
54	+ (GM)	64	-	128	House	Yes	May	6 y.	F	U	No	No	Cats
57	-	-	-	128	House	Yes	May	<1 y.	F	U	No	No	Gat, dogs
61	+ (GM)	-	-	128	House	No	June	1.8 y.	F	U	No	No	No
67	-	-	-	128	Street	Yes	June	2 y.	F	R	Fleas	No	Cats, dogs
68	+ (GM,GC)	64	-	128	Street	Yes	July	8 y.	F	R	No	No	Cats, dogs
73	-	-	-	128	House	Yes	May	1.2 y.	F	R	No	No	Cats
77	-	-	-	128	Apartment	No	July	9 y.	F	U	No	No	No
83	ND	-	-	128	House	No	September	6 y.	F	U	No	No	-
103	+ (GM,GC)	-	-	128	House	Yes	March	<1 y.	F	U	No	No	No
181	ND	-	-	128	Street	Yes	June	≥1 y.	F	U	No	No	Cats
219	-	-	-	128	Unknown	-	September	5 m.	F	U	Fleas	F, C, L	Cats
260	-	-	256	128	House	No	July	7 m.	M	SU	No	No	Cats
4	ND[e]	-	-	64	Apartment	No	January	5 y.	M	U	No	No	No
7	+ (GM,GC)	-	-	64	House	Yes	January	2 y.	M	U	No	No	Cats
8	ND	-	-	64	House	No	February	3 y.	M	U	No	No	Cats
24	+ (GM)	-	-	64	Street	Yes	February	<1 y.	F	U	Fleas	No	Cats, dogs
33	-	-	-	64	Apartment	No	March	13 y.	F	U	No	No	Dogs
47	+ (GM,GC)	64	64	64	House	No	May	<1 y.	F	U	No	No	Cats
53	-	-	-	64	House	Yes	May	<1 y.	M	U	Fleas	No	Cats
66	+	64	-	64	Street	Yes	June	<1 y.	F	R	No	No	Cats, dogs
69	-	-	-	64	Street	Yes	July	2 y.	F	R	Fleas	Ov Inf	Cats, dogs
76	-	-	-	64	House	Yes	July	4 y.	M	U	No	No	Cats
98	+ (GM)	-	-	64	House	No	December	1.4 y.	F	U	No	No	Cats
105	-	-	-	64	House	No	March	2.6 y.	M	U	No	No	-
111	+ (GM,GC)	-	-	64	Street	Yes	April	1 y.	F	U	No	No	Cats
183	ND	-	-	64	Street	Yes	June	≥1 y.	M	U	Ticks	No	Cats
207	-	-	-	64	House	Yes	April	7 m.	F	SU	Fleas	No	Cats
209	GM	-	-	64	Apartment	No	April	11 m.	M	SU	No	No	Cats, dogs
216	-	-	-	64	Apartment	No	May	9 m.	M	U	Fleas	-	No
217	+ (GM,GC)	-	-	64	House	No	May	8 m.	M	R	Fleas	No	Cats
233	ND	-	-	64	Street	Yes	May	≥1 y.	F	U	RS	Res Dis	Cats
243	ND	-	64	64	Street	Yes	May	≥1 y.	M	U	RS	Res Dis	Cats
247	ND	-	-	64	Street	Yes	May	≥1 y.	M	U	RP	Res Dis	Cats
266	-	-	-	64	Apartment	Yes	June	9 y.	M	. SU	Fleas	FIV	Cats, dogs
275	+ (GM)	-	-	64	Apartment	No	October	7 m.	F	U	No	No	No
13	+ (GM)	-	64	-	House	No	January	3 y.	M	SU	Fleas	No	No
42	+ (GC)	64	**128**	-	Apartment	No	April	7 y.	M	U	No	No	No
52	+ (GM,GC)	64	-	-	Apartment	No	May	3 y.	M	U	No	No	No
58	+	-	64	-	Apartment	No	May	<1 y.	M	U	No	No	No
94	-	64	64	-	House	No	November	<1 y.	F	U	No	No	Cats, dogs
97	-	64	-	-	House	Yes	December	3 y.	F	SU	Fleas	No	Cats, dogs
170	-	-	64	-	Street	Yes	March	≥1 y.	M	U	Fleas	Res Dis	Cats
171	+ (GM,GC)	64	64	-	Street	Yes	March	≥1 y.	F	U	No	No	Cats
175	ND	64	-	-	Street	Yes	May	≥1 y.	F	U	Ticks	NR	Cats
179	ND	-	64	-	Street	Yes	June	≥1 y.	F	U	No	No	Cats
180	ND	-	64	-	Street	Yes	June	≥1 y.	F	U	No	No	Cats
193	-	-	64	-	Apartment	No	January	9 y.	F	U	No	Res Dis	gos
198	+ (GM,GC)	-	64	-	House	No	February	13 y.	F	SU	No	An, Deh	Cats, dogs
237	ND	64	-	-	Street	Yes	May	≥1 y.	F	U	RS,RT	Ging	Cats
240	ND	-	64	-	Street	Yes	May	≥1 y.	F	U	Fleas	No	Cats
252	ND	-	64	-	Street	Yes	May	≥1 y.	F	U	Fleas	No	Cats
274	ND	-	64	-	House	No	October	7 y.	F	U	No	Diab	No
272	ND	-	64	-	House	Yes	July	1 y.	M	U	No	No	Cats

[a]Sequence homology are shown in brackets. GM: identical to those sequences joined as group-M in Table 1; GC: identical to those ones joined as Group-C. [b]y: years; m: months. [c]F: female, M: male. [d]U: urban, SU: suburban; R: rural. [e]RT: *Rhipicephalus turanicus*, RS: *Rhipicephalus sanguineus*, RP: *Rhipicephalus pusillus*. [f]Bact: Bacteraemia; F: Fever; C: cough; L: listlessness: Ov Inf: Ovarian infection; Res Dis: Respiratory disease; FIV: Feline Immunodeficiency; NR: Cat ill but disease not reported An: Anaemia, Deh: dehydration; Ging: Gingivitis; Diab: Diabetes. [g]ND: Not done.

Molecular detection

Whole blood samples had been collected in EDTA-vacutainers in 42 of the 59 seropositive cats. No amplification was obtained when PCRs targeting genes *omp* A, *rick* A, and *omp* B were performed. When a 17 kDa PCR assay was carried out, positive amplifications were observed in 23 cats (Table 3). The amplification products were sequenced. The amount of DNA amplified was not enough to analyse it by sequencing in two cats (numbers 58, and 66). Low copy number of rickettsial DNA amplified as well as the short length of amplicon (141 nucleotides) allowing us to obtain good short sequences. Thus, the sequence consensus for each cat was defined as that fragment in which two or more sequences obtained align to each other.

As 17 kDa PCR assay was the only PCR with positive results, in order to be sure of the amplifications, DNA from 29 seronegative cats was extracted and this PCR was performed using those DNAs as templates. No amplification was obtained in these 29 samples.

The 17 kDa PCR amplifies a fragment of 114 nucleotides. All *Rickettsia* strains that belonged to the same species had identical sequences into this fragment. For this study, sequences were joined into groups (Group-M and Group-C) when they were identical among them (Table 1). Figure 1 shows alignment of the different *Rickettsia* sequences found in this region, as well as all consensus sequences obtained from the cats. All sequences obtained were similar to Group-M or Group-C rickettsiae and different to the other ones. One nucleotide allows differentiating Group-M and Group-C. Nine cats had this nucleotide included in their consensus sequences. One cat had a 'C' like Group-C. Eight cats had an 'A' as Group-M. In 11 cats, it was not possible to define the different nucleotide between Group-M and Group-C. Table 4 showed the results of comparing consensus sequences of each cat with those in the GenBank by Nucleotide BLAST program.

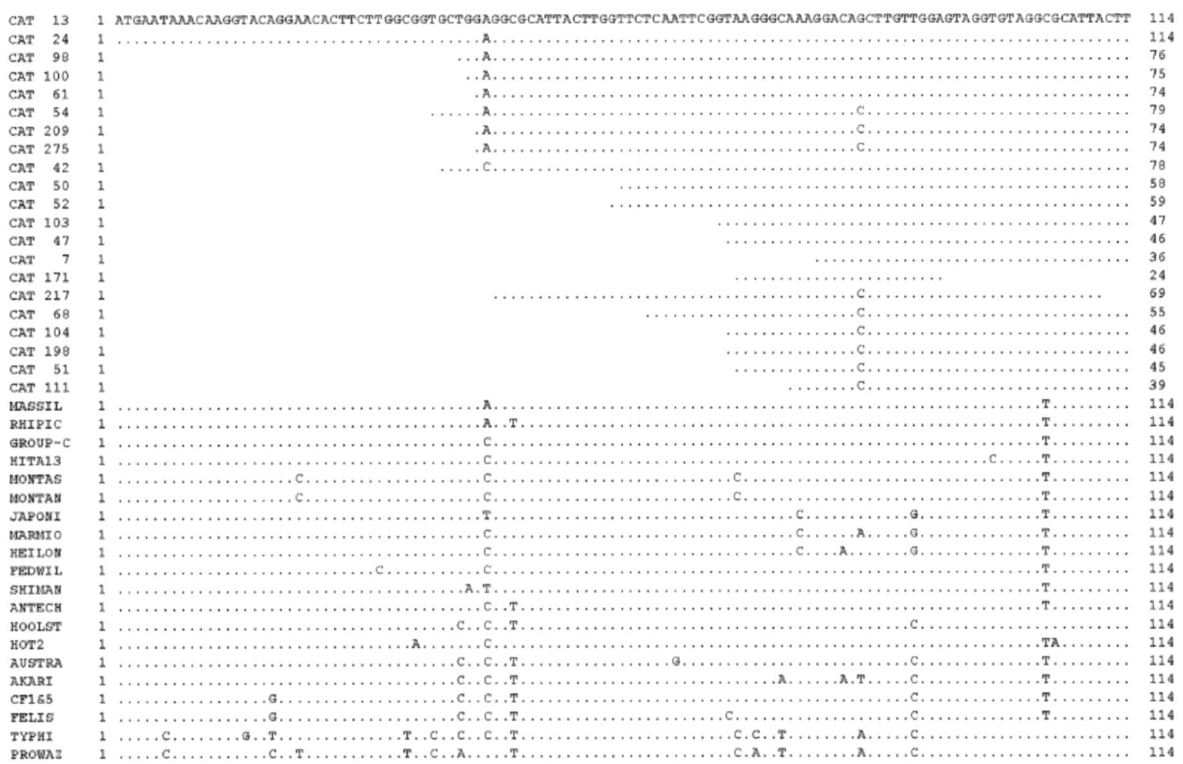

Figure 1: Alignment of the fragments amplified by 17 kDa PCR. MASSIL: Massiliae Group-M (see Table 1) RHIPIC: R. rhipicephali Group-C (group of sequences identical among them, see Table 1) HITA13: Rickettsia sp. HymargITA13, MONTAS: R. montanensis, MONTAN: R. montana, JAPONI: R. japonica, MARMIO: R. marmionii, HEILON: R. heilongjiangensis, FEDWIL: Uncultured Rickettsia sp. clone FedWild17.12, SHIMAN: Uncultured Rickettsia sp. clone Shimane042, ANTECH: Candidatus R. antechini, HOOLST: Candidatus R. hoogstraalii, HOT2: Rickettsia sp. HOT2, AUSTRA: R. australis, AKARI: R. akari, CF1&5: Rickettsia sp. cf1and5, FELIS: R. felis, TYPHI: R. typhi, PROWAZ: R. prowazekii.

Table 4: Results obtained using database of Basic Local Alignment Search Tool (BLAST)

Cat	Sequence length	Highest homology[a]	Score	Max. Identity	Identities
13	114	Group-M	201	99%	113/114 (99%)
24	114	Group-M	201	99%	113/114 (99%)
98	76	Group-M	132	99%	75/76 (99%)
100	75	Group-M	131	99%	74/75 (99%)
61	74	Group-M	129	99%	73/74 (99%)

54	79	Group-M	134	97%	77/79 (97%)
209	74	Group-M	125	97%	72/74 (97%)
275	74	Group-M	125	97%	72/74 (97%)
42	78	Group-C	139	99%	77/78 (99%)
50	58	Group-C or Group-M	102	98%	57/58 (98%)
52	59	Group-C or Group-M	102	98%	58/59 (98%)
103	47	Group-C or Group-M	85.7	98%	46/47 (98%)
47	46	Group-C or Group-M	83.8	100%	45/46 (98%)
7	36	Group-C or Group-M	63.9	100%	35/36 (97%)
171	24	Group-C or Group-M	48.1	100%	24/24 (100%)
217	69	Group-C or Group-M	116	97%	67/69 (97%)
68	55	Group-C or Group-M	91.5	96%	53/55 (96%)
104	46	Group-C or Group-M	75.8	96%	44/46 (96%)
198	46	Group-C or Group-M	75.8	96%	44/46 (96%)
51	45	Group-C or Group-M	73.8	100%	43/45 (96%)
111	39	Group-C or Group-M	61.9	100%	37/39 (95%)

[a]Group-M: those sequences in GenBank identical to *R. massiliae;* Group-C: sequences in GenBank that belong to different *Rickettsia* sequences (including *R. conorii*) and are identical among them (Table 1).

Culture

Cats selected were those in which rickettsial DNA was detected in blood samples, or whose titres of antibodies against *R. conorii*, *R. felis*, or *R. massiliae*- Bar29 were$\geq$1/128. Among them, cultures were carried out in those cats whose heparin whole-blood samples were available (Cats: 181, 198, 260, and 275). All six SVs of cats 275 and 181 were incubated at 32°C. Three SVs of cats 198 and 260 were incubated at 28°C, whereas three other ones were incubated at 32°C. After 3 weeks of incubation in a 25 cm^2 flask, all cultures were negative by molecular detection and IFA.

DISCUSSION

Cats can be the reservoir of many pathogens. A considerable percentage of cats are pets, which are in close contact with humans. Therefore, it is important to perform serological as well as molecular studies of pathogens in cats. It was suggested that cats can be sentinels for rickettsiae [30]. However, their role in maintaining and transmitting these microorganisms to humans has not been entirely elucidated [37]. Our data showed a substantial percentage (27.1%) of SFG seropositive cats, even with high titres and molecular detection in blood. Some studies have also shown that cats can be seroreactive to SFG rickettsiae [29, 30, 31, 38, 39]. For instance, more than 50% of cats studied in Australia were SFG seroreactive [38]. Cross-reaction among SFG rickettsiae has been well described and it is a limitation of seroprevalence studies. We used antigens of those SFG rickettsiae described in our area [2, 3, 5, 8, 28, 32, 33]. In our study, a proportion of cats were seropositive exclusively against one of the SFG rickettsiae studied. Therefore, although actual seroprevalences couldn't be established, data do show seroreactivity of cats against each antigen. Taking into account cross-reactions, *R. massiliae*-Bar29 seroprevalence was 15.6% - 19.5%, *R. conorii* seroprevalence was 1.9% - 6.2%, and *R. felis* seroprevalence was 5.2% - 7.5%.

Interestingly, *R. massiliae*-Bar29 seroprevalence was the highest, even if cats with antibodies exclusively against this strain were considered (15.6%). Moreover, highest titres were observed against *R. massiliae*-Bar29 antigen, most of them in cats without cross-reactions. The majority of studies are focused on the presence of *R. massiliae* strains in ticks. In fact, *R. massiliae* has been detected in *Rhipicephalus sanguineus, R. turanicus, R. pusillus, R. guilhoni, R muhsamae, R. lunulatus, R. sulcatus* collected on humans, dogs, cats, donkeys, cows, hedgehogs, horses, red foxes, roe deer, goat, cattle and sheep and wild boars or by flagging [6, 8, 12, 14, 15, 16, 17, 18, 19, 20, 21, 24, 25]. Moreover, it has been found in other genera such as *Ixodes tasmani* (collected on Tasmanian devils) [22], *Ixodes ricinus*[16], and *Dermacentor marginatus* (collected on dogs) [23]. Association between ticks and human cases has been observed [12, 16, 24]. The transstadial and trasovarial transmission of *Rickettsia massiliae*- Bar29 have been observed in *R. sanguineus* group. In addition, this microorganism does not have any effect on viability of *R. sanguineus* and its reproductive fitness [6, 25, 40]. Therefore, these ticks are considered a reservoir.

On the other hand, in spite of the fact that mammals can be reservoirs for many *Rickettsia* species, little is known about the role of them in the *R. massiliae* cycle. Since *Rhipicephalus* spp. is described mainly as a dog tick, most studies are focused on dogs. For instance, association between *R. massiliae*- Bar29 seropositivity in humans and contact with dogs had been observed in our previous serological study [9]. *R. massiliae* infection had been detected by serum cross-absorption and Western blot in dogs from California [25]. To our knowledge, this is the first study focused on *R. massiliae*- Bar29 infection in cats.

Tick infestation was observed in our cats. All of the ticks identified belonged to the genus *Rhipicephalus (R. sanguineus, R. pusillus*, and *R. turanicus),* whose members can use cats as possible hosts [26]. Cats showed lower infestation by ticks than by fleas. On the one hand, the lower infestation by ticks could be due to the host specificity because of *Rhipicephalus* spp. tends to infest mainly dogs. On the other hand, some authors explain the low infestation by ticks as a consequence of the grooming habits of cats [41]. In addition, since most cats in our study were pets, they were probably disinfested by their owner. In fact, all cats infested by ticks were stray cats surveyed by municipal veterinarians. Considering our area as an endemic area for the *R. massiliae*- Bar29 strain [7, 8, 9], it can be suspected that this microorganism may infect some of the ticks on the cats. In fact, *R. massiliae* had been detected in one *R. turanicus* collected on a cat in the Camargue [14]. Some studies have described cats not only as transport hosts of ticks, but also as susceptible and seroreactive to infection of SFG rickettsiae [30, 31]. According to our results, cats can be infected and produce antibodies against *R. massiliae*- Bar29. More than fifteen percent of our cats were seroreactive against *R. massiliae*-Bar29, exclusively. Moreover, high titres were observed. For instance, cat number 102 had titres higher than 512 (more than two-fold of its *R. conorii* titre) and cat number 100 had antibodies against exclusively *R. massiliae*- Bar29 at titres higher than 512.

The role of *R. sanguineus* in the transmission of *R. conorii* has been widely described since 1930 [1]. A transstadial and trasovarial transmission of *R. conorii* takes place in this tick. Therefore, *R. sanguineus* cannot only act as a vector but also as a reservoir [30]. However, unlike *R. massiliae, R. conorii* can negatively affect the survival and fecundity of *R. sanguineus*[6, 40]. For this reason, *R. conorii* in ticks declines gradually each generation [40]. This could explain why the prevalence of *R. conorii* is usually low in ticks. In fact, whereas *R. massiliae* has been detected, *R. conorii* has not been found in ticks from areas where both species have been described [8, 16, 17]. As a consequence, the role of the mammals as reservoir hosts is important. Epidemiological surveys have demonstrated the role of dogs, sheep and hedgehogs as vertebrate reservoirs for *R. conorii*[2]. High seroprevalence in dogs has been observed in MSF endemic areas [4]. Dogs are considered reservoirs and sentinels of *R. conorii*[28, 42]. Recently, *R. conorii* has been detected in blood samples of dogs by PCR and sequencing [43]. On the other hand, some studies have shown that cats can be seroreactive to *R. conorii*[29, 38]. A Spanish study showed that 44% of cats were seroreactive against *R. conorii*antigen. Titres ranged from 64 to 8192 [31]. In a study carried out in Zimbabwe and South Africa, 34% and 19% of cats had antibodies against *R. conorii*[30]. We did not use only *R. conorii* antigen but antigens of other SFG rickettsiae of our area. Almost 2% of our cats had antibodies against *R. conorii,* exclusively. Therefore, seroreactivity of cats to *R. conorii* is confirmed.

Seroprevalence studies suggest the exposure of the animal to microorganisms. However, the infection needs to be shown by the detection of the microorganisms within the animal. DNA of SFG rickettsiae were detected in blood of our cats. Three PCR assays that amplify SFG rickettsiae were used (17 kDa, *rick* A, and *omp* A). Positive results were only obtained using real time PCR targeting the 17 kDa gene. The latter incorporated a probe while *rick* A and *omp* A used SYBGreen as intercalant. Real time PCR using probes instead of SYBGreen are much more sensitive. The amount of *Rickettsia* in blood may have been very low as it was only detected by 17 kDa PCR. In fact, in two cases, sequencing was not possible due to the low amount of DNA amplified. In order to be sure of these results, DNA from 29 seronegative cats was used as a template for 17 kDa assays and no amplification was obtained.

The sequence amplified by 17 kDa assay is not able to distinguish among all SFG rickettsia. This is a limitation of the study. DNA detected belonged to two groups of SFG rickettsiae. In some cats, rickettsiae closely related to *R. massiliae* were identified pointing towards the presence of its infection in cats. It is important to highlight that most cats, in which rickettsia DNA were detected, were pets. Therefore, SFG rickettsiae may be in close contact with humans through the cats. However, the role of cats as reservoirs of these microorganisms needs further studies to focus on the cats' ability to acquire the microorganisms from vectors, maintain or amplify them, and transmit them again to vectors.

Ctenocephalides felis is the main vector of *R. felis,* although this microorganism has been detected in other fleas [32]. In addition, fleas act as a reservoir for *R. felis* because vertical transmission has been observed [27]. Experimental infection of cats has been demonstrated when they have been exposed to fleas infected with *R. felis.* The experimentally infected cats became seroreactive by the fourth month after exposure, had a very short bacteraemia, and *R. felis* DNA was detected in blood transiently [27]. However, the role of the cat in the epidemiology of *R. felis* has not been determined yet. *R. felis* was detected in 43.6% of fleas (*Ctenocephalides felis*) from our area [32]. In our study, a quarter of cats had fleas. *R. felis* seroprevalence in cats ranged from 5.2% to 7.5%. Likewise, some studies found serum antibody responses to *R. felis* in naturally infected cats [37, 39]. Therefore, naturally infected cats are susceptible to *R. felis* infection and produce antibodies against it.

Interestingly, whereas DNA closely related to other species of SFG rickettsiae was detected in blood samples, no DNA related to *R. felis* was identified. Amplification was obtained by PCR targeting 17 kDa using a probe. Although this PCR amplifies a short fragment of DNA, its sequencing would allow the identification of *R. felis.*However, no sequence obtained was similar to those of *R. felis* in GenBank. In the same way, *R. felis*-specific PCRs targeting the *ompB* gene were negative. Quite a few studies have failed to detect this microorganism in blood [37, 44, 45, 46]. For instance, whereas *R. felis* was detected in 18% of fleas from Ontario, molecular detection was negative in cats [45]. When pairs of feline blood and fleas were analyzed by Hawley *et al.*, 67.4% of fleas were infected with *R. felis*; however, no cat was positive [46]. Bayliss *et al.* studied cats with and without fever. Although both cat populations were seropositive, no *R. felis* was detected in any blood sample [37]. There are some hypotheses about the lack of *R. felis* amplification in blood. It could be related to a rapid immune response [37]; a low concentration of *R. felis* in blood, lower than the detection limit of PCR assays [44, 46]; an intermittent bacteraemia that could be missed when the sample is taken [47]; and a sequestration of *R. felis* in other tissues such as endothelial cells, spleen, and dermal tissues [44, 46]. In this way, Lappin *et al.* analyzed the presence of *Rickettsia* DNA in blood, oral cavity, skin, and claw beds of 83 dead cats using the same PCR of Hawley's study. *R. felis* DNA was detected in skin and gingival samples [47]. In the same way, *R. felis* were detected in renal, hepatic and pulmonary tissues of opossums while PCR of blood samples were negative [48]. Therefore, although cats can be susceptible to *R. felis* infection, probably they may not be an effective reservoir. A high percentage of our cats were pets in close contact with humans. In our area, *R. felis*prevalence in fleas is much higher that *R. felis* seroprevalence in the human population [32, 33] *R. felis* may be maintained in a cycle away from humans who were sporadically infected. Moreover, cats may be an unlikely reservoir host and may not have an important role in its transmission.

Overall, there were no significant associations between seropositivity and either habitat or outdoor activities, even though stray cats or cats with outdoor activities might be more exposed to infection. Similar results have been described in rickettsiae as well as other pathogens infecting cats [39, 44]. Our results may be due to the fact that our area is a predominantly urban area, in which stray cats are very controlled, and most of them are sterilized. On the other hand, there were more pets than stray cats in our survey. As a consequence, seropositive cats, even cats in which rickettsiae have been directly detected, lived in close contact with humans.

Like other studies [31], sex and age were not associated to SFG seropositivity. No statistically significant association was found between SFG seroprevalence and health status. Therefore, cats may present a SFG rickettsiae subclinical infection. Likewise, experimentally *R. felis* infection in cats was asymptomatic [27]. Moreover, those cats, in which *R. felis* had been detected in oral cavity or skin by PCR, did not have clinical evidence of skin disease or gingivitis [47]. Bayliss *et al.* did not find statistically significant association between fever and both *R. felis* and *R. rickettsii* seropositivity [37]. In the same way, there was no association between health status and *R. conorii* seroprevalence in the Solano's study [31]. Izzard *et al.* did not find statistical correlation between illness and SFG seropositivity [38]. These authors also suggested that clinical symptoms could be so early and mild that they may not warrant veterinary attention.

Even though the highest percentage of infested cats and stray cats were surveyed between March and July, there was no statistically significant association between month of the year and SFG seropositivity. On the one hand, it could be due to the persistence of antibodies over time. On the other hand, larvae and nymphs can also be vectors of SFG rickettsiae [1]. Eggs, larvae, nymphs and unfed adults have also been collected in the winter [40]. Taking into account ticks feed at each life stage as well as transstadial and transovarial transmission [1], rickettsiae can be transmitted to the host in each season. Moreover, early stages are smaller than adults and could go unnoticed. Finally, although *R. sanguineus* is active from spring to autumn, the climate change could be influencing its activity.

CONCLUSIONS

In conclusion, cats can be infected by SFG rickettsiae and produce antibodies against them. In spite of cross-reaction, some cats have reacted exclusively against one of the species studied: *R. conorii, R. massiliae*- Bar29, and *R. felis*. Although a good identification of species was not possible by molecular detection, infection by SFG rickettsiae has been observed; even a strain closely related to *R. massiliae*- Bar29. Therefore, cats may have a role in the transmission cycle of these microorganisms, particularly in those such as *R. conorii,* which can be decline gradually in tick populations. *R. felis* has not been detected in cat blood samples, pointing towards *R. felis* being found in other tissues, in addition, cats may not have a main role in its transmission cycle. Further studies will be necessary to study in depth the importance of cats as reservoirs of SFG rickettsiae. This fact is particularly important because many of them live in close contact with humans, and could be infected in spite of their habitat, infestation, month of year, or health status.

DECLARATIONS

Acknowledgments

This study was supported by Ministerio de Sanidad y Consumo grant FIS06/0433 and supported partially by Catalan society of infectious diseases and clinical microbiology.

Authors' contribution

FS conceived of the study, participated in the design of the study, analysed the results, and reed the manuscript. IP performed laboratory experiments. JM, JP, and AO contributed to acquisition of data. MMN conceived and design of the study, coordinated the study, performed laboratory experiments and statistical analysis, analysed the results, and wrote the manuscript. All authors read and approved the final version of the manuscript.

REFERENCES

1. Parola P, Paddock CD, Socolovschi C, Labruna MB, Mediannikov O, Kernif T, Abdad MY, Stenos J, Bitam I, Fournier PE, Raoult D: Update on tick-borne rickettsioses around the world: a geographic approach. Clin Microbiol Rev. 2013, 26: 657-702.
2. Segura F, Diestre G, Ortuño A, Sanfeliu I, Font B, Muñoz T, Mateu E, Casal J: Prevalence of antibodies to spotted fever group rickettsiae in human beings and dogs from an endemic area of Mediterranean spotted fever in Catalonia. Eur J Epidemiol. 1998, 14: 395-398.
3. Cardeñosa N, Roux V, Font B, Sanfeliu I, Raoult D, Segura F: Isolation and identification of two spotted fever group rickettsial strains from patients in Catalonia. Am J Trop Med Hyg. 2000, 62: 142-144.
4. Nicholson WL, Allen KE, Mc Quiston JH, Breitschwerdt EB, Little SE: The increasing recognition of rickettsial pathogens in dogs and people. Trends Parasitol. 2010, 26: 205-212.
5. Antón E, Font B, Muñoz T, Sanfeliu I, Segura F: Clinical and laboratory characteristics of 144 patients with mediterranean spotted fever. Eur J Clin Microbiol Infect Dis. 2003, 22: 126-128.
6. Eremeeva ME, Bosserman EA, Demma LJ, Zambrano ML, Blau DM, Dasch GA: Isolation and identification of *Rickettsia massiliae* from *Rhipicephalus sanguineus* ticks collected in Arizona. Appl Environ Microbiol. 2006, 72: 5569-5777.
7. Cardeñosa N, Segura F, Raoult D: Serosurvey among

Mediterranean spotted fever patients of a new spotted fever group rickettsial strain (Bar29). Eur J Epidemiol. 2003, 18: 351-356.

8. Beati L, Roux V, Ortuño A, Castella J, Segura F, Raoult D: Phenotypic and genotypic characterization of spotted fever group rickettsiae isolated from Catalan rhipicephalus sanguineus ticks. J Clin Microbiol. 1996, 34: 2688-2694.

9. Cardeñosa N, Nogueras MM, Font B, Muñoz T, Sanfeliu I, Segura F: Serological evidence of human infection with rickettsial strain Bar29 in Catalonia, northeastern Spain. Eur J Clin Microbiol Infect Dis. 2006, 25: 541-543.

10. Bernabeu-Wittel M, del Toro MD, Nogueras MM, Muniain MA, Cardeñosa N, Segura F, Pachón J: Presence of human past infections due to the Bar29 rickettsial strain in Southern Spain. J Infect. 2006, 52: e117-119.

11. Vitale G, Mansuelo S, Rolain JM, Raoult D: *Rickettsia massiliae* human isolation. Emerg Infect Dis. 2006, 12: 174-175.

12. García-García JC, Portillo A, Núñez MJ, Santibáñez S, Castro B, Oteo JA: A patient from Argentina infected with *Rickettsia massiliae*. Am J Trop Med Hyg. 2010, 82: 691-692.

13. Parola P, Socolovschi C, Jeanjean L, Bitam I, Fournier PE, Sotto A, Labauge P, Raoult D: Warmer weather linked to tick attack and emergence of severe rickettsioses. PLoS Negl Trop Dis. 2008, 2: e338.

14. Socolovschi C, Reynaud P, Kernif T, Raoult D, Parola P: Rickettsiae of spotted fever group, *Borrelia valaisiana*, and *Coxiella burnetii* in ticks on passerine birds and mammals from the Camargue in the south of France. Ticks Tick Borne Dis. 2012, 3: 355-360.

15. Mediannikov O, Diatta G, Fenollar F, Sokhna C, Trape JF, Raoult D: Tick-borne rickettsioses, neglected emerging diseases in rural Senegal. PLoS Negl Trop Dis. 2010, 4: e821.

16. Fernández-Soto P, Pérez-Sánchez R, Díaz Martín V, Encinas-Grandes A, Alamo Sanz R: *Rickettsia massiliae* in ticks removed from humans in Castilla y León, Spain. Eur J Clin Microbiol Infect Dis. 2006, 25: 811-813.

17. Márquez FJ, Rodríguez-Liébana JJ, Soriguer RC, Muniaín MA, Bernabeu-Wittel M, Caruz A, Contreras-Chova F: Spotted fever group *Rickettsia* in brown dog ticks *Rhipicephalus sanguineus* in southwestern Spain. Parasitol Res. 2008, 103: 119-122.

18. Khaldi M, Socolovschi C, Benyettou M, Barech G, Biche M, Kernif T, Raoult D, Parola P: Rickettsiae in arthropods collected from the North African Hedgehog (*Atelerix algirus)* and the desert hedgehog (*Paraechinus aethiopicus*) in Algeria. Comp Immunol Microbiol Infect Dis. 2012, 35: 117-122.

19. Fornadel CM, Smith JD, Zawada SE, Arias JR, Norris DE: Detection of *Rickettsia massiliae* in *Rhipicephalus sanguineus*from the eastern United States. Vector Borne Zoonotic Dis. 2013, 13: 67-69.

20. Keysary A, Eremeeva ME, Leitner M, Din AB, Wikswo ME, Mumcuoglu KY, Inbar M, Wallach AD, Shanas U, King R, Waner T: Spotted fever group rickettsiae in ticks collected from wild animals in Israel. Am J Trop Med Hyg. 2011, 85: 919-923.

21. Psaroulaki A, Ragiadakou D, Kouris G, Papadopoulos B, Chaniotis B, Tselentis Y: Ticks, tick-borne rickettsiae, and *Coxiella burnetii* in the Greek Island of Cephalonia. Ann N Y Acad Sci. 2006, 1078: 389-399.

22. Vilcins IM, Old JM, Deane E: Detection of a Hepatozoon and spotted fever group Rickettsia species in the common marsupial tick (Ixodestasmani) collected from wild Tasmanian devils (*Sarcophilus harrisii*), Tasmania. Vet Parasitol. 2009, 162: 23-31.

23. Hornok S, Fuente J, Horváth G, de Mera IG F, Wijnveld M, Tánczos B, Farkas R, Jongejan F: Molecular evidence of *Ehrlichia canis* and *Rickettsia massiliae* in ixodid ticks of carnivores from South Hungary. Acta Vet Hung. 2013, 61: 42-50.

24. Renvoisé A, Delaunay P, Blanchouin E, Cannavo I, Cua E, Socolovschi C, Parola P, Raoult D: Urban family cluster of spotted fever rickettsiosis linked to *Rhipicephalus sanguineus* infected with *Rickettsia conorii* subsp. caspia and *Rickettsia massiliae*. Ticks Tick Borne Dis. 2012, 3: 389-392.

25. Beeler E, Abramowicz KF, Zambrano ML, Sturgeon MM, Khalaf N, Hu R, Dasch GA, Eremeeva ME: A focus of dogs and *Rickettsia massiliae*-infected *Rhipicephalus sanguineus* in California. Am J Trop Med Hyg. 2011, 84: 244-249.

26. Mendes-de-Almeida F, Crissiuma AL, Gershony LC, Willi LM, Paiva JP, Guerrero J, Labarthe N: Characterization of ectoparasites in an urban cat (*Felis catus* Linnaeus, 1758) population of Rio de Janeiro, Brazil. Parasitol Res. 2011, 108: 1431-1435.

27. Wedincamp J, Foil LD: Infection and seroconversion of cats exposed to cat fleas (*Ctenocephalides felis* Bouché) infected with *Rickettsia felis*. J Vector Ecol. 2000, 25: 123-126.

28. Ortuño A, Pons I, Nogueras MM, Castellà J, Segura F: The dog as epidemiological marker of *R. conorii* infection. Clin Microbiol Infect. 2009, 15: 241-242.

29. Alves AS, Milhano N, Santos-Silva M, Santos AS, Vilhena M, de Sousa R: Evidence of *Bartonella* spp., *Rickettsia* spp. and *Anaplasma phagocytophilum* in domestic, shelter and stray cat blood and fleas, Portugal. Clin Microbiol Infect. 2009, 15: 1-3.

30. Matthewman L, Kelly P, Hayter D, Downie S, Wray K, Bryson N, Rycroft A, Raoult D: Domestic cats as indicators of the presence of spotted fever and typhus group rickettsiae. Eur J Epidemiol. 1997, 13: 109-111.

31. Solano-Gallego L, Hegarty B, Espada Y, Llull J, Breitschwerdt E: Serological and molecular evidence of exposure to arthropod-borne organisms in cats from northeastern Spain. Vet Microbiol. 2006, 118: 274-277.

32. Nogueras MM, Pons I, Ortuño A, Lario S, Segura F: *Rickettsia felis* in Fleas from Catalonia. Northeastern Spain. Vector Borne Zoonotic Dis. 2011, 11: 479-483.

33. Nogueras MM, Cardeñosa N, Sanfeliu I, Muñoz T, Font B, Segura F: Serological evidence of infection with

*Rickettsia typhi*and *Rickettsia felis* among the population of Catalonia, Northeast of Spain. Am J Trop Med Hyg. 2006, 74: 123-126.

34. Henry KM, Jiang J, Rozmajzl PJ, Azad AF, Macaluso KR, Richards AL: Development of quantitative real-time PCR assays to detect *Rickettsia typhi* and *Rickettsia felis*, the causative agents of murine typhus and flea-borne spotted fever. Mol Cell Probes. 2007, 21: 17-23.
35. Jiang J, Chan TC, Temenak JJ, Dasch GA, Ching WM, Richards AL: Development of a quantitative real-time polymerase chain reaction assay specific for *Orientia tsutsugamushi*. Am J Trop Med Hyg. 2004, 70: 351-356.
36. Balraj P, Vestris G, Raoult D, Renesto P: Comparison of *Rickettsia conorii* growth within different cell lines by real-time quantitative PCR. CMI. 2009, 15: 294-295.
37. Bayliss DB, Morris AK, Horta MC, Labruna MB, Radecki SV, Hawley JR, Brewer MM, Lappin MR: Prevalence of *Rickettsia*species antibodies and *Rickettsia* species DNA in the blood of cats with and without fever. J Feline Med Surg. 2009, 11: 266-270.
38. Izzard L, Cox E, Stenos J, Waterston M, Fenwick S, Graves S: Serological prevalence study of exposure of cats and dogs in Launceston, Tasmania, Australia to spotted fever group rickettsiae. Aust Vet J. 2010, 88: 29-31.
39. Case JB, Chomel B, Nicholson W, Foley JE: Serological survey of vector-borne zoonotic pathogens in pet cats and cats from animal shelters and feral colonies. J Feline Med Surg. 2006, 8: 111-117.
40. Socolovschi C, Gaudart J, Bitam I, Huynh TP, Raoult D, Parola P: Why are there so few *Rickettsia conorii conorii*-infected *Rhipicephalus sanguineus* ticks in the wild?. PLoS Negl Trop Dis. 2012, 6: e1697.
41. Kelly PJ, Lucas H, Eremeeva ME, Dirks KG, Rolain JM, Yowell C, Thomas R, Douglas T, Dasch GA, Raoult D: *Rickettsia felis,*West Indies. Emerg Infect Dis. 2010, 16: 570-571.
42. Levin ML, Killmaster LF, Zemtsova GE: Domestic dogs (*Canis familiaris*) as reservoir hosts for *Rickettsia conorii*. Vector Borne Zoonotic Dis. 2012, 12: 28-33.
43. Kamani J, Baneth G, Mumcuoglu KY, Waziri NE, Eyal O, Guthmann Y, Harrus S: Molecular detection and characterization of tick-borne pathogens in dogs and ticks from Nigeria. PLoS Negl Trop Dis. 2013, 7: e2108.
44. Barrs VR, Beatty JA, Wilson BJ, Evans N, Gowan R, Baral RM, Lingard AE, Perkovic G, Hawley JR, Lappin MR: Prevalence of *Bartonella* species, *Rickettsia felis*, haemoplasmas and the *Ehrlichia* group in the blood of cats and fleas in eastern Australia. Aust Vet J. 2010, 88: 160-165.
45. Kamrani A, Parreira VR, Greenwood J, Prescott JF: The prevalence of *Bartonella*, hemoplasma, and *Rickettsia felis*infections in domestic cats and in cat fleas in Ontario. Can J Vet Res. 2008, 72: 411-419.
46. Hawley JR, Shaw SE, Lappin MR: Prevalence of *Rickettsia felis* DNA in the blood of cats and their fleas in the United States. J Feline Med Surg. 2007, 9: 258-262.
47. Lappin MR, Hawley J: Presence of *Bartonella* species and *Rickettsia* species DNA in the blood, oral cavity, skin and claw beds of cats in the United States. Vet Dermatol. 2009, 20: 509-514.
48. Manfredi MT, Dini V, Piacenza S, Genchi C: Tick species parasitizing people in an area endemic for tick-borne diseases in north-western Italy. Parassitologia. 1999, 41: 555-560.

CHAPTER 49 TICK-BORNE RICKETTSIOSES, NEGLECTED EMERGING DISEASES IN RURAL SENEGAL

Oleg Mediannikov, Georges Diatta, Florence Fenollar, Cheikh Sokhna, Jean-Franc¸ois Trape, Didier Raoult

INTRODUCTION

Cases of tick-borne rickettsiosis have been regularly reported in North [1] and South Africa [2], [3] since 1910. Despite Pijper's suggestions [4], all cases of spotted fevers in sub-Saharan Africa were considered to be Mediterranean spotted fever (MSF) with *Rickettsia conorii* as an agent [5]. *Rickettsia conorii* was isolated in Tunisia in 1932 [6]. Since that time, multiple cases of the disease and isolations of the agent have been reported, mostly in countries in the Mediterranean region. *R. conorii conorii* has also been detected in ticks in Kenya, Somalia, South Africa, and Chad [7]. In 1992, however, a case of another spotted fever group (SFG) rickettsiosis in a 36-year-old woman presenting with tick bite fever at a hospital in Zimbabwe was described [8]. Authors succeeded in isolating the etiological agent. By PCR and restriction fragment length polymorphism they proved that the obtained strain differed from all other SFG rickettsiae, including *Rickettsia conorii*. The new strain was not, however, absolutely unique. It was indistinguishable from the strains isolated earlier from the Ixodid tick, *Amblyomma variegatum*, collected in Ethiopia [9] and from isolates recovered from another tick of the same genus, *Amblyomma hebraeum*, collected in Zimbabwe in the 1980s [10]. *Rickettsia africae*, a SFG rickettsia that causes African tick-bite fever (ATBF) officially received its name in 1996 [11]. *R. africae* seems to be very widely distributed in the continent. It has been either isolated or found by PCR in a number of African countries, including Niger, Mali, Burundi, Sudan [12], Chad, Ethiopia [13], and in most countries of equatorial and Southern Africa [14]. The majority of strains and cases are reported in South Africa [11], [15]. Recently, we have reported the high prevalence of *R. africae* in *A. variegatum* in Senegal [16].

Moreover, many proven and potential rickettsial pathogens were discovered in Africa [14], mostly in ticks. *Rickettsia sibirica mongolitimonae*, the agent of lymphangitis-associated rickettsiosis (LAR) was identified in ticks in Niger 10 years after its first isolation in China in 1991 [12]. *Rickettsia slovaca*, which causes tick-borne lymphadenopathy (TIBOLA) in Europe, was found in *Dermacentor marginatus* ticks in Morocco by PCR [17]. Two *Ixodes*-associated rickettsiae, *Rickettsia helvetica* and *Rickettsia monacensis*, were also detected in ticks in North Africa [17], [18]. Both were reported several times as probable human pathogens, although more information is required regarding their pathogenicity [14]. Beginning in 1994, another SFG rickettsia, *Rickettsia massiliae*, was repeatedly detected in *Rhipicephalus* spp. ticks in Central African Republic, Mali, Algeria and Morocco [12],[17],[19],[20]. The first human case of spotted fever caused by this rickettsia was identified in 2005 [21]. *Rickettsia aeschlimannii* was first isolated in Morocco in 1992 from the *Hyalomma marginatum marginatum* tick [22]. Genotypically similar or identical strains were reported in many regions, including Kazakhstan, Southern Europe, Zimbabwe, Mali, Niger, and Algeria [14], [19]. These strains are almost always associated with almost always associated with *Hyalomma* ticks. Several human cases have been reported in Africa, including the sub-Saharan regions [14]. Many other SFG rickettsiae not previously associated with human diseases have been reported in Ixodid ticks in Africa. Some of them are genetically described and registered under *Candidatus* status [23]. Tick-borne rickettsioses play a very important role in public health. A recent worldwide report demonstrated a 5.6% incidence of rickettsial infection in a group of travelers who developed acute febrile infections after returning from sub-Saharan Africa. It is one of the most frequently identified etiology for systemic febrile illness among travelers, following

Citation: Mediannikov O, Diatta G, Fenollar F, Sokhna C, Trape J-F, Raoult D (2010) Tick-Borne Rickettsioses, Neglected Emerging Diseases in Rural Senegal. PLoS Negl Trop Dis 4(9): e821. doi:10.1371/journal.pntd.0000821.

malaria [24], [25]. The precise serological identification of the etiological agent of spotted fever in humans may be difficult because of the strong cross-reactivity in serological studies [26]. In some cases, cross-absorption studies and western blots may help [27], but these techniques may only work in cases in which the suspected agent is known and isolated. In all cases of new and emerging rickettsioses, the serological study may indicate only the group etiology (SFG). One of the first studies performed with *R. conorii* antigen showed the strikingly high incidence of rickettsial antibodies is human sera from many African countries, including Angola, Burkina Faso, Central African Republic, Mali, Cote d'Ivoire [28], Zambia [29], and other countries [30]–[40]. The percentage of seroprevalence found in different studies is shown in Figure 1.

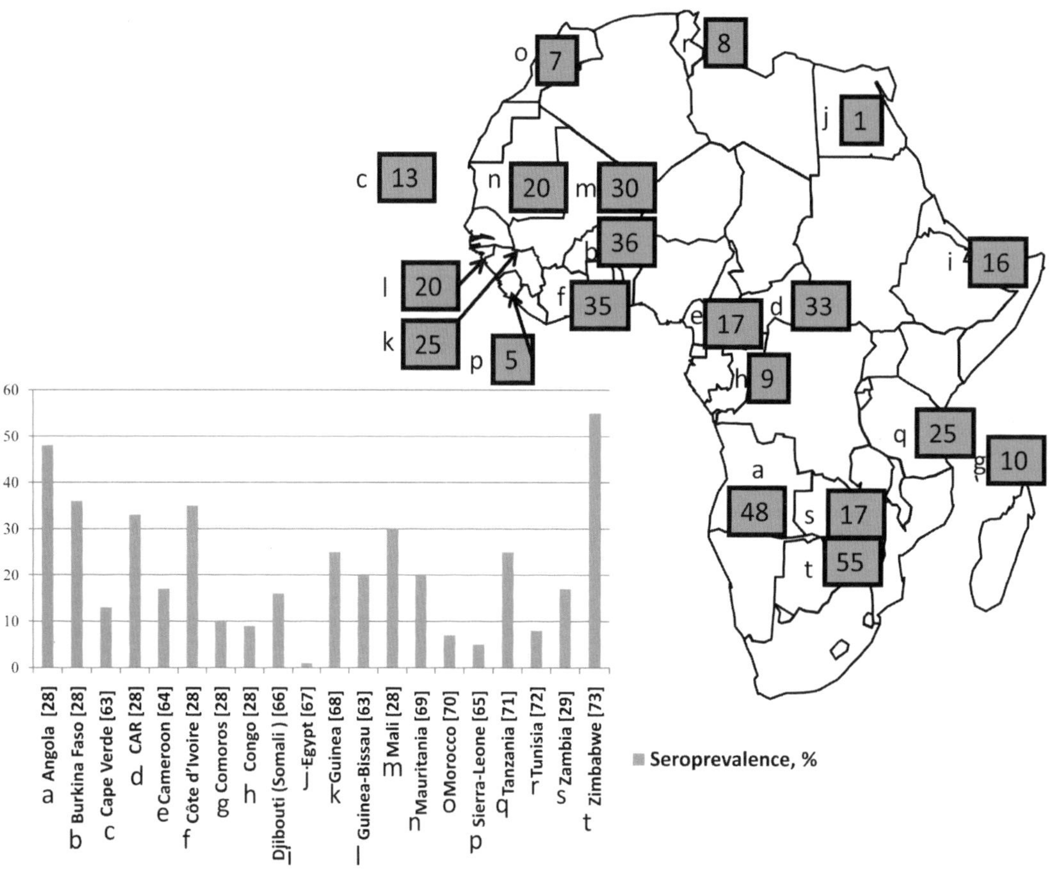

Figure 1: Map of Africa showing the countries where serological studies for SFG rickettsioses were performed before our study.

The numbers on the map indicate seroprevalence in %. The diagram represents relative seroprevalence in different countries and reference [in square brackets].

The growing number of newly discovered rickettsial species outlines the indispensable role of molecular methods in microbiology. However, the studies are still in early stages because the distribution of many agents of rickettsioses is incompletely described. West Africa, including Senegal, remains incompletely studied in terms of tick-borne rickettsioses. Despite recent reports of high rates of infection of *A. variegatum* ticks in Senegal [16], other tick species were never studied for the presence of rickettsial agents. Thirty-three species of Ixodid ticks are known in Senegal [41]; many of them are associated with domestic animals and readily bite humans.

The present work was performed in order to enlarge the scant knowledge about tick-borne rickettsioses in Senegal.

MATERIALS AND METHODS

Human sample collection and treatment

The study was performed in two Senegalese villages, Dielmo (13°43′N;16°24′W) and Ndiop (13°41′N;16°22′W), situated in the Sine-Saloum region. Since 1990, a longitudinal study of malaria and tick-borne relapsing fever has been ongoing in these villages [42], [43]. The project consists of long-term investigations of host-parasite relationships in the entire village population, which was enrolled in a longitudinal prospective study. The project was approved by the National Ethics Committee of Senegal [42] and the Local Ethics Committee (Marseille, France). Written individual informed consent was obtained from each participant, including the parents or legal guardians of all children, at the beginning of the current study. Dielmo and Ndiop villagers are settled agricultural workers. Millet and peanut crops are cultivated during the rainy season, and market gardening is the main agricultural activity during the dry season.

Here we used the serological techniques to detect immune response to different rickettsial species. We tested the samples from the serological bank created for the above-mentioned longitudinal study and collected in 2008. In total, 238 serum samples collected in Dielmo in 2008 (mean age 26±18, range from 3 to 78, 117 men and 121 women) and 241 samples from Ndiop (mean age 25±17, range from 5 to 82, 112 men and 129 women) were tested.

Another part of the study was to investigate the role of tick-borne rickettsiae as the causes of acute non-malarial febrile disease in rural populations of the same villages. Interviews and sampling were conducted in the same two villages from December 2008 through June 2009. During the period between November 2008 and July 2009, a total of 204 samples from 134 patients (62M and 72F) were included in this study. In this study, we included patients who came into the dispensary with a recent fever and had negative test results for malaria; 103 (77%) were from Dielmo (468 inhabitants) and 31 (23%) from Ndiop (628 inhabitants); 90 (67.2%) were younger than 10 years, including 64 (47.8%) under five years. No one died during the study.

Medical examinations were performed by a medical attendant for each individual with fever (defined by an axillary temperature >37.5°C). A questionnaire was completed for each individual. Whole blood was collected from the fingertip by lancet stick and then applied to glass microscope slides. Thick and thin blood smears were stained with Giemsa and analyzed by microscopy for the trophozoites and gametocytes of malaria. If the malaria test was negative, 200 µl of whole blood (3–4 drops) were collected for DNA extraction. The first stages of DNA extraction (digesting, binding and washing) was performed directly in the village dispensary using the QIAamp kit (QIAGEN, Hilden, Germany). The columns with the bound and dry DNA inside were then stored at 4°C before transportation and final elution, which was performed in URMITE, Marseilles, France.

Ticks

In November-December 2008, ticks were collected from domestic animals (cows, goats, sheep, horses, donkeys) in two regions of Senegal: Sine-Saloum and Niakhar (Table 1, Figure 2). A total of 406 ticks were collected from four villages in the Sine-Saloum region and 2361 ticks from the Niakhar region. They were stored in 70% ethanol. Twenty adult *Hyalomma truncatum* ticks were preserved alive in a flask at 90–95% of relative humidity. The species and sex were identified according to standard taxonomic keys for adult ticks [44], [45].

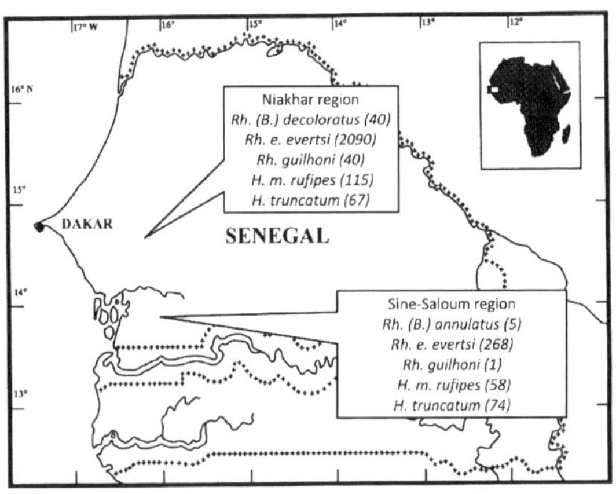

Figure 2: Map of Senegal with indicated locations of tick collection, species of ticks and a quantity collected.

Table 1: Geographic coordinates of tick collection sites

Region	Village	Coordinates
Sine-Saloum	Dielmo	13°43′N;16°24′W
	Ndiop	13°41′N;16°22′W
	Medina	13°42′N;16°24′W
	Passi	13°42′N;16°23′W
Niakhar	Ngangarlame	14°34′N-16°29′W
	Poudaye	14°32′N-16°28′W
	Toucar	14°32′N-16°28′W
	Poultok Diohine	14°31′N-16°29′W
	Ngonine	14°34′N-16°31′W
	Logdir	14°29′N-16°29′W
	Ngayokheme	14°31′N-16°26′W
	Diokoul	14°29′N-16°26′W
	Sob	14°29′N-16°26′W
	Diohine	14°30′N-16°30′W
	Kalom	14°31′N-16°25′W
	Sass-Ndiafadji	14°30′N-16°24′W
	Mboyene	14°31′N-16°27′W
	Ngan-Fissel	14°30′N-16°26′W
	Ngardiame	14°29′N-16°27′W
	Ngonine	14°34′N-16°31′W

doi:10.1371/journal.pntd.0000821.t001

Culture

Live *H. truncatum* ticks were used for bacterial culture and were not included in the overall statistics. Each was washed in a 10% water solution of a commercial disinfectant-detergent (Amphomousse, Hydenet S.A., Sainghin-en-Melantois, France), then rinsed in sterile water and placed in a 1% solution of sodium hypochlorite for 10 min. After rinsing with distilled water, they were incubated in 70% ethanol for 15 min. A final rinse in sterile phosphate buffer saline preceded inoculation. Ticks were placed in a sterile 1.5 ml plastic tube, where they were triturated with a sterile micropestle in 300 μl of Minimum Essential Medium (MEM) supplied with 4% of fetal bovine serum (FBS). Isolation was done according to the well-known shell-vial technique with modifications [46]. We used 300 μl of whole tick suspension for inoculation of a vial with a monolayer of L929 cells. After centrifugation, the supernatant was removed and conserved. The cells were covered with culture media (MEM, 4% FBS). Antibiotics were not used during the cultivation.

Molecular biology

DNA from homogenized ticks that were conserved in ethanol, supernatants collected after shell-vial inoculation, as well as supernatants of cell culture were extracted using the BioRobot MDx Workstation (Qiagen, Courtaboeuf, France) with a customized extraction protocol following the manufacturer's instructions. DNA was stored at 4°C until use in PCR amplifications. Rickettsial DNA was initially detected by *Rickettsia* genus-specific quantitative PCR (qPCR) reactions that were performed using LightCycler 2.0 equipment and software (Roche Diagnostics GmbH, Mannheim, Germany). Master mixtures were prepared by following the instructions of the manufacturer with primers RKND03F and RKND03R and a probe, whose sequences are specific for the sequence of the rickettsial citrate synthase gene. PCR cycling and melting curve conditions have been described previously [47]. A new qPCR system based on rickettsial *sca1* gene and specific for *R. aeschlimannii* was designed and tested for specificity and sensitivity. The sequences of the primers and probe are as follows: forward primer R_aesSca1_F 3′-AAGCGGCACTTTAGGTAAAGAAA-5′, reverse primer R_aesSca1_R 3′-CATGCTCTGCAAATGAACCA-5′, probe 6-FAM®-TGGGGAAATATGCCGTATACGCAAGC-TAMRA®. Specificity was tested with 26 species and strains of different rickettsiae and sensitivity was compared with RKND03 by serial dilutions [47].

Chosen positive samples were subjected to simple PCR using primers manufactured by Eurogentec, Seraing, Belgium. They amplified almost the complete genetic sequence of rickettsial citrate synthase (*gltA*), as previously described [48], [49]. Additionally, a 632 bp fragment of the *ompA* gene was amplified using Rr. 190.70 and Rr. 190.701 primers [50].

The screening of DNA from human samples for SFG rickettsiae was also performed with the Rickettsia genus-specific RKND03 qPCR system. The positive results were then confirmed by the "1029 system" based on the RC0338 gene (referenced by *R. conorii* genome AE006914) coding for hypothetical protein and present in all rickettsiae of spotted fever group [51]. A nested PCR was later used to obtain the larger portion of the rickettsial *gltA* gene for the subsequent sequencing of the amplicons derived from positive samples. For the nested PCR, CS2d and CSendR primers were used to amplify most of the full-length *gltA* gene, and the primers RpCS409p and RpCS877p were subsequently used as described above.

We used the amplification of the beta actin gene by specific qPCR [51] as the control for appropriate handling and extraction of DNA from human samples.

DNA extracted from uninfected ticks from colonies at the Unité des Rickettsies, Marseille, France and sterile cardiac valve biopsies were used as negative controls, and DNA extracted from the cell culture supernatant of *Rickettsia bellii* served as a positive control. Polymerase chain reactions were performed in automated DNA thermal cyclers (GeneAmp 2400 and 9700; Applied Biosystems, Foster City, CA, USA). PCR products were visualized by electrophoresis on a 1.5% agarose gel, stained with ethidium bromide, and examined using an ultraviolet transilluminator. The PCR products were purified using a QIAquick Spin PCR Purification Kit (Qiagen) according to the manufacturer's instructions. Sequencing of amplicons was performed using the BigDye Terminator Cycle Sequencing Kit (Perkin Elmer Applied Biosystems) with an ABI automated sequencer (Applied Biosystems). Obtained sequences were assembled (ChromasPro 1.49 beta, Technelysium Pty Ltd, Tewantin, Australia), edited by BioEdit Sequence alignment editor v. 7.0.9.0 [52], and compared with those available in GenBank by NCBI BLAST (http://blast.ncbi.nlm.nih.gov/Blast.cgi). Sequences of *gltA* genes from *Rickettsiae* species chosen in GenBank for comparison were concatenated and aligned with the ClustalW program, and a neighbor-joining phylogenetic tree was constructed with Geneious 4.7.6 software (Biomatters Ltd, Australia).

Serological studies

Titers of IgG and IgM antibodies in serum samples obtained from each person were determined using an indirect immunofluorescence assay with antigens generated in-house. We tested sera with the following antigens: *R. conorii conorii* strain Malish (ATCC VR-613), *R. africae* strain ESF-5, *R. aeschlimanni* strain MC16, *Rickettsia sibirica mongolitimonae* strain HA-91 (ATCC VR-1526), *Rickettsia felis* strain Marseille (ATCC VR-1525), and *R. typhi* strain Wilmington. All serum samples were diluted at ratios of 1:25, 1:50, and 1:100 and were screened for total immunoglobulin. If the serological screening with any rickettsial antigen was positive, final titers for IgG and IgM were determined for all anti-rickettsial antibodies.

Statistical analysis

Data were analyzed using Epi Info software, version 3.4.1 (Centers for Disease Control and Prevention, Atlanta, GA, USA). Non-parametric values were compared using a $\chi 2$ test. Statistical significance was defined as $p<0.05$.

RESULTS

Human samples

We have found that that 51/238 (21.4%) and 123/241 (51%) of randomly screened healthy population of the Dielmo and

Ndiop villages of Sine-Saloum region of Senegal, respectively, had serological evidence of contact with rickettsiae (Table 2). We have noted that the prevalence of anti-rickettsial antibodies in sera was higher in young villagers, with the positive ratio declining with age. This tendency was always true for Ndiop; however, in Dielmo only inhabitants older than 40 showed a higher seroprevalence compared with the younger population (Table 2). In most cases, sera reacted with several rickettsial antigens, and the titers of total Ig were low and did not exceed 1/100 (94.1% of positive results in Dielmo and 88% in Ndiop). We found IgM in 2 out of 3 sera with high antibody levels from Dielmo and in 13 of 15 from Ndiop, indicating recent infection. The highest titers for IgG and IgM were 1/256, and both sera were from Ndiop. We identified the antibodies against *R. typhi* in 6 cases (2.4%) from Dielmo and in 7 cases (2.9%) from Ndiop, but in all cases sera also reacted with rickettsiae of SFG with at least the same titers. Only one patient from Dielmo had low titer (1/50) antibodies against *R. felis*. His serum also reacted with *R. typhi* and all SFG rickettsiae. We noted that among all antigens tested, *R. africae* reacted most often with the tested sera; 49 of 51 (96%) and 110 of 123 (89%) reacted with its antigen in Dielmo and Ndiop respectively; it constitutes 20.6% and 45.6% of tested villagers, respectively. The second most commonly reactive rickettsia was *R. sibirica mongolitimonae* with 35 sera of 51 (68.6% and 14.7% of tested villagers) positive sera from Dielmo and 93 sera of 123 (75.6% and 35.6% of tested villagers) positive sera from Ndiop.

Table 2: Results of serological screening of the generally healthy population of two villages (Dielmo and Ndiop) of the Sine-Saloum region of Senegal

Dielmo				Ndiop				P value
Population screened, number of participants								
238				241				
Positive with at least one SFG rickettsial antigen at titer of **1/50 minimum**, number (% of screened)								
51 (21.4%)				123 (51%)				$<10^{-3}$
Age	No. of positives	% among screened of the same age	% among positives	Age	No. of positives	% among screened of the same age	% among positives	
3–5	3	33.3	5.9	3–5	4	66.7	3.3	
6–10	11	25.6	21.6	6–10	26	57.8	21.1	
11–15	6	13.3	11.8	11–15	23	59.0	18.7	
16–20	4	14.3	7.8	16–20	22	52.4	17.9	
21–40	8	14.	15.7	21–40	27	43.5	22.0	
>40	19	33.9	37.3	>40	21	44.7	17.1	
Positive with *R. typhi* antigen at titer of 1/50 minimum, number (% of screened)								
6 (2.4%)				7 (2.9%)				0.8
Positive with *R. africae* antigen at titer of 1/50 minimum, number (% of screened; % of overall positive with rickettsial antigens)								
49 (20.6%; 96%)				110 (45.6%; 89%)				$<10^{-3}$ (0.1)
Positive with *R. sibirica mongolitimonae* antigen at titer of 1/50 minimum, number (% of screened; % of overall positive with rickettsial antigens)								
35 (14.7%; 68.6%)				93 (35.6%; 75.6%)				$<10^{-3}$ (0.3)
Positive with at least one SFG rickettsial antigen at titer of higher than 1/50, number (% of screened; % of overall positive with rickettsial antigens)								
3 (1.3%; 5.9%)				15 (6.2%; 12%)				0.004 (0.2)

doi:10.1371/journal.pntd.0000821.t002

As for rickettsial DNA, nine patients who presented in the dispensary with acute fever of non-malarial origin were positive. We considered patients positive only in samples in which the qPCRs for both rickettsial genes were positive and the subsequent standard PCR/sequencing produced the rickettsial *gltA* gene. Data for eight of the patients positive for the DNA of *R. felis*were already reported [51]. In one patient, we have successfully amplified the DNA of *Rickettsia conorii conorii*. The patient was a 4-year-old girl with tachycardia and a fever that appeared on the same day (27 March 2009). No rash or eschar was noticed during her examination. Paracetamol was prescribed and the girl was sent home. The fever resolved within several days without antibiotics.

Ticks

We have collected ticks of seven different species on domestic animals (Table 3), 491 ticks from four villages in the Sine-Saloum region and 2494 ticks from 16 villages of the Niakhar region. The results of studies of *Amblyomma variegatum* ticks have already been reported (74/85 (87.1%) and 101/133 (79.7%) positive for *R. africae*, respectively, for both regions) [16]. The majority of ticks in both regions (268 of 406 (66%) and 2090 of 2361 (88.5%)) were represented by *Rhipicephalus evertsi evertsi* (Figure 3). In our study, *Rhipicephalus guilhoni*was the predominantly collected species in the Niakhar region (49 of 50 ticks collected). Most of the ticks (85.7%) were collected from donkeys. We have collected only five *Rhipicephalus (Boophilus) annulatus* ticks and these ticks were all collected in the Sine-Saloum region. Another species, *Rhipicephalus (B.) decoloratus*, was only collected in the Niakhar region. Two species of the *Hyalomma* genus were collected in both regions. *Hyalomma marginatum rufipes*was less common than *Hyalomma truncatum* in Sine-Saloum (58 ticks collected versus 74) when compared with Niakhar (115 versus 67).

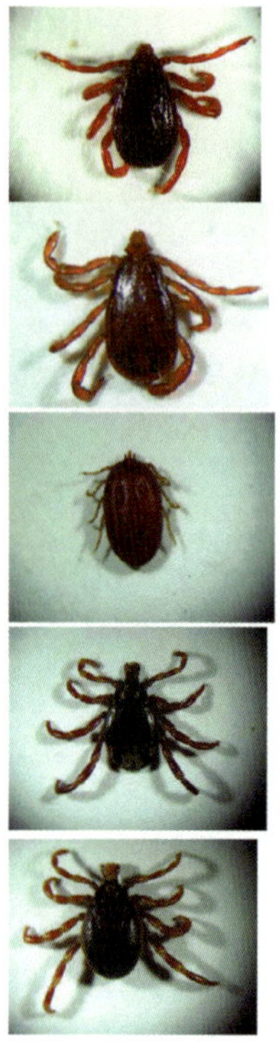

Figure 3: Photos of ticks studied with indication of rickettsiae found by PCR.

Table 3: Tick species collected in Senegal and studied for SFG rickettsiae

Species	Collected	Positive for rickettsiae: number (%)			Species of rickettsial identified	Animals from which positive ticks were collected
Niakhar region						
Rhipicephalus (Boophilus) decoloratus	40	0			-	-
Hyalomma marginatum rufipes	115	60 (51.3%)			*Rickettsia aeschlimannii*	Cows, donkeys, sheep, goats, horses
Hyalomma truncatum	67	4 (6%)			*Rickettsia aeschlimannii*	Cows, donkeys, sheep, goats, horses
Rhipicephalus evertsi evertsi	2090	14 (0.7%) 10 (0.5%)			*Rickettsia africae* *Rickettsia aeschlimannii*	Cows, donkeys, sheep, goats, horses
Rhipicephalus guilhoni	49	11 (22.4%)			*Rickettsia massiliae*	Predominantly donkeys (9), cows (2)
Sine-Saloum region						
		In total in region	Dielmo	Ndiop		
Rhipicephalus (Boophilus) annulatus	5	1 (20%)	0/1 (0%)	0/2 (0%)	*Rickettsia africae*	Cow
Hyalomma marginatum rufipes	58	26 (44.8%)	0/2 (0%)	19/43 (44%)	*Rickettsia aeschlimannii*	Cows, donkeys, sheep, goats, horses
Hyalomma truncatum	74	5 (6.8%)	1/25 (4%)	1/30 (3%)	*Rickettsia aeschlimannii*	Cows, donkeys, sheep, goats, horses
		10 (13.5%)	5/25 (20%)	3/30 (10%)	*Rickettsia sibirica mongolitimonae*	Cows, donkeys, sheep, goats, horses
Rhipicephalus evertsi evertsi	268	1 (0.4%)	0/21 (0%)	0/151 (0%)	*Rickettsia conorii* ssp.	Horse
		1 (0.4%)	0/21 (0%)	1/151 (0,7%)	*Rickettsia africae 99%*	Sheep
Rhipicephalus guilhoni	1	0	0	0	-	-

Separate columns represent data for two villages in the Sine-Saloum region (Dielmo and Ndiop) where serological and molecular studies in humans were performed.
doi:10.1371/journal.pntd.0000821.t003

Molecular identification of rickettsiae in ticks

We found three different rickettsial species in *Rh. e. evertsi*, with a low rate of infection from 0.4 to 0.7% (Table 3). In the Sine-Saloum region, one tick collected from the horse was infected with *R. conorii conorii*, the agent of MSF. One tick from Sine-Saloum and 14/2090 (0.7%) total were infected with *R. africae*, the agent of African tick-bite fever. This finding represents the first time that it was found in *Rh. e. evertsi*. In the Niakhar region, 10 (0.5%) ticks were infected by *R. aeschlimannii*. In both regions we were able to amplify and sequence almost complete *gltA* gene (all samples positive by qPCR were subjected to standard PCR and sequencing). The *gltA* sequence was not absolutely identical to the *R. africae* reference strain (ESF-5), the clonality of which was previously based on analysis of strains isolated from patients and *A. variegatum* ticks [53]. Moreover, the sequence of the *gltA* gene of *R. aeschlimannii* found in *Rh. e. evertsi* differed slightly from all GenBank records. The phylogenetic positions of these rickettsiae are shown in Figure 4.

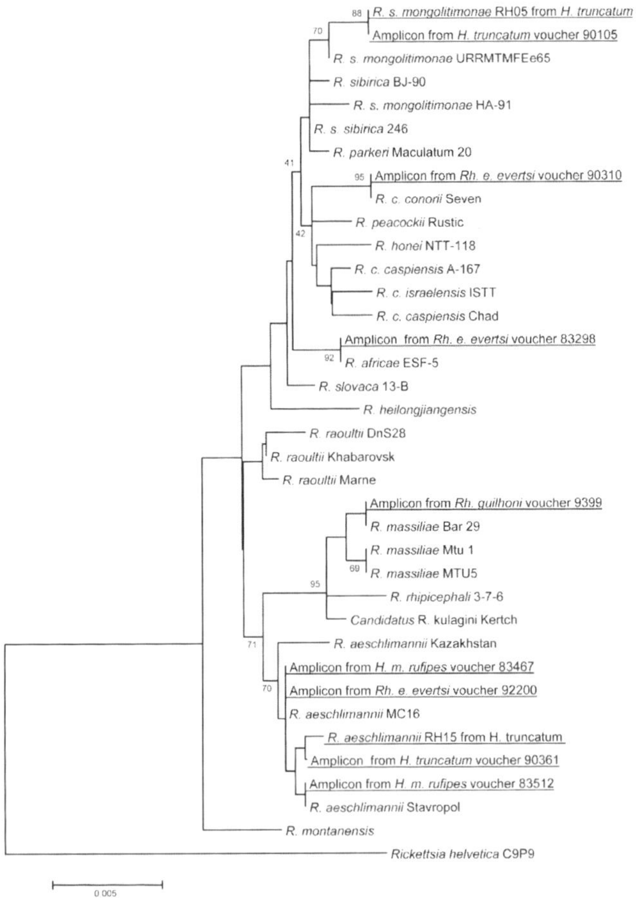

Figure 4: Phylogenetic tree based on aligned complete sequences of *gltA* **gene and constructed by neighbor-joining method. Numbers in nodes represent bootstrap values.**

The tree shows the position of isolates and amplicons from ticks collected in Senegal.

We have identified only one rickettsia in *Rh. guilhoni* and only in the Niakhar region. All samples positive by qPCR were subjected to a standard PCR (*ompA* and *gltA* genes) and amplicons were sequenced. Both genes showed 100% identity with *R. massiliae* strain Bar29 isolated from *Rh. sanguineus* from Spain. The rate of infection in the Niakhar region is 22.4%; in Sine-Saloum the only collected tick was negative by PCR.

We have also tested two species of *Rhipicephalus (Boophilus)* ticks; *R. africae* was also detected in one *Rh. (B.) annulatus* tick from Sine-Saloum. The *gltA* and *ompA* sequences were identical to the reference strain, ESF-5. All of our *Rhipicephalus (B.) decoloratus* ticks were negative when tested by rickettsial genus-specific qPCR. We found that 44.8% and 51.3% of *H. marginatum rufipes* ticks in the Sine-Saloum and Niakhar regions, respectively, are infected with *R. aeschlimannii*. In our study, it was the only species of rickettsiae identified in this species of tick. All ticks positive by genus-specific qPCR were subjected to a *R. aeschlimannii*-specific qPCR and all were found to be positive. In 6.8% and 4.6% of *H. truncatum* ticks from the Sine-Saloum and Niakhar regions, respectively, we found a variant of *R. aeschlimannii* that insignificantly differed from the one found in *Rh. e. evertsi* and *H. m. rufipes* (Figure 4). We also identified *R. s. mongolitimonae* in 13.5% of ticks, but only in the Sine-Saloum region. All ticks positive by genus-specific qPCR were tested for *R. aeschlimannii*-specific qPCR. Positive ticks were considered to harbor *R. aeschlimannii* and all negative ticks were subjected to a standard PCR with sequencing. The *gltA* gene of *R. s. mongolitimonae* was identified in all positive ticks.

Rickettsial strains

We have also succeeded in isolating two strains of rickettsiae from *Hyalomma truncatum*collected in Dielmo village, in the region of Sine-Saloum. Both strains were deposited in official collection of Unité des Rickettsies, Medical Faculty, Marseilles, France (http://ifr48.timone.univ-mrs.fr/portail2/index.php?option=com_content&task=view&id=96) under the following references: CSUR R175 for *R. s. mongolitimonae* strain RH05 and CSUR R176 for *R. aeschlimannii* strain RH15. Sequences of the *rrs, gltA, ompA, ompB*, and *sca4*genes of *R. sibirica mongolitimonae*, strain RH05, were deposited in GenBank under the accession numbers HM050271, HM050296, HM050272, HM050273, and HM050295, respectively. Sequences of the *rrs, gltA, ompA, ompB*, and *sca4* genes of *R. aeschlimannii*, strain RH15, were deposited in GenBank under the accession numbers HM050274, HM050276, HM050277, HM050278, and HM050275, respectively. According to the proposed criteria for species definition in rickettsiology [54], the isolated bacteria do not belong to a new species. Strain RH05 was close but not identical to *R. s. mongolitimonae*. Strain RH15 was also close but not identical to *R. aeschlimannii*. The degree of divergence of the five above-mentioned genes from the closest relative (*R. s. mongolitimonae* for RH05 and *R. aeschlimannii* for RH15) was less than that required for the definition of a new species. Genes of both strains were almost completely identical with sequenced amplicons from *H. truncatum* ticks.

Sequenced amplicons from the ticks were registered in GenBank under the following accession numbers: *gltA* and *ompA* genes of *R. s. mongolitimonae* from *H. truncatum* voucher #90105 (HM050279 and HM050280); *gltA* and *ompA* genes of *R. aeschlimannii* from *H. truncatum* voucher #90361 (HM050282 and HM050281); *gltA* and *ompA* genes of *R. aeschlimannii* from *H. m. rufipes* voucher #83512 (HM050283 and HM050284); voucher #83467 (HM050285 and HM050286); *gltA* and *ompA* genes of *R. africae* from *Rh. e. evertsi* voucher #83298 (HM050288 and HM050287); *gltA* and *ompA* genes of *R. aeschlimannii* from *Rh. e. evertsi* voucher #92200 (HM050289 and HM050290); *gltA* and *ompA* genes of *R. massiliae*from *Rh. guilhoni* voucher #93995 (HM050293 and HM050294); and *gltA* and *ompA* genes of *R conorii* from *Rh. e. evertsi*.voucher#90310 (HM050292 and HM050291).

DISCUSSION

Entomological studies performed in two regions of Senegal confirmed that Ixodid ticks, the potential vectors of spotted fevers in Senegal, are highly prevalent in domestic animals and that the close contact of humans with ticks is continual and permanent. Seven different tick species of 33 known in Senegal were collected in the studied regions. The most abundant species, *Rhipicephalus evertsi evertsi*, is one of the most common ticks that feed not only on domestic animals, but also many species of wild animals in Africa [41], [55]. The species is confined to the Afrotropical zoogeographical region in sub-Saharan Africa [44]. This species, although very common and prevalent, has not been frequently studied as the vector of agents of humans and animal diseases. To date, it has been known to transmit the protozoa *Babesia bigemina* [56], Crimean-Congo hemorrhagic fever virus (CCHFV) [57], and *Ehrlichia ruminantium* [58]. Rickettsial agents have not been previously reported in these ticks, although tick hemolymph tests showed the presence of rickettsial-like organisms [10]. Here, we report the first identification of *R. conorii* in Senegal and in this tick. This report also provides the first evidence of the role of this tick species in the epidemiology of MSF. Despite its very low infection rate (that is, in fact, always very low for all vectors of MSF [7]), the abundance of this tick and its close contact with humans who take care of and often live close to animals increases the probability of infection. Two other rickettsial species, *R. africae* and *R. aeschlimannii*, were not previously reported in *Rh. e. evertsi*.

Rh. guilhoni is a member of the *Rhipicephalus sanguineus* group. It can be a common tick in the drier areas in a horizontal band south of the Sahara. Cattle, sheep, horses, and dogs, as well as wild carnivores and birds are the preferred hosts of adult *Rh. guilhoni* [44]. The only previously known pathogenic agent associated with this species is CCHFV [57], although the disease itself has never been reported to result from a bite by this tick. *R. massiliae*, a recently emerged pathogen [21], was found in our study of this tick. Interestingly, this rarely studied species was collected from donkeys and ruminants and not from dogs, which are the usual hosts for ticks of the *R. sanguineus* group.

Ticks of the *Boophilus* sub-genus of *Rhipicephalus* are one-host ticks with a monotropic type of behavior. *Rhipicephalus (Boophilus) annulatus* transmits the protozoans *Babesia bigemina*and *Babesia bovis* to cattle, both of which cause bovine babesiosis. It also transmits *Anaplasma marginale* and *Eh. ruminantium* to cattle [44]. *R. africae* has also been found in the closely related species, *Rhipicephalus (B.) microplus* [59]. *Rhipicephalus (B.) decoloratus* was already shown to harbor *R. africae* in Botswana [60]. Our finding of typical *R. africae* in *Rh. (B.) annulatus* is not surprising. The low percentage of infection compared with *A. variegatum*collected in the same region from the same animals may be explained by lower genus/species susceptibility to *R. africae*.

H. marginatum rufipes is the most widespread *Hyalomma* in Africa and is notorious as a vector of the CCHF virus [61]. The feeding of adults on cattle often causes large lesions at the attachment sites, leading to the formation of severe abscesses. It has also been identified as a host of *R. aeschlimannii* [22], which our data supported. *H. truncatum* is found predominantly in sub-Saharan Africa where it may be the most common *Hyalomma*. This species of tick is notorious for causing many types of direct damage to its hosts. Certain strains of *H. truncatum*have a toxin in their saliva that causes the skin disease known as sweating sickness in cattle [62], particularly calves. *H. truncatum* also transmits the protozoan *Babesia caballi* to horses [44]. Rickettsia-like organisms have been previously observed microscopically in this species [10]. We found *R. s. mongolitimonae*, which causes lymphangitis-associated rickettsiosis, in this aggressive tick that readily bites humans. Interestingly, the reported clinical picture of the illness caused by this rickettsia strikingly resembles the description of the disease of "young shepherds" mentioned by the village chiefs. The theory that rickettsiae are responsible for this disease is also supported by the highest seroprevalence in the younger members of the village population.

Finally, we have identified five different pathogenic rickettsial species in tick vectors with an incidence up to 51.3% (*R. aeschlimannii* in *H. marginatum* rufipes). *R. africae* is a pathogen known to be responsible for African tick-bite fever. The high incidence (87.1%) of this rickettsia in *A. variegatum* ticks was previously reported. We have found that, although to a lesser degree, two other species of ticks, *Rh. e. evertsi* and *Boophilus (Rhipicephalus) annulatus*, may harbor this pathogen. *R. aeschlimannii* is a recently recognized pathogen [63]. The properties of aggressivity, abundance, and the high rate of infection of vectors that are characteristic of ticks of the *Hyalomma* genus may enhance the probability of this infection.

We suppose that ticks in Senegal may play an important role in the transmission of vector-borne diseases, primarily because of the elevated probability of contact with humans and because of high levels of rickettsial infection in ticks. Indirect evidence of the role of Ixodid ticks in vector-borne diseases may be obtained from local populations. The village chiefs of Dielmo and Ndiop told us, for instance, that the beginning of the field activities of children coincides with the appearance of multiple eschar-like lesions on the child›s ankles that is often associated with a fever. This description perfectly corresponds with many rickettsial diseases, including African tick-bite fever (Table 4). Several publications from other regions confirm that Ixodid ticks, and especially tick larvae, may be a serious pest, causing "skin disease" [64], [65]. Here and in previous works [16], we have shown that A. variegatum, *H. marginatum rufipes, H. truncatum*, and *Rh. evertsi evertsi* are among the most important species that may have a contact with humans.

Table 4: Clinical and epidemiological characteristics of spotted fevers caused by rickettsiae found in this study

Species	Disease	Tick species associated (literature data)	Tick species associated (present study)	Fever, %	Diffuse rash, %	Eschar, %	Lymphadenopathy	Lymphangitis	Reported mortality rates,%
R. conorii conorii	Mediterranean spotted fever	*Rh. sanguineus, Rh. simus* (?)	*Rh. e. evertsi*	100	97	72	Rare	No	1–5
R. africae	African tick-bite fever	*A. variegatum, A. hebraeum, Rh. (B.) microplus, Rh. (B.) decoloratus*	*Rh. e. evertsi, Rh. (B.) annulatus*	92	43	98%, often multiple	Yes	No	Very low
R. sibirica mongolitimonae	Lymphangitis-associated rickettsiosis	*H.truncatum, H. asiaticum, H. anatolicum excavatum, Rh. pusillus*	*H.truncatum*	100	78	89%	55%	Yes, up to 44%	0
R. aeschlimannii	Unnamed	*H. m. marginatum, H. m. rufipes, H. aegyptium, Haemaphysalis inermis*	*H.truncatum,H. m. rufipes, Rh. e. evertsi*	Yes	Yes	Yes	?	?	0
R. massiliae	Unnamed (one case)	*Rh. sanguineus, Rh. turanicus, Rh. muhsamae, Rh. lunulatus, Rh. sulcatus*	*Rh. guilhoni*	Yes	Yes	Yes	?	?	0

doi:10.1371/journal.pntd.0000821.t004

The results of the serological screening confirmed our assumption. They showed a very high prevalence (21.4% and 51% in Dielmo and Ndiop, respectively) of sera that react with rickettsial antigens (spotted fever group) in a generally healthy population of rural Senegal. Generally, our results correspond with the previous data from Burkina Faso, Central African Republic, Mali, Cote d'Ivoire, and Guinea-Bissau where an incidence of rickettsial antibodies in human sera of up to 36% was shown [28]. Preliminary results show that two rickettsial species, *R. africae* and *R. sibirica mongolitimonae*, which show a greater affinity with human sera may play a more important role in human pathology in the studied regions. *R. aeschlimannii*, which is most prevalent in ticks, is not as pathogenic as two above-mentioned rickettsiae, however, because of cross-reactivity among rickettsiae of spotted-fever group and *R. felis*, based on performed serological studies we may not say exactly which species of rickettsia play the most important role in elevated seroprevalence in West Africa.

We have also studied the role of rickettsial infections as possible causes of acute fevers in the indigenous population of rural Senegal. It was found that rickettsioses may be responsible for up to 6.7% of cases of recent acute non-malarial fever in the rural dispensary. Although most of the cases were found to be caused by flea-borne rickettsiosis caused by *R. felis* [51], in 0.7% the origin of the fever was tick-borne rickettsia. The identified case was from Dielmo village, and the tick positive for R. *conorii* (*Rh. e. evertsi*) was collected in Medina, a small village not far from Ndiop. Despite the very low percentage of infected ticks, we succeeded in the identification of this rickettsia in the blood of a febrile girl that was evidently ill with Mediterranean spotted fever.

The prevalence of five tick-borne and one flea-borne rickettsiae in the same region poses a question about cross-protection. To the best of our knowledge, no other region in the world has yet been found to present such a variety of pathogenic rickettsiae. The model studies that have been performed in animals since the beginning of 20th century often showed opposite results (Table 5), even when the same animals and rickettsiae were tested, for instance *R. conorii* and *R. africae* on guinea pigs [66], [67]. Usually, broader cross-protection was seen when sublethal doses of live rickettsiae were used for immunization [68], [69] when compared with inactivated bacteria. No studies in humans have been performed. In Senegal, the natural condition favors simultaneous contact of the rural population with different rickettsiae, so further studies on the dynamics of antibody levels over several years and their protective significance should be performed. Moreover, the prevalence Q fever in humans and its causative agent, *C. burnetii*, in ticks in the same regions [70] shows that these regions of rural Senegal present a natural reservoir of at least several emerging zoonoses.

Table 5: Selected literature data on serological cross-protection among different spotted fever group rickettsiae in animal models

Compared rickettsiae	Animal model	Antigen	Results of the study	Reference
R. africae vs. *R. conorii*	Guinea pigs	Sublethal doses alive rickettsiae	Absence of cross-immunity	[66]
	Guinea pigs	Sublethal doses alive rickettsiae	Reciprocal cross-protection	[67]
R. conorii vs. *R. rickettsii*	Guinea pigs	Sublethal doses alive rickettsiae	Reciprocal cross-protection	[69,73]
R. rickettsii vs. *R. australis*	Guinea pigs	Sublethal doses alive rickettsiae	Absence of cross-immunity	[74]
R. parkeri vs. *R. rickettsii* vs. *R. conorii*	Guinea pigs	Sublethal doses alive rickettsiae	Reciprocal cross-protection	[75]
R. sibirica vs. *R. heilongjiangensis* vs. *R. conorii*	Guinea pigs	Sublethal doses alive rickettsiae	Absence of cross-immunity	[76]
R. rickettsii vs. *R. montanensis*	Guinea pigs	Sublethal doses alive rickettsiae	Reciprocal cross-protection	[77]

doi:10.1371/journal.pntd.0000821.t005

In conclusion, we have to emphasize that the pathogenic spotted fever rickettsiae are very common in rural Senegal. Both occasional travelers and local villagers have a very high probability of being infected. Unfortunately, the modern reader is familiar almost exclusively with rickettsioses as the cause of returning travelers' fever [25]. The fevers in returning travelers are easy to identify, because these people are usually intently observed after returning. In contrast, little is known about rickettsioses in the local indigenous African population. The only known report is from Cameroon [71], where seven cases were described based on the molecular identification of *R. africae* in the blood of febrile patients. The integral approach applied in our work (studies of vectors, seroprevalence, and causes of acute fevers) allowed us to reveal the important role of rickettsial diseases in public health in Western Africa.

Our results are compatible with previously reported data, and the very high prevalence of spotted fevers may be explained by the surprising number of pathogenic rickettsiae identified in the studied region (*R. conorii conorii, R. africae, R. sibirica mongolitimonae, R. aeschlimannii*, and *R. massiliae*). We have summarized the clinical and epidemiological data concerning spotted fevers caused by all five tick-borne rickettsiae (Table 4). In addition, our study contributes to the discovery of the origin of unexplained fevers in Africa. We showed that up to 6.7% (9 of 134) of acute non-malarial fevers in rural Africa may have rickettsial (*R. felis*and *R. conorii*) origin.

Based on these data, we concluded that tick-borne rickettsioses together with Q fever [70], flea-borne rickettsiosis caused by *R. felis* [51], *Tropheryma whipplei* infection [72], and tick-borne relapsing fever [43] are major public health problems in West Africa. Taking into consideration that the role of tick-borne fevers in West Africa was previously underestimated, it is very important to perform long-term surveys on the distribution of vector ticks and rickettsiae, as well as screening targeted groups, both tourists and the indigenous population. We suggest implementing diagnostic procedures and adapted treatments in the field to enhance the health of the people living in rural sub-Saharan Africa.

ACKNOWLEDGMENTS

We thank Denis Pyak and Geetha Subramanian for the technical assistance.

AUTHOR CONTRIBUTIONS

Conceived and designed the experiments: OM GD FF J-FT DR. Performed the experiments: OM GD. Analyzed the data: OM GD FF CS J-FT. Contributed reagents/materials/analysis tools: CS J-FT DR. Wrote the paper: OM DR.

REFERENCES

1. Conor A, Bruch A (1910) Une fièvre eruptive observée en Tunisie. Bull Soc Pathol Exot Filial 8: 492–496.
2. McNaught JG (1911) A tick-bite in the Union of South Africa. J R Army Med Corps 16: 505.
3. Sant'Anna JF (1912) On a disease in man following tick-bites and occurring in Lourenco Marques. Parasitology 4: 87–88.
4. Pijper A (1936) Etude expérimentale comparée de la Fièvre boutonneuse et de la Tick-Bite-Fever. Arch Inst Pasteur Tunis 25: 388–401.
5. Gear JHS (1938) South African typhus. S Afr J Med Sci 3: 134–160.
6. Blanc G, Caminopetros J (1932) Etudes épidémiologiques et expérimentales sur la fièvre boutonneuse, faites a l'Institut Pasteur d'Athénes. Arch Inst Pasteur Tunis 20(4): 343–394.
7. Rovery C, Raoult D (2008) Mediterranean spotted fever. Infect Dis Clin North Am 22: 515–530. S0891-5520(08)00022-6 [pii];10.1016/j.idc.2008.03.003 [doi].
8. Kelly PJ, Matthewman LA, Beati L, Raoult D, Mason P, et al. (1992) African tick-bite fever: a new spotted fever group rickettsiosis under an old name. Lancet 340: 982–983.
9. Philip CB, Hoogstraal H, Reiss-Gutfreund R, Clifford CM (1966) Evidence of rickettsial disease agents in ticks from Ethiopian cattle. Bull World Health Organ 35: 127–131.
10. Beati L, Kelly PJ, Matthewman LA, Mason P, Raoult D (1995) Prevalence of Rickettsia-like organisms and spotted fever group Rickettsiae in ticks (Acari : Ixodidae) from Zimbabwe. J Med Entomol 32: 787–792.
11. Kelly PJ, Beati L, Mason PR, Matthewman LA, Roux V, et al. (1996) Rickettsia africae sp. nov., the etiological agent of African tick bite fever. Int J Syst Bacteriol 46: 611–614.
12. Parola P, Inokuma H, Camicas JL, Brouqui P, Raoult D (2001) Detection and identification of spotted fever group Rickettsiae and Ehrlichiae in African ticks. Emerg Infect Dis 7: 1014–1017.
13. Mura A, Socolovschi C, Ginesta J, Lafrance B, Magnan S, et al. (2008) Molecular detection of spotted fever group rickettsiae in ticks from Ethiopia and Chad. Trans R Soc Trop Med Hyg 102: 945–949. S0035-9203(08)00113-2 [pii];10.1016/j.trstmh.2008.03.015 [doi].
14. Cazorla C, Socolovschi C, Jensenius M, Parola P (2008) Tick-borne diseases: tick-borne spotted fever rickettsioses in Africa. Infect Dis Clin North Am 22: 531–544. S0891-5520(08)00016-0 [pii];10.1016/j.idc.2008.03.009 [doi].
15. Raoult D, Fournier PE, Fenollar F, Jensenius M, Prioe T, et al. (2001) Rickettsia africae, a tick-borne pathogen in travelers to sub-Saharan Africa. N Engl J Med 344: 1504–1510.
16. Mediannikov O, Trape JF, Diatta G, Parola P, Fournier PE, et al. (2010) Rickettsia africae, Western Africa. Emerg Infect Dis 16: 571–573.
17. Sarih M, Socolovschi C, Boudebouch N, Hassar M, Raoult D, et al. (2008) Spotted fever group rickettsiae in ticks, Morocco. Emerg Infect Dis 14: 1067–1073.
18. Dib L, Bitam I, Bensouilah M, Parola P, Raoult D (2009) First description of Rickettsia monacensis in Ixodes ricinus in Algeria. Clin Microbiol Infect. CLM2277 [pii];10.1111/j.1469-0691.2008.02277.x [doi].
19. Bitam I, Parola P, Matsumoto K, Rolain JM, Baziz B, et al. (2006) First molecular detection of R. conorii, R. aeschlimannii, and R. massiliae in ticks from Algeria. Ann N Y Acad Sci 1078: 368–372. 1078/1/368 [pii];10.1196/annals.1374.073 [doi].
20. Dupont HT, Cornet JP, Raoult D (1994) Identification of rickettsiae from ticks collected in the Central African Republic using the polymerase chain reaction. Am J Trop Med Hyg 50: 373–380.
21. Vitale G, Mansueto S, Rolain JM, Raoult D (2005) Rickettsia massiliae human isolation. Emerg Infect Dis 12: 174–175.
22. Beati L, Meskini M, Thiers B, Raoult D (1997) Rickettsia aeschlimannii sp. nov., a new spotted fever group rickettsia associated with Hyalomma marginatum ticks. Int J Syst Bacteriol 47: 548–554.
23. Matsumoto K, Parola P, Rolain JM, Jeffrey I, Raoult D (2006) Detection of "Candidatus Rickettsia uilenbergi" and "Candidatus Rickettsia davousti" in Amblyomma tholloni ticks from elephants in Africa. BMC Microbiol In revision.
24. Freedman DO, Weld LH, Kozarsky PE, Fisk T, Robins R, et al. (2006) Spectrum of disease and relation to place of exposure among ill returned travelers. N Engl J Med 354: 119–130. 354/2/119 [pii];10.1056/NEJMoa051331 [doi].
25. Jensenius M, Davis X, von SF, Schwartz E, Keystone JS, et al. (2009) Multicenter GeoSentinel analysis of rickettsial diseases in international travelers, 1996-2008. Emerg Infect Dis 15: 1791–1798.
26. Raoult D, Roux V (1997) Rickettsioses as paradigms of new or emerging infectious diseases. Clin Microbiol Rev 10: 694–719.
27. Jensenius M, Fournier PE, Vene S, Ringertz SH, Myrvang B, et al. (2004) Comparison of immunofluorescence, Western blotting, and cross-adsorption assays for diagnosis of African tick bite fever. Clin Diagn Lab Immunol 11: 786–788.

28. Tissot-Dupont H, Brouqui P, Faugere B, Raoult D (1995) Prevalence of antibodies to Coxiella burnetii, Rickettsia conorii, and Rickettsia typhi in seven African countries. Clin Infect Dis 21: 1126–1133.

29. Okabayashi T, Hasebe F, Samui KL, Mweene AS, Pandey SG, et al. (1999) Short report: prevalence of antibodies against spotted fever, murine typhus, and Q fever rickettsiae in humans living in Zambia. Am J Trop Med Hyg 61: 70–72.

30. Kovacova E, Sixl W, Stunzner D, Urvolgyi J, Kazar J (1996) Serological examination of human and animal sera from six countries of three continents for the presence of rickettsial antibodies. Eur J Epidemiol 12: 85–89.

31. Maurice Y, Fernagut R, Gerome R (1968) [Rickettsial diseases of North Cameroon; epidemiological study]. Rev Elev Med Vet Pays Trop 21: 341–349.

32. Redus MA, Parker RA, McDade JE (1986) Prevalence and distribution of spotted fever and typhus infections in Sierra Leone and Ivory Coast. Int J Zoonoses 13: 104–111.

33. Gray GC, Rodier GR, Matras-Maslin VC, Honein MA, Ismail EA, et al. (1995) Serologic evidence of respiratory and rickettsial infections among Somali refugees. Am J Trop Med Hyg 52: 349–353.

34. Botros BA, Soliman A, Darwish M, el Said S, Morill JC, et al. (1989) Seroprevalence of murine typhus and Fièvre Boutonneuse in certain human populations in Egypt. J Trop Med Hyg 92: 373–378.

35. Kalivogi S (1986) Epidemiology and prophylaxis of Q fever and spotted fever group rickettsioses in Guinea [dissertation]. Gamaleya Institute of Epidemiology and Microbiology. Moscow: 134 p.

36. Niang M, Parola P, Tissot-Dupont H, Baidi L, Brouqui P, et al. (1998) Prevalence of antibodies to Rickettsia conorii, Rickettsia africae, Rickettsia typhi and Coxiella burnetii in Mauritania. Eur J Epidemiol 14: 817–818.

37. Meskini M, Beati L, Benslimane A, Raoult D (1995) Seroepidemiology of rickettsial infections in Morocco. Eur J Epidemiol 11: 655–660.

38. Anstey NM, Tissot-Dupont H, Hahn CG, Mwaikambo ED, McDonald MI, et al. (1997) Seroepidemiology of Rickettsia typhi, spotted fever group rickettsiae, and Coxiella burnetii infection in pregnant women from urban Tanzania. Am J Trop Med Hyg 57: 187–189.

39. Letaief AO, Yacoub S, Tissot-Dupont H, Le Cam C, Ghachem L, et al. (1995) Seroepidemiological survey of rickettsial infections among blood donors in central Tunisia. Trans R Soc Trop Med Hyg 89: 266–268.

40. Kelly PJ, Mason PR, Matthewman LA, Raoult D (1991) Seroepidemiology of spotted fever group rickettsial infections in human in Zimbabwe. J Trop Med Hyg 94: 304–309.

41. Dione , M M (2004) Contribution a l'etude des tiques vectrices d'agents pathogenes au Senegal: distribution et identification de zones a risque de la fievre hemorrhagique de Crimee-Congo (FCHH) et la cowdriose [dissertation]. Faculte de Medecine, de Pharmacie et d'Odonto-Stomatologie de Dakar. 120 p.

42. Trape JF, Rogier C, Konate L, Diagne N, Bouganali H, et al. (1994) The Dielmo project: a longitudinal study of natural malaria infection and the mechanisms of protective immunity in a community living in a holoendemic area of Senegal. Am J Trop Med Hyg 51: 123–137.

43. Vial L, Diatta G, Tall A, Ba eH, Bouganali H, et al. (2006) Incidence of tick-borne relapsing fever in west Africa: longitudinal study. Lancet 368: 37–43. S0140-6736(06)68968-X [pii];10.1016/S0140-6736(06)68968-X [doi].

44. Walker AR, Bouattour A, Camicas JL, Estrada-Pena A, Horak IG, et al. (2003) Ticks of domestic animals in Africa. Edinburgh, UK. Bioscience Reports.

45. Hoogstraal H (1956) African Ixodoidea: I. Ticks of the Sudan (With special reference to Equatoria Province and with preliminary reviews of the genera Boophilus, Margaropus, and Hyalomma). Washington, DC.

46. Kelly PJ, Raoult D, Mason PR (1991) Isolation of spotted fever group rickettsias from triturated ticks using a modification of the centrifugation-shell vial technique. Trans R Soc Trop Med Hyg 85: 397–398.

47. Rolain JM, Sthul L, Maurin M, Raoult D (2002) Evaluation of antibiotic susceptibilities of three Rickettsial species including Rickettsia felis by a quantitative PCR DNA assay. Antimicrob Agents Chemother 46: 2747–2751.

48. Roux V, Rydkina E, Eremeeva M, Raoult D (1997) Citrate synthase gene comparison, a new tool for phylogenetic analysis, and its application for the rickettsiae. Int J Syst Bacteriol 47: 252–261.

49. Mediannikov OY, Sidelnikov Y, Ivanov L, Mokretsova E, Fournier PE, et al. (2004) Acute tick-borne rickettsiosis caused by Rickettsia heilongjiangensis in Russian Far East. Emerg Infect Dis 10: 810–817.

50. Fournier PE, Roux V, Raoult D (1998) Phylogenetic analysis of spotted fever group rickettsiae by study of the outer surface protein rOmpA. Int J Syst Bacteriol 48: 839–849.

51. Socolovschi C, Mediannikov O, Sokhna C, Tall A, Diatta G, et al. (2010) Rickettsia felis, a common cause of uneruptive fever in rural Senegal. Emerg Infect 2010 Jul; 16(7): 1140–2.

52. Hall TA (1999) BioEdit: a user-friendly biological sequence alignment editor and analysis program for Windows 95/98/NT. Nucl Acids Symp Ser 41: 95–98.

53. Fournier PE, El KK, Leroy Q, Robert C, Giumelli B, et al. (2009) Analysis of the Rickettsia africae genome reveals that virulence acquisition in Rickettsia species may be explained by genome reduction. BMC Genomics 10: 166. 1471- 2164-10-166[pii];10.1186/1471-2164-10-166 [doi].

54. Fournier PE, Dumler JS, Greub G, Zhang J, Wu Y, et al. (2003) Gene sequence-based criteria for identification of new rickettsia isolates and description of Rickettsia heilongjiangensis sp. nov. J Clin Microbiol 41: 5456–5465.

55. Swai ES, Mtui PF, Chang'a AK, Machange GE (2008)

The prevalence of serum antibodies to Ehrlichia ruminantium infection in ranch cattle in Tanzania: a cross-sectional study. J S Afr Vet Assoc 79: 71–75.

56. Hove T, Sithole N, Munodzana D, Masaka S (1998) Isolation and characterization of a Babesia species from Rhipicephalus evertsi evertsi ticks picked off a sable antelope (Hippotragus niger) which died of acute babesiosis. Onderstepoort J Vet Res 65: 75–80.

57. Zeller HG, Cornet JP, Diop A, Camicas JL (1997) Crimean-Congo hemorrhagic fever in ticks (Acari: Ixodidae) and ruminants: field observations of an epizootic in Bandia, Senegal (1989-1992). J Med Entomol 34: 511–516.

58. Allsopp MT, van Strijp MF, Faber E, Josemans AI, Allsopp BA (2007) Ehrlichia ruminantium variants which do not cause heartwater found in South Africa. Vet Microbiol 120: 158–166. S0378-1135(06)00425-1 [pii];10.1016/j.vetmic.2006.10.026 [doi].

59. Robinson JB, Eremeeva ME, Olson PE, Thornton SA, Medina MJ, et al. (2009) New approaches to detection and identification of Rickettsia africae and Ehrlichia ruminantium in Amblyomma variegatum (Acari: Ixodidae) ticks from the Caribbean. J Med Entomol 46: 942–951.

60. Portillo A, Perez-Martinez L, Santibanez S, Blanco JR, Ibarra V, et al. (2007) Detection of Rickettsia africae in Rhipicephalus (Boophilus) decoloratus ticks from the Republic of Botswana, South Africa. Am J Trop Med Hyg 77: 376–377. 77/2/376 [pii].

61. Camicas JL, Cornet JP, Gonzalez JP, Wilson ML, Adam F, et al. (1994) [Crimean-Congo hemorrhagic fever in Senegal. Latest data on the ecology of the CCHF virus]. Bull Soc Pathol Exot 87: 11–16.

62. Spickett AM, Burger DB, Crause JC, Roux EM, Neitz AW (1991) Sweating sickness: relative curative effect of hyperimmune serum and a precipitated immunoglobulin suspension and immunoblot identification of proposed immunodominant tick salivary gland proteins. Onderstepoort J Vet Res 58: 223–226.

63. Mokrani N, Parola P, Tebbal S, Dalichaouche M, Aouati A, et al. (2008) Rickettsia aeschlimannii infection, Algeria. Emerg Infect Dis 14: 1814–1815.

64. Nduaka O, Ikeme MM (1973) Human skin lesions in East Central State, Nigeria due to the larvae of Amblyomma variegatum (Fabricius, 1794). Niger Med J 3: 140–143.

65. Nakamura-Uchiyama F, Komuro Y, Yoshii A, Nawa Y (2000) Amblyomma testudinarium tick bite : one case of engorged adult and a case of extraordinary number of larval tick infestation. J Dermatol 27: 774–777.

66. Pijper A (1936) Etude expérimentale comparée de la Fièvre boutonneuse et de la Tick-Bite-Fever. Arch Inst Pasteur Tunis 25: 388–401.

67. Bozeman FM, Humphries JW, Campbell JM, O'Hara PL (1960) Laboratory studies of the spotted fever group of rickettsiae. In: Wisseman CLJ, editor. Symposium on the spotted fever group of rickettsiae. Washington, D.C.: Walter Reed Army Medical Center. pp. 7–11.

68. Philip RN, Casper EA, Burgdorfer W, Gerloff RK, Hugues LE, et al. (1978) Serologic typing of rickettsiae of the spotted fever group by micro immunofluoresence. J Immunol 121: 1961–1968.

69. Davis GE (1934) Comparative experiments on spotted fever and boutonneuse fever. Pub Health Rep 49: 423.

70. Mediannikov O, Fenollar F, Socolovschi C, Diatta G, Bassene H, et al. (2010) Coxiella burnetii in humans and ticks in rural Senegal. PLoS Negl Trop Dis 2010 Apr 6; 4(4): e654.

71. Ndip LM, Fokam EB, Bouyer DH, Ndip RN, Titanji VP, et al. (2004) Detection of Rickettsia africae in patients and ticks along the coastal region of Cameroon. Am J Trop Med Hyg 71: 363–366. 71/3/363 [pii].

72. Fenollar F, Trape JF, Bassene H, Sokhna C, Raoult D (2009) Tropheryma whipplei in fecal samples from children, Senegal. Emerg Infect Dis 15: 922–924.

73. Badger LF (1933) Rocky Mountain spotted fever and boutonneuse fever. A study of their immunological relationships. Public Health Rep 48: 507.

74. Plotz H, Smadel JE, Bennet BI (1946) North Queensland tick typhus: studies of the aetiological agent and its relation to other rickettsial diseases. Med J Aust 263–268.

75. Parker RR, Kohls GM, Cox GW, Davis GE (1939) Observations on an infectious agent from Amblyomma maculatum. Public Health Rep 54: 1482–1484.

76. Korshunova OS (1943) About etiology of Far Eastern tick-borne typhus. Part I [In Russian]. Zh Mikrobiol Epidemiol Immunobiol 1-2: 51–55.

77. Feng WC, Waner JL (1980) Serological cross-reaction and cross-protection in guinea pigs infected with Rickettsia rickettsii and Rickettsia montana. Infect Immun 28: 627–629.

SECTION XIV: ANAPLASMA AND EHRLICHIA – TICK-BORNE DISEASES

CHAPTER 50

GUIDELINE FOR VETERINARY PRACTITIONERS ON CANINE EHRLICHIOSIS AND ANAPLASMOSIS IN EUROPE

Ángel Sainz, Xavier Roura, Guadalupe Miró, Agustín Estrada-Peña, Barbara Kohn, Shimon Harrus and Laia Solano-Gallego

Keywords: Canine ehrlichiosis, canine anaplasmosis, *Ehrlichia canis, Anaplasma phagocytophilum, Anaplasma platys*consensus

INTRODUCTION

Canine ehrlichiosis and anaplasmosis are important tick-borne diseases with a worldwide distribution.

Ehrlichia canis was first identified in 1935 in Algeria; dogs infested with ticks showed fever and anemia [1]. Later, during the Vietnam War, many military working dogs brought to Vietnam by the US army exhibited a severe disease called Tropical Canine Pancytopenia [2]. Later, it was renamed canine monocytic ehrlichiosis (CME).

In 1978, an ehrlichial infection that affected platelets was first identified in the US. It was caused by *Anaplasma platys* (initially identified as *Ehrlichia platys*), and it caused a clinical syndrome known as canine infectious cyclic thrombocytopenia [3]. In 1982, a natural infection of granulocytic anaplasmosis, caused by *Ehrlichia phagocytophila,* was first identified in dogs in California. Currently, this species is called *Anaplasma phagocytophilum* [4].

Over the 1980's and 90's, several species closely related to *E. canis* were found in infected dogs. Improvements in molecular techniques indicated that they were phylogenetically distant from *E. canis*, and therefore, they were reclassified under the genera *Anaplasma* or *Neorickettsia* [5].

In 2002, a large amount of information on ehrlichial infections was gathered by the *American College of Veterinary Internal Medicine* (ACVIM) *Infectious Disease Study Group*. That group published a *Consensus Statement* on diseases caused by *Ehrlichia* spp. in small animals [6]. Over the years, and probably as a result of globalization, urbanization, global warming, increased trade, and travel, these diseases have spread to new niches. Recently, diseases caused by *Ehrlichia* spp have been reported in many countries that had not previously detected them. Information has been continuously collected on these infections, and publications have increased in recent years. This document was intended to answer common questions of interest on this group of infections, with a special focus on the situation in Europe.

REVIEW

What species of *Ehrlichia* and/or *Anaplasma* can infect dogs in Europe?

To date, three species have been clearly identified in dogs in Europe; *E. canis*, *A. phagocytophilum*, and *A. platys*.

Ehrlichia canis

Ehrlichia canis is the only *Ehrlichia* species that has been isolated in dogs from Europe [7,8]. To our knowledge, other *Ehrlichia* species (*E. chaffeensis*, *E. ewingii*, *E. muris*, and *E. ruminantium*) have not been detected in dogs from Europe. However, *E. muris* has been described in *Ixodes* ticks from Russia and Slovakia [9,10]. All European countries bordering the Mediterranean Sea are endemic for *E. canis*. Some surveys have indicated that the infectious agent is spreading to countries north of the Mediterranean (i.e., Switzerland, Germany) [11-13]. Table 1 shows the prevalence of *E. canis* infections in dogs from Europe.

Citation: Ángel SainzEmail author, Xavier Roura, Guadalupe Miró, Agustín Estrada-Peña, Barbara Kohn, Shimon Harrus and Laia Solano-Gallego, Guideline for veterinary practitioners on canine ehrlichiosis and anaplasmosis in Europe, DOI: 10.1186/s13071-015-0649-0.

Table 1: Prevalence of *E. canis* infections in dogs of different European countries

Country	Number of dogs (n)	Prevalence (%)	Test methods	Reference
Albania	30	50.0/17.0	IFAT/Blood smear	[14]
Finland	340	0.3	4DX ELISA	[15]
France	919	0.3	4DX ELISA	[16]
Germany	106[a]	0.9	IFAT	[17]
	997[a]	3.1/0	IFAT/PCR	[18]
	4681[a]	10.1	IFAT	[19]
Hungary	1305	0.2	4DX ELISA	[20]
Italy	249[b]	46.0	IFAT	[21]
	135	44.0/6.0	IFAT/PCR	[22]
	51	0	PCR	[23]
	131[b]	22.9	IFAT	[24]
	601	6.4	PCR	[25]
	1000	46.7	IFAT	[26]
	423	20.0	IFAT	[27]
Portugal	557	4.1	4Dx ELISA	[28]
	55	22.0	PCR	[29]
	104	50.0	IFAT	[30]
Romania	1146	2.1	4DX ELISA	[31]
Russia	442[c] 82[d]	0 2.4	4DX ELISA	[32]
Spain	1100	5.0	4DX ELISA	[33]
	131	5.3	4DX ELISA	[34]
	153	4.0[e]	PCR	[35]
	479	3.1	IFAT	[36]
	466	16.7 4.5	IFAT 3DX ELISA	[37]
	200	6.5	IFAT	[38]
	308	19.2	IFAT	[39]
Switzerland	996[a]	2.2	IFAT	[13]
Turkey	284	20.7	IFAT	[40]

[a]Travelled/imported dogs.

[b]Kenelled dogs.

[c]Dogs with external antiparasitary treatment.

[d]Dogs without external antiparasitary treatment.

[e]Using primers for *Ehrlichia/Anaplasma.*

Anaplasma phagocytophilum

Infections of *A. phagocytophilum* have been described mainly in northern and Europe. Epidemiological studies performed in Europe (Table 2) that evaluated the seroprevalence (rarely a DNA-based analysis) showed that 3 to 57% of dogs carried *A. phagocytophilum*. However, the different studies investigated different dog populations (i.e., healthy and sick), and they used different tests (i.e., immunofluorescent antibody test [IFAT] or enzyme-linked immunosorbent assay [ELISA]). In addition, serological cross-reactivity with other *Anaplasma* spp. (e.g., *A. platys*) can potentially cause an overestimation of the true seroprevalence.

Table 2: Prevalence of infections with *A. phagocytophilum* in dogs of different European countries

Country	Number of dogs (n)	Prevalence (%)	Test methods	Reference
Austria	1470	56.5	IFAT	[41]
Albania	30	40.0/0	IFAT/Blood smear	[14]
Finland	340	5.3	4Dx ELISA[a]	[15]
France	919	2.7	4Dx ELISA[a]	[16]

Germany	1124	50.1	IFAT	[42]
	111	43.2 / 6.3	IFAT/PCR	[43]
	245	19.2	IFAT	[44]
	5881	21.5	4Dx ELISA[a]	[45]
	522	43.0 / 5.7	IFAT/PCR	[46]
	448	19.4	4Dx ELISA[a]	[47]
Hungary	1305	7.9	4Dx ELISA[a]	[20]
Italy	344	0	PCR	[48]
	460	0	PCR	[25]
	5634	33.0	IFAT	[49]
	1232	8.8	IFAT	[50]
	249	38.0	IFAT	[21]
	215	15.0 / 0.02	IFAT/PCR	[51]
Latvia	470	11.4	4Dx ELISA[a]	[52]
Poland	192	1.0	PCR	[53]
Portugal	55	55.0/0	IFAT/PCR	[54]
Romania	1146	5.5	4DX ELISA[a]	[31]
Russia	442[b] 82[c]	1.1 34.1	4Dx ELISA[a]	[32]
Sweden	611	17.7	IFAT	[55]
	248	20.7	IFAT	[56]
Switzerland	996	7.5	IFAT	[13]
Spain	649	15.6	IFAT	[36]
	466	11.5	IFAT	[37]
	1100	3.1	4Dx ELISA[a]	[33]
United Kingdom	120	0.8	PCR	[57]

[a]This test cannot differentiate between *A. phagocytophilum* and *A. platys.*

[b]Dogs with external antiparasitary treatment.

[c]Dogs without external antiparasitary treatment.

Anaplasma platys

Anaplasma platys has been diagnosed in dogs, particularly from countries in the Mediterranean basin, including Italy [48], Spain [58], Portugal [59], France [60], Turkey [61], Greece [62], Croatia [63], and Romania [64]. Information is limited regarding the prevalence *of A. platys* infections in dogs from Europe, based on a molecular analysis (Table 3).

Table 3: Prevalence of infections with *A. platys* in dogs in Europe

Country	Number of dogs (n)	Prevalence (%)	Test methods	Reference
Italy	34[a]	52.9	PCR	[65]
	34[a]	70.5	PCR	[66]
	109[a]	27.5	PCR	[67]
	344	4	PCR	[48]
	100[a]	23	RLB-PCR	[68]
Portugal	55[b]	9	IFAT/PCR	[54]

[a]Kenelled dogs.

[b]Dogs with suspected tick-borne diseases.

What are the vectors and geographic distributions of vectors for these infections in dogs in Europe?

Ehrlichia canis

The main, and probably the only, vector for *E. canis* in Europe is the tick *Rhipicephalus sanguineus* sensu lato, known as the brown dog-tick. This tick was shown experimentally to be a competent vector for *E. canis*[69,70]. A recent study has shown that transmission of *E. canis* by *R. sanguineus* ticks starts within 3 h after tick attachment to the dog [71]. The tick vector is currently considered a complex of species [72]. The details of this vector's morphology and molecular biology have been published, and it has been identified in wide areas of the world. However, it is difficult to ascertain which "species" comprise the actual vector, because the description of the original specimen type has been lost [72].

Rhipicephalus sanguineus is abundant in the Mediterranean basin. When introduced to colder areas, due to movements of the host (i.e., dogs travelling to and returning from the Mediterranean region), it can survive in kennels and other protected areas provided by man-made constructions (Figure 1). The latitude at which the tick can be established is currently unknown [72,73]. Protected environments, such as a house, a kennel, or the den of a wild carnivore, provide an ideal environment for the reproduction and survival of tick populations. It has been reported that even a single tick female was sufficient to engorge and oviposit on a dog inside an apartment, which then could give rise to the development of subadults [74]. *Rhipicephalus sanguineus* populations can reach very high numbers in sheltered environments, because the blood supply necessary for their development is guaranteed by the presence of hosts in close proximity. In dogs without appropriate protection, parasitic loads can reach hundreds of ticks per animal, with ticks in all developmental stages.

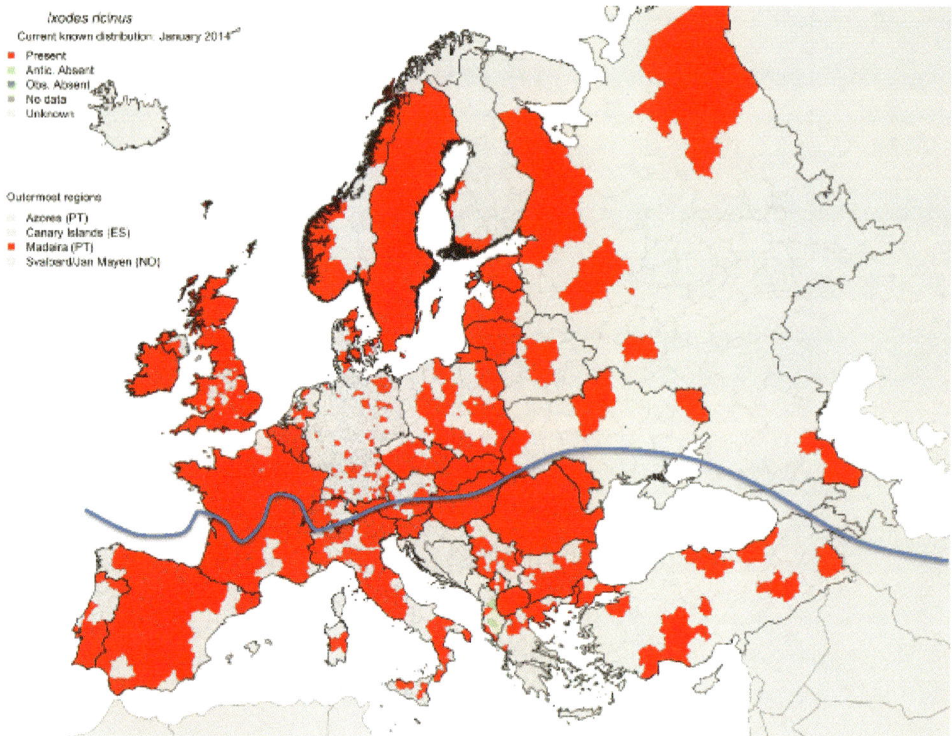

Figure 1: Distribution of *Ixodes ricinus* and *Rhipicephalus sanguineus* in Europe. The reported distribution of *I. ricinus* was officially recorded by the European Center for Disease Control (ECDC) in January, 2014 (red areas). The map includes only records with reliable, accurate data that can be ascribed to one of the NUTS (statistical regions of Europe). Many reports in the literature only mention the presence of one species in a country. Some of the areas in the Mediterranean region might be based on identified collections that do not have permanent populations (i.e., casual introduction without further survival) or based on small areas of suitability. The line shows the northern range of the distribution of ticks that belong to the *R. sanguineus* complex. Due to the confusion surrounding the morphology and systematics of this complex group, many records cannot be confidently tracked as "true" *R. sanguineus*. This northern limit is also an educated guess for the current distribution, because persistent populations may live in northern latitudes, protected in shelters, burrows, or private gardens, where adequate conditions for survival may exist.

The tick requires a minimum temperature of about 6°C for adequate survival, and when temperatures drop below this value, it may hibernate during winter, sheltered in the cracks of kennels and buildings. Ticks also require a certain level of humidity, which is provided by the high environmental moisture in the kennels (cleaned with water) or in gardens that receive artificial watering. Ticks are common and can reach significant population densities on riverbanks of the Mediterranean region, which are temperate and hold moisture. The tick is mainly active from spring to early autumn, when the highest infestations occur. The regional weather or the local conditions of some buildings may result in a different phenology or in different seasonal dynamics for the tick [72]. The impact of climate trends on the tick is unknown, although preliminary results have shown that their area of distribution is increasing, due to the increase in urbanized areas surrounding cities, and due to the warmer environment observed in autumn and winter at progressively higher latitudes.

Anaplasma phagocytophilum

Ixodes ricinus is the only known vector for *A. phagocytophilum* in Europe. This tick is widely distributed in most European regions, including western Norway and in Sweden; it has been collected in mixed forests, open pastures, and other areas with high humidity (Figure 1). The driving feature of the northern distribution is the temperature required for tick development. In the northern areas of Sweden, the tick was found at an approximate latitude of 68°N, but some tick populations have spread even farther north [75]. *Ixodes ricinus* is present in Ireland, the United Kingdom, and in southern Finland. It is also present in almost every territory in Europe, and the eastern limit seems to be along the Baltic countries and Ukraine. At its present limit to the east, it coexists with the closely-related, species *Ixodes persulcatus*, with which there is a certain degree of sympatry. In the south, the tick is present in parts of the Mediterranean region, commonly in mixed or deciduous forests [76,77]. It has been detected in Portugal, Spain (only in northern areas of the country and isolated points in southern hills), and Italy. It is also common in the northern belt of humid forests in Turkey [76,77]. It is hypothesized that the driving feature of its southern distribution is the atmospheric water vapour, which must be relatively high (around 80%) to support permanent populations.

In the eastern regions of Europe, *I. ricinus* is replaced with *I. persulcatus*, a closely related species. The habitats of *I. persulcatus* extend to the east and into Japan [78]. This well-known parasite inhabits a wide range of domestic animals, and it acts as a vector for different pathogens. It is probably best known as the main vector for *Borrelia* spp. and for tick-borne encephalitis virus in the territories it colonizes [79]. *I. persulcatus* was found to be infected by *Ehrlichia* spp. in the Baltic region [80] and by *A. phagocytophilum* in Ukraine [81]. Members of the Anaplasmataceae family (without further description) have also been found in *I. persulcatus* collected in Moldova [82].

Anaplasma platys

The probable vector of *A. platys* in Europe is *R. sanguineus*. Experimental transmission has not been achieved [83]. Nevertheless, molecular studies have detected *A. platys* DNA in *R. sanguineus* ticks, which suggested that these ticks act as the vector for *A. platys* [84].

Are there other routes of transmission for these infections in dogs?

Outside the European continent (on which this guideline is focused), other species of ticks have been shown to be responsible for the transmission of *E. canis* [85]. However, to date, *R. sanguineus* appears to be the main vector for this pathogen.

In general, another route of transmission is through blood transfusion. Due to the potential transmission of these pathogens via infected blood, screening canine blood products for bacterial DNA with a polymerase chain reaction (PCR) assay is recommended in highly endemic areas to ensure the safety of blood products [86]. This route of transmission has been described for *E. canis* [69], *A. phagocytophilum* [87-89], and *A. platys*[90].

Are *Ehrlichia* and *Anaplasma* species present in dogs in Europe able to affect other hosts?

Ehrlichia canis

Other wild canids (foxes, wolves, jackals) can become infected with *E. canis* [91-93]. However, experimental infection has only been reproduced in dogs. In addition, *E. canis*-like DNA was claimed to be detected in cat samples with PCR [94]. Moreover, several studies reported the presence of *E. canis* DNA in cats and wild felids from Brazil and Portugal [95-97]. However, to the best of our knowledge, *E. canis* has not been isolated from cats or other felids to date.

Anaplasma phagocytophilum

Anaplasma phagocytophilum can infect humans and several animals other than dogs, including cats, sheep, goats, cows, equines, rodents, roe deer, deer, other wild mammals, and birds [98-100].

Anaplasma platys

Anaplasma platys DNA was also recently found in cats in non-European continents [101,102].

What is the public health importance of *E. canis, A. phagocytophilum*, and *A. platys*?

Ehrlichia canis

An organism closely related to *E. canis* has been described in humans in Venezuela [103]. To date, it is not considered an agent with important zoonotic potential.

Anaplasma phagocytophilum

Anaplasma phagocytophilum has important zoonotic potential, because humans can acquire the infection through a bite from a tick infected with the pathogen. *Anaplasma phagocytophilum* causes human granulocytic anaplasmosis, a febrile illness that closely resembles the disease in dogs. After infection (1-2 weeks), a syndrome frequently occurs of malaise, low-back pain, fever, and/or gastrointestinal disorders. Other, less frequent symptoms include arthralgia, lymphadenomegaly, conjunctivitis, dysuria, and peripheral edema [104,105].

The first infection by *A. phagocytophilum* in humans was described by Bakken *et al* in 1994 in the USA [106]. After that description, numerous human cases from different European countries were described [107]. Dogs may act as sentinels for human exposure, because infected ticks on their coats may travel to humans. Blood from infected dogs should be handled with caution [107,108].

Anaplasma platys

Anaplasma platys DNA was recently detected in two family members in the USA [109] and two women from Venezuela [110].

Other *Ehrlichia/Anaplasma* spp. that have not been described in Europe can also infect humans. *Ehrlichia ewingii* has been described as a cause of infection in immune-suppressed patients [111], but there is no evidence of direct or tick-mediated transmission from dogs to human beings. *Ehrlichia ruminantium*, which typically infects wild ruminants, is also able to cause a disease in dogs [112] and humans [112,113]. *Ehrlichia chaffeensis* is the etiologic agent of human monocytic ehrlichiosis [99]. *Amblyomma americanum* acts as a vector for *E. chaffeensis* in the USA. Its hosts include white-tailed deer, goats, domestic dogs, red foxes, and birds. This *Ehrlichia* sp. has also been described in dogs [114,115], and DNA of *E. chaffeensis* has been found in ticks collected from dogs [116]. Finally, it has been shown that *E. muris* can infect both humans and dogs [117,118].

Is there a breed, age, or sex predisposition for canine ehrlichiosis or anaplasmosis?

Ehrlichia canis

All breeds are prone to CME. However, German Shepherd dogs and Siberian Huskies are predisposed to develop more severe clinical signs of ehrlichiosis; therefore, these breeds have a worse prognosis [119,120]. This fact was corroborated in experimental studies, which showed that the cell-mediated immune response to a challenge with *E. canis* was reduced in German Shepherd dogs compared to Beagle dogs [119].

Canine ehrlichiosis may appear at any age. No sex predisposition has been detected in the development of CME. Some studies have found higher seropositivity in males, but this may be explained by a higher exposure to vectors than females, due to behavioral characteristics [121]. Similarly, in epidemiological studies, higher seropositivity rates were found in older dogs [121-123]; this observation may be attributed to a higher probability of exposure to *E. canis* as the dog ages, rather than an increase in susceptibility with age.

Anaplasma phagocytophilum

No breed predisposition has been confirmed for *A. phagocytophilum* infections. In a few studies, Retriever breeds were overrepresented; however, this might reflect the popularity of taking these dogs along for outdoor activities [124]. No sex or age predisposition has been documented for clinical cases. Older dogs were more often seropositive compared to younger dogs, probably due to an increased opportunity for exposure over time [46,55].

Anaplasma platys

No breed, age, or sex predisposition has been described for *A. platys* infections.

What stages of disease can be identified during infections with *Ehrlichia* and/or *Anaplasma*spp. in dogs?

Ehrlichia canis

Following an incubation period of 1 to 3 weeks, three typical phases of the disease may develop sequentially: acute, subclinical, and chronic [2,125]. The acute phase can last 2 to 4 weeks; then, clinical signs may vary or disappear spontaneously, even without treatment. However, some dogs that show clinical improvement may remain persistent subclinical carriers for months and years [126]. The subclinical phase follows the acute stage. Dogs in this stage present no clinical signs; therefore, they may not seem to require veterinary attention. However, when screened for hematological abnormalities, these dogs may have subnormal platelet concentrations [127]. Some, but not all infected dogs may advance to a chronic phase. In the chronic phase, the clinical signs are more severe. Unfortunately, the acute and chronic phases are not always easy to distinguish in clinical practice, because many of the clinical signs are similar. A complete blood count and bone marrow aspiration may assist in diagnosing the chronic severe form of the disease. Dogs in the chronic phase exhibit bone marrow hypoplasia and severe pancytopenia [128]. No studies have fully elucidated the different responses of dogs to infection or the factors that induce some dogs to develop the chronic severe form of the disease.

Anaplasma phagocytophilum

The incubation period for an *A. phagocytophilum* infection lasts 1 to 2 weeks. Thereafter, the dog may develop a self-limiting febrile illness [87]. The main difference between *A. phagocytophilum* and *E. canis* is that most *A. phagocytophilum* cases present in the acute stage of the disease. Indeed, most dogs naturally infected with *A. phagocytophilum* probably remain healthy, as indicated by the high number of healthy seropositive dogs relative to dogs with the clinical disease [46]. The extent to which *A. phagocytophilum* can persist in tissues and contribute to subclinical/chronic disease manifestations in dogs has been a controversial issue [129]. Three dogs experimentally inoculated with *A. phagocytophilum* were monitored for 4 to 6 months to determine whether the organisms persisted. Rickettsial DNA was detected intermittently in two dogs, when PCR was performed on blood samples throughout the study [129].

Anaplasma platys

The incubation period for an *A. platys* infection is similar to that of an *A. phagocytophilum* infection (1 to 2 weeks). After that, alternate periods of thrombocytopenia and fever are observed, which appear and disappear cyclically every 1-2 weeks [130].

After an experimental inoculation of dogs with *A. platys*, parasitized platelets were detected in the peripheral blood after 8 to 15 days. The dogs developed severe thrombocytopenia within 7 days post inoculation [90]. After a reduction in the number of circulating bacteria, the platelet concentration increased within 3-4 days. These episodes of bacteremia and thrombocytopenia occurred at 1-2 week intervals. Chronic infection is associated with low-level bacteremia and mild thrombocytopenia, which may reflect a process where the host attempts to adapt to the *A. platys* infection [131].

What clinical signs are associated to *Ehrlichia* spp. and *Anaplasma* spp. infections in dogs?

Ehrlichia canis

Clinical signs of an *E. canis* infection can be variable, depending on the strain, the immune response of the dog, and the presence of concomitant infections with other tick- or flea-borne pathogens. It must be kept in mind that some dogs may not show clinical or laboratory signs associated with an *Ehrlichia* infection, and others may show severe signs. In general, *E. canis* seems to cause more severe clinical signs than anaplasmosis [3,35,87,120,124,132-142].

Clinical signs of ehrlichiosis can vary, and it may include nonspecific signs, like fever, weakness, lethargy, anorexia, lymphadenomegaly, splenomegaly, hepatomegaly, or weight loss. Other signs have also been described, including vomiting, diarrhea, pain, exercise intolerance, edema (in hind legs, tail, or scrotum), cough and/or dyspnea (associated with pneumonia), serous or mucopurulent oculonasal discharge, abortion or neonatal death, and skin ulcers. Although some older studies have included lameness, due to polyarthritis, as a sign of CME [143,144], no evidence-based studies have supported this sign. Therefore, in cases of lameness and/or polyarthritis in dogs infected with *E. canis*, it is advisable to rule out coinfections with other pathogens, such as *A. phagocytophilum* or *B. burgdorferi*. Common clinical signs of ehrlichiosis include pale mucous membranes, due to anemia, epistaxis, petechiae, ecchymoses, prolonged bleeding during estrus, hematuria or melena associated with thrombocytopenia, thrombocytopathy, or vasculitis. Ocular signs are also common in CME. The most common are anterior uveitis, corneal opacity, hyphema, retinal vessel tortuosity, chorioretinal lesions, subretinal hemorrhage, retinal detachment, or blindness. Neurological signs are less commonly described (typically secondary to meningitis).

Anaplasma phagocytophilum

The most common clinical signs of *A. phagocytophilum* are non-specific; they include lethargy, inappetence/anorexia, and fever. Other findings are pale mucous membranes, a tense abdomen, and gastrointestinal signs (vomiting/diarrhea). Lameness may result from secondary immune-mediated (neutrophilic) polyarthritis. Mildly enlarged lymph nodes, tachypnea, and surface bleeding (petechiae, melena, epistaxis) may occur. Rare signs include collapse, mild cough, scleral injection, uveitis, limb edema, and polydipsia/polyuria [145-151]. It is controversial whether nervous system signs are associated with this infection [152-154]. In a few cases, an association was suggested between steroid-responsive meningitis/arteritis and *A. phagocytophilum* infection [155]. *A. phagocytophilum* infection may trigger some immunopathies, such as immune-mediated thrombocytopenia/anemia. Splenomegaly diagnosed with radiography and ultrasonography is a very common finding [147].

Anaplasma platys

Clinical signs of *A. platys* infection have been described both experimentally and in naturally infected dogs in Greece, Spain, Portugal, and Israel. These signs included fever, lethargy, anorexia, weight loss, pale mucous membranes, petechiae, nasal discharge, and lymphadenomegaly. Furthermore, single case studies have described bilateral uveitis and epistaxis. However, not all studies used PCR to exclude co-infections with other vector-transmitted diseases that produce the same clinical signs [54,62,63,66,146,156-158].

What abnormal laboratory findings can be found in dogs with ehrlichiosis and/or anaplasmosis?

Abnormal laboratory findings in canine ehrlichiosis or anaplasmosis are variable and nonspecific. However, the most common finding in ehrlichiosis and anaplasmosis is thrombocytopenia; this finding should alert clinicians. Other common abnormal laboratory findings are shown in Table 4 [54,147,148,159].

Table 4: Laboratory abnormal findings in ehrlichiosis caused by *Ehrlichia canis* and anaplasmosis caused by *Anaplasma platys* and*Anaplasma phagocytophilum*

Clinical disease	Species	Laboratory abnormal findings
Canine monocytyc ehrlichiosis	*E. canis*	• Mild to moderate normocytic normochromic non regenerative anemia
		• Neutropenia
		• Neutrophilia
		• Lymphopenia
		• Monocytosis
		• Granular lymphocytosis (uncommon)
		• Thrombocytopenia
		• Thrombocytopathy
		• Pancytopenia: medullary hypoplasia or aplasia (chronic forms, 15-20% of clinical cases)
		• Hyperproteinemia
		• Hyperglobulinemia
		• Hypergammaglobulinemia, usually polyclonal
		• Hypoalbuminemia
		• Proteinuria
		• Renal azotemia
		• Mild increase in hepatic enzymes (ALT, ALP)
		• Mononuclear or neutrophilic pleocytosis

Canine granulocytic anaplasmosis	*A. phagocytophilum*	• Non regenerative mild to moderate normocytic normochromic anemia
		• Regenerative anemia (rare)
		• Lymphopenia
		• Neutropenia, neutrophilia (sometimes left shift) or normal neutrophil concentration
		• Thrombocytopenia
		• Hyperglobulinemia
		• Hypoalbuminemia
		• Increased ALP
		• Mild hyperbilirubinemia
		• Neutrophilic inflammation in synovial fluid
		• Sometimes direct Coombs' test/platelet-bound antibody test positive
Canine thrombocytotrophic anaplasmosis	*A. platys*	• Thrombocytopenia
		• Non regenerative mild to moderate normocytic normochromic anemia
		• Hyperglobulinemia
		• Hypoalbuminemia

Is microscopic evaluation of a blood smear or another tissue sample useful for the diagnosis of ehrlichiosis and anaplasmosis?

The diagnostic usefulness of evaluating a blood smear depends on the pathogen species that has infected the dog.

Ehrlichia canis

It is rare to detect an *E. canis* morula (an aggregate of *E. canis* organisms; Figure 2) in a blood smear. It occurs in about 4-6% of clinical cases [160]. The highest likelihood of detecting morulae can be achieved by performing a buffy coat smear [160]. Because the direct detection method has low sensitivity, further diagnostic tests must be conducted, such as serology or molecular techniques (PCR). The highest rates of detecting morulae (50%) seem to be achieved when lymph node aspirates are examined by expert cytologists that evaluate a large number of oil immersion fields [160,161].

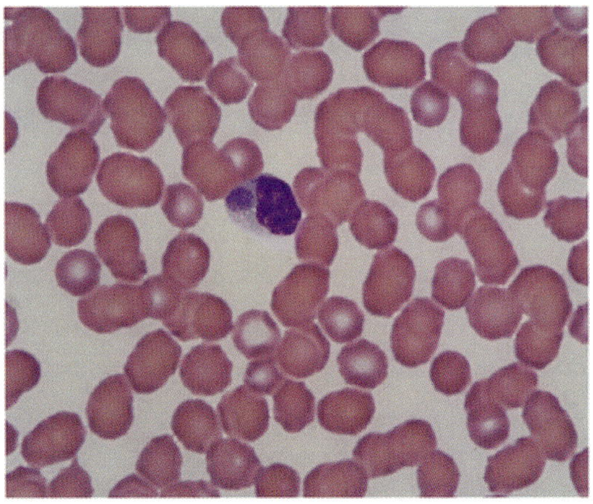

Figure 2: Microscopic image of a morula of *Ehrlichia canis* in the cytoplasm of a monocyte (x100).

Anaplasma phagocytophilum

The direct blood smear detection method seems to have higher sensitivity for detecting *A. phagocytophilum*than for detecting *E. canis* in dogs. Morulae can be observed in neutrophils in up to 60% of clinical cases [147] (Figure 3). In experimentally infected dogs, morulae appear as early as 4 days after inoculation and persist for 4-8 days [129]. However, the morulae cannot be distinguished from those of other *Ehrlichia* spp. that infect neutrophils (e.g., *Ehrlichia ewingii*); therefore, the finding should be confirmed by PCR in areas where both organisms are likely to occur.

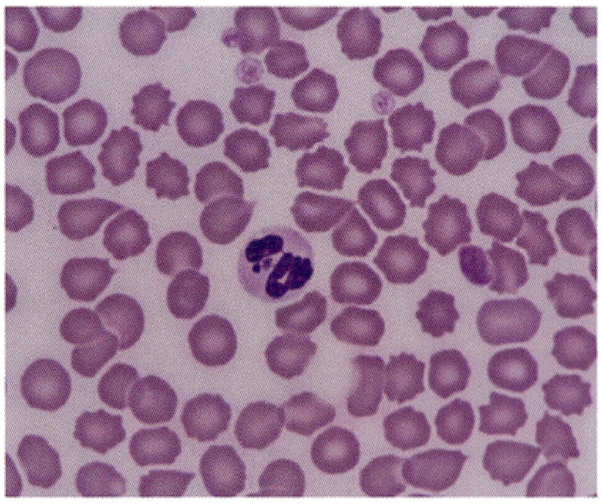

Figure 3: Microscopic image of a morula of *Anaplasma phagocytophilum* in the cytoplasm of a neutrophil (x100).

Anaplasma platys

The method of detecting morulae in platelets during an *A. platys* infection also appears to have a low sensitivity (Figure 4) [57], but some studies suggest that this method may have higher sensitivity during the early phase of the infection [162]. It was recently reported that *A. platys* were found in megakaryocytes [163], but the sensitivity of bone marrow cytology remains to be evaluated.

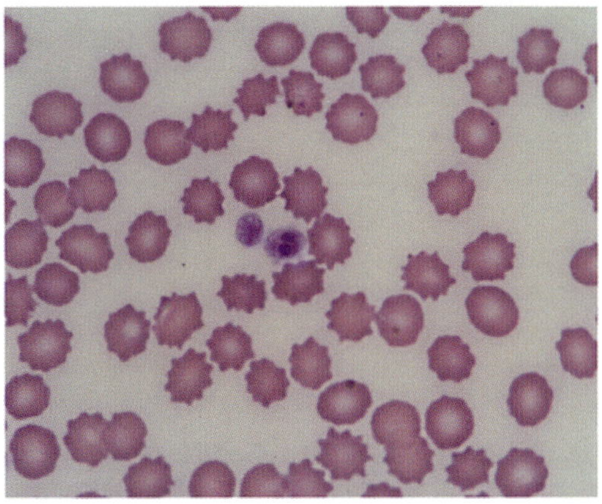

Figure 4: Microscopic image of a morula of *Anaplasma platys* in a platelet (x100).

What serological techniques can be used in the diagnosis of ehrlichiosis and/or anaplasmosis?

Ehrlichiosis and/or anaplasmosis can be diagnosed with the IFAT or ELISA [142,164,165]. These tests require specific equipment and trained technicians. One of the advantages of these tests is that they allow determination of antibody levels and their changes over time. Therefore, it is important to conduct quantitative serologic tests and to determine either the final antibody titer with the IFAT or the optical density with the ELISA for a quantitative evaluation (negative, low, or high signals). Quantitative laboratory techniques are more sensitive and specific than rapid tests [164]. Some commercial in-house dot-ELISA kits are qualitative, and show only a positive or negative result, without providing the dog's antibodies levels. Other dot-ELISA kits are semi-quantitative and provide some information on antibody levels. However, an accurate, reliable serological diagnosis is limited by the lack of standardization among different diagnostic laboratories and tests.

How should we interpret a positive serologic result for *Ehrlichia* and/or *Anaplasma*?

A positive serologic result indicates a past or current infection, but it does not always denote an ongoing disease condition. A single positive titer result may only reflect a past infection that may be resolved, because antibody titers may persist for several months or years [46,90,126]. Moreover, seroprevalence is high in endemic areas. In dogs naturally infected with *E. canis*, some authors have found that animals with high IFAT titers were more likely to show PCR positivity than negativity; this finding suggested that there may be a relationship between antibody titer and active infection [166]. Nevertheless, this information must be confirmed. We suggest that suspected cases should be evaluated based on the performance of two or more serological tests conducted in 2-4 weeks intervals. This approach can provide information on antibody kinetics (an increase, no change, or a decrease), which may point to the current status of infection. It has been suggested that a four-fold increase in IgG antibodies over time can be taken as evidence of an ongoing infection [165]. Recent research has suggested that the combination of serology and PCR was preferable for the diagnosis of *Ehrlichia* and *Anaplasma* spp. infections [167]. Presently, we recommend performing molecular tests to support any positive serological case, because the presence of bacterial DNA is a sign of active infection.

Could a seronegative dog be infected with *Ehrlichia* and/or *Anaplasma* spp.?

A dog can be seronegative, despite harboring an infection, with some species of *Ehrlichia* or *Anaplasma*. This is particularly common during the incubation period and in the early stages of the acute disease, when bacterial loads are low, for example:

- In the case of *E. canis*, antibody production typically does not occur before 12 -14 days post-infection [126,168].
- After experimentally infecting dogs with *A. phagocytophilum*, IgG antibodies may first be detectable 8 days after the initial exposure and 2 to 5 days after the appearance of morulae [129].
- After experimentally infecting dogs with *A. platys*, antibodies were first detected on day 16 [90].

Consequently, seroconversion can be used as a serologic technique to corroborate signs that suggest an acute infection with *Ehrlichia* or *Anaplasma*. Thus, an initial quantitative serology is conducted to detect acute antibody levels, when the dog shows clinical signs and/or abnormal laboratory findings; then, another quantitative serology is conducted to detect convalescent antibody levels after 2-4 weeks. Positive antibody levels in the convalescent stage confirm the infection for some species of *Ehrlichia* and/or *Anaplasma* at disease onset. It should be noted that the administration of doxycycline will take effect over days and weeks; therefore, it will have no impact on the production of antibodies or the seroconversion [90,168-171].

Do serological cross reactions exist among *E. canis*, *A. phagocytophilum*, and *A. platys*?

It is generally accepted that no important cross reaction exists between *Ehrlichia* and *Anaplasma*. However, a potential cross reaction has been described between *E. canis* and *A. phagocytophilum*, particularly when one of the pathogens is present at very high titers or when the follow up is prolonged [37,165]. Apparently, there is no serological cross reaction between *E. canis* and *A. platys*; however, only a few, limited serologic studies have investigated this possibility [172].

When antibodies cross-react with more than one antigen/pathogen, the antibody titers that are highest indicate the most probable infecting pathogen in the dog [37]. However, a cross reaction was described between *A. phagocytophilum* and *A. platys* [37,173]. Moreover, *A. phagocytophilum* might cross react with other non-ehrlichial species (e.g., *Coxiella burnettii*) [54,145]. As serological cross reactions may occur between different *Ehrlichia* and *Anaplasma* species, the serology should be complemented with molecular techniques, such as PCR and DNA sequencing.

Why is a polymerase chain reaction assay useful in the diagnosis of these diseases?

PCR is very useful in diagnosing these infectious diseases for several reasons. First, PCR detection is more sensitive than a direct microscopic examination. Second, the detection of DNA for a specific pathogen in a clinical setting should be considered evidence of an active infection. Third, real-time PCR permits quantification of bacterial loads. Finally, PCR allows one to investigate specific gene fragments after amplification. Sequencing the gene fragment/s amplified by PCR may reveal the identification of the specific *Ehrlichia*/*Anaplasma* species that infected the dog.

Real-time PCR assays that were developed for detecting infections of *Ehrlichia* or *Anaplasma* in peripheral blood have provided high sensitivity, similar to the sensitivity previously obtained with splenic samples [169,174]. Several third-party laboratories provide various PCR assays for detecting *Ehrlichia* and/or *Anaplasma* spp. However, the results depend on the experience and quality of the laboratory. The use of non-specific primers and low annealing temperatures in some PCR assays can result in non-specific amplification; thus, the evaluation may provide misleading, false-positive results.

Finally, it must be kept in mind that false-negative results can also occur due to the absence of pathogens in the sample. For example, bacteremia may be intermittent in some dogs or in specific diseases (e.g., *A. platys*infection); it may be present below the minimal detection level of the assay [174,175]; or it may be absent, due to previous administration of antibiotics, such as doxycycline. Therefore, a negative PCR result should be interpreted as "no detection of the tested pathogen-DNA in the sample", rather than "the sample is free of the tested pathogen". Thus, to improve the usefulness of PCR and obtain as much information as possible from the results, it is important to submit samples to reliable laboratories and to assess the results in combination with an evaluation of antibody titers, clinical signs, and abnormal laboratory findings.

What samples should be chosen to perform a molecular diagnosis of *Ehrlichia* and/or *Anaplasma* spp. infections?

The sample of choice for a PCR assay is peripheral blood, buffered with EDTA. Some studies have suggested that splenic aspirates seem to be optimal specimens for the diagnosis of *E. canis* infections based on PCR [176]. When microscopic examination reveals structures suggestive of morulae in the cytoplasm of neutrophils or mononuclear cells in any tissue or fluid, PCR can be used to corroborate the diagnosis.

Are coinfections common in dogs infected with Ehrlichia and/or Anaplasma spp.?

Coinfections with *Ehrlichia* and/or *Anaplasma* spp. are common, because some species are transmitted in the same arthropod vector [145,177]. Accordingly, coinfection of *E. canis* with *A. platys* should occur frequently.

Currently, many other vector-borne diseases have been shown to coexist in the same dog, including other tick-borne pathogens (*Babesia* and *Hepatozoon* spp.), Culicidae mosquito-borne pathogens (*Dirofilaria* and other filariae), sand fly-borne pathogens (*Leishmania infantum*) [33,162], and even intestinal parasites [178]. In the Mediterranean basin, the most common coinfecting agents are *L. infantum* and *Babesia* spp. Less common are coinfections with *Hepatozoon* spp.

Due to the shared arthropod vectors and/or concurrent exposure to multiple vector-carrying ticks, co-infections may occur with other tick-borne pathogens (e.g., *Borrelia*, *Bartonella*, *Rickettsia*, *Babesia*, and arboviral spp.), which can complicate the clinical picture [179]. Because *Borrelia burgdorferi* and *A. phagocytophilum* are transmitted by the same ixodid tick species, coinfections with these two pathogens are frequently detected. Moreover, the two organisms may enhance one another's pathogenicity [180]. In northern California, dogs that are seroreactive to *A. phagocytophilum* were 18 times more likely to be seropositive for *Bartonella vinsonii* subs. *berkhoffii* than dogs seronegative for *A. phagocytophilum* [181].

What is the clinical significance of a coinfection during the course of the disease?

Coinfections tend to worsen some conditions and mask others, which could complicate the diagnosis [131]. Most vector-borne diseases have the special feature of causing similar clinical signs and abnormal laboratory findings in dogs (e.g., epistaxis and uveitis are signs that can be due to ehrlichiosis and/or leishmaniosis). This similarity complicates the diagnosis and increases the list of differential diagnoses. In one study, a coinfection with CME and *Leishmania* sp. delayed clinical improvement compared to dogs with either CME or leishmaniosis alone [182]. In another study, more clinical signs were noticed in dogs with dual infections (*E. canis* and *L. infantum*), which supported the notion that the pathogens may have synergistic pathological effects [183]. Furthermore, the occurrence of *A. platys* together with other infectious agents (e.g., *E. canis*, *Babesia vogeli*, or *Rickettsia conorii)* may potentiate the clinical disease and the laboratory abnormalities [54,66,90].

Therefore, when an infection of one specific species is diagnosed, a comprehensive work-up is necessary to rule out coinfections with other vector-borne pathogens [177].

What is the treatment of choice for *Ehrlichia* spp. and *Anaplasma* spp. infections?

Ehrlichia canis

CME is usually successfully treated with antibiotics that belong to the tetracycline family. The treatment of choice is doxycycline at 5 mg/kg twice daily or 10 mg/kg once daily for 4 weeks. This regime guarantees a complete response in the majority of cases [125,168,176]. Some reports described experimentally infected dogs that remained infected and became subclinical carriers after shorter treatments with doxycycline, even at the recommended doses [125,166,170]. Therefore, the more prolonged treatment of 4 weeks is recommended.

Although clinical improvement is achieved in most cases, it can be difficult to ensure treatment effectiveness regarding the total elimination of *Ehrlichia* spp. in naturally infected dogs. The clinician should not target seronegativity with treatment, but rather, negative PCR results [6,142,166,168].

Doxycycline, unlike other tetracyclines, does not seem to cause enamel discoloration in puppies. Moreover, one of the most common side effects of tetracyclines, vomiting, can be eliminated by splitting the antibiotic dose into two half-doses every 12 h (q12h) or by administering the antibiotic after feeding. When the dog has liver problems, the use of doxycycline should be reconsidered. In any case, liver function tests should be performed before and during treatment; when liver parameters increase, the treatment regime should be stopped [6,142,166,168].

Other drugs have been historically used for treating CME. Chloramphenicol has been used in dogs under 1 year of age, but its use is not recommended when doxycycline is available. Imidocarb dipropionate has also been described as a potential treatment for ehrlichiosis in dogs [171,184,185]. Recent studies performed *in vitro* and in experimentally infected dogs showed that imidocarb dipropionate was not effective against *E. canis* [186,187]. It should only be used in cases of co-infection with *Babesia canis* or *Hepatozoon canis*. Other antibiotics, such as rifampicin or levofloxacin, have been effective in *in vitro* studies [188]. However, recent studies have shown that, in experimental infections, rifampicin contributed to improving laboratory findings, but it was not effective in eliminating the infection [189].

A. phagocytophilum

Doxycycline (for 2-3 weeks) at the dosage described above for *E. canis* is apparently effective in treating *A. phagocytophilum* infections. However, several parameters remain to be established, including the most effective or optimal dose; the length of doxycycline treatment; and the value of adding other antibiotics [145,146,174,175,190]. Rifampin and levofloxacin have also shown *in vitro* effects against *A. phagocytophilum*[190]. Chloramphenicol has been mentioned as an alternative for treating puppies [191].

When dogs with circulating *Anaplasma* organisms have moderate to severe clinical disease or do not rapidly respond to doxycycline therapy, they should probably be tested for other tick-borne diseases [146].

Anaplasma platys

Anaplasma platys infections can be treated with tetracyclines (e.g., doxycycline 5-10 mg/kg q12-24h for 8-10 days). Alternatively, they can be treated with enrofloxacin at 5 mg/kg, q12h for 14-21 days [131,192].

Are there other supportive therapies that could be used for ehrlichiosis and/or anaplasmosis?

In severe or chronic ehrlichiosis and/or anaplasmosis, other therapeutic agents or treatments may be needed, particularly for *E. canis* infections. For cases with hemorrhage or organic lesions, the dog may require admission to a hospital for a more intensive treatment. In general, according to the seriousness determined in the clinic, dogs may need blood transfusions when the packed cell volume (PCV) is very low; fluid therapy when dehydration or secondary kidney disease is present; or antipyretic and analgesic drugs [138,142,146].

In some cases of chronic ehrlichiosis, when aplasia of all cell lines occurs, other treatments have been used. For example, growth factors, like granulocyte colony stimulating factor or erythropoietin have been used; however, scientific evidence of effectiveness is scarce. One case of chronic ehrlichiosis was treated successfully with a combination of hematopoietic growth factors, low dose vincristine, doxycycline, and glucocorticoids [193].

Is it necessary to use steroids for treating ehrlichiosis and/or anaplasmosis?

Treatment of ehrlichiosis or anaplasmosis should not be initiated with glucocorticoids combined with antibiotics. Steroids should only be considered when no satisfactory response is noticed, or when immune-mediated complications arise. *Ehrlichia* and *Anaplasma* species may mediate an immune response, typically indicated by hemolytic anemia, thrombocytopenia, uveitis, glomerulonephritis, vasculitis, etc. In those cases, treatment with glucocorticoids (usually prednisone or prednisolone) may be indicated; doses of prednisone should range from 0.5 to 2 mg/kg/day, and the treatment duration should vary according to the type and seriousness of the associated immune-mediated condition [133,147,152,194-196]. However, the use of immunosuppressive glucocorticoids for treatment of secondary immune-mediated diseases must be considered very carefully. Of note, the administration of immunosuppressive doses of glucocorticoids or other drugs to subclinically infected dogs may result in the re-emergence of bacteremia, although the dog may not show clinical signs [6,129,142,174,175].

What is the expected clinical response following the treatment of ehrlichiosis and/or anaplasmosis?

Doxycycline is an effective drug against ehrlichiosis and/or anaplasmosis in dogs [120,145,146]. When dogs are treated in the acute phase of ehrlichiosis and anaplasmosis, they improve quickly, within 24-48 h, and their prognosis is good when the whole course of therapy is administered [120,147,197].

However, the prognosis of dogs with the chronic severe form of ehrlichiosis is grave [120,197]. Shipov and colleagues (2008) investigated prognostic indicators for mortality and survival in canine ehrlichiosis [198]. They found that pronounced pancytopenia (white blood cells [WBC] $<4 \times 10^3/\mu L$; PCV<25%; and platelet concentration [PLT] $<50 \times 10^3/\mu L$) was a risk factor for mortality. In that study, they found that severe leucopenia (WBC $<0.93 \times 10^3/\mu L$), severe anemia (PCV<11.5%), prolonged activated partial thromboplastin time (APTT>18.25 s), and hypokalemia (K<3.65 mmol/L) could each predict mortality with a probability of 100%. Conversely, a WBC $>5.18 \times 10^3/\mu L$, PLT $>89.5 \times 10^3/\mu L$, PCV>33.5%, APTT<14.5 s, or K>4.75 mmol/L could each predict survival with a probability of 100%.

When the clinical response in canine ehrlichiosis or anaplasmosis is not rapid, or when clinical signs persist after treatment with doxycycline, the dog must be re-examined for other infectious diseases or diseases with similar clinical signs (neoplasia or immune-mediated diseases) [6,142,146].

How do abnormal laboratory findings evolve in dogs infected with ehrlichiosis/anaplasmosis after the treatment?

Ehrlichia canis

Laboratory abnormalities in canine ehrlichiosis typically resolve in dogs after treatment with acute disease. In general, both the complete blood count and the alterations in serum protein electrophoresis should normalize within 10-15 days after therapy initiation [6,142].

Chronic changes, such as mild or moderate hyperglobulinemia, anemia, or thrombocytopenia may persist as long as the infectious agent has not been completely eliminated, or when some other associated conditions exist [171]. In naturally infected dogs, despite evident clinical improvement, it is difficult to guarantee treatment effectiveness and complete elimination of the involved pathogens [6,142]. When the dog no longer produces specific antibodies to the pathogen, it can be assumed that complete elimination of the *Ehrlichia*species has been achieved [120].

Quantification of acute phase proteins in serum has been assessed for its value in monitoring and evaluating the prognosis of dogs with ehrlichiosis. Although quantification of acute phase proteins may be a useful indicator of the clinical stage, it has no predictive value for the final clinical outcome [199].

Finally, it must be recognized that prior infections with *E. canis* do not confer permanent immunity to dogs. Therefore, dogs can be re-infected with the same pathogen or with other species after re-exposure to infected ticks [6,142].

Anaplasma phagocytophilum

Similar to canine ehrlichiosis, after treating anaplasmosis, laboratory alterations in the complete blood cell count and in serum protein electrophoresis should be resolved in most dogs [146,147].

Anaplasma platys

Thrombocytopenia in dogs infected with *A. platys* typically disappears around one week after starting therapy [192].

How do antibody titers evolve following treatment?

Ehrlichia canis

Antibody titers may persist for months. Then, in most *E. canis* infections, they decrease gradually over 6-9 months post treatment. Sometimes, antibodies are no longer detectable at 12 months. However, frequently, some cases remain seropositive for several years after the treatment [194], particularly when starting with very high antibody titers [171].

Anaplasma phagocytophilum

Information regarding the persistence of *A. phagocytophilum* antibody titers is limited. However, some studies have described persistence of seropositivity for up to one year after the treatment [200].

Anaplasma platys

Information regarding antibody titers in dogs naturally infected with *A. platys* is scarce. A steady decline of antibody titers after therapy has been described in dogs experimentally infected with *A. platys* [90].

Why is PCR useful after treatment?

PCR testing, when conducted several weeks after termination of doxycycline treatment, allows clinicians to be more confident that the treatment has been effective and that the dog did not enter the subclinical stage [6,142,146,186,201]. Yet, it must be recognized that a negative PCR result does not guarantee that the animal is "free of infection" (see above).

There are two goals for performing PCR some weeks after the completion of treatment. One is to minimize the probability of obtaining false-negative results, due to antibiotic effects on bacteremia. The second is to minimize the chance of detecting DNA of dead pathogens that continue to circulate during the treatment period [6,132,142,174,175].

In conclusion, PCR is useful for monitoring dogs treated for these diseases, because it can detect the presence of pathogen DNA, regardless of the serologic antibody titers. However, although this technique is more sensitive than serology in confirming an infection, its effectiveness may be limited for detecting pathogens in subclinically infected dogs, because the organisms may circulate intermittently in peripheral blood. Therefore, a PCR analysis should not be considered a definitive method for conclusively excluding subclinical infection in clinically normal dogs that remain seropositive after treatment [6,142,145,146].

Can canine ehrlichiosis and/or anaplasmosis be cured?

In general, most acutely ill dogs infected with *Ehrlichia* or *Anaplasma* species heal after a specific, effective treatment of appropriate length. This finding has been corroborated with multiple clinical and experimental trials [166,168,170]. However, a recent work conducted with dogs experimentally infected with *E. canis*suggested that some dogs may remain persistently infected and may not eliminate the infection even after acceptable treatment [125].

Can dogs be re-infected by *Ehrlichia* and/or *Anaplasma* spp.?

Ehrlichia canis

Re-infections of canine ehrlichiosis are possible, because no persistent or effective immunity develops to defend against re-infection with these pathogens [120]. In most cases, after treatment, the dogs return to the habitat they lived in prior to the infection; therefore, their exposure to infected ticks remains feasible. When no proper tick-control measures are employed, and the dogs are re-exposed, they can easily become re-infected. Moreover, mainly in cases of canine ehrlichiosis, it is difficult to distinguish a re-infection from recurrence of an established persistent subclinical condition [177].

Anaplasma phagocytophilum

It is not known whether a natural infection can provide long term protection against the development of clinical anaplasmosis. Re-infection following the therapeutic elimination of the organism has not been reported in dogs; however, in human medicine, one re-infection case was documented [202]. Conversely, horses have been shown to resist re-infection after recovery from an initial infection with *A. phagocytophilum*[200].

Anaplasma platys

The possibility of *A. platys* re-infections in dogs living in endemic areas and exposed to ticks has not been fully evaluated, but cannot be ruled out.

What prophylactic measures can be implemented to prevent infection by *Ehrlichia* and/or *Anaplasma* spp. in dogs?

The prevention of ehrlichiosis and/or anaplasmosis infections in dogs must be focused on tick control. Ticks of the *R. sanguineus* complex are mainly found indoors, but other populations of the tick may be common in gardens, pastures, and fields in the Mediterranean basin. Therefore, dogs may become infected with the most common tick present in infested private gardens or kennels, but also, whenever they are engaged in an activity that involves contact with natural green areas. Nevertheless, to prevent transmission, actions must focus mainly on:

- preventing dogs from becoming infested in the field, which is the source of peridomestic parasitism. This infestation can introduce ticks to indoor habitats (kennels, etc.), which will result in a large population, due to their high reproductive capacity.
- preventing dogs from becoming infested with ticks, even when they live in a peridomestic environment with abundant ticks. This objective is more difficult to achieve than the former, due to the high parasitism pressure that can arise from those populations of ticks [203].

To appropriately control tick infestations in dogs requires knowledge of tick seasonality. This seasonality is usually strict under natural conditions, and each stage of the life cycle of the tick follows the previous stage with regularity. However, these patterns can be lost in areas with large infestations in a peridomestic environment. Under those conditions, all stages can be active simultaneously, due to the presence of several infestations in the kennel.

Outdoor populations of *R. sanguineus* can be active and, therefore infest dogs, when the average temperature is 10-12°C. Below this temperature, it is very rare that dogs acquire infestations from outdoor populations of that tick; consequently, during winter, it may be appropriate to reduce the treatment pressure against ticks. However, it must be noted that indoor populations of the ticks may be active year round, which adds extra risk for dogs living in kennels or dogs that spend time in dog day care centers. In Europe, tick control should be continuous between spring and autumn in areas where ticks are present. This pattern may vary according to the local weather and the historic weather particularities. Clearly, measures against *R. sanguineus* must follow extended schedules in the Mediterranean basin, because winters are shorter, and therefore, the periods of *R. sanguineus* activity are prolonged.

In the case of *I. ricinus*, the activation temperature for the ticks may be around 6°C. Therefore, adequate measures of control should be strictly followed to limit contact of dogs with ticks in infested areas [72].

Various antiparasitic treatments are registered in Europe that have activity against ticks and can be prescribed for dogs [204]. The specific product can be selected according to the preferences of use (collar, pour-on, or spot on) and the therapeutic needs for each case. Some compounds, such as the pyrethroids or some preparations of diazinon, are registered as repellents.

Apart from appropriate epidemiological measures, the best prevention against dog tick infestation is based on the use of ectoparasiticides. In general, these are active molecules that act against ticks, and they must also provide some degree of appropriate control within a short period of time [205]. Rapid action could contribute to the elimination of attached ticks before they are able to transmit pathogens. To optimize efficacy, preventive chemicals must be applied at the recommended time intervals, based on the length of efficacy claimed by the manufacturer. Although knowledge may be lacking for some diseases, most tick-borne pathogens require 4 to 48 h to complete their development in the salivary gland and enter the bloodstream [100]. However, a recent report showed that transmission of *E. canis* can occur within shorter periods of time (e.g., 3 h) [71].

Are there vaccines available to prevent ehrlichiosis and/or anaplasmosis in dogs?

Currently, no commercial vaccines are available to protect against infections with *E. canis*, *A. phagocytophilum*, or *A. platys*. A recent study showed that an attenuated *E. canis* strain may serve as an effective future vaccine for CME [206].

CONCLUSIONS

Information on canine ehrlichiosis and anaplasmosis in Europe has significantly increased in the last few years. This guideline aimed to answer common questions of interest on the etiology, transmission, epidemiology, clinical signs, laboratory findings, diagnosis, therapy, and prophylaxis of infections caused by *Ehrlichia* and *Anaplasma* spp. This guideline contributes to the understanding of the current status of these diseases on the European continent. However, these pathogens are spreading to new niches, and reports have described infections in many countries where they were not detected previously.

DECLARATIONS

Acknowledgements

The authors would like to acknowledge Merial Laboratorios (Spain), the sponsor of the manuscript publication, and we extend special thanks to Marta León for providing assistance.

Competing interests

Five authors of this guideline (AS, XR, GM, AEP and LSG) are members of the ENTRA group. The ENTRA group is supported by Merial Laboratorios (Spain), but it is a scientifically independent body.

Authors' contributions

AS, XR, GM, AEP, and LSG designed the initial structure of the guideline, and wrote the first version of the manuscript. BK reviewed the manuscript and made substantial contributions to the structure and content, particularly parts related to *A. phagocytophilum* infections. SH reviewed the manuscript and made substantial contributions to the structure and content, particularly parts related to *E. canis* and *A. platys* infections. AS participated as the coordinator of the group. All authors read and approved the final manuscript.

Authors' information

About the ENTRA group

The ENTRA group (abbreviation in Spanish for "*Grupo de Estudio de Enfermedades Transmitidas por Artrópodos*" – Arthropod-Borne Disease Experts Group) is composed of Spanish veterinary scientists, whose careers have focused on research on arthropods and arthropod-borne diseases.

The main goal of this group is to process and report the most significant information on this variety of diseases. This work is deemed useful for small animal veterinary practitioners. Based on those premises, the ENTRA group decided to publish a practical guideline regarding ehrlichiosis and anaplasmosis in dogs, given the high prevalence rates described in Spain and the multiple studies recently conducted on these diseases in that country. Subsequently, the group decided that this guideline could have greater relevance by broadening the scope to the European continent. Consequently, we invited other European scientists working on these diseases to participate in this project. This guideline was the result of a complete review of the literature. The experience of all the authors has been included, and a consensus among them was reached.

The questions included in this document are intended to address the most common concerns about these diseases, and we provided answers from a practical point of view.

The authors Member of ENTRA group are Ángel Sainz, Xavier Roura, Guadalupe Miró, Agustín Estrada-Peña and Laia Solano-Gallego.

REFERENCES

1. Donatien A, Lestoquard F. Existence en Algerie d'une Rickettsia du chien. Bull Soc Pathol Exot. 1935;28:418–9.
2. Huxsoll DL, Hildebrandt PK, Nims RM, Walker JS. Tropical canine pancytopenia. J Am Vet Med Assoc. 1970;157(11):1627–32.
3. Harvey JW, Simpson CF, Gaskin JM. Cyclic thrombocytopenia induced by a Rickettsia-like agent in dogs. J Infect Dis. 1978;137(2):182–8.
4. Madewell BR, Gribble DH. Infection in two dogs with an agent resembling Ehrlichia equi. J Am Vet Med Assoc. 1982;180(5):512–4.
5. Dumler JS, Barbet AF, Bekker CP, Dasch GA, Palmer GH, Ray SC, et al. Reorganization of genera in the families Rickettsiaceae and Anaplasmataceae in the order Rickettsiales: unification of some species of Ehrlichia with Anaplasma, Cowdria with Ehrlichia and Ehrlichia with Neorickettsia, descriptions of six new species combinations and designation of Ehrlichia equi and 'HGE agent' as subjective synonyms of Ehrlichia phagocytophila. Int J Syst Evol Microbiol. 2001;51(Pt 6):2145–65.
6. Neer TM, Breitschwerdt EB, Greene RT, Lappin MR. Consensus statement on ehrlichial disease of small animals from the infectious disease study group of the ACVIM. American College of Veterinary Internal Medicine. J Vet Intern Med. 2002;16(3):309–15.
7. Keysary A, Waner T, Rosner M, Warner CK, Dawson JE, Zass R, et al. The first isolation, in vitro propagation, and genetic characterization of Ehrlichia canis in Israel. Vet Parasitol. 1996;62(3–4):331–40.
8. Aguirre E, Sainz A, Dunner S, Amusategui I, Lopez L, Rodriguez-Franco F, et al. First isolation and molecular characterization of Ehrlichia canis in Spain. Vet Parasitol. 2004;125(3–4):365–72.
9. Shpynov SN, Fournier PE, Rudakov NV, Samoilenko IE, Reshetnikova TA, Yastrebov VK, et al. Molecular identification of a collection of spotted Fever group rickettsiae obtained from patients and ticks from Russia. Am J Trop Med Hyg. 2006;74(3):440–3.
10. Spitalska E, Boldis V, Kostanova Z, Kocianova E, Stefanidesova K. Incidence of various tick-borne microorganisms in rodents and ticks of Slovakia. Acta Virol. 2008;52(3):175–9.
11. Dongus H, Zahler M. Gothe R: [The brown dog tick, Rhipicephalus sanguineus (Ixodidae), in Germany: an epidemiologic study and control measures]. Berl Munch Tierarztl Wochenschr. 1996;109(6–7):245–8.
12. Gothe R. [Ehrlichia canis infections of dogs in Germany. Epidemiology, diagnosis, therapy and prophylaxis]. Tierarztl Prax Ausg K Kleintiere Heimtiere. 1998;26(6):396–401.
13. Pusterla N, Pusterla JB, Deplazes P, Wolfensberger C, Muller W, Horauf A, et al. Seroprevalence of Ehrlichia canis and of canine granulocytic Ehrlichia infection in dogs in Switzerland. J Clin Microbiol. 1998;36(12):3460–2.
14. Hamel D, Silaghi C, Knaus M, Visser M, Kusi I, Rapti D, et al. Detection of Babesia canis subspecies and other arthropod-borne diseases in dogs from Tirana, Albania. Wien Klin Wochenschr. 2009;121 Suppl 3:42–5.
15. Perez Vera C, Kapiainen S, Junnikkala S, Aaltonen K, Spillmann T, Vapalahti O. Survey of selected tick-borne diseases in dogs in Finland. Parasit Vectors. 2014;7:285.
16. Pantchev N, Schaper R, Limousin S, Norden N, Weise M, Lorentzen L. Occurrence of Dirofilaria immitis and tick-borne infections caused by Anaplasma phagocytophilum, Borrelia burgdorferi sensu lato and Ehrlichia canis in domestic dogs in France: results of a countrywide serologic survey. Parasitol Res. 2009;105 Suppl 1:S101–14.
17. Hamel D, Silaghi C, Pfister K. Arthropod-borne infections in travelled dogs in Europe. Parasite. 2013;20:9.
18. Hamel D, Rohrig E, Pfister K. Canine vector-borne disease in travelled dogs in Germany–a retrospective evaluation of laboratory data from the years 2004–2008. Vet Parasitol. 2011;181(1):31–6.
19. Menn B, Lorentz S, Naucke TJ. Imported and travelling

dogs as carriers of canine vector-borne pathogens in Germany. Parasit Vectors. 2010;3:34.

20. Farkas R, Gyurkovszky M, Lukacs Z, Aladics B, Solymosi N. Seroprevalence of some vector-borne infections of dogs in Hungary. Vector Borne Zoonotic Dis. 2014;14(4):256–60.
21. Pennisi MG, Capri A, Solano-Gallego L, Lombardo G, Torina A, Masucci M. Prevalence of antibodies against Rickettsia conorii, Babesia canis, Ehrlichia canis, and Anaplasma phagocytophilum antigens in dogs from the Stretto di Messina area (Italy). Ticks Tick Borne Dis. 2012;3(5–6):315–8.
22. Trotta M, Fogliazza A, Furlanello T, Solano-Gallego L. A molecular and serological study of exposure to tick-borne pathogens in sick dogs from Italy. Clin Microbiol Infect. 2009;15 Suppl 2:62–3.
23. Torina A, Vicente J, Alongi A, Scimeca S, Turla R, Nicosia S, et al. Observed prevalence of tick-borne pathogens in domestic animals in Sicily, Italy during 2003-2005. Zoonoses Public Health. 2007;54(1):8–15.
24. Corrain R, Di Francesco A, Bolognini M, Ciucci P, Baldelli R, Guberti V. Serosurvey for CPV-2, distemper virus, ehrlichiosis and leishmaniosis in free-ranging dogs in Italy. Vet Rec. 2007;160(3):91–2.
25. Solano-Gallego L, Trotta M, Razia L, Furlanello T, Caldin M. Molecular survey of Ehrlichia canis and Anaplasma phagocytophilum from blood of dogs in Italy. Ann N Y Acad Sci. 2006;1078:515–8.
26. Cocco R, Sanna G, Cillara MG, Tola S, Ximenes L, Pinnaparpaglia ML, et al. Ehrlichiosis and rickettsiosis in a canine population of Northern Sardinia. Ann N Y Acad Sci. 2003;990:126–30.
27. Buonavoglia D, Sagazio P, Gravino EA, De Caprariis D, Cerundolo R, Buonavoglia C. Serological evidence of Ehrlichia canis in dogs in southern Italy. New Microbiol. 1995;18(1):83–6.
28. Cardoso L, Mendao C. Madeira de Carvalho L: Prevalence of Dirofilaria immitis, Ehrlichia canis, Borrelia burgdorferi sensu lato, Anaplasma spp. and Leishmania infantum in apparently healthy and CVBD-suspect dogs in Portugal--a national serological stud. Parasit Vectors. 2012;5:62.
29. Alexandre N, Santos AS, Nuncio MS, Sousa R, Boinas F, Bacellar F. Detection of Ehrlichia canis by polymerase chain reaction in dogs from Portugal. Vet J. 2009;181(3):343–4.
30. Bacellar F, Dawson JE, Silveira CA, Filipe AR. Antibodies against Rickettsiaceae in dogs of Setubal. Portugal Cent Eur J Public Health. 1995;3(2):100–2.
31. Mircean V, Dumitrache MO, Gyorke A, Pantchev N, Jodies R, Mihalca AD, et al. Seroprevalence and geographic distribution of Dirofilaria immitis and tick-borne infections (Anaplasma phagocytophilum, Borrelia burgdorferi sensu lato, and Ehrlichia canis) in dogs from Romania. Vector Borne Zoonotic Dis. 2012;12(7):595–604.
32. Volgina NS, Romashov BV, Romashova NB, Shtannikov AV. Prevalence of borreliosis, anaplasmosis, ehrlichiosis and Dirofilaria immitis in dogs and vectors in Voronezh Reserve (Russia). Comp Immunol Microbiol Infect Dis. 2013;36(6):567–74.
33. Miro G, Montoya A, Roura X, Galvez R, Sainz A. Seropositivity rates for agents of canine vector-borne diseases in Spain: a multicentre study. Parasit Vectors. 2013;6:117.
34. Couto CG, Lorentzen L, Beall MJ, Shields J, Bertolone N, Couto JI, et al. Serological study of selected vector-borne diseases in shelter dogs in Spain using point-of-care assays. Vector Borne Zoonotic Dis. 2010;10(9):885–8.
35. Tabar MD, Francino O, Altet L, Sanchez A, Ferrer L, Roura X. PCR survey of vectorborne pathogens in dogs living in and around Barcelona, an area endemic for leishmaniasis. Vet Rec. 2009;164(4):112–6.
36. Amusategui I, Tesouro MA, Kakoma I, Sainz A. Serological reactivity to Ehrlichia canis, Anaplasma phagocytophilum, Neorickettsia risticii, Borrelia burgdorferi and Rickettsia conorii in dogs from northwestern Spain. Vector Borne Zoonotic Dis. 2008;8(6):797–803.
37. Solano-Gallego L, Llull J, Osso M, Hegarty B, Breitschwerdt E. A serological study of exposure to arthropod-borne pathogens in dogs from northeastern Spain. Vet Res. 2006;37(2):231–44.
38. Sainz A, Amusategui I, Tesouro MA. Canine ehrlichiosis in the Comunidad de Madrid in Spain. Ann N Y Acad Sci. 1998;849:438–40.
39. Sainz A, Delgado S, Amusategui I, Tesouro MA, Carmenes P. Seroprevalence of canine ehrlichiosis in Castilla-Leon north-west Spain. Prev Vet Med. 1996;29(1):1–7.
40. Batmaz H, Nevo E, Waner T, Senturk S, Yilmaz Z, Harrus S. Seroprevalence of Ehrlichia canis antibodies among dogs in Turkey. Vet Rec. 2001;148(21):665–6.
41. Kirtz B, Czettel B, Thum D, et al. Anaplasma phagozytophilum in einer österreichischen Hundepopulation: eine Prävalenz-Studie (2001-2006). Kleintierpraxis. 2007;52:562–8.
42. Barutzki D, De Nicola A, Zeziola M. Reule M: [Seroprevalence of Anaplasma phagocytophilum infection in dogs in Germany]. Berl Munch Tierarztl Wochenschr. 2006;119(7–8):342–7.
43. Jensen J, Simon D, Murua Escobar H, Soller JT, Bullerdiek J, Beelitz P, et al. Anaplasma phagocytophilum in dogs in Germany. Zoonoses Public Health. 2007;54(2):94–101.
44. Schaarschmidt-Kiener D, Müller W. Labordiagnostische und klinische Aspekte der caninen Anaplasmose und Ehrlichiose. Tierarztl Prax. 2007;35:129–36.
45. Krupka I, Pantchev N, Lorentzen L, Weise M, Straubinger RK. Tick-transmitted, bacterial infections in dogs: seroprevalences of Anaplasma phagocytophilum, Borrelia burgdorferi sensu lato and Ehrlichia canis in Germany. Prakt Tierarzt. 2007;88(10):776–88.
46. Kohn B, Silaghi C, Galke D, Arndt G, Pfister K. Infections with Anaplasma phagocytophilum in dogs in Germany. Res Vet Sci. 2011;91(1):71–6.

47. Barth C, Straubinger RK, Sauter-Louis C, Hartmann K. Prevalence of antibodies against Borrelia burgdorferi sensu lato and Anaplasma phagocytophilum and their clinical relevance in dogs in Munich, Germany. Berl Munch Tierarztl Wochenschr. 2012;125(7–8):337–44.

48. de la Fuente J, Torina A, Naranjo V, Nicosia S, Alongi A, La Mantia F, et al. Molecular characterization of Anaplasma platys strains from dogs in Sicily, Italy. BMC Vet Res. 2006;2:24.

49. Torina A, Caracappa S. Dog tick-borne diseases in Sicily. Parassitologia. 2006;48(1–2):145–7.

50. Ebani V, Cerri D, Fratini F, Ampola M, Andreani E. Seroprevalence of Anaplasma phagocytophilum in domestic and wild animals from Italy. New Microbiol. 2008;31(3):371–5.

51. Ebani VV, Bertelloni F, Turchi B, Cerri D. Serological and molecular survey of Anaplasma phagocytophilum in Italian hunting dogs. Ann Agric Environ Med. 2013;20(2):289–92.

52. Berzina I, Matise I. Seroprevalence against Borrelia burgdorferi sensu lato and occurence of antibody co-expression with Anaplasma phagocytophilum in dogs in Latvia. Ir Vet J. 2013;66(1):9.

53. Skotarczak B, Adamska M, Rymaszewska A, Supron M, Sawczuk M. Maciejewska A: [Anaplasma phagocytophila and protozoans of Babesia genus in dogs from endemic areas of Lyme disease in north-western Poland]. Wiad Parazytol. 2004;50(3):555–61.

54. Santos AS, Alexandre N, Sousa R, Nuncio MS, Bacellar F, Dumler JS. Serological and molecular survey of Anaplasma species infection in dogs with suspected tickborne disease in Portugal. Vet Rec. 2009;164(6):168–71.

55. Egenvall A, Bonnett BN, Gunnarsson A, Hedhammar A, Shoukri M, Bornstein S, et al. Sero-prevalence of granulocytic Ehrlichia spp. and Borrelia burgdorferi sensu lato in Swedish dogs 1991-94. Scand J Infect Dis. 2000;32(1):19–25.

56. Jaderlund KH, Egenvall A, Bergstrom K, Hedhammar A. Seroprevalence of Borrelia burgdorferi sensu lato and Anaplasma phagocytophilum in dogs with neurological signs. Vet Rec. 2007;160(24):825–31.

57. Shaw SE, Binns SH, Birtles RJ, Day MJ, Smithson R, Kenny MJ. Molecular evidence of tick-transmitted infections in dogs and cats in the United Kingdom. Vet Rec. 2005;157(21):645–8.

58. Aguirre E, Tesouro MA, Ruiz L, Amusategui I, Sainz A. Genetic characterization of Anaplasma (Ehrlichia) platys in dogs in Spain. J Vet Med B Infect Dis Vet Public Health. 2006;53(4):197–200.

59. Cardoso L, Tuna J, Vieira L, Yisaschar-Mekuzas Y, Baneth G. Molecular detection of Anaplasma platys and Ehrlichia canis in dogs from the North of Portugal. Vet J. 2010;183(2):232–3.

60. Beaufils JP, Inokuma H, Martin-Granel J, Jumelle P, Barbault-Jumelle M, Brouqui P. *Anaplasma platys* (*Ehrlichia platys*) infection in a dog in France: description of the case, and characterization of the agent. Rev Med Vet. 2002;153:85–90.

61. Ulutas B, Bayramli G, Karangec T. First case of Anaplasma (Ehrlichia) platys infection in a dog in Turkey. Turk J Vet Anim Sci. 2007;31:279–82.

62. Kontos VI, Papadopoulos O, French TW. Natural and experimental canine infections with a Greek strain of Ehrlichia platys. Vet Clin Pathol. 1991;20(4):101–5.

63. Dyachenko V, Pantchev N, Balzer HJ, Meyersen A, Straubinger RK. First case of Anaplasma platys infection in a dog from Croatia. Parasit Vectors. 2012;5:49.

64. Andersson M, Turcitu MA, Stefanache M, Tamba P, Barbuceanu F, Chitimia L. First evidence of Anaplasma platys and Hepatozoon canis co-infection in a dog from Romania–a case report. Ticks Tick Borne Dis. 2013;4(4):317–9.

65. Ramos RA, Latrofa MS, Giannelli A, Lacasella V, Campbell BE, Dantas-Torres F, et al. Detection of Anaplasma platys in dogs and Rhipicephalus sanguineus group ticks by a quantitative real-time PCR. Vet Parasitol. 2014;205(1-2):285–8.

66. de Caprariis D, Dantas-Torres F, Capelli G, Mencke N, Stanneck D, Breitschwerdt EB, et al. Evolution of clinical, haematological and biochemical findings in young dogs naturally infected by vector-borne pathogens. Vet Microbiol. 2011;149(1–2):206–12.

67. Otranto D, de Caprariis D, Lia RP, Tarallo V, Lorusso V, Testini G, et al. Prevention of endemic canine vector-borne diseases using imidacloprid 10% and permethrin 50% in young dogs: a longitudinal field study. Vet Parasitol. 2010;172(3–4):323–32.

68. Sparagano OA, de Vos AP, Paoletti B, Camma C, de Santis P, Otranto D, et al. Molecular detection of Anaplasma platys in dogs using polymerase chain reaction and reverse line blot hybridization. J Vet Diagn Invest. 2003;15(6):527–34.

69. Groves MG, Dennis GL, Amyx HL, Huxsoll DL. Transmission of Ehrlichia canis to dogs by ticks (Rhipicephalus sanguineus). Am J Vet Res. 1975;36(7):937–40.

70. Smith RD, Sells DM, Stephenson EH, Ristic MR, Huxsoll DL. Development of Ehrlichia canis, causative agent of canine ehrlichiosis, in the tick Rhipicephalus sanguineus and its differentiation from a symbiotic Rickettsia. Am J Vet Res. 1976;37(2):119–26.

71. Fourie JJ, Stanneck D, Luus HG, Beugnet F, Wijnveld M, Jongejan F. Transmission of Ehrlichia canis by Rhipicephalus sanguineus ticks feeding on dogs and on artificial membranes. Vet Parasitol. 2013;197(3–4):595–603.

72. Gray J, Dantas-Torres F, Estrada-Pena A, Levin M. Systematics and ecology of the brown dog tick, Rhipicephalus sanguineus. Ticks Tick Borne Dis. 2013;4(3):171–80.

73. Gray JS, Dautel H, Estrada-Pena A, Kahl O, Lindgren E. Effects of climate change on ticks and tick-borne diseases in europe. Interdiscip Perspect Infect Dis. 2009;2009:593232.

74. Uspensky I, Ioffe-Uspensky I. The dog factor in brown

dog tick Rhipicephalus sanguineus (Acari: Ixodidae) infestations in and near human dwellings. Int J Med Microbiol. 2002;291 Suppl 33:156–63.

75. Jaenson TG, Jaenson DG, Eisen L, Petersson E, Lindgren E. Changes in the geographical distribution and abundance of the tick Ixodes ricinus during the past 30 years in Sweden. Parasit Vectors. 2012;5:8.

76. Medlock JM, Hansford KM, Bormane A, Derdakova M, Estrada-Pena A, George JC, et al. Driving forces for changes in geographical distribution of Ixodes ricinus ticks in Europe. Parasit Vectors. 2013;6:1.

77. Estrada-Pena A, Farkas R, Jaenson TG, Koenen F, Madder M, Pascucci I, et al. Association of environmental traits with the geographic ranges of ticks (Acari: Ixodidae) of medical and veterinary importance in the western Palearctic. A digital data set. Exp Appl Acarol. 2013;59(3):351–66.

78. Yasyukevich VV, Kazakova EV, Popov IO, Semenov SM. Distribution of Ixodes ricinus L., 1758 and Ixodes persulcatus Shulze, 1930 (Parasitoformes, Ixodidae) in Russia and adjacent countries in view of observable climate changes. Dokl Earth Sci. 2009;427(2):1030–4.

79. Ecker M, Allison SL, Meixner T, Heinz FX. Sequence analysis and genetic classification of tick-borne encephalitis viruses from Europe and Asia. J Gen Virol. 1999;80(Pt 1):179–85.

80. Alekseev AN, Dubinina HV, Van De Pol I, Schouls LM. Identification of Ehrlichia spp. and Borrelia burgdorferi in Ixodes ticks in the Baltic regions of Russia. J Clin Microbiol. 2001;39(6):2237–42.

81. Hamel D, Silaghi C, Zapadynska S, Kudrin A, Pfister K. Vector-borne pathogens in ticks and EDTA-blood samples collected from client-owned dogs, Kiev. Ukraine Ticks Tick Borne Dis. 2013;4(1–2):152–5.

82. Movila A, Toderas I, Uspenskaia I, Conovalov J. Molecular detection of tick-borne pathogens in Ixodes ricinus from Moldova collected in 1960. Ticks Tick Borne Dis. 2013;4(4):359–61.

83. Simpson RM, Gaunt SD, Hair JA, Kocan KM, Henk WG, Casey HW. Evaluation of Rhipicephalus sanguineus as a potential biologic vector of Ehrlichia platys. Am J Vet Res. 1991;52(9):1537–41.

84. Sanogo YO, Davoust B, Inokuma H, Camicas JL, Parola P, Brouqui P. First evidence of Anaplasma platys in Rhipicephalus sanguineus (Acari: Ixodida) collected from dogs in Africa. Onderstepoort J Vet Res. 2003;70(3):205–12.

85. Johnson EM, Ewing SA, Barker RW, Fox JC, Crow DW, Kocan KM. Experimental transmission of Ehrlichia canis (Rickettsiales: Ehrlichieae) by Dermacentor variabilis (Acari: Ixodidae). Vet Parasitol. 1998;74(2–4):277–88.

86. McQuiston JH, Childs JE, Chamberland ME, Tabor E. Transmission of tick-borne agents of disease by blood transfusion: a review of known and potential risks in the United States. Transfusion. 2000;40(3):274–84.

87. Egenvall A, Bjoersdorff A, Lilliehook I, Olsson Engvall E, Karlstam E, Artursson K, et al. Early manifestations of granulocytic ehrlichiosis in dogs inoculated experimentally with a Swedish Ehrlichia species isolate. Vet Rec. 1998;143(15):412–7.

88. Wardrop KJ, Reine N, Birkenheuer A, Hale A, Hohenhaus A, Crawford C, et al. Canine and feline blood donor screening for infectious disease. J Vet Intern Med. 2005;19(1):135–42.

89. Kohn B. Anaplasma phagocytophilum in the dog – update on epidemiology and clinical disease. In: *Canine vector-borne disease world forum*. New York: Bayer HealthCare Animal Health; 2010. p. 36–43. *12-15 April*.

90. Gaunt S, Beall M, Stillman B, Lorentzen L, Diniz P, Chandrashekar R, et al. Experimental infection and co-infection of dogs with Anaplasma platys and Ehrlichia canis: hematologic, serologic and molecular findings. Parasit Vectors. 2010;3(1):33.

91. Ebani VV, Verin R, Fratini F, Poli A, Cerri D. Molecular survey of Anaplasma phagocytophilum and Ehrlichia canis in red foxes (Vulpes vulpes) from Italy. J Wildl Dis. 2011;47(3):699–703.

92. Fishman Z, Gonen L, Harrus S, Strauss-Ayali D, King R, Baneth G. A serosurvey of Hepatozoon canis and Ehrlichia canis antibodies in wild red foxes (Vulpes vulpes) from Israel. Vet Parasitol. 2004;119(1):21–6.

93. Torina A, Blanda V, Antoci F, Scimeca S, D'Agostino R, Scariano E, et al. A Molecular survey of Anaplasma spp., Rickettsia spp., Ehrlichia canis and Babesia microti in foxes and fleas from Sicily. Transbound Emerg Dis. 2013;60 Suppl 2:125–30.

94. Breitschwerdt EB, Abrams-Ogg AC, Lappin MR, Bienzle D, Hancock SI, Cowan SM, et al. Molecular evidence supporting Ehrlichia canis-like infection in cats. J Vet Intern Med. 2002;16(6):642–9.

95. Andre MR, Adania CH, Machado RZ, Allegretti SM, Felippe PA, Silva KF, et al. Molecular and serologic detection of Ehrlichia spp. in endangered Brazilian wild captive felids. J Wildl Dis. 2010;46(3):1017–23.

96. Braga Mdo S, Andre MR, Freschi CR, Teixeira MC, Machado RZ. Molecular and serological detection of Ehrlichia spp. in cats on Sao Luis Island, Maranhao, Brazil. Rev Bras Parasitol Vet. 2012;21(1):37–41.

97. Maia C, Ramos C, Coimbra M, Bastos F, Martins A, Pinto P, et al. Bacterial and protozoal agents of feline vector-borne diseases in domestic and stray cats from southern Portugal. Parasit Vectors. 2014;7:115.

98. Groen J, Koraka P, Nur YA, Avsic-Zupanc T, Goessens WH, Ott A, et al. Serologic evidence of ehrlichiosis among humans and wild animals in The Netherlands. Eur J Clin Microbiol Infect Dis. 2002;21(1):46–9.

99. Ismail N, Bloch KC, McBride JW. Human ehrlichiosis and anaplasmosis. Clin Lab Med. 2010;30(1):261–92.

100. Nicholson WL, Allen KE, McQuiston JH, Breitschwerdt EB, Little SE. The increasing recognition of rickettsial pathogens in dogs and people. Trends Parasitol. 2010;26(4):205–12.

101. Lima ML, Soares PT, Ramos CA, Araujo FR, Ramos RA, Souza II, et al. Molecular detection of Anaplasma platys in a naturally-infected cat in Brazil. Braz J Microbiol. 2010;41(2):381–5.

102. Qurollo BA, Balakrishnan N, Cannon CZ, Maggi RG, Breitschwerdt EB. Co-infection with Anaplasma platys, Bartonella henselae, Bartonella koehlerae and 'Candidatus Mycoplasma haemominutum' in a cat diagnosed with splenic plasmacytosis and multiple myeloma. J Feline Med Surg. 2014;16(8):713–20.
103. Perez M, Rikihisa Y, Wen B. Ehrlichia canis-like agent isolated from a man in Venezuela: antigenic and genetic characterization. J Clin Microbiol. 1996;34(9):2133–9.
104. Fishbein DB, Dawson JE, Robinson LE. Human ehrlichiosis in the United States, 1985 to 1990. Ann Intern Med. 1994;120(9):736–43.
105. Ganguly S, Mukhopadhayay SK. Tick-borne ehrlichiosis infection in human beings. J Vector Borne Dis. 2008;45(4):273–80.
106. Bakken JS, Dumler JS, Chen SM, Eckman MR, Van Etta LL, Walker DH. Human granulocytic ehrlichiosis in the upper Midwest United States. A new species emerging? JAMA. 1994;272(3):212–8.
107. Parola P, Davoust B, Raoult D. Tick- and flea-borne rickettsial emerging zoonoses. Vet Res. 2005;36(3):469–92.
108. Dumler JS, Choi KS, Garcia-Garcia JC, Barat NS, Scorpio DG, Garyu JW, et al. Human granulocytic anaplasmosis and Anaplasma phagocytophilum. Emerg Infect Dis. 2005;11(12):1828–34.
109. Maggi RG, Mascarelli PE, Havenga LN, Naidoo V, Breitschwerdt EB. Co-infection with Anaplasma platys, Bartonella henselae and Candidatus Mycoplasma haematoparvum in a veterinarian. Parasit Vectors. 2013;6:103.
110. Arraga-Alvarado CM, Qurollo B, Parra OC, Berrueta MA, Hegarty BC, Breitschwerdt EB. Molecular Evidence of Anaplasma platys Infection in Two Women from Venezuela. Am J Trop Med Hyg. 2014;91(6):1161–5.
111. Buller RS, Arens M, Hmiel SP, Paddock CD, Sumner JW, Rikhisa Y, et al. Ehrlichia ewingii, a newly recognized agent of human ehrlichiosis. N Engl J Med. 1999;341(3):148–55.
112. Allsopp MT, Louw M, Meyer EC. Ehrlichia ruminantium: an emerging human pathogen? Ann N Y Acad Sci. 2005;1063:358–60.
113. Allsopp MT, Allsopp BA. Novel Ehrlichia genotype detected in dogs in South Africa. J Clin Microbiol. 2001;39(11):4204–7.
114. Gutierrez CN, Martinez M, Sanchez E, De Vera M, Rojas M, Ruiz J, et al. Cultivation and molecular identification of Ehrlichia canis and Ehrlichia chaffeensis from a naturally co-infected dog in Venezuela. Vet Clin Pathol. 2008;37(3):258–65.
115. Beall MJ, Alleman AR, Breitschwerdt EB, Cohn LA, Couto CG, Dryden MW, et al. Seroprevalence of Ehrlichia canis, Ehrlichia chaffeensis and Ehrlichia ewingii in dogs in North America. Parasit Vectors. 2012;5:29.
116. Ndip LM, Ndip RN, Esemu SN, Walker DH, McBride JW. Predominance of Ehrlichia chaffeensis in Rhipicephalus sanguineus ticks from kennel-confined dogs in Limbe. Cameroon Exp Appl Acarol. 2010;50(2):163–8.
117. Pritt BS, Sloan LM, Johnson DK, Munderloh UG, Paskewitz SM, McElroy KM, et al. Emergence of a new pathogenic Ehrlichia species, Wisconsin and Minnesota, 2009. N Engl J Med. 2011;365(5):422–9.
118. Hegarty BC, Maggi RG, Koskinen P, Beall MJ, Eberts M, Chandrashekar R, et al. Ehrlichia muris infection in a dog from Minnesota. J Vet Intern Med. 2012;26(5):1217–20.
119. Nyindo M, Huxsoll DL, Ristic M, Kakoma I, Brown JL, Carson CA, et al. Cell-mediated and humoral immune responses of German Shepherd Dogs and Beagles to experimental infection with Ehrlichia canis. Am J Vet Res. 1980;41(2):250–4.
120. Harrus S, Kass PH, Klement E, Waner T. Canine monocytic ehrlichiosis: a retrospective study of 100 cases, and an epidemiological investigation of prognostic indicators for the disease. Vet Rec. 1997;141(14):360–3.
121. Costa Jr LM, Rembeck K, Ribeiro MF, Beelitz P, Pfister K, Passos LM. Sero-prevalence and risk indicators for canine ehrlichiosis in three rural areas of Brazil. Vet J. 2007;174(3):673–6.
122. Rodriguez-Vivas RI, Albornoz RE, Bolio GM. Ehrlichia canis in dogs in Yucatan, Mexico: seroprevalence, prevalence of infection and associated factors. Vet Parasitol. 2005;127(1):75–9.
123. Watanabe M, Okuda M, Tsuji M, Inokuma H. Seroepidemiological study of canine ehrlichial infections in Yamaguchi prefecture and surrounding areas of Japan. Vet Parasitol. 2004;124(1–2):101–7.
124. Egenvall AE, Hedhammar AA, Bjoersdorff AI. Clinical features and serology of 14 dogs affected by granulocytic ehrlichiosis in Sweden. Vet Rec. 1997;140(9):222–6.
125. McClure JC, Crothers ML, Schaefer JJ, Stanley PD, Needham GR, Ewing SA, et al. Efficacy of a doxycycline treatment regimen initiated during three different phases of experimental ehrlichiosis. Antimicrob Agents Chemother. 2010;54(12):5012–20.
126. Harrus S, Waner T, Aizenberg I, Foley JE, Poland AM, Bark H. Amplification of ehrlichial DNA from dogs 34 months after infection with Ehrlichia canis. J Clin Microbiol. 1998;36(1):73–6.
127. Waner T, Harrus S, Bark H, Bogin E, Avidar Y, Keysary A. Characterization of the subclinical phase of canine ehrlichiosis in experimentally infected beagle dogs. Vet Parasitol. 1997;69(3–4):307–17.
128. Mylonakis ME, Koutinas AF, Breitschwerdt EB, Hegarty BC, Billinis CD, Leontides LS, et al. Chronic canine ehrlichiosis (Ehrlichia canis): a retrospective study of 19 natural cases. J Am Anim Hosp Assoc. 2004;40(3):174–84.
129. Egenvall A, Lilliehook I, Bjoersdorff A, Engvall EO, Karlstam E, Artursson K, et al. Detection of granulocytic Ehrlichia species DNA by PCR in persistently infected dogs. Vet Rec. 2000;146(7):186–90.
130. Gaunt SD, Baker DC, Babin SS. Platelet aggregation studies in dogs with acute Ehrlichia platys infection. Am J Vet Res. 1990;51(2):290–3.

131. Harvey JW. Thrombocytotrophic anaplasmosis (A.platys [E.platys] infection). In: Greene CG, editor. Infectious diseases of the dog and cat. 3rd ed. St. Louis: Saunders Elsevier; 2006. p. 229–31.

132. Greig B, Asanovich KM, Armstrong PJ, Dumler JS. Geographic, clinical, serologic, and molecular evidence of granulocytic ehrlichiosis, a likely zoonotic disease, in Minnesota and Wisconsin dogs. J Clin Microbiol. 1996;34(1):44–8.

133. Varela F, Font X, Valladares JE, Alberola J. Thrombocytopathia and light-chain proteinuria in a dog naturally infected with Ehrlichia canis. J Vet Intern Med. 1997;11(5):309–11.

134. Breitschwerdt EB, Hegarty BC, Hancock SI. Sequential evaluation of dogs naturally infected with Ehrlichia canis, Ehrlichia chaffeensis, Ehrlichia equi, Ehrlichia ewingii, or Bartonella vinsonii. J Clin Microbiol. 1998;36(9):2645–51.

135. Goldman EE, Breitschwerdt EB, Grindem CB, Hegarty BC, Walls JJ, Dumler JS. Granulocytic ehrlichiosis in dogs from North Carolina and Virginia. J Vet Intern Med. 1998;12(2):61–70.

136. Lilliehöök I, Egenvall A, Twedten HW. Hematopathology in dogs experimentally infected with a Swedish granulocytic Ehrlichia species. Vet Clin Pathol. 1998;27(4):116–22.

137. Neer TM. Canine monocytic and granulocytic ehrlichiosis. In: Greene CE, editor. Infectious Diseases of the Dog and Cat. 2nd ed. Philadelphia: W.B. Saunders Co; 1998. p. 139–47.

138. Breitschwerdt EB. Obligate intracellular pathogens. In: Ettinger SJ, Feldman EC, editors. Textbook of Veterinary Internal Medicine. 6th ed. Philadelphia, PA: W.B. Saunders Co; 2005. p. 631–2.

139. Komnenou AA, Mylonakis ME, Kouti V, Tendoma L, Leontides L, Skountzou E, et al. Ocular manifestations of natural canine monocytic ehrlichiosis (Ehrlichia canis): a retrospective study of 90 cases. Vet Ophthalmol. 2007;10(3):137–42.

140. Leiva M, Naranjo C, Pena MT. Ocular signs of canine monocytic ehrlichiosis: a retrospective study in dogs from Barcelona. Spain Vet Ophthalmol. 2005;8(6):387–93.

141. Diniz PP, de Morais HS, Breitschwerdt EB, Schwartz DS. Serum cardiac troponin I concentration in dogs with ehrlichiosis. J Vet Intern Med. 2008;22(5):1136–43.

142. Little SE. Ehrlichiosis and anaplasmosis in dogs and cats. Vet Clin North Am Small Anim Pract. 2010;40(6):1121–40.

143. Bellah JR, Shull RM, Selcer EV. Ehrlichia canis-related polyarthritis in a dog. J Am Vet Med Assoc. 1986;189(8):922–3.

144. Cowell RL, Tyler RD, Clinkenbeard KD, Meinkoth JH. Ehrlichiosis and polyarthritis in three dogs. J Am Vet Med Assoc. 1988;192(8):1093–5.

145. Greig B, Armstrong PJ. Canine granulocytotrophic anaplasmosis (A.phagocytophilum infection). In: Greene CG, editor. Infectious diseases of the dog and cat. 3rd ed. St. Louis: Saunders Elsevier; 2006. p. 219–24.

146. Alleman R, Heather W: An update on anaplasmosis in dogs. *Vet Med* 2008, April:212-220.

147. Kohn B, Galke D, Beelitz P, Pfister K. Clinical features of canine granulocytic anaplasmosis in 18 naturally infected dogs. J Vet Intern Med. 2008;22(6):1289–95.

148. Granick JL, Armstrong PJ, Bender JB. Anaplasma phagocytophilum infection in dogs: 34 cases (2000-2007). J Am Vet Med Assoc. 2009;234(12):1559–65.

149. Ravnik U, Tozon N, Strasek K, Avsic Zupanc T. Clinical and haematological features in Anaplasma phagocytophilum seropositive dogs. Clin Microbiol Infect. 2009;15 Suppl 2:39–40.

150. Mazepa AW, Kidd LB, Young KM, Trepanier LA. Clinical presentation of 26 anaplasma phagocytophilum-seropositive dogs residing in an endemic area. J Am Anim Hosp Assoc. 2010;46(6):405–12.

151. Eberts MD. Vissotto de Paiva Diniz PP, Beall MJ, Stillman BA, Chandrashekar R, Breitschwerdt EB: Typical and atypical manifestations of Anaplasma phagocytophilum infection in dogs. J Am Anim Hosp Assoc. 2011;47(6):e86–94.

152. Maretzki CH, Fisher DJ, Greene CE. Granulocytic ehrlichiosis and meningitis in a dog. J Am Vet Med Assoc. 1994;205(11):1554–6.

153. Jaderlund KH, Bergstrom K, Egenvall A, Hedhammar A. Cerebrospinal fluid PCR and antibody concentrations against Anaplasma phagocytophilum and Borrelia burgdorferi sensu lato in dogs with neurological signs. J Vet Intern Med. 2009;23(3):669–72.

154. Barber RM, Li Q, Diniz PP, Porter BF, Breitschwerdt EB, Claiborne MK, et al. Evaluation of brain tissue or cerebrospinal fluid with broadly reactive polymerase chain reaction for Ehrlichia, Anaplasma, spotted fever group Rickettsia, Bartonella, and Borrelia species in canine neurological diseases (109 cases). J Vet Intern Med. 2010;24(2):372–8.

155. Lazzerini K, Tipold A, Kornberg M, Silaghi C, Mietze A, Lübke-Becker A, et al. Meningitis and meningoencephalitis of unknown etiology in dogs – are canine vector borne diseases (CVBD) triggering the diseases? In: *Proceedings of 26th Symposium ESVN-ECVN2013; Paris*. J Vet Intern Med. 2014;28(3):968–969.

156. Glaze MB, Gaunt SD. Uveitis associated with Ehrlichia platys infection in a dog. J Am Vet Med Assoc. 1986;189(8):916–7.

157. Harrus S, Aroch I, Lavy E, Bark H. Clinical manifestations of infectious canine cyclic thrombocytopenia. Vet Rec. 1997;141(10):247–50.

158. Sainz A, Amusategui I, Tesouro MA. Ehrlichia platys infection and disease in dogs in Spain. J Vet Diagn Invest. 1999;11(4):382–4.

159. Cohn LA. Ehrlichiosis and related infections. Vet Clin North Am Small Anim Pract. 2003;33(4):863–84.

160. Mylonakis ME, Koutinas AF, Billinis C, Leontides LS, Kontos V, Papadopoulos O, et al. Evaluation of cytology in the diagnosis of acute canine monocytic ehrlichiosis

(Ehrlichia canis): a comparison between five methods. Vet Microbiol. 2003;91(2–3):197–204.

161. Mylonakis ME, Borjesson DL, Leontides L, Siarkou VI, Theodorou K, Koutinas AF. Cytologic patterns of lymphadenopathy in canine monocytic ehrlichiosis. Vet Clin Pathol. 2011;40(1):78–83.

162. Otranto D, Testini G, Dantas-Torres F, Latrofa MS, Diniz PP, de Caprariis D, et al. Diagnosis of canine vector-borne diseases in young dogs: a longitudinal study. J Clin Microbiol. 2010;48(9):3316–24.

163. De Tommasi AS, Baneth G, Breitschwerdt EB, Stanneck D, Dantas-Torres F, Otranto D, et al. Anaplasma platys in Bone Marrow Megakaryocytes of Young Dogs. J Clin Microbiol. 2014;52(6):2231–4.

164. Harrus S, Alleman AR, Bark H, Mahan SM, Waner T. Comparison of three enzyme-linked immunosorbant assays with the indirect immunofluorescent antibody test for the diagnosis of canine infection with Ehrlichia canis. Vet Microbiol. 2002;86(4):361–8.

165. Waner T, Harrus S, Jongejan F, Bark H, Keysary A, Cornelissen AW. Significance of serological testing for ehrlichial diseases in dogs with special emphasis on the diagnosis of canine monocytic ehrlichiosis caused by Ehrlichia canis. Vet Parasitol. 2001;95(1):1–15.

166. Wen B, Rikihisa Y, Mott JM, Greene R, Kim HY, Zhi N, et al. Comparison of nested PCR with immunofluorescent-antibody assay for detection of Ehrlichia canis infection in dogs treated with doxycycline. J Clin Microbiol. 1997;35(7):1852–5.

167. Maggi RG, Birkenheuer AJ, Hegarty BC, Bradley JM, Levy MG, Breitschwerdt EB. Comparison of serological and molecular panels for diagnosis of vector-borne diseases in dogs. Parasit Vectors. 2014;7:127.

168. Harrus S, Waner T, Aizenberg I, Bark H. Therapeutic effect of doxycycline in experimental subclinical canine monocytic ehrlichiosis: evaluation of a 6-week course. J Clin Microbiol. 1998;36(7):2140–2.

169. Baneth G, Harrus S, Ohnona FS, Schlesinger Y. Longitudinal quantification of Ehrlichia canis in experimental infection with comparison to natural infection. Vet Microbiol. 2009;136(3–4):321–5.

170. Breitschwerdt EB, Hegarty BC, Hancock SI. Doxycycline hyclate treatment of experimental canine ehrlichiosis followed by challenge inoculation with two Ehrlichia canis strains. Antimicrob Agents Chemother. 1998;42(2):362–8.

171. Sainz A, Tesouro MA, Amusategui I, Rodriguez F, Mazzucchelli F, Rodriguez M. Prospective comparative study of 3 treatment protocols using doxycycline or imidocarb dipropionate in dogs with naturally occurring ehrlichiosis. J Vet Intern Med. 2000;14(2):134–9.

172. French TW, Harvey JW. Serologic diagnosis of infectious cyclic thrombocytopenia in dogs using an indirect fluorescent antibody test. Am J Vet Res. 1983;44(12):2407–11.

173. Chandrashekar R, Mainville CA, Beall MJ, O'Connor T, Eberts MD, Alleman AR, et al. Performance of a commercially available in-clinic ELISA for the detection of antibodies against Anaplasma phagocytophilum, Ehrlichia canis, and Borrelia burgdorferi and Dirofilaria immitis antigen in dogs. Am J Vet Res. 2010;71(12):1443–50.

174. Alleman AR, Wamsley HL, Abbott J, et al. Experimental Anaplasma phagocytophilum infection of dogs by intravenous inoculation of human and canine isolates and treatment with doxycycline. Vet Pathol. 2007;44:19.

175. Alleman A, Chandrashekar R, Beall M, Cyr K, Barbet A, Lundgren A, et al. Experimental inoculation of dogs with a human isolate (NY18) of Anaplasma phagocytophilum and demonstration of persistent infection following doxycycline therapy. J Vet Intern Med. 2006;20:763.

176. Harrus S, Kenny M, Miara L, Aizenberg I, Waner T, Shaw S. Comparison of simultaneous splenic sample PCR with blood sample PCR for diagnosis and treatment of experimental Ehrlichia canis infection. Antimicrob Agents Chemother. 2004;48(11):4488–90.

177. Sainz A. Ehrlichiosis/Anaplasmosis. In: Miró G, Solano-Gallego L, editors. Enfermedades Vectoriales del perro y del gato. 1st ed. Madrid: Ed. Achalantis; 2011. p. 203–26.

178. Gal A, Harrus S, Arcoh I, Lavy E, Aizenberg I, Mekuzas-Yisaschar Y, et al. Coinfection with multiple tick-borne and intestinal parasites in a 6-week-old dog. Can Vet J. 2007;48(6):619–22.

179. Beall MJ, Chandrashekar R, Eberts MD, Cyr KE, Diniz PP, Mainville C, et al. Serological and molecular prevalence of Borrelia burgdorferi, Anaplasma phagocytophilum, and Ehrlichia species in dogs from Minnesota. Vector Borne Zoonotic Dis. 2008;8(4):455–64.

180. Grab DJ, Nyarko E, Barat NC, Nikolskaia OV, Dumler JS. Anaplasma phagocytophilum-Borrelia burgdorferi coinfection enhances chemokine, cytokine, and matrix metalloprotease expression by human brain microvascular endothelial cells. Clin Vaccine Immunol. 2007;14(11):1420–4.

181. Foley JE, Brown RN, Gabriel MW, Henn J, Drazenovich N, Kasten R, et al. Spatial analysis of the exposure of dogs in rural north-coastal California to vectorborne pathogens. Vet Rec. 2007;161(19):653–7.

182. Cortese L, Pelagalli A, Piantedosi D, Cestaro A, Di Loria A, Lombardi P, et al. Effects of therapy on haemostasis in dogs infected with Leishmania infantum, Ehrlichia canis, or both combined. Vet Rec. 2009;164(14):433–4.

183. Mekuzas Y, Gradoni L, Oliva G, Foglia Manzillo V, Baneth G. Ehrlichia canis and Leishmania infantum co-infection: a 3-year longitudinal study in naturally exposed dogs. Clin Microbiol Infect. 2009;15 Suppl 2:30–1.

184. Matthewman LA, Kelly PJ, Brouqui P, Raoult D. Further evidence for the efficacy of imidocarb dipropionate in the treatment of Ehrlichia canis infection. J S Afr Vet Assoc. 1994;65(3):104–7.

185. Price JE, Dolan TT. A comparison of the efficacy of imidocarb dipropionate and tetracycline hydrochloride in the treatment of canine ehrlichiosis. Vet Rec. 1980;107(12):275–7.

186. Eddlestone SM, Neer TM, Gaunt SD, Corstvet R, Gill A,

Hosgood G, et al. Failure of imidocarb dipropionate to clear experimentally induced Ehrlichia canis infection in dogs. J Vet Intern Med. 2006;20(4):840–4.

187. Kelly PJ, Matthewman LA, Brouqui P, Raoult D. Lack of susceptibility of Ehrlichia canis to imidocarb dipropionate in vitro. J S Afr Vet Assoc. 1998;69(2):55–6.

188. Schaefer JJ, Kahn J, Needham GR, Rikihisa Y, Ewing SA, Stich RW. Antibiotic clearance of Ehrlichia canis from dogs infected by intravenous inoculation of carrier blood. Ann N Y Acad Sci. 2008;1149:263–9.

189. Theodorou K, Mylonakis ME, Siarkou VI, Leontides L, Koutinas AF, Koutinas CK, et al. Efficacy of rifampicin in the treatment of experimental acute canine monocytic ehrlichiosis. J Antimicrob Chemother. 2013;68(7):1619–26.

190. Maurin M, Bakken JS, Dumler JS. Antibiotic susceptibilities of Anaplasma (Ehrlichia) phagocytophilum strains from various geographic areas in the United States. Antimicrob Agents Chemother. 2003;47(1):413–5.

191. Diniz PPVP, Breitschwerdt E. Canine granulocytotropic anaplasmosis (A. phagocytophilum infection). In: Greene CE, editor. Infectious diseases of the dog and cat. 4th ed. Philadelphia: Saunders; 2011. p. 244–54.

192. Chang WL, Su WL, Pan MJ. Two-step PCR in the evaluation of antibiotic treatment for Ehrlichia platys infection. J Vet Med Sci. 1997;59(9):849–51.

193. Aroch I, Harrus S. The use of recombinant human colony stimulating factor and recombinant human erythropoietin in the treatment of severe pancytopenia due to canine monocytic ehrlichiosis. Israel J Vet Med. 2001;56(2):65–9.

194. Perille AL, Matus RE. Canine ehrlichiosis in six dogs with persistently increased antibody titers. J Vet Intern Med. 1991;5(3):195–8.

195. Massa KL, Gilger BC, Miller TL, Davidson MG. Causes of uveitis in dogs: 102 cases (1989-2000). Vet Ophthalmol. 2002;5(2):93–8.

196. Heeb HL, Wilkerson MJ, Chun R, Ganta RR. Large granular lymphocytosis, lymphocyte subset inversion, thrombocytopenia, dysproteinemia, and positive Ehrlichia serology in a dog. J Am Anim Hosp Assoc. 2003;39(4):379–84.

197. van Heerden J. A retrospective study on 120 natural cases of canine ehrlichiosis. J S Afr Vet Assoc. 1982;53(1):17–22.

198. Shipov A, Klement E, Reuveni-Tager L, Waner T, Harrus S. Prognostic indicators for canine monocytic ehrlichiosis. Vet Parasitol. 2008;153(1–2):131–8.

199. Mylonakis ME, Ceron JJ, Leontides L, Siarkou VI, Martinez S, Tvarijonaviciute A, et al. Serum acute phase proteins as clinical phase indicators and outcome predictors in naturally occurring canine monocytic ehrlichiosis. J Vet Intern Med. 2011;25(4):811–7.

200. Carrade DD, Foley JE, Borjesson DL, Sykes JE. Canine granulocytic anaplasmosis: a review. J Vet Intern Med. 2009;23(6):1129–41.

201. Martin AR, Brown GK, Dunstan RH, Roberts TK. Anaplasma platys: an improved PCR for its detection in dogs. Exp Parasitol. 2005;109(3):176–80.

202. Horowitz HW, Aguero-Rosenfeld M, Dumler JS, McKenna DF, Hsieh TC, Wu J, et al. Reinfection with the agent of human granulocytic ehrlichiosis. Ann Intern Med. 1998;129(6):461–3.

203. Dantas-Torres F. The brown dog tick, Rhipicephalus sanguineus (Latreille, 1806) (Acari: Ixodidae): from taxonomy to control. Vet Parasitol. 2008;152(3–4):173–85.

204. Therapy Tables [www.esccap.org]

205. Pereira CP, Oliveira PR, Furquim KC, Bechara GH, Camargo-Mathias MI. Effects of fipronil (active ingredient of Frontline) on salivary gland cells of Rhipicephalus sanguineus females (Latreille, 1806) (Acari: Ixodidae). Vet Parasitol. 2009;166(1–2):124–30.

206. Rudoler N, Baneth G, Eyal O, van Straten M, Harrus S. Evaluation of an attenuated strain of Ehrlichia canis as a vaccine for canine monocytic ehrlichiosis. Vaccine. 2012;31(1):226–33.

CHAPTER 51

FIRST CASE OF ANAPLASMA PLATYS INFECTION IN A DOG FROM CROATIA

Viktor Dyachenko, Nikola Pantchev, Hans-Joerg Balzer, Ariane Meyersen and Reinhard K Straubinger

Keywords: *Anaplasma platys, Babesia vogeli,* CRP, Infectious canine cyclic thrombocytopenia, Croatia

BACKGROUND

Anaplasma platys (formerly *Ehrlichia platys*) was first identified and described in 1978 in Florida (USA) as a *Rickettsia*-like, platelet-specific organism in dogs with infectious canine cyclic thrombocytopenia (ICCT) [1]. Based on morphology and serological cross-reactions with *Ehrichia canis*, the microorganism was first proposed as *E. platys*[2]. Sequencing and phylogenic analysis of the 16S rRNA gene and GroESL operon showed that the pathogen was related to *A. phagocytophilum* and *A. marginale*, which led to reclassification and designation as *A. platys*[3, 4].

In dogs *A. platys* organisms infect peripheral blood platelets and form basophilic inclusions in the cells, so-called morulae, which contain one or more subunits [1, 5]. Both, the appearance of the pathogen in the platelets and the following thrombocytopenia are cyclic [1]. The initial thrombocytopenias may develop primarily as a consequence of direct injury to platelets by replicating organisms. However, immune-mediated mechanisms of thrombocytopenia become more important in subsequent thrombocytopenic episodes [1]. The fraction of infected platelets decreases dramatically in successive parasitaemias, but the associated thrombocytopenic episodes remain severe [6]. In general, the infection is accompanied by unspecific and mild clinical manifestation including anorexia, depression, generalized lymph node enlargement, pale mucous membranes and elevated rectal temperatures [1, 7, 8, 9]. Nevertheless, a severe course of *A. platys* infection with ecchymotic haemorrhagia was reported to be caused by a Greek strain [10]. The pathogen is assumed to be transmitted by *Rhipicephalus sanguines*, as in several studies *A. platys*-DNA was detected in this tick species and co-infections in dogs with *E. canis* and *B. vogeli*, two pathogens that share the same vector, reinforce this speculation [11, 12, 13]. The vector competence of *R. sanguineus*, however, could not be proven so far [14]. Currently, *A. platys* has been described in both American continents (USA [2], Venezuela [15], Brazil [16]), Asia (China [17], Thailand [12], Taiwan [18], Japan [19]), Australia [20] and Africa [21]. In Europe the occurrence of *A. platys* has been shown in Mediterranean countries: Italy [22], France [23], Spain [8], Portugal [24], Turkey [25] and Greece [10]. Here the first case of a presumed autochthonous *A. platys* infection is described in a dog from Croatia.

Citation: Viktor Dyachenko, Nikola Pantchev, Hans-Joerg Balzer, Ariane Meyersen and Reinhard K Straubinger, First case of Anaplasma platys infection in a dog from Croatia, DOI: 10.1186/1756-3305-5-49.

CASE REPORT

A one-year-old male dog was imported from Croatia to Germany in May 2010 and, according to the owner declaration, has never been outside Croatia before. The dog was presented to a local veterinarian in Germany one month after the import due to intermittent/recurrent diarrhoea. Diagnostic tests for infections uncommon for the German area were requested (CBC with blood smear re, complete serum chemistry analysis as well as a "travel disease profile"). No abnormalities were found during the clinical assessment.

Blood analysis indicated anaemia with erythrocytes at 4.20 T/L (reference range 6-9 T/L), haemoglobin of 9.4 g/dL (reference range 15-19 g/dL) and haematocrit of 32% (reference range 38-55%). The anaemia was classified as normocytic at the upper limit to macrocytic (MCV of 75 fL; reference range 60-75 fL) as well as hypochromic due to a mean corpuscular hemoglobin concentration (MCHC) lower than the reference range (30 g/dL; reference range 31-34 g/dL). Thrombocytopenia was registered as well (62×10^9/L; reference range $150\text{-}500 \times 10^9$/L). The differential and absolute white blood cell (WCB) counts were within the usual range (Table 1). Biochemistry parameters were within the reference range apart from a total protein at the lower limit of the reference range (53 g/L; 53-77 g/L), decreased albumin values of 2.70 g/dL (3.2-4.7 g/dL) as well as increased urea nitrogen of 34.7 mg/dL (10-25 mg/dL) and phosphorus at 2.0 mmol/L (0.7-1.6 mmol/L). A subsequent immunological examination revealed an elevated C-reactive protein (CRP, 38.2 mg/L; reference range 0-9.7 mg/L). In addition, the examination of a blood smear revealed basophilic inclusions in thrombocytes resembling *A. platys* (Figure 1). The following *A. phagocytophilum* and *A. platys*- specific PCRs confirmed the *A. platys* infection. The *A. platys*-positive PCR result (cycle threshold (Ct) value 19.1) was accompanied by a *B. vogeli*-positive PCR (Ct value 35.8). PCR testing for other Babesia (including *B. canis, B. rossi, B. gibsoni, B. conradae*), *Hepatozoon canis, Ehrlichia* spp. (including *E. canis, E. chaffeensis, E. ewingii)*and *Leishmania* spp. were negative. Serological assays as the SNAP 4Dx test (antibodies to *A. phagocytophilum, E. canis, Borrelia burgdorferi* and antigen of *Dirofilaria immitis*), microplate ELISA for antibodies against *Leishmania infantum* and IFA on *A. phagocytophilum, E. canis*, and *Leishmania*-antigen produced negative results. In contrast, a *B. canis*- specific ELISA was positive (a low level of antibodies at 20.2 test units was detected).

Table 1: Patient's haematological and serum biochemical parameters at the time of clinical examination

haematological parameters	**found values**	**reference values**	**SI units**
white blood cells	11.7	(6-12)	10^9/L
red blood cells	4.20	(6-9)	10^{12}/L
haemoglobin	9.4	(15-19)	g/dL
hematocrit	32	(38-55)	%
mean corpuscular volume	75	(60-77)	fL
haemoglobin E	22	(17-23)	pg
mean corpuscular haemoglobin concentration	30	(31-34)	g/dL
platelets	62	(150-500)	10^9/L
basophil granulocytes	0	(0-1)	%
	0		
eosinophil granulocytes	1	(0-6)	%
	0.117	(0 - 0.6)	10^9/L
neutrophil granulocytes (band)	0	(0-3)	%
	0	(0 - 0.3)	10^9/L
neutrophil granulocytes (segmented)	70	(55-75)	%
	8.176	(3-10)	10^9/L
lymphocytes	24	(12-30)	%
	2.803	(1-4)	10^9/L
monocytes	4	(0-4)	%
	0.467	(0-0.5)	10^9/L
atypical cells	1	(0)	
serum biochemical parameters			
protein	53	(53-77)	g/L
albumin	27	(32-47)	g/L
globulin	26	(15-35)	g/L
urea nitrogen	34.7	(10-25)	mg/dL
phosphorus	2.0	(0.7-1.6)	mmol/L
CRP	38.2	(0-9.7)	mg/L
creatinine	0.9	(< 1.4)	mg/dL

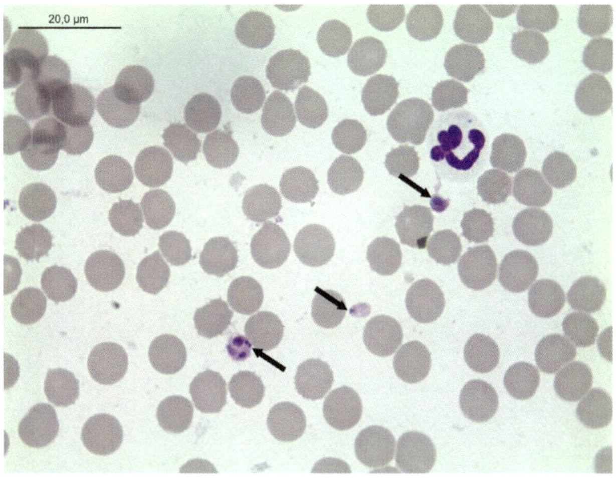

Figure 1: *A. platys* inclusion in blood platelets (arrows); Giemsa-stained blood smear of the dog presented in this report.

Based on abnormal clinicopathological findings in conjunction with the positive PCR results, specific therapy with doxycycline (10 mg/kg, orally, SID) was initiated for four weeks. After three weeks of Doxycycline therapy, a single injection of imidocarb dipropionate (6 mg/kg) was administered subcutaneously. In the following hours after the application the general health condition of the dog worsened, described as an anaphylactic reaction by the in-clinic veterinarian. Despite the immediate use of infusions and the administration of parenteral atropine, the dog died the next day.

METHODS

Blood analysis

Blood was collected on the day of the presentation in the clinic. CBC with blood smear re was performed on the sample paying particular attention to blood parasites and hemotropic bacteria, as was complete serum chemistry (IDEXX Vet Med Lab). CRP concentrations were measured by means of a validated CRP immunoturbidimetric assay.

DNA extraction and diagnostic PCRs

Total DNA was extracted from whole blood by using QIAamp DNA Blood Mini kit (QIAGEN, Germany) according to the manufacturer's instructions. Real-time PCR at IDEXX Vet Med Lab was performed using the LightCycler 480 (Roche) with proprietary forward and reverse primers and hydrolysis probes. Target genes for pathogen detection using real-time PCR were as follows: *A. platys* (groEL), *A. phagocytophilum* (msp2), *B. vogeli, B. canis, B. rossi, B. gibsoni* (hsp 70), *B. conradae* (ITS2), *H. canis* (18S rRNA), *Leishmania* spp. (GP63), *E. canis, E. chaffeensis, E. ewingii* (dsb).

Serological examinations

Serological examinations for antibody detection were performed using an *A. phagocytophilum* IFA (MegaScreen FLUOANAPLASMA ph., cut-off = 1:50, MegaCor, Hoerbranz, Austria), a microplate *L. infantum*ELISA (*Leishmania*-ELISA Dog, Afosa GmbH Dahlewitz, Germany; reference range: negative < 7, borderline 7-12 and positive > 12), an *E. canis* IFA (MegaScreen FLUOEHRLICHIA c., cut-off = 1:40, MegaCor, Hoerbranz, Austria), and a microplate *B. canis* ELISA (*Babesia*-ELISA Dog, Afosa GmbH Dahlewitz, Germany; reference range: negative < 14, borderline 14-19 and positive > 19). In regard to *B. vogeli*, positive reactions were documented earlier utilizing a *B. canis* IFA test [26]. Furthermore, a rapid enzyme immunoassay assay test system (IDEXX SNAP® 4Dx®) was used as described elsewhere [27] following the manufacturer›s directions. The IDEXX SNAP® 4Dx® detects antibodies against *A. phagocytophilum* (p44), *Borrelia burgdorferi* sensu lato (C6), *E. canis* (p30, p30-1) as well as antigen of *Dirofilaria immitis*.

Sequencing of 16S ribosomal RNA gene and sequence analysis

A 1,400-bp fragment of the 16S ribosomal RNA gene was amplified from total blood DNA by using forward (AGAGTTTGATCCTGGCTCAG) and reverse (CGGCTACCTTGTTACGACTT) Anaplasmataceae-specific primers, which were modified according to a study published elsewhere [28]. The reactions were prepared in total volumes of 50 µl with 15 pmol each primer, 0.2 mM each dNTP and 2 U Pwo DNA-polymerase in a 1× polymerase specific buffer complemented with $MgSO_4$. After an initial denaturation step at 94°C the reactions cycled 30 times at 94°C for 30 sec, 58°C for 45 sec, 68°C for 90 sec and finally incubated at 68°C for 5 min in a Mastercycler pro (Eppendorf, Hamburg, Germany). The PCR products were purified with a peqGOLD Gel extraction Kit (PEQLAB, Erlangen, Germany) and submitted for sequencing to Eurofins MWG Operon (Ebersberg, Germany). The PCR product was sequenced three times in both directions. A 1,348-bp partial ribosomal RNA sequence was deposited to GenBank™ under accession number JQ396431.

RESULTS AND DISCUSSION

With the exception of intermittent/recurrent diarrhoea the dog had no clinical signs, but anaemia and thrombocytopenia were evident in the haemogram (Table 1). Both are common, major abnormal clinicopathological findings observed in *A. platys* and *B. vogeli*- co-infected dogs [13] and are in concordance with the positive PCR results for *A. platys* and *B. vogeli* found in the dog. Infections with *A. platys* are difficult to detect, as in most cases the clinical manifestations are not clearly evident. *B. vogeli* infections usually cause subclinical to mild or moderate changes in adult dogs, however, concomitant conditions or additional pathogens present at the same time can exacerbate the course of infection [29].

Thrombocytopenia due to a monoinfection with *A. platys* has a cyclic character and is considered the result of the destruction of blood platelets by the proliferating pathogen during initial phase of infection, which probably triggers immunologic mechanisms in the subsequent course of the infection [6]. In *B. vogeli*- infected dogs, regenerative haemolytic anaemia is a well-known feature, but not all naturally infected dogs become anaemic. Furthermore, *B. vogeli* infections do not show a homogenous clinicopathological pattern [29, 30]. Indeed, thrombocytopenia was reported to also be a haematological abnormality of *B. vogeli* infections, even though the decrease of platelets in blood is a consistent haematological abnormality in *B. canis* infections [30, 31]. The thrombocytopenia can be enhanced by mixed *A. platys* and *B. vogeli* infections leading to significantly lower numbers of platelets compared to single pathogen infection [20]. Both, thrombocytopenia (2.5 fold below lower limit of normal range) and anaemia (low value of RBC count, haemoglobin and haematocrit), were found in the presented case (Table 1). Based on data generated with additional PCR and serology tests there was no evidence of co-infections with other pathogens such as *A. phagocytophilum, H. canis, Ehrlichia*spp. and *Leishmania* spp., which may occur also in Croatia and could take further influence on haematological parameters [32, 33, 34]. On the other hand, at the moment there are no available reports confirming the occurrence of *E. canis* in Croatia.

As representatives for acute phase proteins C-reactive protein (CRP, belonging to positive acute phase proteins) and albumin (negative acute phase protein) were evaluated, which in fact showed abnormal values. While CRP was elevated to up to 38.2 mg/L (reference range 0-9.7 mg/L), the serum albumin was decreased to 2.7 g/dL (reference range 3.2-4.7 g/dL) indicating systemic involvement likely due to a co-infection of *A. platys*and *B. vogeli*. Acute phase response as a part of the innate host defence system is linked to early innate responses for any pathological processes or diseases as reed elsewhere [35, 36]. In dogs, CRP is known to show the highest response among acute phase proteins and has been used as an early unspecific marker [35]. An increase of CRP in dogs has been reported for many diseases caused for example by *B. canis*[31], *E. canis*[37], *L. infantum*[38] and *A. phagocytophilum*[39]. Thus far, no comprehensive investigations of acute phase response in tick-borne concurrent infections such as *A. platys* and *B. vogeli* exist.

The serological tests (IFA and SNAP 4Dx) based on *A. phagocytophilum* antigen failed to detect antibodies in the present case, but an ELISA based on *B. canis* antigen produced a positive result. However, the antibody level was low. It is known, that IFA tests with *B. canis* as a substrate cross-react with antibodies against *B. vogeli* and *B. rossi*, but homologous species antigens will cause stronger reactions [40]. Furthermore, that exact time point of seroconversion is not known for a natural *B. vogeli* infection and follow-up serological examinations after initial PCR-positive results, as shown previously [26], was not possible in the present case. The attempt to detect antibodies against *A. platys* was based on cross-reaction with *A. phagocytophilum*antigen. It has previously been shown, that the serum samples from naturally infected *A. platys* dogs from USA and China react positively with *A. phagocytophilum* antigen on the SNAP 4Dx [41, 42]. Furthermore serum samples from *A. platys* infected animals in Portugal react well by means of IFA with *A. phagocytophilum*antigen [43]. Therefore, strain differences do not appear be a reason for the negative serological tests in the present study. According to the literature, seroconversion as a consequence of an *A. platys* mono-infection occurs between 13 to 19 days post infection as shown with strains collected in US and Greece [2, 10]. As the dog was imported approx. 30 days before sampling to Germany and it is unlikely that the infection was acquired in Germany, an unusually long seronegative period can be inferred. It can be speculated that the tested blood samples were collected during the acute phase of infection probably before seroconversion occurred. This would be in concordance with negative IFA results as well as with high C-reactive protein and severe thrombocytopenia as described in *A. phagocytophilum*-infections previously [39]. The other possible reason for the seronegativity could be the dual infection. In case of a simultaneous infection with *A. platys* and *E. canis* it was documented, that *A. platys*-specific antibodies were detectable for the first time on average 27 days (range 14-35 days) post infection [42]. Consequently, the concurrent infections of *A. platys* and *B. vogeli*might have induced a delay in the humoral immunological response in this patient.

Intermittent diarrhoea was a reason for the presentation of the dog. The possible cause for the diarrhoea remains unknown, as no faecal sample was examined. But, it seems unlikely that intermittent diarrhoea alone could have led to hypoalbuminemia in the dog due to substantial gastrointestinal loss of fluids.

The dog died shortly after imidocarb dipropionate administration. However, the cause of death stays speculative, because no post-mortem examination was performed. An anaphylactoid reaction was observed in this case. Such reactions were described after imidocarb dipropionate administration in rare cases [44], while side effects of the drug (hypotension, hypersalivation, nasal discharge, lacrimation, diarrhoea, vomiting) can be reduced by atropine pretreatment. Furthermore, occasional renal tubular necrosis and hepatotoxicity after treatment have been described also [45, 46]. In this case the elevated urea nitrogen of 34.7 mg/dL (reference range 10-25 mg/dL) and creatinine within the reference range (0.9; reference range < 1.4 mg/dl) are indicative for azotaemia but not for a strong renal involvement, which could exacerbate the side effects of imidocarb dipropionate therapy. In a group of seven dogs with *B. canis* infection, which had been preselected due to renal involvement and treated with imidocarb dipropionate, four dogs died spontaneously and the kidneys of all animals of the group showed degenerative changes of mainly the proximal convoluted tubules as well as necrosis of the whole tubule in some cases [47]. The authors reported that the histological alterations seen in the dogs were similar in dogs treated with imidocarb dipropionate and in the untreated animal. Hence, the pathological changes observed in the kidneys cannot be explained exclusively by the potential nephrotoxicity of imidocarb dipropionate [47]. In the case presented here it remains open, whether the dog died because of the side effects or as a result of the combined impact of the observed *B. vogeli* and *A. platys* infections. Nevertheless, it is recommended to treat simultaneously even mildly azotaemic dogs with proper intravenous fluid therapy when imidocarb dipropionate is applied and lower the dose of the drug (e.g. 3 mg/kg) in patients suspected to have renal involvement, in order to decrease the risk of renal insufficiency [47].

Sequencing of the 16S rRNA gene produced a 1,348-bp sequence, which was identical to other *A. platys* 16S rRNA sequences generated in Thailand (EF139459), Japan (AY077619) and France (AF303467). The analysis of 16S rRNA sequences confirms the previous results, in which little genetic diversity was observed in 16S rRNA sequences of *A. platys* strains from different geographic locations [8, 22, 48].

The mixed *A. platys* and *B. vogeli* infection is well known from previous reports and represents a large fraction of co-infections among tick borne pathogens in dogs [20, 26, 49]. The examination of free-roaming dogs associated with remote Aboriginal communities in Australia showed 11% of dogs co-infected with both *A. platys* and *B. vogeli*[20]. The occurrence of *B. vogeli* in Croatia and other southern European countries is well documented [32]. The natural occurrence of *A. platys* in moderate climate zones and simultaneous coinfections with *Babesia* spp. allow the assumption that *Rhipicephalus* sp. e.g. *Rhipicephalus sanguineus*ticks may serve as the natural vector. On the other hand, this tick species has a wide genetic diversity [50] making it difficult to find the definitive vector for *A. platys*. The detection of *A. platys* in non-engorged questing adult *Rhipicephalus turanicus* tick in Israel [51] raises the question, whether other *Rhipicephalus* species actually serve as vectors for this agent.

To our knowledge this is the first report of *A. platys* infection in a dog imported from Croatia. Based on the owner's declaration, the dog has never travelled abroad before importation to Germany and the dog was presumably infected in Croatia. The infection in Germany is unlikely due to the following reasons: the vectors *Rhipicephalus* spp. ticks are commonly not present in Germany, even though ticks imported from abroad with travelled dogs can survive in homes with moderate temperatures [52]. The dog owners in Germany, however, did not report any tick infestation and so far there are no reports of autochthonous occurrences of *B. vogeli*and *A. platys* from the region where the dog spent its final days.

CONCLUSIONS

A. platys infection was detected for the first time in a dog imported from Croatia. A co-infection with *B. vogeli*probably induced the untypical serological results. The major clinical manifestations were thrombocytopenia, anaemia and elevated values of C-reactive protein. *A. platys* infection should be considered in dogs living in or returning after travel from this area and showing abnormal clinicopathologic findings described in this report.

DECLARATIONS

Authors' contributions

VD wrote the manuscript and performed sequencing and analysis of 16S rRNA. NP performed serological and clinicopathologic examinations, case consultation and correction of manuscript. H-JB performed diagnostic PCRs and correction of manuscript. AM performed anamnesis, clinical examination and treatment. RKS supervised and revised the manuscript. All authors read and approved the final version of the manuscript.

REFERENCES

1. Harvey JW, Simpson CF, Gaskin JM: Cyclic thrombocytopenia induced by a *Rickettsi*-like agent in dogs. J Infect Dis. 1978, 137: 182-188. 10.1093/infdis/137.2.182.
2. French TW, Harvey JW: Serologic diagnosis of infectious cyclic thrombocytopenia in dogs using an indirect fluorescent antibody test. Am J Vet Res. 1983, 44: 2407-2411.
3. Yu XJ, Zhang XF, McBride JW, Zhang Y, Walker DH: Phylogenetic relationships of *Anaplasma marginal* and '*Ehrlichia platy*' to other *Ehrlichi* species determined by GroEL amino acid sequences. Int J Syst Evol Microbiol. 2001, 51: 1143-1146. 10.1099/00207713-51-3-1143.
4. Dumler JS, Barbet AF, Bekker CP, Dasch GA, Palmer GH, Ray SC, Rikihisa Y, Rurangirwa FR: Reorganization of genera in the families Rickettsiaceae and Anaplasmataceae in the order Rickettsiales: unification of some species of *Ehrlichi* with *Anaplasm, Cowdri* with *Ehrlichi* and *Ehrlichi* with *Neorickettsi*, descriptions of six new species combinations and designation of *Ehrlichia equ* and 'HGE agent' as subjective synonyms of *Ehrlichia phagocytophil*. Int J Syst Evol Microbiol. 2001, 51: 2145-2165. 10.1099/00207713-51-6-2145.
5. Arraga-Alvarado C, Palmar M, Parra O, Salas P: *Ehrlichia platy*(*Anaplasma platy*) in dogs from Maracaibo, Venezuela: an ultrastructural study of experimental and natural infections. Vet Pathol. 2003, 40: 149-156. 10.1354/vp.40-2-149.
6. French TW, Harvey JW: Canine Infectious Cyclic Thrombocytopenia (*Ehrlichia platy* Infection in Dogs). Rickettsial and chlamydial diseases of domestic animals. Edited by: Woldehiwet Z, Ristic M. 1993, New York: Pergamon Press, 195-208.
7. Harrus S, Aroch I, Lavy E, Bark H: Clinical manifestations of infectious canine cyclic thrombocytopenia. Vet Rec. 1997, 141: 247-250. 10.1136/vr.141.10.247.
8. Aguirre E, Tesouro MA, Ruiz L, Amusategui I, Sainz A: Genetic characterization of *Anaplasm*(*Ehrlichi*)*platy* in dogs in Spain. J Vet Med B Infect Dis Vet Public Health. 2006, 53: 197-200. 10.1111/j.1439-0450.2006.00937.x.
9. Baker DC, Simpson M, Gaunt SD, Corstvet RE: Acute *Ehrlichia platy* infection in the dog. Vet Pathol. 1987, 24: 449-453.

10. Kontos VI, Papadopoulos O, French TW: Natural and experimental canine infections with a Greek strain of *Ehrlichia platy*. Vet Clin Pathol. 1991, 20: 101-105. 10.1111/j.1939-165X.1991.tb00867.x.

11. Inokuma H, Raoult D, Brouqui P: Detection of *Ehrlichia platy* DNA in brown dog ticks (*Rhipicephalus sanguineu*) in Okinawa Island, Japan. J Clin Microbiol. 2000, 38: 4219-4221.

12. Suksawat J, Pitulle C, Arraga-Alvarado C, Madrigal K, Hancock SI, Breitschwerdt EB: Coinfection with three *Ehrlichi*species in dogs from Thailand and Venezuela with emphasis on consideration of 16S ribosomal DNA secondary structure. J Clin Microbiol. 2001, 39: 90-93. 10.1128/JCM.39.1.90-93.2001.

13. de Caprariis D, Dantas-Torres F, Capelli G, Mencke N, Stanneck D, Breitschwerdt EB, Otranto D: Evolution of clinical, haematological and biochemical findings in young dogs naturally infected by vector-borne pathogens. Vet Microbiol. 2011, 149: 206-212. 10.1016/j.vetmic.2010.10.006.

14. Simpson RM, Gaunt SD, Hair JA, Kocan KM, Henk WG, Casey HW: Evaluation of *Rhipicephalus sanguineu* as a potential biologic vector of *Ehrlichia platy*. Am J Vet Res. 1991, 52: 1537-1541.

15. Huang H, Unver A, Perez MJ, Orellana NG, Rikihisa Y: Prevalence and molecular analysis of *Anaplasma platy* in dogs in Lara, Venezuela. Braz J Microbiol. 2005, 36: 211-216. 10.1590/S1517-83822005000300002.

16. Ferreira RF, Figueiredo Cerqueira AdM, Pereira AM, Guimaraes CM, Sa AG, Abreu FdS, Massard CL, Pereira Almosny NR: *Anaplasma platy* diagnosis in dogs: Comparison between morphological and molecular tests. Int J Appl Res Vet Med. 2007, 5: 113-119.

17. Hua P, Yuhai M, Shide T, Yang S, Bohai W, Xiangrui C: Canine ehrlichiosis caused simultaneously by *Ehrlichia cani* and *Ehrlichia platy*. Microbiol Immunol. 2000, 44: 737-739.

18. Chang AC, Chang WL, Lin CT, Pan MJ, Lee SC: Canine infectious cyclic thrombocytopenia found in Taiwan. J Vet Med Sci. 1996, 58: 473-476. 10.1292/jvms.58.473.

19. Inokuma H, Fujii K, Matsumoto K, Okuda M, Nakagome K, Kosugi R, Hirakawa M, Onishi T: Demonstration of *Anaplasm*(*Ehrlichi*)*platy* inclusions in peripheral blood platelets of a dog in Japan. Vet Parasitol. 2002, 110: 145-152. 10.1016/S0304-4017(02)00289-3.

20. Brown GK, Canfield PJ, Dunstan RH, Roberts TK, Martin AR, Brown CS, Irving R: Detection of *Anaplasma platy* and *Babesia canis vogel* and their impact on platelet numbers in free-roaming dogs associated with remote Aboriginal communities in Australia. Aust Vet J. 2006, 84: 321-325. 10.1111/j.1751-0813.2006.00029.x.

21. Sanogo YO, Davoust B, Inokuma H, Camicas JL, Parola P, Brouqui P: First evidence of *Anaplasma platy* in *Rhipicephalus sanguineu*(Acari: Ixodida) collected from dogs in Africa. Onderstepoort J Vet Res. 2003, 70: 205-212.

22. de la Fuente J, Torina A, Naranjo V, Nicosia S, Alongi A, La MF, Kocan KM: Molecular characterization of *Anaplasma platy*strains from dogs in Sicily. Italy. BMC Vet Res. 2006, 2: 24-10.1186/1746-6148-2-24.

23. Beaufils JP, Inokuma H, Martin-Granel J, Jumelle P, Barbault-Jumelle M, Brouqui P: *Anaplasma platy*(*Ehrlichia platy*) infection in a dog in France: description of the case, and characterization of the agent. Revue de Medecine Veterinaire. 2002, 153: 85-90.

24. Cardoso L, Tuna J, Vieira L, Yisaschar-Mekuzas Y, Baneth G: Molecular detection of *Anaplasma platy* and *Ehrlichia cani* in dogs from the North of Portugal. Vet J. 2010, 183: 232-233. 10.1016/j.tvjl.2008.10.009.

25. Ulutas B, Bayramli G, Karagenc T: First case of *Anaplasm* (*Ehrlichi*)*platy* infection in a dog in Turkey. Turk J Vet Anim Sci. 2007, 31: 279-282.

26. Otranto D, Testini G, Dantas-Torres F, Latrofa MS, Diniz PP, De CD, Lia RP, Mencke N, Stanneck D, Capelli G: Diagnosis of canine vector-borne diseases in young dogs: a longitudinal study. J Clin Microbiol. 2010, 48: 3316-3324. 10.1128/JCM.00379-10.

27. Pantchev N, Schaper R, Limousin S, Norden N, Weise M, Lorentzen L: Occurrence of *Dirofilaria immiti* and tick-borne infections caused by *Anaplasma phagocytophilu, Borrelia burgdorfer* sensu lato and *Ehrlichia cani* in domestic dogs in France: results of a countrywide serologic survey. Parasitol Res. 2009, 105 (Suppl 1): S101-S114.

28. Schouls LM, Van DPI, Rijpkema SG, Schot CS: Detection and identification of *Ehrlichi, Borrelia burgdorfer* sensu lato, and *Bartonell* species in Dutch *Ixodes ricinu* ticks. J Clin Microbiol. 1999, 37: 2215-2222.

29. Solano-Gallego L, Baneth G: Babesiosis in dogs and cats-expanding parasitological and clinical spectra. Vet Parasitol. 2011, 181: 48-60. 10.1016/j.vetpar.2011.04.023.

30. Solano-Gallego L, Trotta M, Carli E, Carcy B, Caldin M, Furlanello T: *Babesia canis cani* and *Babesia canis vogel*clinicopathological findings and DNA detection by means of PCR-RFLP in blood from Italian dogs suspected of tick-borne disease. Vet Parasitol. 2008, 157: 211-221. 10.1016/j.vetpar.2008.07.024.

31. Matijatko V, Mrljak V, Kis I, Kucer N, Forsek J, Zivicnjak T, Romic Z, Simec Z, Ceron JJ: Evidence of an acute phase response in dogs naturally infected with *Babesia cani*. Vet Parasitol. 2007, 144: 242-250. 10.1016/j.vetpar.2006.10.004.

32. Beck R, Vojta L, Mrljak V, Marinculic A, Beck A, Zivicnjak T, Caccio SM: Diversity of Babesia and Theileria species in symptomatic and asymptomatic dogs in Croatia. Int J Parasitol. 2009

33. Vojta L, Mrljak V, Curkovic S, Zivicnjak T, Marinculic A, Beck R: Molecular epizootiology of canine hepatozoonosis in Croatia. Int J Parasitol. 2009, 39: 1129-1136. 10.1016/j.ijpara.2009.02.007.

34. Zivicnjak T, Martinkovic F, Marinculic A, Mrljak V, Kucer N, Matijatko V, Mihaljevic Z, Baric-Rafaj R: A seroepidemiologic survey of canine visceral leishmaniosis among apparently healthy dogs in Croatia. Vet Parasitol. 2005, 131: 35-43. 10.1016/j.vetpar.2005.04.036.

35. Ceron JJ, Eckersall PD, Martynez-Subiela S: Acute phase proteins in dogs and cats: current knowledge and future perspectives. Vet Clin Pathol. 2005, 34: 85-99. 10.1111/j.1939-165X.2005.tb00019.x.

36. Eckersall PD, Bell R: Acute phase proteins: Biomarkers of infection and inflammation in veterinary medicine. Vet J. 2010, 185: 23-27. 10.1016/j.tvjl.2010.04.009.

37. Rikihisa Y, Yamamoto S, Kwak I, Iqbal Z, Kociba G, Mott J, Chichanasiriwithaya W: C-reactive protein and alpha 1-acid glycoprotein levels in dogs infected with *Ehrlichia cani*. J Clin Microbiol. 1994, 32: 912-917.

38. Martinez-Subiela S, Strauss-Ayali D, Ceron JJ, Baneth G: Acute phase protein response in experimental canine leishmaniasis. Vet Parasitol. 2011, 180: 197-202. 10.1016/j.vetpar.2011.03.032.

39. Pantchev N: C-reactive protein as a marker in canine granulocytic anaplasmosis. Vet Rec. 2010, 166: 632-10.1136/vr.c2546.

40. Jongejan F, Fourie JJ, Chester ST, Manavella C, Mallouk Y, Pollmeier MG, Baggott D: The prevention of transmission of Babesia canis canis by Dermacentor reticulatus ticks to dogs using a novel combination of fipronil, amitraz and (S)-methoprene. Vet Parasitol. 2011, 179: 343-350. 10.1016/j.vetpar.2011.03.047.

41. Wong SS, Teng JL, Poon RW, Choi GK, Chan KH, Yeung ML, Hui JJ, Yuen KY: Comparative evaluation of a point-of-care immunochromatographic test SNAP 4Dx with molecular detection tests for vector-borne canine pathogens in Hong Kong. Vector Borne Zoonotic Dis. 2011, 11: 1269-1277. 10.1089/vbz.2010.0265.

42. Gaunt S, Beall M, Stillman B, Lorentzen L, Diniz P, Chandrashekar R, Breitschwerdt E: Experimental infection and co-infection of dogs with *Anaplasma platy* and *Ehrlichia cani*: hematologic, serologic and molecular findings. Parasit Vectors. 2010, 3: 33-10.1186/1756-3305-3-33.

43. Santos AS, Alexandre N, Sousa R, Nuncio MS, Bacellar F, Dumler JS: Serological and molecular survey of *Anaplasm*species infection in dogs with suspected tickborne disease in Portugal. Vet Rec. 2009, 164: 168-171. 10.1136/vr.164.6.168.

44. Steuber S, Kroker R: Antiprotozoika. Pharmakotherapie bei Haus- und Nutztieren. Edited by: Löscher W, Ungemach F-R, Kroker R. 2006, Stuttgart: Parey, 410-433.

45. Green C, Calpin J: Antimicrobal Drug Formulary. Infectious Diseases of Dog and Can. Edited by: Green CE. 2012, St. Louis: Elsevier, 1207-1320. Fourthth

46. Kock N, Kelly P: Massive hepatic necrosis associated with accidental imidocarb dipropionate toxicosis in a dog. J Comp Pathol. 1991, 104: 113-116. 10.1016/S0021-9975(08)80093-X.

47. Mathe A, Voros K, Nemeth T, Biksi I, Hetyey C, Manczur F, Tekes L: Clinicopathological changes and effect of imidocarb therapy in dogs experimentally infected with *Babesia cani*. Acta Vet Hung. 2006, 54: 19-33. 10.1556/AVet.54.2006.1.3.

48. Pinyoowong D, Jittapalapong S, Suksawat F, Stich RW, Thamchaipenet A: Molecular characterization of Thai *Ehrlichia cani* and *Anaplasma platy* strains detected in dogs. Infect Genet Evol. 2008, 8: 433-438. 10.1016/j.meegid.2007.06.002.

49. Abd Rani PA, Irwin PJ, Coleman GT, Gatne M, Traub RJ: A survey of canine tick-borne diseases in India. Parasit Vectors. 2011, 4: 141-10.1186/1756-3305-4-141.

50. Dantas-Torres F: The brown dog tick, *Rhipicephalus sanguineu* (Latreille, 1806) (Acari: Ixodidae): from taxonomy to control. Vet Parasitol. 2008, 152: 173-185. 10.1016/j.vetpar.2007.12.030.

51. Harrus S, Perlman-Avrahami A, Mumcuoglu KY, Morick D, Eyal O, Baneth G: Molecular detection of *Ehrlichia canis, Anaplasma bovi, Anaplasma platy*, Candidatus *Midichloria mitochondri* and *Babesia canis vogel* in ticks from Israel. Clin Microbiol Infect. 2011, 17: 459-463. 10.1111/j.1469-0691.2010.03316.x.

52. Dongus H, Zahler M, Gothe R: The brown dog tick, *Rhipicephalus sanguineu* (Ixodidae), in Germany: an epidemiologic study and control measures. Berl Munch Tierarztl Wochenschr. 1996, 109: 245-248.

SECTION XV: CORYNEBACTERIUM SPP.- AN EMERGING BACTERIA

CHAPTER 52

FIRST REPORT OF CORYNEBACTERIUM PSEUDOTUBERCULOSIS FROM CASEOUS LYMPHADENITIS LESIONS IN BLACK ALENTEJANO PIG (SUS SCROFA DOMESTICUS)

Manuela Oliveira, Cynthia Barroco, Carla Mottola, Raquel Santos, Abdelhak Lemsaddek, Luis Tavares and Teresa Semedo-Lemsaddek

Keywords: Antimicrobial resistance, Black Alentejano pig, Caseous lymphadenitis, Corynebacterium pseudotuberculosis, Pulsed Field Gel Electrophoresis

BACKGROUND

Corynebacterium pseudotuberculosis is an important animal pathogen, being the etiological agent of caseous lymphadenitis (CLA) or cheesy gland disease in small ruminants [1]. CLA is frequently detected in major sheep and goat production areas around the world. It is characterized by abscess formation in the skin, internal and external lymph nodes and internal organs. This disease causes significant economic impact on the small ruminant industry through decreased meat yield, damaged wool and leather, decreased reproductive efficiency, culling of affected animals and increased morbidity and mortality rates [2]. CLA can become endemic in a herd or flock and once established it is difficult to eradicate due to its poor response to therapeutics, ability to persist in the environment and difficulties in detecting subclinical infected animals [1]-[3]. It is also easily spread amongst animals due to direct contact with superficial wounds or draining abscesses [3]. Nowadays, the most common treatment for CLA is abscess drainage followed by disinfection with an iodine solution and antibiotic therapy.

C. pseudotuberculosis is a relatively homogenous taxonomic group that can be distinguished from most *Corynebacterium* species by the production of Phospholipase D (PLD) and urease and the inability to ferment starch. The importance of *C. pseudotuberculosis* as an animal pathogen has prompted characterization studies on its toxins, particularly the haemolytic toxin PLD [4]. The differentiation between biovars is also important for infection epidemiology, as they are host specific. Evaluation of the ability to reduce nitrates allows discriminating between the negative isolates from biovar ovis, usually related with CLA in sheeps and goats, and the positive members of biovar equi, found in horses and bovines [3],[4].

Other species belonging to the *Corynebacterium* genus have already been related to CLA. *Corynebacterium ulcerans* was isolated from abscessed lymph nodes in wild boar (*Sus scrofa*) [5],[6]. However, to our understanding, there is only one report available regarding *C. pseudotuberculosis* isolation from asymptomatic swine [7]. In this work we describe the first phenotypic and genotypic characterization of *C. paratuberculosis* clinical isolates from caseous lymphadenitis lesions in the Black Alentejano pig (*Sus scrofa domesticus*), Alentejo region, South Portugal.

CASE PRESENTATION

Data presented refers to two "Alentejana" breed swine farms, A and B, located in "Odemira" district, "Alentejo" region, South Portugal, where purulent lymphadenitis cases were detected (Figure 1). In farm A and B, respectively with 700-800 and 400-500 animals, piglets are maintained in camping with the sows until weaning at 5 weeks, and afterwards are reared in extensive system, in lots with around 200 animals each. Farms

Citation: Manuela Oliveira, Cynthia Barroco, Carla Mottola, Raquel Santos, Abdelhak Lemsaddek, Luis Tavares and Teresa Semedo-Lemsaddek, First report of Corynebacterium pseudotuberculosis from caseous lymphadenitis lesions in Black Alentejano pig (Sus scrofa domesticus), DOI: 10.1186/s12917-014-0218-3.

only reared swine, but they were not isolated, as animals' movement could be observed. There was no commercial relationship between farms A and B. In both farms, CLA was detected in piglets from weaning until 10 month of age, in all rearing lots, affecting up to 10% of the animals. Lesions were observed mainly in the mandibular and retropharyngeal lymphnodes, but were also found in other locations. About 1% of the animals died as a consequence of polyarthritis and/or infection dissemination to other organs. In the remaining cases, infection was controlled and was not responsible for rejections at slaughter.

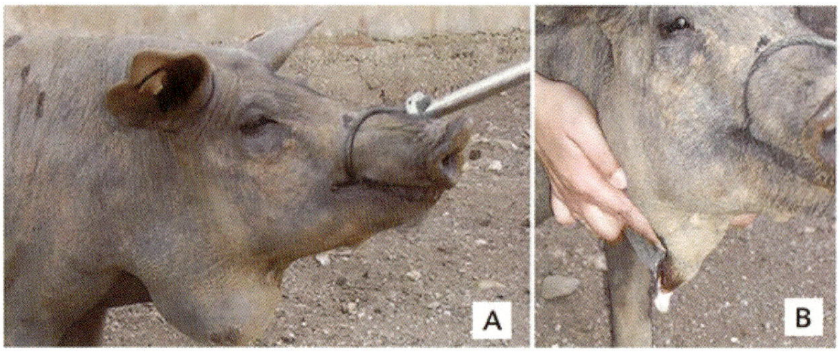

Figure 1: Caseous lymphadenitis lesions in Black Alentejano pig (*Sus scrofa domesticus*) from a farm located in the Odemira district, «Alentejo» region, south Portugal; A) Mandibular abscess; B) Abscess purulent content.

Ten bacterial isolates were obtained from ten swabs collected from abscesses in ten Black Alentejano pigs (*Sus scrofa domesticus*). Samples were collected as part of routine diagnostics, from live animals using sterile materials and after performing the asepsis of the abscess skin, and kept refrigerated at 4°C until transport to the laboratory. Samples were plated on Columbia Agar (COS) (43041, bioMérieux, Basingstoke, UK) and incubated aerobically at 37°C for 24 h. Isolates were initially checked for Gram staining, morphology and production of cytochrome c oxidase. From the swine samples it was possible to obtain pure cultures, formed by Gram-positive, oxidase negative, pleomorphic rods. Identification was performed using biochemical identification galleries (12136A, API Coryne®, bioMérieux, Basingstoke, UK) according to the manufacturer›s instructions. Subsequently, in order to distinguish between *C. pseudotuberculosis* biovar equi and biovar ovis, the ability to reduce nitrates was also evaluated [3]. Isolates were identified as *C. pseudotuberculosis* by Api Coryne®, all of which were nitrate reductase negative, hence identified as *C. pseudotuberculosis* biovar ovis. Although other microorganisms have already been related to lymphadenitis in several animals, such as *Actinomyces hyovaginalis* in goats, sheeps and pigs [8],[9], *Francisella tularensis* in humans [10], *Staphylococcus aureus* ssp. *anaerobius* in lambs [11] and *C. ulcerans* in wild boars and roe deer [5],[6], *C. pseudotuberculosis* is the main bacterial species responsible for CLA [1]. Results from this study confirm that this bacterial species is also the main responsible for CLA development in the Black Alentejano pig (*Sus scrofa domesticus*) at the sampled farms, as it was possible to isolate this agent from all collected samples, in pure cultures.

As *C. pseudotuberculosis* is frequently related to CLA in small ruminants but not in pigs, we included in this study nine *C. pseudotuberculosis* caprine isolates belonging to a collection of clinical isolates from the Bacteriology Laboratory from the Faculty of Veterinary Medicine from the University of Lisbon, Portugal, for comparison purposes.

PLD production by the 19 isolates was determined by observation of haemolytic antagonism with β haemolysin from *Staphylococcus aureus* and haemolytic synergism with *Streptococcus agalactiae*, according to Literák et al. [12]. cAMP phenotypic assay demonstrated that all, except one swine isolate, were PLD positive.

For assessment of the antimicrobial resistance profile, 13 antimicrobial compounds (Oxoid, Basingstoke, Hampshire, UK) commonly used in veterinary medicine were selected, as follows: Amoxycillin/Clavulanic acid (AMC, CT0223B, 30 μg), Ampicillin (AMP, CT0003B, 10 μg), Chloramphenicol (C, CT0013B, 30 μg), Cephalexin (CL, CT0007B, 30 μg), Gentamicin (CN, CT0024B, 10 μg), Cefotaxime (CTX, CT0166B, 30 μg), Enrofloxacin (ENR, CT0639B, 5 μg), Nalidixic acid (NA, CT0031B, 30 μg), Penicillin G (P, CT0043B, 10 units), Streptomycin (S, CT0047B, 10 μg), Sulfamethoxazole/Trimethoprim (SXT, CT0052B, 25 μg), Tetracycline (TE, CT0054B, 30 μg) and Vancomycin (VA, CT0058B, 30 μg). The compounds were tested by the Disk Diffusion (DD) Method, according to the Clinical and Laboratory Standards Institute [13] guidelines. Isolates were susceptible to the majority of the antimicrobial compounds tested. All *C. pseudotuberculosis*, except one, were resistant to nalidix acid and streptomycin. Although isolates were susceptible to most antimicrobial compounds tested, CLA infections are difficult to eradicate, as the bacterial agent remains enclosed in caseous abscesses, where the penetration of therapeutic drugs is extremely difficult.

Isolate molecular characterization was performed by Multiplex PCR and Pulsed Field Gel Electrophoresis (PFGE). For DNA isolation, 4-5 bacterial colonies of 48 hour cultures were resuspended in 100 μL TE [10 mM Tris-Cl (pH 8.0), 1 mM EDTA (pH 8.0)]. Afterwards, samples were incubated at 96°C for 5-7 minutes and centrifuged at 15000 g during 5 minutes. Supernatants were stored at -20°C.

Primers targeting the 16S rRNA, *rpoB* and *pld* genes of *C. pseudotuberculosis* previously described by other authors were used [14]-[16]. Reference strain *C. pseudotuberculosis* CECT 808 was included as positive control.

Multiplex PCR was performed in a final reaction volume of 25 μL containing 2.5 U NZYTaq 2x Green Master Mix (NZYTech, Portugal), and 10 μM of each of the primers 16S-F/16S-R, *rpoB*-F/*rpoB*-R and *pld*-F/*pld*-R. Reactions were carried out in a thermal cycler (MyCycler; Bio-Rad laboratories, Hemel Hempstead, UK), using the conditions described by Pacheco et al. 2007 [16].

All *Corynebacterium* isolates under analysis generated the amplicons of ~446 bp and ~816 bp, corresponding respectively to the *rpoB* and 16S RNA genes. Regarding the *pld* gene product (200 bp) it was detected in only 14 isolates. This discrepancy between PLD phenotypic and genotypic assays (18 vs. 14 positive isolates) led us to perform another PCR amplification using the primers directed to the *pld* gene described by Pacheco et al. but in a single reaction, i.e., 16S-F/16S-R, *rpoB*-F/*rpoB*-R were excluded. In this PCR amplification the 19 isolates under analysis showed a positive result. Thus, the false negative results obtained in the previous multiplex PCR were probably due to reagent consumption, which prevented *pld* amplification. Since the other multiplex targets were 16S rRNA, *rpoB* (two housekeeping genes present in more than one copy in the bacterial genome) this is not totally surprising. These findings highlight the need of performing both phenotypic and genotypic PLD analysis and, in case of discrepancy, converting the multiplex in a PCR directed to a single target to further confirm the negative results.

For PFGE analysis, isolates were grown in Brain-Heart Infusion broth with 0.1% Tween 20 for 48 hour at 37°C and DNA plugs were prepared as previously described by Connor et al. [17]. Macrorestrition was carried overnight with 20 U of the endonuclease *Sfi*I (Takara BIO INC, Saint-Germain-en-Laye, France) at 50°C. PFGE was performed using a Chef DRII system (Bio-Rad laboratories, Hemel Hempstead, UK), and gels consisted of 1% agarose (Sigma-Aldrich Química, S.L) in 0.5X Tris-borate-EDTA buffer (Bio-Rad laboratories, Hemel Hempstead, UK). The Lambda Ladder PFG Marker (New England Biolabs, Ipswich, USA) was used as a molecular weight marker. Electrophoresis was performed at 6 V/cm at 14°C for 23 hour with an initial switch time of 5 s and final switch time of 20 s. After staining with ethidium bromide, gel images were acquired with the ImageMaster (PharmaciaBiotech, GE Healthcare, UK).

BioNumerics 6.5 software (Applied Maths, Belgium) was used to register PFGE macrorestriction patterns and clustering analysis performed using the Dice similarity coefficient and the unweighted-pair group method with arithmetic mean (UPGMA).

As *C. pseudotuberculosis* is often related with CLA in small ruminants, goat isolates (n = 9) from caseous lymphadenitis lesions, belonging to a large collection of clinical isolates from the Laboratory of Microbiology and Immunology of the Faculty of Veterinary Medicine of the University of Lisbon, Portugal, were used in this study for comparison and genotypic characterization, as previously mentioned.

From the PFGE macrorestriction profiles obtained for the nineteen isolates under analysis (ten *C. pseudotuberculosis* from pigs and nine from goats) a similarity dendogram was built using the Bionumerics software (Figure 2). Above 55%, isolates grouped in two clusters: cluster I, including eight swine isolates (four from each farm) and one caprine isolate; and cluster II, with eight caprine and two swine isolates (one from each farm). The higher similarity index observed within each cluster reveals the clonal relationship between the *C. pseudotuberculosis* under analysis, despite animal host species and farm of origin. Similar results were reported by other authors who also found high genomic similarities between *C. pseudotuberculosis* isolated from distinct animal species [3],[17],[18].

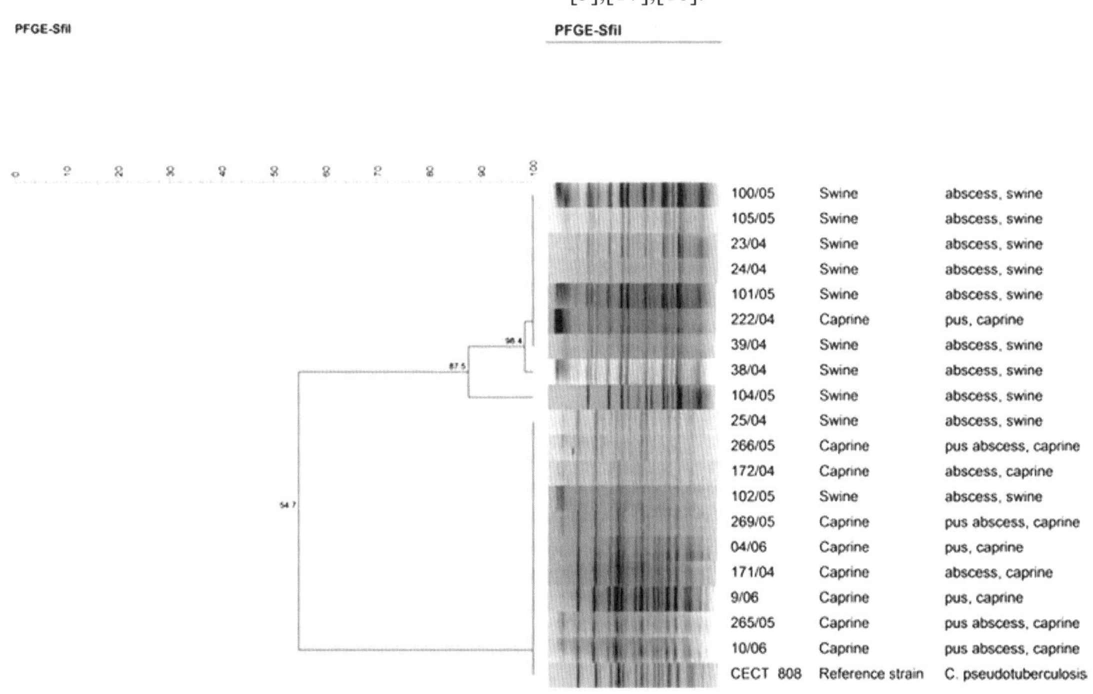

Figure 2: Dendrogram based on PFGE patterns from *C. pseudotuberculosis* strains analyzed using the endonuclease *Sfi* I.Similarity was calculated with Dice correlation coefficient -r- and clustering was performed with UPGMA.

Overall, our study suggests the prevalence of dominant clones and a putative cross-dissemination between swine and goats. As the farms under study only rear this swine breed, animals could have been infected by pigs coming from other farms that also have sheep and goats, as the production system was not closed.

CONCLUSIONS

This work represents the first report of *Corynebacterium pseudotuberculosis* from caseous lymphadenitis lesions in Black Alentejano pig (*Sus scrofa domesticus*). It also alerts for the importance of the establishment of suitable control and sanitary management practices to control the infection and avoid further dissemination of this important pathogen to other animal hosts. The presence of this microorganism in the two farms studied confirms its spreading ability, as well as their clonal relationships established by PFGE analysis. Further studies including a larger number of isolates should be performed in order to fully characterize these agents and identify possible routes of transmission.

AUTHORS' CONTRIBUTIONS

MO conceived the study and participated in its coordination, helped to draft the manuscript, having also participated in bacterial isolation and in the phenotypic assays; CB carried out the phenotypic assays and the molecular genetic studies; CM participated in the molecular genetic studies; RS participated in results analysis and helped to draft the manuscript; AL participated in the sequence alignment; LT participated in the study design and coordination; TSL participated in the design, coordination and execution of the molecular genetic studies and helped to draft the manuscript. All authors read and approved the final manuscript.

DECLARATIONS

Acknowledgements

Authors would like to acknowledge Lina Cavaco, DVM, PhD and Filipe Nunes, DVM, PhD, for all the help in isolates collection and identification and Diogo Costa, DVM, for allowing access to the farms. This work was supported by CIISA ("Centro de Investigação Interdisciplinar em Sanidade Animal") from the Faculty of Veterinary Medicine, University of Lisbon, Project PEst-OE/AGR/U10276/2014, funded by "Fundação para a Ciência e Tecnologia" (FCT), Lisbon, Portugal.

REFERENCES

1. Dorella FA, Pacheco LC, Oliveira SC, Miyoshi A, Azevedo V: *Corynebacterium pseudotuberculosis*: microbiology, biochemical properties, pathogenesis and molecular studies of virulence. Vet Res. 2006, 37: 1-18. 10.1051/vetres:2005056.
2. Williamson LH: Caseous lymphadenitis in small ruminants. Vet Clin North Am Food Anim Pract. 2001, 17: 359-371.
3. Soares SC, Silva A, Trost E, Blom J, Ramos R, Carneiro A, Ali A, Santos AR, Pinto AC, Diniz C, Barbosa EG, Dorella FA, Aburjaile F, Rocha FS, Nascimento KK, Guimarães LC, Almeida S, Hassan SS, Bakhtiar SM, Pereira UP, Abreu VA, Schneider MP, Miyoshi A, Tauch A, Azevedo V: The pan-genome of the animal pathogen *Corynebacterium pseudotuberculosis* reveals differences in genome plasticity between the biovar ovis and equi strains. PLoS ONE. 2013, 8: e53818-10.1371/journal.pone.0053818.
4. Coyle MB, Lipsky BA: Coryneform bacteria in infectious diseases: Clinical and laboratory aspects. Clin Microbiol Rev. 1990, 3: 227-246.
5. Contzen M, Sting R, Blazey B, Rau J: *Corynebacterium ulcerans* from Diseased Wild Boars. Zoonoses Public Health. 2011, 58: 479-488. 10.1111/j.1863-2378.2011.01396.x.
6. Eisenberg T, Kutzer P, Peters M, Sing A, Contzen M, Rau J: Nontoxigenic tox-bearing *Corynebacterium ulcerans* infection among game animals, Germany. Emerg Infect Dis. 2014, 20: 448-452.
7. Zhao HK, Yonekawa K, Takahashi T, Kikuchi N, Hiramune T, Yanagawa R: Isolation of *Corynebacterium pseudotuberculosis* from the cervical canal of clinically normal sows. Res Vet Sci. 1993, 55: 356-359. 10.1016/0034-5288(93)90107-Q.
8. Schumacher VL, Hinckley L, Gilbert K, Risatti GR, Londoño AS, Smyth JA: *Actinomyces hyovaginalis*-associated lymphadenitis in a Nubian goat. J Vet Diagn Invest. 2009, 21: 380-384. 10.1177/104063870902100315.
9. Foster G, Wragg P, Koylass MS, Whatmore AM, Hoyles L: Isolation of *Actinomyces hyovaginalis* from sheep and comparison with isolates obtained from pigs. Vet Microbiol. 2012, 157: 471-475. 10.1016/j.vetmic.2012.01.003.
10. Markoc F, Koseoglu RD, Koc S, Gurbuzler L: Tularemia in differential diagnosis of cervical lymphadenopathy: cytologic features of tularemia lymphadenitis. Acta Cytol. 2014, 58: 23-28. 10.1159/000355869.
11. Møller K, Agerholm JS, Ahrens P, Jensen NE, Nielsen TK: Abscess disease, caseous lymphadenitis, and pulmonary adenomatosis in imported sheep. J Vet Med B Infect Dis Vet Public Health. 2000, 47: 55-62. 10.1046/j.1439-0450.2000.00310.x.
12. Literák I, Horváthová A, Jahnová M, Rychlík I, Skalka B: Phenotype and genotype characteristics of the Slovak and Czech *Corynebacterium pseudotuberculosis* strains isolated from sheep and goats. Small Rumin Res. 1999, 32: 107-111. 10.1016/S0921-4488(98)00174-6.
13. Performance Standards for antimicrobial Susceptibility Testing; Seventeenth Informational Supplement. CLSI document M100-S17. 2007
14. Çetinkaya B, Karahana M, Atila E, Kalina R, De Baereb T, Vaneechoutteb M: Identification of *Corynebacterium pseudotuberculosis* isolates from sheep and goats by PCR. Vet Microbiol. 2002, 88: 75-83. 10.1016/S0378-1135(02)00089-5.
15. Khamis A, Raoult D, La Scola B: *rpoB* gene sequencing for identification of *Corynebacterium* species. J

Clin Microbiol. 2004, 42: 3925-3931. 10.1128/JCM.42.9.3925-3931.2004.

16. Pacheco LG, Pena RR, Castro TL, Dorella FA, Bahia RC, Carminati R, Frota MN, Oliveira SC, Meyer R, Alves FS, Miyoshi A, Azevedo V: Multiplex PCR assay for identification of *Corynebacterium pseudotuberculosis* from pure cultures and for rapid detection of this pathogen in clinical samples. J Med Microbiol. 2007, 56: 480-486. 10.1099/jmm.0.46997-0.

17. Connor KM, Fontaine MC, Rudge K, Baird GJ, Donachie W: Molecular genotyping of multinational ovine and caprine *Corynebacterium pseudotuberculosis* isolates using pulsed-field gel electrophoresis. Vet Res. 2007, 38: 613-623. 10.1051/vetres:2007013.

18. Dorneles EM, Santana JA, Ribeiro D, Dorella FA, Guimarães AS, Moawad MS, Selim SA, Garaldi AL, Miyoshi A, Ribeiro MG, Gouveia AM, Azevedo V, Heinemann MB, Lage AP: Evaluation of ERIC-PCR as genotyping method for *Corynebacterium pseudotuberculosis* isolates. PLoS ONE. 2014, 9: e98758-10.1371/journal.pone.0098758.

CHAPTER 53

TOXIGENIC CORYNEBACTERIUM ULCERANS IN WOMAN AND CAT

Anja Berger, Ingrid Huber, Sophie-Susann Merbecks, Ingrid Ehrhard, Regina Konrad, Stefan Hörmansdorfer, Michael Hogardt, and Andreas Sing

Diphtheria and diphtheria-like illness are caused by *Corynebacterium* spp. that harbor the diphtheria toxin–encoding *tox* gene. Recently in many industrialized countries, cases of diphtheria-like infection caused by toxigenic *C. ulcerans* have outnumbered those caused by toxigenic *C. diphtheriae* (*1,2*). *C. ulcerans*infection was originally associated with consumption of raw milk and dairy products or contact with cattle, but *C. ulcerans* has increasingly been isolated from domestic animals such as pet dogs and cats (*3–5*). So far, isolation of an identical toxigenic *C. ulcerans* strain from an animal and its owner has been documented only for dogs (*3,4*) and a pig (*6*). We report the isolation of an identical toxigenic *C. ulcerans* strain from an asymptomtic pet cat and a person with pharyngeal diphtheria-like illness; therefore, it might be speculated that the woman has acquired her infection from the cat.

In November 2010, an 86-year-old woman with arterial hypertension and rheumatoid arthritis was admitted to an ear, nose, and throat clinic in Dresden, Germany, with a 3-day history of sore throat, hoarseness, and nasal respiratory obstruction. Fever was not reported. Because the patient had visible fibrinous rhinitis, a nasal and pharyngeal swab was obtained before treatment with amoxicillin was begun. The patient had no history of recent travel abroad or contact with livestock. Her complete vaccination status against diphtheria was unknown, but she had received a vaccination booster in 2006.

Toxigenic *C. ulcerans* grew from culture of the nasal swab specimen; it was identified by biochemical differentiation (API Coryne code 0111326; bioMèrieux, Nürtingen, Germany), *rpoB* sequencing (*6*), and MALDI-TOF analysis (MALDI Biotyper; Bruker Daltonics, Bremen, Germany) (*7*). Toxigenicity was verified by real-time PCR (*8*) and a modified Elek test (*6*).

Because the microbiological result suggested diphtheria-like illness, the patient was transferred to an infectious diseases department in an academic hospital, where she was isolated and treated with amoxicillin for 12 days. Because the patient's condition was stable and no severe complications occurred during her hospital stay, she was not given diphtheria antitoxin. Her predominant symptoms, such as sore throat and earache, improved after antimicrobial drug therapy, and she recovered quickly. Electrocardiogram performed before discharge from hospital showed no signs of myocarditis or other toxin-related effects, such as neurologic disorder.

Although person-to-person transmission of *C. ulcerans* has not yet convincingly been demonstrated, an outbreak investigation involving the patient's close contacts (6 family members, the physician, and 19 nurses and other health care workers) was conducted. Although all close contacts had completed the series of diphtheria toxoid vaccinations, they were all given postexposure prophylaxis with erythromycin.

Because of the zoonotic potential of human *C. ulcerans* infections, nasal and pharyngeal swab samples were collected from the patient's asymptomatic pet cat. Strains of *tox*-positive *C. ulcerans* (which we named KL251 and KL252) grew on culture; the API Coryne code was identical to that of the human isolate KL246. In contrast to the human isolate, which yielded a weakly positive Elek result, both isolates from the cat showed Elek-negative results.

Antimicrobial drug susceptibility testing of the 3 isolates was performed on Mueller-Hinton blood agar (supplemented with 5% sheep blood) by using the Etest system after overnight incubation at 37°C and in 5% CO_2. In the absence of standardized breakpoints for *C. ulcerans*, susceptibility

Citation: Anja Berger, Ingrid Huber, Sophie-Susann Merbecks, Ingrid Ehrhard, Regina Konrad, Stefan Hörmansdorfer, Michael Hogardt, and Andreas Sing, Toxigenic Corynebacterium ulcerans in Woman and Cat, http://dx.doi.org/10.3201/eid1709.110391.

was determined by using the Clinical Laboratory Standards Institute criteria for broth microbouillon dilution susceptibility testing for *Corynebacterium* spp (*9*). All *C. ulcerans* strains were susceptible to amoxicillin, benzyl penicillin, ceftriaxone, erythromycin, and tetracycline (MICs 0.19–0.5 μg/mL) but less susceptible to clindamycin in vitro (MIC 2 μg/mL).

Sequencing of *rpoB* and *tox* showed 100% homology between the strains from the woman and the cat. Ribotyping revealing a U3-like ribotype (*5*), and multilocus sequence typing (*10*) confirmed the clonal identity of the strains.

The cat was given a combined preparation of benzyl penicillin and streptomycin. After completion of therapy, *C. ulcerans* no longer grew from nasal swab specimens from the woman or the cat.

Our findings of transmission of toxigenic *C. ulcerans* between a woman and her cat underline the zoonotic potential of this organism and highlight the need for more studies investigating the carrier status of companion animals such as cats and dogs. Although clindamycin is not a first-line drug for diphtheria therapy, the intermediate susceptibility of *C. ulcerans* against clindamycin underscores the necessity of standardized susceptibility testing for diphtheria cases because clindamycin-resistant toxigenic *C. ulcerans* strains in human infections have been recently reported (*6*). Toxigenic *C. ulcerans* strains are rare, but the numbers of human wound infections or diphtheria-like disease caused by *C. ulcerans* have increased in the past few years. However, detection of toxigenic *C. ulcerans* is often still incidental, often resulting in delayed specific therapy, including patient isolation or contact tracing.

ACKNOWLEDGMENTS

We thank Wolfgang Schmidt, Karola Grünwald, Marzena Maggipinto, and Daniela Sebah for cultivation and microbiological and molecular characterization of the *Corynebacteria*.

The study was partially supported by the Bavarian State Ministry of the Environment and Public Health, by the European Commission's Directorate General for Health and Consumer Policy through the Diphtheria Surveillance Network, and by the German Federal Ministry of Health through the Robert Koch-Institute and its National Reference Laboratories Network.

REFERENCES

1. Bonmarin I, Guiso N, Le Flèche-Matéos A, Patey O, Patrick AD, Levy-Bruhl D. Diphtheria: a zoonotic disease in France? Vaccine. 2009;27:4196–200.
2. Wagner KS, White JM, Crowcroft NS, De Martin S, Mann G, Efstratiou A. Diphtheria in the United Kingdom, 1986–2008: the increasing role of *Corynebacterium ulcerans*. Epidemiol Infect. 2010;138:1519–30.
3. Lartigue MF, Monnet X, Le Flèche A, Grimont PA, Benet JJ, Durrbach A, *Corynebacterium ulcerans* in an immunocompromised patient with diphtheria and her dog. J Clin Microbiol. 2005;43:999–1001.
4. Hogg RA, Wessels J, Hart J, Efstratiou A, De Zoysa A, Mann G, Possible zoonotic transmission of toxigenic *Corynebacterium ulcerans* from companion animals in a human case of fatal diphtheria. Vet Rec. 2009;165:691–2.
5. De Zoysa A, Hawkey PM, Engler K, George R, Mann G, Reilly W, Characterization of toxigenic *Corynebacterium ulcerans* strains isolated from humans and domestic cats in the United Kingdom. J Clin Microbiol. 2005;43:4377–81.
6. Schuhegger R, Schoerner C, Dlugaiczyk J, Lichtenfeld I, Trouillier A, Zeller-Peronnet V, Pigs as source for toxigenic *Corynebacterium ulcerans*. Emerg Infect Dis. 2009;15:1314–5.
7. Konrad R, Berger A, Huber I, Boschert V, Hörmansdorfer S, Busch U, Matrix-assisted laser desorption/ionisation time-of-flight (MALDI-TOF) mass spectrometry as a tool for rapid diagnosis of potentially toxigenic *Corynebacterium* species in the laboratory management of diphtheria-associated bacteria. Euro Surveill. 2010;15:pii:19699.
8. Schuhegger R, Lindermayer M, Kugler R, Heesemann J, Busch U, Sing A. Detection of toxigenic *Corynebacterium diphtheriae* and *Corynebacterium ulcerans* strains by a novel real-time PCR. J Clin Microbiol. 2008;46:2822–3.
9. Clinical Laboratory Standards Institute. Methods for antimicrobial dilution and disk susceptibility testing of infrequently isolated or fastidious bacteria; approved guideline. 2nd ed. Wayne (PA): The Institute; 2006. p. M45–A2.
10. Bolt F, Cassiday P, Tondella ML, Dezoysa A, Efstratiou A, Sing A, Multilocus sequence typing identifies evidence for recombination and two distinct lineages of *Corynebacterium diphtheriae*. J Clin Microbiol. 2010;48:4177–85.

SECTION XVI: ZOONOSES

CHAPTER 54 ZOONOSES IN PET BIRDS: REVIEW AND PERSPECTIVES

Geraldine Boseret, Bertrand Losson, Jacques G Mainil, Etienne Thiry and Claude Saegerman

INTRODUCTION

The term "Pet bird" designates birds housed and bred for an exclusively ornamental use. This category includes and will refer later in this paper to mainly passeriformes (e.g. canaries, finches, sparrows: see Table 1), also called songbirds, and psittaciformes (parrots, parakeets, budgerigars, love birds: see Table 1) [1, 2, 3]. It is a rather unknown vet's clientship fraction. A statistical study made by the American Veterinary Medicine Association (AVMA) recorded 11 to 16 million companion and exotic birds in the United States in 2007 [4]. In 2010, following a study made by the FACCO (*chambre syndicale des Fabricants d'Aliments préparés pour Chiens, Chats, Oiseaux et autres animaux familiers*), 6 million pet birds are owned by French people [5]. In Belgium, every bred bird has to be identified by a ring sharing a number directly connected to the breeder's owner (Arrêté du Gouvernement wallon fixant des dérogations aux mesures de protection des oiseaux, AM 2003-11-27). In 2011, the Association Ornithologique de Belgique (AOB) registered 249 ornithological societies authorized to identify their birds by an official ring.

Table 1: Main pet bird species according to the International Ornithologic Congress (IOC) classification 3.1 (2012)

Order	Family	Genus	Species	English name	French name
Passeriforms	Fringillidae	*Serinus*	*S. canaria*	Canary	Canari/serin des canaries
		Carduelis	*C. carduelis*	Gold finch	Chardonneret
			C. chloris	Green finch	Verdier
			C. spinus	siskin	Tarin
		Pyrrhula	*P. pyrrhula*	Bullfinch	Bouvreuil
		Fringilla	*F. coelebs*	Chaffinch	Pinson des arbres
	Estrildidae	*Taeniopygia*	*T. guttata*	Zebra finch	Moineau man-darin
		Poephila	*P. acuti-cauda*	Long-tailed finch	Diamant à longue queue
		Erythrura	*E. gouldiae*	Gouldian Finch	Diamant de Gould

Citation: Geraldine Boseret, Bertrand Losson, Jacques G Mainil, Etienne Thiry and Claude Saegerman, Zoonoses in pet birds: review and perspectives, DOI: 10.1186/1297-9716-44-36.

		Lonchura	*L. striata*	Bengalese finch	Bengali/moineau du japon
	Sturnidae	*Gracula*	*G. religiosa*	Mynah	Mainate
		Sturnus	*S. vulgaris*	Starling	Etourneau
Psittaciforms	Psittacidae	*Melopsittacus*	*M. undulatus*	Budgerigar	Perruche ondulée
		Agapornis	*A spp*	Lovebird	Inséparable
		Psittacula	*P. eupatria*	Alexandrine parakeet	Perruche alexandrine
		Lorius	*L. spp*	Lories	Loris
		Psittacus	*P. erithacus*	African or Timneh grey parrot	Gris du Gabon
		Poicephalus	*P.senegalus*	Senegal parrot	Perroquet Youyou
		Ara	*A spp*	Macaw	Ara
		Aratinga	*A spp*	Conure	Conure
		Amazona	*A. aestiva*	Amazon	Amazone
	Cacatuidae	*Cacatua*	*C. alba*	Cockatoo	Cacatoës
		Nymphicus	*N. hollandicus*	Cockatiel	Calopsitte

Many families own their "kitchen pet bird", which represents a lucrative business for pet shops or local breeders, since a single male canary is sold around 30 euros in Belgium and a female around 20 euros. Prices are about the same for zebra finches or budgerigars, and 50% to 100% higher for "special" finches like Gould diamonds. Bird fairs and live bird markets also gather a lot of people. In addition, some species are bred for their very high value; for example, in the case of canaries, male and female breeding stock reproducers with recognized genetic potential are presented in national and international contests for their posture (the Bossu Belge), their color (red mosaic) or for their song (Harzer). As a consequence, their offspring could be sold at high for rising prices. Finally, exotic birds like greater psittaciforms (parrots, e.g. ara or cockatoo), legally or illegally traded from for example Asia or South America, remain high in the ranking of popular pets and are also profusely represented in zoos and parks.

Notwithstanding these socio-economic facts, these animals are potential carriers and/or transmitters of zoonotic diseases. Some of these pathologies could have an important impact on human health, like chlamydophilosis, salmonellosis or even highly pathogenic avian influenza A H5N1, but also have an economic impact if some of these pathogens are spread via carriers or vectors like wild birds, human beings, insects or mites to poultry breeding units or cattle facilities [6], then entering the food chain. The aim of this re is to enlighten and discuss the risks encountered by bird handlers (including children), professional workers (e.g. veterinarians, traders or shop owners) in particular and the human population in general, and to assess the eventual health and economic consequences, and propose some guidelines to prevent transmission from such birds to humans.

MAIN TRANSMISSION ROUTES

Note: main transmission routes of diseases are summarized in Table 2.

Table 2: Main transmission routes of diseases

Transmission route	**Contagious diseases**				**Non contagious diseases**	
Direct contact	yes	yes	no	no	no	no
Indirect contact	yes	yes	yes	yes	no	no
Vector-borne	yes	no	yes	no	yes	no
Example in pet birds	Chlamydophilosis	Tuberculosis	West Nile Fever	Cryptosporidiosis	Lyme disease	Genetic disorders

Direct contact

Households

Passeriforms and psittacines are housed under different conditions, due to their respective behavior. Indeed, psittacines, especially parrots, are more aggressive than passerines and would then rather be kept in pairs than groups [2, 3]. However, relatively high numbers of budgerigars can be gathered temporarily in the same cage for example in pet shop facilities or markets.

Besides the "kitchen-housing", which is usually a single cage typically containing a couple of canaries or budgerigars for example, passeriform species are rather kept in captivity in two different types of aviaries [2]: mixed ornamental aviaries and breeding facilities. The first type is usually a big wire-netting space (up to 10 m^3) located outside and sometimes with different species kept together, mostly for ornamental purposes [2]. In the second type, relatively large numbers of the same species, depending on the breeding size and breeding purpose (pet shops versus competitions) are maintained in pairs, mostly indoors (but sometimes with a partial access to the outside). In both types, new individuals are regularly introduced, in the first case with a purpose of ornamental diversification and in the second, to bring new blood into the genetic diversity of birds. These movements are supposed to be preceded by a quarantine of the new incomers.

Several times a year, performing birds are brought to shows and competitions, where exchange or selling could occur, and by the same way, transmission of pathogens, as this has been well illustrated by several authors [7, 8]. In the case of the "kitchen-canary", it could be interesting to mention that in the summer, the cages can be moved outside, in order to allow the bird to sunbathe. This could be a condition favoring contact between wild and captive passerines (Boseret, personal observations). It is also not rare for canaries to escape from their cage, with a potential risk of disseminating pathogens into a wild avian population, pathogens which they could have contracted in their original breeding facility or from humans (for example, chlamydophilosis [8]). Predators, like cats, could also be infected. The question whether bird predators could eventually become sentinels has to be raised and needs to be further investigated. Finally, one should not forget other potential zoonotic pathogens shedders, like arthropods or rodents, which could also find an easily reachable source of food in cages (Boseret, personal observations) or directly on birds themselves, as this could be the case for haematophagous insects [9, 10].

Pet shops, bird fairs and markets

In direct relationship with local breeders, housing of birds in pet shop facilities enhances the risk of transfer of several zoonoses, like for example chlamydophilosis [8]. Cages are indeed often overcrowded, filled with birds of mixed origin [8]. The overcrowding also induces intense stress to the birds due to fighting for females, territory (which is extremely limited in this case) or food. This will cause quick debilitation of the weakest individuals and higher sensitivity to infections [11]. This situation is particularly true in live animal markets as represented in numerous studies performed in Asian countries [12, 13]. Unfortunately, no data are available for European countries. But it is frequently observed that pet birds share the same space as poultry, making transmission of pathogens and parasites easier (e.g. *Dermanyssus gallinae*).

Finally, bird fairs are a final example of possible contamination. In these regional, national or international gatherings, breeders meet each other and present their production, in a context of championships. Cases of transmission of *Chlamydophila psittaci* from birds-to-humans in France and The Netherlands in such conditions have recently been related by respectively Belchior et al. and Berk et al. [7, 14]. In both cases, clinical symptoms were developed by patients and led in several cases to hospitalization.

International trade

As illustrated by several authors, controlled as well as non-controlled movements of birds could enhance the introduction of zoonotic pathogens (like chlamydophilosis or highly pathogenic avian influenza A) and their vectors (like *D. gallinae*) in non-endemic countries [15, 16, 17, 18]. Indeed it is still difficult to obtain an accurate estimation of wildlife trade since most of the time it is conducted through non-official and non-legal routes [19, 20, 21]. It must be pointed out that illegal wildlife trade for e.g. companion or ornamental pets, ranks second in terms of economic activities as compared to illegal narcotic trade [22]. In addition to this huge financial impact, this situation also reflects a non-negligible threat for human health since it facilitates multiplication and circulation of zoonotic pathogens and could facilitate adaptation of these pathogens to new hosts [16, 22]. However, controlling movement is not the absolute way to prevent pathogen transmission. Roy and Burnonfosse have illustrated this fact through their study on nuclear and sequence data analysis of pest species [18] wherein the authors showed that commercial exchanges could have an impact on international gene flow in populations of *D. gallinae*, even in a highly controlled context (for example, quarantine measures in industrial layer farms).

Vector borne transmission

Mites

Vector-borne diseases represent a major problem for public health. Bird ectoparasites, especially mesostigmatic mites belonging to Dermanyssidae and Macronyssidae, are well known for their heavy potential to transmit diseases to poultry. *Dermanyssus gallinae* in particular, even if exhaustively described in poultry breeding, is also an underestimated pet bird pathogen. This mite is often found in both the pet bird family household and intensive breeding. *D. gallinae* is a nocturnal haematophagous ectoparasite and has been described to cause an important debilitation by exsanguination, involving high mortality rate in newborns, and sometimes in hens. *D. gallinae* has also been proven to transmit zoonotic pathogens [23, 24, 25], such as *C. psittaci*[26], *Coxiella burnetii*[24, 25], *Salmonella spp.*[27, 28, 29], *Erysipelothrix rhusiopathiae*[30, 31], *Listeria monocytogenes*[24, 25] and viruses like Fowl pox virus [24]. Moreover, evidence of transmission to humans has been described, with subsequent apparition of skin lesions and a dermatological pruritic syndrome. [32, 33, 34, 35, 36, 37, 38] *D. gallinae* is characterized by a specific thigmotactic behavior and spends most of its life in the bird's environment rather than on the host itself, especially in narrow interstices like perches, feeding bowls and sand tray anfractuosities; it acts more like a mosquito or a bed bug than like other parasites, since it only occasionally bites its hosts to take a blood meal [39]. In addition to complicating early detection of the mite (on the contrary to other parasites spending most of their life on the bird, like e.g. the blood-sucking mite *Ornithonyssus silviarum*-see also below), this particular life trait makes the parasite hard to eliminate by antiparasitic spray treatment (e.g. organo-phosphorus, pyrethrinoids) [40]. A topic treatment, with application of a long-term remanent antiparasitic spot-on product (e.g. 0.1% ivermectine) directly on the birds' skin, has been suggested by Dorrestein [41]; this alternative may not, however, be easily applicable in large breeding and big facilities.

D. gallinae could be considered as an invasive species presenting a wide host spectrum, of more than 40 bird families (including passeriforms [39, 40]). The hypothesis has been formulated that these parasites could be easily transmitted horizontally, from one infested bird nest to another close one [42] or in the case of mixed colonies [43]) or from wild birds (e.g. passerines) feeding in open air together with domestic species [40]. This could also represent a way of transmission to humans. Indeed it has been shown that pigeons do nest in the vicinity of humans (such as city buildings, including hospitals [44]) and several case studies have presented the evidence of *D. gallinae* populations close to abandoned pigeons perches or nests, near windows or aeration circuitry [2, 35]. Such infestations are in direct relationship with dermatologic clinical syndromes in humans ("pseudo-scabies"), associated with pruritic syndrome [32, 33, 34, 35, 36, 37, 38]. Since *D. gallinae* has been provento shed zoonotic pathogens [28, 37] and since birds like pigeons have been found to be perching alongside hospital walls [35], one could point out the eventual risks encountered by immunocompromised humans, like hospitalized people, if they experience such a situation.

Ornithonyssus sylviarum (Macronissidae), also named Northern Fowl mite or white poultry mite is another blood-sucking arthropod identified in pet birds. Clinical symptoms are similar to those developed by a *D. gallinae* infestation: depression, anemia, newborn mortality [41]. However, *O. sylviarum* behavior is notably different from *D. gallinaes*, since it spent its entire life on the host's body, making pest detection in some way easier [41, 45]. *O. sylviarum* has been isolated in wild avifauna and pet birds; it has the ability to leave its host and reach birds even housed in other cages. However, its capacity to resist from starvation (i.e. living in the absence of any host) in the environment is significantly shorter than the red mite's (resp. 3 weeks and 24 weeks [45]). Only a few cases of zoonotic transmission to humans have been reported, with clinical signs restricted to dermatologic symptoms associated with pruritus [46]. Nonetheless, *O. sylviarum* is considered to be emergent in Europe and to present an increasing problem in aviaries [41] and should therefore not be neglected.

Mosquitoes

Different species of mosquitoes (*Diptera*, especially *Culex* species) are responsible for horizontal and reciprocal transmission of arboviruses like West Nile fever Virus (WNV; [47, 48]) or Usutu virus [49]. These diseases will be discussed further in the next section.

Dipterae act as bridging vectors between two host categories: amplificators (e.g. birds) and incidental/dead-end (e.a. humans). According to Turell et al., Sardelis et al. [50, 51], cited in [47], an infected vertebrate must present a viremia of 10^5 pfu/mL (pfu: plate forming unit) to be efficient as an amplification host. Studies have shown that house sparrows develop WNV viremia superior to 10^{10} pfu/mL after experimental infection, and maintain it above 10^5 pfu/mL for five days [47, 52, 53] and they are indeed good amplificatory hosts and, moreover overwintering hosts [48] for at least one arbovirus, the WNV. Beside these effects of amplification and seasonal resistance, international exchanges, trade and migration are factors enhancing the emergence of these viral diseases, as shown by the increasing number of diagnosed infections acquired during stays in tropical countries. Interestingly, Pfeffer and Dobler [53] pointed out the fact that no attention is actually paid on accompanying pet animals and the parasites that these pets could be carrying. Pet birds are also important since a large number of companion birds are obtained by sellers from trade with exotic countries [15, 53].

Ticks

Ticks from the genus *Ixodes* (e.g. *I. ricinus*, *I. scapularis*), are carried by birds and then have the ability to transmit pathogens like *Borrelia burgdoferi*, the causative agent of Lyme disease, and the flavivirus louping ill virus. Migrating birds could also be carriers of infected ticks and then contribute to long distance dispersal of both vectors and spirochetes [54]. Mathers et al. recently published an interesting study on the potential role of wild birds and the ticks that feed on them in the introduction of the Lyme disease agent to emergent areas [55]. No evidence, however, has been reported on transmission from wild to domestic pet birds even housed in open air aviaries.

MOST IMPORTANT DISEASES

Note: Tables 3 and 4 summarize the main diseases described below in terms of clinical signs and gross lesions presented by birds, recommended diagnostic tools and treatment, and symptomatology reported in humans.

Table 3: Summary of main pet bird zoonotic diseases

Disease	Pathology	Clinical issue	Asymptomatic shedding	Transmission route	OIE listed disease	Risk for humans*
Chlamydophilosis	Systemic	Fatal	yes	D/I/V	Yes	high
Salmonellosis	Digestive to systemic	Treatable	yes	D/I/V	No	moderate

Tuberculosis	Respiratory to systemic	Fatal	no	D/I/V	Yes	high
Campylobacteriosis	Digestive to systemic	Treatable	yes	D/I/V	No	moderate
Lyme disease		None	no	V	No	low
Avian Influenza	Systemic	Fatal	no	D/V?	Yes	high
West Nile fever and other arboviruses	Respiratory to systemic	Fatal	yes	V	Yes (WNF)	moderate
Avian Bornavirus	Digestive/nervous to systemic	Fatal	no	D	No	null
Newcastle disease	Ocular To Systemic	Mild to fatal	yes	D/I/V	Yes	low
Toxoplasmosis	Digestive	Digestive	yes	I	No	Null to low
Giardiosis *(G. duodenalis)*	Digestive to systemic	Treatable	yes	I	No	moderate
Cryptosporidiosis	Digestive	Treatable	yes	I	No	moderate
Cryptococcosis	Digestive	Treatable	yes	I	No	moderate

*when handling a bird without hygienic precautions.

Legend: D = direct contact; I = Indirect contact; V = vector-mediated contact.

Table 4: Summary of clinical data associated with main pet bird zoonotic diseases [[41]]

Disease	Sensitive species	Clinical signs	Necroptic lesions	Diagnostic (sample/analysis)	Remarks and Pitfalls	Treatment	Human symptoms
Blood-sucking mites	All	*Nestlings*: weakness, anemia, death *Adults*: AA, respiratory distress, depression	None	Direct examination	*Dermanyssus gallinae*: hide in cages anfractuosities and could not be found on birds themselves	Ivermectine, permethrins in spray. Total disinfection of cages and facilities (see also chapter 4)	Dermatitis, pruritus
Chlamydophilosis	Psittacines – canaries – finches	AA, SBS, diarrhea, nasal discharge, dehydration, Ocular signs	Air sac lesions, hepato-splenomegaly	CSw, OSw, FE/BC, serology (paired serology 2 weeks apart),IMF, PCR	Asymptomatic carriage (up to 40%), false negative	Tetracyclins (1st of 2d generation)	Flu-like syndrome, genital, articular, skin symptoms
Salmonellosis	All (open-air aviaries)	AA, WL, diarrhea, mild respiratory symptoms	Congestive gastro-intestinal tract, hepato-splenomegaly	CSw, FE	Mostly in winter and in outdoor aviaries; hard to differentiate from pseudo-tuberculosis	Not recommended (high probability of antibio-resistance)	Gastro-intestinal infection
Tuberculosis	Psittacines (canaries?)	Progressive AA, WL, respiratory symptoms, long bone lesions	Cachexia, osteolysis spots in long bones, lung lesions (non caseous)	RX (bone lesions), OSw/MO (Ziehl-Nielsen), BC, HP	Chronic development, sometimes during months to years; human origin infection	Not recommended (high probability of antibio-resistance)	Chronic pulmonary symptoms (caseous lung knots), generalized infection

Campylo-bacteriosis	Estrildidae mostly.	Apathy, yellow feces (solid or liquid)	Cachexia, congestive gastro-intestinal tract, containing a yellow amylum or undigested seeds.	FE/MO (curved rods in stained smears), BC	Canaries and psittacines are asymptomatic carriers	Not recommended (high probability of antibio-resistance)	Gastro-intestinal infection, Gillain-Barré syndrome
Avian Influenza	Passerines	Sudden death, SBS, respiratory and neurological signs	Dehydration, respiratory lesions	OSw, CSw, BS/HP, PCR	Mostly in outdoor aviaries	None	Mild to severe respiratory and systemic infection
West Nile fever	All	Ocular and neurological signs		OSw, CSw/PCR	Mostly asymptomatic carriage	None: prevention based on limitation of exposure to mosquitoes (vectors)	Mild to severe respiratory and systemic infection, encephalitis, septicaemia, death
Newcastle disease	All	SBS, AA, ocular, respiratory and neurological signs	Dehydration, respiratory lesions	OSw, CSw/serology		None; prevention by vaccination	Cunjunctivitis, mild flu-like symptoms
Toxoplasmosis	Canary, finch, budgerigar minah	SBS, AA, respiratory and neurological signs, blindness	iridocyclitis, panophthalmia, catarrhal pneumonia, hepato-splenomegaly	CSw/MO, serology, HP, PCR	Systemic symptoms sometimes unseen; detection of the disease 3 months later (blindness)	Trimetoprim-sulfamids	Mostly asymptomatic. Abortion, congenital malformation.
Giardiosis (G. duodenalis)		None	None				Sometimes asymptomatic. WL, diarrhoea, abdominal pain
Crypto-sporidiosis	All	Rare; acute diarrhoea	Gastro-enteric lesions	CsW/MO		Ronidazole	Gastro-intestinal symptoms; liver, pancreas, respiratory tract lesions
Cryptococcosis	Parrots, little pet birds	Rare	None	CSw/MO	Possible aerosol-borne contamination		Mostly asymptomatic. Respiratory and nervous symptoms.

AA apathy-Anorexia, *WL* weight loss, *FE* feces examination, *BC* bacterial culture, *MO* microscopic observation, *SBS* sick bird signs (ruffled feathers, standing at the bottom of the cage, depression), *HP* histopathology (including immunocytochemistry), *BS* blood sample, *CSw* cloacal swab, *OSw* oral swab, *IMF* Immunofluorescence, *PCR* polymerase chain reaction.

Bacterial diseases

Chlamydophilosis

One of the most threatening zoonotic diseases transmitted by birds to humans is chlamydophilosis (also known as chlamydiosis, ornithosis, psittacosis or parrot fever), caused by the intracellular bacterium *Chlamydophila psittaci*. Psittacine species are highly sensitive to this pathogen, but passerines are not excluded [26, 41, 56]. Human symptoms come from mild respiratory signs to severe pneumonia, with localization in several organs leading to diarrhea, conjunctivitis, arthritis and genital organ infection. The first people susceptible to be infected appear to be, as expected, veterinarians and birds breeders; this has been e.g. enlightened by the two following studies. The first reported an accidental contamination of a vet by infected turkeys [57]; the second, an epidemiological study made by Ghent university, pointed out a high percentage of human infection in owners and vets working in breeding psittacine facilities [8]. On 39 breeding facilities, which represent 308 birds (most of them are psittacines (e.g.): cockatoos, parrots, parakeets or lories) and 46 humans, 19.2% of birds tested positive for *C. psittaci* by nested PCR/EIA, 13% of pet owners (and the vet student in charge of the study) also tested positive after swap pharyngeal sampling. Sixty-six percent of the positive people presented mild respiratory symptoms, in association with viable *C. psittaci* isolation. Van Rompay et al. concluded their investigation with an important observation: on 18 breeding facilities, despite a broad spectrum-antibiotherapy, 60.6% were still positive for *C. psittaci* through culture and PCR (16.6% and 44% respectively) [8]. This raises the point of antibiotic resistance and development of drug-resistant strains in some facilities.

Another interesting case was described in a Liège hospital (Belgium), where a 10-year old child was admitted for persistent fever, acute abdomen, pneumonia and neurologic symptoms [58]. The pathogen, further identified as *C. psittaci*, was cefotaxime-resistant. Two budgerigars (the second most popular pet bird) were housed in the child's living place; the elder brother of this child presented a high level of anti-*C. psittaci* IgA, which suggested a non-symptomatic chlamydophilosis.

Direct transmission of *C. psittaci* from birds to humans is underlined in a compendium of security measures about avian chlamydophilosis edited by the Centre of Diseases Control and Prevention in 1998, warning bird owners (43% of infected people in the USA between 1987 and 1996) but also professionals working with birds like e.g. veterinarians, breeders, zoo workers… to be aware of a real risk of zoonotic transmission [59]. Bird fairs are a good illustration of the occupational risk presented by a high concentration of people and birds in the same space for a relatively long period of time. Belchior et al. and Berk et al. reported recently two similar events in respectively France and The Netherlands, where chlamydophilosis outbreaks occurred during bird fairs. In Belchior's study, 68% of the exhibitors tested positive for *C. psittaci* infection [7, 14].

Finally, one has to mention a case of illegally imported *C. psittaci*-positive psittacine occurring at the Antwerp custom office, that led to the hospitalization of custom officers after handling infected parakeets [15, 17].

This points out the real threat pet birds could represent when little information on biosecurity is provided to the people breeding and/or handling them. *D. gallinae* could moreover transfer this pathogen [24, 25, 26]. This reinforces the urgent need for hygienic measures to be applied in places of risk, i.e. at bird fairs, pet shop facilities and small familial breeding units. The CDC compendium of measures to control *C.psittaci* would be of great help [59].

Salmonellosis

Salmonella species were isolated from several captive passerine or psittacine birds, in relation or not (asymptomatic carriage) to clinical symptoms: diarrhea, multisystem disease, septicaemia, osteomyelitis, depression, crop stasis, dehydration, anorexia [56, 60, 61, 62, 63]. The serovar Typhimurium, a well-known zoonotic agent, was described in passerine birds in such clinical manifestations as granulomas (liver, ceca, spleen), multisystemic symptoms, ocular lesions and osteomyelitis [61, 64]. Transmission to humans was reported in different cases [63, 65, 66]. Smith et al. also reported two cases of *Salmonella typhimurium*outbreaks in elementary schools related to owl pellet dissection [67]. Even if these cases are more anecdotal than quite frequent, people should be careful (and at least respect elementary hygienic rules) when manipulating bird products such as wild bird pellets, which could be in a somehow comprehensive way undertaken as a didactical manner to teach nature to kids. Another point of is the problematic of wild reservoirs. Indeed, wild songbirds have been repeatedly documented as *Salmonella spp.* carriers [68, 69] and implicated in the transmission of these pathogens to humans and mammals. Starlings in particular, have been shown to be potential spread agents of salmonellosis in cattle feeding operations [6]. In addition, bovine herds have been demonstrated to be reservoirs of many gastro-intestinal pathogens being of concern to humans, especially professionals like livestock producers or veterinarians [70], as well as consumers [71].

Finally, as discussed in the chapters above, *D. gallinae* seems to play a significant role in *Salmonella spp.* Transmission in layer farms, as developed by Valiente Moro et al. [23, 27, 28, 29].

Tuberculosis

Isolation of zoonotic agents from the *Mycobacterium* species is not so rare in pet birds, especially in psittacines. The most commonly isolated species are respectively *Mycobacterium genavense* and *Mycobacterium avium*[56, 72]. The main species causing tuberculosis in humans, i.e. *M. tuberculosis*, has only rarely been reported in birds, and essentially in parrots. In this particular bird family, an interesting observation should to be pointed out, especially since it seems that the main route of infection was of human origin. Well documented examples are the green-winged macaws (*Ara chloroptera*) diagnosed positive for *Mycobacterium tuberculosis*, the first in New York City [73] and the second in Switzerland [74]. Both birds developed a panel of clinical signs associated with tuberculosis: lethargy, osteomyelitis, multifocal granulomatous panniculitis and granulomatous hepatitis. In both cases, the bird owners had a history of culture-confirmed pulmonary tuberculosis and confessed real close contact with their birds (mouth-to-beak feeding). Moreover, in the Swiss case, two veterinarians in charge of the case showed a positive reaction to tuberculin skin test after handling the sick bird [74]. One observation made by the authors is that these parrots have lived a sufficiently long time while incubating the disease to become themselves a potential source of infection for other humans. Data are lacking on the susceptibility of non psittacine pet birds to *M. tuberculosis*, since the authors found only one study reporting such an infection in a canary, diagnosed with a lung knot positive for *M. tuberculosis*[75].

It is, however, a fact that infection with zoonotic *Mycobacterium spp* in pet birds is rare. Regarding the susceptibility of birds to *Mycobacterium bovis*, to date, only experimental infections have been reported as being responsible for clinical signs. A recent study focusing on the experimental infection of budgerigars by several species of *Mycobacterium* reported that the only clinical signs were seen 70 days after inoculation with *M. bovis*, while no clinical signs were observed following the challenge with the other species [76]. *M. bovis* is also a zoonotic agent, considered to be responsible for 1 to 2% of human cases of tuberculosis in industrialized countries, while this proportion is susceptible to be much more important in developing countries (until 8% of human cases, depending on the region) [77, 78].

Nevertheless, infected/carrying/untreated birds could become a potential reservoir for humans, and then have consequences on public health. In an ideal situation, surveillance and early diagnosis of zoonotic mycobacteria should be performed in every imported bird bunch [79, 80] including animals captured from the wild [81]. Mycobacterial culture or PCR analyses would be the most sensitive and specific laboratory tests for a definitive diagnosis [82]. However, the long-term onset of the disease, the pathogen's intracellular localization and the difficulty to dispose of not expensive highly sensitive diagnostic tests makes systematic and/or regular check-ups difficult to perform in routine conditions.

Campylobacteriosis

Campylobacter spp., and in particular *Campylobacter jejuni* are responsible for food-borne diseases in many countries, responsible in humans for debilitating symptoms such as gastro-enteritis (diarrhea, vomiting), headaches, and depression, leading sometimes to death. Campylobacteriosis was the most frequent zoonotic disease reported in 2009 in the European Union [71]. But *Campylobacter spp.* is not exclusively a food-borne disease. Even if little information is available on the role of other avian species (like pet birds) in the epidemiology of the disease, this pathogen is shed by an important bird variety, among which are "hobby birds" including estrildidae, canaries and psittacines [41, 83, 84]. Moreover, an Italian study showed a high occurrence of *C. jejuni* in migrating passeriforms [85], and concluded that these birds constitute a reservoir and a possible transmission route from birds to humans and domesticated animals, including cattle. This observation was also made by Adhikari et al. in 2004 [86], in a study dealing with dairy cows and sparrow fecal matters in New Zealand. However, other reports and experimental protocols tend to demonstrate that *C. jejuni* infection is highly host-specific and that transmission from birds to humans, *a fortiori* from pet birds, although not impossible, is likely to play a minor role [87, 88]. Nevertheless, one still has to consider the potential role of pet birds in *C. jejuni* shedding and consequently apply elementary hygienic precautions while manipulating birds and/or feces.

Lyme disease

Different strains of *Borrelia burgdorferi sensu lato* were isolated from ticks collected on songbirds in different areas of the world, including Europe [54]. Olsen et al. [89] showed that canaries presentrelatively quickly a mild spirochetemia after experimental infection with *B. burgdorferi,* but without or few clinical symptoms. This suggests that passerines may be of little importance as long-term amplifying reservoirs for borreliosis. Moreover, ticks are usually quickly detected in the feathers of bred birds, as well as in kitchen-canaries, diminishing then the risk of wild-to-captive bird transmission and a fortiori to humans.

Concerning psittacines, no evidence of Lyme disease seems to have been shown.

Others

There are numerous other potential zoonotic bacteria also identified in pet birds, including multiple gram-negative bacteria such as *Pasteurella* spp, *Klebsiella* spp, *Yersinia* spp, *Pseudomonas spp.*, and *Escherichia coli*[41, 56, 90, 91]. Indeed, *Escherichia coli* O157:H7 strains transmitted from wild passerines (European starlings mostly) to cattle and then introduced into the food chain has been reported in several studies [92, 93, 94]. Lack of hygiene and the absence of quarantine (especially concerning imported birds), and dirty food and water sources seem to be the most probable origin of infection with these zoonotic pathogens. Besides, the potential transmission from wild birds to open-air aviaries hosted pet birds (via fecal drops) should be considered (Boseret, personal observations). However, reports of transmission of these bacteria from pet birds to humans still lack in the literature.

Viral diseases

Avian influenza

Highly pathogenic avian influenza A H5N1 has been in the world health focus since the year 2000's outbreaks. Perkins and Swayne [95], demonstrated in 2003 that the avian influenza A virus H5N1 after intranasal administration was able to induce clinical symptoms leading to death in pet bird species like zebra finches and common budgerigars, which are very common hosts of domestic ornamental aviaries, as well as in wild species like house sparrows and European starlings, usually living close to human habitations [95]. Several studies demonstrated the important role of migrating birds as pathogen vehicles all over the world [21, 96, 97], being putatively able to infect wild indigenous birds (house sparrows, European starlings), these latter possibly contaminating pet birds living in open air aviaries [2]. This virus could also spread from endemic countries [12, 16] to other locations through international trade of exotic birds [15, 16, 22]. In relation with this fact, markets where live birds are sold appear to represent a great risk for zoonotic transmission as demonstrated by several authors [12, 13]. This is indeed noticeable that Asian owners seem to be, even at the peak of the H5N1 outbreak, unaware of the zoonotic risks this kind of business could cause [12, 13] and this was also the case in Western countries as hybrids between canaries and different wild passerines were and are still sold on public markets (Boseret, personal information). Illegal bird importation can also induce a risk as suggested by Van Borm et al. [16].

Arboviruses

West Nile Fever is an emergent vector-borne zoonosis in which birds, e.g. house sparrows, play a key role as main and amplifying reservoir hosts [48]. The virus responsible for this disease is a flavivirus (*Flaviviridae*) known under the name of the West Nile Fever Virus (WNV) which was isolated from numerous passeriform species, including canaries [48], as well as psittacines [98]. Most of the time Birds are sub-clinically affected, but can, however, develop a clinical form of the disease with ocular and neurologic symptoms [56]. Usutu virus (USUV) is another mosquito-borne flavivirus of African origin. This avian virus is transmitted by arthropod vectors (mainly mosquitoes of the *Culex pipiens* complex). Since 2001, the death of birds especially passerines, has been associated with infection by USUV [99, 100]. It is well known that free-living birds, including migratory species, have the potential to disperse certain pathogenic microorganisms [53]. Usutu virus has recently been detected in Europe and is spreading through Austria, Hungary, Italy, Spain and Switzerland, causing disease in birds and humans [49]. Following the same pattern as the West Nile Fever virus, USUV is a candidate as an emerging pathogen in Europe and the consequences for human health safety have to be considered [49, 53]. Open air aviaries are common in our countries and could be an important feeding source for mosquitoes, which could then inoculate the virus to humans.

Others

Proventricular dilation disease (PDD) is a disease in pet birds and, since it could be frequently lethal, PDD is considered as a major threat to aviculture [101]. This syndrome is associated with inflammation of the nervous system and gastrointestinal dysfunction as well as neurologic changes like seizures. Recently, the cause of this disease has been attributed to a novel bornavirus, the Avian Borna Virus (ABV) [102]. However, there is no evidence of ABV cross-species transmission and the zoonotic potential of this family of viruses remains unclear [103].

Newcastle disease, caused by avian paramyxovirus (APMV) has also been described in pet birds [56, 91, 104]. Transmission to humans is also possible, with conjunctivitis [56] but the most important consequence would be spreading the infection among poultry breeding by the intermediary of humans, wild birds (especially pigeons) or maybe insect mechanical vectors like the house fly (*Musca domestica*) [105].

Parasitic/fungal diseases

Toxoplasmosis

Toxoplasmosis is a well-known human disease, responsible for abortion or congenital malformations in humans. Although less documented than through the cat-cycle transmission, *Toxoplasma gondii* has also been described as an important pathogen for canaries, finches and budgerigars [106, 107], inducing blindness among other symptoms. However, transmission to humans appears to be most unlikely, since the birds do not excrete *T. gondii* in feces (implying no risk of contamination by lack of hygiene or fecal matter manipulation). Indeed, *Toxoplasma gondii* should be found in internal organs and muscles, but since these birds are not usually bred for food purposes, this then eliminates the possibility of contamination by raw or undercooked flesh eating (Losson, personal communication).

Cryptococcosis

Pigeons are known to be reservoirs of pathogenic yeasts, like *Cryptococcus neoformans*, which is described to cause opportunistic infections in humans [108]. However less is known on the role that pet birds might play in such zoonotic transmission. Several studies have demonstrated the presence of *C. neoformans* in parrots, little pet birds like canaries, budgerigars or lovebirds and cockatiels [109, 110]. As discussed above, pet birds, housed in outdoor aviaries could be a potential health hazard for humans as *C. neoformans* reservoirs since they could be in contact with wild pigeon droppings.

Others

Despite a relatively poor documentation on pet bird parasitic diseases, giardiosis, aspergillosis and cryptosporidiosis have been reported in these avian populations, both in chronic and in acute infections. Favorizing conditions could be high-density populations, stress, and adaptation to a new environment or prolonged periods in confined housing [111]. Transmission to humans often results from feces manipulation or lack of hygiene [41, 56, 90].

Avian giardiasis is caused by two different *Giardia* species: *G. ardeae* and *G. psittaci*. *G. psittaci* has been demonstrated to be responsible for fatal infections in budgerigars [112], but is not transmissible to humans. The species responsible for zoonotic infections is *G. duodenalis*, generally causing a self-limited illness, sometimes asymptomatic, characterized by diarrhoea, abdominal pain and weight loss [112]. *G. duodenalis* is divided into eight genotypes or "Assemblages", among which the Assemblages A and B appear to be responsible for human infections [113]. Interestingly, these genotypes have been isolated in the feces of different avian species, without leading to the development of clinical symptoms. Birds then seem more likely to serve as mechanical vectors of cysts and oocysts [111].

In birds, *Cryptosporidium* infection leads to intestinal, respiratory or nephrotic symptoms and could be caused by three distinct species: *C. galli*, *C. meleagridis* and *C. baylei*. The latter two have been described as possible zoonotic agents, though in a low frequency in comparison with other species such as *C. hominis* or *C. parvum*[114]. The main human population at risk is very young children (first exposure, lack of hygiene) and immunocompromised individuels such as HIV-positive patients, who will develop gastro-intestinal lesions but also infections of other organs such as the pancreas, liver and occasionally the respiratory tract [115]. *C. parvum* has been isolated in feces of various avian species, corroborating the possibility of zoonotic parasite shedding and transmission by birds [116].

Aspergillosis has been frequently isolated from pet birds [56, 117], in both acute (severe respiratory condition with lethargy and changes in vocalization) and chronic forms (more often fatal because of its long-term development). However, human infection would rather come from environmental origin, and therefore be considered as a minor zoonotic threat, apart from human immunocompromised patients [117].

GUIDELINES TO PREVENT TRANSMISSION FROM BIRDS TO HUMANS

One interesting document to start with is the "Compendium of Measures To Control *Chlamydia psittaci*Infection Among Humans (Psittacosis) and Pet Birds (Avian Chlamydiosis), 1998" edited by the Centre for Disease Control in 1998 [59].

Household hygiene

The transmission of zoonotic pathogens from animals to humans could be easily decreased by applying some elementary hygiene principles. A few recommendations could be delivered to the owner by the bird seller:

- Clean clothing and shoes after any contact with other birds (bird club meeting, bird fair, live poultry).
- Wash hands before and after handling birds (including cage cleanings).
- Check cages, food and water every day to be sure they are clean (including perches, feeding cups, etc.…).
- When giving fruits or vegetables to birds, discard the rotten remainings.
- Change bath pots every day and make them available to birds only one hour/day (to avoid the bathing waste water to become a reservoir for pathogens).
- Wash cages once a week.
- Preserve food in clean and sealed containers.
- Clean and disinfect every aviary item before use.

Usually, bird breeders are correctly aware of these precautions; the risk is, however, higher in the case of family pets bought for the first time in a decorative purpose or as present for children, especially when either parents or children have not been informed about the cited above elementary advice.

Bird origin traceability

In the case of birds bred in the country where they are sold (e.g. little birds like canaries, finches, budgerigars), they are usually provided without any certificate or identification (apart from a leg band with the breeding identification number). Sellers are supposed to keep an accurate traceability of their stocks, but as far as we know there is no legal obligation for the seller to give any documents to the buyer.

For exotic pet birds issued from importation, laws differ from countries, but in a general , a vet certificate, a passport and an importation authorization have to be delivered with the birds. As said before, smuggled birds represent a high risk of introducing zoonoses. In Europe, exotic bird importation from non EU countries is forbidden and animals imported from other EU-member countries should have an international passport, a correct identification and a veterinary certificate of good health (Directive 91/496/CE).

However from the owner's point of , there are some recommendations to be aware of after buying a new pet bird:

- If the bird comes from another country, request certification from the seller that these were legally imported (eventually ask for official documents) and were healthy prior to shipment (certified by an official veterinarian).
- Schedule an appointment with a veterinarian.
- Isolate new birds from other birds for a quarantine time determined by the veterinarian.
- Restrict access to birds from people owning birds too.
- Keep birds away from other birds (e.g. in the gardens).

Awareness of sickness signs

Breeders usually know signs of sickness in a bird, even if they could be somehow difficult to detect. But for non-initiated people, like sellers in animal shops or new owners, this could be difficult to see whether their birds are healthy or ill. Prevention tools and information should then be provided by the breeders to people to whom they are selling/giving their animals. Veterinarians should also better inform owners for example by providing documentation on warning signs of infectious bird diseases. If unusual signs of disease or if unexpected deaths occur in a breeding, the owners should then warn their avian veterinarian.

Biosecurity and hygiene precautions in big facilities

When of sufficient size, a Hazard Analysis and Critical Control Points (HACCP) plan could be applied in breeding facilities and in selling facilities. To quarantine newly incoming birds is an absolutely necessary precaution. These animals should be kept in clean cages for a duration estimated by the sanitary veterinarian, and pathogens and/or pest absence (including *D. gallinae*) should be carefully checked. CDC recommends at least a quarantine of 30–45 days when *C. psittaci* infection is suspected [59]. For example, one should check these different control points:

1. Direct bird environment:

    - Presence/absence of *D. gallinae* in the quarantine cages after at least one week, which is the time needed by the parasite to accomplish a complete reproduction cycle, from egg to egg [40]. For example, the acarids could be easily found on feed balls, perches or on the removable bottom sand tray. An easy test is to push strongly with the thumb on dirty spots pasted on the reverse face of this tray and scratch them from left to right (or vice versa). If a bloody smear does appear, this would be an efficient sign that blood-fed parasites did begin to colonize cage anfractuosities (Boseret, personal observations).
    - Color/consistency/quantity of droppings: for example, a yellow stain could suggest campylobacteriosis, a liquid consistency could refer to salmonellosis or other entero-bacteriaceae infections [41].
    - Transport cages: were they soiled or clean? Presence of dead birds?

2. Birds: general examination
    - o Presence/absence of other pest species living most of their time on the host, e.g. at the calamus of the feathers (like *O. sylviarum)*, at the edge of the beak or in the leg's scales (like *Knemidokoptes pilae,* which is a non-zoonotic mange agent*)* or in another part of the body (e.g. ticks, lice). Broken feathers or feather-loss could indicate pruritus and discomfort, other indicators of ectoparasite infestation [41]. Ectoparasites are considered by many breeders to be a good indicator of inadequate hygiene and management and their detection therefore could awaken attention of the owner to the health status of their infested incoming birds.
    - o General state of the birds (good/bad)
        - ▪ Perching/lying at the bottom of the cage,
        - ▪ Normal activity/apathy, rolled in ruffled feathers,
        - ▪ In social groups/isolated,
        - ▪ Bright eyes/exophthalmia,
        - ▪ Good respiratory state/nasal-ocular discharge, open beak.
    - o Plumage aspect: are the birds in a molting period? How is the molting: homogenous and bilateral/heterogenous and asymmetric.
3. Quarantine facilities hygienic state:
    - o Frequency and efficiency of cages/walls/floor/shells disinfection,
    - o Food storage (access to mice, rats?),
    - o Environmental conditions: temperature, humidity, duration of light hours.

This list is not exhaustive and a complete list of adequate control points has to be determined as a function of the kind and size of breeding, facility conformation, season, frequence of bird movements, etc. The above recommendations should, however, constitute a basis of elementary examinations to be performed in every case.

In case of a high level of risk or when a doubt emerges relative to the birds' health state, the following laboratory analyses could be performed:

1. Individual level: necropsy of a dead or a sacrificed sick bird, performed along with bacterial analyses of intestinal content or other organs presenting lesions.
2. Group level: Bacterial analyses of cloacal and/or oral swabs of a bird's sample bunch (one-to-ten, one-to-fifteen…).
3. Vector level: molecular analyses of vectors found on birds and/or in the cages, to specifically detect zoonotic agents: *C. psittaci*, West Nile fever, etc.…

The first two types of analyses could be an interesting investment and should not be too expensive (less than 100 euros/bird's bunch).

However, molecular analyses are on another financial level. One should recommend them in particular cases, first when birds are about to be handled by owners, like parrots, parakeets or cockatiels, second when the pathogen targeted is of zoonotic non negligible importance. For example, tuberculosis detection has to be carried out with a critical mind, as false negatives do occur. On the contrary, since surveillance of zoonoses is a European legal obligation (Directive 2003/99/EC), testing birds could be systematically included in national surveillance programs, a fortiori when human health is estimated to be put at risk. Then the breeders would be able to obtain an official intervention budget.

Another suggestion to diminish the costs at a local level would be to perform such tests in multiplex series, allowing breeders to somehow share elevated costs. But all these possibilities involves a complete change of mind and implies a broader transparency in these kinds of breeding, which still lacks even in our high-controlled countries (Boseret, personal information).

When birds are proven to be healthy, then they could be introduced in their definitive facilities. Outcoming birds should undergo similar sanitary systematic checking.

Moreover, the precaution of an all-in/all-out replacement system, already applied in poultry exploitations, should be carried out in pet bird breeding too. For example, only birds of the same age should be kept in the same location, and when moved, the facility should be disinfected carefully before welcoming a new flock.

In selling facilities, where birds from different origins could be mixed up, only replace them when the whole flock has been sold and the cages cleaned with ad hoc disinfectants. One interesting initiative would be to create a certificate of "good health" to moving flocks, but since many animals are sold in non-official ways (e.g. private breeding, markets), this would not be so easy to set up.

Control point should also be implemented on bird fairs. Sanitary certificates could be an obligatory document to be provided to authorities to allow the breeder to attend any fair.

CONCLUSIONS

This re aimed to present a non-exhaustive panorama of data relative to pet bird-human pathogen transmission. Different situations have been illustrated in this short re: familial households, breeding or selling facilities, bird fairs, international trade and the wild birds' problematic of reservoirs. Although this represents a minor part of the companion animal vet clientship, pet bird diseases with zoonotic potential should not be neglected or underestimated, considering the major health impact on the population, including children. Referring to Pastoret and Vallat's zoonoses classification, pet bird zoonoses are responsible for the most threatening disease types: 2 and 2+ (see Table 5; [118]). Vets could then play an important role in educating pets (including bird) owners.

Table 5: Classification of emerging zoonoses [[106]]

Transmission	Wild to humans	Humans to humans	Wild to domestic	Domestic to humans	Example in pet birds
1	Yes	No	No	No	None
1+	Yes	Yes	No	No	None
2	Yes	No	Yes	No	West Nile fever
					Newcastle disease
2+	Yes	Yes	Yes	Yes	Avian Influenza
					Salmonellosis
					Chlamydophilosis
					Tuberculosis

On another point of , pathogen shedding by wild passerine birds could be responsible of maintaining infection in domestic bird pools, such as open-air aviaries or poultry breeding, and could have important economic impact. The presence of *Salmonella* species in starling feces and in cattle feeding operations reported e.g. by Carlson et al. is a good example of an under-known reservoir phenomenon [6]. Another example is the role of birds, including passerines, as amplifying hosts for some vector-borne zoonotic emerging viruses. Open air aviaries are not protected from mosquitoes, and ornamental birds have been shown to be able to act in the same way as their wild counterparts. Migrating birds are also a sanitary concern, since these birds can spread a high variety of pathogens by solely defecating above outdoor aviaries wherein pet birds are housed. Thus this bird concentration could become a non-negligible reservoir of pathogens, contributing to maintain and spread infection in the human population. Referring to vectors, *D. gallinae* according to the author's advice, is an underestimated concern – probably too many times misdiagnosed - in pet bird medicine as well as in small avian breeding, since the parasite could be carried and transferred from one species to another, mostly by inert materials such as cages, perches, water or feed bowls, etc.… and eventually by man. Threatening pathogens like *C. psittaci* or *Salmonella ssp.* were reported to be carried by the mite and transmitted to pet birds, which could then infect either their owners or their cage mates. In addition, the sanitary state of pet bird owning and trade is rather unclear in many countries. HACCP or other quality control plans (ISO, AFNOR…) are applied by the Federal Agency for Food Safety Chain (FAFSC) in Belgian poultry breeding, but not in "backyard poultry flocks" or in local passerine breeding. Legislation does exist e.g. on international trade but despite this, illegal introduction of birds in our countries still remains a threat for human health when considering the highly pathogenic agents that could be brought in through our frontiers (avian influenza A virus H5N1, chlamydophilosis…).

Therefore, investigating the health status of pet birds, facilities, avian exploitations and owners should be an interesting starting point to define human health risks encountered (from family to breeding scale), to propose economic and sanitary prevention measures (e.g. biosecurity, prophylaxis, hygiene) in an interest of health protection and economic improvement. This investigation could be a good picture illustrating the concept of "Animals+Humans=One Health".

AUTHORS' INFORMATION

GB is a doctor in veterinary medicine and defended a PhD on songbird behavior and health status. She is currently studying zoonoses transmitted by birds, especially pet birds, in a CS research unit. BL, ET, JGM and CS are professors and heads respectively of parasitology, virology, bacteriology and epidemiology and risk analysis sections of the department of infectious and parasitic diseases, (Faculty of Veterinary Medicine, University of Liège, Belgium) and therefore provided the author with expert advice on diseases discussed in this manuscript.

DECLARATIONS

Acknowledgments

We would like to acknowledge the team of the UREAR-ULg unit for their kind support in this redacting process, Drs Dal Pozzo, Humblet and Martinelle.

Authors' contributions

GB and CS fixed the design of the study; GB realized the literature research and analysis; BL, ET, JM and CS were involved in critically revising the manuscript for important intellectual content; CS gave final approval of the version to be published. All authors read and approved the final manuscript.

REFERENCES

1. Tully TN: Birds. Manual of exotic pet practice. Edited by: Elsevier. 2009, St. Louis, Missouri (USA): Elsevier, 250-298.
2. Dorrestein Gerry M: 8 - Passerines. Handbook of avian medicine. Edited by: Thomas NTJr, Ecams G, Alan KJ. 2009, Edinburgh: W.B. Saunders, 169-208. Second
3. Harcourt–Brown Nigel H: Chapter 6 - psittacine birds. Avian medicine. edn. Edited by: Thomas NTJ, Martin PCL, Dorrestein GM. 2000, Oxford: Butterworth-Heinemann, 112-143.
4. U.S Pet ownership & demographics sourcebook (2007 edition). 2007, Schaumburg, Illinois (USA): American Veterinary Medical Association, [https://www.avma.org/KB/Resources/Statistics/Pages/Market-research-statistics-US-Pet-Ownership-Demographics-Sourcebook.aspx]

5. Enquête FACCO/TNS SOFRES 2010 sur le parc des animaux familiers français: Chambre syndicale des fabricants d'aliments préparés pour chien, chats, oiseaux et autres animaux familiers. 2010, Paris (France), [http://www.facco.fr/-Population-animale-]
6. Carlson JC, Engeman RM, Hyatt DR, Gilliland RL, DeLiberto TJ, Clark L, Bodenchuk MJ, Linz GM: Efficacy of European starling control to reduce Salmonella enterica contamination in a concentrated animal feeding operation in the Texas panhandle. BMC Vet Res. 2011, 7: 9-10.1186/1746-6148-7-9.
7. Belchior E, Barataud D, Ollivier R, Capek I, Laroucau K, De Barbeyrac B, Hubert B: Psittacosis outbreak after participation in a bird fair, Western France, December 2008. Epidemiol Infect. 2011, 139: 1637-1641. 10.1017/S0950268811000409.
8. Vanrompay D, Harkinezhad T, Van De Walle M, Beeckman D, Van Droogenbroeck C, Verminnen K, Leten R, Martel A, Cauwerts K: Chlamydophila psittaci transmission from pet birds to humans. Emerg Infect Dis. 2007, 13: 1108-1110. 10.3201/eid1307.070074.
9. Lindeborg M, Barboutis C, Ehrenborg C, Fransson T, Jaenson TG, Lindgren PE, Lundkvist A, Nyström F, Salaneck E, Waldenström J, Olsen B: Migratory birds, ticks, and crimean-congo hemorrhagic fever virus. Emerg Infect Dis. 2012, 18: 2095-2097. 10.3201/eid1812.120718.
10. Loye J, Carroll S: Birds, bugs and blood: avian parasitism and conservation. Trends Ecol Evol. 1995, 10: 232-235. 10.1016/S0169-5347(00)89072-2.
11. Boseret G, Carere C, Ball GF, Balthazart J: Social context affects testosterone-induced singing and the volume of song control nuclei in male canaries (Serinus canaria). J Neurobiol. 2006, 66: 1044-1060. 10.1002/neu.20268.
12. Amonsin A, Choatrakol C, Lapkuntod J, Tantilertcharoen R, Thanawongnuwech R, Suradhat S, Suwannakarn K, Theamboonlers A, Poovorawan Y: Influenza virus (H5N1) in live bird markets and food markets, Thailand. Emerg Infect Dis. 2008, 14: 1739-1742. 10.3201/eid1411.080683.
13. Wang M, Di B, Zhou DH, Zheng BJ, Jing H, Lin YP, Liu YF, Wu XW, Qin PZ, Wang YL, Jian LY, Li XZ, Xu JX, Lu EJ, Li TG, Xu J: Food markets with live birds as source of avian influenza. Emerg Infect Dis. 2006, 12: 1773-1775. 10.3201/eid1211.060675.
14. Berk Y, Klaassen CHW, Mouton JW, Meis JFGM: An outbreak of psittacosis in a bird-fanciers fair in the Netherlands. Neth J Med. 2008, 152: 1889-1892.
15. Chomel BB, Belotto A, Meslin FX: Wildlife, exotic pets, and emerging zoonoses. Emerg Infect Dis. 2007, 13: 6-11. 10.3201/eid1301.060480.
16. Van Borm S, Thomas I, Hanquet G, Lambrecht B, Boschmans M, Dupont G, Decaestecker M, Snacken R, Van Den Berg T: Highly pathogenic H5N1 influenza virus in smuggled Thai eagles, Belgium. Emerg Infect Dis. 2005, 11: 702-705. 10.3201/eid1105.050211.
17. De Schrijver K: A psittacosis outbreak in customs officers in Antwerp (Belgium). Bull Inst Marit Trop Med Gdynia. 1998, 49: 97-99.
18. Roy L, Buronfosse T: Using mitochondrial and nuclear sequence data for disentangling population structure in complex pest species: a case study with *dermanyssus gallinae*. PLoS One. 2011, 6: e2230-
19. Karesh WB, Cook RA, Bennett EL, Newcomb J: Wildlife trade and global disease emergence. Emerg Infect Dis. 2005, 11: 1000-1002.
20. Karesh WB, Cook RA, Gilbert M, Newcomb J: Implications of wildlife trade on the movement of avian influenza and other infectious diseases. J Wildl Dis. 2007, 43 (Suppl 3): S55-S59.
21. Fèvre EM, Bronsvoort BMDC, Hamilton KA, Cleaveland S: Animal movements and the spread of infectious diseases. Trends Microbiol. 2006, 14: 125-131. 10.1016/j.tim.2006.01.004.
22. Brooks-Moizer F, Roberton SI, Edmunds K, Bell D: Avian influenza H5N1 and the wild bird trade in Hanoi, Vietnam. Ecol Soc. 2009, 14: 1-20.
23. Valiente Moro C, Thioulouse J, Chauve C, Normand P, Zenner L: Bacterial taxa associated with the hematophagous mite Dermanyssus gallinae detected by 16S rRNA PCR amplification and TTGE fingerprinting. Res Microbiol. 2009, 160: 63-70. 10.1016/j.resmic.2008.10.006.
24. Valiente Moro C, Chauve C, Zenner L: Vectorial role of some dermanyssoid mites (Acari, Mesostigmata, Dermanyssoidea). Parasite. 2005, 12: 99-109. 10.1051/parasite/2005122099.
25. Valiente Moro C, De Luna CJ, Tod A, Guy JH, Sparagano OAE, Zenner L: The poultry red mite (Dermanyssus gallinae): a potential vector of pathogenic agents. Exp Appl Acarol. 2009, 48: 93-104. 10.1007/s10493-009-9248-0.
26. Circella E, Pugliese N, Todisco G, Cafiero MA, Sparagano OAE, Camarda A: Chlamydia psittaci infection in canaries heavily infested by Dermanyssus gallinae. Exp Appl Acarol. 2011, 55: 329-338. 10.1007/s10493-011-9478-9.
27. Valiente Moro C, Chauve C, Zenner L: Experimental infection of Salmonella Enteritidis by the poultry red mite, Dermanyssus gallinae. Vet Parasitol. 2007, 146: 329-336. 10.1016/j.vetpar.2007.02.024.
28. Valiente Moro C, Desloire S, Chauve C, Zenner L: Detection of Salmonella sp. in Dermanyssus gallinae using an FTA® filter-based polymerase chain reaction. Med Vet Entomol. 2007, 21: 148-152. 10.1111/j.1365-2915.2007.00684.x.
29. Valiente Moro C, Desloire S, Vernozy-Rozand C, Chauve C, Zenner L: Comparison of the VIDAS® system, FTA® filter-based PCR and culture on SM ID for detecting Salmonella in Dermanyssus gallinae. Lett Appl Microbiol. 2007, 44: 431-436. 10.1111/j.1472-765X.2007.02119.x.
30. Chirico J, Eriksson H, Fossum O, Jansson D: The poultry red mite, Dermanyssus gallinae, a potential vector of Erysipelothrix rhusiopathiae causing erysipelas in hens. Med Vet Entomol. 2003, 17: 232-234. 10.1046/j.1365-2915.2003.00428.x.

31. Brännström S, Hansson I, Chirico J: Experimental study on possible transmission of the bacterium Erysipelothrix rhusiopathiae to chickens by the poultry red mite, Dermanyssus gallinae. Exp Appl Acarol. 2010, 50: 299-307. 10.1007/s10493-009-9317-4.

32. Akdemir C, Gülcan E, Tanritanir P: Case report: dermanyssus gallinae in a patient with pruritus and skin lesions. Act parasitol. 2009, 33: 242-244.

33. Cafiero MA, Camarda A, Circella E, Galante D, Lomuto M: An urban outbreak of red mite dermatitis in Italy. Int J Dermatol. 2009, 48: 1119-1121. 10.1111/j.1365-4632.2009.04107.x.

34. Cafiero MA, Galante D, Camarda A, Giangaspero A, Sparagano O: Why dermanyssosis should be listed as an occupational hazard. Occup Environ Med. 2011, 68: 628-10.1136/oemed-2011-100002.

35. Bellanger AP, Bories C, Foulet F, Bretagne S, Botterel F: Nosocomial dermatitis caused by Dermanyssus gallinae. Infect Control Hosp Epidemiol. 2008, 29: 282-283. 10.1086/528815.

36. Cafiero MA, Camarda A, Circella E, Santagada G, Schino G, Lomuto M: Pseudoscabies caused by Dermanyssus gallinae in Italian city dwellers: a new setting for an old dermatitis. J Eur Acad Dermatol. 2008, 22: 1382-1383. 10.1111/j.1468-3083.2008.02645.x.

37. Dogramaci AC, Culha G, Özçelik S: Dermanyssus gallinae infestation: an unusual cause of scalp pruritus treated with permethrin shampoo. J Dermatol Treat. 2010, 21: 319-321. 10.3109/09546630903287437.

38. Haag-Wackernagel D, Bircher AJ: Ectoparasites from feral pigeons affecting humans. Dermatology. 2010, 220: 82-92. 10.1159/000266039.

39. Roy L, Dowling APG, Chauve CM, Lesna I, Sabelis MW, Buronfosse T: Molecular phylogenetic assessment of host range in five Dermanyssus species. Exp Appl Acarol. 2009, 48: 115-142. 10.1007/s10493-008-9231-1.

40. Roy L: Ecologie évolutive d'un genre d'acarien hématophage: approche phylogénétique des délimitations interspécifiques et caractérisation comparative des populations de cinq espèces du genre Dermanyssus (Acari: Mesostigmata). articles. 2009, Lyon, France: Ecole nationale Vétérinaire de Lyon

41. Dorrestein GM: Bacterial and parasitic diseases of passerines. Vet Clin North Am Exot Anim Pract. 2009, 12: 433-451. 10.1016/j.cvex.2009.07.005.

42. Clayton DH, Tompkins DM: Ectoparasite virulence is linked to mode of transmission. Proc Biol Sci. 1994, 256: 211-217. 10.1098/rspb.1994.0072.

43. Valera F, Casas-Crivillé A, Hoi H: Interspecific parasite exchange in a mixed colony of birds. J Parasitol. 2003, 89: 245-250. 10.1645/0022-3395(2003)089[0245:IPEIAM]2.0.CO;2.

44. Haag-Wackernagel D, Geigenfeind I: Protecting buildings against feral pigeons. Eur J Wildl Res. 2008, 54: 715-721. 10.1007/s10344-008-0201-z.

45. Roy L, Chauve CM, Buronfosse T: Contrasted ecological repartition of the northern fowl mite ornithonyssus sylviarum (mesostigmata: Macronyssidae) and the chicken red mite dermanyssus gallinae (mesostigmata: Dermanyssidae). Acarologia. 2010, 50: 207-219. 10.1051/acarologia/20101958.

46. Orton DI, Warren LJ, Wilkinson JD: Avian mite dermatitis. Clin Exp Dermatol. 2000, 25: 129-131.

47. Blitvich BJ: Transmission dynamics and changing epidemiology of West Nile virus. Anim Health Res Rev. 2008, 9: 71-86. 10.1017/S1466252307001430.

48. Nemeth N, Young G, Ndaluka C, Bielefeldt-Ohmann H, Komar N, Bowen R: Persistent West Nile virus infection in the house sparrow (Passer domesticus). Arch Virol. 2009, 154: 783-789. 10.1007/s00705-009-0369-x.

49. Vázquez A, Jiménez-Clavero MA, Franco L, Donoso-Mantke O, Sambri V, Niedrig M, Zeller H, Tenorio A: Usutu virus: potential risk of human disease in Europe. Euro Surveill. 2011, 16 (31): :pii=19935. Available online: http://www.eurosurveillance.org/Article.aspx?ArticleId=19935

50. Turell MJ, O'Guinn M, Oliver J: Potential for New York mosquitoes to transmit West Nile virus. Amer J Trop Med Hyg. 2000, 62: 413-414.

51. Sardelis MR, Turell MJ, O'Guinn ML, Andre RG, Roberts DR: Vector competence of three North American strains of Aedes albopictus for West Nile virus. J Am Mosq Control Assoc. 2002, 18: 284-289.

52. Komar N, Langevin S, Hinten S, Nemeth N, Edwards E, Hettler D, Davis B, Bowen R, Bunning M: Experimental infection of North American birds with the New York 1999 strain of West Nile virus. Emerg Infect Dis. 2003, 9: 311-322. 10.3201/eid0903.020628.

53. Pfeffer M, Dobler G: Emergence of zoonotic arboviruses by animal trade and migration. Parasit Vectors. 2010, 3: 35-10.1186/1756-3305-3-35.

54. Comstedt P, Bergström S, Olsen B, Garpmo U, Marjavaara L, Mejlon H, Barbour AG, Bunikis J: Migratory passerine birds as reservoirs of Lyme borreliosis in Europe. Emerg Infect Dis. 2006, 12: 1087-1095. 10.3201/eid1207.060127.

55. Mathers A, Smith RP, Cahill B, Lubelczyk C, Elias SP, Lacombe E, Morris SR, Vary CP, Parent CE, Rand PW: Strain diversity of Borrelia burgdorferi in ticks dispersed in North America by migratory birds. J Vector Ecol. 2011, 36: 24-29. 10.1111/j.1948-7134.2011.00137.x.

56. Evans EE: Zoonotic diseases of common pet birds: psittacine, passerine, and columbiform species. Vet Clin North Am Exot Anim Pract. 2011, 14: 457-476. 10.1016/j.cvex.2011.05.001.

57. Van Droogenbroeck C, Beeckman DSA, Verminnen K, Marien M, Nauwynck H, Boesinghe LT, Vanrompay D: Simultaneous zoonotic transmission of Chlamydophila psittaci genotypes D, F and E/B to a veterinary scientist. Vet Microbiol. 2009, 135: 78-81. 10.1016/j.vetmic.2008.09.047.

58. Henrion E, Trippaerts M, Lepage P: Severe multiorgan psittacosis in a 10-year-old boy. Arch Pediatr. 2002, 9: 810-813. 10.1016/S0929-693X(01)00993-9. (in French)

59. (CDC) CfDCap: Compendium of measures to control chlamydia psittaci infection among humans (psittacosis)

and pet birds (avian chlamydiosis), 1998. MMWR. 1998, 47 (No.RR-10): 1-15.

60. Hoelzer K, Moreno Switt AI, Wiedmann M: Animal contact as a source of human non-typhoidal salmonellosis. Vet Res. 2011, 42: 34-10.1186/1297-9716-42-34.

61. Panigrahy B, Clark FD, Hall CF: Mycobacteriosis in psittacine birds. Avian Dis. 1983, 27: 1166-1168. 10.2307/1590218.

62. Ward MP, Ramer JC, Proudfoot J, Garner MM, Juan-Sallés C, Wu CC: Outbreak of salmonellosis in a zoologic collection of lorikeets and lories (Trichoglossus, Lorius, and Eos spp.). Avian Dis. 2003, 47: 493-498. 10.1637/0005-2086(2003)047[0493:OOSIAZ]2.0.CO;2.

63. Madewell BR, McChesney AE: Salmonellosis in a human infant, a cat, and two parakeets in the same household. J Am Vet Med Assoc. 1975, 167: 1089-1090.

64. Joseph V: Infectious and parasitic diseases of captive passerines. Semin Avian Exot Pet. 2003, 12: 21-28. 10.1053/saep.2003.127878.

65. Harris JM: Zoonotic diseases of birds. Vet Clin North Am Small Anim Pract. 1991, 21: 1289-1298.

66. Grimes JE: Zoonoses acquired from pet birds. Vet Clin North Am Small Anim Pract. 1987, 17: 209-218.

67. Smith KE, Anderson F, Medus C, Leano F, Adams J: Outbreaks of Salmonellosis at elementary schools associated with dissection of owl pellets. Vector Zoon Dis. 2005, 5: 133-136. 10.1089/vbz.2005.5.133.

68. Morishita TY, Aye PP, Ley EC, Harr BS: Survey of pathogens and blood parasites in free-living passerines. Avian Dis. 1999, 43: 549-552. 10.2307/1592655.

69. Refsum T, Vikøren T, Handeland K, Kapperud G, Holstad G: Epidemiologic and pathologic aspects of Salmonella Typhimurium infection in passerine birds in Norway. J Wildl Dis. 2003, 39: 64-72.

70. Wells SJ, Fedorka-Cray PJ, Dargatz DA, Ferris K, Green A: Fecal shedding of Salmonella spp. by dairy cows on farm and at cull cow markets. J Food Prot. 2001, 64: 3-11.

71. Lahuerta A, Westrell T, Takkinen J, Boelaert F, Rizzi V, Helwigh B, Borck B, Korsgaard H, Ammon A, Mäkelä P: Zoonoses in the European Union: origin, distribution and dynamics - the EFSA-ECDC summary report 2009. Euro Surveill. 2011, 16 (13): :pii=19832. Available online: http://www.eurosurveillance.org/Article.aspx?ArticleId=19832

72. Hoop RK, Ehrsam H, Ossent P, Salfinger M: Mycobacteriosis of ornamental birds–frequency, pathologo-anatomic, histologic and microbiologic data. Berl Munch Tierarztl. 1994, 107: 275-281. (in German)

73. Washko RM, Hoefer H, Kiehn TE, Armstrong D, Dorsinville G, Frieden TR: Mycobacterium tuberculosis infection in a green-winged macaw (Ara chloroptera): report with public health implications. J Clin Microbiol. 1998, 36: 1101-1102.

74. Steinmetz HW, Rutz C, Hoop RK, Grest P, Bley CR, Hatt JM: Possible human-avian transmission of Mycobacterium tuberculosis in a green-winged macaw (Ara chloroptera). Avian Dis. 2006, 50: 641-645. 10.1637/7609-041906R.1.

75. Hoop RK: Mycobacterium tuberculosis infection in a canary (Serinus canaria L.) and a blue-fronted Amazon parrot (Amazona amazona aestiva). Avian Dis. 2002, 46: 502-504. 10.1637/0005-2086(2002)046[0502:MTIIAC]2.0.CO;2.

76. Ledwón A, Szeleszczuk P, Zwolska Z, Augustynowicz-Kopeć E, Sapierzyński R, Kozak M: Experimental infection of budgerigars (Melopsittacus undulatus) with five Mycobacterium species. Avian Pathol. 2008, 37: 59-64. 10.1080/03079450701802255.

77. Grange JM: Mycobacterium bovis infection in human beings. Tuberculosis. 2001, 81: 71-77. 10.1054/tube.2000.0263.

78. O'Reilly LM, Daborn CJ: The epidemiology of mycobacterium bovis infections in animals and man: a re. Tubercle Lung Dis. 1995, 76 (Suppl 1): 1-46.

79. Shitaye EJ, Grymova V, Grym M, Halouzka R, Horvathova A, Moravkova M, Beran V, Svobodova J, Dvorska-Bartosova L, Pavlik I: Mycobacterium avium subsp. hominissuis infection in a pet parrot. Emerg Infect Dis. 2009, 15: 617-619. 10.3201/eid1504.081003.

80. Shitaye JE, Halouzka R, Svobodova J, Grymova V, Grym M, Skoric M, Fictum P, Beran V, Slany M, Pavlik I: First isolation of mycobacterium genavense in a blue headed parrot (Pionus menstruus) imported from surinam (South America) to the Czech Republic: a case report. Vet Med Czech. 2010, 55: 339-347.

81. Skoric M, Fictum P, Frgelecova L, Kriz P, Slana I, Kaevska M, Pavlik I: Avian tuberculosis in a captured ruppell's griffon vulture (Gyps ruppellii): a case report. Vet Med Czech. 2010, 55: 348-352.

82. Dahlhausen B, Tovar DS, Saggese MD: Diagnosis of mycobacterial infections in the exotic pet patient with emphasis on birds. Vet Clin North Am Exot Anim Pract. 2012, 15: 71-83. 10.1016/j.cvex.2011.11.003.

83. Yogasundram K, Shane SM, Harrington KS: Prevalence of Campylobacter jejuni in selected domestic and wild birds in Louisiana. Avian Dis. 1989, 33: 664-667. 10.2307/1591142.

84. Wedderkopp A, Madsen AM, Jørgensen PH: Incidence of Campylobacter species in hobby birds. Vet Rec. 2003, 152: 179-180. 10.1136/vr.152.6.179.

85. Sensale M, Cuomo A, Dipineto L, Santaniello A, Calabria M, Menna LF, Fioretti A: Survey of Campylobacter jejuni and Campylobacter coli in different taxa and ecological guilds of migratory birds. Ital J An Sci. 2006, 5: 291-294.

86. Adhikari B, Connolly JH, Madie P, Davies PR: Prevalence and clonal diversity of Campylobacter jejuni from dairy farms and urban sources. N Z Vet J. 2004, 52: 378-383. 10.1080/00480169.2004.36455.

87. Colles FM, Dingle KE, Cody AJ, Maiden MCJ: Comparison of Campylobacter populations in wild geese with those in starlings and free-range poultry on the same farm. Appl Environ Microbiol. 2008, 74: 3583-3590. 10.1128/AEM.02491-07.

88. Waldenström J, Axelsson-Olsson D, Olsen B, Hasselquist

D, Griekspoor P, Jansson L, Teneberg S, Svensson L, Ellström P: Campylobacter jejuni colonization in wild birds: results from an infection experiment. PLoS One. 2010, 5: e9082-10.1371/journal.pone.0009082.

89. Olsen B, Gylfe A, Bergström S: Canary finches (Serinus canaria) as an avian infection model for Lyme borreliosis. Microb Pathog. 1996, 20: 319-324. 10.1006/mpat.1996.0030.

90. Rosskopf WJ: Common conditions and syndromes of canaries, finches, lories and lorikeets, lovebirds, and macaws. Semin Avian Exot Pet. 2003, 12: 131-143. 10.1053/seap.2003.00023-9.

91. Jorn KS, Thompson KM, Larson JM, Blair JE: Polly can make you sick: pet bird-associated diseases. Clev Clin J Med. 2009, 76: 235-243. 10.3949/ccjm.76a.08018.

92. Kauffman MD, LeJeune J: European starlings (sturnus vulgaris) challenged with escherichia coli O157 can carry and transmit the human pathogen to cattle. Lett Appl Microbiol. 2011, 53: 596-601. 10.1111/j.1472-765X.2011.03163.x.

93. Williams ML, Pearl DL, LeJeune JT: Multiple-locus variable-nucleotide tandem repeat subtype analysis implicates European starlings as biological vectors for Escherichia coli O157:H7 in Ohio, USA. J Appl Microbiol. 2011, 111: 982-988. 10.1111/j.1365-2672.2011.05102.x.

94. Gaukler SM, Linz GM, Sherwood JS, Dyer NW, Bleier WJ, Wannemuehler YM, Nolan LK, Logue CM: Escherichia coli, salmonella, and mycobacterium avium subsp. paratuberculosis in Wild European starlings at a Kansas cattle feedlot. Avian Dis. 2009, 53: 544-551. 10.1637/8920-050809-Reg.1.

95. Perkins LEL, Swayne DE: Varied pathogenicity of a Hong Kong-origin H5N1 avian influenza virus in four passerine species and budgerigars. Vet Pathol. 2003, 40: 14-24. 10.1354/vp.40-1-14.

96. Fereidouni SR, Ziegler U, Linke S, Niedrig M, Modirrousta H, Hoffmann B, Groschup MH: West Nile virus monitoring in migrating and resident water birds in Iran: are common coots the main reservoirs of the virus in wetlands?. Vector Borne Zoonotic Dis. 2011, 11: 1377-1381. 10.1089/vbz.2010.0244.

97. Rutz C, Dalessi S, Baumer A, Kestenholz M, Engels M, Hoop R: Avian influenza: wildbird monitoring in Switzerland between 2003–2006. Schweiz Arch Tierheilkd. 2007, 149: 501-509. 10.1024/0036-7281.149.11.501. (in German)

98. Carboni DA, Nevarez JG, Tully TN, Evans DE: West Nile virus infection in a sun conure (Aratinga solstitialis). J Avian Med Surg. 2008, 22: 240-245. 10.1647/2005-016.1.

99. Chvala S, Bakonyi T, Bukovsky C, Meister T, Brugger K, Rubel F, Nowotny N, Weissenböck H: Monitoring of Usutu virus activity and spread by using dead bird surveillance in Austria, 2003–2005. Vet Microbiol. 2007, 122: 237-245. 10.1016/j.vetmic.2007.01.029.

100. Chvala S, Kolodziejek J, Nowotny N, Weissenböck H: Pathology and viral distribution in fatal Usutu virus infections of birds from the 2001 and 2002 outbreaks in Austria. J Comp Pathol. 2004, 131: 176-185. 10.1016/j.jcpa.2004.03.004.

101. Doneley RJT, Miller RI, Fanning TE: Proventricular dilatation disease: an emerging exotic disease of parrots in Australia. Aust Vet J. 2007, 85: 119-123. 10.1111/j.1751-0813.2007.00109.x.

102. Honkavuori KS, Shivaprasad HL, Williams BL, Quan PL, Hornig M, Street C, Palacios G, Hutchison SK, Franca M, Egholm M, Briese T, Lipkin WI: Novel Borna virus in psittacine birds with proventricular dilatation disease. Emerg Infect Dis. 2008, 14: 1883-1886. 10.3201/eid1412.080984.

103. Staeheli P, Sauder C, Hausmann J, Ehrensperger F, Schwemmle M: Epidemiology of Borna disease virus. J Gen Virol. 2000, 81: 2123-2135.

104. Pearson GL, McCann MK: The role of indigenous wild, semidomestic, and exotic birds in the epizootiology of velogenic viscerotropic Newcastle disease in Southern California, 1972–1973. J Am Vet Med Assoc. 1975, 167: 610-614.

105. Barin A, Arabkhazaeli F, Rahbari S, Madani SA: The housefly, Musca domestica, as a possible mechanical vector of Newcastle disease virus in the laboratory and field. Med Vet Entomol. 2010, 24: 88-90. 10.1111/j.1365-2915.2009.00859.x.

106. Dubey JP: A re of toxoplasmosis in wild birds. Vet Parasitol. 2002, 106: 121-153. 10.1016/S0304-4017(02)00034-1.

107. Dubey JP, Hamir AN: Experimental toxoplasmosis in budgerigars (Melopsittacus undulatus). J Parasitol. 2002, 88: 514-519.

108. Wu Y, Du PC, Li WG, Lu JX: Identification and molecular analysis of pathogenic yeasts in droppings of domestic pigeons in Beijing, China. Mycopathologia. 2012, 174: 203-214. 10.1007/s11046-012-9536-9.

109. Brilhante RSN, Castelo-Branco DSCM, Soares GDP, Astete-Medrano DJ, Monteiro AJ, Cordeiro RA, Sidrim JJC, Rocha MFG: Characterization of the gastrointestinal yeast microbiota of cockatiels (Nymphicus hollandicus): a potential hazard to human health. J Med Microbiol. 2010, 59: 718-723. 10.1099/jmm.0.017426-0.

110. Lugarini C, Goebel CS, Condas LAZ, Muro MD, De Farias MR, Ferreira FM, Vainstein MH: Cryptococcus neoformans isolated from Passerine and Psittacine bird excreta in the state of Paraná, Brazil. Mycopathologia. 2008, 166: 61-69. 10.1007/s11046-008-9122-3.

111. Papini R, Girivetto M, Marangi M, Mancianti F, Giangaspero A: Endoparasite infections in pet and zoo birds in Italy. Sci World J. 2012, 2012: 253127-

112. Filippich LJ, McDonnell PA, Munoz E, Upcroft JA: Giardia infection in budgerigars. Aust Vet J. 1998, 76: 246-249. 10.1111/j.1751-0813.1998.tb10148.x.

113. Yaoyu F, Xiao L: Zoonotic potential and molecular epidemiology of Giardia species and giardiasis. Clin Microbiol Rev. 2011, 24: 110-140. 10.1128/CMR.00033-10.

114. Joachim A: Human cryptosporidiosis: an update with special emphasis on the situation in Europe. J Vet Med B.

2004, 51: 251-259. 10.1111/j.1439-0450.2004.00765.x.

115. Farthing MJ: Clinical aspects of human cryptosporidiosis. Contrib Microbiol. 2000, 6: 50-74.

116. Quah JX, Ambu S, Lim YAL, Mahdy MAK, Mak JW: Molecular identification of Cryptosporidium parvum from avian hosts. Parasitology. 2011, 138: 1-5.

117. Cray C: Infectious and zoonotic disease testing in pet birds. Clin Lab Med. 2011, 31: 71-85. 10.1016/j.cll.2010.10.008.

118. Bernard PP-PV: A global veterinary education to cope with societal needs. Proceedings of the OIE global conference on evolving veterinary education for a safer world OIE, 12–14 October 2009. 2009, Paris (France): Office International des Epizooties, 15-22.

CHAPTER 55

ONE HEALTH: THE IMPORTANCE OF COMPANION ANIMAL VECTOR-BORNE DISEASES

Michael J Day

ONE HEALTH: HISTORY AND SCOPE

The 'One Health' concept states simply that there should be a seamless interaction between veterinary and human medicine with clinicians, researchers, agencies and governments working together for the benefit of domestic and wild animal and human health and the global environment. Such interactions may take place at many levels - from management of zoonotic infectious disease outbreaks in the field, to joint research programmes to integrated policy making and funding decisions.

The concept of One Health is nothing new. Dunlop and Williams in their *History of Veterinary Medicine*[1] catalogue the early recognition of the significance of zoonotic infectious disease. The ancient Mesopotamians collated laws into codes and the Eshuna Code of 2300 BC makes the owner of a rabid dog responsible for the containment of that animal. The Babylonian king Adad-apla-iddina (1068-1047 BC) constructed a temple to the healing goddess Gula who was represented with or as a dog and was worshiped as a healer and protector from rabies. It is also believed that the role of the dog as an adjunct to healing was recognized through the ability of these animals to provide comfort to patients. The ancient Egyptians provide the first documentation of animal diseases in the Kahun papyrus (1900 BC) and in the context of the present re; it is believed that this civilization had awareness of vector-borne disease through their use of mosquito netting. There is a rich history of comparative medicine within the ancient Chinese dynasties in which there were organized specialities of physicians, surgeons, dieticians and veterinarians - clearly emphasizing the importance of animals to this society. The principles of yin-yang as practiced through acupuncture applied equally to human and animal patients. In ancient Greece, Aristotle (384-322 BC) continued the tradition of Hippocrates (460-367 BC) and promoted comparative medicine through his extensive studies of animal anatomy and the pathology of animal diseases. This tradition of comparative anatomy was continued in ancient Roman civilization with the most prominent contribution made by Galen (130-200 AD). The Hippocratic-Galenic principles continued throughout Medieval Europe to the Renaissance where the comparative anatomical legacy of Leonardo da Vinci (1452-1519) laid the way for future developments. Later, John Hunter (1728-1793) became a true practitioner of comparative medicine and was tutor to Edward Jenner (1749-1823) whose development of vaccination was a classical example of the One Health principle. The formalization of One Health is often attributed to Claude Bourgelat, the founder of the first veterinary school in Lyon in 1761, precisely 250 years ago. In writing on the relationship between human and animal medicine, Bourgelat stated that 'either medicine will mutually enlighten and perfect the other when we discard a derisory, harmful prejudice'. The greats of the golden era of infectious disease research - Louis Pasteur (1822-1895), Robert Koch (1843-1910), Rudolf Virchow (1821-1902) and John M'Fadyean (1853-1941), were all proponents of One Health and many of their advances were based in studies of animal disease [1, 2, 3].

It was perhaps in the 20th century that the medical and veterinary professions became slightly distant, a fact that was recognized by Calvin Schwabe (1927-2006) who promoted a ‹re-unification› from the 1960s and is attributed with coining the term ‹One Medicine› or One Health [3, 4]. It was however, not until the past five years, that the One Health concept has truly gathered international momentum. Collaborative ventures between the British Medical Association and the British Veterinary Association [5] and the American Medical Association and the American Veterinary Medical Association [6] paved the way for the seminal concept note produced following a meeting of the World Organization for Animal

Citation: Michael J Day, One health: the importance of companion animal vector-borne diseases, DOI: 10.1186/1756-3305-4-49.

Health (OIE), the World Health Organization (WHO), the Food and Agriculture Organization (FAO), the United Nations Children›s Fund (UNICEF) and the World Bank http://www.oie.int/fileadmin/Home/eng/Current_Scientific_Issues/docs/pdf/FINAL_CONCEPT_NOTE_Hanoi.pdf. A number of organizations have endorsed the One Health concept (e.g. the Federation of Veterinarians of Europe) and One Health groups have been established; including the One Health Commission http://www.onehealthcommission.org/, the One Health Initiative http://www.onehealthinitiative.com/index.php and the Comparative Clinical Science Foundation http://www.onemedicine.org.uk/. These initiatives have culminated recently in the First International One Health Conference, held in Melbourne, Australia.

COMPANION ANIMALS IN ONE HEALTH

From the beginnings summarized above, One Health has now expanded rapidly with endorsement by numerous medical and veterinary organizations. The major focus of these proponents has been the very high-impact interactions between human and production animal and wildlife health with global zoonotic disease pandemics and 'emerging' infectious diseases deemed to have arisen in these animal species. Many of the best examples of such infections are viral, where virus mutation or re-assortment permits extension of the target host range (e.g. SARS coronavirus, H5N1 and H1N1 influenza virus, Nipah virus, Hendra virus, human immunodeficiency virus [HIV]), but the role of parasitic diseases in One Health has also been discussed [7, 8]. The impact of environmental change (e.g. climate change, deforestation and urbanization) and lifestyle change including the increase in global human and animal movement [9] has also become part of the One Health concept.

Perhaps less often considered has been the enormous potential role of companion animals, and particularly the domesticated dog and cat, in One Health. In developed nations, pet ownership has reached unprecedented levels and these animals play a significant role in family life. In 2006, there were 72 million pet dogs in the USA (in 37% of households) and 81 million pet cats (in 32% of households) (2007 US Pet Ownership and Demographics Sourcebook). Estimates for 2010 in the UK are for 8 million pet dogs (in 23% of households) and 8 million pet cats (in 19% of households) http://www.pfma.org.uk. Increasingly over past decades, the small companion animal spends a majority of its life within the indoor domestic environment in very close physical association with its owners. Although many of these animals will enjoy a very high standard of healthcare with increasing longevity, there are a number of zoonotic infectious diseases that may be transmitted directly or indirectly from these species. Transmission of such diseases is dependent upon the lifestyle of the pet and is influenced by factors such as vaccination and parasite control, exposure to other domestic animals or wildlife (including urban wildlife such as foxes or small rodents) or exposure to particular environments (e.g. exercise in wooded areas with questing tick populations). The keeping of domestic companion or working small animals is not solely linked to affluence - in most developing nations there is individual or communal village ownership of dogs and cats, and in most of these countries there are extraordinary numbers of feral dogs and cats that have intensive contact with the human urban environment. In contrast, the majority of these animals may never receive veterinary attention and remain significant reservoirs of zoonotic infection.

There is no better example of this than rabies infection, which despite its long historical documentation, remains as much an issue today as at any time in history. Recent WHO estimates suggest that at least 55,000 people die each year from rabies infection; that 95% of these deaths occur in the developing nations of Asia and Africa and that 99% of cases are transmitted by dogs [10]. The significance of rabies virus infection is promoted through initiatives such as World Rabies Day http://www.worldrabiesday.org/ and the Afya vaccination programme in Africa http://www.afya.org/ and in September 2011 the OIE, WHO and FAO will host a Global Conference on Rabies Control in Seoul, Republic of Korea.

Less well-publicized are the remaining infectious diseases shared by man and dogs and cats that are well-summarized in a new text edited by Rabinowitz and Conti [11]. The present re is written in association with the 6th World Forum on Canine Vector-Borne Diseases and those of zoonotic potential will be highlighted in the section following.

COMPANION ANIMAL VECTOR-BORNE DISEASES IN ONE HEALTH

The major vector-borne infectious diseases of dogs and cats that also infect man are summarized in Table 1. Of single greatest significance is zoonotic visceral leishmaniosis caused by *Leishmania infantum* (*L. chagasi*) for which the domestic dog is the major reservoir for human infection via sandfly transmission. The disease is endemic in many countries throughout southern Europe, the Americas, northern Africa and Asia and high proportions of dogs in these areas are exposed to and often infected by the pathogen. Recent WHO estimates suggest that worldwide up to 12 million people are infected, with 2 million new cases identified annually and a population of some 350 million people at risk of infection; the risk of infection is significantly enhanced in HIV-infected individuals [12]. Control of leishmaniosis represents one of the greatest challenges for One Health and provides a clear example for the necessity of human and veterinary medicine to work together to develop strategies for management and elimination of this disease. Such measures have already occurred in the endemic focus of disease occurring in Brazil where the Ministry of Health oversees a programme of serologically testing dogs and culling positive animals [13]. Two commercially available vaccines for dogs have become available in Brazil and should form an important part of the control strategy. Data have already been published that show that where vaccination is widely practiced, the prevalence of both canine and human infection decreases due to reduced transmission of the organism [14].

Table 1: Canine and feline vector-borne diseases that also infect man

Disease	Vector
Leishmaniosis	Sand fly
Borreliosis	Tick
Bartonellosis	Flea Tick
Ehrlichiosis	Tick
Rickettsiosis	Tick Flea
Anaplasmosis	Tick
Dirofilariosis	Mosquito
Yersiniosis	Flea
Tularaemia	Tick
Coxiellosis	Tick
Tick-borne encephalitis	Tick
Louping ill	Tick
West Nile virus encephalitis	Mosquito
Trypanosomiosis	*Triatoma* bugs

A major concern is the extension of traditional endemic areas for *Leishmania* infection, which is now reported as autochthonous disease in northern European countries and North America [15, 16, 17, 18]. This is associated directly with the increased mobility of pet animals across borders [16]. Pet travel has been responsible for establishment of reservoirs of Leishmania-infected dogs in these non-endemic areas and has incidentally contributed to the widening geographical range of arthropod vectors (e.g. the establishment of *Rhipicephalus sanguineus* in northern Europe). The unprecedented scale of global companion animal travel is readily demonstrated by the success of the European pet passport scheme. Since its inception in 2000 and up to August 2010, the number of pet animals entering or re-entering the UK alone was 717, 965 http://www.defra.gov.uk/. The focus of attention for health certification for international pet travel has been rabies vaccination (with some countries also requiring evidence of seroconversion after vaccination); however, apart from certain national requirements for tick and tapeworm treatment there has been little consideration of the spread of other zoonotic infectious diseases. Some exceptions to this rule exist; for example importation of dogs into Australia requires testing for monocytic ehrlichiosis, brucellosis, leishmaniosis and leptospirosis, but without such controls there is clear evidence of importation of infection from endemic to non-endemic areas [15]. Global pet travel therefore creates the potential for rapid dissemination of zoonotic infection and represents another major challenge for One Health.

Borreliosis (Lyme disease) is a significant disease of people in endemic areas (particularly in Europe and North America) associated with avian and wildlife reservoirs and *Ixodes* spp. ticks. The major species infecting man and companion animals are *Borrelia burgdorferi* sensu stricto (in North America) and *B. garinii* and *B. afzelii*(in Europe) [19]. Infected dogs and cats pose minimal threat to man, but do provide a means by which infected ticks can be carried into the domestic environment. There is also a risk of human infection should ticks be crushed during removal from a pet animal and tick salivary gland material be exposed to wounds on the hands of an owner. The dog in particular might be employed as a 'sentinel' for monitoring the risk of human disease in an endemic area [20].

Bartonellosis should be regarded as one of the major potential emerging infections of man. Most is known about 'cat scratch disease' caused primarily by *Bartonella henselae* acquired directly from an infected cat and mostly likely transmitted between cats by the cat flea *Ctenocephalides felis*[21, 22, 23]. This infection becomes particularly significant in immunocompromised individuals (e.g. HIV-infected individuals with acquired immunodeficiency syndrome [AIDS], those receiving cancer chemotherapy or immunosuppression for transplantation or immune-mediated disease). The scale of the potential problem can be estimated by considering the extraordinary numbers of pet household cats (see above) and their very close physical association with owners, coupled with knowledge that in developing countries the prevalence of seropositivity amongst cats is on average 27% and the presence of active bacteraemia around 10% [24]. The major canine pathogen of these taxa is the tick-transmitted *B. vinsonii* subsp. *berkhoffii*, but a range of other *Bartonella*species are also reported from cats and dogs (and potential arthropod vectors) associated with a spectrum of clinical diseases. Attention is now focussed on these organisms due to a series of investigations showing that they may be associated with a wide range of human syndromes that were often considered chronic idiopathic diseases [21, 25]. There remains much to learn about the transmission of *Bartonella* from companion animals to man, but veterinary professionals have an occupational exposure risk due to their frequency of exposure to animal bites, arthropods, arthropod faeces and animal bodily fluids [21]. A target for One Health programmes should be further exploration of the significance of these pathogens in animal and human medicine.

A number of ehrlichial and rickettsial infections are shared by man and companion animals [26]. The cause of canine monocytic ehrlichiosis (*Ehrlichia canis* transmitted by *Rhipicephalus sanguineus*) is not considered an organism with significant zoonotic potential (although human cases of infection are reported); however, human and canine infections with *E. chaffeensis* and *E. ewingii* (transmitted by *Amblyoma americanum*) are well-documented although it is not clear whether the dog acts as a reservoir for human infection. Of increasing significance in human, canine and feline populations is the *Ixodes*-transmitted cause of granulocytic 'ehrlichiosis' (*Anaplasma phagocytophilum*). The reservoir species for this infection are wild rodents and wild and domestic ruminants, but human and companion animal infections are emerging as a significant problem in Europe and North America. The spotted fever group of rickettsiosis are also significant problems for man and dogs. In the Americas, Rocky Mountain spotted fever caused by *Rickettsia rickettsii*(transmitted by *Dermacentor andersoni*, *D. variablis*, *R. sanguineus* and *Amblyomma cajennese*) is the most important of this group, while in Europe, Asia and Africa, Mediterranean spotted fever caused by *R. conorii*(transmitted by *R. sanguineus*) is of greatest concern. The role of the dog in these human infections is again in transporting infected ticks into the domestic environment and the risk to owners of removing infected ticks from their pets. The early diagnosis of canine rickettsiosis by the veterinarian is of importance as this may precede the recognition of the pathogen in in-contact people. The flea-transmitted rickettsioses (*R. typhi* and *R. felis*) also fall into this group [23]. The reservoir potential for domestic pets for *R. typhi* is not proven, but there is much recent interest in the emergence of *R. felis* which is found in dogs, cats and cat fleas (*Ct. felis*) [23, 27]. As *R. felis* may be transmitted transovarially and trans-stadially, the domestic pet may introduce infected fleas into the home environment, which then become the means for human infection.

Table 1 also lists a range of other vector-transmitted diseases shared by man and companion animals, a number of which are relatively uncommon causes of human infection, but are important in animal species (e.g. dirofilarasis, West Nile fever).

In summary, the overall challenges for the One Health agenda in addressing these vector-borne diseases are several: (1) promoting awareness and ability to recognize these diseases by the human and veterinary medical professions, (2) undertaking ‹joined-up› research programmes that investigate the agents, their vectors and epidemiology, geographical distribution, clinical significance and pathogenesis, (3) developing robust diagnostic tests and surveillance systems for mapping these infectious agents and their vectors globally, (4) identifying diseases for which domestic pet animals are true reservoirs of human infection (e.g. leishmaniosis) and formulating public health strategies that effectively control the disease in the reservoir (e.g. stray dog control, ectoparasiticide treatment, vaccination) in addition to the human patient, (5) investigating the contact between pet animals and peridomestic wildlife species that may act as true reservoirs of these diseases and developing strategies to minimize such contact, (6) promoting awareness of these diseases in the pet-owning public and the importance of regular ectoparasite control programmes for their pets and their domestic environment, and (7) identifying the risks and challenges imposed by increasing global mobility of pet animals and developing strategies to minimize the associated movement of zoonotic infectious disease.

COMPANION ANIMAL ONE HEALTH: THE WSAVA ONE HEALTH COMMITTEE

Given the growing importance of the One Health concept the World Small Animal Veterinary Association (WSAVA) has recently established a One Health Committee, which has as its remit the firm positioning of small companion animals within the global One Health programme [28]. The committee is chaired by the author and includes academic experts on small animal zoonotic infection (including rabies, leishmaniosis and vector-borne diseases), first opinion veterinary practitioner representation and delegates from the OIE and Centers for Disease Control and Prevention (CDC) in the USA. The committee is funded by the WSAVA Foundation through sponsorship by a consortium of the pet food and small animal pharmaceutical industry and commenced a three year programme of work in January 2011.

Although a major focus of the work of the One Health Committee will be zoonotic infectious disease, including those reed in this paper, there are two further key areas in One Health in which small companion animals should play a major role. The first of these is in the field of comparative and translational research. The historical perspective given earlier indicates clearly how throughout history human medicine has benefitted from comparative veterinary studies. To an extent, we seem to have forgotten this legacy and over recent decades research efforts have been polarized and veterinary science been very much the 'poor relation' of its larger brother. It is unquestionable that studies of spontaneously arising disease in relatively outbred and long-lived animals that so closely share our domestic environment must provide information of benefit to human medicine. The availability of the canine and feline genomes [29, 30] and the development of microarray genomic screening tools [31, 32] provide us with unprecedented ability to explore the basis of canine and feline diseases that so closely mimic those that occur in man. Promoting comparative clinical research will be the second major focus of the WSAVA One Health Committee.

The final aspect of the work of this group will be in supporting the most visible and simple aspect of the interaction between man and companion animals. The ancient Mesopotamians recognized the psychological benefit of companion animal interaction for human healing and in recent decades the 'human - companion animal bond' has been widely explored. This touches not only on 'pets as therapy' in hospitals or care homes but the widespread psychological and social impact of pets in society [33].

DECLARATIONS

Acknowledgements

Publication of the CVBD6 thematic series has been sponsored by Bayer Animal Health GmbH

Competing interests

The author is a member of the Bayer CVBD World Forum. The WSAVA One Health Committee is funded through the WSAVA Foundation by a consortium of industry sponsors (Bayer Animal Health, Dechra, Hills Pet Nutrition, Intervet-Schering Plough Animal Health, Merial, Nestlé Purina, Novartis Animal Health, Pfizer Animal Health and Waltham).

REFERENCES

1. Dunlop RH, Williams DJ: Veterinary Medicine: an Illustrated History. 1996, St Louis, Mosby-Year Book, Inc
2. Day MJ: One Health and the legacy of John M'Fadyean. J Comp Pathol. 2008, 139: 151-153. 10.1016/j.jcpa.2008.07.007.
3. Monath TP, Kahn LH, Kaplan B: Introduction: one health perspective. ILAR J. 2010, 51: 193-198.
4. Cardiff RD, Ward JM, Barthold SW: 'One medicine - one pathology': are veterinary and human pathology prepared?. Lab Invest. 2008, 88: 18-26. 10.1038/labinvest.3700695.
5. Alder M, Easton G: One medicine!. Vet Rec. 2005, 157: 699-
6. King LJ, Anderson LR, Blackmore CG, Blackwell MJ, Lautner EA, Marcus LC, Meyer TE, Monath TP, Nave JE, Ohle J, Pappaioanou M, Sobota J, Stokes WS, Davis RM, Glasser JH, Mahr RK: Executive summary of the AVMA One Health Initiative Task Force report. J Am Vet Med Assoc. 2008, 233: 259-261. 10.2460/javma.233.2.259.
7. Kaplan B, Kahn LH, Monath TP, Woodall J: One Health' and parasitology. Parasites Vectors. 2009, 2: 36-10.1186/1756-3305-2-36.
8. Paul M, King L, Carlin EP: Zoonoses of people and their pets: a US perspective on significant pet-associated parasitic diseases. Trends Parasitol. 2010, 26: 153-154. 10.1016/j.pt.2010.01.008.
9. Brown C: Emerging diseases: the global express. Vet Pathol. 2010, 47: 9-14. 10.1177/0300985809354351.
10. Bourhy H, Dautry-Varsat A, Hotez PJ, Salomon J: Rabies, still neglected after 125 years of vaccination. PLoS Negl Trop Dis. 2010, 4: 11-
11. Rabinowitz PM, Conti LA: Human - Animal Medicine: Clinical Approaches to Zoonoses, Toxicants and other Shared Health Risks. 2010, Maryland Heights, Saunders Elsevier
12. WHO: Report of the 5th Consultative Meeting on Leishmania/HIV Co-infection. 2007, Addis Ababa, Ethiopia
13. Nunes CM, Pires MM, Marques da Silva K, Assis FD, Filho JG, Perri SHV: Relationship between dog culling and incidence of human visceral leishmaniasis in an endemic area. Vet Parasitol. 2010, 170: 131-133. 10.1016/j.vetpar.2010.01.044.
14. Palatnik-de-Sousa CB, Silva-Antunes I, de Aguiar Morgado A, Menz I, Palatnik M, Lavor C: Decrease of the incidence of human and canine visceral leishmaniosis after dog vaccination with Leishmune® in Brazilian endemic areas. Vaccine. 2009, 27: 3505-3512. 10.1016/j.vaccine.2009.03.045.
15. Shaw SE, Binns SH, Birtles RJ, Day MJ, Smithson R, Kenny MJ: Molecular evidence of tick-transmitted infections in dogs and cats in the United Kingdom. Vet Rec. 2005, 157: 646-648.
16. Shaw SE, Langton DA, Hillman TJ: Canine leishmaniosis in the United Kingdom: a zoonotic disease waiting for a vector?. Vet Parasitol. 2009, 163: 281-285. 10.1016/j.vetpar.2009.03.025.
17. Gaskin AA, Schantz P, Jackson J, Birkenheuer A, Tomlinson L, Gramiccia M, Levy M, Steurer F, Kollmar E, Hegarty BC, Ahn A, Breitschwerdt EB: Visceral leishmaniasis in a New York foxhound kennel. J Vet Intern Med. 2002, 16: 34-44. 10.1111/j.1939-1676.2002.tb01604.x.
18. Boggiatto PM, Ramer-Tait AE, Metz K, Kramer EE, Gibson-Corley K, Mullin K, Hostetter JM, Gallup JM, Jones DE, Petersen CA: Immunologic indicators of clinical progression during canine *Leishmania infantum* infection. Clin Vaccine Immunol. 2010, 17: 267-273. 10.1128/CVI.00456-09.
19. Little SE, Heise SR, Blagburn BL, Callister SM, Mead PS: Lyme borreliosis in dogs and humans in the USA. Trends Parasitol. 2010, 26: 213-218. 10.1016/j.pt.2010.01.006.
20. Hamer SA, Tsao JI, Walker ED, Mansfield LS, Foster ES, Hickling GJ: Use of tick surveys and serosurveys to evaluate pet dogs as a sentinel species for emerging Lyme disease. Am J Vet Res. 2009, 70: 49-56. 10.2460/ajvr.70.1.49.
21. Breitschwerdt EB, Maggi RG, Chomel BB, Lappin MR: Bartonellosis: an emerging infectious disease of zoonotic importance to animals and human beings. J Vet Emerg Crit Care. 2010, 20: 8-30. 10.1111/j.1476-4431.2009.00496.x.
22. Guptill L: Bartonellosis. Vet Microbiol. 2010, 140: 347-359. 10.1016/j.vetmic.2009.11.011.
23. McElroy KM, Blagburn BL, Breitschwerdt EB, Mead PS, McQuiston JH: Flea-associated zoonotic diseases of cats in the USA: bartonellosis, flea-borne rickettsioses, and plague. Trends Parasitol. 2010, 26: 197-204. 10.1016/j.pt.2010.01.001.
24. Birtles R: Bartonellosis. Arthropod-Borne Infectious Diseases of the Dog and Cat. Edited by: Shaw SE, Day MJ. 2005, London, Manson Publishing Ltd, 110-119.
25. Chomel BB, Boulouis HJ, Maruyama S, Breitschwerdt EB: *Bartonella* spp. in pets and effect on human health. Emerg Inf Dis. 2006, 12: 389-394.
26. Nicholson WL, Allen KE, McQuiston JH, Breitschwerdt EB, Little SE: The increasing recognition of rickettsial pathogens in dogs and people. Trends Parasitol. 2010, 26: 205-212. 10.1016/j.pt.2010.01.007.
27. Kenny MJ, Birtles RJ, Day MJ, Shaw SE: *Rickettsia felis* in the United Kingdom. Emerg Infect Dis. 2003, 9: 1023-1024.

28. Day MJ: One health: the small companion animal dimension. Vet Rec. 2010, 167: 847-849. 10.1136/vr.c6492.

29. Lindblad-Toh K, Wade CM, Mikkelsen TS, Karlsson EK, Jaffe DB, Kamal M, Clamp M, Chang JL, Kulbokas EJ, Zody MC: Genome sequence, comparative analysis and haplotype structure of the domestic dog. Nature. 2005, 438: 803-819. 10.1038/nature04338.

30. Pontius JU, Mullikin JC, Smith DR: Initial sequence and comparative analysis of the cat genome. Genome Res. 2007, 17: 1675-1689. 10.1101/gr.6380007.

31. Shearin AL, Ostrander EA: Leading the way: canine models of genomics and disease. Dis Models and Mech. 2010, 3: 27-34. 10.1242/dmm.004358.

32. Wilbe M, Jokinen P, Truve K, Seppala EH, Karlsson EK, Biagi T, Hughes A, Bannasch D, Andersson G, Hansson-Hamlin H, Lohi H, Lindblad-Toh K: Genome-wide association mapping identifies multiple loci for a canine SLE-related disease complex. Nature Genet. 2010, 42: 250-254. 10.1038/ng.525.

33. Johnson RA: Psychosocial and therapeutic aspects of human-animal interaction. Human-Animal Medicine: Clinical Approaches to Zoonoses, Toxicants and Other Shared Health Risks. Edited by: Rabinowitz PM, Conti LA. 2010, Maryland Heights, Saunders Elsevier, 24-36.

INDEX